Medicinal Plants of the World

Medicinal Plants
of the
World

Chemical Constituents,
Traditional and Modern
Medicinal Uses

Volume 3

Ivan A. Ross

HUMANA PRESS ✸ TOTOWA, NEW JERSEY

© 2005 Humana Press Inc.
999 Riverview Drive, Suite 208
Totowa, New Jersey 07512

www.humanapress.com

All papers, comments, opinions, conclusions, or recommendations are those of the author(s), and do not necessarily reflect the views of the publisher.

The author assumes no responsibility for, makes no warranty with respect to results that may be obtained from the uses or dosages listed, and does not necessarily endorse such uses or dosages and procedures. The author is not liable to any person whatsoever for and damage resulting from reliance on any information contained herein, whether with respect to plant identification, uses, procedures, dosages or by reason of any misstatement or error contained in this work. The author recognized that there are differences in varieties of plants, the geographical location in which they are grown, growing conditions, stage of maturity, and method of harvesting and preparation.

This publication is printed on acid-free paper. ∞
ANSI Z39.48-1984 (American Standards Institute)
Permanence of Paper for Printed Library Materials.

Production Editor: Amy Thau

Cover design by Patricia F. Cleary

Cover Illustrations: Background figure from Chapter 11, "*Oryza sativa.*" Foreground figures from Chapter 3, "*Cocos nucifera;*" Chapter 4, "*Coffea arabica;*" Chapter 6, "*Ferula assafoetida;*" and Chapter 12, "*Plantago ovata.*"

For additional copies, pricing for bulk purchases, and/or information about other Humana titles, contact Humana at the above address or at any of the following numbers: Tel.: 973-256-1699; Fax: 973-256-8341; E-mail: orders@humanapr.com; or visit us at www.humanapress.com

Printed in the United States of America. 10 9 8 7 6 5 4 3 2 1
eISBN: 1-59259-887-0

Library of Congress Cataloging-in-Publication Data

Ross, Ivan A.
    Medicinal plants of the world: chemical constituents, traditional and modern medicinal
    uses / by Ivan A. Ross.
      p.cm.
    Includes bibliographical references and index.
      ISBN 1-58829-129-4 (alk. paper)   eISBN 1-59259-887-0
      1. Medicinal plants--Encyclopedias. I. Title.

RS164.R676 2005
615'.32--dc21

2002032933

Preface

This volume of the series *Medicinal Plants of the World: Chemical Constituents, Modern and Traditional Medicinal Uses* contains information on 16 plant species and follows the same format as volumes 1 and 2. Some of the plants discussed in volume 3 may be considered controversial in their classification as "medicinal." However, the Paracelsian dictum that "sola dosis fecit venenum" has been appreciated since ancient times, and throughout the ages many highly toxic materials used for lethal purposes have also found applications in modern medicine. It has been recognized that plants contain substances that are either harmful or toxic. However, it is wrong to think that there are plant toxins that are known or that are likely to have adverse effects on any and every form of life. A common feature of most toxic plants is that they are also known for their curative properties, and although they may provide the cure for an individual's disease at one dose, they may cause the death of the same individual at another.

Poisons are widespread in plants, and humans have tried to either get rid of them or convert them to their own advantage. By their very nature, poisons are biodynamic substances because they affect, or are intended to affect, the functioning of the victim's body. This also means that they have been, and continue to be, important sources of medicine. With such potentially dangerous substances, care in medication is essential, which raises the question of the relationship between the toxic dose and the therapeutic dose. For full advantage to be taken of their properties, a combination of reliable sources of materials and effective methodologies is required to enable not only isolation of the substances responsible, but also the investigation of their mechanisms of action. As more sophisticated methods evolve to elucidate the chemical and pharmacological natures of these substances, it will be possible to target more precisely their use as possible templates to produce medicinal agents.

I am very grateful to a number of individuals for their valuable cooperation in this work. I owe sincere appreciation to Professor Ron Olowin of St. Mary's College of California for granting me permission to use his photograph of *Plantago ovata* and Mr. Gary Monroe of Reno, Nevada for sharing his picture of *Larrea tridentata*.

In work of this nature there is always room for improvement. Suggestions from readers are welcome and will be gratefully received.

Ivan A. Ross

Acknowledgments

I am very grateful to Dr. Diana E. Dyrda of the University of Agriculture, Lublin, Poland for her contribution in collecting data and working on the manuscript, and to Yvonne Gordon for editing this work. Also, thanks are due to our families for enduring our absence in their lives.

Contents

List of Plants Covered in *Medicinal Plants of the World Volumes 1 and 2*

Volume 1

1. *Abrus precatorius*
2. *Allium sativum*
3. *Aloe vera*
4. *Annona muricata*
5. *Carica papaya*
6. *Cassia alata*
7. *Catharanthus roseus*
8. *Cymbopogon citratus*
9. *Cyperus rotundus*
10. *Curcuma longa*
11. *Hibiscus rosa-sinensis*
12. *Hibiscus sabdariffa*
13. *Jatropha curcas*
14. *Lantana camara*
15. *Macuna pruriens*
16. *Mangifera indica*
17. *Manihot esculenta*
18. *Momordica charantia*
19. *Moringa pterygosperma*
20. *Persea americana*
21. *Phyllathus niruri*
22. *Portulaca oleracea*
23. *Psidium guajava*
24. *Punica granatum*
25. *Syzygium cumini*
26. *Tamarindus indica*

Volume 2

List of Color Plates

Color plates appear as an insert following page 270.

Abbreviations Used in Chemical Constituents Sections

Aer	Aerial parts
An	Anther
As	Ash
Bd	Bud
Bk	Bark
Bu	Bulb
Call Tiss	Callus tissue
Cr	Crown
Ct	Coat
Cx	Calyx
Cy	Cotyledon
Em	Embryo
EO	Essential oil
Ep	Epidermis
Fl	Flower
Fr	Fruit
Gel	Jell
Hu	Hull
Ju	Juice
Lf	Leaf
Lx	Latex
Pc	Pericarp
Pe	Peel
Pl	Plant
Pn	Panicle
Pt	Part
Pu	Pulp
Rh	Rhizome
Rt	Root
Sd	Seed
Sh	Shoot
St	Stem
Tr	Trunk
Tu	Tuber
Tw	Twig

1 | Camellia sinensis

L.

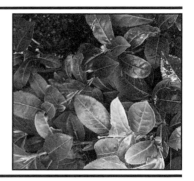

Common Names

Aisiksikimi	United States	Te	Denmark
Caj	Albania	Te	Faroe Islands
Caj	Croatia	Te	France
Caj	Czech Republic	Te	Italy
Caj	Hawaii	Te	Norway
Caj	Serbia	Te	Spain
Cay	Turkey	Te	Surinam
Ceai	Romania	Te	Switzerland
Cha	Brazil	Te	Wales
Cha	China	Tea plant	England
Cha	Hawaii	Tea	Australia
Cha	Japan	Tea	England
Cha	Pacific Islands	Tea	Guyana
Cha	Portugal	Tea	Hungary
Chai	Bulgaria	Tea	United States
Chai	Mozambique	Tebusk	Denmark
Chai	Russia	Tebuske	Sweden
Chai	Tanzania	Tee	Finland
Chai	Ukraine	Tee	Germany
Chai	Zaire	Tee	Netherlands
Chaj	Macedonia	Tee	South Africa
Chayna roslina	Ukraine	Teepensas	Finland
Chinesischer tea	Germany	Tey	The Isle of Man (Manx)
Cunuc yacu	Ecuador	Teye	Northern Sotho
Eaj	Czech Republic	The	France
Eajovnik	Czech Republic	The	Indonesia
Herbata	Poland	The	Malaysia
Icayi	Rwanda	Thee	Netherlands
Ilitye	Africa	Theesoort	Netherlands
Itiye	Africa	Theestrauch	Germany
Oti	United States	Theestruik	Netherlands
Taa	Germany	Theler	France
Tae	Ireland	Ti	Congo
Te	Cornwall	Ti	Samoa

From: *Medicinal Plants of the World, vol. 3: Chemical Constituents, Traditional and Modern Medicinal Uses*
By: I. A. Ross © Humana Press Inc., Totowa, NJ

Ti	Scotland	Tra	Vietnam
Tii	Greenland	Tsa	Philippines
Tii	New Zealand	Yaku-q'oniwan	Ecuador
Tii	Northwest Territories, Canada	Zaya	Turkmenistan

BOTANICAL DESCRIPTION

Camellia sinensis is an evergreen tree or shrub of the THEACEAE family that grows to 10–15 m high in the wild, and 0.6–1.5 m under cultivation. The leaves are short-stalked, light green, coriaceous, alternate, elliptic-obovate or lanceolate, with serrate margin, glabrous, or sometimes pubescent beneath, varying in length from 5 to 30 cm, and about 4 cm wide. Young leaves are pubescent. Mature leaves are bright green in color, leathery, and smooth. Flowers are white, fragrant, 2.5–4 cm in diameter, solitary or in clusters of two to four. They have numerous stamens with yellow anthers and produces brownish-red, one- to four-lobed capsules. Each lobe contains one to three spherical or flattened brown seeds. There are numerous varieties and races of tea. There are three main groups of the cultivated forms: China, Assam, and hybrid tea, differing in form. *Camellia sinensis assamica*, the source of much of the commercial tea crop of Ceylon is a tree that, unpruned, may attain a height of 15 m and has proportionally longer, thinner leaves than typical species.

ORIGIN AND DISTRIBUTION

The cultivation and enjoyment of tea are recorded in Chinese literature of 2700 BC and in Japan about 1100. Through the Arabs, tea reached Europe about 1550. Native to Assam, Burma, and the Chinese province of Yunnan, it is highly regarded in southern Asia and planted in India, southern Russia, East Africa, Java, Ceylon, Sumatra, Argentina, and Turkey. China, India, Indonesia, and Japan produced about a half of the total world production.

TRADITIONAL MEDICINAL USES

India. Decoctions of the dried and fresh buds and leaves are taken orally for headache and fever[CS145]. Powder or decoction of the dried leaf is applied to teeth to prevent tooth decay[CS146]. Fresh leaf juice is taken orally for abortion[CS155], and as a contraceptive and hemostatic[CS147].

Mexico. Hot water extract of the leaf is taken orally by nursing mothers to increase milk production[CS148].

Turkey. Leaves are taken orally to treat diarrhea[CS149].

China. Hot water extract of the dried leaf is taken orally as a sedative, an antihypertensive, and anti-inflammatory[CS108].

Guatemala. Hot water extract of the dried leaf is used as eyewash for conjunctivitis[CS154].

Kenya. Water extract of the dried leaf is applied ophthalmically to treat corneal opacities[CS150]. The infusion is used for chalzion and conjunctivitis[CS151].

Thailand. Hot water extract of the dried leaf is taken orally as a cardiotonic and neurotonic[CS152]. Hot water extract of the dried seed is taken orally as an antifungal[CS153].

CHEMICAL CONSTITUENTS

(ppm unless otherwise indicated)
Acetaldehyde, phenyl: Sh 1.52–1.78%[CS100]
Acetaldehyde: Lf[CS073]
Acetamide, N-ethyl: Lf[CS027]
Acetic acid: Lf[CS086]
Acetoin: Lf[CS068]
Acetone: Lf[CS091]
Acetophenone, 2-4-dimethyl: Lf[CS027]
Acetophenone, 3-4-dimethoxy: Lf[CS027]
Acetophenone, para-ethyl: Lf[CS027]

Acetophenone: Headspace volatile[CS044]

Actinidiolide, dihydro: Lf EO[CS132]

Afzelechin, epi, (–): Lf 350[CS084]

Afzelechin, epi, 3-O-gallate (–): Lf 37[CS005]

Afzelechin, epi, 3-O-gallate (4-b-6)-epi, gallocatechin-3-O-gallate: Lf 5.6[CS008]

Allantoic acid: Pl[CS033]

Allantoin: Pl[CS033]

Aluminium inorganic: Lf[CS028]

Amyrin, α: Sd oil[CS095]

Amyrin, β: Sd oil 76[CS095]

Aniline, N-ethyl: Lf[CS027]

Aniline, N-methyl: Lf[CS027]

Aniline: Lf[CS027]

Apigenin: Lf[CS108]

Apigenin-6-8-di-C-β-D-arabinopyranosyl: Lf 20[CS156]

Apigenin-6-8-di-C-glucoside: Sh[CS096]

Arbutin: Lf 0.2[CS078]

Aromadenrin: Sh[CS094]

Ascorbic acid: Sh[CS038], Lf 0.257%[CS048]

Assamicain A: Lf 58.2[CS007]

Assamicain B: Lf 76.6[CS007]

Assamicain C: Lf 33.6[CS007]

Assamsaponin A: Sd 0.01%[CS021]

Assamsaponin B: Sd 28.3[CS021]

Assamsaponin C: Sd 36.5[CS021]

Assamsaponin D: Sd 26.1[CS021]

Assamsaponin E: Sd 11.1[CS021]

Assamsaponin F: Sd 14.1[CS021]

Assamsaponin G: Sd 79.1[CS021]

Assamsaponin H: Sd 13.4[CS021]

Assamsaponin I: Sd 98.5[CS021]

Astragalin: Lf[CS139]

Avicularin: Lf[CS058]

Barrigenol, A-1: Pl[CS118]

Barringtogenol C, 3-O-β-D-galacto-pyranosyl(1-2) β-D-xylopyranosyl (1-2)α-l-arabinopyranosyl(1-3)β-D-glucuronopyranosyl-21-O-cinnamoyl-16-22-di-O-acetyl: Lf[CS013]

Benzene, 1-2-3-trimethoxy: Lf[CS077]

Benzene, 1-2-3-trimethoxy-5-ethyl: Lf[CS077]

Benzene, 1-2-3-trimethoxy-5-methyl: Lf[CS077]

Benzene, 1-2-4-trihydroxy: Lf[CS003]

Benzene, 1-2-5-trihydroxy: Lf[CS003]

Benzene, 1-2-dimethoxy: Lf[CS077]

Benzene, 1-2-dimethoxy-4-ethyl: Lf[CS3077]

Benzene, 1-2-dimethoxy-4-methyl: Lf[CS077]

Benzene, 1-3-diacetyl: Lf[CS027]

Benzene, 1-4-diacetyl: Lf[CS027]

Benzoic acid: Headspace volatile[CS044]

Benzothiazole, 2-methyl: Lf[CS036]

Benzothiazole: Lf[CS036]

Benzoxazole: Lf[CS036]

Benzyl alcohol: Lf EO 1.01–1.6%[CS136], Headspace volatile[CS044], Lf[CS091], Sh 0.09–0.14%[CS100]

Benzyl butyrate: Lf[CS002]

Benzyl ethyl ketone: Lf[CS002]

Benzylaldehyde, 2-methyl: Lf[CS002]

Benzylaldehyde, 4-methoxy: Lf[CS002]

Benzylaldehyde: Headspace volatile[CS044], Lf[CS077], Sh 0.21–0.23%[CS100]

Benzylamine: N-N-dimethyl: Lf[CS027]

Bicyclo(4.3.0)non-8-en-7-one, 1-5-5-9-tetramethyl: Lf[CS002]

Brassicasterol: Sd oil[CS134]

Brassinolide, 28-homo, 6-keto: Lf[CS135]

Brassinolide, 28-nor, 6-keto: Lf[CS135]

Brassinolide, 28-nor: Lf[CS135]

Brassinolide, 6-keto: Lf[CS135]

Brassinolide: Lf 0.0046 ppb[CS089]

Brassinone, 24(S)-ethyl: Lf 30 ng/65 kg[CS110]

Brassinone, 24-ethyl: Lf[CS089]

Brassinone: Lf 130 ng/65 kg[CS110]

Butan-2-ol: Lf[CS068]

Butyrate, ethyl-3-hydroxy: Lf[CS068]

Butyroin: Lf[CS068]

Butyrospermol: Sd oil[CS095]

Caffeine: Lf 0.381–9.9%[CS114,CS049], Sh[CS038], Pl, Call Tiss[CS050], Sd[CS093], Sd Ct, Peduncle, Pc[CS102], Fl bud, Stamen, Pistil, Fl[CS107], An 0.05–6.77 ppt, Stem call 0.64 ppt[CS099], Petal[CS117], Fr[CS037]

Camellia galactoglucan: Lf[CS067]

Camellia polysaccharide: Lf[CS122]

Camellia saponin B, deacyl: Lf[CS081]

Camellia sinensis polysaccharide TSA: Lf[CS012]

Camellianin A: Lf[CS108]

Camellianin B: Lf[CS108]
Camelliaside A: Sd 656–2733.3[CS011,CS119]
Camelliaside B: Sd 291–3026.6 [CS011,CS119]
Camelliaside C: Sd 2.5[CS011]
Campesterol: Sd oil[CS134]
Carvacrol: Lf[CS002]
Castasterone: Lf 7.2 mg/65 kg[CS110]
Catechin-(4-α-8)-epi-gallocatechin:
    Lf 45.4[CS008]
Catechin-(4-α-8)-epi-gallocatechin-3-
    gallate: Lf 45.4[CS008]
Catechin-(4-β-8)-epi-gallocatechin-3-
    gallate, epi: Lf 20.8[CS008]
Catechin, (+): Lf 0.0017–2.9%[CS053,CS049],
    Call Tiss[CS060]. St call[CS099], Sh[CS038],
    An, St[CS099]
Catechin, epi (–): Lf 0.004–6.8%[CS053,CS049],
    Call Tiss[CS060], Sh[CS038], St call 0.07 ppt[CS099]
Catechin, epi, 3-O-para-hydroxy-benzoate
    (–): Lf 3.6[CS005]
Catechin, epi, epi-gallo-catechin(4-β-8)-
    3-O-galloyl: Lf 50[CS092]
Catechin, epi-gallo (–), 3-O-para-
    coumaroate: Lf 83.3[CS140]
Catechin, epi-gallo (–): Lf 3269[CS140]
Catechin, epi-gallo, 3-3'-di-O-gallate(–):
    Lf[CS140]
Catechin, epi-gallo, 3-4'-di-O-gallate(–):
    Lf[CS140]
Catechin, epi-gallo, 3-O-gallate (–):
    Lf 0.8718%[CS140]
Catechin, epi-gallo, gallate(–): St call 0.02
    ppt[CS099], Lf[CS109]
Catechin, epi-gallo: Lf[CS140]
Catechin-3-O-(3'-O-methyl)-gallate,
    epi(–): Lf 0.08%[CS010]
Catechin-3-O-(3-O-methyl)-gallate,
    epi(–): Lf 70.6-96.2[CS005,CS140]
Catechin-3-O-(4-O-methyl)-gallate,
    epi(–): Lf 16[CS005]
Catechin-3-O-gallate-(4-β-6)-epi-
    gallocatechin-3-O-gallate, epi:
    Lf 5.8[CS008]
Catechin-3- O-gallate-(4-β-8)-epi-
    gallocatechin-3-O-gallate, epi: Lf 3.6[CS008]
Catechin-3-O-gallate, (+): Lf 0.011%[CS084]

Catechin-3-O-gallate, epi(–): Lf 0.0086–
    6.6%[CS053,CS049]
Catechin-gallate, (+): Lf[CS082]
Catechin-gallate: Lf[CS042]
Catechol, (+): Pl[CS138]
Catechol, epi(–): Sh[CS128], Pl[CS138]
Catechol, epi, gallate(–): Sh[CS128]
Catechol, epi-gallo(–): Sh[CS128]
Catechol, epi-gallo, gallate(–): Sh[CS128]
Catechol, gallo, (+): Sh[CS128]
Chasaponin: Pl[CS035]
Chlorogenic acid: Call Tiss[CS087], Lf[CS139]
Chondrillasterol: Sd oil[CS130]
Citric acid: Lf[CS086]
Cresol, meta: Lf[CS003]
Cresol, ortho: Lf[CS003]
Cresol, para: Lf[CS003]
Cyclocitral, β: Sh 0.08–0.1%[CS100], Lf[CS002]
Cyclohex-2-en-1-4-dione, 2-6-6-trimethyl:
    Lf[CS002]
Cyclohex-2-en-1-one, 2-6-6-trimethyl:
    Lf[CS002]
Damascenone, β: Lf[CS002]
Damascone, α: Lf[CS002]
Damascone, β: Lf[CS002]
Dammaridienol: Sd oil 30[CS095]
Deca-trans-2-cis-4-dien-1-al: Lf[CS002]
Deca-trans-2-en-1-al: Lf[CS002]
Dehydrogenase, NADP-dependent-alco-
    hol: Sd[CS031]
Demmarenol, 24-methylene: Sd oil[CS095]
Diphenylamine: Lf 0.013–1.17%[CS098]
Dodeca-trans-2-trans-6-10-trien-1-al,
    4-ethyl-7-11-dimethyl: Lf[CS002]
Erucid acid: Sd oil Lf[CS134]
Ethyl acetate: Lf[CS091]
Ethyl lactate: Lf[CS068]
Eugenol: Fr EO[CS030]
Euphol: Sd oil[CS095]
Farnesene, α, trans-trans: Lf EO[CS115]
Farnesol: Lf[CS091]
Fluoride inorganic: Lf 188[CS143]
Fluorine, inorganic: Lf[CS043]
Furan, 2-acetyl: Lf[CS002]
Furan-3-one, tetrahydro, 2-methyl: Lf[CS068]
Furocoumarin, angular, 4-hydroxy-2'-
    methoxy: Lf[CS014]

Gadoleic acid: Sd oil[CS134]

Gallic acid: Lf[CS051]

Gallocatechin gallate, (−): Lf 0.188%[CS112]

Gallocatechin gallate, (+): Lf[CS082]

Gallocatechin gallate, epi(−): Lf[CS125]

Gallocatechin gallate, epi(+): Lf[CS123]

Gallocatechin-(4-α-8)-epi-catechin:
Lf 36.6[CS008]

Gallocatechin, (−): Lf[CS056]

Gallocatechin, (+): Lf 0.01–12.8%[CS053,CS049]

Gallocatechin, epi(+): Lf 1.1%[CS083]

Gallocatechin, epi, (−): Lf 0.088-
16.8%[CS005,CS049], Sh[CS038]

Gallocatechin, epi, (4-β-8)-epi-catechin-
3-)-gallate: Lf 27.6[CS008]

Gallocatechin, epi, 3-O-cinnamate(−):
Lf 13.2[CS005]

Gallocatechin, epi, 3-3'-di-O-gallate(−):
Lf 9[CS005]

Gallocatechin, epi, 3-4'-di-O-gallate(−):
Lf 9[CS005]

Gallocatechin, epi, 3-O-gallate(−):
Lf 0.714%[CS005]

Gallocatechin, epi, 3-O-gallate-(4-β-6)-
epi-catechin-3-O-gallate: Lf 4.2[CS008]

Gallocatechin, epi, 3-O-gallate-(4-β-8)-
epi-catechin-3-O-gallate: Lf 44[CS008]

Gallocatechin, epi, 3-O-para-
coumaroate(−): Lf 38.4[CS005]

Gallocatechin, epi, 8-C-ascorbyl-3-O-
gallate: Lf 11.2[CS008]

Gallocatechin, epi: Lf 1.0867%[CS101]

Gallocatechin-3-5'-di-O-gallate, epi(−):
Lf 0.06%[CS008]

Gallocatechin-3-O-(3'-O-methyl)-gallate,
epi(−):Lf 38[CS084]

Gallocatechin-3-O-gallate (−): Lf[CS079]

Gallocatechin-3-O-gallate (+): Lf[CS157]

Gallocatechin-3-O-gallate (4-β-8) epi-
catechin-gallate, epi: Lf 0.06%[CS010]

Gallocatechin-3-O-gallate, epi(−):
Lf 0.0328–21.3%[CS053,CS049], Sh[CS038]

Gallocatechin-3-O-para-coumaroate, epi
(−): Lf[CS010]

Gallocatechin-gallate, (−): Lf[CS042]

Gallocateuchin-3-O-gallate, epi (−):
Lf 5.33%[CS010]

Galloyl-β-D-glucose, 1-4-6-tri-O:
Lf 0.01%[CS010]

Galloylcatechin, epi (−): Lf[CS054]

Geranic acid, *trans*: Lf[CS002]

Geraniol β-D-glucopyranoside: Sh[CS113]

Geraniol: Sh[CS113], Lf EO 3.16-25.46%[CS136],
Lf[CS109]

Geranyl-β-primeveroside, 8-hydroxy:
Lf 2.08[CS018]

Germanicol: Sd oil 25[CS095]

Germanicum inorganic: Lf[CS120]

Gibberellin A-1: Endosperm[CS004]

Gibberellin A-19: Endosperm[CS004]

Gibberellin A-20: Endosperm[CS004]

Gibberellin A-3, iso: Endosperm[CS004]

Gibberellin A-3: Endosperm[CS004]

Gibberellin A-38: Endosperm[CS004]

Gibberellin A-44: Endosperm[CS004]

Gibberellin A-8: Endosperm[CS004]

Gibberellin A-S: Endosperm[CS004]

Glucogallin, β: Lf 28.4[CS008]

Glucose, β-D, 1-O-galloyl-4-6-(−)-
hexahyroxy-diphenoyl: Lf 30[CS092]

Glucose, β-D, 1-4-6-tri-O-galloyl: Lf 5[CS092]

Glutamic acid: *N*-para-coumaryl: Lf[CS133]

Heptan-1-al: Sh 0.02–0.03%[CS100]

Heptan-2-ol: Lf[CS068]

Heptan-2-one, 5-iso-propyl: Lf[CS002]

Heptan-2-one: Lf[CS002]

Heptan-3-ol: Lf[CS068]

Hepta-*trans*-2-*trans*-4-dien-1-al:
Sh 0.06–0.1%[CS100]

Hept-*trans*-2-en-1-al: Lf[CS002]

Hex-1-en-3-ol: Lf[CS068]

Hex-2-en-1-al, 5-methyl-2-phenyl: Lf[CS002]

Hex-5-en-4-olide, 4-methyl: Lf[CS002]

Hexadecane, N: Lf[CS091]

Hexan-1-al: ChloroplastCS129,
Sh 0.55–1.03%[CS100]

Hexan-1-ol, 2-ethyl: Lf[CS002]

Hexan-2-ol: Lf[CS068]

Hexa-*trans*-2-*cis*-4-dien-1-al: Lf[CS002]

Hex-*cis*-3-en-1-al: Lf 370[CS034]

Hex-*cis*-3-en-1-ol acetate: Lf[CS091]

Hex-*cis*-3-en-1-ol butyrate: Lf[CS091]

Hex-*cis*-3-en-1-ol caproate: Lf[CS091]

Hex-*cis*-3-en-1-ol formate: Lf[CS002]

Hex-*cis*-3-en-1-ol hexanoate: Sh 0.02–0.03%[CS100]

Hex-*cis*-3-en-1-ol hex-*trans*-2-enoate: Lf[CS002]

Hex-*cis*-3-en-1-ol propionate: Lf[CS002]

Hex-*cis*-3-en-1-ol, β-D-glucoside: Lf[CS076]

Hex-*cis*-3-en-1-ol: Lf[CS025], Lf EO 2.15–15%[CS136], Sh 0.09–0.13%[CS100]

Hex-*trans*-2-en-1-al: Lf[CS065], Lf EO 1.13–25.48%[CS136], Sh 2.09–3.1%[CS100]

Hex-*trans*-2-en-1-ol: Sh 0.04–0.06%[CS100]

Hex-*trans*-2-enyl acetate: Lf[CS002]

Hex-*trans*-2-enyl butyrate: Lf[CS002]

Hex-*trans*-2-enyl formate: Lf[CS002]

Hex-*trans*-2-enyl hexanoate: Lf[CS002]

Hex-*trans*-2-enyl propionate: Lf[CS002]

Hex-*trans*-3-enyl butyrate: Lf[CS002]

Hex-*trans*-3-enyl hex-*cis*-3-enoate: Lf[CS002]

Hex-*trans*-3-enyl propionate: Lf[CS002]

Hex-*trans*-3-enyl-2-methyl butyrate: Lf[CS002]

Hexyl butyrate: Lf[CS002]

Hexyl formate: Lf[CS002]

Hyperoside: Lf[CS058]

Indole: Lf[CS109]

Indole-3-methyl-ethanolate: Lf[CS015]

Inositol, myo, 2-O-β-L-arabinopyranosyl: Lf 0.4%[CS116]

Inositol, myo, 2-O-β-L-arabinopyranoside: Lf 0.4%[CS106]

Inositol, myo, 2-O-β-L-arabinoside: Lf[CS077]

Ionone, α: Sh 0.03–0.05%[CS100], Lf[CS068]

Ionone, β, 1'-2'-dihydro, 1'-2'-epoxy: Lf EO[CS132]

Ionone, β, 1'-2'-dihydroxy, 1'-2'-threo: Lf EO[CS132]

Ionone, β, 3'-oxo: Lf EO[CS132]

Ionone, β: Lf EO 0.02–0.31%[CS136], Sh 0.17–0.29%[CS100]

Jasmonate, dihydro, methyl-*trans*: Lf[CS002]

Jasmone, *cis*: Lf EO 0.05–0.2%[CS136]

Jasmone: Lf[CS091]

Jasmonic acid, (1R, 2R), (–): Lf[CS080]

Jasmonic acid, (1R, 2S), (+): Lf[CS080]

Jasmonic acid: Pollen[CS137], An[CS137], Lf[CS091]

Kaempferitin: Lf[CS139]

Kaempferol: Lf[CS026], Sh[CS094]

Kaempferol-3-O-galactosyl-rhamnosyl-glucoside: Lf[CS058]

Kaempferol-3-O-glucosyl(1-3)rhamnosyl(1-6)galactoside: Lf[CS009]

Kaempferol-3-O-glucosyl-rhamnoside: Lf[CS058]

Kaempferol-3-O-glucosyl-rhamnosyl-galactoside: Lf[CS058]

Lauric acid: Sd oil[CS134]

Ligustrazine: Lf[CS027]

Limonene: Lf[CS068]

Linalool β-D-glucopyranoside: Sh[CS113]

Linalool oxide A: Lf[CS091]

Linalool oxide B: Lf[CS091]

Linalool oxide C: Lf[CS091]

Linalool oxide I: Lf[CS077]

Linalool oxide II: Lf[CS077]

Linalool oxide III: Lf[CS077]

Linalool oxide IV: Lf[CS077]

Linalool oxide: Headspace volatile[CS044]

Linalool, (R): Lf[CS074]

Linalool, *cis*, oxide (furanoid): Lf[CS074]

Linalool, *cis*, oxide (pyranoid): Lf[CS074]

Linalool, *cis*, oxide: Sh 0.06–0.16%[CS100]

Linalool, *trans*, oxide (furanoid): Lf[CS074]

Linalool, *trans*, oxide (pyranoid): Lf[CS074]

Linalool, *trans*, oxide: Lf EO 3.18–4.23%[CS136], Sh 0.15–0.43%[CS100]

Linalool: Lf[CS121], Headspace volatile[CS044], Sh[CS113], Lf EO 8.2–19.84%[CS136]

Linoleic acid: Sd oil[CS134], Lf[CS069]

Linolenic acid: Lf[CS069]

Loliolide: Lf EO[CS132]

Lupeol: Sd oil[CS062]

Malic acid: Lf[CS086]

Malonic acid: Lf[CS086]

Menthol: Lf[CS068]

Methionine, S-methyl: Lf 7–24.5 mg%[CS158]

Methylamine: Lf 50[CS141]

Morine: Lf[CS045]

Myrcene: Lf[CS091]

Myricetin: Lf[CS026]

Myristic acid: Sd oil[CS134], Lf[CS069]

Naringenin: Sh[CS094]

Naringenin-fructosyl-glucoside: Lf[CS063]

Neral: Lf[CS002]

Nerolidol: Lf[CS109], Sh 0.08–0.12%[CS100]

NH₃ inorganic: Lf 400[CS111]

Nicotiflorin: Lf[CS133]

Nicotine: Lf 15.5 ng/g[CS047]

Nonal-1-al: Sh 0.04–0.06%[CS100]

Nonal-2-ol: Lf[CS068]

Nonan-2-one: Lf[CS002]

Nona- trans-2-cis-4-dien-1-al: Lf[CS002]

Nona- trans-2-cis-6-dien-1-al: Lf[CS002]

Nona-trans-2-en-1-al: Lf[CS002]

Nona-trans-2-trans-4-dien-1-al: Lf[CS002]

Oct-1-en-3-ol: Lf[CS068]

Octa-1-5-7-trien-3-ol, 3(S)-7-dimethyl: Lf EO[CS132]

Octa-1-5-diene-3-7-diol, 3(S)-7-dimethyl, (+): Lf EO[CS132]

Octan-2-one: Lf[CS002]

Octan-3-ol: Lf[CS068]

Octanoate, ethyl: Lf[CS002]

Octanoate, methyl: Lf[CS002]

Octa-trans-2-cis-4-dien-1-al: Lf[CS002]

Octa-trans-2-trans-4-dien-1-al: Lf[CS002]

Octa-trans-3-cis-5-dien-2-one: Lf[CS002]

Oct-trans-2-enoic acid: Lf[CS002]

Oleic acid: Sd oil[CS134], Lf[CS069]

Oolonghomobisflavan A: Lf 10.6[CS008]

Oolonghomobisflavan B: Lf 7.2[CS008]

Oolongtheanin: Lf 1.8[CS006]

Oxalic acid: Lf 1.0%[CS144]

Palmitic acid: Sd oil[CS134], Lf[CS069]

Pedunculagin: Lf[CS041]

Pent-1-en-3-ol: Lf[CS068], Sh 0.21–0.23%[CS100]

Pent-2-en-1-al, 4-methyl-2-phenyl: Lf[CS002]

Pentadecane, 2-6-10-14-tetramethyl: Lf[CS091]

Pentan-1-ol: Sh 0.06–0.11%[CS100]

Pentan-2-ol, methyl: Lf[CS068]

Pentan-3-ol, methyl: Lf[CS068]

Pentanoic acid: 2-amino-5-(N-ethyl-carboxamido): Lf 120[CS105]

Pent-cis-2-en-1-ol: Sh 0.1-0.14%[CS100]

Pent-cis-3-en-1-al: Lf[CS002]

Phenol: Lf[CS003]

Phenyl, acetate, ethyl: Lf[CS002]

Phenyl, acetate, hexyl: Lf[CS002]

Phenylacetic acid: Lf[CS002]

Phenylethanol, 2: Lf[CS091]

Phenylethyl alcohol, 2: Sh 0.1–0.13%[CS100]

Phenylethyl alcohol: Headspace volatile[CS044]

Pheophytin A: Lf[CS088]

Pheophytin B: Lf[CS088]

Pinene, a: Lf[CS068]

Pipecolic acid, L: Fr[CS030]

Pipecolic acid: Lf[CS037], Fr[CS037]

Polysaccharide T-B: Lf[CS111]

Procyanidin B-2 3'-O-gallate: Lf 166.7[CS140]

Procyanidin B-2, 3-3'-di-O-gallate: Lf 0.00084–0.13%[CS008,CS010]

Procyanidin B-2: Lf 5.8[CS008]

Procyanidin B-3, 3-O-gallate: Lf[CS070]

Procyanidin B-3: Lf 0.21%[CS010]

Procyanidin B-4, 3'-O-gallate: Lf 141[CS140]

Procyanidin B-4: Lf 46.6[CS008]

Procyanidin B-5, 3-3'-di- O-gallate: Lf 2.6[CS008]

Procyanidin C-1: Lf[CS010]

Prodelphinidin A-2, 3'-O-gallate: Lf 4.4[CS008]

Prodelphinidin B-2, 3'-O-gallate: Lf 238[CS008]

Prodelphinidin B-2, 3-3'-di-O-gallate: Lf 18.4[CS008]

Prodelphinidin B-2,3'-O-gallate: Lf 147.4[CS140]

Prodelphinidin B-4, 3'-O-gallate: Lf 63.8–1200[CS008,CS010]

Prodelphinidin B-4: Lf 56.8–800[CS008,CS010]

Prodelphinidin B-5, 3-3'-di-O-gallate: Lf 29.8[CS008]

Proline, hydroxy: Lf[CS037], Fr[CS037]

Propionamide, N-ethyl: Lf[CS027]

Propiophenone, 2-4-dimethyl: Lf[CS027]

Propiophenone, para-ethyl: Lf[CS027]

Prunasin: Lf[CS059]

Pyrazine, 2-3-dimethyl: Lf[CS027]

Pyrazine, 2-5-dimethyl: Lf[CS027]

Pyrazine, 2-6-dimethyl: Lf[CS027]

Pyrazine, 2-ethyl-3-5-dimethyl: Lf[CS027]

Pyrazine, 2-ethyl-3-6-dimethyl: Lf[CS036]

Pyrazine, 2-ethyl-5-methyl: Lf[CS027]

Pyrazine, 2-ethyl-6-methyl: Lf[CS027]

Pyrazine, ethyl: Lf[CS027]

Pyrazine, methyl: Lf[CS027]

Pyrazine, trimethyl: Lf[CS027]

Pyridine, 2-5-dimethyl: Lf[CS027]

Pyridine, 2-6-dimethyl: Lf[CS027]
Pyridine, 2-acetyl: Lf[CS036]
Pyridine, 2-ethyl: Lf[CS027]
Pyridine, 2-ethyl-5-methyl: Lf[CS036]
Pyridine, 2-ethyl-6-methyl: Lf[CS036]
Pyridine, 2-methyl: Lf[CS027]
Pyridine, 2-phenyl: Lf[CS027]
Pyridine, 3-ethyl: Lf[CS027]
Pyridine, 3-methoxy: Lf[CS036]
Pyridine, 3-methyl: Lf[CS027]
Pyridine, 3-N-butyl: Lf[CS036]
Pyridine, 3-phenyl: Lf[CS027]
Pyridine, 4-methyl: Lf[CS027]
Pyridine, 4-vinyl: Lf[CS036]
Pyridine: Lf[CS027]
Quercetin: Lf[CS026], Sh[CS094]
Quercetin-3-glucosyl(1-3)rhamnosyl (1-6)galactoside: Lf[CS009]
Quercetin-fructosyl-glucoside: Lf[CS063]
Quercimeritrin: Lf[CS026]
Quercitrin, iso: Lf[CS133]
Quercitrin: Lf[CS058]
Quinic acid, (−): Lf[CS104]
Quinoline, 2-4-dimethyl: Lf[CS027]
Quinoline, 2-6-dimethyl: Lf[CS027]
Quinoline, 2-methyl: Lf[CS036]
Quinoline, 3-N-butyl: Lf[CS027]
Quinoline, 3-N-propyl: Lf[CS027]
Quinoline, 4-8-dimethyl: Lf[CS027]
Quinoline, 6-methyl: Lf[CS036]
Rutin: Lf[CS058]
Safranal: Lf[CS002]
Safrole: Lf[CS002]
Salicylic acid: Headspace volatile[CS044]
Sesquiphelandrene, b: Lf[CS109]
Sitosterol, β: Sd oil[CS134]
Spinasterol, 22-23-dihydro: Sd oil[CS131]
Spinasterol, α, β-D-glucoside: Rt[CS039]
Spinasterol, α: Rt[CS039]
Spinasterol: Sd oilCS131
Spinasterone, 22-23-dihydro: Sd oil[CS131]
Spinasterone: Sd oil[CS131]
Stearic acid: Sd oil[CS134]
Stigmasterol: Sd oil[CS134]
Strictinin: Lf 0.01%[CS010]
Succinic acid: Lf[CS086]

Tannic acid: Lf [CS126]
Tannin: Lf[CS024]
Taraxasterol, Pseudo: Sd oil[CS095]
Taraxerol: Sd oil 20[CS095]
Tartaric acid: Lf[CS086]
Tea polysaccharides: Lf[CS055]
Teasaponin B-1: Lf[CS057]
Teasaponin B-2: Lf[CS040]
Teasaponin B-3: Lf[CS040]
Teasaponin B-4: Lf[CS040]
Teasterone: Lf[CS090]
Tectoquinone: Rt[CS039]
Terpineol, 4: Lf[CS002]
Terpineol, α: Sh 0.07–0.1%[CS100], Lf[CS068]
Theacitrin A: Lf 0.08%[CS016]
Theaflagallin, epi, 3-O-gallate: Lf 17[CS008]
Theaflagallin-3-O-gallate, epi: Lf 0.02%[CS010]
Theaflavate B: Lf[CS019]
Theaflavic acid, epi, gallate: Lf[CS064]
Theaflavic acid, epi: Lf[CS064]
Theaflavin, digallate: Lf[CS071]
Theaflavin, iso: 3'-O-gallate: Lf 25[CS019]
Theaflavin, monogallate A: Lf[CS071]
Theaflavin, monogallate B: Lf[CS071]
Theaflavin, monogallate: Lf[CS124]
Theaflavin, neo: 3-O-gallate: Lf 30[CS019]
Theaflavin: Lf[CS046], Sh 1.12–1.40%[CS100], Fl[CS159]
Theaflavin-3'-gallate: Lf[CS046]
Theaflavin-3'-O-gallate: Fl[CS159], Lf 18.6–800[CS008,CS010]
Theaflavin-3-3'- digallate: Fl[CS159]
Theaflavin-3-3'-di-O-gallate: Lf 18.2–300[CS008,CS010]
Theaflavin-3-gallate: Lf[CS046]
Theaflavin-3-O-gallate: Fl[CS159], Lf 6-700[CS008,CS010]
Theaflavin-monogallate A: Lf[CS085]
Theaflavin-monogallate B: Lf[CS085]
Theaflavonin, degalloyl: Lf 17.5[CS010]
Theaflavonin: Lf 11.5[CS010]
Theanaphthoquinone: Lf[CS023]
Theanine: Lf[CS052], Call Tiss[CS066], Seedling Rt 109, Sh 63, Cy 577 mg%[CS097], St Call 0.37 ppt, An 1.6-2.9%, St 34.9 ppt[CS099]
Thearubigin: Sh 13.56–15.74%[CS100], Lf[CS139]

Theasapogenol A, 22-O-angeloyl: Sd[CS020]
Theasapogenol B, 22-O-angeloyl: Sd[CS020]
Theasapogenol E, 22-O-angeloyl: Sd[CS020]
Theasaponin B-1: Lf[CS081]
Theasaponin E-1: Sd 75[CS017]
Theasaponin E-2: Sd 10[CS017]
Theasaponin, gluco: Sd[CS061]
Theasaponin: Sd[CS127], Lf[CS142]
Theasinensin A: Lf 0.01866–4.8718%[CS006,CS140]
Theasinensin B: Lf 128.2–600[CS140,CS010]
Theasinensin C: Lf 70.2[CS006]
Theasinensin D: Lf 17.6[CS006]
Theasinensin E: Lf 14.4[CS006]
Theasinensin F: Lf 19.6[CS006]
Theasinensin G: Lf 8[CS006]
Theaspirane, dihydro, 6-7-epoxy: Lf[CS002]
Theaspirane, dihydro, 6-hydroxy: Lf[CS002]
Theaspirane: Lf[CS002]
Theaspirone: Lf EO[CS132]
Theobromine: Lf[CS029], Call Tiss[CS050], Sd,
    Pc[CS102], Fl Bd, Fl[CS107], Petal, Pistil,
    Stamen[CS117], An, St, St Call[CS099], Pl[CS033],
    Seedcoat[CS102]
Theogallin: Lf 6-55.5[CS008,CS010]
Theophylline: Sd[CS093]
Thiazole, 2-4-5-trimethyl: Lf[CS036]
Thiazole, 2-4-dimethyl: Lf[CS036]
Thiazole, 2-4-dimethyl-4-ethyl: Lf[CS036]
Thiazole, 2-5-dimethyl: Lf[CS036]
Thiazole, 5-methyl: Lf[CS036]
Thymol: Lf[CS002]
Tirucalla-7-24-dien-3-β-ol, 5-α:
    Sd oil 12[CS062]
Tirucalla-7-24-dien-3-β-ol: Sd oil[CS095]
Tirucallol: Sd oil[CS095]
Toluidine, ortho: Lf[CS027]
Triacontan-1-ol: Lf[CS075]
Tricetin: Sh[CS094]
Tricetinidin: Lf[CS139]
Trifolin: Lf[CS058]
Tr-saponin A: Rt 2.2[CS022]
Tr-saponin B: Rt 5.9[CS022]
Tr-saponin C: Rt 2.8[CS022]
Typhasterol: Lf[CS090]
Umbelliferone: Lf[CS032]
Undeca-2-one, 6-10-dimethyl: Lf[CS002]

Undeca-*trans*-2-en-1-al: Lf[CS002]
Urea: Pl[CS033]
Vitamin K-1: Lf 3.1-16.5[CS072],
Vitexin, iso, 2''-O-glucoside: Lf[CS103]
Vitexin: Sh[CS096]
Vomifeliol, dehydro: Lf EO[CS132]

PHARMACOLOGICAL ACTIVITIES AND CLINICAL TRIALS

Antibacterial activity. Alcohol extract of black tea, assayed on *Salmonella typhi* and *Salmonella paratyphi* A, was active on all strains of Salmonella paratyphi A, and only 42.19% of Salmonella typhi strains were inhibited by the extract[CS048]. Hot water extract of the dried entire plant and the tannin fraction, on agar plate, were active on *Escherichia coli*, *Pseudomonas aeruginosa*, and *Staphylococcus aureus*[CS160].

Anticancer activity. Catechin, administered to pheochromocytoma cells in cell culture, was active. The cells were incubated with different concentrations of catechin at short-term (2 days) and long-term (7 days) in Dulbecco's modified Eagle medium. The activity of superoxide dismutase was measured and its mRNA assayed by Northern blotting. After incubation for 2 days, catechin significantly increased the activity of copper/zinc superoxide dismutase. However, it did not produce significant effect at 7 days. The magnesium superoxide dismutase activity produced significant changes in both short- and long-term treatment groups. The amount of mRNA also showed similar changes[CS040].

Anticarcinogenic activity. The anticarcinogenic activity of tea phenols has been demonstrated in rats and mice transplantable tumors, carcinogen-induced tumors in digestive organs, mammary glands, hepatocarcinomas, lung cancers, skin tumors, leukemia, tumor promotion, and metastasis. The mechanisms of this effect indicated that the inhibition of tumors may be the result of both extracellular and intracellular mechanisms indicating the modulation of metabolism, blocking or suppression, modulation of DNA replication and repair effects, promotion, inhibition of invasion and metastasis, and induction of novel mechanisms[CS002]. The association of green tea and cancer has been investigated in 8552 Japanese women 40 years of age. After 9 years of follow-up study, 384 cases of cancer were identified. There was a negative association between cancer incidence and green tea consumption, especially among females consuming more than 10 cups of tea a day. A slow down in increases of cancer incidence with age was observed among females who consumed more than 10 cups daily[CS010]. Tea, taken by lung cancer patients at a dose of two or more cups per day, reduced the risk by 95%. The protected effect was more evident among Kreyberg I tumors (squamous cell and small cells) and among light smokers[CS011]. The green tea polyphenols, epi-gallocatechin-3-gallate, applied topically to human skin, prevented penetration of ultraviolet (UV) radiation. This was demonstrated by the absence of immunostaining for cyclobutane pyrimidine dimers in the reticular dermis. Topical administration to the skin of mice inhibited UVB-induced infiltration of CDIIb⁺ cells. The treatment also results in reduction of the UVB-induced immunoregulatory cytokine interleukin (IL)-10 in the skin and draining lymph nodes, and an elevated amount of IL-12 in draining lymph nodes[CS015]. Green tea extract, in human umbilical vein endothelial cells, did not affect cell viability but significantly reduced cell proliferation dose-dependently and produced a dose-dependent accumulation of cells in the gastrointestinal phase. The decrease of the expression of vascular endothelial growth factor receptors fms-like tyrosine kinase and fetal liver kinase-I/ kinase insert domain containing receptor in the cell culture by the extract was detected with immunohistochemical and Western blotting methods[CS020]. Green and black tea, administered orally to hairless mice in the absence of any chemical initiators or promoters, resulted in significantly fewer skin papillomas and tumors induced by UVA and UVB light. Black tea however, provided better protection against UVB-induced tumors than green tea. Black tea consumption was associated with a reduction in the number of sunburn cells in the epidermis of mice 24 hours after irradiation, although there was no effect of green tea. Other indices of early damage such as necrotic cells or mitotic figures were not affected. Neutrophil infiltration as a measure of skin redness was slightly lowered by tea consumption in the UVB group[CS023]. Epigallocatechin-3-gallate, in cell culture, activated proMMP-2 in U-87 glioblastoma cells in the presence of concanavalin A or cytochalasin D, two potent activators of MT1-MMP, resulted in proMMP-2 activation that was correlated with the cell surface proteolytic processing of Mt1-MMP to it's inactive 43 kDa form. Addition of epigallocatechin-3-gallate strongly inhibited the MT1-MMP-driven migration in the cells. The treatment of cells with non-cytotoxic doses of epigallocatechin-3-gallate significantly reduced the amount of secreted pro MMP-2, and led to a concomitant increase in intracellular levels of that protein. The effect was similar to that observed using well-characterized secretion inhibitors such as brefeldin A and manumycin, indicative that epigallocatechin could also potentially act on intracellular secretory pathways[CS044]. Green tea polyphenols, at a dose of 30 mg/mL, inhibited the photolabeling of P-glycoprotein (P-gp) by 75% and increased the accumulation of rhodamine-123 in the multidrug-resistant cell line CH(R)C5. This result indicated that green tea polyphenols interact with P-gp and inhibited its transport activity. The modulation of P-gp was a reversible process. Epigallocatechin-3-gallate potentiates the cytotoxicity of vinblastine in CH(R)C5 cells. The inhibitory effect on P-gp was also observed in human Caco-2 cells[CS045].

Anticataract activity. Tea, administered in culture to enucleated rat lens, reduced the incidence of selenite cataract in vivo. The rat lenses were randomly divided into normal, control and treated groups and incubated for 24 hours at 37°C. Oxidative stress was induced by sodium selenite in the culture medium of the two groups (except the normal group). The medium of the treated group was additionally supplemented with tea extract. After incubation, lenses were subjected to glutathione and malondialdehyde estimation. Enzyme activity of superoxide dismutase, catalase, and glutathione peroxidase were also measured in different sets of the experiment. In vivo cataract was induced in 9-day-old rat pups of both control and treated groups by a single subcutaneous injection of sodium selenite. The treated pups were injected with tea extract intraperitoneally prior to selenite challenge and continued for 2 consecutive days thereafter. Cataract incidence was evaluated on 16 postnatal days by slit lamp examination. There was positive modulation of biochemical parameters in the organ culture study. The results indicated that tea act primarily by preserving the antioxidant defense system[CS039].

Antidiarrheal activity. Hot water extract of tea, administered orally to rats, was effective in all the models of diarrhea used. Naloxone (0.5 mg/kg, ip) and loperamide significantly inhibited the antidiarrheal activity of the extract[CS029].

Antifungal activity. Ethanol (50%) extract of the entire plant, in broth culture at a concentration of 1 mg/mL, was inactive on *Aspergillus fumigatus* and *Trichophyton mentagrophytes*[CS161]. Hot water extract of the leaf on agar plate at a concentration of 1.0% was active on *Alternaria tenuis*, *Pythium apha-*nidermatum, and *Rhizopus stolonifer*[CS162]. Saponin fraction of the leaf on agar plate was active on *Microsporum audonini*, minimum inhibitory concentration (MIC) 10 mg/mL; *Epidermophyton floccosum* and *Trichophyton mentagrophytes*, MICs 25 µg/mL[CS165].

Antihypercholesterolemic activity. Tea supplemented with vitamin E, administered to male Syrian hamsters, reduced plasma low-density lipoprotein (LDL) cholesterol concentrations, LDL oxidation, and early atherosclerosis compared to the consumption of tea alone by the hamsters. The antioxidant action of vitamin E is through the incorporation of vitamin E into the LDL molecule. The hamsters were fed a semipurified hypercholesterolemic diet containing 12% coconut oil, 3% sunflower oil, and 0.2% cholesterol (control), control and 0.625% tea, control and 1.25% tea or control and 0.044% tocopherol acetate for 10 weeks. The hamsters fed the vitamin E diet compared to the different concentrations of tea significantly lower plasma LDL cholesterol concentrations, –18% ($p < 0.007$), –17% ($p < 0.02$), and –24% ($p < 0.0001$), respectively. Aortic fatty streak areas were reduced in the vitamin E diet group compared to the control, –36% ($p < 0.04$) and low tea –45% ($p < 0.01$) diets. Lag phase of conjugated diene production was greater in the vitamin E diet compared to the control, low tea, and high tea diets, 41% ($p < 0.0004$), 40% ($p < 0.0004$), and 39% ($p < 0.0008$), respectively. Rate of conjugated diene production was reduced in the vitamin E diet compared to the control, low tea, and high tea diets, –63% ($p < 0.002$), –57% ($p < 0.005$), and –59% ($p < 0.02$), respectively[CS005]. Infusion of black tea leaves was taken by 31 men (ages 47 ± 14) and 34 females (ages 35 ± 13) in a 4-week study. Six mugs of tea were taken daily vs placebo (water, caffeine, milk, and sugar) and blood lipids, bowel habit, and blood pressure measured during a run-in period and at the end weeks 2, 3, and 4 of the test period. Compliance was established by adding a known amount of *p*-aminobenzoic acid to selected tea bags and then measure it excretion in the urine. Mean serum cholesterol values during run-in, placebo and on tea drinking were 5.67 ± 1.05, 5.76 ± 1.11, and 5.69 ± 1.09 mmol/L ($p = 0.16$). There were also no significant changes in diet, LDL-cholesterol, high-density lipoprotein (HDL) cholesterol, triacylglycerols, and blood pressure in the tea intervention period compared with placebo. Stool consistency was softened with tea compared with the placebo, and no other differences were observed in bowel habit. The results were unchanged within 15 "noncompliers" whose *p*-aminobenzoic acid excretion indicated that fewer than six tea bags had been used, were excluded from the analysis, and when differenced between run-in and tea periods were considered separately for those who were given tea first or second[CS167].

Anti-inflammatory effect. Epigallocatechin-3-gallate was shown to mimic its antiinflammatory effects in modulating the IL-I β-induced activation of mitogen activated protein kinase in human chondrocytes. It inhibited the IL-I β-induced phosphorylation of c-Jun N-terminal kinase (JNK) isoforms, accumulation of phospho-c-Jun and DNA-binding activity of AP-1 in osteoarthritis chondrocytes, IL-I β but not epigallocatechin-3-gallate, and induced the expression of JNK p46 without modulating the expression of JNK p54 in osteoarthritis chondrocytes. In immune complex kinase assays, epigallocatechin-3-gallate completely blocked the substrate phosphorylating activity of JNK but not p38-mitogen activated protein kinase (MAPK). Epigallocatechin-3-gallate had no inhibitory effect on the activation of extracellular signal-regulated kinase p44/p42 (ERKp44/p42) or

p38-MAPK in chondrocytes. Epigallocatechin-3-gallate did not alter the total nonphosphorylated levels of either p38-MAPK or ERKp44/p42 in osteoarthritis chondrocytes[CS033]. Epigallocatechin-3-gallate administered to primary human osteoarthritis chondrocytes at a concentration of 100 µM in cell culture, inhibited the IL-I β-induced production of nitric oxide by interfering with the activation of nuclear factor (NF)κB[CS042]. Tea, in culture with bovine nasal and metacarpophalangeal cartilage and human nondiseased osteoarthritis and rheumatoid cartilage with and without reagents known to accelerate cartilage matrix breakdown, produced chondroprotective effect that may be beneficial for the arthritis patient by reducing inflammation and the slowing of cartilage breakdown. Individual catechins were added to the cultures and the amount of released proteoglycan and type II collagen were measured by metachromatic assay and inhibition enzyme-linked immunosorbent assay (ELISA), respectively. Possible nonspecific or toxic effects of the catechins were assessed by lactate output and proteoglycan synthesis. Catechins, particularly those containing a gallate ester, were effective at micromolar concentrations at inhibiting proteoglycan and type II collagen breakdown[CS043].

Antimutagenic activity. The anticarcinogenic activity of tea phenols has been demonstrated in rats and mice, transplantable tumors, carcinogen-induced tumors in digestive organs, mammary glands, hepatocarcinomas, lung cancers, skin tumors, leukemia, tumor promotion, and metastasis. The mechanisms of this effect indicated that the inhibition of tumors maybe the result of both extracellular and intracellular mechanisms indicting the modulation of metabolism, blocking or suppression, modulation of DNA replication and repair effects, promotion, inhibition of invasion and

Metastasis, and induction of novel mechanisms[CS002]. Green and black teas, administered orally to human adults, were effective. Between 60 and 180 minutes after the teas were administered, the antimutagenic active compounds were recovered from the jejunal compartment by means of dialysis. The dialysate appeared to inhibit the mutagenicity of the food mutagen 2-amino-3,8-dimethylimidazo[4,5-f]quinoxaline on *Salmonella typhimurium*. The maximum inhibition was measured at 2 hours after administration and was comparable for black and green teas. The maximum inhibition observed with black tea was reduced by 22, 42, and 78% in the presence of whole milk, semi-skimmed milk, and skimmed milk, respectively. Whole milk and skimmed milk abolished the antimutagenic activity of green tea by more than 90% and semi-skimmed milk by more than 60%. When a homogenized breakfast was taken with black tea, the antimutagenic activity was eliminated. When tea and mutagen 2-amino-3,8-dimethylimidazo[4,5-f]quinoxaline were added to the system, 2-amino-3,8-dimethyl-imidazo[4,5-f]quinoxaline mutagenicity was efficiently inhibited, with green tea showing a slightly stronger antimutagenic activity than black tea. The addition of milk had only a small inhibiting effect on the antimutagenicity. The antimutagenic activity corresponded with reduction in antioxidant capacity and with a decrease of concentration of catechin, epigallocatechin gallate, and epigallocatechin[CS014]. Chinese white tea, tested on rat liver S9 in assay for methoxyresorufin O-demethylase, inhibited methoxyresorufin O-demethylase activity and attenuated the mutagenic activity of 3-methylimidazo[4,5-f]quinoline (IQ) in absence of S9. Nine of the major constituents found in green and white teas were mixed to produce artificial teas according to their relative levels in white and green teas. The complete tea exhibited higher antimu-

tagenic potency compared with the corresponding artificial tea[CS019]. Green and black tea polyphenols, applied to the surfaces of ground beef before cooking, inhibited the formation of the mutagens in a dose-related fashion[CS025]. Green or black tea polyphenols sharply decreased the mutagenicity of a number of aryl- and heterocyclic amines, of aflatoxin B_1, benzo[a]pyrene, 1,2-dibromoethane, and more selectively of 2-nitropropane, all involving an induced rat liver S9 fraction. Good inhibition was found with two nitrosamines that required a hamster S9 fraction for biochemical activation. No effect was found with 1-nitropyrene and with the direct-acting (no S9) 2-chloro-4-methyl-thiobutanoic acid[CS027]. Hot water extract on the leaf was evaluated in cell cultures on various systems vs decaffeinated and caffeinated teas. On mouse mammary gland vs decaffeinated and caffeinated teas, ICs_{50} were 10 mg/mL and 10 µg/mL on CA-A427, IC_{50} 27 mg/mL and 31 µg/mL, and on epithelial cells, IC_{50} 0.01 ng/mL and 0.3 ng/mL[CS169]. Hot water extract of the leaf, on agar plate at a concentration of 1 mg/plate, was active on Salmonella typhimurium TA98 vs 2-amino-3-methylimidazo[4,5-f]quinoline-induced mutagenesis and produced weak activity vs benzo[a]pyrene-induced mutagenesis[CS168]. Infusion of the leaf, on agar plate at a concentration of 0.7 mg/plate, was active on *Salmonella typhimurium* TA98 and TA100 vs 2-amino-3-methylimidazo[4,5-f]quinoline-; 3-amino-1,4-dimethyl-5H-pyrid[4,3-b]indole(Trp-1); aflatoxin B1-; 2-amino-6-methyl-dipyrido[1,2-A:3,2-d]imidazole-, and benzo[a]pyrene-induced carcinogenesis[CS170]. Infusion of the leaf, on agar plate at a concentration of 50 mg/plate, was active on *Salmonella typhimurium* TA98 vs 2-amino-3-methylimidazo[4,5-f]quinoline-; 2-amino-3,4-dimethyl-imidazo[4,5-f]quinoline-;2-amino-3,8-dimethylimidazo[4,5-f]quinoxaline-;

2-amino-1-methyl-6-phenylimidazo[4,5-b]-pyridine-; 2-amino-3,7,8-trimethylimidazo[4,5-f]quinoxaline-; 2-amino-3,4,7,8-tetramethyl-3H-imidazo-[4,5-f]quinoxaline-inoxaline-; 3-amino-1,4-dimethyl-5H-pyrid[4,3-b]indole (Trp-P-I)- and 3-amino-1-methyl-5H-pyrido [4,3-b]indole-induced mutagenesis. Metabolic activation was required for positive results[CS171].

Anti-neoplastic effect. Green tea, administered orally at a dose of 6 g per day in six doses to 42 patients who were asymptomatic and had manifested, progressive prostate specific antigen elevation with hormone therapy, produced limited anti-neoplastic activity. Continued use of luteinizing hormone-releasing hormone agonist was permitted. However, patients were ineligible if they had received other treatments for their disease in the preceding 4 weeks or if they had received a long-acting antiandrogen therapy in the preceding 6 weeks. The patients were monitored monthly for response and toxicity. Tumor response, defined as a decline of 50% or greater in the baseline prostate-specific antigen (PSA) value, occurred in a single patient, or 2% of The cohort (95% confidence interval [CI], 1–14%). This one response was not sustained beyond 2 months. At the end of the first month, the median change in the PSA value from baseline for the cohort increased by 43%[CS031]. Infusion of the leaf, administered in the drinking of female mice at a concentration of 1.25%, was active vs UV radiation-induced papillomas and tumors[CS172]. Leaves in the drinking water of female mice at a dose of 0.6% reduced lung tumor multiplicity and volume in 4-(methylnitrosamine)-1-(3-pyridyl)-1-butanone (NNK) treated mice[CS173].

Antioxidative effect. Tea, administered orally to rats, decreased the thiobarbituric acid reactive substances (TBARS) contents

in urine and lowered the esterified and total cholesterol contents in plasma as compared with a control group. TBARS contents in liver, plasma, and cholesterol levels in the liver were not affected. The lower plasma cholesterol concentration could not be explained by increased fecal excretion of cholesterol or bile acids. On the other hand, a relationship between decreased plasma cholesterol and significantly higher acetate concentrations in the cecum, colon, and portal blood of rats was assumed. Copper absorption was significantly increased while iron absorption was not affected[CS007]. Epigallocatechin gallate, tea polyphenols, and tea extract were added to human plasma and lipid peroxidation induced by the water-soluble radical generator 2,2'-azobis (2-amidinopropane) dihydrochloride. Following a lag phase, lipid peroxidation was initiated and it occurred at a rate that was lower in a dose that was lowered in a dose-dependent manner by the polyphenols. Similarly, epigallocatechin gallate and the extract added to plasma strongly inhibited 2,2'-azobis(2-amidinopropane) dihydrochloride-induced lipid peroxidation. The lag phase preceding detectable lipid peroxidation was the result of the antioxidant activity of endogenous ascorbate, which was more effective at inhibiting lipid peroxidation than the tea polyphenols and was not spared by these compounds. When eight volunteers consumed the equivalent of six cups of tea, the resistance of their plasma to lipid peroxidation did not increase over a period of 3 hours[CS009]. Black tea leaves, administered to human red blood cells, was effective against damage by oxidative stress induced by inducers such as phenylhydrazine, Cu^{2+}-ascorbic acid, and xanthine/xanthine oxidase systems. Lipid peroxidation of pure erythrocyte membrane and of whole red blood cell was completely prevented by black tea extract. Similarly, the tea provided total protection against degradation of membrane proteins. Membrane fluidity studies as monitored by the fluorescent probe 1,6-diphenyl hexa 1,3,5-triene showed considerable disorganization of its architecture that could be restored back to normal on addition of black tea or free catechins. The tea extract in comparison to free catechin seemed to be a better protecting agent against various types of oxidative stress[CS013]. Ethanol/water (7:3) extract of green tea, tested on 2,2-azino-di-3-ethylbenzthiazoline sulphonate, produced antioxidant activity compared with that of ascorbic acid (10 mmol/L)[CS018]. The Nonpolyphenolic fraction of residual green tea (after hot water extraction) produced a significant suppression against hydroperoxide generation from oxidized linoleic acid in a dose-dependent manner. Using silica gel TLC plate, chlorophylls a and b, pheophytins a and b, β-carotene, and lutein were isolated. All of these constituents exhibited significant antioxidant activites, the ranks of suppressive activity against hydroperoxide generation were chlorophyll a > lutein > pheophytin a > chlorophyll b > b-carotene > pheophytin b[CS047].

Antiproliferative activity. Green tea fractions, tested on human stomach cancer (MK-1) cells, indicated six active flavan-3-ols, epicatechin, epigallocatechin, epigallocatechin gallate, gallocatechin, epicatechin gallate, and gallocatechin gallate. Among the six active flavan-3-ols, epigallocatechin gallate and gallocatechin gallate produced the highest activity. Epigallocatechin, gallocatechin, and epicatechin gallate followed next, and the activity of epicatechin was lowest. This suggests that the presence of the three adjacent hydroxyl groups (pyrogallol or galloyl group) in the molecule would be a key factor for enhancing the activity[CS032].

Antiprotozoan activity. Ethanol (50%) extract of the entire plant, in broth culture at a concentration of 125 μg/mL, was inactive on *Entamoeba histolytica*[CS161].

Antispasmodic activity. Hot water extract and tannin fraction of the dried entire plant were active on the rabbit and rat intestines vs pilocarpine-induced spasms and barium-induced contractions[CS160].

Antiviral activity. Epigallocatechin-3-gallate, administered to Hep2 cells in culture, produced a therapeutic index of 22 and an IC_{50} of 25 μM. The agent was the most effective when added to the cells during the transition from the early to the late phase of viral infection suggesting that the polyphenol inhibits one or more late steps in virus infection[CS016]. Ethanol (50%) extract of the entire plant, in broth culture at a concentration of 50 μg/mL, was inactive on Raniket and Vaccinia viruses[CS161]. Hot water extract of the leaf in cell culture was active on Coxsackie A9, B1, B2, B3, B4, and B6 viruses, Echo type 9 virus, herpes simplex virus, poliovirus III, vaccinia virus, and REO type 1 virus[CS163].

Anti-yeast activity. Ethanol (50%) extract of the entire plant, in broth culture at a concentration of 1 mg/mL, was inactive on *Candida albicans*, *Cryptococcus neoformans*, and *Sporotrichum schenckii*[CS161]. Ethanol extract of the leaf on agar plate produced MIC 9.3 mg/mL on *Candida albicans*[CS164].

Coronary heart disease prevention. Tea, taken by men and women age 30 to 70 years at a dose of 480.0 mL per day, produced a positive dose–response effect[CS008].

Cytochrome P50 expression. Fresh leaves of green, black, and decaffeinated black tea enhanced lauric acid hydroxylation. The decaffeinated black tea produced no significant effect. Green tea and black tea but not decaffeinated black tea, stimulated the O-dealkylations of methoxy-, ethoxy-, and pentoxy-resorufin indicating upregulation of cytochrome P50 (CYP)1A and CYP2B. Immunoblot analysis revealed that green and black tea, but not decaffeinated black tea, elevated the hepatic CYP1A2 apoprotein levels. Hepatic microsomes from green and black tea-treated rats, but not those from the decaffeinated black tea-treated rats, were more effective than controls in converting IQ into mutagenic species in the Ames test[CS001].

Dental enamel erosion. Herbal tea and conventional black tea, tested on teeth, resulted in erosion of dental enamel. After exposure to tea, sequential profilometric tracings of the specimens were taken, superimposed, and the degree of enamel loss calculated as the area of disparity between the tracings before and after exposure. Tooth surface loss resulted from herbal tea (mean 0.05 mm^2) was significantly greater than that which resulted from exposure to conventional black tea (0.01 mm2), and water (0.00 mm^2)[CS022]. Tannin, catechin, caffeine, and tocopherol, tested in vitro on tooth enamel, demonstrated that these components possess the property of increasing the acid resistance of tooth enamel. The effects increased dramatically when the components were used in combination with fluoride. A mixture of tannic acid and fluoride showed the highest inhibitory effect (98%) on calcium release to an acid solution. Tannin in combination with fluoride inhibited the formation of artificial enamel lesions in comparison with acidulated phosphate fluoride (APF) as determined by electron probe microanalysis, polarized-light microscopy, and Vickers microhardness measurement[CS024].

DNA effect. Green tea extract, in cell culture at a dose of 10 mg/L corresponding to 15 mmol/L EGCg for 24 hours, did not protect Jurkat cells against H_2O_2-induced DNA damage. The DNA damage, evaluated by the Comet assay, was dose-dependent. However, it reached plateau at 75 mmol/L of H_2O_2 without any protective effect exerted by the extract. The DNA repair process, completed within 2 hours, was unaffected by supplementation[CS021].

Fluoride retention. Tea, used as a mouth rinse, demonstrated strong avidity of enamel for tea and salivary pellicle components. Thirty-four percent of the fluoride was retained in the oral cavity. Differences in retention at the tooth surface in the presence and absence of an acquired pellicle were not statistically significant at incisor or molar sites. Fluoride from tea showed strong binding to enamel particles, which was only partially dissociated by solutions of ionic strength considerably greater than that of saliva[CS012].

Gastrointestinal effect. Green tea, administered to rats fasted for 3 days, reverted to normal the mucosal and villous atrophy induced by fasting. Black tea ingestion had no effect. Ingestion of black tea, green tea, and vitamin E before fasting protected the intestinal mucosa against atrophy[CS003]. Characterization of melanin extracted from tea leaves proved similarity of the original compound to standard melanin. The Langmuir adsorption isotherms for gadolinium (Gd) binding were obtained using melanin. Melanin–Gd preparation demonstrated low acute toxicity. LD50 for the preparation was in a range of 1.25–1.50 g/kg in mice. Magnetic resonance imaging (MRI) properties of melanin itself and melanin-Gd complexes have been estimated. Gadolinium-free melanin fractions possess slighter relaxivity compared with its complexes. The relaxivity of lower molecular weight fraction was 2 times higher than relaxivity of Gd(DTPA) standard. Postcontrast images demonstrated that oral administration of melanin complexes in concentration of 0.1 mM provides essential enhancement to longitudinal relaxation times (T[1])-weighted spin echo image. The required contrast and delineation of the stomach wall demonstrated uniform enhancement of MRI with proposed melanin complex[CS049].

Hypocholesterolemic effect. Green tea, in human HepG2 cell culture, increased both LDL receptor-binding activity and protein. The ethyl acetate extract, containing 70% (w/w) catechins, also increased

LDL receptor-binding activity, protein, and mRNA, indicating that the effect was at the receptor level of gene transcription and that the catechins were the active constituents. The mechanism by which green tea upregulated the LDL receptor was investigated. Green tea decreased the cell cholesterol concentration (–30%) and increased the conversion of the sterol-regulated element binding protein (SREBP-1) from the inactive precursor form to the active transcription-factor form. Consistent with this, the mRNA of 3-hydroxy-3-methylglutaryl coenzyme-A reductase, the rate limiting enzyme in cholesterol synthesis, was also increased by green tea[CS050].

Immunomodulatory effect. To determine the effects of tea on transplant-related immune function in vitro lymphocyte proliferation tests using phytohemagglutinin, mixed lymphocytes culture assay, IL-2, and IL-10 production from mixed lymphocyte proliferation were performed. Tea had immunosuppressive effects and decreased alloresponsiveness in the culture. The immunosuppressive effect of tea was mediated through a decrease in IL-2 production[CS038]. Tea, assayed in cell culture, enhanced neopterin production in unstimulated peripheral mononuclear cells, whereas an effective reduction of neopterin formation in cells stimulated with concanavalin A, phytohemagglutinin or interferon (IFN)-γ was observed[CS041]. Theaflavins potently suppressed IL-2 secretion, IL-2 gene expression, and the activation of NF-κB in murine spleens enriched for CD4(+) T-cells. Theaflavins also inhibited the induction of IFN-γ mRNA. However, the expression of the T(H2) cytokines IL-4 and IL-5, which lack functional NF-κB sites within their promoters was unexpectedly suppressed by theaflavins as well[CS046].

Insulin-enhancing effect. Tea, as normally consumed, was shown to increase insulin activity more than 15-fold in vitro in an epididymal fat cell assay. The majority of the insulin-potentiating activity for green and oolong teas was owing to epigallocatechin gallate. For black tea, the activity was present in addition to epigallocatechin gallate, tannins, theaflavins, and other undefined compounds. Several known compounds found in tea were shown to enhance insulin with the greatest activity due to epigallocatechin gallate followed by epicatechin gallate, tannins, and theaflavins. Caffeine, catechin, and epicatechin displayed insignificant insulin-enhancing activities. Addition of lemon to the tea did not affect the insulin-potentiating activity. Addition of 5 g of 2% milk per cup decreased the insulin-potentiating activity one-third, and addition of 50 g of milk per cup decreased the insulin-potentiating activity approx 90%. Non-dairy creamers and soymilk also decreased the insulin-potentiating activity[CS034].

Iron absorption. Tea, administered by gastric intubation to rats, did not affect iron absorption when tea was consumed for 3 days but when delivered in tea the absorption was decreased. Rats maintained on a commercial diet were fasted overnight with free access to water and then gavaged with 1 mL of ^{59}Fe labeled FeCl3 (0.1 mM or 1 mM) and lactulose (0.5 M) in water or black tea. Iron absorption was estimated from Fe retention. Intestinal permeability was evaluated by lactulose excretion in the urine. Iron absorption was lower with given with tea at both iron concentrations but tea did not affect lactulose excretion[CS004].

Lipid peroxidation activity. Solubilized green tea, administered orally to rats for 5 weeks, reduced lipid peroxidation products. The treatment produced increased activity of glutathione (GSH) peroxidase and GSH reductase, increased content of reduced GSH, a marked decrease in lipid hydroperoxides and malondialdehyde in the liver, an increase in the concentration of vitamin A by about 40%. A minor change in the measured parameters was observed in the blood serum. GSH content increased slightly, whereas the index of the total antioxidant status increased significantly. In contrast, the lipid peroxidation products, particularly malondialdehyde, was significantly diminished. In the central nervous tissue, the activity of superoxide dismutase and glutathione peroxidase decreased, whereas the activity of GSH reductase and catalase increased after drinking green tea. Moreover, the level of lipid hydroperoxides, 4-hydroksynonenal, and malondialdehyde decreased significantly[CS036].

Neuromuscular-blocking action. Thearubigin fraction of black tea was investigated for neuromuscular-blocking action of botulinum neurotoxin types A, B, and E in the mouse phrenic nerve-diaphragm preparations. On binding, A (1.5 nM), B (6 nM), and E (5 nM) abolished indirect twitches within 50, 90, and 90 minutes, respectively. Thearubigin fraction mixed with each toxin protected against the neuromuscular-blocking action of botulinum neurotoxin types A, B, and E by binding with the toxins[CS037].

Oral submucousal fibrosis effect. Tea, administered orally to 39 patients with oral submucous fibrosis, indicated that the treatment was effective for patients with abnormal hemorheology. The patients were divided into control and experimental groups. The control group included 22 oral submucous fibrosis patients who were treated by oral administration of vitamins A and D, vitamin B complex, and vitamin E. The experimental group included 17 patients who were treated with vitamins and tea pigment after their examination of hemorheology. The results showed that 7 of 12 patients in the experimental group with abnormal hemorheology had average 7.9 mm improvement on the open degree (58.3%), and the open degree of the other five patients whose hemorheology was normal only increased 2 mm (20%). The therapeutical results of the experimental group (58.3%) were significantly better than that of the control group (13.6%) ($p <$ 0.005)[CS035].

P-glycoprotein activity. Green tea polyphenols (30 µg/mL) inhibited the photolabeling of P-gp by 75% and increased the accumulation of rhodamine-123 threefold in a multidrug-resistant cell line CH(R)C5, indicating that the polyphenols interact with P-gp and inhibit its transport activity. The modulation of P-gp transport by polyphenols was a reversible process[CS045].

Photoprotection effect. Tea extracts, administered topically, produced a dose-dependent inhibition of the erythema response evoked by UV radiation. The (–)-epigallocatechin-3-gallate and (–)-epicatechin-3-gallate polyphenolic fractions were most efficient at inhibiting erythema, whereas (–)-epigallocatechin and (–)-epicatechin had little effect. On histological examination, skin treated with the extracts reduced the number of sunburn cells and protected epidermal Langerhans cells from UV damage. The extract also reduced damage that formed after UV radiation[CS006]. Green tea polyphenols, applied topically to the human skin, prevented UVB-induced cyclobutane pyrimidine dimers, which are considered to be mediators of UVB-induced immune suppression and skin cancer induction. The treatment, prior to exposure to UVB, protected against UVB-induced local as well as systemic immune suppression in laboratory animals. Additionally, treatment of mouse skin inhibited UVB-induced infiltration of CD11b cells. CD11b is a cell-surface marker for activated macrophages and neutrophils, which are associated with induction of UVB-induced suppression of contact hypersensitivity responses. The treatment also resulted in reduction of the UVB-induced immunoregulatory cytokine IL-10 in skin as well as in draining lymph nodes, and an elevated amount of IL-12 in draining lymph nodes[CS026].

Protease inhibition. Epigallocatechin-3-gallate, in cell culture at a concentration of 100 μM, reduced virus yield by 2 orders of magnitude producing an IC_{50} of 25 μM and a therapeutic index of 22 in Hep2 cells. The agent was the most effective when added to the cells during the transition from the early to the late phase of viral infection, suggesting that it inhibited one or more late steps in virus infection. One of these steps appears to be virus assembly, because the titer of infectious virus and the production of physical particles were much more affected than the synthesis of virus proteins. Another step might be the maturation cleavages carried out by adenain. When tested on adenain, epigallocatechin-3-gallate produced an IC_{50} of 109 μM[CS017].

Radical scavenging activity. Green tea, evaluated using the 1,1-diphenyl-2-picryl-hydrazyl radical, indicated that the galloyl moiety showed more potent activity. The contribution of the pyrogallol moiety in the B-ring to the scavenging activity seemed to be less than that of the galloyl moiety[CS032].

Tetanus toxin protection. Thearubigin fraction of black tea was investigated for neuromuscular-blocking action on tetanus toxin in the mouse phrenic nerve-diaphragm preparations and on binding of this toxin to the synaptosomal membrane preparations of rat cerebral cortices. Tetanus toxin (4 μg/mL) abolished indirect twitches in the mouse phrenic nerve–diaphragm preparations within 150 minutes. Thearubigin fraction mixed with tetanus toxin blocked the inhibitory effect of the toxin[CS030].

Toxicity. Green tea, administered orally at a dose of 6 g per day in six doses to 42 patients who were asymptomatic and had manifested, progressive prostate specific antigen elevation with hormone therapy, produced grade 1 or 2 toxicity in 69% of the patients and included nausea, emesis, insomia, fatigue, diarrhea, abdominal pain, and confusion. However, six episodes of grade 3 toxicity and one episode of grade 4 toxicity also occurred, with the latter manifesting as severe confusion[CS051].

Toxicity assessment. Ethanol (50%) extract of the entire plant, administered intraperitoneally to mice produced lethal dose $(LD)_{50}$ 316 mg/kg[CS161]. Ethanol (95%) extract of the leaf, administered by gastric intubation to mice, produced LD_{50} 10 g/kg. Intraperitoneal administration produced CD_{90} 0.7 g/kg[CS166].

REFERENCES

CS001 Vincent, D., G. Segonzae and R. Issandou-Carles. Action of purine alkaloids and caffeine-containing drugs on hyaluronidase. **C R Seances Soc Biol Ses Fil** 1954; 148: 1075.

CS002 Renold, W., R. Naf-Muller, U. Keller, B. Willhalm and G. Ohloff. An investigation of the tea aroma. Part I. New volatile black tea constituents. **Helv Chim Acta** 1974; 57: 1301.

CS003 Kaiser, H. E. Cancer-promoting effect of phenols in tea. Cancer (Philadelphia) 1967; 20: 361.

CS004 Koshioka, M., S. Yamaguchi, T. Nishima, H. Yamazaaki, D. O. Ferraren and L. N. Mander. Endogenous gibberellins in the developing liquid endosperm of tea. **Biosci Biotech Biochem** 1993; 57(9): 1586–1588.

CS005 Hashimoto, F., G. I. Nonaka and I. Nishioka. Tannins and related compounds. LVI. Isolation of four new acylated flavan-3-ols from oolong tea. **Chem Pharm Bull** 1987; 35(2): 611–616.

CS006 Hashimoto, F., G. I. Nonaka and I. Nishioka. Tannins and related compounds. LXIX. Isolation and structure elucidation of B,B'-linked bisflavanoids, theasinensis D-G and oolongtheanin from oolong tea. **Chem Pharm Bull** 1988; 36(5): 1676–1684.

CS007 Hashimoto, F., G. Nonaka and I. Nishioka. Tannins and related compounds. LXXVII. Novel chalcan–flavan dimmers, assamicains A, B and C, and a new flavan-3-ol and proanthocyanidins from the fresh leaves of *Camellia sinensis* L. *var. assamica Kita-*

mura. **Chem Pharm Bull** 1989; 37(1): 77–85.

CS008   Hashimoto, F., G. I. NAnaka and I. Nishioka. Tannins and related compounds. XC. 8-C-ascorbyl (–)-epogalocatechin 3-O-gallate and novel dimeric flavan-3-ols, oolonghomobisflavans A and B, from oolong tea. (3). **Chem Pharm Bull** 1989; 37(12): 3255–3263.

CS009   Finger, A., U. H. Engelhadt and V. Wray. Flavonol triglycosides containing galactose in tea. **Phytochemistry** 1991; 30(6): 2057–2060.

CS010   Hashimoto, F., G. I. Nonaka and I. Nishioka. Tannins and related compounds. CXIV. Structure of novel fermentation products, theogallinin, theaflavonin and desgalloyl theaflavonin from black tea and changes of tea leaf polyphenols during fermentation. **Chem Pharm Bull** 1992; 40(6): 1383–1389.

CS011   Sekine, T., Y. Arai, F. Ikegami, Y. Fujii, S. Shindo, T. Yanagisawa, Y. Ishida, S. Okonogi and I. Murakoshi. Isolation of camelliaside C from "tea seed cake" and inhibitory effects of its derivatives on arachidonate 5-lipoxygenase. **Chem Pharm Bull** 1993; 41(6): 1185–1187.

CS012   Fang, J. N., Z. H. Zhang, G. Q. Song and B. N. Liu. Structural features of a polysaccharide from the leaves of *Thea sinensis*. **Chin J Chem** 1991; 9(6): 547–551.

CS013   Sagesak, Y. M., T. Uemura, N. Watanabe, K. Sakata and J. Uzawa. A new glucuronide saponin from tea leaves (*Camellia sinensis var. sinensis*). **Biosci Biotech Biochem** 1994; 58(11): 2036–2040.

CS014   Banerjee, J. and S. N. Ganguly. A new furocoumarin from the leaves of *Camellia sinensis* (L.) O. Kuntze. **Nat Prod Sci** 1997; 3(1): 11–13.

CS015   Roy, M. and S. N. Ganguly. Isolation and characterization of indole-3-methylethanoate from *Camellia sinensis* (L.) O. Kuntz and its biological activity. **Nat Prod Sci** 1997; 3(2): 106–107.

CS016   Davis, A. L., J. R. Lewis, Y. Cai, C. Powell, A. P. Davis, J. P. G. Wilkins, P. Pudney and M. N. Clifford. A polyphenolic pigment from black tea. **Phytochemistry** 1997; 46(8): 1397–1402.

CS017   Kitagawa, I., K. Hori, T. Motozawa, T. Murakami and M. Yoshikawa. Structures of new acylated oleanene–type triterpene oligoglycosides, teasaponins E-I and E-2, from the seeds of tea plant, *Camellia sinensis* (L.) O. Kuntze. **Chem Pharm Bull** 1998; 46(12): 1901–1906.

CS018   Moon, J. H., N. Watanabe, Y. Ijima, A. Yagi and K. Sakata. Cis-and trans-linalool 3,7-oxides and methyl salicylate glycosides and (Z)-3-hexenyl beta-D-glucopyranoside as aroma precursors from tea leaves of oolong tea. **Biosci Biotech Biochem** 1996; 60(11): 1815–1819.

CS019   Lewis, J. R., A. L. Davis, Y. Cai, A. P. Davies, J. P. G. Wilkins and M. Pennington. Theaflavate B, isotheaflavin-3'-O-gallate and neotheaflavin-3-O-gallate: three polyphenolic pigments from black tea. **Phytochemistry** 1998; 49(8): 2511–2519.

CS020   Wei, J. X., Q. Y. Zuo and Y. Zhu. Studies on the chemical constituents of seeds of *Camellia sinensis var. assamica*. **Zhongguo Zhongyao Zazhi** 1997; 22(4): 228–230.

CS021   Murakami, T., J. Nakamura, H. Matsuda and M. Yoshikawa. Bioactive saponins and glycosides. XV. Saponin constituents with gastroprotective effect from the seeds of tea plant, *Camellia sinensis* L. var. *assamica* Pierre, cultivated in Sri Lanka: structures of assamsaponins A, B, C, D and E. **Chem Pharm Bull** 1999; 47(12): 1759–1764.

CS022   Lu, Y., T. Umeda, A. Yagi, K. Sakata, T. Chaudhuri, D. K. Ganguly and S. Sarma. Triterpenoid saponins from the roots of tea plant (*Camellia sinensis var. assamica*). **Phytochemistry** 2000; 53(8): 941–946.

CS023   Tanaka, T., Y. Betsumiya, C. Mine and I. Kouno. Theanaphthoquinone, a novel pigment oxidatively derived from theaflavin during tea–fermentation. **Chem Commun** 2000; 2000(15): 1365–1366.

CS024   Zarnadze, D. N., L. G. Lominadze and G. I. Kharebava. Rapid method for determination of tannin. **Subtrop Kult** 1974; 1974(4): 21–24.

CS025 Saijo, R. and T. Takeo. Increase of cis-3-hexen-1-ol content in tea leaves following mechanical injury. **Phytochemistry** 1975; 14: 181–182.

CS026 Mikaberidze, K. G. and I. I. Moniava. Flavonoids of tea leaves. **Chem Nat Comp** 197; 10(4): 527.

CS027 Vitzthum, O. G., P. Werkhoff and P. Hubert. New volatile constituents of black tea aroma. **J Agr Food Chem** 1975; 23(5): 999.

CS028 Lancaster, L. A. and B. Rajadurai. An automated procedure for the determination of aluminum in soil and plant digest. **J Sci Food Agr** 1974; 25: 381.

CS029 Suzuki, T. and E. Takahashi. Biosynthesis of caffeine b tea leaf extracts. Enzymic formation of theobromine from 7–mehylxanthine and of caffeine from theobromine. **Biochem J** 1975; 146: 87.

CS030 Fuit, Y., S. Fujita and H. Yoshikawa. Comparative biochemical and chemical–taxonomical studies of the plants of Theaceae. I. Essential oils of *Camelliasasanqua, C. japonica* and *Thea sinensis*. **Osaka Kogyo Gijutsu Shikensho Kiho** 1974; 25: 198.

CS031 Sekya, J., W. Kawasaki, T. Kajiwara and A. Hatanaka. NADP-dependent alcohol dehydrogenase from tea seeds. **Agr Biol Chem** 1975; 39: 1677.

CS032 Mikaberidze, K. G. ad I. I. Moniawa. Umbelliferone from tea leaves. Chem Nat Comp 1974; 10(1): 81.

CS033 Suzuki, T. and E. Takahashi. Metabolism of xanthine and hypoxnthine in the tea plant (*Thea sinensis*). **Biochem J** 1975; 146: 79.

CS034 Kajiwara, T., T. Harada and A. Hatanaka. Isolation of Z-3-hexenal in tea leaves, *Thea sinensis*, and synthesis thereof. **Agr Biol Chem** 1975; 39: 243.

CS035 Yamahara, J., Y. Shintani, T. Konoshima, T. Sawada and H. Fujimura. Biological active principles of the crude drugs. II. Antiulcerogenic and anti-inflammatory actions of the crude drugs contained saponin. **Yakugaku Zasshi** 1975; 95: 1179.

CS036 Vitzhum, O. G., P. Werkhoff and P. Hubert. New volatile constituents of black tea aroma. **J Agr Food Chem** 1975; 23(5): 999.

CS037 Higuchi, K., T. Suzuki and H. Ashihara. Pipecolic acid from the developing fruits (pericarp and seeds) of *Coffea arabica* and *Camellia sinensis*. **Colloq Sci Int Café(C. R.)** 1995; 16: 389–395.

CS038 Yoshida, Y., M. Kiso, H. Ngashima and T. Goto. Alterations in chemical constituents of tea shoot during its development. **Chagyo Kenkyu Hokoku** 1996; 83: 9–16.

CS039 Chaudhuri, T., S. K. Das, J. R. Vedasiromoni and D. K. Ganguly. Phytochemical investigation of the roots of *Camellia sinensis* L. (O. Kuntze). **J Indian Chem Soc** 1997; 74(2): 166.

CS040 Akagi, M., N. Fukuishi, T. Kan, Y. M. Sagesaka and R. Akagi. Anti-allergic effect of tea-saponin (TLS) from tea leaves (*Camellia sinensis* var. *sinensis*). **Biol Pharm Bull** 1997; 20(5): 565–567.

CS041 Ooishi, K., J. Kato and K. Hayamizu. Topoisomerase inhibitors conaining tannins, especially pedunculagin, for treatment of cancer. Patent-Japan Kokai Tokkyo Koho-06 72,885 1994; 7 pp.

CS042 Sakanaka, S., S. Maaku, S. Shu and B. Kin. Isolation and characterization of anticancer polyphenols from tea. Patent-Japan Kokai Tokkyo Koho-07 238,078 1995; 6 pp.

CS043 Sha, J. Q. and D. Zheng. Fluorine content in fresh leaves of tea plant in Fijian province. **Chaye Kexue** 1994; 14(1): 37–42.

CS044 Omata, A., K. Yomogida, S. Nakamura, T. Ota and Y. Izawa. Volatile compounds of *Camellia*flowers. **Engei Gakkai Zasshi** 1989; 58(2): 429–434.

CS045 Wang, D. X., M. Zhou and Y. A. Chen. Effect of tea polyphone and morin on oxidative modification of LDL (ox-LDL) in prevention of artherosclerosis. **Tianjin Yiyao** 1995; 23(6): 354–355.

CS046 Yang, G. Y., Z. J. Liu, D. N. Seril, Lioa, W. Ding, S. B. Kim, F. Bondoc and C. S. Yang. Black tea constituents, theaflavins, inhibit 4-(methylnitrosamino)-1-(3-pyridyl)-1-butanone (NNK)-induced lung tumorigenesis in A/J mice. **Carcinogenesis** 1997; 18(12): 2361–2365.

CS047 Davis, R. A., M. F. Stiles, J. D. de Bethizy and J. H. Reynolds. Dietary nicotine: a source of urinary cotinine. **Food Chem Toxicol** 1991; 29(12): 821–827.

CS048   Yen, G. C. and H. Y. Chen. Relationship between antimutagenic activity and major components of various teas. **Mutagenesis** 1996; 11(1): 37–41.

CS049   Miyagawa, C., C. Wu, D. O. Kennedy, T. Nakatani, K. Ohtani, S. Sakanaka, M. Kim and I. Matsui-Yuasa. Protective effect of green tea extract and tea polyphenols against the cytotoxicity of 1,4-naphthoquinone in isolated rat hepatocytes. **Biosci Biotech Biochem** 1997; 61(11): 1901–1905.

CS050   Shervington, A., L. A. Shervington, F. Afifi and M. A. El-Omari. Caffeine and theobromine formation by tissue cultures of *Camellia sinensis*. **Phytochemistry** 1998; 47(8): 1535–1536.

CS051   Apostolides. Z. and J. H. Weisburger. Catechins of *Camellia sinensis* for treatment of periodontosis. Patent-Japan Kokai Tokkyo Koho-04 77,424 1992; 7 pp.

CS052   Horie, H. and K. Kohata. Application of capillary electrophoresis to tea quality estimation. **J Chromatogr A** 1998; 802(1): 219–223.

CS053   Ahn, Y. J., T. Kawamura, M. Kim, T. Yamamoto and T. Mitsuoka. Tea polyphenols: selective growth inhibitors of *Clostridium ssp.* **Agr Biol Chem** 1991; 55(5): 1425–1426.

CS054   Sakanaka, S., Y. Ito, B. Kin and N. Yamazaki. Dental caries and periodontosis-treating agents containing catechins. Patent-Japan Kokai Tokkyo Koho-01 90,124: 6 pp.

CS055   Mori, M., N. Morita and K. Ikegaya. Polysaccharides from tea for manufacture of hypoglycemics, antidiabetics, and health foods. Patent-Japan Kokai Tokkyo Koho-63,308,001 1988; 8 pp.

CS056   Lin, J. K., C. L. Lin, Y. C. Liang, S. Y. Lin-Shiau and I. M. Juan. Survey of catechins, gallic acid, and methylxanthines in green, oolong, pu-erh, and black teas. **J Agr Food Chem** 1998; 46(9): 3635–3642.

CS057   Sagesaka, Y. M., T. Uemura, Y. Suzuki, T. Sugiura, M. Yoshida, K. Yamaguchi and K. Kyuki. Antimicrobial and anti-inflammatory actions of tea-leaf saponin. **Yakugaku Zasshi** 1996; 116(3): 238–243.

CS058   Price, K. R., M. J. C. Rhodes and K. A. Barnes. Flavonol glycoside content and composition of tea infusions made from commercially available teas and tea products. **J Agr Food Chem** 1998; 46(7): 2517–2522.

CS059   Guo, W. F., N. Sasaki, M. Fukuda, A. Yagi, N. Watanabe and K. Sakata. Isolation of an aroma precursor of bnzaldehyde from tea leaves (*Camellia sinensis var. sinensis* cv. Yabukita). **Biosci Biotech Biochem** 1998; 62(10): 2052–2054.

CS060   Koetskaya, T. F. and M. N. Zaprometov. Phenolic compounds in the tissue culture of *Camellia sinensis* and effect of light on their formation. **Fiziol Rast(Moscow)** 1975; 22: 941.

CS061   Sokol'skii, I. N., A. I. Ban'kovskii and E. P. Zinkevich. The structure of glucotheasaponin. **Chem Nat Comp** 1975; 11(1): 119–120.

CS062   Itoh, T., T. Tamura and T. Matsumoto. Tirucalla-7,24-dienol: a new triterpene alcohol from tea seed oil. **Lipids** 1975; 11: 434.

CS063   Imperato, F. D-fructose in flavonol and flavanone gly$_{co}$sides from *Camellia sinensis*. **Phytochemistry** 1976; 15: 439–440.

CS064   Cattell, D. J. and H. E. Nursten. Fractionation and chemistry of ethyl acetate-soluble thearubigins from black tea. **Phytochemistry** 1976; 15: 1967–1970.

CS065   Hatanaka, A., T. Kajiwara and J. Sekiya. Biosynthesis of trans-2-hexenal in chloroplasts from *Thea sinensis*. **Phytochemistry** 1996; 15: 1125.

CS066   Matsura, T., T. Tsunoda and M. Arai. Theanine manufacture with tissue cultures of tea. Patent-Japan Kokai Tokkyo Koho-03 187,388 1991; 7 pp.

CS067   Takeo, C., H. Kinugass, H. Oosu, T. Kawasaki, N. Takakuwa, M. Shimizu and H. Kondo. Extraction of hyperglycemics from tea. Patent-Japan Kokai Tokkyo Koho-04 124,139 1992; 8 pp.

CS068   Stalcup, A. M., K. H. Ekborg, M. P. Gasper and D. W. Armstron. Enantiomeric separation of chiral components reported to be in coffee, tea or cocoa. **J Agr Food Chem** 1993; 41(10):1684–1689.

CS069 Katiyar, S. K. and A. K. Bhatia. Epicatechin derivatives and fatty acid composition of a traditional product made in Sikkim from leaves of *Camellia sinensis*. **J Sci Food Agr** 1992; 60(2): 271–273.

CS070 Cho, Y. J., B. J. An and C. Choi. Isolation and enzyme inhibition of tannins from Korean green tea. **Han'guk Saenghwa Hakhoe Chi** 1993; 26(3): 216–223.

CS071 Shiraki, M., Y. Hara, T. Osawa, H. Kumon, T. Nakayama and S. Kawakishi. Antioxidative and antimutagenic effects of theaflavins from black tea. **Mutat Res** 1994; 323 (1/2): 29–34.

CS072 Booth, S. L., H. T. Madabushi, K. W. Davidson and J. A. Sadowski. Tea and coffee brews are not dietary sources of vitamin K-1 (phylloquinone). **J Amer Diet Ass** 1995; 95(1): 82–83.

CS073 Miyake, T. and T. Shibamoto. Quantitative analysis of acetylaldehyde in foods and beverages. **J Agr Food Chem** 1993; 41(11): 1968–1970.

CS074 Wang, D. M., K. Ando, K. Morita, K. Kubota and A. Kobayashi. Optical isomers of linalool and linalool oxides in tea aroma. **Biosci Biotech Biochem** 1994; 58(1): 2050–2053.

CS075 Narayan, M. S., B. Bhattacharya, N. Dhanaraj and R. Seshadri. Free and bound triacontanol in tea leaves. **J Agr Food Chem** 1988; 43(3): 229–233.

CS076 Kobayashi, A., K. Kubota, Y. Joki, E. Wada and M. Wakabayashi. (Z)-3-hexenyl-beta-D-glucopyranoside in fresh tea leaves as a precursor of green odor. **Biosci Biotech Biochem** 1994; 58(3): 592–593.

CS077 Gong, Z. L., N. Watanabe, A. Yagi, H. Etoh, K. Sakata, K. Ina and Q. J. Liu. Compositional change of Pu-Erh tea during processing. **Biosci Biotech Biochem** 1993; 57(10): 1745–1746.

CS078 Deisinger, P. J., T. S. Hills and J. C. English. Human exposure to naturally occurring hydroquinone. **J Toxicol Environ Health** 1996; 47(1): 31–46.

CS079 Yokozawa, T., H. Oura, H. Nakagawa, S. Sakanaka and M. Kim. Effects of a component of green tea on the proliferation of vascular smooth muscle cells. **Biosci Biotech Biochem** 1995; 59(11): 2134–2136.

CS080 Wang, D. M., K. Kubota and A. Kobayashi. Optical isomers of methyl jasmonate in tea aroma. **Biosci Biotech Biochem** 1996; 60(3): 508–510.

CS081 Kitagawa, I., S. Kobayashi, H. Sagesaka and T. Uemura. Extraction of saponins from tea leaves. Patent-Japan Kokai Tokkyo Koho-07 61,998 1995; 9 pp.

CS082 Goto, T., Y. Yoshida, M. Kiso and H. Nagashima. Simultaneous analysis of individual catechins and caffeine in green tea. **J Chromatogr A** 1996; 749(1/2): 295–299.

CS083 Lin, Y. L., I. M. Juan, Y. L. Chen, Y. C. Liang and J. K. Lin. Composition of polyphenols in fresh tea leaves and associations of their oxygen-radical-absorbing capacity with antiproliferative actions in fibroblast cells. **J Agr Food Chem** 1996; 44(6): 1387–1394.

CS084 Davis, A. L., Y. Cai, A. P. Davies and J. R. Lewie. ^{1}H and ^{13}C NMR assignments of some green tea polyphenols. **Magn Reson Chem** 1996; 34(11): 887–890.

CS085 Shiragami, T., Y. Shobu, M. Morino and C. Yoshikumi. Polyphenols and extraction of the compounds from *Camellia sinensis* (l.) O. Kuntze for use as anticancer agent-resistance inhibitors. Patent–Japan Kokai Tokkyo Koho–07 330,599 1995; 6 pp.

CS086 Ding, M. Y., P. R. Chen and G. A. Luo. Simultaneous determination of organic acids and inorganic anions in tea by ion chromatography. **J Chromatogr A** 1997; 764(2): 341–345.

CS087 Zaprometov, M. N., N. V. Zagoskina and T. F. Koretskaya. Effect of some precursors on the formation of phenolic compounds in tea plant tissue cultures. **Fiziol Rast** 1976; 23: 1274.

CS088 Higashi-Okai, K., S. Otani and Y. Okai. Potent suppressive activity of pheophytin A and B from the non-polyphenolic fraction of green tea (*Camellia sinensis*) against tumor promotion in mouse skin. **Cancer Lett** 1998; 129(2): 223–228.

CS089 Ikekawa, N., S. Takatsuto, T. Kitsuwa, H. Saito, T. Morishita and H. Abe. Analysis of natural brassinosteroids by gas chromatography and gas chromatography-mass spectrometry. **J Chromatogr** 1984; 290(1): 289–302.

CS090 Abe, H., T. Morishita, M. Uchiyama, S. Takatsuto and N. Ikekawa. A new brassinolide-related steroid in the leaves of *Thea sinensis*. **Agr Biol Chem** 1984; 1984(1): 2127–2172.

CS091 Lin, Z. K., Y. F. Hua and Y. H. Gu. Analysis of the aroma of Sichuan oolong tea. **You-ji Hua Hsueh** 1984; 1984(1): 21–24.

CS092 Nonaka, G. I., R. Sakai and I. Nishioka. Hydrolysable tannins and proanthocyanidins from green tea. **Phytochemistry** 1984; 23(8): 1753–1755.

CS093 Skhiladze, N. R. and V. Y. Vachnadze. Isolation of caffeine and theophylline from ripe tea seeds. **Chem Nat Comp** 1984; 20(5): 641.

CS094 Chkhikvishivili, I. D., V. A. Kurkin and M. N. Zaprometov. Flavonoids of *Camellia sinensis*. **Chem Nat Comp** 1984; 20(5): 629–630.

CS095 Itoh, O., T. Uetsuki, T. Tamura and A. Matsumoto. Characterization of triterpene alcohols of seed oils from some species of *Theaaceae*, *Phytolaccaceae* and *Sapotaceae*. **Lipids** 1980; 15(6): 407–411.

CS096 Chkhikvishivili, I. D., V. A. Kurkin and M. N. Zaprometov. Flavonids of *Camellia sinensis*. II. Components of a methanolic extract. **Khim Prir Soedin** 1985; 21(1): 118–119.

CS097 Tsushida, T. and T. Takeo. Occurrence of theanine in *Camellia japonica* and *Camellia sasanqua* seedlings. **Agr Biol Chem** 1984; 48(11): 2861–2862.

CS098 Karawya, M. S., S. M. A. Wahab, M. M. El-Olemy and N. M. Farrrag. Diphenylamine, an antiyperglycemic agent from onion and tea. **J Nat Prod** 1984; 47(5): 775–780.

CS099 Tsushida, T. and Y. Doi. Caffeine, theanine and catechin content in calluses of tea stem and anther. **Nippon Nogei Kagaku Kaishi** 1984; 58(11): 1131–1133.

CS100 Barruah, S., M. Hhazarika, P. K. Mahanta, H. Horita and T. Mutai. Effect of plucking intervals on the chemical constituents of CTC black tea. **Agr Biol Chem** 1986; 50(4): 1039–1041.

CS101 Anon. Extraction of tannins especially catechins. Patent-Japan Kokai Tokkyo Koho-59 216,884 1984; 3 pp.

CS102 Suzuki, T. and G. R. Waller. Purine alkaloids of the fruis of *Camellia sinensis* L. and of *Coffea arabica* L. during fruit development. **Ann Bot (London)** 1985; 56(4): 537–542.

CS103 Chaboud, A., J. Rayaud, L. Debourcieu and J. Reynaud. The presence of apigenin-2''-O-glucosyl-6-C-glucosylapigenin or 2'')-glucosylisovitexin in the leaves of *Thea sinensis* Sims. *var. macrophylla*. **Pharmazie** 1986; 41(10): 745–746.

CS104 Sakata, K., S. Sakuraba, A. Yagi, K. Ina, T. Hara and T. Takeo. Isolation and identification of (–)-quinic acid as an unidentified major tea–component. **Agr Biol Chem** 1986; 50(7): 1919–1921.

CS105 Afzal, M., N. al-Sweedan, L. A. Massih, K. Takahashi and S. Shibata. 2-amino-5-(N-ethylcarboxamido)-pentanoic acid from green tea leaves. **Planta Med** 1987; 53(1): 109–110.

CS106 Sakata, K., H. Yamaguchi, A. Yagi and K. Ina. A new inositol glycoside, 2-O-beta-L-arabinopyranosyl-myo-inositol, as a major tea component. **Agr Biol Chem** 1987; 51(6): 1737–1739.

CS107 Suzuki, T. Purine alkaloids in *Camellia sinensis* flowers. **Agr Biol Chem** 1985; 49(9): 2803–2805.

CS108 Cheng, G. R., J. L. Jin and Y. X. Wen. The structures of two new flavonoid glycosides from bai-shui-cha, a kind of *Camellia sinensis* L. **Yao Hsueh Hsueh Pao** 1987; 22(3): 203–207.

CS109 Lee, M. H. and C. T. Lin. Changes of flavor components of ti-kuan-yin tea during manufacturing. **Chung-Kuo Nung Yeh Hua Hsueh Hui Chin** 1985; 23(1/2): 127–132.

CS110 Abe, H., T. Morishita, M. Uchiyama, S. Takatsuto, N. Ikekawa, M. Ikeda, T. Sassa, T. Kitsuwa and S. Marumo. Occurrence of three new brassinosteroids: brassinone, (24S)-24-etylbrassinone ad 28–norbrassinolide, in higher plants. **Experientia** 1983; 39(4): 351–353.

CS111 Shimizu, M., S. Wada, T. Hayashi, M. Arisawa, K. Ikegaya, S. Ogakum, S. Yano and N. Morita. Studies on hypoglycemic constituents of Japanese tea. **Yakugaku Zasshi** 1988; 108(10): 964–970.

CS112 Taniguchi, S., Y. Miyashita, T. Ueyama, K. Haji, Y. Hirase, T. Takemoto and S. Arihara. Isolation of (–)-gallocatechin gallate from tea and pharmaceutical compositions containing it. Patent-Japan Kokai Tokkyo Koho-63 30,418 1988; 5 pp.

CS113 Skobeleva, N. I., T. A. Petrova, A. A. Bezzubov and M. A. Bokuchava. Beta-D-glucosides of monoterpene alcohols in tea shoots. **Soobshch Akad Nauk Gruz SSR** 1988; 131(2): 397–400.

CS114 Tanizawa, H., S. Toda, Y. Sazuka, T. Taniyama, T. Hayashi, S. Arichi and Y. T. Akino. Natural antioxidants. I. Antioxidative components of tea leaf (*Thea sinensis* L.). **Chem Pharm Bull** 1984; 32(5): 2011–2014.

CS115 Nobumoto, Y., K. Kubota, A. Kobayashi and T. Yamanishi. Structure of alpha-farnesen in the essential oil of oolong tea. **Agr Biol Chem** 1990; 54(1): 247–248.

CS116 Sakata, K., H. Yamauchi, A. Yagi, K. Ina, L. Parkanyi and J. Clardy. 2-O-(beta-L-arabinopyranosyl)-myo-inositol as a main constituent of tea (*Camellia sinensis*). **Agr Biol Chem** 1989; 53(1): 2975–2979.

CS117 Fujimori, N. and H. Ashihara. Adenine metabolism and the synthesis of purine alkaloids in flowers of *Camellia*. **Phytochemistry** 1990; 29(11): 3513–3516.

CS118 Furuya, T., Y. Orihara and Y. Tsuda. Caffeine and theanine from cultured cells of *Camellia sinensis*. **Phytochemistry** 1990; 29(8): 2539–2543.

CS119 Sekine, T., J. Arita, A. Yamaguchi, K. Saito, S. Oknogi, N. Morisaki, S. Iwasaki and I. Murakoshi. Two flavonol glycosides from seeds of *Camellia sinensis*. **Phytochemistry** 1991; 30(3): 991–995.

CS120 Lin, W. Y., Y. H. He, J. H. Luo, L. J. Huang, K. Lin, S. R. Wu and J. H.

Chen. Determination of trace germanium in herbal medicine by graphite furnace atomic absorption spectrometry. **Fenxi Shiyanshi** 1991; 10(1): 30–31, 34.

CS121 Owuoe, P. O. Differentiation of teas by the variations of linalool and geraniol contents. **Bull Chem Soc Ethiopia** 1989; 3(1): 31–35.

CS122 Wang, D. G. and S. R. Wang. Isolation, purification, analysis and anti-hyperlipidemia effect of green tea polysaccharide. **Zhongguo Yaoke Daxue Xuebao** 1991; 22(4): 225–228.

CS123 Mukoyama, A., H. Ushijima, S. Nishimura, H. Koike, M. Toda, Y. Hara and T. Shimamura. Inhibition of rotavirus AND ENTEROVirus infections by tea extracts. **Jap J Med Sci Biol** 1991; 44(4): 181–186.

CS124 Namiki, K. Platelet aggregation inhibitory components of tea. **Fragrance J** 1990; 18(11): 67–70.

CS125 Park, S. N. and Y. C. Boo. Flavonoids for protection of cells against chemically active species of oxygen, their extraction from plants, and their use in cosmetics. Patent-Fr Demende-2,651,132 1991; 17 pp.

CS126 Wheeler, S. R. Tea and tannins. **Science** 1978; 204: 6.

CS127 Anisimov, M. M., E. B. Shentsova, V. V. Shcheglov, Y. N. Shumilov, V. A. Rasskazov, L. I. Strigina, N. S. Chetyrina and G. B. Elyakov. Mechanism of cytotoxic action of some triterpene glycosides. **Toxicon** 1978; 16: 207–218.

CS128 Dzhavelidze, T. A. Phenolic compounds in various parts of tea shoots. **Subtrop Kult** 1978; 1978: 154–155.

CS129 Hatanaka, A., T. Kajiwara and J. Sekiya. Biosynthesis of leaf alcohol: the oxygenative cleavage of linolenic acid to cis-3-hexenal and 11-formyl-cis-9-undecenoic acid from linolenic acid in tea chloroplasts. Symp Chem Nat Prod-22nd- Fukuoka, Japan 1979; 657–664.

CS130 Iida, T., T. M. Jeong, T. Tamura and T. Matsumoto. Identification of chondrillasterol in two *Cucurbitaceae* seed oils by proton nuclear magnetic resonance spectroscopy. **Lipids** 1980; 15: 66–68.

CS131 Itoh, T., Y. Kikuchi, T. Tamura and T. Matsumoto. Two 3-oxo-steroids in Thea sinensis seeds. **Phytochemistry** 1981; 20: 175–176.

CS132 Etoh, Hina, K. and M. Iguchi. Studies on the aroma of tea. Part IV. 3S-(+)-3,7-dimethyl-1,5-octadiene-3,7-diol and ionone derivatives from tea. **Agr Biol Chem** 1980; 44: 2999–3000.

CS133 Imperato, F. N-P-coumarylglutamic acid, an unusual hydroxycinnamic acid–aminoacid derivative from black tea. **Chem Ind (London)** 1980; 388.

CS134 Huq, M. S., B. K. Mondal and M. S. Khan. Investigation on tea seed. Part I. Studies on the composition of the oil. **Bangladesh J Sci Ind Res** 1980; 15(1): 125–129.

CS135 Takatsuto, S., N. Ikekawa, H. Abe, T. Morishita, M. Uchiyama, M. Ikeda, T. Sasa, S. Marumo and T. Kitsuwa. Microanalysis of brassinolide and its application to the identification of new brassinosteroids in plants. Proc 25th Symp on the Chem of Nat Prod Tokyo 1982; 290–297.

CS136 Lin, Z., Y. Hua, Y. Gu, J. Ma, P. Chen and Y. Xiao. Study on the chemical constituents on the volatile oils from the fresh leaves of Camellia sinensis. **Chih Wu Hsueh Pao** 1982; 24: 440–450.

CS137 Yamane, H., H. Abe and N. Takahashi. Jasmonc acid and methyl jasmonate in pollens and anthers of three Camelliaspecies. **Plant Cell Physiol** 1982; 23: 1125–1127.

CS138 Bagratishvili, D. G. and M. N. Zaprometov. Effect of light on the formation of phenolic compounds in a suspension of a tea plant cells. **Akad Nauk Gruz** 1982; 105: 581–584.

CS139 Ozawa, T. Separation of the components in black tea infusion by chromatography on toyopearl. **Agr Biol Chem** 1982; 46(4): 1079–1081.

CS140 Nonaka, G. I., O. Kawahara and I. Nishioka. Tannins and related compounds. XV. A new class of dimeric flavan-3-ol gallates, theasinensins A and B, and proanthocyanidin gallates from green tea leaf. **I. Chem Pharm Bull** 1983; 31(11): 3906–3914.

CS141 Neurath, G. B., M. Dunger, F. G. Pein, D. Ambrosius and O. Schreiber. Primary and secondary amines in the human environment. **Food Cosmet Toxicol** 1977; 15: 275–282.

CS142 Shecheglov, V. V., S. I. Baranova, M. M. Anisimov, S. Antonov, S. S. Afiyatullov, E. V. Levina, V. F. Sharypov, V. A. Stonik and G. B. Elyakov. Antimicrobial spectrum of some triterpene and steroid glycosides. **Antibiotiki (Moscow)** 1979; 24: 270–273.

CS143 Sakai, T., K. Kobashi, M. Tsunezuka, M. Hattori and T. Namba. Studies on dental caries prevention by traditional Chinese medicine (part VI). On the fluoride contents in crude drugs. **Shoyakugaku Zasshi** 1985; 39(2): 165–169.

CS144 Nakahara, K. Oxalic acid content of vegetable foods. **Eiyo To Shokuryo** 1974; 27(1): 33–36

CS145 John, D. One hundred useful raw drugs of the Kani tribes of Trivandrum forest division, Kerala, India. **Int J Crude Drug Res** 1984; 22(1): 17–39.

CS146 Patel, V. K. and H. Venkatakrishna-Bhatt. Folklore therapeutic indigenous plants in periodontal disorders in India (Review, experimental and clinical approach). **Int J Clin Pharmacol Ther Toxicol** 1988; 26(4): 176–184.

CS147 Jamir, N. S. Some interesting medicinal plants used by Nagas. **J Res Edu Ind Med** 1990; 9(2): 81–87.

CS148 Latorre, D. L. and F. A. Latorre. Plants used by the Mexican Kickapoo Indians. **Econ Bot** 1977; 31: 340–357.

CS149 Yesilada, E., G. Honda, E. Sezike, M. Tabata, T. Fujita, T. Tanaka, Y. Takeda and Y. Takaishi. Traditional medicine in Turkey. V. Folk medicine in the inner Taurus Mountains. **J Ethnopharmacol** 1995; 46(3): 133–152.

CS150 Loewenthal, R. and J. Pe'er. Traditional methods used in the treatment of ophthalmic diseases among the Turkana tribe in North West Kenya. **J Ethnopharmacol** 1991; 33(3): 227–229.

CS151 Klauss, V. and H. S. Adala. Traditional herbal eye medicine in Kenya. **World Health Forum** 1994; 15(9): 138–143.

CS152 Wasuwat, S. A list of Thai medicinal plants, ASRCT, Bangkok, Report No. 1 on Res. Project. 17. Res Report,

A.S.R.C.T., No 1 on Research Project 17. 1067; 22 pp.

CS153 Laohapaiboon, P. and P. Tosukhowong. Antifungal activity of tea seed cake and tea seed extract. **Chulalongkorn Med J** 1981; 24(4): 953–959.

CS154 Caceres, A., L. M. Giron, S. R. Alvarado and M. F. Torres. Screening of antimicrobial activity of plants popularly used in Guatemala for the treatment of dermatomucosal diseases. **J Ethnopharmacol** 1987; 20(3): 223–237.

CS155 Rao, R. R. and N. S. Jamir. Ethnobotanical studies on Nagaland. **I. Medicinal Plants. Econ Bot** 1982; 36: 176–181.

CS156 Chaboud, A., J. Raynaud and L. Debourcieu. 6,8-Di-C-beta-D-arabinopyranosyl apigenin from *Thea sinensis* var. *macrophylla*. **J Nat Prod** 1986; 49(6): 1145.

CS157 Sugita-Konishi, Y., Y. Hara-Kudo, F. Amano, T. Okubo, N. Aoi, M. Iwaki and S. Kumagai. Epicallocatechin gallate and gallocatechin gallate in green tea catechins inhibit extracellular release of vero toxin from enterohemorrhagic *Escherichia coli* O157:H7. **Biochim Biophys Acta** 1999; 1472 (1/2): 42–50.

CS158 Ohtsuki, K., M. Kawabata, K. Taguchi, H. Kokura and S. Kawamura. Determination of S-methylmethionine, vitamin U, in various teas. **Agr Biol Chem** 1984; 48(10): 2471–2475.

CS159 Lin, Y. L., S. H. Tsai, S. Y. Lin-Shiau, C. T. Ho and J. K. Lin. Theaflavin-3-3-digallate from black tea blocks the nitric oxide synthase by down-regulating the activation of NF-KB in macrophages. **Eur J Pharmacol** 1999; 367 (2/3): 379–388.

CS160 Riso, P., D. Erba, F. Criscuoli and G. Testolin. Effect of green tea extract on DNA repair and oxidative damage due to H_2O_2 in Jurkat T cells. **Nutrition Research** 2002; 22(10): 1143–1150.

2 | Cannabis sativa
L.

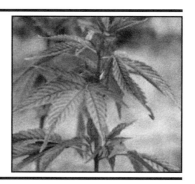

Common Names

Almindelig hamp	Denmark	Harilik kanep	Slovenia
Asa	Japan	Haschischpflanze	Germany
Bang	Egypt	Hash	United Kingdom
Bhaang	India	Hashas	Turkey
Bhaango	Nepal	Hashish	Morocco
Canamo indico	Spain	Hemp	United Kingdom
Canapa indica	Italy	Hennep	Netherlands
Canhamo	Portugal	Hind kinnabi	Turkey
Cares	Nepal	Huo ma cao	China
Chanvre cultive	France	Huo ma	China
Chanvre de l'Inde	France	Indian hemp	United Kingdom
Chanvre	France	Indische hennep	Netherlands
Chanvrier sauvage	France	Indischer hanf	Germany
Charas	India	Indisk hamp	Sweden
Churras	India	Kannabis	Finland
Da ma cao	China	Kannabisu	Japan
Da ma ren	China	Kerp	Albania
Da ma	China	Kinnab	Turkey
Dagga	South Africa	Konopie siewne	Poland
Dansk pot	Denmark	Konopie	Poland
Echter hanf	Germany	Konoplja	Slovenia
Esrar	Turkey	Kultur hanf	Germany
Gaanjaa	Nepal	Maconha	Portugal
Gajiimaa	Nepal	Marihana	Netherlands
Ganja	Guyana	Marihouava	Greece
Ganja	India	Marihuana	Poland
Grifa	Spain	Marihuana	Bulgaria
Hachis	Spain	Marihuana	Croatia
Hamp	Denmark	Marihuana	Czech Republic
Hamp	Norway	Marihuana	Denmark
Hampa	Sweden	Marihuana	France
Hampjurt	Iceland	Marihuana	Germany
Hamppu	Finland	Marihuana	Hungary
Hanf	Germany	Marihuana	Mexico

From: *Medicinal Plants of the World, vol. 3: Chemical Constituents, Traditional and Modern Medicinal Uses*
By: I. A. Ross © Humana Press Inc., Totowa, NJ

Marihuana	Russia	Porkanchaa	Thailand
Marihuana	Serbia	Pot	Denmark
Marihuana	Spain	Qinnib	Arabic countries
Marihuana	Ukraine	Riesen hanf	Germany
Marihuana	United States	Seruma erva	Portugal
Marijuana	France	Taima	Japan
Marijuana	Italy	Til	Arabic countries
Marijuana	Mexico	Vrai chanvre	France
Marijuana	Portugal	Weed	Guyana
Marijuana	Sweden	Xian ma	China
Mashinin	Japan	Ye ma	China
Navadna konoplja	Slovenia		

BOTANICAL DESCRIPTION

Cannabis sativa is an annual herb of the MORACEAE family that grows to 5 m tall. It is usually erect; stems variable, with resinous pubescence, angular, sometimes hollow, especially above the first pairs of true leaves; basal leaves opposite, the upper leaves alternate, stipulate, long petiolate, palmate, with 3–11, rarely single, lanceolate, serrate, acuminate leaflets up to 10 cm long, 1.5 cm broad. Flowers are monoecious or dioecious, the male in axillary and terminal panicles, apetalous, with five yellowish petals and five poricidal stamens; the female flowers germinate in the axils and terminally, with one single-ovulate ovary. Fruit is brown, shining achene, variously marked or plain, tightly embraces the seed with its fleshy endosperm and curved embryo; late summer to early fall; year-round in tropics. Drug-producing selections grow better and produce more drugs in the tropics; oil- and fiber-producing plants thrive better in the temperate and subtropical areas. The form of the plant and the yield of fiber from it vary according to climate and particular variety. Varieties cultivated for their fibers have long stalks, branch very little, and yield only small quantities of seed. Oil seed varieties are small, mature early, and produce large quantities of seed. Varieties grown for the drugs are small, much branched with smaller dark-green leaves. Between these three main types of plants are numerous varieties that differ from the main one in height, extent of branching, and other characteristics.

ORIGIN AND DISTRIBUTION

Native to Central Asia and long cultivated in Asia, Europe, and China. Now a widespread tropical, temperate, and subarctic cultivar. *Cannabis sativa* has been cultivated for more than 4500 years for different purposes, such as fiber, oil, or narcotics. The oldest use of hemp is for fiber, and later the seeds were used for culinary purposes. Plants yielding the drug were discovered in India, cultivated for medicinal purposes as early as 900 BC. In medieval times, it was brought to North Africa, where currently it is cultivated exclusively for hashish or kif.

TRADITIONAL MEDICINAL USES

Afghanistan. Hot water extract of the resin is taken orally to induce abortion[CS235].
China. Hot water extract of the inflorescence is taken orally for wasting diseases, to clear the blood, to cool the temperature, to relieve fluxes, for rheumatism, to discharge pus, and to stupefy and produce hallucinations[CS035]. The seed is taken orally as an emmenagogue[CS014]. Decoction of the seed is taken orally as an anodyne, an emmenagogue, a febrifuge, for migraine, and for cancer[CS112]. It is taken orally as a hallucinogen and externally for rheumatism[CS109].
Guatemala. The leaves are used externally to relieve muscular pains[CS106].

India. Hot water extract of the dried entire plant is taken orally as a narcotic and to relieve pain of dysmenorrhea[CS210]. Hot water extract of the dried flower and leaf is taken orally for dyspepsia and gonorrhea and as a nerve stimulant[CS217]. Hot water extract of the inflorescence of female plants is taken orally as an abortifacient[CS010]. Hot water extract of the leaf is taken orally to relieve menstrual pain[CS086]. For cuts, boils, and blisters, leaf paste is applied topically for 4 days[CS098]. Hot water extract of the bark is taken orally for hydrocele and other inflammation[CS125]. Extract of the leaves is used as an insect repellant[CS246]. Hot water extract of the seed is taken orally as an emmenagogue[CS010]. The powdered seed is taken orally as an aid in conception. One gram of seeds is powdered, then mixed with water, and given to women in the morning before breakfast for 7 days after menstruation. The use of pepper and cane sugar is avoided. Paste of dried leaves is applied over the anus in the morning and evening for piles[CS099]. The dried leaf juice is used externally on cuts and piles and taken orally as an anthelmintic[CS143]. To eliminate cough, bronchitis, and other respiratory ailments, a half tablespoonful of powdered dried leaves is mixed with an equal amount of honey and taken orally three times daily[CS193]. Seed oil is used externally for burns. The oil is extracted by roasting the seeds[CS213]. Seeds are taken orally for diabetes, hysteria, and sleeplessness[CS127]. The aerial parts are smoked to decrease nausea and vomiting induced by anticancer drugs[CS061]. Hot water extract of the aerial parts is taken orally by males as an aphrodisiac[CS123]. The dried aerial parts are smoked by women to increase their amorous prowess[CS181]. The fresh leaves are taken orally for hemorrhoids[CS108]. Hot water extract of the dried leaf and seed is taken orally for stomach troubles and indigestion[CS217]. Fresh leaf juice is administered intraural to treat earache[CS143]. The fruit is used externally for skin diseases[CS227]. The unripe fruit is taken orally to induce sleep[CS192].

Iran. Fluidextract of the dried flowering top or the dried fruit is taken orally for abdominal pain associated with indigestion, for pain associated with cancer, for rheumatoid arthritis, for gastric cramps or neuralgia, for coughing, and as a hypnotic. Fluidextract of the dried fruit is taken orally for whooping cough, as a hypnotic, and a tranquilizer[CS034]. The dried seed is taken orally as a diuretic. An infusion is taken orally as an analgesic in rheumatism or rheumatoid arthritis, a sedative, a diaphoretic, and for hysteric conditions, gout, epilepsy, and cholera. The seed oil is administered *per rectum* to reduce cramps associated with lead poisoning associated with constipation and vomiting. To reduce breast engorgement or reduce milk secretion, the seed oil is applied topically. In some cases, it would completely stop milk secretion. One to 2 g of seed oil is taken orally several times a day for urinary incontinency[CS034].

Jamaica. Hot water extract of the flower, leaf, and twig is taken orally as an antispasmodic and anodyne[CS238]. Hot water extract of the resin is taken orally for diabetes[CS198].

Mexico. The aerial parts are smoked as a hallucinogen[CS117].

Morocco. The aerial parts are taken orally as a narcotic[CS111].

Nepal. Decoction of the leaf is taken orally by adults as an anthelmintic[CS090]. The powdered leaf is mixed with cattle feed as a treatment for diarrhea[CS105]. For headache, the dried leaves are ground with *Datura stramonium* leaves and *Picrorhiza schrophulariflora* stem and water then applied externally[CS222]. The leaf juice is used externally as an antiseptic, as a hemostat on cuts and wounds, and to treat swelling of sprained joints[CS110]. The seeds are crushed, mixed with curd, and taken orally for dysentery[CS090]. Decoction of the seed is taken orally as an anthelmintic[CS104]. To aid in parturition, 2 teaspoonfuls of powdered seeds are made into a paste with sesame oil (*Sesamum indicum* L.) and applied intra-vaginally during labor[CS100].

Pakistan. Hot water extract of the entire plant is taken orally as a parturifacient[CS002]. Infusion of the leaf is taken orally for general weakness[CS113].

Saudi Arabia. The aerial parts, mixed with honey, sugar, and nutmeg, are taken orally as a psychotropic[CS248].

Senegal. The seed is taken orally as an emmenagogue[CS011].

South Africa. Hot water extract of the entire plant is taken orally for asthma[CS107]. Hot water extracts of the root and seed are taken orally to induce abortion, labor, and menstruation[CS234, CS219].

United States. Fluidextract of the inflorescence is taken orally as a narcotic, antispasmodic, analgesic, and aphrodisiac[CS015]. Hot water extract of the flowering top is taken orally as a potent antispasmodic, anodyne, and narcotic. One teaspoon of plant material is steeped in 2 cups of boiling water, and 1 tablespoonful is taken two to four times a day[CS247]. The dried aerial parts are smoked by both sexes as an aphrodisiac[CS166].

Vietnam. The seeds are taken orally as an emmenagogue[CS013].

West Indies. Hot water extract of the entire plant is taken orally as an antispasmodic[CS161].

Yugoslavia. Hot water extract of the seed is taken orally for diabetes[CS169].

Zimbabwe. Hot water extract of the aerial parts is taken orally as a treatment for malaria[CS238].

CHEMICAL CONSTITUENTS

(*ppm unless otherwise indicated*)
Acetaldehyde: Pl[CS172]
Acetone: Pl[CS172]
Actinidiolide, dihydro: EO[CS156], Pl[CS172]
Alanine: Pl[CS172]
Aldotetronic acid, 2-C-methyl: Pl[CS172]
Aldotetronolactone, 2-C-methyl: Pl[CS172]
Anethole, *cis*: EO[CS156], Pl[CS172]
Anethole, *trans*: EO[CS156], Pl[CS172]

Apigenin glycoside: Pl[CS172]
Apigenin-7-O-para-coumaroyl-glucoside: Pl[CS172]
Arabinic acid: Pl[CS172]
Arabinose: Pl[CS172]
Arabitol: Pl[CS172]
Arachidic acid: Pl[CS172], Sd[CS134]
Arginine: Pl[CS172] Aromadendrene, allo: Pl[CS172]
Aspartic acid: Pl[CS172]
Azelaic acid: Pl[CS172]
Behenic acid: Pl[CS172]
Benzaldehyde, para-ethyl: EO[CS156], Pl[CS172]
Benzene, 1-methyl-4-iso-propenyl: Pl[CS068, CS172]
Benzo-(A)-anthracene: Lf Smoke 3.3 μg/100 Cig[CS088]
Benzo-(A)-pyrene: Lf Smoke 4.2 μg/100 Cig[CS088]
Benzo-(F)-fluoranthene: Lf Smoke 3 μg/100 Cig[CS088]
Benzo-(G-H-I-)-perylene: Lf Smoke 0.7 μg/100 Cig[CS088]
Benzo-(K)-fluoranthene: Lf Smoke 1.1 μg/100 Cig[CS088]
Benzoic acid, 4-hydroxy methyl ester: Pl[CS033]
Benzoic acid, 4-hydroxy-N-propyl ester: Pl[CS033]
Benzoic acid, 4-hydroxy: Pl[CS172]
Benzoxocin-5-methanol, 2-(H)-1, 3-4-5-6-tetrahydro, 7-hydroxy-α-2-trimethyl-9-N-propyl-2-6-methano: Pl[CS172]
Benzyl acetate, para-ethyl: EO[CS156], Pl[CS172]
Benzyl acetate: EO[CS156,CS172]
Bergamotene, α, *trans*: Lf EO[CS062], Resin[CS069], Inflorescence[CS036], Pl[CS172]
Bergamotene, α: Lf EO[CS196]
Betaine, iso-leucine, L-(+): Pl[CS172]
Bibenzyl, 3-4-5-trihydroxy: Resin 596.5[CS202]
Bibenzyl, 3-4-dihydroxy-5-5-dimethoxy-3-(3-methyl-but-2-enyl): Aer[CS155]
Bibenzyl, 3-4-dihydroxy-5-methoxy: Aer[CS155], Lf 2[CS157]
Bibenzyl,3-3-dihydroxy-4-5-dimethoxy: Lf 5[CS157], Aer[CS155]
Bisabolene: Pl[CS068]
Bisabolol, α: Pl[CS172], Fl EO[CS196]
Borneol acetate: Pl[CS172], EO[CS156]
Borneol, (−): Pl[CS068]
Borneol: Resin[CS069], EO[CS156]
Bornesitol, D, (+): Pl[CS172]
Butylamine, iso: Pl[CS172]
Butylamine, N: Pl[CS172]
Butylamine, sec: Pl[CS172]

Butyraldehyde, iso: Pl[CS172]
Cadaverine: Pl[CS172]
Cadinene, Δ: Pl[CS172], EO[CS156]
Cadinene, γ: Pl[CS172], EO[CS156]
Calamenene: Pl[CS172], Lf EO[CS062]
Campest-4-en-3-one: Pl[CS172]
Campest-5-en-3-β-ol-7-one: Pl[CS172]
Campestanol: Sd[CS076]
Campesterol: Sd[CS076], Call Tiss[CS083], Rt[CS050]
Camphene hydrate: EO[CS156], Pl[CS172]
Camphene: Inflorescence EO[CS036], Lf EO[CS062], Resin[CS069]
Camphor: Lf EO[CS062], Pl[CS172]
Canabispiran: Lf[CS091]
Cannabamine B: Lf[CS070]
Cannabamine C: Lf[CS070]
Cannabamine D: Lf[CS070]
Cannabamine: Lf[CS070]
Cannabicclovarin: Pl[CS172]
Cannabichromanone, C-3: Resin[CS132]
Cannabichromanone: Resin 59[CS150]
Cannabichromene, propyl: Resin[CS137]
Cannabichromene: Rt[CS145], Resin[CS009], Aer[CS049,CS206]
Cannabichromenic acid: Inflorescence[CS218], Resin[CS055], Lf[CS073]
Cannabichromevarin: Pl[CS172]
Cannabichromevarinic acid: Pl[CS172]
Cannabicitran: Pl[CS172]
Cannabicoumaronic acid: Resin 84[CS150]
Cannabicoumaronone: Pl[CS172]
Cannabicyclol: Aer[CS064], Lf[CS057], Fl[CS074], Resin[CS043]
Cannabicyclolic acid: Inflorescence[CS218]
Cannabidihydrophenanthrene: Lf 20[CS001]
Cannabidiol monomethyl ether: Pl[CS172]
Cannabidiol, C-4: Pl[CS172]
Cannabidiol, propyl: Resin[CS137]
Cannabidiol: Lf[CS040], Aer[CS039], Resin[CS045], Inflorescence[CS052]
Cannabidiolic acid: Pl[CS172]
Cannabidiolic acid-tetrahydro-cannabitriol ester: Pl[CS172]
Cannabidiorcol: Pl[CS172]
Cannabidivarin: Pl[CS172]
Cannabidivarol: Pl[CS146,CS172]
Cannabidivarolic acid: Pl[CS146]
Cannabielsoic acid A: Pl[CS172], Resin[CS056]
Cannabielsoic acid B, C-3: Pl[CS172], Resin[CS132]
Cannabielsoic acid B: Pl[CS172], Resin[CS056]
Cannabielsoic acid, C-3: Pl[CS172]
Cannabielsoin I, dehydro: Resin[CS239]

Cannabielsoin, C-3: Resin[CS132]
Cannabielsoin: Pl[CS172]
Cannabifuran, dehydro: Resin[CS239], Pl[CS172]
Cannabifuran: Pl[CS172], Resin[CS239]
Cannabigerol monomethyl ether: Pl[CS172]
Cannabigerol: Resin[CS084], Pl[CS044]
Cannabigerolic acid monoethyl ether: Lf 20[CS004], Pl[CS172]
Cannabigerolic acid: Lf 40[CS032], Pl[CS172], Inflorescence[CS218]
Cannabigerovarin: Pl[CS172]
Cannabigerovarinic acid: Pl[CS172]
Cannabinerolic acid: Lf 7.6[CS032]
Cannabinodiol: Resin[CS020]
Cannabinodivarin: Pl[CS172]
Cannabinol methyl ether: Resin[CS018]
Cannabinol monomethyl ether: Pl[CS172]
Cannabinol, Δ-6(A)-10(A)-tetrahydro, 10-oxo: Resin[CS239], Pl[CS172]
Cannabinol, Δ-6(A)-10(A)-tetrahydro, 8-9-dihydroxy (DL): Aer[CS158]
Cannabinol, Δ-6(A)-10(A)-tetrahydro, 9-10-dihydroxy (DL): Aer[CS158]
Cannabinol, Δ-6(A)-10(A)-tetrahydro, 9-hydroxy-10-ethoxy: Aer[CS118]
Cannabinol, Δ-6(A)-10(A)-tetrahydro, *cis*: Pl[CS172]
Cannabinol, Δ-8-tetrahydro, *trans* (−): Aer[CS064]
Cannabinol, Δ-8-tetrahydro, *trans*: Pl[CS172]
Cannabinol, Δ-8-tetrahydro: Pl[CS038], Resin[CS055], Rt[CS145], Inflorescence[CS218]
Cannabinol, Δ-9-tetrahydro, 6(A)-7-10(A)-trihydroxy: Pl[CS172]
Cannabinol, Δ-9-tetrahydro, *cis*: Lf 2[CS114], Lf/Fl[CS074]
Cannabinol, Δ-9-tetrahydro, methyl ether: Resin[CS137]
Cannabinol, Δ-9-tetrahydro, propyl: Resin[CS137]
Cannabinol, Δ-9-tetrahydro, *trans* (−): Pl[CS172]
Cannabinol, Δ-9-tetrahydro, *trans*: Fl/Lf[CS074], Pl[CS172], Resin[CS137]
Cannabinol, Δ-9-tetrahydro: Pl[CS041], Resin[CS048], Bk[CS046], Sd 16.5[CS126], Call Tiss 65[CS188], Fr 0.5653%[CS089], Fl tops 4%[CS136], Lf[CS060], Rt[CS145]
Cannabinol, Δ-9-tetrahydroxylic acid: Resin[CS019]
Cannabinol, hexahydro: Aer[CS064]
Cannabinol, propyl: Resin[CS137]
Cannabinol, tetrahydro, iso, propyl: Resin[CS137]

Cannabinol, tetrahydro, iso: Resin[CS137]
Cannabinol, tetrahydro: Pl[CS133]
Cannabinol: Resin[CS009], Sd 8[CS148],
  Fr 0.1275%[CS089], Pl[CS038]
Cannabinol-C-4, Δ-9-tetrahydro, *trans*:
  Pl[CS172]
Cannabinol-C-4: Pl[CS172]
Cannabinolic acid A, Δ-9-tetrahydro, *trans*
  (−): Aer[CS064]
Cannabinolic acid A, Δ-9-tetrahydro, *trans*:
  Pl[CS172]
Cannabinolic acid A, Δ-9-tetrahydro: Lf[CS004]
Cannabinolic acid B, Δ-9- tetrahydro, *trans*
  (−): Aer[CS064]
Cannabinolic acid B, Δ-9-tetrahydro, *trans*:
  Pl[CS172]
Cannabinolic acid B, Δ-9-tetrahydro:
  Resin[CS055]
Cannabinolic acid, Δ-1-tetrahydro:
  Lf 1.4333%[CS032]
Cannabinolic acid, Δ-8-tetrahydro, *trans*:
  Pl[CS172]
Cannabinolic acid, Δ-8-tetrahydro:
  Inflorescence[CS218]
Cannabinolic acid, Δ-9-tetrahydro:
  Inflorescence[CS218], Lf[CS151,CS179]
Cannabinolic acid, tetrahydro: Lf[CS179], Pl[CS041],
  Pollen[CS067]
Cannabinolic acid: Lf[CS004], Resin[CS055],
  Inflorescence[CS218], Pl[CS172]
Cannabinolic acid-C-4, Δ-9-tetrahydro, *trans*:
  Pl[CS172]
Cannabiol, Δ-6(A)-10(A)-tetrahydro, 9-10-
  dihydroxy (DL): Pl[CS172]
Cannabiorcol, Δ-9-tetrahydro, *trans*: Pl[CS172]
Cannabiorcol: Pl[CS172]
Cannabiorcolic acid, Δ-9-tetrahydro, *trans*:
  Pl[CS172]
Cannabipinol: Pl[CS172]
Cannabiprene: Lf 26.8[CS091]
Cannabiripsol: Pl[CS172], Aer[CS165]
Cannabisativine, anhydro: Pl[CS172]
Cannabisativine: Rt 2[CS085]
Cannabiscoumaranone: Resin 140[CS150]
Cannabisin A: Fr 74[CS029]
Cannabisin B: Fr 812[CS030]
Cannabisin C: Fr 0.267%[CS030]
Cannabisin D: Fr 59.8[CS030]
Cannabisin E: Fr 120[CS031]
Cannabisin F: Fr 45[CS031]
Cannabisin G: Fr 20[CS031]
Cannabisiradienone: Pl[CS172]

Cannabisperenone, iso: Pl[CS172]
Cannabispiradienone: Lf 5–6[CS185, CS001]
Cannabispiran, dehydro: Lf 2.3[CS091, CS209]
Cannabispiran, iso: Lf[CS180]
Cannabispiran: Lf 20–245.7[CS080, CS209]
Cannabispiranol, α: Lf 0.3[CS185]
Cannabispiranol, β: Lf 8–80[CS209, CS091]
Cannabispiranol: Lf 18[CS157]
Cannabispirenone A, (−): Lf 30[CS185]
Cannabispirenone A, (DL): Lf 30[CS185]
Cannabispirenone B: Lf[CS185]
Cannabispirenone: Lf 210[CS185]
Cannabispirenone: Lf 61[CS157], Aer 10[CS124]
Cannabispirol, acetyl: Pl[CS172]
Cannabispirone: Aer 30[CS124], Pl[CS172],
  Lf 40[CS157]
Cannabistilbene I: Lf 0.4[CS204]
Cannabistilbene II: Lf[CS204]
Cannabitetrol: Pl[CS205]
Cannabithrene I: Lf 4[CS185]
Cannabithrene II: Lf 8[CS185]
Cannabitriol, (+): Aer[CS118], Pl[CS172]
Cannabitriol, (+): Pl[CS172]
Cannabitriol, (DL): Lf 2.7[CS203]
Cannabitriol, *trans* (DL): Lf[CS194]
Cannabitriol: Aer 250[CS079]
Cannabivarichromene: Resin[CS017]
Cannabivarin, Δ-9-tetrahydro, *trans* (−):
  Pl[CS172], Aer[CS064]
Cannabivarin, Δ-9-tetrahydro, *trans*: Pl[CS172]
Cannabivarin, tetrahydro: Fl/Lf[CS074]
Cannabivarin: Pl[CS172]
Cannabivarinic acid, Δ-9-tetrahydro, *trans* (−):
  Aer[CS064]
Cannabivarinic acid, Δ-9-tetrahydro, *trans*:
  Pl[CS172]
Cannabivarol, Δ-9-tetrahydro: Pl[CS146]
Cannabivarol, tetrahydro: Pl[CS041]
Cannabivarol: Fl tops[CS211]
Cannabivarolic acid, tetrahydro: Pl[CS041]
Cannflavin A: Aer 190[CS028]
Cannflavin B: Aer 30[CS028]
Cannflavin: Lf 138.5[CS027]
Cannflavone 2: Aer[CS226]
Canniflavone 1: Lf 0.8[CS185]
Canniflavone 2: 6[CS185]
Canniprene: Lf 27-1490[CS209, CS182], Pl[CS172]
Car-3-ene: Inflorescence[CS036], EO[CS156], Pl[CS172]
Car-4-ene: Pl[CS172, CS068]
Carbazole: Lf (smoke)[CS054]
Carvacrol: Lf EO[CS062], Pl[CS172]
Carveol acetate, dihydro: Pl[CS172], EO[CS156]

Carvone, dihydro: Rt[CS122], EO[CS156], Pl[CS172]

Carvone: Rt[CS122], EO[CS156], Pl[CS172]

Caryophyllene alcohol, α: EO[CS156], Pl[CS068]

Caryophyllene epoxide, β: Lf EO, Fl EO[CS196]

Caryophyllene epoxide: Lf EO[CS062]

Caryophyllene oxide: Fl tops[CS211], Lf EO[CS053], Pl[CS172]

Caryophyllene, α: Pl[CS172, CS068]

Caryophyllene, β: Pl[CS172], Resin[CS069], Fl EO[CS196], Inflorescence[CS036]

Caryophyllene, iso: Pl[CS172], Inflorescence EO[CS036]

Caryophyllene: Lf EO[CS062]

Caryophyllenol: Pl[CS172]

Castasterone: Sd[CS071]

Cedrene, α: Pl[CS172], EO[CS156]

Cellulose, hemi: Pl[CS172]

Cholest-4-en-3-one, 24-methyl: Sd[CS077]

Cholestan-3-one, 5-α, 24-methyl: Sd[CS077]

Cholesterol: Sd[CS076]

Choline: Rt, Fl tops[CS070], Lf[CS177], Pl[CS172]

Chrysene: Lf (smoke) 5 μg/100 Cig[CS088]

Cineol, 1-4: Pl[CS172], Lf EO[CS062]

Cineol, 1-8: Lf EO[CS062], Pl[CS172]

Cinnamic acid, *trans*: Lf[CS006], Pl[CS172]

Cinnamide, N-(para-hydroxy-β-phenylethyl)-para-hydroxy-(*trans*): Pl[CS172]

Citric acid, iso: Pl[CS172]

Citric acid: Pl[CS172]

Citronellol: EO[CS156], Pl[CS172]

Copaene, α: Lf EO[CS062], Pl[CS172]

Cosmosioside: Pl[CS172]

Coumaric acid, para: Pl[CS172]

Cubebene, α: Pl[CS172], EO[CS156]

Curcumene, α: Pl[CS172], Lf EO[CS062]

Curcumene, β: Pl[CS172,CS068]

Curcumene: EO[CS156]

Cyclocitral, β: Pl[CS172], EO[CS156]

Cyclohex-5-enone, 2-2-6-trimethyl: Pl[CS172], EO[CS156]

Cyclohexanone, 2-2-6-trimethyl: EO[CS156], Pl[CS172]

Cyclolanost-24-methylene-3-β-acetate: Pl[CS033]

Cymen-8-ol, para: EO[CS156], Pl[CS172]

Cymene, para: Pl[CS172, CS068], EO[CS156], Inflorescence[CS036]

Cystine: Pl[CS172]

Dec-3-en-5-one: EO[CS156], Pl[CS172]

Decan-1-al: Pl[CS172], EO[CS156]

Decan-2-one: EO[CS156], Pl[CS172]

Decane, N: Pl[CS172]

Dibenz-(A-1)-anthracene: Lf (smoke) 0.3 μg/Cig[CS088]

Docosane, N: Pl[CS172]

Dodecan-1-al: EO[CS156], Pl[CS172]

Dodecan-2-one: Pl[CS172], EO[CS156]

Dodecane, N: Pl[CS172]

Dotriacontane, 2-methyl: Pl[CS172]

Dotriacontane, N: Pl[CS172]

Edestin: Pl[CS172]

Edestinase: Pl[CS172]

Eicosadienoic acid: Pl[CS172]

Eicosane, N: Pl[CS172]

Eicosenoic acid: Pl[CS172]

Elemene,γ: EO[CS156], Fl EO, Lf EO[CS196], Pl[CS172]

Ereptase (peptidase): Pl[CS172]

Ergostan-3-one, 5-α: Call Tiss[CS083]

Ergosterol: Pl[CS172]

Erythritol: Pl[CS172],

Essential oil: Aer 0.09–0.11%[CS156], Lf 0.15%[CS062], Inflorescence[CS036]

Ethanol: Pl[CS172]

Ethanolamine: Pl[CS172]

Ethylamine, (DL): Pl[CS172]

Ethylamine: Pl[CS172]

Eudesmol,γ: EO[CS156], Pl[CS172]

Eugenol methyl ether: EO[CS156], Pl[CS172]

Eugenol, iso: EO[CS156], PL[CS172]

Eugenol: EO[CS156], Pl[CS172]

Farnesene, α *trans*, *trans*: EO[CS156], Pl[CS172]

Farnesene, α: Fl EO, Lf EO[CS196]

Farnesene, β, *cis*: Pl[CS172]

Farnesene, β, *trans*: Fl EO[CS196], Lf EO[CS062, CS196]

Farnesene, β: Resin[CS069], Inflorescence EO[CS036], EO[CS156], Pl[CS172]

Farnesene: Pl[CS172]

Farnesol: Pl[CS172], EO[CS156]

Farnesyl-acetone: EO[CS156], Pl[CS172]

Fatty acids: Sd[CS059]

Fenchol: Lf EO[CS062], Pl[CS068]

Fenchone: EO[CS156], Pl[CS172]

Fenchyl alcohol: Resin[CS069], EO[CS156], Pl[CS172]

Ferulic acid: Pl[CS172]

Flavocannabiside: Aer[CS121]

Flavone, 4-5-7-trihydroxy-3-methoxy-6-geranyl: Lf 6[CS182]

Flavosativaside: Aer[CS121]

Friedelanol, epi: Pl[CS172, CS068]

Friedelin: Pl[CS172, CS033, CS068], Rt[CS122]

Friedelinol, epi: Pl[CS172], Rt[CS122]

Fructose: Pl[CS172]

Furfural, 5-methyl: EO[CS156]

Furo-(1,2,A)-4-N-pentyl-7-7-10-trimethyl-dibenzopyran, 2-methyl: Lf (smoke)[CS195]

Furo-(1,2,A)-4-N-pentyl-7-7-10-trimethyl-dibenzopyranyl: Lf (smoke)[CS195]

Furo-(1,2-A)-4-N-pentyl-7-7-10-trimethyl-dibenzopyran, 2-3-dimethyl: Lf (smoke)[CS195]

Galactitol: Pl[CS172]

Galactosamine: Pl[CS172], Lf/St 1.9%[CS081]

Galactose: Pl[CS172]

Galacturonic acid: Pl[CS172]

Geraniol: Lf EO[CS062], Pl[CS172]

Geranyl acetone: Pl[CS172], EO[CS156]

Glucaric acid: Pl[CS172]

Gluconic acid: Pl[CS172]

Glucosamine: Pl[CS172]

Glucose, α (D): Pl[CS172]

Glucose, β(D): Pl[CS172]

Glutamic acid: Pl[CS172]

Glyceric acid: Pl[CS172]

Glycerol, (D), D-manno-octulose: Pl[CS172]

Glycerol: Pl[CS172]

Glycine: Pl[CS172]

Glycoprotein (*Cannabis sativa*): Lf[CS119]

Grossamide: Fr 8[CS029]

Guaiol: Pl[CS172]

Gurjunene,α: Fl EO[CS196], Resin[CS069], Pl[CS172]

Heneicosane, 3-methyl: Pl[CS172]

Heneicosane, N: Pl[CS172]

Hentriacontane, 2-methyl: Pl[CS172]

Hentriacontane, 3-methyl: Pl[CS172]

Hentriacontane, N: Pl[CS172]

Hept-2-3n-6-one, 2-methyl: Pl[CS172]

Hept-5-en-2-one, 6-methyl: EO[CS156]

Heptacosane, 3-methyl: Pl[CS172]

Heptacosane, N: Aer[CS063], Pl[CS172]

Heptadecane, 3-6-dimethyl: Pl[CS172]

Heptadecane, 3-7-dimethyl: Pl[CS172]

Heptadecane, N: Pl[CS172]

Heptan-1-al: Pl[CS172], EO[CS156]

Heptan-2-one: EO[CS156], Pl[CS172]

Heptatriacontane, N: Pl[CS172]

Heptulose, sedo: Pl[CS172]

Hexacosane, 2-methyl: Pl[CS172]

Hexacosane, N: Pl[CS172]

Hexadecanamide: Resin[CS116]

Hexadecane, N: Pl[CS172]

Hexadecane-1-ol: Pl[CS172], EO[CS156]

Hexan-1-al: EO[CS156], Pl[CS172]

Hexan-1-ol acetate: Pl[CS172]

Hexan-1-ol butyrate: Pl[CS172]

Hexan-1-ol caproate: Pl[CS172]

Hexan-1-ol iso-butyrate: Pl[CS172]

Hexatriacontane, N: Pl[CS172]

Hex-*cis*-3-en-1-ol caproate: EO[CS156]

Hex-*cis*-3-enol caproate: Pl[CS172]

Hexyl acetate: EO[CS156]

Hexyl iso-butyrate: EO[CS156]

Histamine: Pl[CS172]

Histidine: Pl[CS172]

Hordenine: Lf[CS051], Pl[CS172]

Humulene oxide I: Pl[CS172]

Humulene oxide II: Pl[CS172]

Humulene oxide: EO[CS156]

Humulene, α: Lf EO, Fl EO[CS196]

Humulene, β: Pl[CS172], Inflorescence EO[CS036], EO[CS156]

Humulene: Lf EO[CS062], Resin[CS069]

Indan-1-spiro-cyclohexane, 5-7-dihydroxy: Resin[CS026]

Indan-1-spiro-cyclohexane, 5-hydroxy-7-methoxy: Resin[CS026]

Indan-1-spiro-cyclohexane, 7-hydroxy-5-methoxy: Resin[CS026]

Indole: Lf (smoke)[CS054]

Inositol, (+): Pl[CS172]

Inositol, myo: Pl[CS172], Fl/Lf[CS082]

Ionone, β: EO[CS172], Pl[CS172]

Kaempferol: Aer[CS241]

Ledol: Pl[CS172], EO[CS156]

Leucine, iso: Pl[CS172]

Leucine: Pl[CS172]

Lignanamide I: Fr[CS093]

Limonene: Pl[CS172], Fl EO[CS196], Resin[CS069], Inflorescence EO[CS036]

Linalool, *cis*, oxide: EO[CS156], Pl[CS172]

Linalool, *trans*, oxide: Pl[CS172]

Linalool: Pl[CS172], Resin[CS069], Lf EO[CS062]

Linoleic acid methyl ester: Pl[CS172]

Linoleic acid: Pl[CS172], Sd[CS134]

Linolenic acid methyl ester: EO[CS156]

Linolenic acid: Pl[CS172], Sd[CS134]

Longifolene, (+): Pl[CS068]

Longifolene: Pl[CS172], EO[CS156], Inflorescence EO[CS036]

Lysine: Pl[CS172]

Malic acid: Pl[CS172]

Malonic acid: Pl[CS172]

Maltose: Pl[CS172]

Mannitol: Pl[CS172]

Mannose: Pl[CS172]

Mentha-1-8(9)-dien-5-ol, meta: Pl[CS172]

Methanol: Pl[CS172]

Methionine: Pl[CS172]

Methyl acetate: Pl[CS172]

Methylamine, di: Pl[CS172]

Methylamine: Pl[CS172]

Muscarine: Pl[CS172]

Myrcene: Fl EO[CS196], Resin[CS069], Inflorescence EO[CS036], Pl[CS068]

Myristic acid: Pl[CS172], EO[CS156]

Nerol: EO[CS062], Pl[CS172]

Nerolidol: Lf EO[CS062], Pl[CS172]

Neurine: Pl[CS172], Rt[CS070]

Nonacosane, *N*: Aer[CS063], Pl[CS172]

Nonadecane, *N*: Pl[CS172]

Nonan-1-al: Pl[CS172], EO[CS156]

Nonan-1-ol: Pl[CS172], EO[CS156]

Nonane, *N*: Pl[CS172]

Nonatriacontane, *N*: Pl[CS172]

Ocimene, β, *cis*: Pl[CS172], EO[CS156]

Ocimene, β, *trans*: Lf EO[CS062], Pl[CS172, CS068]

Ocimene, *cis*: Inflorescence EO[CS036]

Ocimene, *trans*: Inflorescence EO[CS036]

Oct-1-en-3-ol: Pl[CS172], EO[CS156]

Octacosane, 2-methyl: Pl[CS172]

Octacosane, 9-methyl: Pl[CS172]

Octacosane, *N*: Pl[CS172]

Octadecane, 3-6-dimethyl: Pl[CS172]

Octadecane, 3-7-dimethyl: Pl[CS172]

Octadecane, *N*: Pl[CS172]

Octan-1-al: EO[CS156], Pl[CS172]

Octan-1-ol caproate: Pl[CS172]

Octan-1-ol: EO[CS156], Pl[CS172]

Octan-3-ol: EO[CS156], Pl[CS172]

Octan-3-one: EO[CS156], Pl[CS172]

Octatriacontane, *N*: Pl[CS172]

Octyl caproate: EO[CS156]

Oleic acid methyl ester: Call Tiss[CS083]

Oleic acid: Pl[CS172], Sd[CS134]

Olivetol: Aer[CS226]

Orientin: Aer[CS121], Pl[CS172]

Orientin-2-O-β-D-glucoside: Pl[CS172], Aer 4.2[CS131]

Orientin-7-O-α-L-rhamnosyl glucoside: Pl[CS172]

Orientin-7-O-β-D-glucoside: Pl[CS172]

Oxidase, polyphenol: Pl[CS172]

Palmitic acid methyl ester: Call Tiss[CS083], EO[CS156], Pl[CS172]

Palmitic acid: Sd[CS134], Pl[CS172]

Palmitoleic acid: Pl[CS172]

Pectin: Pl[CS172]

Pentacosane, 3-methyl: Pl[CS172]

Pentacosane, *N*: Pl[CS172]

Pentadecan-2-one, 6-10-14-trimethyl: Pl[CS172], EO[CS156]

Pentadecan-2-one: EO[CS156], Pl[CS172]

Pentadecane, *N*: Pl[CS172]

Pentan-1-al: EO[CS156], Pl[CS172]

Pentatriacontane, *N*: Pl[CS172]

Perillene: EO[CS156], Pl[CS172]

Peroxidase: Pl[CS172]

Perylene: Lf (smoke) 0.9 μg/Cig[CS088]

Phellandrene, α: Inflorescence EO[CS036], Pl[CS172]

Phellandrene, β: Lf EO[CS062], Pl[CS172]

Phenethylamine, β: Pl[CS172]

Phenol, 2-6-di-tert-butyl-4-methyl: EO[CS156]

Phenol, 3-[2-(3-hydroxy-4-methoxy-phenyl)-ethyl]-5-methoxy: Pl[CS172]

Phenol, 3-[2-(3-hydroxy-4-methoxy-phenyl)-ethyl]-ethyl-5-methoxy: Pl[CS172]

Phenol, 3-[2-(3-iso-prenyl-4-hydroxy-5-methoxy-phenyl)-ethyl]-5-methoxy: Pl[CS172]

Phenol, 3-[2-(4-hydroxy-phenyl)-ethyl]-5-methoxy: Pl[CS172]

Phenol, 4-vinyl: Aer[CS159]

Phenol, 5-methoxy-3-[2-(3-hydroxy-4-methoxy-phenyl)-ethyl]: Lf 1.9[CS209]

Phenylalanine: Pl[CS172]

Phloriglucinol, β-D-glucoside: St[CS102]

Phosphatase, adenosine-5: Pl[CS172]

Phosphoric acid: Pl[CS172]

Phthalate, *N*-butyl: EO[CS156]

Phthalate, *N*-propyl: EO[CS156]

Phytol: EO[CS156], Pl[CS172]

Pinene, α, oxide: EO[CS172], Pl[CS172]

Pinene, α: Resin[CS069], Inflorescence EO[CS036], Lf EO[CS062], Pl[CS172]

Pinene,β: Lf EO[CS062], Resin[CS069], Inflorescence EO[CS036], Pl[CS172]

Pinocarveol: EO[CS156], Pl[CS172]

Pinocarvone: EO[CS156], Pl[CS172]

Piperidine: Fl top, Lf[CS070], Pl[CS172]

Piperitenone oxide: EO[CS156], Pl[CS172]

Piperitenone: Resin[CS069], EO[CS156], Pl[CS172]

Piperitone oxide: EO[CS156], Pl[CS172]

Proline, L: Rt[CS070]

Proline: Pl[CS172]

Prop-1-ene, 3-phenyl-2-methyl: Pl[CS172], EO[CS156]

Prospylamine, *N*: Pl[CS172]

Pulegone: EO[CS156], Pl[CS172]

Pyrano-(3-4-B)-benzofuran, 1-4 5-hydroxy-7-pentyl-1-(A)-α-3-3-trimethyl-ethano-1-(H): Aer[CS115]

Pyrene: Lf (smoke) 6.6 μg/Cig[CS088]

Pyroglutamic acid: Pl[CS172]

Pyrrolidine: Pl[CS172]

Quebrachitol, (+): Pl[CS172]

Querachitol: Fl/Lf[CS082]

Quercetin: Aer[CS241]

Raffinose: Pl[CS172]

Rhamnose: Pl[CS172]
Ribitol: Pl[CS172]
Ribose: Pl[CS172]
Sabinene, *trans*: Pl[CS172], EO[CS156]
Sabinene: EO[CS156], Pl[CS172]
Safranal: EO[CS156], Pl[CS172]
Salicyclic acid methyl ester: EO[CS156], Pl[CS172]
Santalene, β, epi: Pl[CS172], EO[CS156]
Sativic acid: Pl[CS172]
Scyllitol: Fl/Lf[CS082]
Selina-3-7(11)-diene: Pl[CS172], Inflorescence EO[CS036]
Selina-4(14)-7(11)-diene: Inflorescence EO[CS036], Pl[CS172]
Selinene,α: Pl[CS172], Inflorescence EO[CS036], EO[CS156]
Selinene,β: Inflorescence EO[CS036], Pl[CS172], EO[CS156]
Serine: Pl[CS172]
Sitostanol: Sd[CS076]
Sitosterol, β: Rt[CS122], Sd[CS076], Call Tiss[CS083], Pl[CS172]
Skatole: Lf (smoke)[CS054]
Sorbitol: Pl[CS172]
Spiro-(cyclohexane-1-3-(4-6-dihydroxy)-indan): Fl top[CS135]
Spiro-(cyclohexane-1-3-(4-hydroxy-6-methoxy)-indan): Fl top[CS135]
Spiro-(cyclohexane-1-3-(6-hydroxy-4-methoxy)-indan): Fl top[CS135]
Stearic acid methyl ester: Call Tiss[CS083]
Stearic acid: Pl[CS172], Sd[CS134]
Stigmast-22-en-3-one, 5-α: Call Tiss[CS083]
Stigmast-4-en, 3-one: Pl[CS172], Rt[CS050]
Stigmast-5-en-3-β-ol-7-one: Rt[CS050], Pl[CS172]
Stigmasta-4-22-diene-3-one: Rt[CS050], Pl[CS172]
Stigmasta-5-22-dien-3-β-ol-7-one: Rt[CS050]
Stigmasta-7-24(28)-dien-3-β-ol, 5-α: Pl[CS172]
Stigmastan-3-one, 5-α: Call Tiss[CS083]
Stigmasterol: Sd[CS076], Pl[CS172]
Stilbene, dihydro 3'-5-dihydroxy-3-4-dimethoxy: Lf[CS185]
Stilbene, dihydro 4'-5-dihydroxy-3-methoxy: Lf[CS185]
Succinic acid: Pl[CS172]
Sucrose: Pl[CS172]
Terpinen-4-ol, α: Pl[CS172]
Terpinen-4-ol: Lf EO[CS062], Pl[CS172]
Terpinene, α: Lf EO[CS062], Pl[CS172], Inflorescence EO[CS036]
Terpinene, γ: Pl[CS172], Resin[CS069], EO[CS156], Inflorescence EO[CS036]

Terpineol, α: Pl[CS172], Resin[CS069], Lf EO[CS062], EO[CS068]
Terpineol, β: EO[CS156], Pl[CS172]
Terpinolene: Fl EO[CS062], Lf EO[CS062], Inflorescence EO[CS036], Pl[CS172]
Tetracosane, 2-methyl: Pl[CS172]
Tetracosane, N: Pl[CS172]
Tetradecane, 2-6-dimethyl: Pl[CS172]
Tetradecane, N: Pl[CS172]
Tetratriacontane, N: Pl[CS172]
Threonic acid: Pl[CS172]
Threonine: Pl[CS172]
Thujene, α: Pl[CS172, CS068], EO[CS156]
Thujol alcohol: Pl[CS172], EO[CS156]
Triacontane, 3-methyl: Pl[CS172]
Triacontane, N: Pl[CS172]
Tricosane, 3-methyl: Pl[CS172]
Tricosane, N: Pl[CS172]
Tridecan-1-al: EO[CS156], Pl[CS172]
Tridecane, 3-6-dimethyl: Pl[CS172]
Tridecane, N: Pl[CS172]
Trigonelline: Pl[CS172], FL top[CS070]
Tritriacontane, N: Pl[CS172]
Tryptophan: Pl[CS172]
Tyramine, feruloyl: Sd 2.5, Rt, Resin, Lf[CS149,CS230]
Tyramine, N-(para-coumaroyl): Fr 111[CS029], Sd 111[CS092]
Tyramine, N-trans-caffeoyl: Fr 47.1[CS029]
Tyramine, N-trans-feruloyl: Fr 78.5[CS029]
Tyramine, para-coumaroyl: Sd 0.5[CS230], Rt, Lf, Resin[CS149,CS230]
Tyramine: Pl[CS172]
Tyrosine: Pl[CS172]
Undecan-1-al: EO[CS156], Pl[CS172]
Undecan-2-one, 6-10-dimethyl: EO[CS156], Pl[CS172]
Undecan-2-one: EO[CS156], Pl[CS172]
Undecane, N: Pl[CS172]
Valine: Pl[CS172]
Vanillic acid: Pl[CS172]
Vitamin K: Pl[CS172]
Vitexin, iso, 7-O-α-L-rhamnosyl-glucoside: Pl[CS172]
Vitexin, iso, 7-O-β-D-glucosyl-arabinoside: Pl[CS172]
Vitexin, iso: Pl[CS172]
Vitexin-2-β-D-glucoside: Pl[CS172], Aer 4[CS131]
Vitexin-7-O-β-D-(6-glucoside): Pl[CS172]
Vomifoliol, dihydroxylan: Pl[CS172]
Vomifoliol: Pl[CS172]
Xylitol: Pl[CS172]

Xylose: Pl[CS172]
Zeatin nucleoside: Pl[CS172]
Zeatin: Pl[CS172]

PHARMACOLOGICAL ACTIVITIES AND CLINICAL TRIALS

Abortifacient activity. Alcohol extract of the dried leaf, administered intragastrically to pregnant rats at a dose of 125 mg/kg, produced teratogenic effects[CS233]. Water extract of the dried leaf, administered intragastrically to pregnant rats at variable dosage levels on days 6–15 of pregnancy was active[CS228].

Acute cardiovascular fatalities. Six cases of possible acute cardiovascular death in young adults were reported where very recent cannabis ingestion was documented by the presence of Δ-9-tetrahydrocannabinol (Δ-9-THC) in postmortem blood samples. A broad toxicological blood analysis could not reveal other drugs[CS392].

Acute panic reaction (Koro). Koro, an acute panic reaction related to the perception of penile retraction, was once considered limited to specific cultures. Over 70 American men responded by telephone to report negative reactions to cannabis. Three of them (Caucasians aged 22–26 years with considerable experience with cannabis) spontaneously mentioned experiencing symptoms of Koro after smoking cannabis. All three cases occurred after the participants had heard about cannabis-induced Koro and used the drug in a novel setting or atypical way. Two of the men had body dysmorphia, which may have contributed to symptoms. All three decreased their cannabis consumption after the Koro experience. Several factors may have interacted to create the symptoms. These include previous knowledge of cannabis-induced Koro, the use of cannabis in a way that might heighten a panic reaction, and poor body image[CS393].

Adverse effects. A causal role of acute cannabis intoxication in motor vehicle and other accidents has been shown by the presence of measurable levels of Δ-9-THC in the blood of drivers in the absence of alcohol or other drugs, by surveys of driving under the influence of cannabis, and by significantly higher accident culpability risk of drivers using cannabis. Evidence demonstrated that cannabis dependence, both behavioral and physical, occurred in about 7–10% of regular users, and that early onset of use—especially of weekly or daily use—is a strong predictor of future dependence. Cognitive impairments of various types are readily demonstrable during acute cannabis intoxication, but there is no suitable evidence yet available to permit a decision as to whether long-lasting or permanent functional losses can result from chronic heavy use in adults[CS265]. The gender effects on progression to treatment entry and on the frequency, severity, and related complications of the *Diagnostic and Statistical Manual of Mental Disorders*, 3rd edition revised drug and alcohol dependence among 271 substance-dependent patients (mean age: 32.6 years; 156 women) was studied. There was no gender difference among patients in the age at onset of regular use of any substance. Women experienced fewer years of regular use of opioids and cannabis and fewer years of regular alcohol drinking before entering treatment. Although the severity of drug and alcohol dependence did not differ by gender, women reported more severe psychiatric, medical, and employment complications[CS285]. In a 3-day, double-blind, randomized, counterbalanced study, the behavioral, cognitive, and endocrine effects of 2.5 and 5 mg intravenous Δ-9-THC were characterized in 22 healthy individuals, who had been exposed to cannabis but had never been diagnosed with a cannabis abuse disorder. Prospective safety data at 1, 3, and 6 months post-study was also analyzed. Δ-9-THC produced schizophrenia-like positive and negative symptoms, altered perception, increased anxiety and plasma cortisol, euphoria, disrupted immediate and delayed word recall, sparing recognition recall, impaired performance on tests of distractibility, verbal fluency, and working memory, but did not impair orientation[CS287]. This study examined the behavioral and neurochemical (cannabinoid *CB1* receptor gene expression) changes induced by spontaneous cannabinoid withdrawal in mice. Cessation of CP-55,940 treatment in tolerant mice induced a spontaneous time-dependent behavioral withdrawal syndrome consisting of marked increases (140%) in motor activity, number of rearings (170%), decreases in grooming (57%), wet-dog shakes (73%), and rubbing behaviors (74%) on day 1, progressively reaching values similar to vehicle-treated mice on day 3. This spontaneous cannabinoid withdrawal resulted in *CB1* gene expression up-regulation (20–30%) in caudate-putamen, ventromedial hypothalamic nucleus, central amygdaloid nucleus, and CA1, whereas in the CA3 field of hippocampus, a significant decrease (15–20%) was detected[CS293].

Alcohol interaction. The complementary DNA and genomic sequences encoding G protein-coupled cannabinoid receptors (CB1 and CB2) from several species were cloned. This has facilitated discoveries of endogenous ligands (endocannabinoids). Two fatty acid derivatives characterized to be arachidonylethanolamide and 2-arachidonylglycerol isolated from both nervous and peripheral tissues mimicked the pharmacological and behavioral effects of Δ-9-THC. The down-regulation of CB1 receptor function and its signal transduction by chronic alcohol was demonstrated. The observed down-regulation of CB1 receptor-binding and its signal transduction resulted from the persistent stimulation of receptors by the endogenous CB1 receptor agonists arachidonylethanolamide and 2-arachidonylglycerol, whose synthesis is increased by chronic alcohol treatment. The deletion of CB1 receptor has been shown to block voluntary alcohol intake in mice[CS255].

Allergenic effect. An "All India Coordinated Project on Aeroallergens and Human Health" was undertaken to discover the quantitative and qualitative prevalence of aerosols at 18 different centers in the country. Predominant airborne pollens were *Holoptelea, Poaceae, Asteraceae, Eucalyptus, Casuarina, Putanjiva, Cassia, Quercus, Cocos, Pinus, Cedrus, Ailanthus, Cheno/Amaranth, Cyperus, Argemone, Xanthium, Parthenium*, and others. Clinical and immunological evaluations revealed some allergenically important taxa. Allergenically important pollens were *Prosopis juliflora, Ricinus communis, Morus, Mallotus, Alnus, Querecus, Cedrus, Argemone, Amaranthus, Chenopodium, Holoptelea, Brassica, Cocos, Cannabis, Parthenium, Cassia*, and grasses[CS317]. In the multitest routine skin-test battery, 78 of 127 patients tested (61%) were cannabis-test positive. Thirty of the 78 patients were randomly selected to determine if they had allergic rhinitis and/or asthma symptoms during the cannabis pollination period. By history, 22 (73%) claimed respiratory symptoms in July through September. All 22 of these subjects were also skin test-positive to weeds pollinating during the same period as cannabis (ragweed, pigweed, cocklebur, Russian thistle, marsh elder, or kochia)[CS411].

Alkaline phosphatase stimulation. Ethanol (95%) extract of the dried resin, administered intraperitoneally to toads at a dose of 10 mg/day for 14 days, was active. The results were significant at $p < 0.01$ level[CS216].

Aminopyrene-*N*-demethylase induction. Ethanol (95%) extract of the dried aerial parts, administered intraperitoneally to rats at a dose of 2 mg/kg for 15 days, was active. A dose of 20 mg/kg for 7 days was also active[CS141].

Amnesic syndrome. A 26-year-old woman suffered disseminated intravascular coagulation (DIC) and a brief respiratory arrest following recreational use of 3,4-methylene-dioxymethamphetamine (MDMA, or "ecstasy") together with amyl nitrate, lysergic acid (LSD), cannabis, and alcohol. She was left with residual cognitive and physical deficits, particularly severe anterograde memory disorder, mental slowness, severe ataxia, and dysarthria. Follow-up investigations have shown that these have persisted, although there has been some improvement in verbal recognition memory and in social functioning. Magnetic resonance imaging and quantified positron emission tomography investigations revealed severe cerebellar atrophy and hypometabolism accounting for the ataxia and dysarthria; thalamic, retrosplenial, and left medial temporal hypometabolism to which the anterograde amnesia can be attributed. There was some degree of frontotemporal–parietal hypometabolism, possibly accounting for the cognitive slowness. The putative relationship of these abnormalities to the direct and indirect effects of MDMA toxicity, hypoxia, and ischemia was considered[CS394].

Amyotrophic lateral sclerosis. One hundred thirty one respondents with amyotrophic lateral sclerosis—13 of whom reported using cannabis in the last 12 months—were examined. The results indicated that cannabis might be moderately effective at reducing symptoms of appetite loss, depression, pain, spasticity, and drooling. Cannabis was reported ineffective in reducing difficulties with speech and swallowing, and sexual dysfunction. The longest relief was reported for depression (approx 2–3 hours)[CS296].

Analgesic activity. Ethanol (50%) extract of the entire plant, administered intraperitoneally to mice at a dose of 250 mg/kg, was active vs tail pressure method[CS007]. Flavonoid fraction of the leaf, administered intraperitoneally to mice, was active[CS242]. The inflorescence, administered orally to male rats, produced weak activity vs paw pressure test,

effective dose $(ED)_{50}$ 35.5 mg/kg and hot plate method, ED_{50} 53 mg/kg[CS052]. Petroleum ether and ethanol (95%) extracts of the dried aerial parts, administered intragastrically to mice, was active vs phenylbenzo-quinone-induced writhing, inhibitory concentration $(IC)_{50}$ 0.013 mg/kg and 0.045 mg/kg, respectively[CS140].

Analgesic effect. Ajulemic acid (AJA, CT-3, or IP-751), administered to healthy human adults and patients with chronic neuropathic pain, demonstrated a complete absence of psychotropic actions. It proved to be more effective than placebo in reducing this type of pain as measured by the visual analog scale. Signs of dependency were not observed after withdrawal at the end of the 1-week treatment period[CS274]. Forty women undergoing elective abdominal hysterectomy were investigated in a randomized, double-blind, placebo-controlled, single-dose trial. Randomization took place when postoperative patient-controlled analgesia was discontinued on the second postoperative day. When patients requested further analgesia, they received a single, identical capsule of either 5 mg of oral Δ-9-THC (n = 20) or placebo (n = 20) in a double-blind fashion. The primary outcome measure was summed pain intensity difference (SPID) at 6 hours after administration of the study medication derived from visual analog pain scores on movement and at rest. Secondary outcome measures were time-to-rescue medication and adverse effects of study medication. Mean (standard deviation [SD]) visual analog scale pain scores before medication in the placebo and Δ-9-THC groups were 6.3(2.6) and 6.4(1.3) cm on movement, and 3.2(1.9) and 3.3(0.9) at rest, respectively. There were no significant differences in mean (95% confidence interval [CI] of the difference) SPID at 6 hours between the groups (placebo 7.9, Δ-9-THC 4.3[–1.8 to 9] cm per hour on movement; placebo 8.8, Δ-9-THC 4.9[–0.2 to 8.1] cm per hour at rest) and time to rescue analgesia (placebo 217, Δ-9-THC 163[–22 to 130] minutes). Increased awareness of surroundings was reported more frequently in patients receiving Δ-9-THC (40 vs 5%, p = 0.04). There were no other significant differences with respect to adverse events[CS326]. THC, morphine, and a THC–morphine combination were administered to 12 healthy subjects using experimental pain models (heat, cold, pressure, and single and repeated transcutaneous electrical stimulation). THC (20 mg), morphine (30 mg), THC–morphine (20 mg THC + 30 mg morphine), or placebo were given orally as single dose. Reaction time, side effects (visual analog scales), and vital functions were monitored. For the pharmacokinetic profiling, blood samples were collected. THC did not significantly reduce pain. In the cold and heat tests, it even produced hyperalgesia, which was completely neutralized by THC–morphine. A slight additive analgesic effect was observed for THC–morphine in the electrical stimulation test. No analgesic effect resulted in the pressure and heat test, with neither THC nor THC–morphine. Psychotropic and somatic side effects (sleepiness, euphoria, anxiety, confusion, nausea, dizziness, etc.) were common, but usually mild[CS330]. Three cannabis-based extracts Δ-9-THC, cannabidiol [CBD], and a 1:1 mixture of them both) were given over a 12-week period in a randomized, double-blind, placebo-controlled, crossover trial. Extracts, which contained THC, proved most effective in symptom control. Regimens for the use of the sublingual spray emerged and a wide range of dosing requirements was observed. Side effects were common, reflecting a learning curve for both patient and study team. These were generally acceptable and little different to those seen when other psychoactive agents are used for chronic pain[CS294]. Over a 6-week period 209 chronic noncancer pain patients

were studied. Seventy-two (35%) subjects reported ever having used cannabis. Thirty-two (15%) subjects reported having used cannabis for pain relief (pain users), and 20 (10%) subjects were currently using cannabis for pain relief. Thirty-eight subjects denied using cannabis for pain relief (recreational users). Compared with nonusers, pain users were significantly younger (p = 0.001) and were more likely to be tobacco users (p = 0.0001). The largest group of patients using cannabis had pain caused by trauma and/or surgery (51%), and the site of pain was predominantly neck/upper body and myofascial (68 and 65%, respectively). The median duration of pain was similar in both pain users and recreational users (8 vs 7 years; p = 0.7). There was a wide range of amounts and frequency of cannabis use. Of the 32 subjects who used cannabis for pain, 17 (53%) used four puffs or less at each dosing interval, eight (25%) smoked a whole cannabis cigarette (joint), and four (12%) smoked more than one joint. Seven (22%) of these subjects used cannabis more than once daily, five (16%) used it daily, eight (25%) used it weekly, and nine (28%) used it rarely. Pain, sleep, and mood were most frequently reported as improving with cannabis use, and "high" and dry mouths were the most commonly reported side effects[CS351]. Patients with chronic pain completed a questionnaire about the type of cannabis used, the mode of administration, the amount used and the frequency of use, and their perception of the effectiveness of cannabis on a set of pain-associated symptoms and side effects. Fifteen patients (10 males) were interviewed (median age, 49.5 years; range, 24–68 years). All patients smoked herbal cannabis for therapeutic reasons (median duration of use, 6 years; range, 2 weeks–37 years). Seven patients only smoked at night (median dose eight puffs, range two to eight puffs), and eight patients used cannabis mainly during the day (median dose of three puffs; range, two to eight puffs); the median frequency of use was four times per day (range, 1 to 16 times/day). Twelve patients reported improvement in pain and mood, whereas 11 reported improvement in sleep. Eight patients reported a "high;" six denied a "high." Tolerance to cannabis was not reported[CS368]. THC was administered to six patients with chronic pain at doses 5–20 mg/day. A sufficient pain relief had been achieved in three patients. The other three suffered from intolerable side effects, such as nausea, dizziness, and sedation without a reduction of pain intensity. In these cases, the treatment was continued with other analgesics[CS391].

Anaphrodisiac effect. Tincture of the resin, administered intraperitoneally to male mice at a dose of 12.5 mg/kg, produced a significant reduction in mounts and attempted mounts. Other behaviorial activities were unaffected[CS153].

Angiotensin-converting enzyme inhibition. Ethanol (100%) extract of the dried leaf at a concentration of 333.3 μg/mL produced weak activity, and the water extract was inactive[CS129].

Ankylosing spondylitis. Ankylosing spondylitis is a systemic disorder occurring in genetically predisposed individuals. The disease course appears to be characterized by bouts of partial remission and flares. There were 214 patients questioned (169 men, 45 women; average disease duration, 25 years; age of disease onset, 22 years). The main symptoms of flare were pain (all groups), immobility (90%), fatigue (80%), and emotional symptoms, such as depression, withdrawal, and anger, (75%). All of patients experienced between one and five localized flares per year. Fifty-five percent of the groups contained patients (n = 85) who experienced a generalized flare. The main perceived triggers of flare were stress (80%) and "overdoing it" (50%). Patients reported

that a flare might last anywhere from a few days to a few weeks and relief from flare were by analgesic injections (including opiates), relaxation, sleep, and cannabis (three individuals). Three-quarters of the groups agreed that there was no long-term effect on the ankylosing sponylitis following a flare[CS378].

Anti-anaphylactic activity. Water extract of the dried fruit, at a concentration of 1 μg/mL, produced weak activity on the rat Leuk-RBL 2H3 vs biotinyl immunoglobulin E-avidin complex-induced degranulation of β-hexosaminidase[CS103].

Anti-androgenic effect. Ethanol (95%) extract of the aerial parts, administered intraperitoneally to castrated mice at a dose of 2 mg/animal, produced strong activity[CS012]. The dried leaf, smoked by 13 male adults for 21 days, was inactive[CS208].

Anti-arthritic effect. Oral administration of AJA, a cannabinoid acid devoid of psychoactivity, reduced joint tissue damage in rats with adjuvant arthritis. Peripheral blood monocytes (PBM) and synovial fluid monocytes (SFM) were isolated from healthy subjects and patients with inflammatory arthritis, respectively, treated with AJA (0–30 mM) in vitro, and then stimulated with lipopolysaccharide. Cells were harvested for messenger RNA (mRNA), and supernatants were collected for cytokine assay. Addition of AJA to PBM and SFM in vitro reduced both steady-state levels of interleukin-1γ (IL-1γ) mRNA and secretion of IL-1γ in a concentration-dependent manner. Suppression was maximal (50.4%) at 10 mM AJA (p < 0.05 vs untreated controls, n = 7). AJA did not influence tumor necrosis factor-α (TNF-α) gene expression in or secretion from PBM[CS358].

Antibacterial activity. Essential oil, on agar plate, was active on *Staphylococcus aureus* and *Streptococcus faecalis*, minimum inhibitory concentration (MIC) 0.5 mg/mL, and produced weak activity on *Pseudomonas fluorescens* and *Escherichia coli*, MIC 10 mg/mL and 5 mg/mL, respectively[CS152].

Anticonvulsant activity. Ethanol (95%) extract of the entire plant, administered subcutaneously to male mice and rats at a dose of 2–4 mL/kg, was active vs metrazole and electroshock, respectively. A dose of 4 mL/kg was inactive vs strychnine convulsions in mice[CS005]. The entire plant, smoked by 29 patients with epilepsy under the age of 30 years, was active. It must be noted that in some species, cannabinoids can precipitate epileptic seizures[CS120]. Tincture of the resin, administered intraperitoneally to mice at a dose of 25 mg/kg, produced 80% protection vs pentylenetetrazole convulsions[CS058].

Antidiuretic activity. After ingesting the aerial parts, a 55-year-old man developed urinary retention that required catheterization for relief[CS154].

Anti-emetic activity. In a qualitative study of self-care in pregnancy, birth, and lactation within a nonrandom sample of 27 women in British Columbia, Canada, 20 women (74%) experienced pregnancy-induced nausea. Ten of these women used antiemetic herbal remedies, which included ginger, peppermint, and cannabis. Only ginger has been subjected to clinical trials among pregnant women, although the three herbs were clinically effective against nausea and vomiting in other contexts, such as chemotherapy-induced nausea and postoperative nausea[CS311]. CBD, a major nonpsychoactive cannabinoid administered by oral infusion to rats with nausea elicited by lithium chloride, and with conditioned nausea elicited by a flavor paired with lithium chloride, was active[CS382]. Oral nabilone, oral dronabinol (THC), and intramuscular levonantradol were administered to 1366 patients. Cannabinoids were more effective antiemetics than prochlorperazine, metoclopramide, chlorpromazine, thiethyl-

perazine, haloperidol, domperidone, or alizapride. Relative risk was 1.38 (95% CI 1.18–1.62), number-needed-to-treat (NNT) was 6 for complete control of nausea; relative risk was 1.28 (CI 1.08–1.51), NNT 8 for complete control of vomiting. Cannabinoids were not more effective in patients receiving very low or very high emetogenic chemotherapy. In crossover trials, patients preferred cannabinoids for future chemotherapy cycles: relative risk 2.39 (2.05–2.78), NNT 3. Some potentially beneficial side effects occurred more often with cannabinoids: "high" 10.6 (6.86–16.5), NNT 3; sedation or drowsiness 1.66 (1.46–1.89), NNT 5; euphoria 12.5 (3–52.1), NNT 7. Harmful side effects also occurred more often with cannabinoids: dizziness 2.97 (2.31–3.83), NNT 3; dysphoria or depression 8.06 (3.38–19.2), NNT 8; hallucinations 6.10 (2.41–15.4), NNT 17; paranoia 8.58 (6.38–11.5), NNT 20; and arterial hypotension 2.23 (1.75–2.83), NNT 7. Patients given cannabinoids were more likely to withdraw because of side effects (relative risk 4.67 [3.07–7.09]; NNT 11)[CS400].

Anti-estrogenic effect. Ethanol (95%) extract of the dried aerial parts, administered intragastric to rats at variable doses was inactive[CS231]. Petroleum ether extract of the dried leaf, administered intraperitoneally to female rats at a dose equivalent to 10 mg/kg tetrahydrocannabinol (THC) on 11–21 days of age, was active[CS175].

Antifertility effect. Petroleum ether extract of the entire plant, administered by gastric intubation to female mice at doses of 75 mg/kg and 150 mg/kg, was active. A dose of 3 mg/kg, produced weak activity[CS170]. Resin, administered by gastric intubation to male mice at variable dosage levels, was inactive[CS189].

Antifungal activity. Ethanol (50%) extract of the dried leaf was active on *Rhizoctonia solani*, mycelial inhibition was 65.99%[CS229]. Water extract of the fresh leaf on agar plate at a concentration of 1:1 was active on *Fusarium oxysporum*[CS096]. The water extract also produced strong activity on *Ustilago maydis* and *Ustilago nuda*[CS212]. Water extract of the fresh shoot on agar plate was inactive on *Helminthosporium turcicum*[CS237].

Antiglaucomic activity. Water extract of the dried entire plant, administered intravenously to Rhesus monkeys and rabbits at a dose of 0.01 µg/animal, was active. The intraocular pressure rose for 24 hours postinjection, then fell for 3 days. A dose of 25 µg/animal, administered intravenously to rabbits, was also active. The effect was not influenced by atropine, scopolamine, methysergide, haloperidol, chlorpromazine, spironolactone, yohimbine or dexamethasone. Partial inhibition was seen when galactose, glucose or mannose were administered intravenously, concurrently[CS232]. Water extract of the dried leaf and stem, applied opthalmically to rabbits was active[CS072].

Antigonadotropin effect. Ethanol (80%) extract of the dried aerial parts, administered intragastrically to male langurs at a dose of 14 mg/kg daily for 90 days produced equivocal effect[CS173].

Anti-inflammatory activity. Petroleum ether and ethanol (95%) extracts of the dried aerial parts, applied externally on mice at a dose of 100 µg/ear, was active vs tissue plasminogen activator-induced erythema of the ear[CS140]. CBD was administered orally to rats at doses of 5–40 mg/kg daily for 3 days after the onset of acute inflammation induced by intraplantar injection of 0.1 mL carrageenan (1% w/v in saline). CBD had a time- and dose-dependent antihyperalgesic effect after a single injection. Edema following carrageenan peaked at 3 hours and lasted 72 hours. A single dose of CBD reduced edema in a dose-dependent fashion and subsequent daily doses produced further time- and dose-related reductions. There were decreases in prostaglandin E2 (PGE2) plasma levels, tissue cyclo-oxygenase activ-

ity, production of oxygen-derived free radicals, and nitric oxide ([NO], nitrite/nitrate content) after three doses of CBD. The effect on NO seemed to depend on a lower expression of the endothelial isoform of NO synthase[CS303].

Antimalarial activity. The dried leaf was inactive on *Plasmodium falciparum* D-6 and W-2, IC_{50} greater than 1000 nmols[CS095].

Antimycobacterial activity. Essential oil, on agar plate, was active on *Antimycobacterium smegmatis*, MIC 0.1 mg/mL[CS152].

Anti-nematodal activity. Water extract of the dried leaf at variable concentrations produced strong activity on *Meloidogyne incognita*[CS200].

Antioxidant activity. Methanol extract of the stem, at concentration 50 µL, produced strong activity[CS101].

Antispasmodic activity. Ethanol (50%) extract of the entire plant was active on the guinea pig ileum vs acetylcholine and histamine-induced spasms[CS007]. The resin antagonized serotonin contractions of the rat intestine and non-pregnant uterus[CS003].

Antispermatogenic effect. Sixteen healthy chronic marijuana smokers were associated with a decline in sperm concentration and total sperm count during the fifth and sixth weeks after 4 weeks of high-dose smoking (8–20 cigarettes/day)[CS164]. The dried aerial part, taken by inhalation daily, decreases the quantity as well as quality of spermatozoa[CS181]. Ethanol (80%) extract of the dried aerial parts, administered intragastrically to langurs at a dose of 14 mg/kg daily for 90 days, was equivocal[CS173]. Ethanol (95%) extract of the dried aerial parts, administered intraperitoneally to mice at a dose of 2 mg/animal daily for 45 days, produced a complete arrest of spermatogenesis. The effect was reversible[CS244].

Antistress activity. The leaf smoke, in combination with hashish smoke, administered to rats housed in a wire cage inside a larger cage with a cat, was equivocal. The rats' brains were dissected and measured for protein and catecholamine levels[CS214].

Anti-tumor activity. Arachidonyl ethanolamide, in three cervical carcinoma (CxCa) cell lines at increasing doses with or without antagonists to receptors to arachidonyl ethanolamide, induced apoptosis of CxCa cell lines via aberrantly expressed vanilloid receptor-1. Arachidonyl ethanolamide-binding to the classical CB1 and CB2 cannabinoid receptors mediated a protective effect. A strong expression of the three forms of arachidonyl ethanolamide receptors was observed in ex vivo CxCa biopsies[CS297]. Three cannabis constituents, CBD, Δ-8-THC, and cannabinol displayed antiproliferative activity in several human cancer cell lines in vitro. They were oxidized to their respective paraquinones 2, 4, and 6. Quinone 2 significantly reduced cancer growth of HT-29 cancer in nude mice[CS275]. Δ-9-THC binds and activates membrane receptors of the 7-transmembrane domain, G protein-coupled superfamily. Several putative endocannabinoids have been identified, including anandamide (AEA), 2-arachidonyl glycerol, and noladin ether. Synthesis of numerous cannabinomimetics has expanded the repertoire of cannabinoid receptor ligands with the pharmacodynamic properties of agonists, antagonists, and inverse agonists. These ligands have proven to be powerful tools both for the molecular characterization of cannabinoid receptors and the delineation of their intrinsic signaling pathways. Much of the understanding of the signaling mechanisms activated by cannabinoids has been derived from studies of receptors expressed by tumor cells[CS318]. Cannabinoids and their derivatives exerted palliative effects in cancer patients by preventing nausea, vomiting, and pain and by stimulating appetite. These compounds have been shown to inhibit the growth of tumor cells in culture and animal models by modulating key cell-signaling pathways.

Cannabinoids are usually well tolerated, and do not produce the generalized toxic effects of conventional chemotherapies[CS328].

Anti-ulcer activity. Petroleum ether extract of the dried aerial parts, administered intraperitoneally to male rats, was active[CS097].

Antiviral activity. Hot water extract of the dried fruit, in vero cell culture at a concentration of 0.5 mg/mL, was inactive on herpes simplex 1 virus, measles virus, and poliovirus 1[CS094].

Anxiolytic activity. AEA, a primary endogenous ligand of the brain cannabinoid receptors, is released in selected regions of the brain and is deactivated through a two-step process consisting of transport into cells followed by intracellular hydrolysis. Pharmacological blockade of the enzyme fatty acid amide hydrolase (FAAH), which is responsible for intracellular AEA degradation, produced anxiolytic-like effects in rats without causing the wide spectrum of behavioral responses typical of direct-acting cannabinoid agonists. These findings suggest that AEA contributes to the regulation of emotion and anxiety, and that FAAH might be the target for a novel class of anxiolytic drugs[CS323].

Aphrodisiac activity. The leaf, smoked by adults of both sexes, was active[CS171].

Attention deficit hyperactivity disorder. Attention deficit hyperactivity disorder has been considered a mental and behavioral disorder of childhood and adolescence. It is being increasingly recognized in adults, who may have psychiatric comorbidity with secondary depression, or a tendency to drug and alcohol abuse. A 32-year-old woman known for years as suffering from borderline personality disorder and drug dependence (including cannabis, LSD, and ecstasy) and alcohol abuse that did not respond to treatment was reported. Only when correctly diagnosed as attention deficit hyperactivity disorder and appropriately treated with the psychotropic stimulant methylphenidate

(Ritalin®), was there significant improvement. She succeeded academically, which had not been possible previously, her craving for drugs diminished, and a drug-free state was reached[CS446].

Auditory function. Eight male subjects (aged 22–30 years) who had previously used cannabis were investigated. They performed air conduction pure tone audiometry in both ears over 0.5–8 kHz. A simple test of frequency selectivity by detecting a 4-kHz tone under two masking noise conditions was also carried out in one ear. Three test sessions at weekly intervals were carried out, at the start of which they ingested a capsule containing either placebo, 7.5, or 15 mg of THC. These were administered in a randomized cross-over, double-blind manner. Auditory testing was carried out 2 hours after ingestion. Blood samples were also obtained at this time point and assayed for Δ-9-THC and 11-hydroxy-THC levels. No significant changes in threshold or frequency resolution were seen with the dosages employed in this study[CS367].

Barbiturate potentiation. Flavonoid fraction of the leaf, administered intraperitoneally to mice, was active[CS242]. Petroleum ether extract of the dried entire plant, administered intraperitoneally to pigs at a dose of 250 mg/kg, was inactive[CS022].

Behavioral effect. A four-page, self-completed questionnaire was designed to determine the drugs used (licit, illicit, and doping substances) along with beliefs about doping and the psychosociological factors associated with their consumption. The questionnaire was distributed to high school students enrolled in a school sports association in eastern France. The completed forms were received from 1459 athletes: 4% stated that they had used doping agents at least once in their life (their main source of supply being peers and health professionals). Thirty-four percent of the sample smoked some tobacco, 66% used alcohol, 19% used cannabis, 4% took ecstasy, 10% took tranquillizers, 9% used hypnotics, 4% used creatine, and 41% used vitamins against fatigue. Beliefs about doping did not differ among doping agent users and nonusers, except for the associated health risks, which were minimized by users. Users of doping agents stated that the quality of the relations that they maintained with their parents was sharply degraded, and they reported that they were susceptible to influence and difficult to live with. More often than nondoping-agent users, these adolescents were neither happy, nor healthy, although paradoxically, they seemed less anxious and were more self-confident[CS302]. Maternal exposure to Δ-9-THC in rats resulted in alteration in the pattern of ontogeny of spontaneous locomotor and exploratory behavior in the offspring. Adult animals exposed during gestational and lactational periods exhibited persistent alterations in the behavioral response to novelty, social interactions, sexual orientation, and sexual behavior. They also showed a lack of habituation and reactivity to different illumination conditions. Adult offspring of both sexes also displayed a characteristic increase in spontaneous and water-induced grooming behavior. Some of the effects were dependent on the sex of the animals being studied, and the dose of cannabinoid administered to the mother during gestational and lactational periods. Maternal exposure to low doses of THC sensitized the adult offspring of both sexes to the reinforcing effects of morphine, as measured in a conditioned place preference paradigm[CS462].

β-Endorphin interaction. Δ-9-THC administered to rats produced large increases in extracellular levels of β-endorphin in the ventral tegmental area and lesser increases in the shell of the nucleus accumbens (Nac). In rats that had learned to discriminate injections of THC from injections of vehicle, the opioid agonist morphine did not produce THC-like discriminative effects, but markedly increased discrimination of THC. The opioid antagonist naloxone reduced the discriminative effects of THC. Bilateral microinjections of β-endorphin directly into the ventral tegmental area, but not into the shell of the Nac, markedly increased the discriminative effects of ineffective threshold doses of THC, but had no effect when given alone. The increase was blocked by naloxone[CS280].

Binocular depth inversion reduction. A study to assess whether the binocular depth inversion illusion (BDII) could detect subtle cognitive impairment owing to regular cannabis use was conducted. Ten regular cannabis users and 10 healthy controls from the same community sources, matched for age, sex, and premorbid intelligence quotient (IQ) were evaluated. The subjects were also compared on measures of executive functioning, memory, and personality. Regular cannabis users were found to have significantly higher BDII scores for inverted images. This was not to the result of a problem in the primary processing of visual information, as there was no significant difference between the groups for depth perception of normal images. There was no relationship between BDII scores for inverted images and time since the last dose, suggesting that the measured impairment of BDII more closely reflected chronic than acute effects of regular cannabis use. There were no significant differences between the groups for other neuropsychological measures of memory or executive function. A positive relationship was found between psychoticism as defined by the revised Eysenck Personality Questionnaire and cannabis, tobacco, and alcohol use. Cannabis users also used significantly larger amounts of alcohol. No relationship was found between BDII scores and drug use other than cannabis or psychoticism[CS332]. Nabilone, a psychoactive synthetic 9-*trans*-ketocannabinoid, CBD, and a combined oral application of both substances on binocular depth inversion and behavioral states were investigated in nine healthy male volunteers. A significant impairment of binocular depth perception was found when nabilone was administered, but combined application with CBD revealed reduced effects on binocular depth inversion[CS414].

Birth-weight effect. A total of 32,483 cannabis-using women giving birth to live-born infants were investigated. The largest reduction in mean birth-weight for any cannabis use during pregnancy was 48 g (95% CI, 83–14 g), with considerable heterogeneity among the five studies. Mean birth-weight was increased by 62 g (95% CI, 8-g reduction – 132-g increase; *p* heterogeneity, 0.59) among infrequent users (≤ weekly), whereas cannabis use at least four times per week had a 131-g reduction in mean birth-weight (95% CI 52–209-g reduction; *p* heterogeneity, 0.25). From the five studies of low birth-weight, the pooled odds ratio for any use was 1.09 (95% CI 0.94–1.27; *p* heterogeneity, 0.19)[CS437]. In a cohort study consisted of a multiethnic population of 7470 pregnant women. Information on the use of drugs was obtained from personal interviews at entry to the study and assays of serum obtained during pregnancy. Pregnancy outcome data (low birth-weight [<2500 g], pre-term birth [<37 weeks gestation], and abruptio placentae) were obtained with a standardized study protocol. A total of 2.3% of the women used cocaine and 11% used cannabis during pregnancy. Cannabis use was not associated with low birth-weight (1.1, 0.9–1.5), pre-term delivery (adjusted odds ratio [OR] 1.1, CI 0.8–1.3), or abruptio placentae (1.3, 0.6–2.8)[CS465].

Bladder dysfunction. Two whole-plant extracts of *Cannabis sativa* were administered to patients with advanced multiple sclerosis (MS) and refractory troublesome lower urinary tract symptoms. The patients took the extracts containing Δ-9-THC and CBD (2.5 mg of each per spray) for 8 weeks followed by THC-only (2.5 mg THC per spray) for a further eight weeks, and then into a long-term extension. Assessments included urinary frequency and volume charts, incontinence pad weights, cystometry, and visual analog scales for secondary troublesome symptoms. Twenty-one patients were recruited and data from 15 were evaluated. Urinary urgency, the number and volume of incontinence episodes, frequency, and nocturia all decreased significantly following treatment ($p <$ 0.05, Wilcoxon's signed rank test). Daily total voided, catheterized and urinary incontinence pad weights also decreased significantly for both extracts. Patient self-assessment of pain, spasticity, and quality of sleep improved significantly ($p < 0.05$, Wilcoxon's signed rank test) with pain improvement continuing up to a median of 35 weeks. There were few troublesome side effects, suggesting that cannabis-based medicinal extracts are a safe and effective treatment for urinary and other problems in patients with advanced MS[CS269].

Blood pressure stress reactivity effect. Data from an ascorbic acid (AA) trial (Cetebe 3 g/day for 14 days, $n = 108$) were compared by substance use level regarding systolic blood pressure (SBP) stress reactivity to the anticipation and actual experience phases of a standardized psychological stressor (10 minutes of public speaking and arithmetic). Self-reported never users of cannabis, persons not currently smoking tobacco, and persons consuming three or more caffeine beverages daily all exhibited AA SBP stress reactivity protection to the actual stressor, but not during the anticipation phase. Self-reported ever cannabis users, current tobacco smokers, and persons consuming less than three caffeine beverages daily exhibited the AA SBP protection during the anticipation phase, but only the lower caffeine consumption group exhibited AA protection during both phases. Covariates (neuroticism, extraversion and depression scores, age, sex, body mass index) were not significant[CS377].

Blood-borne sexually transmitted infections. Substance use, including alcohol and illicit drugs, increases the risk for the acquisition and transmission of sexually transmitted infection (STI). The prevalence of blood-borne STI including human immunodeficiency virus (HIV), human T-cell lymphotrophic virus type 1, hepatitis B virus, and syphilis in residents of a detoxification and rehabilitation unit in Jamaica were investigated. The demographic characteristics and the results of laboratory investigations for STI in 301 substance abusers presented during a 5-year period were reviewed. The laboratory results were compared with those of 131 blood donors. The substances used by participants were alcohol, cannabis, and cocaine. None of the clients was an intravenous drug user. Female substance abusers were at higher risk for STI. The prevalence of STI in substance abusers did not differ significantly from that in blood donors (12% vs 10%). The prevalence of syphilis in substance abusers was significantly higher than that in blood donors (6% vs 3%, $p < 0.05$). The prevalence of syphilis was dramatically increased in female substance abusers and female blood donors (30%, $p < 0.001$ and 13%, $p < 0.05$, respectively). An excess of human T-cell lymphotrophic virus type 1 was also observed in female compared with male substance abusers. Unemployment was identified also as a risk factor for sexually transmitted disease in substance abusers[CS401].

Brain aging effect. The impact of duration of education, cannabis addiction and smoking on cognition and brain aging was studied in 211 healthy Egyptian volunteers with mean age of 46.4 ± 3.6 years (range, 20–76 years). The subjects were classified into two groups: Gr I (n = 174; mean age, 49.9 ± 3.8 years; range, 20–76 years), nonaddicts, smokers, and nonsmokers, educated and noneducated, and Gr II cannabis addicts (n = 37; mean age, 43.6 ± 2.6 years; range, 20–72 years) all smokers, educated and noneducated. Outcome measures included the Paced Auditory Serial Addition test for testing attention and the Trailmaking test A and Trailmaking test B (TMb) for testing psychomotor performance. Age correlated positively with score of TMb in the nonaddict group and in the addict group (Trailmaking test A and TMb). Years of education correlated negatively with scores of TMb in the nonaddict group (Gr I) but not the addict group (Gr II). Cannabis addicts (Gr II) had significantly poorer attention than nonaddict normal volunteers (Gr I). It was determined that impairment of psychomotor performance is age related whether in normal nonaddicts or in cannabis addicts. A decline in attention was detected in cannabis addicts and has been considered a feature of pathological aging[CS448].

Brain cannabinoid receptor. In humans, psychoactive cannabinoids produce euphoria, enhancement of sensory perception, tachycardia, antinociception, difficulties in concentration, and impairment of memory. The cognitive deficiencies persist after withdrawal. The toxicity of cannabis has been underestimated for a long time, since recent findings revealed that Δ-9-THC-induced cell death with shrinkage of neurons and DNA fragmentation in the hippocampus. The acute effects of cannabinoids, as well as the development of tolerance, are mediated by G protein-coupled cannabinoid receptors. The CB1 receptor and its splice variant, CB1A, are found predominantly in the brain with highest densities in the hippocampus, cerebellum, and striatum. The CB2 receptor is found predominantly in the spleen and in hemopoi-

etic cells and has only 44% overall nucleotide sequence identity with the CB1 receptor. The existence of this receptor provided the molecular basis for the immunosuppressive actions of cannabis. The CB1 receptor mediates inhibition of adenylate cyclase, inhibition of N- and P/Q-type calcium channels, stimulation of potassium channels, and activation of mitogen-activated protein kinase. The CB2 receptor mediates inhibition of adenylate cyclase and activation of mitogen-activated protein kinase. The discovery of endogenous cannabinoid receptor ligands, AEA (N-arachidonyl-ethanolamine), and 2-arachidonylglycerol made the notion of a central cannabinoid neuromodulatory system plausible. AEA is released from neurons on depolarization through a mechanism that requires calcium-dependent cleavage from a phospholipid precursor in neuronal membranes. The release of AEA is followed by rapid uptake into the plasma and hydrolysis by fatty-acid amidohydrolase. The psychoactive cannabinoids increase the activity of dopaminergic neurons in the ventral tegmental area–mesolimbic pathway. Because these dopaminergic circuits are known to play a pivotal role in mediating the reinforcing (rewarding) effects of the most drugs of abuse, the enhanced dopaminergic drive elicited by the cannabinoids is thought to underlie the reinforcing and abuse properties of cannabis. Thus, cannabinoids share a final common neuronal action with other major drugs of abuse such as morphine, ethanol, and nicotine in producing facilitation of the mesolimbic dopamine system[CS423]. Hippocampal slices from humans, guinea pigs, rats, and mice, and cerebellar, cerebrocortical, and hypothalamic slices from guinea pigs were incubated with [³H] noradrenaline and then superfused. Tritium overflow was evoked either electrically (0.3 or 1 Hz) or by introduction of Ca^{2+} ions (1.3 μM) into Ca^{2+}-free, K^+-rich medium (25 μM) containing 1 μM of tetrodotoxin. The cyclic adenosone monophosphate (cAMP) accumulation stimulated by 10 μM of forskolin was determined in guinea pig hippocampal membranes. The following drugs were used: the cannabinoid receptor-agonists (-)-cis-3-[2-hydroxy-4-(1,1-dimethylheptyl)phenyl]-trans-4-(3-hydroxypropyl)cyclo-hexanol (CP-55,940) and R(+)-[2,3-dihydro-5-methyl-3-[(morpholinyl)methyl]pyrrolo[1,2,3-de]-1,4-benzoxazinyl]-(1-naphthalenyl)methanone (WIN 55,212-2 [WIN]), the inactive S(-)-enantiomer of the latter (WIN 55,212-3) and the CB1 receptor antagonist N-piperidino-5-(4-chlorophenyl)-1-(2,4-dichlorophenyl)-4-methyl-3-pyrazole-carboxamide (SR 141716). The electrically evoked tritium overflow from guinea pig hippocampal slices was reduced by WIN (peak inhibitory concentration 30%, 6.5) but not affected by WIN 55,212-3 up to 10 mM. The concentration–response curve of WIN was shifted to the right by SR 141716 (0.032-μM) (apparent pA2 8.2), which by itself did not affect the evoked overflow. WIN (1 μM) also inhibited the Ca^{2+}-evoked tritium overflow in guinea pig hippocampal slices and the electrically evoked overflow in guinea pig cerebellar, cerebrocortical, and hypothalamic slices, as well as in human hippocampal slices, but not in rat and mouse hippocampal slices. SR 141716 (0.32 μM) markedly attenuated the WIN-induced inhibition in guinea pig and human brain slices. SR 141716 (0.32 μM) by itself increased the electrically evoked tritium overflow in guinea pig hippocampal slices, but failed to do so in slices from the other brain regions of the guinea pig and in human hippocampal slices, but failed to do so in slices from the other brain regions of the guinea pig and in human hippocampal slices. The cAMP accumulation stimulated by forskolin was reduced by CP-55,940 and WIN. The concentration-response curve of CP-55,940 was shifted to the right by SR

141716 (0.1 μM; apparent pA2 8.3), that by itself did not affect cAMP accumulation. In conclusion, cannabinoid receptors of the CB1 subtype occur in the human hippocampus, where they may contribute to the psychotropic effects of cannabis, and in the guinea pig hippocampus, cerebellum, cerebral cortex, and hypothalamus. The CB1 receptor in the guinea pig hippocampus is located presynaptically, was activated by endogenous cannabinoids, and may be negatively coupled to adenylyl cyclase[CS442]. The acute administration of AEA or THC in rats increased the maximum binding capacity (B_{max}) of cannabinoid receptors in the cerebellum and, particularly, in the hippocampus. This effect was also observed after 5 days of a daily exposure to AEA or THC. The increase in the B_{max} after the acute treatment seemed to be caused by changes in the receptor affinity (high K_d). The increase after the chronic exposure may be attributed to an increase in the density of receptors. The [^{3}H]CP-55,940 binding to cannabinoid receptors in the striatum, the limbic forebrain, the mesencephalon, and the medial basal hypothalamus was not altered after the acute exposure to AEA or THC. The chronic exposure to THC significantly decreased the B_{max} of these receptors in the striatum and nonsignificantly in the mesencephalon. This effect was not elicited after the chronic exposure to AEA and was not accompanied by changes in the K_d[CS463].

Bronchoconstrictor activity. Water extract of seed, administered by inhalation to human adults, was active[CS147].

Bronchodilator activity. Petroleum ether extract of the aerial parts, administered orally to adults of both sexes, was inactive[CS078].

Cannabinoid hyperemesis. Nineteen patients were identified with chronic cannabis abuse and a cyclical vomiting illness. Follow-up was provided with serial urine drug screen analysis and regular clinical consultation to chart the clinical course. Of the 19 patients, five refused consent and were lost to follow-up, and five were excluded based on cofounders. In all cases, chronic cannabis abuse predated the onset of the cyclical vomiting illness. Cessation of cannabis abuse led to cessation of the cyclical vomiting illness in seven cases. Three cases did not abstain and continued to have recurrent episodes of vomiting. Three cases rechallenged themselves after a period of abstinence and suffered a return to illness. Two of these cases abstained again and became, and remain, well. The third case did not and remains ill. A novel finding was that 9 of the 10 patients, including the previously published case, displayed an abnormal washing behavior during episodes of active illness[CS258].

Cannabinoid-induced Fos expression. Cannabinoid CB1 receptor agonist CP-55,940 in Lewis and Wistar rats was investigated. A moderate (50 µg/kg) and a high (250 µg/kg) dose level were used. The 250-µg/kg dose caused locomotor suppression, hypothermia, and catalepsy in both strains, but with a significantly greater effect in Wistar rats. The 50-µg/kg dose provoked moderate hypothermia and locomotor suppression but in Wistar rats only. CP-55,940 caused significant Fos immunoreactivity in 24 out of 33 brain regions examined. The most dense expression was seen in the paraventricular nucleus of the hypothalamus, the islands of Calleja, the lateral septum (ventral), the central nucleus of the amygdala, the bed nucleus of the stria terminalis (lateral division), and the ventrolateral periaqueductal gray. Despite having a similar distribution of CP-55,940-induced Fos expression, Lewis rats showed less overall Fos expression than Wistar rats in nearly every brain region counted. This held equally true for anxiety-related brain structures (e.g., central nucleus of the amygdala, periaqueductal gray, and the paraventricular nucleus of the hypothalamus) and reward-related sites (Nac and pedunculopontine tegmental nucleus). In a further experiment, Wistar rats and Lewis rats did not differ in the amount of Fos immunoreactivity produced by cocaine (15 mg/kg). These results indicate that Lewis rats are less sensitive to the behavioral, physiological and neural effects of cannabinoids[CS396].

Cannabis withdrawal effect. A 35-year-old male was cognitively assessed prior to cessation of 18 years of daily cannabis use and monitored for several weeks postcessation. Brain event-related potential measures of selective attention reflecting a difficulty in filtering out complex irrelevant information showed no indication of improvement over 6 weeks of abstinence. When tested in the acutely intoxicated state prior to cessation of use, a dramatic normalization of the event-related potential signature was observed. A treatment program based on supportive–expressive psychotherapy was administered and depression, anxiety, and general psychological health were monitored over the course of withdrawal from cannabis[CS466].

Cannabis–amphetamine interaction. Cannabinoid–amphetamine interactions were studied as follows:

1. 30 minutes after acute injection of (-)-Δ-9-THC (0.1 or 6.4 mg/kg, intraperitoneally).

2. 30 minutes after the last injection of 14-daily treatment with (-)-Δ-9-THC (0.1 or 6.4 mg/kg).

3. 24 hours after the last injection of 14-daily treatment with (-)-Δ-9-THC (6.4 mg/kg).

Acute cannabinoid exposure antagonized the amphetamine-induced dose-dependent increase in locomotion, exploration, and the decrease in inactivity. Chronic treatment with (-)-Δ-9-THC resulted in tolerance to this antagonistic effect on locomotion and inactivity but not on exploration, and potentiated amphetamine-induced stereotypes. Lastly, 24 hours of withdrawal after 14 days of cannabinoid treatment resulted in sensitization to the effects of D-amphetamine on locomotion, exploration, and stereotypes[CS431].

Cannabis-induced coma. Two cases of cannabis-induced coma were reported following accidental ingestion of cannabis cookies. The possibility of cannabis ingestion should be considered in cases of unexplained coma in a previously healthy young child if signs of conjunctival hyperemia, pupillary dilatation, and tachycardia were present and other causes, such as central nervous system infection or trauma were unlikely[CS458].

Cannabis-related arteritis. A 19-year-old man who presented with plantar claudication associated with necrosis in a toe underwent diagnostic arteriography and surgery for popliteal artery entrapment type III was studied. Surgical clearance resolved the popliteal artery entrapment but left the clinical symptoms unchanged. Closer questioning disclosed a history of cannabis consumption and intravenous vasodilatory therapy was started. After the 21-day course of vasodilator agents, the pain disappeared and the toe necrosis regressed. The patient stopped taking cannabis and had no signs of recurrence[CS308]. A 24-year-old woman who was a heavy cannabis smoker with progressive Raynauld's phenomenon and digital necrosis, was investigated. Systemic sclerosis and other connective tissue disorders, as well as arteriosclerosis and arterial emboli were excluded with appropriate laboratory examinations. Arteriography revealed multiple forearm, palmar and digital occlusions with corkscrew-shaped vessels. Based on the characteristic arteriography and clinical findings, the diagnosis of cannabis arteritis was retained. With careful necrectomy,

conservative wound dressings and secondary prostacyclin therapy a complete healing of digital necrosis was observed. There was no recurrence during the 6-month follow-up[CS336]. Young men were presented with distal arteriopathy of the lower limbs in three cases, and of the left upper limb in the remaining patient. Symptoms occurred progressively, distal pulses had disappeared, and distal necrosis was constant. Three patients suffered from Raynauld's phenomenon, none of them presented with venous thrombosis. Radiological evaluation revealed distal abnormalities in all cases, and proximal arterial thrombosis in one case. The four patients were cannabis smokers for at least four years. With cannabis interruption and symptomatic treatment, lesions improved for three patients. For one of them, recurrence of arteriopathy occurred when he resumed smoking cannabis. For the fourth who never stopped cannabis, an amputation was necessary[CS349]. Ten male moderate tobacco smokers and regular cannabis users with a median age of 23.7 years, developed subacute distal ischemia of the lower or upper limbs, leading to necrosis in the toes and/or fingers and sometimes to distal limb gangrene. Two of the patients also presented with venous thrombosis and three patients were suffering from a recent Raynauld's phenomenon. Biological test results did not show evidence of the classical vascular risk factors for thrombosis. Arteriographic evaluation in all of the cases revealed distal abnormalities in the arteries of feet, legs, forearms, and hands resembling those of Buerger's disease. A collateral circulation sometimes with opacification of the vasa nervorum was noted. In some cases, arterial proximal atherosclerotic lesions and venous thrombosis were observed. Despite treatment with ilomedine and heparin in all cases, five amputations were necessary in four patients. The vasoconstrictor effect of cannabis on the vascular system has been known for a long time. It has been shown that Δ-8-THC and Δ-9-THC may induce peripheral vasoconstrictor activity. Cannabis arteritis resembles Buerger's disease, but patients were moderate tobacco smokers and regular cannabis users[CS406].

Cannabis-related flashback. A young man who offended a friend without any objective reason was reported. The report of the forensic psychiatrist demonstrated that the offense was committed under the influence of a cannabis flashback. The last time the offender had consumed cannabis was 2 weeks before the acts. A plasmatic detection was realized and showed a level of 6 ng/mL, 30 minutes after the beginning of the flashback[CS383].

Capgras syndrome. A report describes an apparently greater incidence of Capgras syndrome among the Maori population compared with the European population. Five cases of Capgras syndrome were identified in the eastern catchment area where 19% of the population identified as Maori, 75% as European, and 6% as other or nonspecified. All of the cases occurred in Maori patients. No cases were identified in the western catchment area where 12% of the population identified as Maori, 87% as European, and 1% as other or nonspecified. Four of five cases were females. Two cases had a history of cannabis use. Three cases had exhibited dangerous behavior towards family members[CS410].

Carcinogenic activity. The dried leaf, administered intraperitoneally to rats of both sexes at a dose of 7 mg/kg/week, was active. The animals were irradiated with γ radiation between 40 and 50 days of age and observed for 78 weeks. There was a greater incidence of tumors in animals given marijuana extract and γ radiation than either marihuana or γ radiation alone[CS223].

Cardiorespiratory effect. Fifty stable patients (25 males, 25 females) with methadone maintenance treatment (MMT) programs were investigated. Forty-six MMT patients were current tobacco smokers, 19 were current cannabis users, and none were currently using opioids other than prescribed methadone. Abnormalities of respiratory function were defined as those results outside the 95% confidence interval of reference values for normal subjects adjusted for age, weight, height, and sex. Thirty-one (62%) MMT patients had reduced carbon monoxide transfer factor; 17 (34%) had elevated single breath alveolar volume, and 43 (86%) had a reduced carbon monoxide transfer factor–alveolar volume ratio. Six patients (12%) had reduced forced expiratory volume in 1 second (FEV1); one (2%) had reduced forced vital capacity (FVC); and nine (18%) had an obstructive ventilatory defect. Ten (20%) patients had arterial CO_2 pressure higher than 45 mmHg and 14 (28%) had alveolar to arterial oxygen gradient higher than 15 mmHg. Chest X-ray, echocardiography, and electrocardiogram showed no significant abnormalities[CS256]. The potent cannabinoid receptor agonists WIN55,212-2 (0.05, 0.5, or 5 pmol/50 nL) and HU-210 (0.5 pmol/50 nL) or the CB1 receptor antagonist/inverse agonist AM281 (1 pmol/100 nL) were microinjected into the rostral ventrolateral medulla oblongata (RVLM) of urethane-anesthetized, immobilized and mechanically ventilated male Sprague–Dawley rats ($n = 22$). Changes in splanchnic nerve activity, phrenic nerve activity, mean arterial pressure, and heart rate in response to cannabinoid administration were recorded. The CB1 receptor gene was expressed throughout the ventrolateral medulla oblongata. Unilateral microinjection of WIN 55,212-2 into the RVLM evoked short-latency, dose-dependent increases in splanchnic nerve activity (0.5 pmol; $175 \pm 8\%$, $n = 5$) and mean arterial pressure (0.5 pmol; $26 \pm 3\%$, $n = 8$), and abolished phrenic nerve activity (0.5 pmol; duration of apnea: 5.4 ± 0.4 seconds, $n = 8$), with little change in heart rate ($p < 0.005$). HU-210, structurally related to Δ-9-THC, evoked similar effects when microinjected into the RVLM (n = 4). Prior microinjection of AM281 produced agonist-like effects, and significantly attenuated the response to subsequent injection of WIN (0.5 pmol, n = 4)[CS331].

Cardiovascular effects. The leaf, smoked by adults of both sexes, at a dose of 600 mg/person (1–1.5% THC), produced no adverse effects on blood pressure, electrocardiogram, and the heart[CS065]. Cannabis and Δ-9-THC increase heart rate, slightly increase supine blood pressure, and on occasion produced marked orthostatic hypotension. Cardiovascular effects in animals are different, with bradycardia and hypotension the most typical responses. Cardiac output increases, and peripheral vascular resistance and maximum exercise performance decrease. Tolerance to most of the initial cardiovascular effects appears rapidly. With repeated exposure, supine blood pressure decreases slightly, orthostatic hypotension disappears, blood volume increases, heart rate slows, and circulatory responses to exercise and Valsalva maneuver are diminished, consistent with centrally mediated, reduced sympathetic, and enhanced parasympathetic activity. Receptor-mediated and probably nonneuronal sites of action account for cannabinoid effects. The endocannabinoid system appears important in the modulation of many vascular functions. Cannabis' cardiovascular effects are not associated with serious health problems for most young, healthy users, although occasional myocardial infarction, stroke, and other adverse cardiovascular events are reported[CS362].

Cataleptic effect. Petroleum ether extract of the dried entire plant, administered intraperitoneally to guinea pigs at a dose of 100 mg/kg, was active[CS022].

CB1 cannabinoid receptor in human placenta. CB1 (G protein-coupled) receptor and FAAH expression in human term placenta were investigated by immunohistochemistry. CB1 receptor was found in all layers of the membrane, with particularly strong expression in the amniotic epithelium and reticular cells and cells of the maternal decidua layer. Moderate expression was observed in the chorionic cytotrophoblasts. The expression of FAAH was highest in the amniotic epithelial cells, chorionic cytotrophoblast, and maternal decidua layer. The results suggest that the human placenta is a likely target for cannabinoid action and metabolism. This is consistent with a placental site of action of endocannabinoids and cannabis being responsible, at least in part, for the poor outcomes associated with cannabis consumption and pathology in the endocannabinoid system during pregnancy[CS327].

Central nervous system depressant activity. Fluidextract of the aerial parts, administered intraperitoneally to rats at a dose of 25 mg/kg, was active. The fluidextract, administered orally to dogs, produced ataxia[CS240]. The leaf, smoked by human adults, produced a decrease in psychomotor performance[CS066].

Central nervous system effect. Δ-9-THC activates the two G protein-coupled receptors CB1 and CB2. The endogenous ligands of these receptors were identified as lipid metabolites of arachidonic acid, named endocannabinoids. The two most studied endocannabinoids are AEA and 2-arachidonyl-glycerol. The CB1 receptor is massively expressed throughout the central nervous system, whereas CB2 expression seems restricted to immune cells. Following endocannabinoid binding, CB1 receptors modulate second messenger cascades (inhibition of adenylate cyclase, activation of mitogen-activated protein kinases and of focal-adhesion kinases), as well as ionic conductances (inhibition of voltage-dependent calcium channels, activation of several potassium channels). Endocannabinoids transiently silenced synapses by decreasing neurotransmitter release. They play major roles in various forms of synaptic plasticity because of their ability to behave as retrograde messengers and activate noncannabinoid receptors (such as vanilloid receptor type-1)[CS305]. Mice strain with a disrupted *CB1* gene (CB1 knockout mice) appeared healthy and fertile, but they had a significantly increased mortality rate. They also displayed reduced locomotor activity, increased ring catalepsy, and hypoalgesia in hotplate and formalin tests. Δ-9-THC-induced ring catalepsy, hypomobility, and hypothermia were completely absent in CB1 mutant mice. In contrast, Δ-9-THC-induced analgesia in the tail-flick test and other behavioral (licking of the abdomen) and physiological (diarrhea) responses after Δ-9-THC administration were found. Results indicate that most, but not all, central nervous system effects of Δ-9-THC are mediated by the CB1 receptor[CS425].

Central nervous system stimulant activity. The resin, ingested by a 4-year-old girl, showed signs of stupor alternating with brief intervals of excitation and foolish laughing with atactic movements. Her temperature, blood pressure, pulse, hemoglobin, leukocytes, serum electrolytes, and serum urea were normal. Respiratory rate was 12 beats per minute. Blood sugar elevated. Recovery was complete within 24 hours with no treatment[CS047].

Cerebellar clock-altering effect. Twelve volunteers who smoked cannabis recreationally about once weekly, and 12 volunteers who smoked daily for a number of years performed a self-paced counting task during positron emission tomography imaging, before and after smoking cannabis and placebo cigarettes. Smoking cannabis increased regional cerebral blood flow in the ventral forebrain and cerebellar cortex in both groups, but resulted in significantly less frontal lobe activation in chronic users. Counting rate increased after smoking cannabis in both groups, as did a behavioral measure of self-paced tapping, and both increases correlated with regional cerebral blood flow in the cerebellum. Results indicate that smoking cannabis appears to accelerate a cerebellar clock-altering self-paced behaviors[CS343].

Clinical endocannabinoid deficiency. Clinical endocannabinoid deficiency, and the prospect that it could underlie the pathophysiology of migraine, fibromyalgia, irritable bowel syndrome, and other functional conditions alleviated by clinical cannabis were studied. Migraine has numerous relationships to endocannabinoid function. AEA potentiated 5-hydroxytrayptamine (HT1A) and inhibited 5-HT2A receptors supporting therapeutic efficacy in acute and preventive migraine treatment. Cannabinoids also demonstrated dopamine-blocking and anti-inflammatory effects. AEA is tonically active in the periaqueductal gray matter, a migraine generator. THC modulated glutamatergic neurotransmission via N-methyl-D-aspartic acid-receptors. Fibromyalgia is now conceived as a central sensitization state with secondary hyperalgesia. Cannabinoids have similarly demonstrated the ability to block spinal, peripheral and gastrointestinal mechanisms that promote pain in headache, fibromyalgia, irritable bowel syndrome and related disorders[CS288].

Cognitive functioning. Cognitive performance was examined in 145 adolescents aged 13–16 years for whom prenatal exposure to cannabis and cigarettes had been ascertained. The subjects were from a low-risk, predominantly middle-class sample participating in an ongoing, longitudinal study. The assessment battery included tests of general intelligence, achievement, memory, and aspects of executive functioning. Consistent with results obtained at earlier ages, the strongest relationship between prenatal maternal cigarette smoking and cognitive variables was seen with overall intelligence and aspects of auditory functioning, whereas prenatal exposure to marijuana was negatively associated with tasks that required visual memory, analysis, and integration[CS344]. A multisite, retrospective, cross-sectional, neuropsychological study was conducted among 102 near-daily cannabis users (51 long-term users: mean, 23.9 years of use; 51 shorter-term users: mean, 10.2 years of use), compared with 33 nonuser controls. Measures from nine standard neuropsychological tests that assessed attention, memory, and executive functioning were administered prior to entry into a treatment program following a median 17-hour abstinence. Long-term cannabis users performed significantly less well than shorter-term users and controls on tests of memory and attention. On the Rey Auditory Verbal Learning Test, long-term users recalled significantly fewer words than either shorter-term users ($p = 0.001$) or controls ($p = 0.005$). There was no difference between shorter-term users and controls. Long-term users showed impaired learning ($p = 0.007$), retention ($p = 0.003$), and retrieval ($p = 0.002$) compared with controls. Both user groups performed poorly on a time estimation task ($p < 0.001$ vs controls). Performance measures often correlated significantly with the duration of cannabis use, being worse with increasing years of use, but were unrelated to withdrawal symptoms and persisted after controlling for recent cannabis use and other drug use[CS388]. A patient with a history of traumatic brain injury along with current mood disorder and cannabis use was reported. The impact of cannabis use appeared to have a detrimental effect on his mood. Treatment of the mood disorder resulted in larger cognitive gains[CS415]. Sixty healthy volunteers (a negative urine drug-screening test was prerequisite) were investigated. On the first day, baseline data were obtained from a physical examination and a psychological test battery for the investigation of visual and verbal memory and cognitive percep-

tual performance. On the second day, subjects received a regular cigarette or one containing 290 mg/kg body weight of THC. Physical and psychological assessments were performed immediately (15 minutes) after subjects smoked their cigarettes. Twenty-four hours later, physical and psychological examinations were repeated. Results suggest that perceptual motor speed and accuracy, two very important parameters of driving ability, seem to be impaired immediately after cannabis consumption[CS420]. The analyses included 1318 participants under age 65 years who completed the Mini-Mental State Examination (MMSE) during three study waves in 1981, 1982, and 1993–1996. Individual MMSE score differences between waves two and three were calculated for each study participant. After 12 years, study participants' scores declined a mean of 1.20 points on the MMSE (standard deviation, 1.90), with 66% having scores that declined by at least one point. Significant numbers of scores declined by three points or more (15% of participants in the 18–29-year-old age group). There were no significant differences in cognitive decline between heavy users, light users, and nonusers of cannabis. There were also no male–female differences in cognitive decline in relation to cannabis use[CS426]. From 250 individuals consuming cannabis regularly, 99 healthy, free of any other past or present drug abuse, or history of neuropsychiatric disease cannabis users were selected. After an interview, physical examination, analysis of routine laboratory parameters, plasma/urine analyses for drugs, and Minnesota Multiphasic Personality Inventory testing, users and respective controls were subjected to a computer-assisted attention test battery comprising visual scanning, alertness, divided attention, flexibility, and working memory. Of the potential predictors of test performance within the user group, including present age, age of onset of cannabis use, degree of acute intoxication (THC + THC–OH plasma levels), and cumulative toxicity (estimated total life dose), an early age of onset turned out to be the only predictor, predicting impaired reaction times exclusively in visual scanning. Early-onset users (onset before age 16; n = 48) showed a significant impairment in reaction times in this function, whereas late-onset users (onset after age 16; n = 51) did not differ from controls (n = 49)[CS428]. Male volunteers (n = 5) with histories of moderate alcohol and cannabis use were administered three doses of alcohol (0.25, 0.5, or 1 g/kg), three doses of cannabis (4.8, or 16 puffs of 3.55% Δ-9-THC), and placebo in random order under double blind conditions in seven separate sessions. Blood alcohol concentration (10–90 mg/dL) and THC levels (63–188 ng/mL) indicated that active drug was delivered to subjects dose dependently. Alcohol and cannabis produced dose-related changes in subjective measures of drug effect. Ratings of perceived impairment were identical for the high doses of alcohol and cannabis. Both drugs produced comparable impairment in digit–symbol substitution and word recall tests, but had no effect in time perception and reaction time tests. Alcohol, but not cannabis, slightly impaired performance in a number recognition test[CS444].

Comorbid dysthymia and substance disorder. A total of 642 patients were assessed. Thirty-nine had substance-related disorder and dysthymia (SRD-dysthymia) and 308 had SRD only. Data on past use were collected by a research associate using a questionnaire. The patients with SRD-dysthymia and SRD did not differ with regard to use of alcohol, tobacco, and benzodiazepines. The patients with SRD-dysthymia started caffeine use at an earlier age, had shorter "use careers" of cocaine, amphetamines, and opiates, and had fewer days of cocaine and cannabis use in the last year. They also had a lower rate of cannabis

abuse/dependence. The results indicated that patients with dysthymia and SRD have exposure to most substances of abuse that was comparable to patients with SRD only. They selectively use certain substances less often than patients with SRD only[CS433]. A course and severity of SRD among 642 patients with comorbid major depressive disorder (MDD) was analyzed by means of both retrospective and concurrent data. Data on course included lifetime use, age at first use, years of use, use in the last year, periods of abstinence, and current diagnosis. Data on severity included two measures of SRD-associated problems, substance abuse vs dependence, self-help activities, and number of substances being abused. SRD-MDD patients tended to manifest lower levels of cannabis, opiate, and cocaine use, and more SRD-only patients were abusing three or more substances. Men with SRD-MDD demonstrated longer mean durations of abstinence compared with men with SRD-only, whereas SRD-MDD women demonstrated shorter mean durations of abstinence, compared with women with SRD-only. MDD-SRD patients showed slightly less substance abuse, but SRD severity was comparable with SRD-only patients[CS441].

Covariation among risk behaviors. A sample of 913 sexually active high school students completed a self-administered questionnaire that required mainly "yes" or "no" answers to questions involving participation in a range of risk behaviors. Contraceptive nonuse was not significantly associated with use of cigarettes, alcohol, or inhalants; perpetration or being a victim of violence; exposure to risk of physical injury; and suicidality. For males only, there was a significant inverse association between contraceptive nonuse and use of cannabis in the previous month. This was not the case for lifetime cannabis use for either gender[CS404].

Cyclo-oxygenase inhibition. Ethanol (100%) extract and essential oil of the aerial parts were active, IC_{50} 6.7 mg/L and 7.5 mg/L, respectively[CS226].

Cytochrome P450 and 2C6 expression. Hashish (cannabis) and heroin effect on the expression of cytochrome P450 2E1 (CYP 2E1) and cytochrome P450 2C6 (CYP 2C6) was measured after single (24 hours) and repeated-dose treatments (four consecutive days). The expression of CYP 2E1 was slightly induced after single-dose treatments and markedly induced after repeated-dose treatments of mice with hashish (10 mg/kg body weight). It is believed that N-nitrosamines are activated principally by CYP 2E1 and the activity of N-nitrosodimethylamine was found to be increased after single- and repeated-dose treatments of mice with hashish by 23 and 41%, respectively. Hashish treatments of mice increased the total hepatic content of CYP by 112 and 206%, respectively; aryl hydrocarbon hydroxylase activity by 110 and 165%, respectively; nicotinamide adenine dinucleotide phosphate–cytochrome c reductase activity by 21 and 98%, respectively, and glutathione level by 81 and 173%, respectively. The level of free radicals (thiobarbituric acid-reactive substances) was potentially decreased after single- or repeated-dose treatments with either hashish or heroin[CS333].

Cytotoxic activity. Ethanol (50%) extract of the entire plant, in cell culture, was inactive on CA-9KB, ED_{50} greater than 20 μg/mL[CS007]. Water extract of the dried seed, in cell culture at a concentration of 500 μg/mL, was inactive on CA-mammary-microalveolar[CS144].

Cytotoxic effect. THC, in leukemic cell lines (CEM, HEL-92, and HL60) and in peripheral blood mononuclear cells, 6 hours after exposure induced apoptosis, even at one times the IC_{50}. THC did not appear to act synergistically with cytotoxic agents, such as cisplatin. THC-induced cell death was preceded by significant changes in the expression of genes involved in the mitogen-activated protein kinase signal transduction pathways. Both apoptosis and gene expression changes were altered independent of p53 and the cannabinoid 1 and 2 receptors (CB1-R and CB2-R)[CS261].

Depressant activity. Heavy cannabis use and depression are associated and evidence from longitudinal studies suggests that heavy cannabis use may increase depressive symptoms among some users[CS321]. Participants ($n = 1920$) were reassessed as part of a follow-up study. The analysis focused on two cohorts: those who reported no depressive symptoms at baseline ($n = 849$) and those with no diagnosis of cannabis abuse at baseline ($n = 1,837$). Symptoms of depression, cannabis abuse, and other psychiatric disorders were assessed with the Diagnostic Interview Schedule. In participants with no baseline depressive symptoms, those with a diagnosis of cannabis abuse at baseline were four times more likely than those with no cannabis abuse diagnosis to have depressive symptoms at the follow-up assessment, after adjusting for age, gender, antisocial symptoms, and other baseline covariates. These participants were more likely to have experienced suicidal ideation and anhedonia during the follow-up period. Among the participants who had no diagnosis of cannabis abuse at baseline, depressive symptoms at baseline failed to significantly predict cannabis abuse at the follow-up assessment[CS395]. The relationship between depressive symptoms and polydrug use (alcohol, cannabis, and cocaine) among blacks in a high-risk community was studied. A street sample ($n = 570$) from four high-risk communities was collected through personal interviews. Interviewers asked respondents about their drug use behavior during the past 30 days and their depressive symptoms during the past week.

Odds ratios and logistic regressions, adjusted for age and sex, were used to assess the relationship between depressive symptoms and drug and polydrug use (drug use involving cocaine). Results showed that depressive symptoms are significantly associated with polydrug use. Depressive symptoms were not associated with alcohol use or with the combination of alcohol and cannabis use[CS440].

Diabetic ketoacidosis. One hundred fifty-eight young adults, aged 16–30 years, with type 1 diabetes, attending an urban diabetes clinic, were sent an anonymous confidential postal questionnaire to determine the prevalence of street drug use. Eighty-five completed responses were received. Twenty-nine percent of respondents admitted to using street drugs. Of those, 68% habitually took street drugs more than once a month. Seventy-two percent of users were unaware of the adverse effects on diabetes. Results indicated that the street drug usage in young adults with type 1 diabetes is common and may contribute to poor glycemic control and serious complications of diabetes[CS299].

Digital necrosis. An 18-year-old woman, with a history of severe anorexia nervosa of 5 years' duration, who acknowledged regular use of tobacco and cannabis, was hospitalized for necrosis of the left index and thumb that had occurred shortly after left radial artery puncture for blood gas analysis. Acrocyanosis of the four limbs had been present since the onset of anorexia nervosa. Arteriography of the upper limbs showed major spasm of the left radial and cubital arteries and thromboses in the left interdigital arteries of the left index and thumb. The distal portions of the arteries were then on the left and on the right. The necrotic lesions healed after intravenous administration of ilomedine and interruption of tobacco and cannabis. Acrocyanosis of the four limbs persisted[CS398].

Discriminative stimulus effect. Rhesus monkeys, trained to discriminate Δ-9-THC from vehicle in a two-lever drug discrimination procedure, were tested with a variety of psychoactive drugs, including cannabinoids or drugs from other classes. The results indicated that Δ-9-THC discrimination showed pharmacological specificity, in that none of the noncannabinoid drugs fully substituted for Δ-9-THC. The classical cannabinoids, Δ-9-THC and Δ-8-THC, and the novel cannabinoids, WIN and 1-butyl-2-methyl-3-(1-naphthoyl)indole, produced full dose-dependent substitution for Δ-9-THC in all monkeys. A heptyl indole derivative failed to substitute for Δ-9-THC, but it also did not displace [^{3}H] CP-55,940 from its binding site[CS461].

DNA synthesis inhibition. Ethanol (95%) extract of the dried resin, administered intraperitoneally to toads at a dose of 10 mg/day for 14 days, was active. The results were significant at $p < 0.01$ level[CS216].

Dopamine metabolism. The effect of repeated administrations of THC or WIN, a synthetic cannabinoid receptor agonist, on dopamine turnover in the prefrontal cortex, striatum, and Nac in rats, was investigated. THC or WIN (twice daily for seven or 14 days) caused a persistent and selective reduction in medial prefrontal cortical dopamine turnover. No significant alterations of dopamine metabolism were observed in the Nac or striatum. These dopaminergic deficits in the prefrontal cortex were observed after a drug-free period of up to 14 days. The cognitive dysfunction produced by heavy, long-term cannabis use may be subserved, in part, by drug-induced alterations in frontal cortical dopamine turnover[CS346]. Two weeks' administration of THC to rats, reduced dopamine transmission in the medial prefrontal cortex, whereas dopamine metabolism in striatal regions was unaffected[CS434].

Dopamine release. A 38-year-old drug-free schizophrenic patient took part in a single photon emission computerized tomographic study of the brain, and smoked cannabis secretively during a pause in the course of an imaging session. Cannabis had an immediate calming effect, followed by a worsening of psychotic symptoms a few hours later. A comparison of the two sets of images, obtained before and immediately after smoking cannabis, indicated a 20% decrease in the striatal dopamine D2 receptor-binding ratio, suggestive of increased synaptic dopaminergic activity[CS399].

Dopamine transmission modulation. The endogenous cannabinoid system is a new signaling system composed by the central (CB1) and the peripheral (CB2) receptors, and several lipid transmitters including AEA and 2-arachidonylglycerol. Cannabinoid CB1 receptors are present in dopamine projecting brain areas. In primates and certain rat strains it is also located in dopamine cells of the A8, A9, and A10 mesencephalic cell groups, as well as in hypothalamic dopaminergic neurons controlling prolactin secretion. CB1 receptors co-localize with dopamine D1/D2 receptors in dopamine projecting fields. Manipulation of dopaminergic transmission is able to alter the synthesis and release of AEA, as well as the expression of CB1 receptors. CB1 receptors can switch their transduction mechanism to oppose to the ongoing dopamine signaling. Acute blockade of CB1 receptor potentiates the facilitatory role of dopamine D2 receptor agonists on movement. CB1 stimulation results in sensitization to the motor effects of indirect dopaminergic agonists[CS291].

Dyskinetic activity. A 4-week dose escalation study was performed to assess the safety and tolerability of cannabis in six patients with Parkinson's disease (PD) with levodopa (L-DOPA)-induced dyskinesia.

Then a randomized, placebo-controlled crossover study was performed, in which 19 patients with PD were randomized to receive oral cannabis extract followed by placebo or vice versa. Each treatment phase lasted for 4 weeks with an intervening 2-week washout phase. The primary outcome measure was a change in Unified Parkinson's Disease Rating Scale (UPDRS) (items 32 to 34) dyskinesia score. Secondary outcome measures included the Rush scale, Bain scale, tablet arm drawing task, and total UPDRS score following a levodopa challenge, as well as patient-completed measures of a dyskinesia activities of daily living scale, the PDQ-39, on–off diaries, and a range of category rating scales. Seventeen patients completed the study. Cannabis was well tolerated and had no pro- or antiparkinsonian action. There was no evidence for a treatment effect on L-DOPA-induced dyskinesia as assessed by the UPDRS, or any of the secondary outcome measures[CS259]. An anonymous questionnaire sent to all patients attending the Prague Movement Disorder Center revealed that 25% of 339 respondents had taken cannabis and 45.9% of these described some form of benefit[CS262]. 2,4,5-Trihydroxyphenethylamine (6-hydroxydopamine)-lesioned rats were treated with the enantiomers of the synthetic cannabinoid 7-hydroxy-Δ6-THC 1,1-dimethylheptyl. Treatment with its (-)-(3R, 4R) enantiomer (code name HU-210), a potent cannabinoid receptor type 1 agonist, reduced the rotations induced by L-DOPA/carbidopa or apomorphine by 34 and 44%, respectively. Treatment with the (+)- (3S, 4S) enantiomer (code name HU-211), an N-methyl-D-aspartate antagonist, and the psychotropically inactive cannabis constituent: CBD and its primary metabolite, 7-hydroxy-cannabinol, did not show any reduction of rotational behavior. The results indicate that activation of the

CB1 stimulates the dopaminergic system ipsilaterally to the lesion, and may have implications in the treatment of PD[CS338].

Dystonic activity. The neural mechanisms underlying dystonia involve abnormalities within the basal ganglia—in particular, overactivity of the lateral globus pallidus. Cannabinoid receptors are located presynaptically on γ-aminobutyric acid receptor (GABA) terminals within the globus pallidus internus, where their activation reduces GABA reuptake. Cannabinoid receptor stimulation may thus reduce overactivity of the globus pallidus, and thereby reduce dystonia. A double-blind, randomized, placebo-controlled, crossover study using the synthetic cannabinoid receptor agonist nabilone in patients with generalized and segmental primary dystonia showed no significant reduction in dystonia following treatment with nabilone[CS390].

Embryotoxic effect. Resin, administered orally to pregnant rabbits at a dose of 1 mL/kg, was active[CS167].

Endocrine effect. Animal models have demonstrated that cannabinoid administration acutely altered multiple hormonal systems, including the suppression of the gonadal steroids, growth hormone, prolactin, and thyroid hormone and the activation of the hypothalamic–pituitary–adrenal (HPA) axis. These effects were mediated by binding to the endogenous cannabinoid receptor in or near the hypothalamus. Despite these findings in animals, the effects in humans have been inconsistent, and discrepancies were likely owing in part to the development of tolerance[CS363]. Intravenous administration of three cannabinoid agonists (AEA, methanandamide, and WIN) to nine castrated male calves under stress-free conditions provoked immediate increases of serum cortisol and respiration rate, and produced rapid hypoalgesia to cutaneous pain and thermal stimuli. AEA and methanandamide did not affect serum prolactin. Administration of WIN increased serum prolactin abruptly. None of the cannabinoid receptor agonists affected serum growth hormone[CS420].

Environmental stress and cannabinoids interaction. Anxiety and panic are the most common adverse effects of cannabis intoxication. Data suggest that cannabinoid CB1 receptor modulation of amygdalar activity contributes to these phenomena. Using Fos as a marker, it was tested the hypothesis that environmental stress and CB1 cannabinoid receptor activity interact in the regulation of amygdalar activation in male mice. Both 30 minutes of restraint and CB1 receptor agonist treatment (Δ-9-THC [2.5 mg/kg]) or CP-55,940 (0.3 mg/kg); by intraperitoneal injection) produced barely detectable increases in Fos expression within the central amygdala (CeA). The combination of restraint and CB1 agonist administration produced robust Fos induction within the CeA, indicating a synergistic interaction between environmental stress and CB1 receptor activation. An inhibitor of endocannabinoid transport, AM404 (10 mg/kg), produced an additive interaction with restraint within the CeA. In contrast, FAAH inhibitor-treated mice (URB597, 1 mg/kg) and FAAH (–/–) mice did not exhibit any differences in amygdalar activation in response to restraint compared with control mice. In the basolateral amygdala (BLA) and medial amygdala, restraint stress produced a low level of Fos induction, which was unaffected by cannabinoid treatment. The CB1 receptor antagonist SR141716 dose-dependently increased Fos expression in the BLA and CeA[CS272].

Epileptic effect. Δ-9-THC at a dose of 1 μM, significantly depressed evoked depolarizing postsynaptic potentials (PSPs) in rat olfactory cortex neurones. A standardized cannabis extract (SCE) and Δ-9-THC-free SCE significantly potentiated evoked PSPs (all results were fully reversed by the CB1 receptor antagonist SR141716A, 1 μM). The potentiation by Δ-9-THC-free SCE was greater than that produced by SCE. On comparing the effects of Δ-9-THC-free SCE on evoked PSPs and artificial PSPs (aPSPs; evoked electrotonically following brief intracellular current injection), PSPs were enhanced, whereas aPSPs were unaffected, suggesting that the effect was not resulting from changes in background input resistance. Similar recordings made using CB1 receptor-deficient knockout mice and wild-type littermate controls revealed cannabinoid or extract-induced changes in membrane resistance, cell excitability and synaptic transmission in wild-type mice that were similar to those seen in rat neurones, but no effect on these properties were seen in CB1 receptor-deficient knockout mice cells. Results indicated that the unknown extract constituent(s) effects over-rode the suppressive effects of Δ-9-THC on excitatory neurotransmitter release, which may explain some patients' preference for herbal cannabis rather than isolated Δ-9-THC (owing to attenuation of some of the central Δ-9-THC side effects) and possibly account for the rare incidence of seizures in some individuals taking cannabis recreationally[CS278]. A SCE with pure Δ-9-THC, at matched concentrations of Δ-9-THC, and a Δ-9-THC-free extract (Δ-9-THC-free SCE) in in vitro rat brain slice model of epilepsy were examined. In the in vitro epilepsy model, in which sustained epileptiform seizures were induced by the muscarinic receptor agonist oxotremorine-M in immature rat piriform cortical brain slices, SCE was a more potent and again more rapidly-acting anticonvulsant than isolated Δ-9-THC. Δ-9-THC-free extract also exhibited anticonvulsant activity. CBD did not inhibit seizures, nor did it modulate the activity of Δ-9-THC in this model. These results demonstrated that not all of the therapeutic actions of cannabis herb might be a result of the Δ-9-THC content[CS312].

Estrogen cycle disruption effect. The dried aerial part, administered by gastric intubation to rats at a dose of 75 mg/kg for 70 days, was active[CS224].

Estrogen receptors stimulating effect. THC, CBD, and desacetyllevonantradol, in estrogen-induced MCF-7 breast cancer cells at concentrations of no more than 10 μM, produced no effect. THC failed to antagonize the response to estradiol under conditions in which the antiestrogen LY156758 (keoxifene; raloxifene) was effective. The phytoestrogen formononetin behaved as an estrogen at high concentrations, and this response was antagonized by LY156758. THC, desacetyllevonantradol, or CBD did not stimulate transcription of an *EREtkCAT* reporter gene transiently transfected into MCF-7 cells[CS452].

Estrogenic effect. Petroleum ether extract of the resin was active on the rat non-pregnant uterus[CS130]. Resin, in the ration of immature and ovariectomized rats at a concentration equivalent to 250 ppm THC/animal, was inactive[CS236,CS162].

Estrous cycle disruption effect. Ethanol (95%) extract of the dried aerial parts, administered intraperitoneally to gerbils at a dose of 2.5 mg/animal daily for 60 days, was active[CS184]. Petroleum ether extract of the dried aerial, administered intraperitoneally to mice and rats at doses of 1 and 5 mg/animal, respectively, for 64 days, was active[CS174]. Petroleum ether extract of the aerial parts, administered intraperitoneally to female rats, produced weak activity[CS016]. Petroleum ether extract of the entire plant, administered by gastric intubation to female mice at doses of 75 mg/kg and 150 mg/kg, was active. A dose of 3 mg/kg produced weak activity[CS170]. Petroleum ether extract of the resin, administered intraperitoneally to female rats at doses of 10 and 20 mg/kg, was active[CS187]. Resin, administered orally to female rats at doses of 3, 15, and 75 mg/kg daily for 72 days, was active[CS168].

Familial Mediterranean fever. A patient with familial Mediterranean fever was presented with chronic relapsing pain and inflammation of gastrointestinal origin. After determining a suitable analgesic dosage, a double-blind, placebo-controlled, crossover trial was conducted using 50 mg of Δ-9-THC daily in five doses in the active weeks and measuring effects on parameters of inflammation and pain. Although no anti-inflammatory effects of Δ-9-THC were detected during the trial, a highly significant reduction ($p < 0.001$) in additional analgesic requirements was achieved[CS447].

Fish poison. Ethanol (95%) extract of the dried aerial parts at a concentration of 1:1 was active. The water extract was inactive[CS243].

Follicle-stimulating hormone release inhibition. Ethanol (95%) extract of the dried resin, administered intraperitoneally to toads at a dose of 10 mg/day for 14 days, was active. The results were significant at $p < 0.01$ level[CS216].

Food intake modulation. *Cannabis sativa* stimulates appetite, especially for sweet and palatable food. Cannabinoid action has proposed a central role of the cannabinoid system in obesity[CS352]. Dronabinol, a commercially available form of a THC, has been used successfully for increasing appetite in patients with HIV wasting disease. Cannabinoid receptor antagonist may reduce obesity[CS353]. To determine the prevalence of substance use in adolescents with eating disorders, the results of a data set of Ontario high school students were compared. One hundred and one female adolescents who met the *Diagnostic and Statistical Manual of Mental Disorders*, 4th edition's criteria for an eating disorder were followed up in a tertiary care pediatric treatment center. They were asked to participate in a cross-sectional study using a self-administered questionnaire assessing substance use and investigating reasons for use and nonuse; 95 agreed to participate and 77 completed the questionnaire (mean age, 15.2 years). The patients were divided into two groups: 63 with

restrictive symptoms only, 17 with purging symptoms. The rates of drug use between subjects and their comparison groups were compared by Z-scores, with the level of significance set at 0.05. During the preceding year, restrictors used significantly less tobacco, alcohol, and cannabis than grade- and sex-matched comparison populations, and purgers used these substances at rates similar to those of comparison subjects. Other drugs seen frequently in the purgers included hallucinogens, tranquilizers, stimulants, LSD, phencyclidine, cocaine, and ecstasy. Both groups used caffeine and laxatives, but few used diet pills. Restrictors said they did not use substances because they were bad for their health, tasted unpleasant, were contrary to their beliefs, and were too expensive. Purgers generally used substances to relax, relieve anger, avoid eating, and "get away" from problems. Female adolescents with eating disorders who have restrictive symptoms use substances less frequently than the general adolescent population but do not abstain from their use. Those with purging symptoms use substances with a similar frequency to that found in the general adolescent population[CS372].

Gastric secretory inhibition. Petroleum ether extract of the dried aerial parts, administered intraperitoneally to male rats, was active[CS097].

Gene expression effect. Cannabinoids can cross the placental barrier and be secreted in the maternal milk. Through this way, cannabinoids affect the ontogeny of various neurotransmitter systems leading to changes in different behavioral patterns. Dopamine and endogenous opioids are among the neurotransmitters that result more affected by perinatal cannabinoid exposure, which, when animals mature, produce changes in motor activity, drug-seeking behavior, nociception, and other processes. These disturbances are likely originated by the capability of cannabinoids to influence the expression of key genes for both neurotransmitters, in particular, the enzyme tyrosine hydroxylase and the opioid precursor proenkephalin. Cannabinoids seem to be able to influence the expression of genes encoding for neuroglia cell adhesion molecules, which supports a potential influence of cannabinoids on the processes of cell proliferation, neuronal migration or axonal elongation in which these proteins are involved. CB1 receptors, which represent the major targets for the action of cannabinoids, are abundantly expressed in certain brain regions, such as the subventricular areas, which have been involved in these processes during brain development. Cannabinoids might also be involved in the apoptotic death that occurs during brain development, possibly by influencing the expression of Bcl-2/Bax system. CB1 receptors are transiently expressed during brain development in different group of neurons which do not contain these receptors in the adult brain[CS254].

Glaucoma effect. Nine patients with glaucoma unresponsive to treatment were treated with orally administered Δ-9-THC capsules or inhaled cannabis in addition to their existing therapeutic regimen. An initial decrease in intraocular pressure was observed in all patients, and the investigator's therapeutic goal was met in four of the nine patients. The decreases in intraocular pressure were not sustained, and the patients elected to discontinue treatment within 1–9 months for various reasons[CS359].

Gliomatous effect. Gliomas, in particular glioblastoma multiform or grade IV astrocytoma, are the most frequent class of malignant primary brain tumors and one of the most aggressive forms of cancer. Cannabinoids and their derivatives slowed the growth of different types of tumors, including gliomas, in laboratory animals. Cannabinoids induced apoptosis of glioma cells in culture via sustained ceramide accumulation, extracellular signal-regulated kinase activation and Akt inhibition. Cannabinoid treatment inhibited angiogenesis of gliomas in vivo. Cannabinoids killed glioma cells selectively and could protect nontransformed glial cells from death[CS273].

Glucosidase inhibition. Ethyl acetate and water-soluble fractions of the dried aerial parts were inactive on the intestine[CS128].

Gynecomastic effect. A retrospective analysis was carried out on 175 men over the age of 16 years who were presented with breast enlargement and/or "lumps" during a 7-year period to a single surgeon. The patients had complete biochemical assessment (liver function tests, γ-glutamyl transferase, prolactin, α-fetoprotein, and β-human chorionic gonadotropin), and mammography and/or ultrasound with fine-needle biopsy if indicated. Thirty-nine of the patients had bilateral true gynecomastia and 88 had unilateral gynecomastia (53% left). Carcinoma of the breast was diagnosed in eight, pseudo-gynecomastia in 18, 13 had physiological pubertal changes only, and 9 had other diagnoses. Adverse drug reactions were possibly implicated in the etiology of 47 patients, alcohol in seven patients, cannabis in one patient, testicular malignancy in four patients, and hepatocellular carcinoma in one patient. Five patients were found to have hyperprolactinemia. Twenty-four percent of patients were reassured without intervention; 18% failed to attend follow-up[CS348].

Hair stimulant effect. Ethanol (50%) extract of the dried seed, applied externally to mice at a dose of 0.33 g/mL for 14 days, was inactive[CS139].

Hemagglutinin activity. Saline extract of the dried seed at a concentration of 10% was inactive on the human red blood cell[CS207].

Hepatitis C risk factor. The study of a dually diagnosed population estimated the prevalence of hepatitis C virus (HCV) to be

29.7% or 16 times higher than that in the general population. A high correlation was found between the use of tobacco and HCV infection. This appears to be beyond the risk factor conveyed by intravenous drug use. Of the patients whose primary diagnoses were cocaine, opiate, amphetamine, or polysubstance dependence (drugs often used intravenously), 42% of the tobacco users were HCV-positive, whereas only 20% of the nontobacco using patients with similar primary diagnoses were HCV-positive. The association of tobacco use with HCV was found to be strong for females with alcohol, sedative/hypnotic, inhalant, or cannabis dependence, as none of the 17 nontobacco using female patients with these diagnoses were HCV-positive, whereas 14 of the 45 (31%) tobacco-using females with these diagnoses did test positive for HCV[CS306].

Hepatotoxic activity. Ethanol (95%) extract of the dried resin, administered intraperitoneally to toads at a dose of 10 mg/day for 14 days, was active. The results were significant at $p < 0.01$ level[CS216].

Histamine release stimulation. Water extract of the seed, administered intradermally to human adults, was active on human basophils[CS147].

HIV involvement. The prevalence, predictors, and patterns of cannabis use—specifically medicinal cannabis use among patients with HIV—were examined. Any cannabis use in the year prior to interview and self-defined medicinal use were evaluated. A cross-sectional multicenter survey and retrospective chart review were conducted to evaluate overall drug utilization in HIV, including cannabis use. HIV-positive adults were identified through the HIV Ontario Observational Database; 104 consenting patients were interviewed. Forty-three percent of the patients reported cannabis use, whereas 29% reported medicinal use. Reasons for use were similar by gender although

a significantly higher number of women used cannabis for pain management. The most commonly reported reason for medicinal cannabis use was appetite stimulation/weight gain. Male gender and history of intravenous drug use were predictive of any cannabis use. Age, gender, HIV clinical status, antiretroviral use, and history of intravenous drug use were not significant predictors of medicinal cannabis use. Despite the frequency of medicinal use, minimal changes in the pattern of cannabis use on HIV diagnosis were reported with 80% of current medicinal users also indicating recreational consumption[CS289]. HIV patients ($n = 252$) were recruited via consecutive sampling in public health care clinics. Structured interviews assessed patterns of recent cannabis use, including its perceived benefit for symptom relief. Associations between cannabis use and demographic and clinical variables were examined using univariate and multivariate regression analyses. Overall prevalence of smoked cannabis in the previous month was 23%. Reported benefits included relief of anxiety and/or depression (57%), improved appetite (53%), increased pleasure (33%), and relief of pain (28%). Recent use of cannabis was positively associated with severe nausea (OR = 4, $p = 0.004$) and recent use of alcohol (OR = 7.5, $p < 0.001$) and negatively associated with being Latino (OR = 0.07, $p < 0.001$). No associations between cannabis use and pain symptoms were observed[CS315]. No safety problems specific to HIV or protease inhibitors were found in a study in which volunteers stayed in a research hospital 24 hours a day and were randomly assigned to either smoke cannabis, take oral THC, or take an oral placebo. Cannabis and THC use was associated with weight gain[CS369].

Hyperglycemic activity. Ethanol (95%) extract of the leaf, administered intravenously to rats at a dose of 300 mg/kg, produced an increase of 40 mg percentage 2 hours postinjection and a corresponding decrease in liver glycogen[CS163]. Ethanol (95%) extract of the dried leaf, administered by gastric intubation to rabbits, produced an increase followed by a gradual decrease in blood sugar levels[CS021]. The dried leaves, smoked by human adults, produced elevated glucose levels in two out of four subjects and no impairment of insulin release or changes in growth hormone levels[CS024].

Hypertensive activity. Ethanol (95%) and water extracts of the dried aerial parts, administered intravenously to cats, were inactive. The ethanol extract stimulated respiration and the water extract had no effect on respiration[CS243].

Hypoglycemic activity. Ethanol (95%) extract of the dried leaf, administered by gastric intubation to rabbits, produced an increase, followed by a gradual decrease, in blood sugar levels[CS021]. Extract of the dried leaf, administered subcutaneously to rabbits at a dose of 0.5 mL/kg (approx 0.6 mg THC) for 9 weeks, further enhanced hypoglycemia induced by insulin. No hypoglycemic effect was seen in normal animals[CS025]. Hot water extract of the resin, administered by gastric intubation to dogs at a dose of 20 g of air-dried resin/animal, produced weak activity[CS198]. The dried leaf, smoked by adults at a dose of 2 g/person, was inactive[CS023].

Hypotensive activity. Ethanol (50%) extract of the entire plant, administered intravenously to dogs at a dose of 50 mg/kg, was active[CS007]. Ethanol (95%) and water extracts of the dried aerial parts, administered intravenously to cats, were inactive. The ethanol extract stimulated respiration, and the water extract had no effect[CS243].

Ilicit drug in plasmapheresis donors. Seventy-five US plasma units from 10 different states in the United States and 75 German plasma units that had been analyzed principally for their protein composition were screened for drugs. Determinations were made, using automated immunoassays, of the presence of cannabis, cocaine, amphetamine, methamphetamine, MDMA, methylenedioxyethylamphetamine (MDE), and opiates. Positive results were confirmed by gas chromatography–mass spectrometry. Eleven US plasma units were found to be positive for cocaine (14.6%), whereas all German samples were cocaine-negative (p = 0.0007). Fifteen US plasma units (20%) and one German unit (1.3%) were confirmed as positive for cannabis (p = 0.0003). Three out of 75 US plasma units were positive for both cannabis and cocaine. In none of the 150 samples were amphetamine, methamphetamine, MDMA, MDE, or opiates detected[CS355].

Immunomodulatory effect. The smoking of cannabis showed a significant local immunosuppression of the bactericidal activity of human alveolar macrophages. In animal studies, cannabinoids were identified as potent modulators of cytokine production, causing a shift from T-helper-1 (Th1) to Th2 cytokines. In consequence, a compromised cellular immunity was observed in these animals, resulting in enhanced tumor growth and reduced immunity to viral infections. In vitro, immunosuppressive effects were shown in all immune cells, but only at high micromolar cannabinoid concentrations not reached under normal clinical conditions. In conclusion, there was no evidence that cannabinoids induce a serious, relevant immunosuppression in humans, with the exception of cannabis smoking, which may affect local bronchoalveolar immunity[CS279]. The immune function in 16 MS patients treated with oral cannabinoids was measured. A modest increase of tumor necrosis factor (TNF)-α in lipopolysaccharide-stimulated whole blood was found during cannabis plant-extract treatment (p = 0.037), with no change in other cytokines. In the subgroup of patients with high adverse event scores, an increase in plasma IL-12p40 was found ($p = 0.002$). The results indicate pro-inflammatory disease-modifying potential of cannabinoids in MS[CS347]. THC and their metabolites inhibited production of IL-1 and γ-interferon, decreased a 33% of the lymphocytes activity and inhibited 66% of the lymphocytes adenylcyclase activity. The consumption of cannabis decreased immunological competence of macrophages, and alternated their essential role of trophicity of the central nervous system. Inhibiting actions of cannabinoids on the cyclo-oxygenase, promoted production of arachidonic acid degradation products. This compound mimics the action of histamine, induced a raise of the vascular permeability and bronchospasm, and contributed at delayed reaction of anaphylaxia[CS427].

Infant mortality. For a period of 11 months, 2964 infants were enrolled and screened at birth for exposure to cocaine, opiate, or cannabinoid by meconium analysis. At birth, 44% of the infants tested positive for drugs, 30.5% positive for cocaine, 20.2% for opiate, and 11.4% for cannabinoids. Compared with the drug-negative group, a significantly higher percentage ($p < 0.05$) of the drug-positive infants had lower weight and smaller head circumference and length at birth and a higher percent of their mothers were single, multigravid, multiparous, and had little to no prenatal care. Within the first 2 years of life, 44 infants died: 26 were drug-negative (15.7 deaths per 1000 live births) and 18 were drug-positive (13.7 deaths per 1000 live births). The mortality rate among cocaine, opiate, or cannabinoid-positive infants were 17.7, 18.4, and 8.9 per 1000 live births, respectively. Among infants with birth-weight of 2500 g or less, infants who were positive for both cocaine and morphine had a higher mortality rate (OR = 5.9, CI = 1.4–24) than drug-negative infants. Eleven infants died from the

sudden infant death syndrome (SIDS); 58% were positive for drugs, predominantly cocaine. The odds ratio for SIDS among drug-positive infants was 1.5 (CI = 0.46–5.01) and 1.9 (CI = 0.58–6.2) among cocaine-positive infants[CS445].

Infant neurobehavioral effect. The subjects and controls in this study were full-term infants of appropriate gestational age with no medical problems. At 1–2 days of age, 20 infants exposed to cocaine, alcohol, cannabis, and cigarettes, 17 infants exposed to alcohol and/or cannabis and cigarettes, and 20 drug-free infants were evaluated by using the Neonatal Intensive Care Unit Network Neurobehavioral Scale. Cocaine-exposed (CE) infants showed increased tone and motor activity, more jerky movements, startles, tremors, back arching, and signs of central nervous system and visual stress than unexposed infants. They also showed poorer visual and auditory following. There were no differences in how the examination was administered to CE and nonexposed infants. Reduced birth-weight and length were also observed in CE infants. Differences attributable to CE infants were related to muscle tone and motor performance, following during orientation, and signs of stress. CE infants were not more difficult to test, nor did they require an alteration in the examination. Both neurobehavioral patterns of excitability and lethargy were observed. The findings may have been a result of the synergistic effects of cocaine with alcohol and cannabis[CS456].

Inflammatory effect. A case of a 17-year-old male regular cannabis user who developed a large swollen uvula (uvulitis) and partial upper airway obstruction after smoking cannabis was evaluated. Symptoms resolved with the administration of corticosteroids and antihistamines[CS380]. A healthy 17-year-old man who inhaled cannabis prior to general anesthesia is described. In the recovery room, after an uneventful general anesthetic, acute uvular edema resulted in postoperative airway obstruction and admission to the hospital. The uvular edema was treated successfully with dexamethasone[CS455].

Information-processing effect. Information processes are thought to represent the basic building blocks of higher order cognitive processes. The inspection time task was used to investigate the effects of acute and subacute cannabis use on information processing in 22 heavy users compared with 22 nonusers. The findings indicated that users in the subacute state display significantly slowed information-processing speeds (longer inspection times) compared with controls. This deficit appeared to be normalized while users were in the acute state. These results may be explained as a withdrawal effect, but may also be owing to tolerance development because of long-term cannabis use[CS276].

Insecticidal activity. Leaf extract, administered to larvae of *Chironomus samoensis*, produced paralysis leading to death. The extract brought a drastic change in the morphology of sensilla trichoidea, the general body cuticle, and a significant reduction in the concentration of magnesium and iron, whereas manganese showed only slight average increase. Because the sensilla trichoidea has nerve connections, it was assumed that the toxic principle of the leaf extract has affected the central nervous system[CS267].

Intestinal motility activity. Rat intestinal epithelia mounted in an Ussing chamber attached with voltage/current clamp were used for measuring changes of the short-circuit current across the epithelia. The intestinal epithelia were activated with current raised by serosal administration of forskolin 5 μM. Ethanol extracts of cannabis augmented the current additively when each was added after forskolin. In subsequent experiments, ouabain, and bumetanide were added prior to ethanol extract of cannabis to determine their effect on Na$^+$ and Cl$^-$ movement. The results suggested that the extract may affect the Cl$^-$ movement more directly than Na$^+$ movement in the intestinal epithelial cells[CS307].

Intraocular pressure reduction. Polysaccharide fraction of the dried entire plant, administered intravenously to rabbits at a dose of 1 μg/animal was active[CS138]. Water extract of the dried aerial parts, administered intravenously to rabbits at a dose of 250 μg/animal, was active[CS142]. A dose of 5 μg/animal was inactive on Rhesus monkeys and active on rabbits. A dose of 10 mg/animal, administered *per rectum* to Rhesus monkeys and rabbits, was inactive[CS191].

IQ effect. Cannabis use for 70 individuals aged 17–20 years was determined through self-reporting and urinalysis. IQ scores were calculated by subtracting each person's IQ score at 9–12 years (before initiation of drug use) from his or her score at 17–20 years. The difference in IQ scores of current heavy users (at least five joints per week), current light users (less than five joints per week), former users (who had not smoked regularly for at least 3 months), and nonusers (who never smoked more than once per week and no smoking in the past 2 weeks) was compared. Current cannabis use was significantly correlated ($p < 0.05$) in a dose-related fashion with a decline in IQ over the ages studied. The comparison of the IQ difference scores showed an average decrease of 4.1 points in current heavy users ($p < 0.05$) compared with gains in IQ points for light current users (5.8), former users (3.5), and nonusers (2.6)[CS385].

Lactate inhibition. The dried leaf, smoked by adults at a dose of 2 g/person, decreased blood lactic acid[CS023].

Leutinizing hormone-release inhibition. The dried aerial part, smoked by menopausal women at a dose of 1 g/person, was inactive[CS225]. When administered to normal and castrated male rats, at a dose of 75 mg/kg, was active[CS215].

Lower limb occlusive arteriopathy. Seventy-three patients (60 males and 13 females less than 50 years of age) were divided into four groups: Buerger's disease (thromboangiitis obliterans [TAO]), atheromatous juvenile peripheral obstructive arterial diseases (POAD), autoimmune POAD, and arteriopathy of undetermined origin. The first symptoms occurred at 38 ± 8 years of age. Fourteen patients (20%) had TAO, 51 (70%) atheromatous POAD, 4 (5%) POAD with systemic or autoimmune disease, and 4 (5%) undetermined POAD. Age of onset was earlier in TAO (35 ± 8 vs 40 ± 8 years, $p = 0.046$), smoking was greater in the atheroma group (33 ± 16 vs 24 ± 14 pack/years, $p = 0.033$). Fifty-three patients with POAD had dyslipidemia and 26% had hypertension. Regular cannabis intake was more frequent in the TAO group (21% vs 8%). At the time of medical care, Fontaine's stage was more frequently stage II in atheroma patients (57% vs 14%) and stage IV in TAO patients (86% vs 35%). TAO was diagnosed in 43% cannabis users and in 19% nonusers. Results indicated that the main etiology of juvenile POAD is atheroma, followed by TAO. Cannabis users accounted for at least 10% of these patients. They were characterized by lower tobacco intake, more distal lesions, more frequent involvement of the upper limbs. They presented more frequently as TAO[CS379]. A case of a 30-year-old woman who smoked cannabis and developed intermittent claudication of the lower limbs was reported. Results indicated that cannabis could be involved not only in the pathogenesis of juvenile obstructive arteriopathy, but also in the development of atheromatous lesions[CS409].

Lung function. A group of over 900 young adults derived from a birth cohort of 1037 subjects were studied at age 18, 21, and 26 years. Cannabis and tobacco smoking were documented at each age using a standardized interview. Lung function, as measured by the FEV1–vital capacity (VC) ratio, was obtained by simple spirometry. A fixed effects regression model was used to analyze the data and to account for confounding factors. When the sample was stratified for cumulative use, there was evidence of a linear relationship between cannabis use and FEV1–VC ($p < 0.05$). In the absence of adjusting for other variables, increasing cannabis use over time was associated with a decline in FEV1–VC with time; the mean FEV1–VC among subjects using cannabis on 900 or more occasions was 7.2, 2.6 and 5% less than nonusers at ages 18, 21, and 26, respectively. After controlling for potential confounding factors (age, tobacco smoking, and weight) the negative effect of cumulative cannabis use on mean FEV1–VC was only marginally significant ($p < 0.09$). Age ($p < 0.001$), cigarette smoking ($p < 0.05$), and weight ($p < 0.001$) were all significant predictors of FEV1–VC. Cannabis use and daily cigarette smoking acted additively to influence FEV1–VC. Results indicated that longitudinal observations over 8 years in young adults revealed a dose-dependent relationship between cumulative cannabis consumption and decline in FEV1–VC. When confounders were accounted for the effect was reduced and was only marginally significant, but given the limited time frame over which observations were made, the trend suggests that continued cannabis smoking has the potential to result in clinically important impairment of lung function[CS371].

Luteolytic effect. The aerial parts, smoked by a chronic high-dose user, were inactive[CS160].

Memory impairment. The effects of combined exposure to ethanol and Δ-9-THC in a memory task was investigated in rats. Ethanol, voluntarily ingested in alcohol-preferring rats, and THC, given by intraperitoneal injection, had a synergic action to impair object recognition when a 15-minute interval was adopted between the sample phase and the choice phase of the test. Ingestion of ethanol, or 2 or 5 mg/kg of THC were not able to modify object recognition in these experimental conditions. When voluntary ethanol ingestion was combined with administration of these doses of THC, object recognition was markedly impaired. THC impaired object recognition only at the dose of 10 mg/kg, when its administration was not combined with that of ethanol. The selective cannabinoid CB1 receptor antagonist SR 141716A (N-(piperidin-1-yl)-5-(4-chlorophenyl)-1(2, 4-dichloro-phenyl)-4-methyl-1H-pyrazole carboxamide HCl) at the dose of 1 mg/kg reversed the amnesic effect of 10 mg/kg of THC. This indicated that the effect is mediated by the receptor subtype. The synergism of ethanol and THC was not detected when an intertrial interval of 1 minute was adopted[CS370].

Memory improvement. Extract from fructus cannabis (EFC), administered intragastrically to mice with drug-induced dysmnesia at doses of 0.2, 0.4, and 0.8 g/kg, for 7 days, prolonged the latency and decreased the number of errors in the step-down test, and enhanced the spatial resolution of amnesic mice in water maze test. EFC at the dose of 0.2 g/kg overcame amnesia of three stages of memory process. EFC activated calcineurin activity at a concentration range of 0.01–100 g/L. The maximal value of EFC on calcineurin activity (35% ± 5 %) appeared at a concentration of 10 g/L[CS320]. EFC with activation of calcineurin, extracted from Chinese traditional medicine, was used to determine the effects on memory and immunity in mice. In the step-down-type passive avoidance test, the plant extract (0.2 g/kg) significantly improved amnesia induced by drugs, and greatly enhanced the ability of cell-mediated type hypersensitivity and nonspecific immune responses in normal mice[CS334].

Mitochondrial function disruption. Δ-9-THC in the pulmonary transformed cell line A549 produced a rapid and extensive depletion of cellular energy stores. Adenosine 5'-triphosphatase levels declined dose dependently with an IC_{50} of 7.5 μg/mL of THC after 24 hours of exposure. Cell death was observed only at concentrations greater than 10 μg/mL. Studies using JC-1, a fluorescent probe for mitochondrial membrane potential, revealed diminished mitochondrial function at THC concentrations as low as 0.5 μg/mL. At concentrations of 2.5 and 10 μg/mL of THC, a decrease in mitochondrial membrane potential was observed 1 hour after THC exposure. Mitochondrial function remained diminished for at least 30 hours after THC exposure. Flow cytometry studies on cells exposed to particulate smoke extracts indicated that JC-1 red fluorescence was fivefold lower in cells exposed to cannabis smoke extract compared with tobacco smoke-exposed cells. Comparison with a variety of mitochondrial inhibitors demonstrated that THC produced effects similar to that of carbonyl cyanide p-trifluoromethoxyphenylhydrazone, suggesting uncoupling of electron transport. Loss of red JC-1 fluorescence by THC was suppressed by cyclosporin A, suggesting mediation by the mitochondrial permeability transition pore. This disruption of mitochondrial function was sustained for at least 24 hours after removal of THC by extensive washing[CS360].

Mitogenic effect. The resin was inactive on the human and rat white blood cells[CS037].

Molluscicidal activity. Ethanol (95%) and water extracts of the dried flowering tops, at a concentration of 1000 ppm, produced weak activity on *Biomphalaria straminea* and *Biomphalaria glabrata*[CS245]. Water saturated with essential oil of the aerial parts, at a concentration of 1:2, produced weak activity on *Biomphalaria glabrata*[CS201].

Motor function. Nine cannabis smokers and 16 controls were studied to determine the attentional areas related to motor function, and primary and supplementary motor cortices. Echo planar images and high-resolution molecular resonance images were acquired. The challenge paradigm included left and right finger sequencing. Group differences in cerebral activation were examined for Brodmann areas (BA) 4, 6, 24, and 32 using region of interests analyses in statistical parametric mapping. Cannabis users, tested within 4–36 hours of discontinuation, exhibited significantly less activation than controls in BA 24 and 32 bilaterally during right- and left-sided sequencing and for BA 6 in all tasks except for left-sided sequencing in the left hemisphere. There were no statistically significant differences for BA 4. None of these regional activations correlated with urinary cannabis concentration and verbal IQ for smokers. The results suggested that recently abstinent chronic cannabis smokers produce reduced activation in motor cortical areas in response to finger sequencing compared with controls[CS250].

Multiple sclerosis. One hundred fifty-seven drug-naïve, first-episode schizophrenic patients were examined. A significantly elevated brain-derived neurotrophic factor (BDNF) serum concentrations in patients with chronic cannabis abuse ($n = 35$, $p < 0.001$) or multiple substance abuse ($n = 20$, $p < 0.001$) prior to disease onset were found. Drug-naïve schizophrenic patients without cannabis consumption showed similar results to normal controls and cannabis controls without schizophrenia. Elevated BDNF serum levels were not related to schizophrenia and/or substance abuse itself but may reflect a cannabis-related idiosyncratic damage of the schizophrenic brain. Disease onset was 5.2 years earlier in the cannabis-consuming group

($p = 0.0111$)[CS257]. A cannabis-based medicinal extract (CBME) was administered to 160 patients with multiple sclerosis experiencing significant problems from at least one of the following: spasticity, spasms, bladder problems, tremor, or pain. The interventions were oromucosal sprays of matched placebo, or whole plant CBME containing equal amounts of Δ-9-THC and CBD at a dose of 2.5–120 mg of each daily, in divided doses. The primary outcome measure was a Visual Analogue Scale (VAS) score for each patient's most troublesome symptom. Additional measures included VAS scores of other symptoms, and measures of disability, cognition, mood, sleep and fatigue. Following CBME the primary symptom score reduced from mean 74.36 (11.1) to 48.89 (22.0) following CBME and from 74.31 (12.5) to 54.79 (26.3) following placebo. Spasticity VAS scores were significantly reduced by CBME (Sativex®) in comparison with placebo ($p = 0.001$). There were no significant adverse effects on cognition or mood and intoxication was generally mild[CS268]. A SCE with pure Δ-9-THC, at matched concentrations of Δ-9-THC, and a Δ-9-THC-free extract (Δ-9-THC-free SCE) in a mouse model of MS, were examined. Although SCE inhibited spasticity in the mouse model of MS to a comparable level, it caused a more rapid onset of muscle relaxation and a reduction in the time to maximum effect compared with Δ-9-THC alone. The Δ-9-THC-free extract or CBD caused no inhibition of spasticity[CS312]. In an experimental allergic encephalomyelitis (EAE), an animal model of MS, it was demonstrated that the cannabinoid system is neuroprotective during EAE. Mice, deficient in the cannabinoid receptor CB1, tolerated inflammatory and excitotoxic insults poorly, and developed substantial neurodegeneration following immune attack in EAE. Exogenous CB1 agonists can provide significant neuroprotection from the consequences of inflammatory central nervous system disease in an experimental allergic uveitis model[CS339].

Mutagenic activity. Petroleum ether extract of the aerial parts, in the ration of *Drosophila* at concentrations of 0.5, 1, and 5% of the diet, was active[CS190]. Petroleum ether extract of the dried leaf, administered by gastric intubation to male mice at a dose of 50 mg/kg, was active[CS183]. Water and methanol extracts of the seed, on agar plate at a concentration of 100 mg/mL, were inactive on *Bacillus subtilis* H-17 (Rec+) and *Salmonella typhimurium* TA100 and TA98. Metabolic activation had no effect on the results[CS199].

Myocardial infarction. A young man who suffered a myocardial infarction after taking Viagra® in combination with cannabis was investigated. Viagra is metabolized predominantly by the CYP450 3A4 hepatic microsomal isoenzyme. Cannabis is a known inhibitor of CYP450 3A4 isoenzyme. The effect of the Viagra was thus potentiated by the effect of cannabis[CS387].

Natural-killer cells effect. Leukemia susceptible BALB/c and resistant C57BL/6 mice were infected with Friend leukemia virus complex and its helper component Rowson-Parr virus. At different time points, their natural-killer cells were separated from spleens and treated with 0–10 μg/mL of THC, subsequently mixed with Yac-1 target cells for 4 and 18 hours. The natural-killer cell activity in both mouse strains infected by either virus complex or helper virus weakened on days 2–4 postinfection, normalized by day 8 and enhanced on days 11–14. Natural-killer cell activity on the effect of low concentration (1–2.5 μg/mL) of THC slightly increased in BALB/c, was unaffected in C57BL/6, especially in the 18 hour assays. In the combined effects of cannabis and retrovirus, damages by cannabis dominated over those of retroviruses. Inhibition or reactive enhancement of natural-

killer cell activity on the effect of viruses were similar to those of infected but cannabis-free counterparts, but on the level of uninfected cells treated with cannabis. The effects of cannabis and retrovirus were additive resulting in anergy of natural-killer cells[CS432].

Neonatal abstinence syndrome. The relationship of maternal drug abuse to symptoms, the effectiveness of pharmacological agents in controlling symptoms, and the length of in-patient stay were investigated in infants with neonatal abstinence syndrome. Pharmacological treatment was oral morphine sulphate (0.2 mg four to six times hourly), phenobarbitone (3–7 mg/kg/day), or combination of the two were administered to infants with a serial Finnegan score greater than 8. The average maternal age was 24.6 years, (18–34 years). Drug use volunteered by the mothers was methadone alone in 6 cases, methadone and benzodiazepines in 14, methadone and heroin and benzodiazepines in 7, methadone and heroin in 10, heroin alone in 2, and other multiple drug use including oral morphine sulphate, dothiepin, and cannabis in 4. Average gestational age was 40.3 (35–42 weeks). The average birth-weight was 2.81 kg (1.89–3.91 kg). Time-to-onset of withdrawal symptoms was 2.8 (1–13) days. The duration of pharmacological treatment (oral morphine sulphate and/or phenobarbitone) was 21.8 (1–62) days. The total hospital stay for the 43 infants was 1011 days[CS424].

Neuroendocrine abnormalities. Prolactin response to D-fenfluramine was assessed in abstinent ecstasy (MDMA) users with concomitant use of cannabis only (13 males, 11 females) and in two control groups: healthy nonusers (13 females) and exclusive cannabis users (seven males). Prolactin response to D-fenfluramine was slightly blunted in female ecstasy users. Both male user samples exhibited a weak prolactin response to D-fenfluramine, but this was weaker in the group of cannabis users. Baseline prolactin and prolactin response to D-fenfluramine were associated with the extent of previous cannabis use. The results indicated that the endocrinological abnormalities of ecstasy users might be closely related to their coincident cannabis use[CS381].

Neurogenic symptoms alleviation. Whole-plant extracts of Δ-9-THC, CBD, 1:1 CBD: THC, or placebo were self-administered by sublingual spray to 24 patients with MS ($n = 18$), spinal cord injury ($n = 4$), brachial plexus damage ($n = 1$), and limb amputation owing to neurofibromatosis ($n = 1$), at doses determined by titration against symptom relief or unwanted effects within the range of 2.5–120 mg/24 hours for 2 weeks. The patients recorded symptoms, well-being, and intoxication scores on a daily basis using visual analog scales. At the end of each two-week period an observer rated severity and frequency of symptoms on numerical rating scales, administered standard measures of disability (Barthel Index), mood, cognition, and recorded adverse events. Pain relief associated with both THC and CBD was significantly superior to placebo. Impaired bladder control, muscle spasms, and spasticity were improved by cannabis medicinal extract (CME) in some patients with these symptoms. Three patients had transient hypotension and intoxication with rapid initial dosing of THC-containing CME. The results indicated that cannabis could improve neurogenic symptoms unresponsive to standard treatments. Unwanted effects were predictable and generally well tolerated[CS354].

Neuropathic pain relief. Forty-eight patients with at least one avulsed root and baseline pain score of four or more on an 11-point ordinate scale participated in a randomized, double-blind, placebo-controlled, three-period crossover study. The patients had intractable symptoms regard-less of current analgesic therapy. They entered a baseline period of 2 weeks, followed by three, 2-week treatment periods; during each period they received one of three oromucosal spray preparations. These were placebo and two whole plant extracts of *C. sativa* L.: GW-1000-02 (Sativex®), containing Δ-9-THC: CBD in an approx 1:1 ratio and GW-2000-02, containing primarily THC. The primary outcome measure was the mean pain severity score during the last 7 days of treatment. Secondary outcome measures included pain related quality of life assessments. The primary outcome measure failed to fall by the two points defined in our hypothesis. Both this measure and measures of sleep showed statistically significant improvements. The study medications were well tolerated with the majority of adverse events, including intoxication type mild to moderate in severity and resolving spontaneous reactions[CS251].

Neuroprotective effect. The effect of cannabidiol on β-amyloid peptide-induced toxicity in cultured rat pheocromocytoma PC12 cells was investigated. Following exposure of cells to β-amyloid peptide (1 μg/mL), a marked reduction in cell survival was observed. This effect was associated with increased reactive oxygen species production and lipid peroxidation, and caspase 3 (a key enzyme in the apoptosis cell-signalling cascade) appearance, DNA fragmentation, and increased intracellular calcium. Treatment of the cells with CBD (10^{-7}–10^{-4} mol) prior to β-amyloid peptide exposure, significantly elevated cell survival, whereas it decreased reactive oxygen species production, lipid peroxidation, caspase 3 levels, DNA fragmentation, and intracellular calcium[CS298]. CBD and other cannabinoids were examined as neuroprotectants in rat cortical neuron cultures exposed to toxic levels of glutamate. The psychotropic cannabinoid receptor agonist Δ-9-THC and cannabidiol, reduced N-methyl-D-aspartate, α-amino-3-hydroxy-5-methyl-4-isoxazole propionic acid and kainate receptor mediated neurotoxicities. Neuroprotection was not affected by cannabinoid receptor antagonist, indicating a (cannabinoid) receptor-independent mechanism of action. CBD demonstrated a reduction in hydroperoxide toxicity in neurons. In this trial of the abilities of various antioxidants to prevent glutamate toxicity, cannabidiol was superior to both α-tocopherol and ascorbate in protective capacity[CS412].

Neuropsychological effect. Cerebral blood flow was measured in 12 long-term cannabis users shortly after cessation of cannabis use (mean 1.6 days). The findings showed significantly lower mean hemispheric blood flow values and significantly lower frontal values in the cannabis subjects compared with normal controls. The results indicated that the functional level of the frontal lobes was affected by long-term cannabis use[CS397].

Neurotransmission inhibition. The BLA or the medial prefrontal cortex (PFC) stimulation in urethane-anesthetized rats induced generation of action potentials in the Nac neurons. This excitatory effect was strongly inhibited by the synthetic cannabinoid agonists WIN (0.062–0.25 mg/kg, iv [intravenously]) and HU-210 (0.125–0.25 mg/kg, iv), or Δ-9-THC (1 mg/kg, iv). D1 or D2 dopamine receptor antagonists (SCH23390 0.5–1 mg/kg, sulpiride 5–10 mg/kg, iv) or the opioid antagonist naloxone (1 mg/kg, iv) were not able to reverse the action of cannabinoids. The selective CB1 receptor antagonist/reverse agonist SR141716A (0.5 mg/kg, iv) fully suppressed the action of cannabinoid agonists, whereas *per se* had no significant effect[CS374].

Nicotine and Δ-9-THC interaction. Δ-9-THC administration to mice significantly decreased the incidence of several nicotine withdrawal signs precipitated by mecamylamine or naloxone, such as wet-dog-shakes, paw tremor, and scratches. In both experimental conditions, the global withdrawal score was significantly attenuated by Δ-9-THC administration. The effect of Δ-9-THC was not to the result possible adaptive changes induced by chronic nicotine on CB1 cannabinoid receptors. The density and functional activity of these receptors were not modified by chronic nicotine administration in the different brain structures investigated. The consequences of Δ-9-THC administration on *c-Fos* expression in several brain structures after chronic nicotine administration and withdrawal were examined. *c-Fos* was decreased in the caudate putamen and the dentate gyrus after mecamylamine precipitated nicotine withdrawal. Δ-9-THC administration did not modify *c-Fos* expression under these experimental conditions. Δ-9-THC also reversed conditioned place aversion associated to naloxone precipitated nicotine withdrawal. The results indicated that Δ-9-THC administration attenuated somatic signs of nicotine withdrawal and this effect was not associated with compensatory changes on CB1 cannabinoid receptors during chronic nicotine administration. Δ-9-THC also ameliorated the aversive motivational consequences of nicotine withdrawal[CS253].

Night vision improvement. In a double-blind study, graduated THC administration at doses of 0–20 mg (as Marinol) on measures of dark adaptometry and scotopic sensitivity was evaluated. Field studies of night vision were performed among Jamaican and Moroccan fishermen, and mountain dwellers with the LKC Technologies Scotopic Sensitivity Tester-1 (SST-1). Improvements in night vision measures were noted after THC or cannabis. The effect was dose-dependent and cannabinoid-mediated at the retinal level[CS286].

Nocturnal sleep effect. Eight healthy volunteers (four males, four females; aged 21–

34 years) were taking placebo, 15 mg Δ-9-THC, 5 mg THC combined with 5 mg CBD, and 15 mg THC combined with 15 mg CBD. These were formulated in 50:50 ethanol to propylene glycol and administered using an oromucosal spray during a 30-minute period from 10 PM. Electroencephalogram was recorded during the sleep period (11 PM to 7 AM). Performance, sleep latency, and subjective assessments of sleepiness and mood were measured from 8:30 AM (10 hours after drug administration). There were no effects of 15 mg THC on nocturnal sleep. With the concomitant administration of the drugs (5 mg THC and 5 mg CBD to 15 mg THC and 15 mg CBD), there was a decrease in stage 3 sleep, and with the higher dose combination, wakefulness was increased. The next day, with a 15-mg THC dose, memory was impaired, sleep latency was reduced, and the subjects reported increased sleepiness and changes in mood. With the lower dose combination, reaction time was faster on the digit recall task, and with the higher dose combination, subjects reported increased sleepiness and changes in mood. Fifteen milligrams of THC appeared to be sedative, and 15 mg CBD appeared to have alerting properties as it increased waking activity during sleep and counteracted the residual sedative activity of the 15 mg THC[CS290].

Occipital stroke. A right occipital ischemic stroke occurred in a 37-year-old Albanese man with a previously uneventful medical history, 15 minutes after smoking a cigarette with approximately 250 mg of cannabis. Clinical manifestations of the stroke were left-sided hemiparesis, hemihypesthesia and blurred vision, which vanished spontaneously and almost completely after 3 days. The patient has been smoking cannabis regularly from the age of 27, with a frequency of two to three cigarettes/cannabis per week during the 6 months that preceded his stroke. Except for cigarette smoking and slight dyslipidemia, classical risk factors for stroke/embolism were absent. The family history for cerebrovascular events, blood pressure, clotting tests, examinations for thrombophilia, vasculitis, extracranial and intracranial arteries, and cardiac investigations were normal or respectively negative; the stroke was attributed to the chronic cannabis consumption[CS271].

Oral cancer. A study of 116 patients aged 45 years and younger, diagnosed with squamous cell carcinoma of the mouth was conducted. Two hundred and seven controls who had never had cancer, matched for age, sex, and area of residence, were recruited. The self-completed questionnaire contained items about exposure to the following risk factors: tobacco products, cannabis, alcohol, and diet. Conditional logistic analyses were conducted adjusting for social class, ethnicity, tobacco, and alcohol habits. All tests for statistical significance were two-sided. The majority of oral cancer patients reported exposure to the major risk factors of tobacco and alcohol even at the younger age. The estimated risks associated with tobacco or alcohol were low (OR range: 0.6–2.5) among both males and females. Only smoking for 21 years or more produced significantly elevated odds ratios (OR = 2.1; 95% CI: 1.1–4). Exposure associated with other major risk factors did not produce significant risks in this sample. Long-term consumption of fresh fruits and vegetables in the diet appeared to be protective for both males and females[CS310].

Oral cytological effect. The effects of cannabis, methaqualone, or tobacco smoking on the epithelial cells in 16 patients were evaluated. The site samples included the buccal mucosa (left and right sides), the posterior dorsum of the tongue, and the anterior floor of the mouth. There was a significant prevalence of bacterial cells in the smears and a greater number of degenerate and atypical squamous cells in cannabis users compared with controls. Epithelial cells in smears taken from cannabis users and tobacco-smoking controls showed koilocytic changes[CS376].

Ovulation inhibition effect. Petroleum ether extract of the aerial parts, administered orally to rats, produced weak activity[CS087].

Pancreatic effect.

A 29-year-old man presented with acute pancreatitis after a period of heavy cannabis smoking. Other causes of the disease were ruled out. The pancreatitis resolved itself after the cannabis was stopped and this was confirmed by urinary cannabinoid metabolite monitoring in the community. There were no previous reports of acute pancreatitis associated with cannabis use in the general population. Drugs of all types are related to the etiology of pancreatitis in approximately 1.4–2% of cases[CS313].

Pancreatic toxicity. The dried leaf, smoked by a 19-year-old woman, was active. The subject was hospitalized with pancreatitis[CS220].

Panic disorder. Sixty-six panic disorder patients were included in a study. All of whom met the DSM-IV diagnosis of panic disorder (n = 45) or panic disorder with agoraphobia ([PDA]; n = 21). Twenty-four patients experienced their first panic attack within 48 hours of cannabis use and then went on to develop panic disorder. All the patients were treated with paroxetine (gradually increased up to 40 mg/day). The two groups responded equally well to paroxetine treatment as measured at the 8 weeks and 12 months follow-up visits. There were no significant effects of age, sex, and duration of illness as covariates with response rates between the two groups. In addition, panic disorder or panic disorder with agoraphobia diagnosis did not affect the treatment response in either group. There were no significant differences in weight gain, sexual side effects, or relapse rates between patients according to gender or comorbid diagnosis[CS300].

Paroxysmal atrial fibrillation. A healthy young subject was observed for paroxysmal atrial fibrillation following cannabis intoxication. The abuse of this substance was the most possible and identifiable risk factor[CS407].

Place conditioning effect. THC was administered to female rats at doses of 1, 5, or 20 mg/kg) during gestation and lactation. Maternal exposure to low doses of THC (1 and 5 mg/kg), relevant for human consumption, produced an increased response to the reinforcing effects of a moderate dose of morphine (350 µg/kg), as measured in the place-preference conditioning paradigm (CPP) in the adult male offspring. These animals also displayed an enhanced exploratory behavior in the defensive withdrawal test. Only females born from mothers exposed to THC at a dose of 1 mg/kg exhibited a small increment in the place conditioning induced by morphine. The possible implication of the HPA was analyzed by monitoring plasma levels of adrenocorticotropic hormone (ACTH) and corticosterone in basal and moderate-stress conditions (after the end of the CPP test). Female offspring perinatally exposed to THC (1 or 5 mg/kg) displayed high basal levels of corticosterone and a blunted adrenal response to the HPA-activating effects of the CPP test. Male offspring born from mothers exposed to THC (1 or 5 mg/kg) displayed the opposite pattern: normal to low basal levels of corticosterone, and a sharp adrenal response to the CPP challenge[CS436]. THC administration to rats at a low dose (1.5 mg/kg) resulted in failing to develop place conditioning, and developing a place aversion at a high dose (15 mg/kg). Administration of the cannabinoid antagonist SR141716A induced a CPP at both a low (0.5 mg/kg) and a high (5 mg/kg) dose[CS451].

Plant germination effect. Methyl chloride extract of the dried seed produced weak activity on *Amaranthus spinosus* (25.8%) inhibition[CS176]. Methyl chloride extract of the dried leaves produced 17.5% inhibition of *Amaranthus spinosus*[CS176].

Plasma norepinephrine concentration. Forty-six newborn infants participated in a prospective study of the neonatal and long-term effects of prenatal cocaine exposure. Based on maternal self-report, maternal urine screening, and infant meconium analysis, 24 infants were classified as CE and 22 as unexposed. Between 24 and 72 hours postpartum, plasma samples for norepinephrine (NE), epinephrine, dopamine, and dihydroxyphenylalanine analysis were obtained. The Neonatal Behavioral Assessment Scale was administered at 1–3 days of age and at 2 weeks of age by examiners masked to the drug exposure status of the newborns. The CE newborns had increased plasma NE concentrations when compared with the unexposed infants (geometric mean, 923 pg/mL vs 667 pg/mL). There were no significant differences in plasma epinephrine, dopamine, or dihydroxyphenylalanine concentrations. Analysis for the effect of potential confounding variables revealed that maternal cannabis use was also associated with increased plasma NE, although birth-weight, gender, and maternal use of alcohol or cigarettes were not. Geometric mean plasma NE was 1164 pg/mL in those infants with *in utero* exposure to both cocaine and cannabis compared to 812 pg/mL in those exposed to only cocaine and 667.0 pg/mL in those exposed to neither. Among the CE infants, plasma NE concentration correlated with an increased score for the depressed cluster ($r = 0.53$) and a decreased score for the orientation cluster ($r = -0.43$) of the Neonatal Behavioral

Assessment Scale administered at 1–3 days of age. Adjusting for cannabis exposure had no effect on these relationships between plasma NE and the depressed and orientation clusters[CS449].

Pneumonic effect. A case–control study was conducted in 7001 individuals. Odds ratios were calculated by conditional logistic regression with substance use and social factors as cofounders. Pneumonia was not associated with kava use. Crude odds ratios = 1.26 (0.74–2.14, $p = 0.386$) increased after controlling for confounders (OR = 1.98, 0.63–6.23, $p = 0.237$) but was not significant. Adjusted odds ratios for pneumonia cases involving kava and alcohol users was 1.19 (0.39–3.62, $p = 0.756$). Crude odds ratios for associations between pneumonia and cannabis use (OR = 2.27, 1.18–4.37, $p = 0.014$) and alcohol use (OR = 1.95, 1.07–3.53, $p = 0.026$) were statistically significant and approached significance for petrol sniffing (OR = 1.98, 0.99–3.95, $p = 0.056$)[CS335].

Postural syncope. Twenty-nine volunteers participated in a randomized, double-blind, placebo-controlled study. Cerebral blood velocity, pulse rate, blood pressure, skin perfusion on forehead and plasma Δ-9-THC levels were quantified during reclining and standing for 10 minutes before and after THC infusions and cannabis smoking. Both THC and cannabis induced postural dizziness, with 28% reporting severe symptoms. Intoxication and dizziness peaked immediately after drug. The severe dizziness group showed the most marked postural drop in cerebral blood velocity and blood pressure and showed a drop in pulse rate after an initial increase during standing. Postural dizziness was unrelated to plasma levels of THC and other indices[CS340].

Prenatal exposure. Data collected from the National Household Survey on Drug Abuse, a nationally representative sample survey of 22,303 noninstitutionalized women aged

18–44 years, of whom 1249 were pregnant, were analyzed. During the 2-year study period, 6.4% of the non-pregnant women of childbearing age and 2.8% of the pregnant women reported that they used illicit drugs. Of the women who used drugs, the relative proportion of women who abstained from illicit drugs after recognition of pregnancy increased from 28% during the first trimester of pregnancy to 93% by the third trimester. However, because of postpregnancy relapse, the net pregnancy-related reduction in illicit drug use at postpartum was only 24%. Cannabis accounted for three-fourths of illicit drug use, and cocaine accounted for one-tenth of illicit drug use. Of those who used illicit drugs, over half of pregnant and two-thirds of non-pregnant women used cigarettes and alcohol. Among the sociodemographic subgroups, pregnant and non-pregnant women who were young (18–30 years) or unmarried, and pregnant women with less than a high school education had the highest rates of illicit drug use[CS357]. Over 12,000 women at 18–20 weeks of gestation were enrolled in an Avon Longitudinal Study of Pregnancy and Childhood. Five percent of the mothers reported smoking cannabis before and/or during pregnancy; they were younger, of lower parity, better educated, and more likely to use alcohol, cigarettes, coffee, tea, and hard drugs. Cannabis use during pregnancy was unrelated to risk of perinatal death or need for special care, but the babies of women who used cannabis at least once per week before and throughout pregnancy were 216 g lighter than those of nonusers, had significantly shorter birth lengths, and smaller head circumferences. After adjustment for confounding factors, the association between cannabis use and birth-weight failed to be statistically significant ($p = 0.056$) and was clearly nonlinear. The adjusted mean birth-weights for babies of women using cannabis at least once per week before and throughout pregnancy were 90 g lighter than the offspring of other women. No significant adjusted effects were seen for birth length and head circumference[CS389]. In two hospitals, 12,885 pregnant women answered questionnaires regarding consumption of alcohol, tobacco, cannabis, and other drugs. The prevalence of cannabis use was 0.8%. Women using cannabis, but no other illicit drugs were each retrospectively matched with four randomly chosen pregnant women in the same period and the same age group and with same parity. Eighty-four cannabis users were included. These women were socioeconomically disadvantaged and had a higher prevalence of present and past use of alcohol, tobacco, and other drugs. No significant difference in pregnancy, delivery, or puerperal outcome was found. Children of women using cannabis were 150 g lighter, 1.2 cm shorter, and had 0.2 cm smaller head circumference than the control infants[CS418]. A 27-year-old woman who smoked a joint (cannabis) and 20 cigarettes (tobacco) daily up to the time of a positive pregnancy test at 7 weeks and 4 days, was evaluated. On day 20 of pregnancy, she had a LSD minitrip. The patient had a spontaneous term delivery. The baby boy weight was between the 5th and the 50th percentile, length between the 50th and the 90th percentile, normal umbilical arterial and venous pH values, and Apgar scores of 7/9/10. There were no visible abnormalities, and behavior was normal[CS419]. Eight hundred seven consecutive positive-pregnancy test urine samples were screened for a range of drugs, including cotinine as an indicator of maternal smoking habits. A positive test for cannabinoids was found in 117 (14.5%) of the samples. Smaller numbers of samples were positive for other drugs: opiates (11), benzodiazepines (4), cocaine (3), and one each for amphetamines and methadone. Polydrug use was detected in nine individuals. Only two samples tested positive for ethanol. The proportion with a urine cotinine level indicative of active smoking was 34.3%. The outcome of the pregnancy was traced for 288 of the subjects. Cannabis use was associated with a lower gestational age at delivery ($p < 0.005$), an increased risk of prematurity ($p < 0.02$), and reduction in birth-weight ($p < 0.002$). Maternal smoking was associated with a reduction in infant birth-weight ($p < 0.05$). This was less pronounced than the effect of other substance misuse[CS422]. A sample of low-income women attending a prenatal clinic was assessed. The majority of the women decreased their use of cannabis during pregnancy. The assessments of child behavior problems included the Child Behavior Checklist, Teacher's Report Form, and the Swanson, Noland, and Pelham checklist. Multiple and logistic regressions were employed to analyze the relations between cannabis use and behavior problems of the children at age 10, while controlling for the effects of other extraneous variables. Prenatal cannabis use was significantly related to increased hyperactivity, impulsivity, and inattention symptoms as measured by the Swanson, Noland, and Pelham, increased delinquency as measured by the Child Behavior Checklist, and increased delinquency and externalizing problems as measured by the Teacher's Report Form. The pathway between prenatal cannabis exposure and delinquency was mediated by the effects of cannabis exposure on inattention symptoms[CS413]. Attention and impulsivity of prenatally substance-exposed 6-year-olds were assessed as part of a longitudinal study. Most of the women were light-to-moderate users of alcohol and cannabis who decreased their use after the first trimester of pregnancy. Tobacco was used by a majority of women and did not change during pregnancy. The women, recruited from a prenatal clinic, were of low socioeconomic status. Attention and impul-

sivity were assessed using a Continuous Performance Task. Second and third trimester of tobacco exposure and first trimester of cocaine use predicted increased omission errors. Second trimester cannabis use predicted more commission errors and fewer omission errors. There were no significant effects of prenatal alcohol exposure. Lower Stanford-Binet Intelligence Scale composite scores, male gender, and an adult male in the household predicted more errors of commission. Lower Standford-Binet Intelligence Scale composite scores, younger child age, maternal work/school status, and higher maternal hostility scores predicted more omission errors[CS429]. The neurophysiological effects of prenatal cannabis exposure on response inhibition were assessed in thirty-one participants aged 18–22. Ottawa Prenatal Prospective Study performed a blocked design Go/No-Go task while neural activity was imaged with functional magnetic resonance imaging. The Ottawa Prenatal Prospective Study is a longitudinal study that provides a unique body of information collected from each participant over 20 years, including prenatal drug history, detailed cognitive/behavioral performance from infancy to young adulthood, and current and past drug usage. The functional magnetic resonance imaging results showed that with increased prenatal cannabis exposure, there was a significant increase in neural activity in bilateral PFC and right premotor cortex during response inhibition. There was also an attenuation of activity in left cerebellum with increased prenatal exposure to cannabis when challenging the response inhibition neural circuitry. Prenatally exposed offspring had significantly more commission errors than non-exposed participants, but all participants were able to perform the task with more than 85% accuracy. The findings were observed when controlling for present cannabis use and prenatal exposure to nicotine, alcohol, and caffeine, and suggest that prenatal cannabis exposure was related to changes in neural activity during response inhibition that last into young adulthood[CS282]. The effects of prenatal cannabis and alcohol exposure on school achievement at 10 years of age were examined. Women were interviewed about their substance use at the end of each trimester of pregnancy, at 8 and 18 months, and at 3, 6, 10, 14, and 16 years. The women were of lower socioeconomic status, high school-educated, and light-to-moderate users of cannabis and alcohol. At the 10-year follow-up, the effects of prenatal exposure to cannabis or alcohol on the academic performance of 606 children were assessed. Exposure to one or more cannabis joints per day during the first trimester predicted deficits in Wide Range Achievement Test-Revised reading and spelling scores and a lower rating on the teachers' evaluations of the children's performance. This relation was mediated by the effects of first-trimester cannabis exposure on the children's depression and anxiety symptoms. Second-trimester cannabis use was significantly associated with reading comprehension and underachievement. Exposure to alcohol during the first and second trimesters of pregnancy predicted poorer teachers' ratings of overall school performance. Second-trimester binge drinking predicted lower reading scores. There was no interaction between prenatal cannabis and alcohol exposure. Each was an independent predictor of academic performance[CS283]. Pregnant rats were treated daily with Δ-9-THC from the fifth day of gestation up to the day before birth (GD21). Then rats were sacrificed and their pups removed for analysis of the neural adhesion molecule L1-mRNA levels in different brain structures. The levels of L1 transcripts were significantly increased in the fimbria, stria terminalis, stria medullaris, corpus callosum, and in gray-matter structures (septum nuclei and the habenula). It remained unchanged in most of the gray-matter structures analyzed (cerebral cortex, BAL nucleus, hippocampus, thalamic and hypothalamic nuclei, basal ganglia, and subventricular zones) and also in a few white-matter structures (fornix and fasciculus retroflexus). The increase in L1-mRNA levels reached statistical significance only in Δ-9-THC-exposed males but not females, where only trends or no effects were detected. The results supported evidence on a sexual dimorphism, with greater effects in male fetuses, for the action of cannabinoids in the developing brain[CS295]. Fetal cannabis exposure has no consistent effect on outcome. Prenatal cocaine exposure has not been shown to have any detrimental effect on cognition, except as mediated through cocaine effects on head size. Although fetal cocaine exposure has been linked to numerous abnormalities in arousal, attention, and neurological and neurophysiological function, most such effects appear to be self-limited and restricted to early infancy and childhood. Opiate exposure elicits a well-described withdrawal syndrome affecting the central nervous, autonomic, and gastrointestinal systems, which is most severe among methadone-exposed infants[CS319]. Executive functioning in cocaine/polydrug (cannabis, alcohol, and tobacco)-exposed infants was assessed in a single session, occurring between 9.5 and 12.5 months of age. In an A-not-B task, infants searched—after performance-adjusted delays—for an object hidden in a new location. The CE infants did not differ from non-CE controls recruited from the same at-risk population. Comparison of heavier-CE ($n = 9$) with the combined group of lighter-CE ($n = 10$) and non-CE ($n = 32$) infants revealed significant differences on A-not-B performance, as well as on global tests of mental and motor development. Covariates investigated included socioeconomic status, marital status, race, maternal age, years of education, weeks of gestation, and birth-weight, as well as severity of prenatal cannabis, alcohol, and tobacco exposure. The relationship of heavier-CE status to motor development was mediated by length of gestation, and the relationship of heavier-CE status to mental development was confounded with maternal gestational use of cigarettes. The relationship of heavier-CE status to A-not-B performance remained significant after controlling for potentially confounded variables and mediators, but was not statistically significant after controlling for the variance associated with global mental development[CS341]. Weight, height, and head circumference were examined in children from birth to early adolescence for whom prenatal exposure to cannabis and cigarettes had been ascertained. The subjects were from a low-risk, predominantly middle-class sample participating in an ongoing longitudinal study. The negative association between growth measures at birth and prenatal cigarette exposure was overcome, sooner in males than females, within the first few years, and by the age of 6 years, the children of heavy smokers were heavier than control subjects. Pre- and postnatal environmental tobacco smoke did not have a negative effect on the growth parameters; however, the choice of bottlefeeding or shorter duration of breastfeeding by women who smoked during pregnancy appeared to play an important positive role in the catch-up observed among the infants of smokers. Prenatal exposure to cannabis was not significantly related to any growth measures at birth, although a smaller head circumference observed at all ages reached statistical significance among the early adolescents born to heavy cannabis users[CS417].

Prolactin inhibition. The dried leaves, smoked by healthy female volunteers at a dose of 1 g/person, produced a decrease in plasma prolactin levels during the luteal phase of the menstrual cycle but not during the follicular phase. The results were significant at $p < 0.01$ level[CS221].

Propiospinal myoclonus. A 25-year-old woman with clusters of myoclonus induced by a single exposure to inhaled cannabis was evaluated. Investigations excluded a structural abnormality of the spine. Multichannel surface electromyogram with parallel frontal electroencephalogram recording confirmed the diagnosis of propriospinal myoclonus[CS284].

Prostaglandin synthetase inhibition. Chromatographic fraction of the aerial parts was active on the bull seminal vesicles[CS159].

Protein synthesis inhibition. Ethanol (95%) extract of the dried resin, administered intraperitoneally to toads at a dose of 10 mg/day for 14 days, was active. The results were significant at $p < 0.01$ level[CS216].

Psoriatic effect. Hot water extract of the dried seed, taken orally by 108 human adults with psoriasis at variable dosage level, was active. After 3–4 weeks of treatment, there was significant improvement. The extract was taken in combination with *Rehmannia glutinosa* (rhizome), *Salvia miltiorrhiza* (root), *Scrophularia ningpoensis* (root), *Isatis tinctoria* (branch and leaf), *Sophora subprostrata* (root), *Dictamnus dasycarpus* (rootbark), *Polygonum bistorta* (rhizome), and *Forsythia suspensa* (fruit)[CS197].

Psychosocial morbidity association. Cannabis dependence is a prevalent comorbid substance use disorder among patients early in the course of a schizophrenia-spectrum disorder. Among 29 eligible patients, 18 participated in the study. First-episode patients with comorbid cannabis dependence ($n = 8$) reported significantly greater childhood physical and sexual abuse compared with those without comorbid cannabis dependence ($n = 10$). The result indicated the preliminary evidence of an association between childhood maltreatment and cannabis dependence among this especially vulnerable population. Childhood physical and sexual abuse may be a risk factor for the initiation of cannabis dependence and other substance use disorders in the early course of schizophrenia[CS249].

Psychotic effect. Thirty five hundred representatives 19 years of age were examined in a cohort study. The subjects completed a 40-item Community Assessment of Psychic Experiences, measuring subclinical positive (paranoia, hallucinations, grandiosity, first-rank symptoms) and negative psychosis dimensions, depression, and drug use. Use of cannabis was associated positively with both positive and negative dimensions of psychosis, independent of each other and of depression. An association between cannabis and depression disappeared after adjustment for the negative psychosis dimensions. First use of cannabis younger than age 16 years was associated with a much stronger effect than first use after age 15 years, independent of lifetime frequency of use. The association between cannabis and psychosis was not influenced by the distress associated with the experiences, indicating that self-medication may be an unlikely explanation for the entire association between cannabis and psychosis[CS264]. Cross-sectional epidemiological studies indicated that individuals with psychosis use cannabis more often than other individuals in the general population. It has long been considered that this association was explained by the self-medication hypothesis, postulating that cannabis is used to self-medicate psychotic symptoms. This hypothesis has been recently challenged. Several prospective studies carried out in population-based samples, showed that cannabis exposure was associated with an increased risk of psychosis. A dose–response relationship was found between cannabis exposure and risk of psychosis, and this association was independent from potential confounding factors, such as exposure to other drugs and preexistence of psychotic symptoms. The brain mechanisms underlying the association have to be elucidated; they may implicate deregulation of cannabinoid and dopaminergic systems. Cannabis exposure may be a risk factor for psychotic disorders by interacting with a preexisting vulnerability for these disorders[CS277].

Refractory neuropathic pain. Seven patients (three women and four men) aged 60 ± 14 years suffering from chronic refractory neuropathic pain, received oral THC titrated to the maximum dose of 25 mg/day (mean dose: 15 ± 6 mg) during an average of 55.4 days (range: 13–128). Various components of pain (continuous, paroxysmal, and brush-induced allodynia) were assessed using visual analog scale scores. Health-related quality of life was evaluated using the Brief Pain Inventory, and the Hospital Anxiety and Depression scale was used to measure depression and anxiety. THC did not induce significant effect on the various pain, health-related quality of life and anxiety and depression scores. Numerous side effects (notably sedation and asthenia) were observed in five out of seven patients, requiring premature discontinuation of the drug in three patients[CS361].

Reproductive effect. Cannabis use during pregnancy in developed nations is estimated to be approx 10%. Recent evidence suggests that the endogenous cannabinoid system, now consisting of two receptors and multiple endocannabinoid ligands, may also play an important role in the maintenance and regulation of early pregnancy and fertility[CS316]. Drugs of abuse, like alcohol, opiates, cocaine, and cannabis, are used by many young people for their presumed aphrodisiac properties. The opioids inhibit the hypothalamus–pituitary–gonads axis (HPG), and increase the prolactin levels, which interferes with the male and female sexual response. Cannabis, at high doses, could inhibit the HPG axis and reduce fertility[CS350]. Cannabis initially increases libido and potency, but chronic use causes sexual inversion[CS364]. Long-term use of cannabis has been found to cause physiological changes that can alter individual reproductive potential. The effects of cannabis depend on the dose and can include death from depression of the respiratory system. Cannabis is absorbed rapidly and eliminated very slowly. Δ-9-THC is highly liposoluble and fixes to the serum proteins, passing to the lungs and liver for metabolization and to the kidneys and liver for excretion. As with estrogens, there is an enterohepatic circuit for reabsorption and elimination. Ninety percent is eliminated in the feces, 65% within 48 hours. Because of the enterohepatic circuit and liposolubility, elimination requires 1 week for completion. The other important biotransformation of the active principle is hydroxylation. The hydroxylated derivatives are responsible for the psychoactivity of cannabis. Cannabis affects both neuroendocrine function and the germ cells. Studies on experimental animals have indicated that THC can cause a decline in the pituitary hormones, follicle stimulating hormone, luteinizing hormone, and prolactin, and in the steroids progesterone, estrogen, and androgens. Human studies have shown that chronic users have decreased levels of serum testosterone. Because steroidogenesis can be restimulated with human chorionic gonadotropin, it appears that THC does not directly affect steroid production by the corpus luteum, but that its action is mediated by the hypothalamus. Because of its potent antigonadotropic action, THC is under study as an anovulatory agent. The same animal studies have shown that ovulation returns to normal 6 months after termination of use. High rates of anovulation and luteal insufficiency have been observed in women smoking cannabis at least three times weekly. THC accumulates in the milk. Animal studies have shown that THC depresses the enzymes necessary for lactation and causes a diminution in the volume of the mammary glands. Significant amounts of the drug have been detected in both mothers' milk and the blood of newborns. Animal studies indicate that THC crosses the placenta, achieving concentrations in the fetus as high as those in the mother. Animal studies also demonstrated increasing frequency of abortions, intrauterine death, and declines in fetal weight. The effects were probably caused by an alteration in placental function. A human study likewise showed that cannabis use during pregnancy was significantly related to poor fetal development, low birth-weight, diminished size, and decreased cephalic circumference. Congenital malformations have been observed in experimental animals exposed to THC. Declines in sperm volume and count and abnormal sperm motility have been observed in chronic cannabis users. In vitro studies show that THC produces a marked degeneration of human sperm[CS365]. Among sexually experienced girls, 39% (n = 123) reported using oral contraceptive pills(OCPs), 5.4% (n = 17) used Depo-Provera® (medroxyprogesterone acetate) or Norplant® (levonorgestrel), and 55.6% (n = 175) used no hormonal method. Logistic regression analysis revealed that the factors most significantly associated with the use of hormonal methods were older age (OR = 1.19; 95% CI, 1.07–1.33), not using a condom at last intercourse (OR = 0.55; CI, 0.34–0.90), and having had a well visit within 1 year (OR = 2.11; CI, 1.12–3.70). OCP users were less likely than Depo-Provera or Norplant users to have used alcohol (p = 0.041), cigarettes (p = 0.002), or cannabis (p = 0.018) in the past 30 days. OCP users were less likely than nonusers of hormonal methods to have smoked cigarettes (p = 0.034) or cannabis (p = 0.052). The school-based clinic had a greater proportion of subjects using long-acting progestins (p < 0.001)[CS443].

Respiratory effect. Smoking a "joint" of cannabis resulted in exposure to significantly greater amounts of combusted material than with a tobacco cigarette. The histopathological effects of cannabis-smoke exposure included changes consistent with acute and chronic bronchitis. Cellular dysplasia has also been observed, suggesting that, like tobacco smoke, cannabis exposure has the potential to cause malignancy. Symptoms of cough and early morning sputum production are common (20–25%) even in young individuals who smoke cannabis alone. Almost all studies indicated that the effects of cannabis and tobacco smoking are addictive and independent[CS342]. A small group of current male cannabis processors with a mean age of 43 years was studied. Questionnaire data, lung function, serial FEV1 and blood were collected from all workers. Seven workers (64%) complained of at least one respiratory symptom (one with byssinosis). The mean percentage predicted FEV1 was 91.5, FVC 97.7, peak expiratory flow 92.1, and forced expiratory flow between 25 and 75% of FVC 79.5. Serial FEV1 measurements in the two workers with work-related respiratory symptoms revealed a mean change in FEV1 on the first working day of –12.9%. This contrasted with +6.25% on the last working day. Respective values for the two workers without work-related symptoms were –1.4 and +3.2%[CS402]. Nine hundred forty-three young adults from a birth cohort of 1037 were studied at age 21 years. Standardized respiratory symptom questionnaires were administered. Spirometry and methacholine challenge tests were undertaken. Cannabis dependence was determined using DSM-III-R criteria. Descriptive analyses and comparisons between cannabis-dependent, tobacco-smoking, and nonsmoking groups were undertaken. Adjusted odds ratios for respiratory symptoms, lung function, and airway hyperresponsiveness (PC20) were measured. Ninety-one subjects (9.7%) were cannabis-dependent and 264 (28.1%) were current tobacco smokers. After controlling for tobacco use, respiratory symptoms associated with cannabis dependence included wheezing apart from colds, exercise-induced shortness of breath, nocturnal wakening with chest tightness, and early morning sputum production. These were increased by 61, 65, 72 (all $p < 0.05$), and 144% ($p < 0.01$) respectively, compared with non-tobacco smokers. The frequency of respiratory symptoms in cannabis-dependent subjects was similar to tobacco smokers of 1–10 cigarettes per day. The proportion of cannabis-dependent study members with an FEV1/FVC ratio of less than 80% was 36% compared with 20% for nonsmokers ($p = 0.04$). These outcomes occurred independently of coexisting bronchial asthma[CS405].

Reversal of cannabinoid addiction. Δ-9-THC was administered orally to mice at a dose of 10 mg/kg twice daily for 6 days to make them dependent on cannabinoids. Other groups of mice were administered orally with a Δ-9-THC and benzoflavone from *Passiflora incarnata* at doses of 10 or 20 mg/kg twice daily for 6 days. Mice receiving the Δ-9-THC and *Passiflora incarnata* extract developed significantly less dependence, worse locomotor activity, and less of typical withdrawal effects like paw tremors and headshakes, compared with mice receiving Δ-9-THC alone. Administration of SR-141716A, a selective cannabinoid-receptor antagonist (10 mg/kg, orally), to all groups on the seventh day resulted in an artificial withdrawal. Administration of 20 mg/kg of the *Passiflora incarnata* benzoflavone moiety to mice showing symptoms of withdrawal owing to administration of SR-141716A produced a marked attenuation of withdrawal effects[CS375].

Schizophrenic effect. The nerve growth factor (NGF) serum levels of 109 consecutive drug-naïve schizophrenic patients were measured and compared with those of healthy controls. The results were correlated with the long-term intake of cannabis and other drugs. Mean (± standard deviation) NGF serum levels of 61 control persons (33.1 ± 31 pg/mL) and 76 schizophrenics who did not consume illegal drugs (26.3 ± 19.5 pg/mL) did not differ significantly. Schizophrenic patients with regular cannabis intake (> 0.5 g per day on average for at least 2 years) had significantly raised NGF serum levels of 412.9 ± 288.4 pg/mL (n = 21) compared with controls and schizophrenic patients not consuming cannabis (p < 0.001). In schizophrenic patients who abused not only cannabis, but also additional substances, NGF concentrations were as high as 2336.2 ± 1711.4 pg/mL (n = 12). On average, heavy cannabis consumers suffered their first episode of schizophrenia 3.5 years (n = 21) earlier than schizophrenic patients who abstained from cannabis. These results indicate that cannabis is a possible risk factor for the development of schizophrenia. This might be reflected in the raised NGF-serum concentrations when both schizophrenia and long-term cannabis abuse prevail[CS304].

Schizotypy correlation. Two hundred eleven healthy adults who used cannabis showed higher scores on schizotypy, borderline, and psychoticism scales than neverusers. Multivariate analysis, covarying lie scale scores, age, and educational level indicated that high schizotypal traits best discriminated subjects who had used cannabis from never-users, whether or not they reported having used other recreational drugs. The results indicated that cannabis use was related to a personality dimension of psychosis-proneness in healthy people[CS457].

Sedative and stimulant effects. A double-blind, placebo-controlled study assessed subjective effects of smoking cannabis with either a long or short breath-holding dura-

tion. During eight test sessions, 55 male volunteers made repeated ratings of subjective "high," sedation, and stimulation, as well as rating their perceptions of motivation and performance on cognitive tests. The long, relative to the short, breath-holding duration increased "high" ratings after smoking cannabis, but not placebo. Cannabis smoking increased sedation and a perception of worsened test performance, and decreased motivation with respect to test performance. Paradoxical subjective effects were observed in those subjects reporting some stimulation, as well as sedation after smoking cannabis, particularly with the long breath-holding duration. Breath-holding duration did not produce any subjective effects that were independent of the drug treatment (i.e., occurred equally after smoking of cannabis and placebo)[CS438].

Sexual headache. Sexual headaches usually develop during orgasm. The case of a young man and heavy cannabis smoker who suffered posterior cerebral artery infarction during his first episode of coital headache was reported[CS386].

Sexual receptivity. The effects of THC on sexual behavior in female rats and its influence on steroid hormone receptors and neurotransmitters in the facilitation of sexual receptivity was examined. Results revealed that the facilitatory effect of THC was inhibited by antagonists to both progesterone and dopamine D(1) receptors. To test further the idea that progesterone receptors (PR) and/or dopamine receptors (D[1]R) in the hypothalamus were required for THC-facilitated sexual behavior in rodents, antisense, and sense oligonucleotides to PR and D(1)R were administered intracerebroventricularly into the third cerebral ventricle of ovariectomized, estradiol benzoate-primed rats. Progesterone- and THC-facilitated sexual behavior was inhibited in animals treated with antisense oligonucleotides to PR or to D(1)R. Antagonists to cannabinoid receptor-1 subtype (CB1), but not to cannabinoid receptor-2 subtype (CB2) inhibited progesterone- and dopamine-facilitated sexual receptivity in female rats[CS408]. Adult female and male rats that had been perinatally exposed to hashish extracts were investigated. Adult males perinatally exposed to hashish extracts exhibited marked changes in the behavioral patterns executed in the sociosexual approach behavior test; these changes did not exist in females. Control males first visited the incentive male and took longer to visit the incentive female, whereas hashish-exposed males followed the opposite pattern. Hashish-exposed males spent more time in the vicinity of the incentive female, whereas they decreased their frequency of visits to, and the time spent in, the male incentive area. This behavior was observed during the first third of the test, but became normalized and even inverted during the last two-thirds. In the social interaction test, the normal reduction in the time spent in active social interaction following the exposure to a neophobic situation (high light levels) in controls did not occur in hashish-exposed males, although these exhibited a response in the dark-light emergence test similar to that of their corresponding controls. No changes were seen in spontaneous locomotor activity in both tests. These behavioral alterations observed in hashish-exposed males were paralleled by a significant decrease in L-3,4-dihydroxyphenylacetic acid contents in the limbic forebrain; this suggests a decreased activity of mesolimbic dopaminergic neurons. No effects were seen in females[CS459].

Smooth muscle relaxant activity. Ethanol (95%) and water extracts of the dried aerial parts, at a concentration of 1:1, produced weak activity on the rabbit duodenum. The ethanol extract was equivocal on the guinea pig ileum[CS243]. Petroleum ether extract of the dried entire plant, administered intraperi-toneally to rats at a dose of 0.89 mg/kg, was active vs corneo-palpebral reflex[CS022].

Smooth muscle stimulant activity. Hot water extract of the dried leaf was active on the rabbit and guinea pig intestine[CS177]. Water extract of the dried aerial parts at a concentration of 1:1 was equivocal on the guinea pig ileum[CS243].

Spasticity treatment. Standardized plant extract was administered orally to 57 MS patients with poorly controlled spasticity, at a dose of 2.5 mg of THC and 0.9 mg of CBD. Patients in group A started with a drug escalation phase from 15 to a maximum of 30 mg of THC by 5 mg per day if well tolerated, being on active medication for 14 days before starting placebo. Patients in group B started with placebo for 7 days, crossed to the active period (14 days), and closed with a three-day placebo period (active drug-dose escalation and placebo sham escalation as in group A). Measures used included daily self-report of spasm frequency and symptoms, Ashworth Scale, Rivermead Mobility Index, 10-meter timed walk, nine-hole peg test, paced auditory serial addition test, and the digit span test. There were no statistically significant differences associated with active treatment compared with placebo, but trends in favor of active treatment were seen for spasm frequency, mobility, and getting to sleep. In the 37 patients (per-protocol set) who received at least 90% of their prescribed dose, improvements in spasm frequency ($p = 0.013$) and mobility after excluding a patient who fell and stopped walking were seen ($p = 0.01$). Minor adverse events were slightly more frequent and severe during active treatment, and toxicity symptoms, which were generally mild, were more pronounced in the active phase[CS270]. Six hundred thirty participants with stable MS and muscle spasticity were treated with oral cannabis extract ($n = 211$), Δ-9-THC ($n = 206$), or placebo ($n = 213$) for 15 weeks. Six hundred eleven of 630 patients were followed up for the primary end point. No treatment effect of cannabinoids on the primary outcome ($p = 0.40$) was noted. The estimated difference in mean reduction in total Ashworth score for participants taking cannabis extract compared with placebo was 0.32 (95% CI, –1.04 to 1.67), and for those taking Δ-9-THC vs placebo it was 0.94 (–0.44 to 2.31). There was an evidence of a treatment effect on patient-reported spasticity and pain ($p = 0.003$), with improvement in spasticity reported in 61% ($n = 121$, 95% CI, 54.6–68.2), 60% ($n = 108$, 52.5–66.8), and 46% ($n = 91$, 39–52.9) of participants on cannabis extract, Δ-9-THC, and placebo, respectively[CS322].

Spatial working memory effect. Functional magnetic resonance imaging was used to examine brain activity in 12 long-term heavy cannabis users, 6–36 hours after last use, and in 10 control subjects while they performed a spatial working memory task. Regional brain activation was analyzed and compared using statistical parametric mapping techniques. Compared with controls, cannabis users exhibited increased activation of brain regions typically used for spatial working memory tasks (such as PFC and anterior cingulate). Users also recruited additional regions not typically used for spatial working memory (such as regions in the basal ganglia). The findings remained essentially unchanged when reanalyzed using the subjects ages as a covariate. Brain activation showed little or no significant correlation with subjects years of education, verbal IQ, lifetime episodes of cannabis use, or urinary cannabinoid levels at the time of scanning[CS281].

Spermicidal effect. Petroleum ether extract of the dried aerial parts at a concentration of 0.74 mmol was active on the human spermatozoa[CS186].

Spontaneous activity reduction. Petroleum ether extract of the dried entire plant, administered intraperitoneally to guinea pigs at a dose of 100 mg/kg, was active[CS022].

Spontaneous pneumomediastinum. Spontaneous pneumomediastinum is defined as pneumomediastinum in the absence of an underlying lung disease. It is the second most common cause of chest pain in young, healthy individuals (<30 years) necessitating hospital visits. Inhalational drug use (cocaine and cannabis) has been associated with a significant number of cases, although cases with no apparent etiological or incriminating factors are well-recognized. A case of an 18-year-old high school student with spontaneous pneumomediastinum was evaluated[CS421].

Sudden cardiac death. An 18-year-old male suffered sudden cardiac death following the use of cocaine, cannabis, and ethanol[CS439].

Sudden infant death syndrome. In a nationwide case–control study of 369 cases and 1558 controls, two-thirds of SIDS deaths occurred at night (between 10 PM and 7:30 AM). The odds ratio (95% CI) for prone sleep position was 3.86 (2.67–5.59) for deaths occurring at night, and 7.25 (4.52–11.63) for deaths occurring during the day; the difference was significant. The odds ratio for maternal smoking and SIDS deaths occurring at night was 2.28 (1.52–3.42), and for the day, 1.27 (0.79–2.03). If the mother was single, the odds ratio was 2.69 (1.29–3.99) for a nighttime death, and 1.25 (0.76–2.04) for a daytime death. Both interactions were significant. The interactions between time of death and bed sharing, not sleeping in a cot or bassinet, ethnicity, late timing of prenatal care, binge drinking, cannabis use, and illness in the baby were also significant. All were more strongly associated with SIDS occurring at night[CS366]. In a nationwide case–control study, 393 cases and 1592 controls were analyzed. Adjusting for ethnicity and maternal tobacco use, the SIDS odds ratio for weekly maternal cannabis use since the infant's birth was 2.23 (95% CI = 1.39, 3.57) compared with nonusers, and the multivariate odds ratio was 1.55 (95% CI = 0.87, 2.75)[CS403].

Suicidal effect. Standardized interview assessments were conducted with 2311 youths aged 8–15 years who used drugs before age 16. Approximately 15 years after recruitment, 1695 persons (mean age = 21 years) were reassessed. One hundred fifty-five of them made suicide attempts (SA) and 218 had onset of depression-related suicide ideation (SI). The relative risk, from survival analysis and logistic regression models, to study early use of tobacco, alcohol, cannabis, and inhalants, with covariate adjustments for age, sex, race/ethnicity, and other pertinent covariates were examined. Early-onset of cannabis use and inhalant use for females, but not for males, signaled a modest excess risk of SA (cannabis-associated RR = 1.9; p = 0.04; inhalant-associated RR = 2.2; p = 0.05). Early-onset of cannabis use by females (but not for males) signaled excess risk for SI (RR = 2.9; p = 0.006). Early-onset alcohol and tobacco use were not associated with later risk of SA or SI[CS252]. Two hundred seventy-seven same-sex twin pairs (median age: 30 years) discordant for cannabis dependence and 311 pairs discordant for early-onset cannabis use (before age 17 years) were examined. Individuals who were cannabis-dependent had odds of SI and SA that were 2.5–2.9 times higher than those of their noncannabis-dependent co-twin. Cannabis dependence was associated with elevated risks of major depressive disorder (MDD) in dizygotic, but not in monozygotic twins. Twins who initiated cannabis use before age 17 years of age had elevated rates of subsequent SA (OR, 3.5, 95% CI, 1.4–8.6) but not of MDD or SI. Early MDD and SI were significantly associated with subsequent risks of cannabis dependence in discordant dizygotic pairs, but not in discordant monozygotic pairs. The results indicated that the comorbidity between cannabis dependence and MDD likely arises through shared genetic and

environmental vulnerabilities predisposing to both outcomes. In contrast, associations between cannabis dependence and suicidal behaviors cannot be entirely explained by common predisposing genetic and/or shared environmental predisposition[CS260].

Synergic cytotoxicity. THC, in A549 lung tumor cells culture at concentrations of less than 5 µg/mL, produced no cytotoxic effect. At higher levels it induced cell necrosis, with a lethal concentration (LC)$_{50}$ of 16–18 µg/mL. Butylated hydroxyanisole ([BHA], a food additive)alone at concentrations of 10–200 µM, produced limited cell toxicity and significantly enhanced the necrotic death resulting from concurrent exposure to THC. In the presence of BHA at 200 µM, the LC$_{50}$ for THC decreased to 10–12 µg/ mL. Similar results were obtained with smoke extracts prepared from cannabis cigarettes, but not with extracts from tobacco or placebo cannabis cigarettes (containing no THC). Experiments were repeated in the presence of either diphenyleneiodonium or dicumarol as inhibitors of the redox cycling pathway. Neither of the compounds protected cells from the effects of combined THC and BHA, but rather enhanced necrotic cell death. Measurements of cellular ATP revealed that both THC and BHA reduced ATP levels in A549 cells, consistent with toxic effects on mitochondrial electron transport. The combination was synergistic in this respect, reducing ATP levels to less than 15% of the control. Exposure to cannabis smoke in conjunction with BHA may promote deleterious health effects in the lung[CS373].

Teratogenic activity. Resin, administered orally to pregnant rabbits at a dose of 1 mL/ kg, was active[CS167]. Alcohol extract of the dried leaves, administered intragastrically to pregnant rats at a dose of 125 mg/kg from days 7 to 16 of gestation, was active. The fetuses showed several gross abnormalities, visceral anomalies, and skeletal malformations[CS233]. Water extract of the dried leaf, administered intragastrically to pregnant rats at doses of 125, 200, 400, and 800 mg/kg, produced various types of malformations in the fetuses[CS228]. Petroleum ether extract of the aerial parts, administered orally to rats and rabbits, was inactive[CS087].

Tourette syndrome. Tourette syndrome (TS) is a complex inherited disorder of unknown etiology, characterized by multiple motor and vocal tics. Involvement of the central cannabinoid (CB1) system was suggested because of therapeutic effects of cannabis consumption and Δ-9-THC-treatment in TS patients. The central cannabinoid receptor (CNR1) gene encoding the CNR1 was considered as a candidate gene for TS and systematically screened by single-strand conformation polymorphism analysis and sequencing. Compared with the published CNR1 sequence, three single-base substitutions were identified: 1326T→A, 1359G→A, 1419 + 1G→C. The change at position 1359 is a common polymor-phism (1359 G/A) without allelic association with TS. 1326T→A was present in only one TS patient and is a silent mutation, which does not change codon 442 (valine). 1419 + 1G→C affects the first nucleotide immediately following the coding sequence. It was first detected in three of 40 TS patients and none of 81 healthy controls. This statistically significant association with TS ($p = 0.034$) could not be confirmed in two subsequent cohorts of 56 TS patients (one heterozygous for 1419 + 1G→C) and 55 controls, and 64 patients and 66 controls (one heterozygous for 1419 + 1G→C), respectively. Transcript analysis of lymphocyte RNA from five 1419 + 1G→C carriers revealed no systematic influence on the expression level of the mutated allele. In addition, segregation analysis of 1419 + 1G→C in affected families gave evidence that 1419 + 1G→C does not play a causal role in the etiology of TS. It was concluded that genetic variations of the CNR1 gene are not a plau-

sible explanation for the clinically observed relation between the cannabinoid system and TS[CS292]. A single-dose, cross-over study in 12 patients, and a 6-week, randomized trial in 24 patients, demonstrated that Δ9-THC, the most psychoactive ingredient of cannabis, reduced tics in TS patients. No serious adverse effects occurred and no impairment on neuropsychological performance was observed[CS329]. In the randomized, double-blind, placebo-controlled study, 24 patients with TS, according to DSM-III-R criteria, were treated over a 6-week period with up to 10 mg/day of THC. Tics were rated at six visits (visit 1, baseline; visits 2–4, during treatment period; visits 5–6, after withdrawal of medication) using the Tourette Syndrome Clinical Global Impressions scale (TS-CGI), the Shapiro Tourette-Syndrome Severity Scale (STSSS), the Yale Global Tic Severity Scale (YGTSS), the self-rated Tourette Syndrome Symptom List (TSSL), and a videotape-based rating scale. Seven patients dropped out of the study or had to be excluded, but only one because of side effects. Using the TS-CGI, STSSS, YGTSS, and video rating scale, there was a significant difference ($p < 0.05$) or a trend toward a significant difference ($p < 0.1$) between THC and placebo groups at visits 2, 3, and/or 4. Using the TSSL at 10 treatment days (between days 16 and 41) there was a significant difference ($p < 0.05$) between both groups. Analysis of variance also demonstrated a significant difference ($p = 0.037$). No serious adverse effects occurred[CS345]. In the randomized, double-blind, placebo-controlled study, the effect of a treatment with up to 10 mg Δ-9-THC over a 6-week period on neuropsychological performance in 24 patients suffering from TS was investigated. During medication and immediately, as well as 5–6 weeks after, withdrawal of Δ-9-THC treatment, no detrimental effect was seen on learning curve, interference, recall and recognition of word lists, immediate visual memory span, and divided attention. A trend towards a significant immediate verbal memory span improvement during and after treatment was found[CS356]. A randomized double-blind placebo-controlled crossover single-dose trial of Δ-9-THC (5, 7.5, or 10 mg) in 12 adult TS patients was performed. Tic severity was assessed using the TSSL and examiner ratings (STSSS, YGTSS, TS-CGS). Using the TSSL, patients also rated the severity of associated behavioral disorders. Clinical changes were correlated to maxi-mum plasma levels of THC and its metabolites 11-OH-THC and 11-nor-Δ-9-tetrahydrocannabinol-9-carboxylic acid. Using the TSSL, there was a significant improvement of tics ($p = 0.015$) and obsessive-compulsive behavior ($p = 0.041$) after treatment with Δ-9-THC compared with placebo. Examiner ratings demonstrated a significant difference for the subscore "complex motor tics" ($p = 0.015$) and a trend towards a significant improvement for the subscores "motor tics" ($p = 0.065$), "simple motor tics" ($p = 0.093$), and "vocal tics" ($p = 0.093$). No serious adverse reactions occurred. Five patients experienced mild, transient side effects. There was a significant correlation between tic improvement and maximum 11-OH-THC plasma concentration[CS384].

Toxic effect. Petroleum ether extract of the dried leaf, administered by gastric intubation to pregnant rats at a dose of 150 mg/kg, produced a reduction of food and water consumption and maternal weight gain. The weight of pups at birth was reduced by approx 10% of the litter size, and pup mortality at birth was not affected significantly[CS178]. Water extract of the aerial parts, administered intravenously to male adults, was active[CS042]. The resin, ingested by a 4-year-old girl, showed signs of stupor alternating with brief intervals of excitation and foolish laughing with atactic movements.

Her temperature, blood pressure, pulse, hemoglobin, leukocytes, serum electrolytes, and serum urea were normal. Respiratory rate was 12 beats per minute. Blood sugar elevated. Recovery was complete within 24 hours with no treatment[CS047]. Four patients suffered gastrointestinal disorders and psychological effects after eating salad prepared with hemp seed oil. The concentration of THC in the oil far exceeded the recommended tolerance dose[CS450]. From January 1998 to January 2002, 213 incidences were recorded of dogs that developed clinical signs following oral exposure to cannabis, with 99% having neurological signs and 30% exhibiting gastrointestinal signs. The cannabis ingested ranged from 0.5 to 90 g. The lowest dose at which signs occurred was 84.7 mg/kg and the highest reported dose was 26.8 g/kg. Onset of signs ranged from 5 minutes to 96 hours, with most signs occurring within 1–3 hours after ingestion. The signs lasted from 30 minutes to 96 hours. Management consisted of decontamination, sedation (with diazepam as drug of choice), fluid therapy, thermoregulation, and general supportive care. All followed animals made full recoveries[CS309]. The suspension prepared from the benzene washing solution of cannabis seeds, administered intravenously to mice at a dose of 3 mg/kg, produced hypothermia, catalepsy, pentobarbital-induced sleep prolongation, and suppression of locomotor activity. These pharmacological activities of benzene washing solution of cannabis seeds were significantly higher than those of Δ-9-THC (3 mg/kg, iv)[CS435].

Toxicity assessment. Ethanol (50%) extract of the entire plant, administered intraperitoneally to mice, produced a maximum tolerated dose of 500 mg/kg[CS007].

Transient global amnesia. A 6-year-old boy became intoxicated after ingesting cookies laced with cannabis. He was presented with retentive memory deficit of sudden onset that was later diagnosed as transient global amnesia. Transient global amnesia owing to cannabis intoxication is an extremely rare event[CS266].

Transient ischemic attack. A 22-year-old man with a 5-year history of drug and alcohol abuse was presented with a left hemiparesis preceded by three transient ischemic attacks. Two of the attacks occurred while smoking cannabis. Substance abuse was the only identifiable risk factor for the cerebrovascular disease[CS454].

Trauma injuries. An association between combat-related posttraumatic stress disorder (C-PTSD) and other mental disorders was studied in co-twin (male monozygotic twin pairs in the Vietnam Era Twin Registry). Logistic regression analyses demonstrated that combat exposure, adjusted for C-PTSD, was significantly associated with increased risk for alcohol and cannabis dependence and that C-PTSD mediated the association between combat exposure and both major depression and tobacco dependence[CS325]. Sera from 111 patients with trauma injuries who presented during a 3-month period were screened for blood alcohol. Urine specimens were analyzed for metabolites of cannabis and cocaine. Sixty-two percent of patients were positive for at least one substance and 20% for two or more. Positivity rates were as follows: cannabis, 46%; alcohol, 32% (with 71% of these having blood alcohol levels >80 mg/dL); and cocaine (6%). Substance usage was most prevalent in the third decade of life. The patients who yielded a positive result were significantly younger than those negatives. There was no significant difference in age or substance usage between the victims of interpersonal violence or road traffic accidents. In the group designated "other accidents," patients were significantly older and had a lower incidence of substance usage than the other two groups. Cannabis was the most prevalent substance in all groups. Fifty and 55% of victims of road

accidents and interpersonal violence, respectively, were positive for cannabis compared with 43 and 27% for alcohol, respectively. There was no significant difference in hospital stay or injury severity score between substance users and non-users[CS416].

Trigeminovascular system effect. Arachidonylethanolamide is believed to be the endogenous ligand of the cannabinoid CB1 and CB2 receptors. Known behavioral effects of AEA are antinociception, catalepsy, hypothermia, and depression of motor activity, similar Δ-9-THC, the psychoactive constituent of cannabis. A role of the CB1 receptor in the trigeminovascular system, using intravital to study the effects of AEA against various vasodilator agents was examined. AEA inhibited dural blood vessel dilation brought about by electrical stimulation by 50%, calcitonin gene-related peptide (CGRP) by 30%, capsaicin by 45%, and NO by 40%. CGRP(8–37) attenuated NO-induced dilation by 50%. The AEA inhibition was reversed by the CB1 receptor antagonist AM251. AEA also reduced the blood pressure changes caused by CGRP injection, this effect was not reversed by AM251[CS314].

Tumor-promoting effect. A 28-year-old man who abused alcohol, nicotine, and cannabis for several years was investigated. He suffered simultaneously from a squamous cell carcinoma of the hypopharynx with bilateral cervical metastases, an adenocarcinoma of the transverse colon and a primary hepatocellular carcinoma. There were occurrences of three separate malignant tumors with different histologies in the aerodigestive tract, which could be related to a chronic abuse of cannabis[CS460].

Turning behavior. Cannabinoid agonists: WIN (1–100 ng/mouse), CP-55,940 (0.1–50 ng/mouse), and AEA (0.5–50 ng/mouse), administered unilaterally into the mouse striatum, dose-dependently induced turning behavior. SR 141716A [N-(piperidin-1-yl)-5-(4-chlorophenyl)-1-(2,4-dichlorophenyl)-4-methyl-1H- pyrazole-3-carboxamide hydrochloride], the selective antagonist of CB1 receptor, antagonized the three cannabinoid receptor agonists-induced turning with similar effective dose$_{50}$ (0.13–0.15 mg/kg, intraperitoneally). Spiroperidol (a D2 receptor blocker), (+)-SCH 23390 (a D1 receptor blocker), or prior 6-hydroxy-dopamine lesions of the striatum blocked WIN- and CP-55,940-induced turning, thus suggesting the involvement of DA transmission in cannabinoid-induced turning[CS464].

Tyrosinase inhibition. Methanol (80%) extract of the dried aerial parts, at a concentration of 100 μg/mL, produced weak activity[CS075].

Uterine stimulant effect. Ethanol (50%) extract of the entire plant was inactive on the rat uterus[CS007]. Ethanol (95%) and water extracts of the dried aerial parts, at a concentration of 1:1, produced strong activity on the non-pregnant rat uterus[CS243]. Water extract of the flowering tops produced strong activity on the rat uterus[CS008].

Ventricular septal defect. A Birth Defect Case–Control Study was used to identify 122 isolated simple ventricular septal defect (VSD) cases and 3029 control infants. Exposure data on alcohol, cigarette, and illicit drug use were obtained through standardized interviews with mothers and fathers. Associations between lifestyle factors and VSD were calculated using maternal self-reports; associations were also calculated using paternal proxy reports of the mother's exposures. Maternal self-report of heavy alcohol consumption and paternal proxy report of the mother's moderate alcohol consumption were associated with isolated simple VSD. A twofold increase in risk of isolated simple VSD was identified for maternal self- and paternal proxy-reported cannabis use. Risk of isolated simple VSD increased with regular (≥3 days per week)

cannabis use for both maternal self- and paternal proxy report, although the association was significant only for maternal self-report[CS301].

Visuospatial memory effect. Twenty-five college students who were heavy cannabis smokers (who had smoked a median of 29 of the last 30 days) were compared with 30 light smokers (1 day in the last 30 days). The subjects were tested after a supervised period of abstinence from cannabis and other drugs lasting at least 19 hours. Differences between the overall groups of heavy and light smokers did not reach statistical significance on the four subtests of attention administered. On examining data for the two sexes separately, marked and significant differences were found between heavy- and light-smoking women on the subtest examining visuospatial memory. On this test, subjects were required to examine a 6 × 6 "checkerboard" of squares in which certain squares were shaded. The shaded squares were then erased and the subject was required to indicate with the mouse which squares had formerly been shaded. Increasing numbers of shaded squares were presented at each trial. The heavy-smoking women remembered significantly fewer squares on this test, and they made significantly more errors than the light-smoking women. These differences persisted despite different methods of analysis and consideration for possible confounding variables[CS453].

Weight loss. The dried leaves, administered by gastric intubation to male rats at a dose of 75 mg/kg, was active[CS215].

Wilson's disease. A patient with generalized dystonia owing to Wilson's disease obtained marked improvement in response to smoking cannabis[CS263].

Winiwarter-Buerger disease. Two young men aged 18 and 20 years with juvenile endarteritis were evaluated. Both developed acute distal ischemia of the lower or upper limbs with arteriographic evidence suggestive of Winiwarter-Buerger disease. Both smoked regularly but not excessively, and both used cannabis regularly. In one case, the therapeutic response to withdrawal of cannabis was good. In the second, use of cannabis continued and arterial disease persisted. The main clinical and radiographical features in this condition are the same as in Winiwarter-Buerger disease[CS430].

REFERENCES

CS001 Crombie, L., W. M. L. Crombie and S. V. Jamieson. Isolation of cannabispirsdienone and cannabidihydrophenanthrene. Biosynthetic relationships between the spirans and dihydrostibenes of Thailand. **Tetrahedron Lett** 1979; 1979: 661.

CS002 Ahmad, Y. S. A Note on the Plants of Medicinal Value Found in Pakistan. Government of Pakistan Press, Karachi, 1957.

CS003 Bose, B. C., A. Q. Saifi and A. W. Bhagwat. Studies on pharmacological actions of *Cannabis indica*. Part III. **Arch Int Pharmacodyn Ther** 1964; 147: 291.

CS004 Shoyama, Y., T. Yamauchi and I. Nishioka. Cannabis. V. Cannabigerolic acid monomethyl ether and cannabinolic acid. **Chem Pharm Bull** 1970; 18: 1327–1332.

CS005 Rousinov, K. S. and S. Athanasova-Shopova. Experimental screening of the anticonvulsive activity of certain plants used in popular medicine in Bulgaria. **C R Acad Bulg Sci** 1966; 19: 333–336.

CS006 Krejci, Z., M. Horak and F. Santavy. Constitution of the cannabidiolic acid, M.P.133, isolated from *Cannabis sativa*. **Acta Univ Palacki Olomuc Fac Med** 1958; 16: 9.

CS007 Dhar, M. L., M. M. Dhar, B. N. Mehrotra, and C. Ray. Screening of Indian plants for biological activity. Part I. **Indian J Exp Biol.** 1968; 6: 232–247.

CS008 Barros, G. S. G., F. J. A. Mathos, J. E. V. Vieira, M. P. Sousa and M. C. Medeiros. Pharmacological screening of some Brazilian plants. **J Pharm Pharmacol** 1970; 22: 116.

CS009 Segelman, A. B., F. H. Pettler and N. R. Farnsworth. *Cannabis sativa* (marihuana). A correction of reported thin-layer chromatography data. **Pharm Wkly** 1970; 105: 1360–1362.

CS010 Saha, J. C., E. C. Savini and S. Kasinathan. Ecbolic properties of Indian medicinal plants. Part 1. **Indian J Med Res** 1961; 49: 130-151.

CS011 Berhault, J. Flore Illustree du Senegal II. Govt. Senegal, Min Rural Dev, Water and Forest Div. **Dakar** 1974; 2.

CS012 Dixit, V. P. and N. K. Lohiya. Effects of cannabis extract on the response of accessory sex organs of adult male mice to testosterone. **Indian J Physiol Pharmacol** 1975; 19: 98–100.

CS013 Perrot, E. and P. Hurrier. **Matiere Medicale Et Pharmacopee Sino-Annamites**. Vigot Freres, Edit. Paris, 1907; 292 pp.

CS014 Soubeiran, J. L. and M. D. Thiersant. **La Matiere Medicale Chez les Chinois**. G. Masson, Paris. 1874.

CS015 Anon. **Lilly's Handbook of Pharmacy and Therapeutics**. 5th Rev, Eli Lilly and Co., Indianapolis, IN, 1898.

CS016 Chakravarty, I. and J. J. Ghosh. *Cannabis* and the oestrous cycle of adult rats. **U N Document St/Soa/Ser S/38** 1973; 38.

CS017 De Zeeuw, R. A., T. B. Vree and D. D. Breimer. Cannabivarichromene, a new cannabinoid with a propyl side chain in *Cannabis*. **Experientia** 1973; 29: 260.

CS018 Bercht, C. A. L., R. J. J. C. Lousberg, F. J. F. M. Kuppers, C. A. Salemink, T. B. Vree, and J. M. van Rossum. *Cannabis*: VIII. Identification of cannabinol methyl ether from hashish. **J Chromatogr** 1973; 81: 163.

CS019 Korte, F., M. Haag and U. Claussen. Tetrahydrocannabinol carboxylic acid, a component of hashish. **Angew Chem Int Ed Engl** 1965; 4: 872.

CS020 Van Ginneken, C. A. M., T. B. Vree, D. D. Breimer, H. W. H. Thijssen and J. M. van Rossum. Cannabinodiol, a new hashish constituent, identified by gas chromatography-mass spectrometry. **Proc Int Symp Gas Chromatogr Mass Spectrom** 1972; 1972: 109.

CS021 Min, P. The drugs employed in Chinese medicine as antidiabetica. III.

Experimental investigation on the influence of the drugs employed in Chinese medicine as antidiabetica on the blood sugar of rabbits. **Nippon Yakurigaku Zasshi** 1930; 11(2): 181–187.

CS022 Carlini, E. A. and R. J. Gagliardi. Comparison of the pharmacological actions of crude extracts of *Olmedioperebia calophyllum* and *Cannabis sativa*. **Ancad Bras Cienc** 1970; 42: 409–412.

CS023 Papadakis, D. P., C. M. Michael, T. A. Kephalas and C. J. Miras. Effects of cannabis smoking in blood lactic acid and glucose in humans. **Experientia** 1974; 30(10): 1183–1184.

CS024 Podolsky, S., C. G. Pattavina and M. A. Amaral. Effect of marijuana in the glucose-tolerance test. **Ann N Y Acad Sci** 1971; 191: 54–60.

CS025 Lukas, M. C., and D. M. Temple. Some effects of chronic cannabis treatment. **Aust J Pharm Sci** 1974; 3(1): 20–22.

CS026 El-Feraly, F. S., M. M. El-Sherei and F. J. Al-Muhtadi. Spiro-indans from *Cannabis sativa*. **Phytochemistry** 1986; 25(8): 1992–1994.

CS027 Barrett, M. L., D. Gordon and F. J. Evans. Isolation from *Cannabis sativa* L. of cannflavin—A novel inhibitor of prostaglandin production. **Biochem Pharmacol** 1985; 34(11): 2019–2024.

CS028 Barrett, M. L., A. M. Scutt and F. J. Evans. Cannflavin A and B, prenylated flavones from *Cannabis sativa* L. **Experientia** 1986; 42(4): 452–453.

CS029 Sakakibara, I., T. Katsuhara, Y. Ikeya, K. Hayashi and H. Mitsuhashi. Cannabisin A, an arylnaphthalene lignanamide from fruits of *Cannabis sativa*. **Phytochemistry** 1991; 30(9): 3013–3016.

CS030 Sakakibara, I., Y. Ikeya, K. Hayashi and H. Mitsuhashi. Three phenyldihydronaphthalene lignanamides from fruits of *Cannabis sativa*. **Phytochemistry** 1992; 31(P): 3219–3223.

CS031 Sakakibara, I., Y. Ikeya, K. Hayashi, M. Okada and M. Maruno. Three acyclic bis-phenylpropane lignanamides from fruits of *Cannabis sativa*. **Phytochemistry** 1995; 38(4): 1003–1007.

CS032 Taura, F., S. Morimoto and Y. Shoyama. Cannabinerolic acid, a cannab-

inoid from *Cannabis sativa*. **Phytochemistry** 1995; 39(2): 457–458.

CS033 Barik, B. R., A. K. Dey and A. B. Kundu. Chemical constituents of *Cannabis sativa*. **J Indian Chem Soc** 1997; 74(8): 652.

CS034 Zagari, A. Medicinal Plants. Vol 4, 5th Ed., Tehran University Publications, No 1810/4, Tehran, Iran, 1992; 4: 969 pp.

CS035 Li, H. L. The origin and use of cannabis in Eastern Asia. Linguistic-cultural implications. **Econ Bot** 1974; 28: 293.

CS036 Hendriks, H., T. M. Malingre, S. Batterman and R. Bos. Mono- and sesqui-terpene hydrocarbons of the essential oil of *Cannabis sativa*. **Phytochemistry** 1975; 14: 814–815.

CS037 Thorburn, M. J. Jamaican bushes and human chromosomes. **Jamaica J** 1975; 8(4): 18.

CS038 Latta, R. P. and B. J. Eaton. Seasonal fluctuations in cannabinoid content of Kansas marijuana. **Econ Bot** 1975; 29: 153.

CS039 Turner, C. E. Active substances in marijuana. **Arch Invest Med (Mex)** 1974; 5S: 135.

CS040 Rasmussen, K. E. and J. J. Herweijer. Examination of the cannabinoids in young cannabis plants. **Pharm Weekl** 1975; 110: 91.

CS041 Paris, M., F. Boucher and L. Cosson. Importance of propyl compounds in cannabis originating in South Africa. **Plant Med Phytother** 1975; 9: 136.

CS042 Payne, R. J. and S. N. Brand. The toxicity of intravenously used marihuana. **JAMA** 1975; 233: 351.

CS043 Stromberg, L. Minor components of *Cannabis* resin: V. Mass spectrometric data and gas chromatographic retention times of cannabinoid components with retention times shorter than that of cannabidiol. **J Chromatogr** 1974; 96: 179.

CS044 Turner, C. E., K. W. Hadley, J. H. Holley, S. Billets and M. L. Mole, Jr. Constituents of *Cannabis sativa*. VIII. Possible biological application of a new method to separate cannabidiol and cannabichromene. **J Pharm Sci** 1975; 64: 810.

CS045   Alessandro, A., F. Mari and G. Mazzi. Rapid method for the identification of the active principles of *Cannabis* by circular thin-layer chromatography. **Boll Chim Farm** 1975; 114: 21.

CS046   Lee, C. K. Constituents of Korean cannabis. **Yakhak Hoe Chi** 1973; 17: 21.

CS047   Bro, P., J. Schou and G. Topp. Cannabis poisoning with analytical verification. **N Engl J Med** 1975; 293: 1049.

CS048   Wheals, B. B. and R. N. Smith. Comparative cannabis analysis. A comparison of high-pressure liquid chromatography with other chromatographic techniques. **J Chromatogr** 1975; 105: 396–400.

CS049   Turner, C. E., P. S. Fetterman, K. W. Hadley and J. E. Urbanek. Constituents of *Cannabis sativa*. X. Cannabinoid profile of a Mexican variant and its possible correlation to pharmacological activity. **Acta Pharm Jugosl** 1975; 25: 7.

CS050   Slatkin, D. J., J. E. Knapp, P. L. Schiff, Jr., C. E. Turner and M. L. Mole, Jr. Steroids of *Cannabis sativa* root. **Phytochemistry** 1975; 14: 580-581.

CS051   El-Feraly, F. S. and C. E. Turner. Alkaloids of *Cannabis sativa* leaves. **Phytochemistry** 1975; 14: 2304–2305.

CS052   Sofia, R. D., H. B. Vassar and L. C. Knobloch. Comparative analgesic activity of various naturally occurring cannabinoids in mice and rats. **Psychopharmacologia** 1975; 40: 285.

CS053   Malingre, T., H. Hendriks, S. Batterman, R. Bos, and J. Visser. The essential oil of *Cannabis sativa*. **Planta Med** 1975; 28: 56.

CS054   Zamir-Ul Hag, M., S. J. Rose, L. R. Deiderich and A. R. Patel. Identification and quantitative measurement of some n-heterocyclics in marijuana smoke condensates. **Anal Chem** 1974; 46: 1781.

CS055   Smith, R. N. High-pressure liquid chromatography after injection of solid plant material and cold trapping. **J Chromatogr** 1975; 115: 101.

CS056   Shani, A. and R. Mechoulam. Cannabielsoic acids: Isolation and synthesis by a novel oxidative cyclization. **Tetrahedron** 1974; 30: 2437.

CS057   Coffman, C. B. and W. A. Gentner. *Cannabis sativa*. Effect of drying time and temperature on cannabinoid profile of stored leaf tissue. **Bull Nar** 1974; 26(1): 67.

CS058   Dwivedi, C. and R. D. Harbison. Anticonvulsant activities of delta-8- and delta-9-tetrahydrocannabinol and uridine. **Toxicol Appl Pharmacol** 1975; 31: 452.

CS059   Romanenko, V. I. Changes in the physical and biochemical properties of hemp seeds during storage. **Tr Vses Nauchno Issled Inst Lum Kuit** 1974; 35: 80.

CS060   Der Marderosian, A. H. and S. N. S. Murthy. Analysis of old samples of *Cannabis sativa*. **J Forensic Sci** 1974; 19: 670.

CS061   Sallan, S. E., N. E. Zinberg and E. Frei. Antiemetic effect of delta-9-tetrahydrocannabinol in patients receiving cancer chemotherapy. **N Engl J Med** 1975; 293: 795–797.

CS062   Bercht, C. A. L. and M. R. Paris. Oil of *Cannabis sativa*. **Bull Tech Gattefosse Sfpa** 1973; 68: 87.

CS063   Rasmussen, K. E. Quantitative determination of heptacosane and nonacosane in Norwegian-grown cannabis plants. **Medd Nor Farm Selsk** 1975; 37: 128.

CS064   Turner, C. E., K. W. Hadley, J. Henry and M. L. Mole, Jr. Constituents of *Cannabis sativa* L. VII: Use of sialyl derivatives in routine analysis. **J Pharm Sci** 1974; 63: 1872–1876.

CS065   Clark, S. C., C. Greene, G. W. Karr, K. L. Mac Cannell and S. L. Milstein. Cardiovascular effects of marihuana in man. **Can J Physiol Pharmacol** 1974; 52: 706.

CS066   Le Vander, S., M. Binder, S. Agurell, A. Bader-Bartfai, B. Gustafsson, K. Leander, J. E. Lindgren, A. Olsson and B. Tobisson. Pharmacokinetics in relation to physiological effects of delta-8-thc (delta-8-thiocarbanidin). **Acta Pharm Suesica** 1974; 11: 662.

CS067   Paris, M., F. Boucher and L. Cosson. The constituents of *Cannabis sativa* pollen. **Econ Bot** 1975; 29: 245-253.

CS068   Hanus, L. The present state of knowledge in the chemistry of substances of *Cannabis sativa*. III. Terpenoid substances. **Acta Univ Palacki Olomuc Fac Med** 1975; 73: 233.

CS069 Stromberg, L. Minor components of cannabis resin. IV. Mass spectrometric data and gas chromatographic retention times of terpenic components with retention times shorter than that of cannabidiol. **J Chromatogr** 1974; 96: 99.

CS070 Hanus, L. The present state of knowledge in the chemistry of substances of *Cannabis sativa*. IV. Nitrogen containing compounds. **Acta Univ Palacki Olomuc Fac Med** 1975; 73: 241.

CS071 Takatsuto, S. R., H. Y. Abe, T. K. Yokota, K. Y. Shimada and K. J. Gamoh. Identification of castasterone and teasterone in seeds on *Cannabis sativa* L. **Nihon Yukagakkaishi** 1996; 45(9): 871–873.

CS072 Kausar, W., A. Muhammad and I. Ul-Haq. Effect of cannabis on intraocular pressure. **Pak J Pharmacol** 1995; 12(2): 43–48.

CS073 Morimoto, S., K. Komatsu, F. Taura and Y. Shoyama. Enzymological evidence for cannabichromenic acid biosynthesis. **J Nat Prod** 1997; 60(8): 854–857.

CS074 Smith, R. M. Identification of butyl cannabinoids in marijuana. **J Forensic Sci** 1997; 42(4): 610–618.

CS075 Shin, N. H., K. S. Lee, S. H. Kang, K. R. Min, S. H. Lee and Y. S. Kim. Inhibitory effects of herbal extracts on dopa oxidase activity of tyrosinase. **Nat Prod Sci** 1997; 3(2): 111–121.

CS076 Takasuto, S., T. Kawashima, T. Noguchi, S. Fujioka and A. Sakurai. Identification of teasterone and phytosterols in the lipid fraction from seeds of *Cannabis sativa* L. **Nihon Yukagakkaishi** 1997; 46(12): 1499–1504.

CS077 Takasuto, S. and T. Kawashima. Identification of 24-methyl-5-alpha-cholestan-3-one and 24-methylcholest-4-en-3-one in the seeds of *Cannabis sativa* L. **Nihon Yukagakkaishi** 1998; 47(8): 783–786.

CS078 Graham, J. D. P., B. H. Davies, A. Seaton and R. M. Weatherstone. Bronchodilator action of extract of cannabis and delta-1-tetrahydrocannabinol. Pharmacol Marihuana Braude MC Szara S (Eds) Raven Press New York 1976; 1: 269–276.

CS079 Chan, W. R., K. E. Magnus and H. A. Watson. The structure of cannabitriol. **Experientia** 1976; 32: 283.

CS080 Ottersen, T., A. Aasen, F. S. El-Feraly and C. E. Turner. X-ray structure of cannabispiran: A novel cannabis constituent. **Chem Commun** 1976; 1976; 580.

CS081 Wold, J. K. and A. Hillestad. The demonstration of galactosamine in a higher plant: *Cannabis sativa*. **Phytochemistry** 1976; 15: 325B–326B.

CS082 Krishnamurty, H. G. and R. Kaushal. Free sugars & cyclitols of Indian marihuana (*Cannabis sativa*). **Indian J Chem** 1976; 14B: 639.

CS083 Itokawa, H., K. Takeya and M. Akasu. Studies on the constituents isolated from the callus of *Cannabis sativa*. **Shoyakugaku Zasshi** 1975; 29: 106–112.

CS084 Stromberg, L. Minor components of cannabis resin. VI. Mass spectrometric data and gas chromatographic retention times of components eluted after cannabinol. **J Chromatogr** 1976; 121: 313.

CS085 Turner, C. E., M. F. H. Hsu, J. E. Knapp, P. L. Schiff, Jr. and D. J. Slatkin. Isolation of cannabisativine, an alkaloid from *Cannabis sativa* root. **J Pharm Sci** 1976; 65: 1084.

CS086 Tatkon, M. The practice of a Jaipur midwife. **Ethnomedicine** 1976; 2; 59.

CS087 Wright, P. L., S. H. Smith, M. L. Keplinger, J. C. Calandra and M. C. Braude. Reproductive and teratologic studies with delta 9-tetrahydrocannabinol and crude marijuana extract. **Toxicol Appl Pharmacol** 1976; 38: 223.

CS088 Novotny, M., M. L. Lee and K. D. Bartle. A possible chemical basis for the higher mutagenicity of marijuana smoke as compared to tobacco smoke. **Experientia** 1976; 32: 280.

CS089 Liu, T. C., Y. Zhang, G. Liu and J. Chen. Determination of delta 9-tetrahydrocannabinol, cannabinol, and cannabinol in Xinjiang cannabis plant by GC. **Chung Ts'ao Yao** 1992; 23(9): 463–464.

CS090 Bhattarai, N. K. Folk use of plants in veterinary medicine in Central Nepal. **Fitoterapia** 1992; 63(6): 497–506.

CS091 Elsohly, H. N. and C. E. Turner. Constituents of *Cannabis sativa* L. XXII:

Isolation of spiro-indan and dihydro-stilbene compounds from a Panamanian variant grown in Mississippi, United States of America. **Bull Nar** 1982; 34(2): 51–56.

CS092 Sakakibara, I., H. Mihashi, T. Fujihashi and A. Okuma. Antitumor agents containing N-(P-coumaroyl)tyramine. Patent-Japan Kokai Tokkyo Koho—04 1992; 26, 622: 6 pp.

CS093 Sakakibara, I., H. Mihashi, J. Hayashi and M. Chin. Novel liganamides and protease inhibitors-containing them. Patent-Japan Kokai Tokkyo Koho—05 1993; 25,110: 10 pp.

CS094 Kurokawa, M., H, Ochiai, K. Nagasaka, M. Neki, H. X. Xu, S. Kadota, S. Sutardio, T. Matsumoto, T. Namba and K. Shiraki. Antiviral traditional medicines against herpes simplex virus (HSV-1), poliovirus, and Measles virus *in vitro* and their therapeutic efficacies for HSV-1 infection in mice. **Antiviral Res** 1993; 22(2/3): 175–188.

CS095 Makler, M. T. The effect of cocaine on the growth of *Plasmodium falciparum in vitro*. **Trans Roy Soc Trop Med Hyg** 1994; 88(4): 444.

CS096 Singh, J., A. K. Dubey and N. N. Tripathi. Antifungal activity of *Mentha spicata*. **Int J Pharmacog** 1994; 32(4): 314–319.

CS097 El-Fickey, M. S., A. A. El-Tomey and S. F. Mahmoud. Effect of cannabis on gastric secretion and on stress-induced gastric ulcers in albino rats. **Exp Clin Gastroenterol** 1993; 3(1): 55–58.

CS098 Singh, K. K. and J. K. Maheshwari. Traditional phytotherapy of some medicinal plants used by the Tharus of the Nainital District, Uttar Pradesh, India. **Int J Pharmacog** 1994; 32(1): 51–58.

CS099 Anis, M. and M. Iqbal. Medicinal plantlore of Aligarh, India. **Int J Pharmacog** 1994; 32(1): 59–64.

CS100 Bhattarai, N. K. Folk herbal remedies for gynaecological complaints in central Nepal. **Int J Pharmacog** 1994; 32(1): 13–26.

CS101 Kim, S. Y., J. H. Kim, S. K. Kim, M. J. Oh and M. Y. Jung. Antioxidant activities of selected Oriental herb extracts. **J Amer Oil Chem Soc** 1994; 71(6): 633–640.

CS102 Hammond, C. T. and P. G. Mahlberg. Phloroglucinol glucoside as a natural constituent of *Cannabis sativa*. **Phytochemistry** 1994; 37(3): 755–756.

CS103 Kataoka, M. and Y. Takagaki. Effect of the crude drugs (standards of natural drugs not in the J. P. XII) on beta-hexosaminidase release from rat basophilic leukemia (RBL-2H3) cells. **Nat Med** 1995; 49(3): 346–349.

CS104 Bhattarai, N. K. Folk anthelmintic drugs of Central Nepal. **Int J Pharmacol** 1992; 30(2): 145–150.

CS105 Manandhar, N. P. Herbal remedies of Surkhet District, Nepal. **Fitoterapia** 1993; 64(3): 266–272.

CS106 Giron, L. M., V. Freire, A. Alonzo and A. Caceres. Ethnobotanical survey of the medicinal flora used by the Caribs of Guatemala. **J Ethnopharmacol** 1991; 34(2/3): 173–187.

CS107 Simon, C. and M. Lamla. Merging pharmacopoeia: Understanding the historical origins of incorporative pharmacopoeial processes among Xhosa healers in Southern Africa. **J Ethnopharmacol** 1991; 33(3): 237–242.

CS108 Singh, V. K., Z. A. Ali and M. K. Siddioui. Ethnomedicines in the Bahraich District of Uttar Pradesh, India. **Fitoterapia** 1996; 67(1): 65–76.

CS109 Li, H. L. Hallucinogenic plants in Chinese herbals. **Bot Mus Leafl Harv Univ** 1977; 25(6): 161–181.

CS110 Bhattarai, N. K. Medical ethnobotany in the Rapti Zone, Nepal. **Fitoterapia** 1993; 64(6): 483–493.

CS111 Bellakhdar, J., R. Claisse, J. Fleurentin and C. Younos. Repertory of standard herbal drugs in the Moroccan pharmacopoeia. **J Ethnopharmacol** 1991; 35(2): 123–143.

CS112 Duke, J. A. and E. S. Ayensu. Medicinal Plants of China. Reference Publications, Inc. Algonac, Michigan 1985; 1(4): 52–361.

CS113 Leporatti, M. L. and E. Lattanzi. Traditional phytotherapy on coastal areas on Makran (Southern Pakistan). **Fitoterapia** 1994; 65(2): 158–161.

CS114 Smith, R. M. and K. D. Kempfert. Delta-1-3,4-cis-tetrahydrocannabinol in Cannabis sativa. **Phytochemistry** 1977; 16: 1088–1089.

CS115 Uliss, D. B., G. R. Handrick, H. C. Dalzell and R. K. Razdan. A novel cannabinoid containing a 1,8-cineol moiety. **Experientia** 1977; 33: 577.

CS116 Smith, R. N., L. V. Jones, J. S. Brennan and C. G. Vaughan. Identification of hexadecanamide in cannabis resin. **J Pharm Pharmacol** 1977; 29(2): 126–127.

CS117 Diaz, J. L. Ethnopharmacology of sacred psychoactive plants used by the Indians of Mexico. **Ann Rev Pharmacol Toxicol** 1977; 17: 647.

CS118 El Sohly, M. A., F. S. El-Feraly and C. E. Turner. Isolation and characterization of (+)-cannabitriol and (-)-10-ethoxy-9-hydroxy-delta 6A(10A)-tetrahydrocannabinol: Two new cannabinoids from *Cannabis sativa* L. extract. **Lloydia** 1977; 40(3): 275.

CS119 Hillestad, A., J. K. Wold and T. Engen. Water-soluble glycoproteins from *Cannabis sativa* (Thailand). **Phytochemistry** 1977; 16: 1953–1956.

CS120 Feeney, D. M. Marihuana and epilepsy. **Science** 1977; 197: 1301.

CS121 Segelman, A. B., F. P. Segelman, S. D. Varma, H. Wagner and O. Seligmann. *Cannabis sativa* L. (marijuana) IX. Lens aldose reductase inhibitory activity of marijuana flavone c-glycosides. **J Pharm Sci** 1977; 66(9): 1358–1359.

CS122 Sethi, V. K., M. P. Jain and R. S. Thakur. Chemical investigation of wild *Cannabis sativa* roots. **Planta Med Suppl** 1977; 32: 378–379.

CS123 Lewis, W. H. and M. P. F. Elvin-Lewis. **Medical Botany**. Wiley-Interscience, New York, 1977.

CS124 Bercht, C. A. L., J. P. C. M. Van Dongen, W. Heerman, R. J. J. C. Lousberg and F. J. E. M. Kuppers. Cannabispirone and cannabispirenone, two naturally occurring spiro-compounds. **Tetrahedron** 1976; 32: 2939.

CS125 Rana, T. S. and B. Datt. Ethnobotanical observation among Jaunsar-Bawar, Dehra Dun (J. P.), India. **Int J Pharmacog** 1997; 35(5): 371–374.

CS126 Matsunaga, T., K. Watanabe, H. Yoshimura and I. Yamamoto. Quantitative analysis and pharmaco-toxicity of cannabinoids in commercially available cannabis seeds. **Yakugaku Zasshi** 1998; 118(9): 408–414.

CS127 Rajurkar, N. S. and B. M. Pardeshi. Analysis of some herbal plants from India used in the control of diabetes mellitus by NAA and AAS techniques. **Appl Radiat Isot** 1997; 48(8): 1059–1062.

CS128 Toda, M., J. Kawabata and T. Kasai. Alpha-glucosidase inhibitors from glove (*Syzygium aromaticum*). **Biosci Biotech Biochem** 2000; 64(2): 294–298.

CS129 Duncan, A. C., A. K. Jager and J. Van Staden. Screening of Zulu medicinal plants for angiotensin converting enzyme (ACE) inhibitors. **J Ethnopharmacol** 1999; 68(1/3): 63–70.

CS130 Rifka, S. M., M. Sauer, R. L. Hawks, G. B. Cutler and D. L. Loriaux. Marijuana as an estrogen. Proc Endocrine Soc 60th Ann Mtg, Miami Beach, Florida, June 14-16, 1978; 1978: 200.

CS131 Segelman, A. B., F. P. Segelman, A. E. Star, H. Wagner and O. Seligmann. *Cannabis sativa*. Part 8. Structure of two-c-diglycosylflavones from *Cannabis sativa*. **Phytochemistry** 1978; 17: 824–826.

CS132 Grote, H. and G. Spiteller. New cannabinoids. II. **J Chromatogr** 1978; 154: 13.

CS133 Gigliano, G. S. Cannabinols in *Cannabis sativa* L. under different cultivation conditions. **Bull Chem Farm** 1984; 123(7): 352–356.

CS134 Lawi-Berger, C. and I. Kapetanidis. Chemotaxonomic study of cannabis (Cannabaceae). Part 2. Quantitative analysis of fatty acids in hemp seeds of *Cannabis sativa* L. **Pharm Acta Helv** 1983; 58(3): 79–81.

CS135 El-Sherei, M. M. and F. S. El-Feraly. New spiroindans from cannabis. Abstr Internat Res Cong Nat Prod Coll Univ Univ N Carolina Chapel Hill NC July 7-12 1985 1985; ABSTR–56.

CS136 El Sohly, M. A., J. H. Holley and C. E. Turner. Constituents of *Cannabis sativa* L. XXVI. The delta-9-tetrahydrocannabinol content of confiscated marijuana, 1974-1983. **Proc Oxford Symp** Cannabis 1985; 1984: 37-42.

CS137 Morita, M. and II. Ando. Analysis of hashish oil by gas chromatography / mass spectrometry. **Kagaku Keisatsu Kenkyusho Hokoku Hokagaku Hen** 1984; 37(2): 137–140.

CS138   Hodges, L. C., H. M Deutsch, K. Green and L. H. Zalkow. Polysaccharides from *Cannabis sativa* active in lowering intraocular pressure. **Carbohydr Polym** 1985; 5(2): 141–154.

CS139   Kubo, M., H. Matsuda, M. Fukui and Y. Nakai. Development studies of cuticle drugs from natural resources. I. Effects of crude drug extracts on hair growth in mice. **Yakugaku Zasshi** 1988; 108(10): 971–978.

CS140   Formukong, E. A., A. T. Evans and F. J. Evans. Analgesic and antiinflammatory activity of constituents of *Cannabis sativa* L. **Inflammation (NY)** 1988; 12(4): 361–371.

CS141   Sethi, N., P. K. Agnihotri and S. Srivastava. Aminopyrine-n-demethylase activity of rat liver after administration of crude cannabis extract. **Indian J Med Res** 1989; 90(1): 36–38.

CS142   Deutsch, H. M., K. Green and L. H. Zalkow. Water soluble high molecular weight components from plants with potent intraocular pressure lowering activity. **Curr Eye Res** 1987; 6(7): 949–950.

CS143   Shah, N. C. and S. K. Jain. Ethnomedico-botany of the Kumaon Himalaya, India. **Social Pharmacol** 1988; 2(4): 359–380.

CS144   Sato, A. Studies on anti-tumor activity of crude drugs. 1. The effects of aqueous extracts of some crude drugs in short-term screening test. **Yakugaku Zasshi** 1989; 109(6): 407–423.

CS145   Ilanus, L. and K. Tesarik. Capillary gas chromatography of natural substances from *Cannabis sativa* L. III. Content of cannabinoids in dried roots. **Acta Univ Palacki Olomuc Fac Med** 1987; 116: 31–35.

CS146   Hanus, L., C. E. Turner and M. A. El Sohly. Isolation and identification of propylcannabinoids from Soviet variety of hemp grown in Mississippi. **Acta Univ Palacki Olomuc Fac Med** 1987; 116: 25–30.

CS147   Vidal, C., R. Fuente, A. Iglesias and A. Saez. Bronchial asthma due to *Cannabis sativa* seed. **Allergy** 1991; 46(8): 647–650.

CS148   Matsunaga, T., H. Nagatomo, I. Yamamoto and H. Yoshimura. Qualitative and quantitative analyses of cannabinoids in cannabis seeds. **Hochudoku** 1990; 8(2): 88–89.

CS149   Matsunaga, T., K. Watanabe, I. Yamamoto and H. Yoshimura. Analyses of nitrogenous constituents in *Cannabis sativa* L. **Hochudoku** 1991; 9(2): 122–123.

CS150   Grote, H. and G. Spitteler. New cannabinoids. III. The structure of cannabicoumaronone. **Tetrahedron** 1978; 34: 3207.

CS151   Kanter, S. L., M. R. Musumeci and L. E. Hollister. Quantitative determination of delta9-tetrahydrocannabinol and delta9-tetrahydrocannabinolic acid in marihuana by high-pressure liquid chromatography. **J Chromatogr** 1979; 171: 504.

CS152   Fournier, G., M. R. Paris, M. C. Fourniat and A. M. Quero. Bacteriostatic effect of essential oil from *Cannabis sativa*. **Ann Pharm Fr** 1978; 36: 603.

CS153   Cutler, M. G., J. H. Mackintosh and M. R. A. Chance. Cannabis resin and sexual behaviour in the laboratory mouse. **Psychopharmacologia** 1975; 45: 129.

CS154   Burton, T. A. Urinary retention following cannabis ingestion. **JAMA** 1979; 242: 351.

CS155   Kettenes-Van Den Bosch, J. J. and C. A. Salemink. Cannabis. XIX. Oxygenated 1,2-diphenylethanes from marihuana. **Recl Trav Chim Pays-Bas** 1978; 97: 221–222.

CS156   Hendriks, H., T. M. Malingre, S. Batterman and R. Bos. The essential oils of *Cannabis sativa*. **Pharm Weekl** 1978; 113: 413–424.

CS157   Crombie, L. and W. M. L. Crombie. Dihydrostilbenes of Thailand cannabis. **Tetrahedron Lett** 1978; 1978: 4711–4714.

CS158   El Sohly, M. A., E. G. Boeren and C. E. Turner. (DL)-9-10-dihydroxy-delta-6(A)(10A)-tetrahydrocannabinol and (DL)-8,9-dihydroxy-delta-6(A)(10A)-tetrahydrocannabinol. Two new cannabinoids from *Cannabis sativa* L. **Experientia** 1978; 34: 1127–1128.

CS159   Burstein, S., P. Taylor, F. S. El-Feraly and C. E. Turner. Prostaglandins and cannabis—V. Identification of para-vinylphenol as a potent inhibitor of prostaglandin synthesis. **Biochem Pharmacol** 1976; 25: 2003–2004.

CS160 Mendelson, J. H., J. Ellingboe and J. C. Kuehnle. Effects of alcohol and marihuana on plasma luteinizing hormone and testosterone. **Probl Drug Depend** 1976; 1976: 525–537.

CS161 Ayensu, E. S. Medicinal Plants of the West Indies. Unpublished Manuscript 1978; 110 pp.

CS162 Okey, A. B. and G. P. Bondy. Is delta-9-tetrahydrocannabinol estrogenic? Comments. **Science** 1977; 195: 904–905.

CS163 Soni, C. M. and M. L. Gupta. Effect of cannabis (bhang) extract on blood glucose and liver glycogen in albino rats. **Indian J Physiol Pharmacol** 1978; 22: 152–154.

CS164 Hembree III, W. C., G. G. Nahas, P. Zeidenberg and H. F. S. Huang. Changes in human spermatozoa associated with high dose marihuana smoking. **Adv Biosci** 1979; 1979: 429–439.

CS165 Boeren, E. G., M. A. El Sohly and C. E. Turner. Cannabiripsol: A novel cannabis constituent. **Experientia** 1979; 35: 1278–1279.

CS166 Waddell, T. G., H. Jones and A. L. Keith. Legendary chemical aphrodisiacs. **J Chem Ed** 1980; 57; 341–342.

CS167 Cozens, D. D., R. Clark, A. K. Palmer, N. Hardy, G. G. Nahas and D. J. Harvey. The effect of a crude marihuana extract on embryonic and fetal development of the rabbit. **Adv Biosci Marihuana Biological Effects** 1978; 22: 469–477.

CS168 Fujimoto, G. I., A. B. Kostellow, R. Rosenbaum, G. A. Morrill and E. Bloch. Effects of cannabinoids on reproductive organs in the female Fischer rat. **Adv Biosci Marihuana Biological Effects** 1978; 22: 441–447.

CS169 Tucakov, J. Ethnophytotherapy of diabetes. **Srp Arh Celok Lek** 1978; 106: 159–173.

CS170 Kostellow, A. B., D. Ziegler, J. Kunar, G. I. Fujimoto and G. A. Morrill. Effect of cannabinoids on estrous cycle, ovulation, and reproduction capacity of female A/J mice. **Pharmacology** 1980; 21: 68–75.

CS171 Gawin, F. H. Drugs and Eros: Reflection on aphrodisiacs. **J Psychodelic Drugs** 1978; 10: 227–236.

CS172 Turner, C. E., M. A. El Sohly and E. G. Boeren. Constituents of Cannabis sativa L. XVII. A review of the natural constituents. **J Nat Prod** 1980; 43(2): 169–234.

CS173 Dixit, V. P. Effects of Cannabis sativa extract on testicular function of Presbytis entellus. **Planta Med** 1981; 41: 288–294.

CS174 Dixit, V. P., M. Arya and N. K. Lohiya. The effect of chronically administered cannabis extract on the female genital tract of mice and rats. **Endokrinologie** 1975; 66: 365–368.

CS175 Chakravarty, I. and D. Sengupta. Effect of cannabis extract on uterine phosphatase activities in prepubertal rats. **IRCS Med Sci Biochem** 1980; 8:25.

CS176 Rizvi, S. J. H., D. Mukerji and S. N. Mathur. A new report of some possible source of natural herbicide. **Indian J Exp Biol** 1980; 18: 777–781.

CS177 Chen, Y. J., C. H. Yu, S. S. Wang, J. Che, Y. Y. Kuo, W. S. Chen, Y. P. Cheng, Y. L. Liu and S. S. Yiu. Studies on the active principles in leaves of Cannabis sativa. **Chung Ts'ao Yao** 1981; 12(3): 44.

CS178 Abel, E. L., B. A. Dintcheff and N. Day. Effects of marihuana on pregnant rats and their offspring. **Psychopharmacology (Berlin)** 1980; 71: 71–74.

CS179 Yotoriyama, M., I. Ito, D. Takashima, Y. Shoyama and I. Nishioka. Plant breeding of cannabis. Determination of cannabinoids by high-pressure liquid chromatography. **Yakugaku Zasshi** 1980; 100: 611–614.

CS180 Turner, C. E. and H. N. El Sohly. Iso-cannabispiran, a new spiro-compound isolated from a Panamanian variant of Cannabis sativa L. Abstr Joint Meeting American Society of Pharmacognosy and Society for Economic Botany Boston July 13-17 1981: 14.

CS181 Nahas, G. G. Marijuana and sex. **Med Aspects Human Sexuality** 1981; 15(12): 30–39.

CS182 Crombie, L., W. M. L. Crombie and S. V. Jamieson. Extractives of Thailand cannabis: Synthesis of canniprene and isolation of new geranylated and prenylated chrysoeriols. **Tetrahedron Lett** 1980; 21: 3607–3610.

CS183　Dalterio, S., F. Badr, A. Bartke and D. Mayfield. Cannabinoids in male mice: Effects on fertility and spermatogenesis. **Science** 1982; 216: 315–316.

CS184　Dixit, V. P., M. Arya and N. K. Lohiya. Mechanism of action of chronically administered cannabis extract on the female genital tract of gerbils. **Indian J Physiol Pharmacol** 1976; 20: 38–41.

CS185　Crombie, L. and W. M. L. Crombie. Natural products of Thailand high delta-1-THC-strain cannabis. The bibenzyl-spiran-dihydrophenanthrene group: Relations with cannabinoids and canniflavones. **J Chem Soc Perkin Trans I** 1982; 1982: 1455–1466.

CS186　Hong, C. Y., D. M. Chaput de Saintonge, P. Turner and J. W. Fairbairn. Comparison of the inhibitory action of delta-9-tetrahydrocannabinol and petroleum spirit extract of herbal cannabis on human sperm motility. **Human Toxicol** 1982; 1: 151–154.

CS187　Lares, A., Y. Ochoa, A. Bolanos, N. Aponte and M. Montenegro. Effects of the resin and smoke condensate of *Cannabis sativa* on the oestrous cycle of the rat. **Bull Nar** 1981; 33(3): 55–61.

CS188　Heitrich, A. and M. Binder. Identification of (3R,4R)-delta-1-(6)-tetrahydrocannabinol as an isolation artifact of cannabinoid acids formed by callus cultures of *Cannabis sativa* L. **Experientia** 1982; 38: 898–899.

CS189　Frischknecht, H. R., B. Sieber and P. G. Waser. Effects of multiple, chronic and early hashish exposure on mating behavior, nest-building, and gestation in mice. **Comp Biochem Physiol** 1982; 77: 363–368.

CS190　El-Zawahri, M. M. and A. F. Khishin. Mutagenic effect of cannabis. **Adv Genet Dev Evol Drosophila (7th Proc Eur** *Drosophila* **Res Conf)** 1982; 1982: 101–107.

CS191　Green, K., L. H. Zalkow, H. M. Deutsch, M. E. Yablonski, N. Oliver, C. M. Symonds and R. D. Elijah. Ocular and systemic responses to watersoluble material. **Curr Eye Res** 1981; 1(2): 65–75.

CS192　Shah, N. C. Herbal folk medicines in Northern India. **J Ethnopharmacol** 1982; 6(3): 293–301.

CS193　Lal, S. D. and B. K. Yadav. Folk medicine of Kurushetra District (Haryana), India. **Econ Bot** 1983; 37(3): 299–305.

CS194　Mc Phail, A. T., H. N. El Sohly, C. E. Turner and M. A. El Sohly. Stereochemical assignments for the two enantiomeric pairs of 9,10-dihydroxy-delta-6-alpha(10-alpha)-tetrahydrocannabinols. X-ray crystal structure analysis of (DL)-trans-cannabitriol. Abstr 24th Annual Meeting American society of Pharmacognosy Univ Mississippi Oxford July 24–28 1983: ABSTR–50.

CS195　Papadakis, D. P., C. A. Salemink, F. J. Alikaridis and T. A. Kephalas. Isolation and identification of new cannabinoids in cannabis smoke. **Tetrahedron** 1983; 39(13): 2223–2225.

CS196　Lemberkovics, E., P. Veszki, G. Verzar-Petri and A. Trka. Study on sesquiterpenes of the essential oil in the inflorescence and leaves of *Cannabis sativa* L. var. **Mexico Sci Pharm** 1981; 49: 401–408.

CS197　Zhu, R. K., M. S. Zhou, B. J. Lee and L. Lee. Clinical study on the treatment of psoriasis with "ke-yin" (anti-psoriasis) prescription. **Chung I Tsa Chih** 1981; 22(4): 22–24.

CS198　Morrison, E. Y. S. A. and M. West. A preliminary study of the effects of some West Indian medicinal plants on blood sugar levels in the dog. **West Indian Med J** 1982; 31: 194–197.

CS199　Morimoto, I., F. Watanabe, T. Osawa, T. Okitsu and T. Kada. Mutagenicity screening of crude drugs with *Bacillus subtilis* rec-assay and *Salmonella*/microsome reversion assay. **Mutat Res** 1982; 97: 81–102.

CS200　Vijayalakshimi, K., S. D. Mishra and S. K. Prasad. Nematicidal properties of some indigenous plant materials against second stage juveniles of *Meloidogyne incognita* (Koffoid and White) Chitwood. **Indian J Entomol** 1979; 41(4): 326–331.

CS201　Rouquayrol, M. Z., M. C. Fonteles, J. E. Alencar, F. Jose De Abreu Matos and A. A. Craveiro. Molluscicidal activity of essential oils from Northeastern Brazilian plants. **Rev Brasil Pesq Med Biol** 1980; 13: 135–143.

CS202 El-Feraly, F. S. Isolation, characterization and synthesis of 3,5,4'-trihydroxybibenzyl from *Cannabis sativa*. **J Nat Prod** 1984; 47(1): 89–92.

CS203 Mc Phail, A. T., H. N. El Sohly, C. E. Turner and M. A. El Sohly. Stereochemical assignments for the two enantiomeric pairs of 9,10-dihydroxy-delta-6A(10A)-tetrahydrocannabinols. X-ray crystal structure analysis of DL-trans-cannabitriol. **J Nat Prod** 1984; 47(1): 138–142.

CS204 El Sohly, H. N., G. E. Ma, C. E. Turner and M. A. El Sohly. Constituents of *Cannabis sativa*. XXV. Isolation of two new dihydrostilbenes from a Panamanian variant. **J Nat Prod** 1984; 47(3): 445–452.

CS205 El Sohly, H. N., E. G. Boeren, C. E. Turner and M. A. El Sohly. Constituents of *Cannabis sativa* L. XXIIII: Cannabitetrol, a new polyhydroxylated cannabinoid. **Cannabinoids Chem Pharmacol Ther Aspects (PAP Meet)** 1984: 89–96.

CS206 El Sohly, M. A., J. H. Holley, G. S. Lewis, M. H. Russell and C. E. Turner. Constituents of *Cannabis sativa* L. XXIV. The potency of confiscated marijuana, hashish, and hash oil over a ten-year period. **J Forensic Sci** 1984; 1984(4): 500–514.

CS207 Hardman, J. T., M. L. Beck and C. E. Owensby. Range forb lectins. **Transfusion** 1983; 23(6): 519–522.

CS208 Mendelson, J. H., J. Ellingboe, J. C. Kuehnle and N. K. Mello. Effects of chronic marihuana use on integrated plasma testosterone and luteinizing hormone levels. **J Pharmacol Exp Ther** 1978; 207: 611–617.

CS209 El Sohly, H. N. and C. E. Turner. Constituents of *Cannabis sativa* L. XXII. Isolation of spiro-indan and dihydrostilbene compounds from a Panamanian variant grown in Mississippi, United States of America. **Bull Nar** 1982; 34(2): 51–56.

CS210 Flint, M. Lockmi: An Indian midwife. Anthropology of Human Birth 1982: 211–219.

CS211 Hendriks, H., S. Batterman, R. Bos, H. J. Huizing and T. M. Malingre. Use of amberlite XAD-2 columns for the separation of cannabinoids from cannabis extracts. **J Chromatogr** 1981; 205: 444—450.

CS212 Singh, K. V. and R. K. Pathak. Effect of leaves extracts of some higher plants on spore germination of *Ustilago maydes* and *U. nuda*. **Fitoterapia** 1984; 55(5): 318–320.

CS213 Jain, S. P. and H. S. Puri. Ethnomedical plants of Jaunsar–Bawar Hills, Uttar Pradesh, India. **J Ethnopharmacol** 1984; 12(2): 213–222.

CS214 Khan, N. A. and S. S. Hasan. Effect of cannabis hemp (hashish) on normal and rats subjected to psychological stress. **Proc Indian Acad Sci Anim Sci** 1984; 93(2): 121–129.

CS215 Fujimoto, G. I., L. C. Krey and L. Macedonia. Effect of chronic cannabinoid treatment on androgenic stimulation of male accessory sex organs in the rat. **Cannabinoids: Chem Pharmacol Ther Aspects (PAP Meet)** 1984: 401–410.

CS216 Dixit, V. P., H. C. Jain, O. P. Verma and A. N. Sharma. Effects of cannabis extract on the testicular function of the toad *Bufo andersonii* Boulenger. **Indian J Exp Biol** 1977; 15: 555–556.

CS217 Sahu, T. R. Less known uses of weeds as medicinal plants. **Ancient Sci Life** 1984; 3(4): 245–249.

CS218 Hanus, L., K. Tesarik and Z. Krejci. Capillary gas chromatography of natural substances from *Cannabis sativa* L. I. Cannabinol and cannabinolic acid—Artefacts. **Acta Univ Palacki Olomuc Fac Med** 1985; 108(52): 29–38.

CS219 Woo, W. S., E. B. Lee, K. H. Shin, S. S. Kang and H. J. Chi. A review of research on plants for fertility regulation in Korea. **Korean J Pharmacol** 1981; 12(3): 153–170.

CS220 Dabby, V. Acute pancreatitis after marijuana smoking: Is there a relationship? **JAMA** 1985; 253(12): 1791.

CS221 Mendelson, J. H., N. K. Mello and J. Ellingboe. Acute effects of marihuana smoking on prolactin levels in human females. **J Pharmacol Exp Ther** 1985; 232(1): 220–222.

CS222   Manandhar, N. P. Ethnobotany of Jumla District, Nepal. **Int J Crude Drug Res** 1986; 24(2): 81–89.

CS223   Montour, J. L., W. Dutz and L. S. Harris. Modification of radiation carcinogenesis by marihuana. **Cancer** 1981; 47(6): 1279–1285.

CS224   O'Connell, M. E., G. A. Morrill, G. I. Fujimoto and A. B. Kostellow. Factors affecting the response of the female rat reproductive system to cannabinoids. **Toxicol Appl Pharmacol** 1987; 88(3): 411–417.

CS225   Mendelson, J. H., P. Cristofaro, J. Ellingboe, R. Benedikt and N. K. Mello. Acute effects of marihuana on luteinizing hormone in menopausal women. **Pharmacol Biochem Behav** 1985; 23(5): 765–768.

CS226   Evans, A. T., E. A. Formukong and F. J. Evans. Actions of cannabis constituents on enzymes of arachidonate metabolism: Anti–inflammatory potential. **Biochem Pharmacol** 1987; 36(12): 2035–2037.

CS227   Rao, R. R. Ethnobotany of Meghalaya: Medicinal plants used by Khasi and Garo tribes. **Econ Bot** 1981; 35(1): 4–9.

CS228   Sethi, N., D. Nath, R. K. Singh and R. K. Srivastava. Antifertility and teratogenic activity of *Cannabis sativa* in rats. **Fitoterapia** 1991; 62(1): 69–71.

CS229   Renu. Fungitoxicity of leaf extracts of some higher plants against *Rhizoctonia solani* Kuehn. **Nat Acad Sci Lett** 1983; 6(8): 245–246.

CS230   Yamamoto, I., T. Matsunaga, H. Kobayashi, K. Watanabe and H. Yoshimura. Analysis and pharmacotoxicity of feruloyltyramine as a new constituent and P-coumaroyltyramine in *Cannabis sativa* L. **Pharm Biochem Behavior** 1991; 40(3): 465–469.

CS231   Sauer, M. A., S. M. Rifka, R. L. Hawks, G. B. Cutler, Jr. and D. L. Loriaux. Marijuana: Interaction with the estrogen receptor. **J Pharmacol Exp Ther** 1983; 224(2): 404–407.

CS232   Green, K., C. M. Symonds, D. R. Elijah, L. H. Zalkow, H. M. Deutsch, K. A. Bowman and T. R. Morgan. Water soluble marihuana-derived material: Pharmacological actions in rabbit and primate. **Curr Eye Res** 1981; 1(10): 599–608.

CS233   Agnihotri, P. K., R. K. Singh and S. N. Sethi. Fototoxic effects of crude alcoholic *Cannabis sativa* extract in rats. **Fitoterapia** 1992; 63(6): 489–492.

CS234   Lee, E. B., H. S. Yun and W. S. Woo. Plants and animals used for fertility regulation in Korea. **Korean J Pharmacog** 1977; 8: 81–87.

CS235   Hunte, P., M. Safi, A. Macey and G. B. Kerr. Indigenous methods of voluntary fertility regulation in Afghanistan. **Natl Demographic Fam Guid Surv Settled Pop Afghanistan** 1975; 4: 1.

CS236   Okey, A. B. and G. S. Truant. *Cannabis* demasculinizes rats but is not estrogenic. **Life Sci** 1976; 17: 1113.

CS237   Nene, Y. L., P. N. Thapliyal and K. Kumar. Screening of some plant extracts for antifungal properties. **Lab Dev J Sci Tech B** 1968; 6(4): 226–228.

CS238   Asprey, G. F. and P. Thornton. Medicinal plants of Jamaica. III. **West Indian Med J** 1955; 4: 69–82.

CS239   Friedrich–Fiechtl, J. and G. Spiteller. New cannabinoids. I. **Tetrahedron** 1975; 31: 479–487.

CS240   Kubena, R. K., H. Barry III, A. B. Selegman, M. Theiner and N. R. Farnsworth. Biological and chemical evaluation of a 43-year old sample of cannabis fluidextract. **J Pharm Sci** 1972; 61(1): 144–145.

CS241   Gellert, M., I. Novak, M. Szell and K. Szendreil. Glycosidic Components of *Cannabis sativa* L. Undocument St/ Soa/Ser. S/50 1974; 50: 8 pp.

CS242   Segelman, A. B., F. P. Segelman, R. D. Sofia and A. E. Star. Some pharmacological effects of certain cannabinoid-free marijuana extracts. **Lloydia** 1974; 37(4): 645A.

CS243   Vieira, J. E. V., G. S. G. Barros, M. C. Medeiros, F. J. A. Matos, M. P. Souza and M. J. Medeiros. Pharmacologic screening of plants from Northeast Brazil. II. **Rev Brasil Farm** 1968; 49:67–75.

CS244   Dixit, V. P., V. N. Sharma and N. K. Lohiya. The effect of chronically administered *cannabis* extract on the testicular function of mice. **Eur J Pharmacol** 1974; 26: 111–114.

CS245   Pinheiro de Sousa, M. and M. Z. Rouquayrol. Molluscicidal activity of plants from Northeast Brazil. **Rev Bras Pesq Med Biol** 1974; 7(4): 389–394.

CS246 Nayar, S. L. Vegetable insecticides. **Bull Natl Inst Sci India** 1955; 4: 137–145.

CS247 Anon. The Herbalist. Hammond Book Company, Hammond Indiana, 1931; 400 pp.

CS248 Anon. Western Arabia and the Red Sea. Geographical Handbook Series B.R.527. Great Britain Naval Intelligence Division 1946: 590–602.

CS249 Compton M. T., A. C. Furman, and N. J. Kaslow. Preliminary evidence of an association between childhood abuse and cannabis dependence among African American first-episode schizophrenia-spectrum disorder patients. **Drug Alcohol Depend** 2004; 76(3): 311–316.

CS250 Pillay, S. S., J. Rogowska, G. Kanayama, et al. Neurophysiology of motor function following cannabis discontinuation in chronic cannabis smokers: a fMRI study. **Drug Alcohol Depend** 2004; 76(3): 261–271.

CS251 Berman, J. S., C. Symonds, and R. Birch. Efficacy of two cannabis based medicinal extracts for relief of central neuropathic pain from brachial plexus avulsion: results of a randomised controlled trial. **Pain** 2004; 112(3): 299–306.

CS252 Wilcox, H. C. and J. C. Anthony. The development of suicide ideation and attempts: an epidemiologic study of first graders followed into young adulthood. **Drug Alcohol Depend** 2004; 76(Suppl): S53–S67.

CS253 Balerio, G. N., E. Aso, F. Berrendero, P. Murtra, and R. Maldonado. Delta9-tetrahydrocannabinol decreases somatic and motivational manifestations of nicotine withdrawal in mice. **Eur J Neurosci** 2004; 20(10): 2737–2748.

CS254 Fernandez-Ruiz, J., M. Gomez, M. Hernandez, R. de Miguel, and J. A. Ramos. Cannabinoids and gene expression during brain development. **Neurotox Res** 2004; 6(5): 389–401.

CS255 Hungund, B. L. and B. S. Basavarajappa. Role of Endocannabinoids and Cannabinoid CB1 Receptors in Alcohol-Related Behaviors. **Ann NY Acad Sci** 2004; 1025: 515–527.

CS256 Teichtahl, H., D. Wang, D. Cunnington, I. Kronborg, C. Goodman, A. Prodromidis, and O. Drummer. Cardio-respiratory function in stable methadone maintenance treatment (MMT) patients. **Addict Biol** 2004; 9(3–4): 247–253.

CS257 Jockers-Scherubl, M. C., H. Danker-Hopfe, R. Mahlberg, et al. Brain-derived neurotrophic factor serum concentrations are increased in drug-naive schizophrenic patients with chronic cannabis abuse and multiple substance abuse. **Neurosci Lett** 2004; 371(1): 79–83.

CS258 Allen, J. H., G. M. de Moore, R. Heddle, and J. C. Twartz. Cannabinoid hyperemesis: cyclical hyperemesis in association with chronic cannabis abuse. **Gut** 2004; 53(11): 1566–1570.

CS259 Carroll, C.B., P. G. Bain, L. Teare, et al. *Cannabis* for dyskinesia in Parkinson disease: a randomized double-blind crossover study. **Neurology** 2004; 63(7): 1245–1250.

CS260 Lynskey, M. T., A. L. Glowinski, A. A. Todorov, et al. Major depressive disorder, suicidal ideation, and suicide attempt in twins discordant for cannabis dependence and early-onset cannabis use. **Arch Gen Psychiatry** 2004; 61(10): 1026–1032.

CS261 Te Poele, R., and J. Shamash, et al. *Cannabis* induced cytotoxicity in leukaemic cell lines: the role of the cannabinoid receptors and the MAPK pathway. **Blood** 2004 Sep 28 (Epub ahead of print).

CS262 Venderova, K., E. Ruzicka, V. Vorisek, and P. Visnovsky. Survey on cannabis use in Parkinson's disease: subjective improvement of motor symptoms. **Mov Disord** 2004; 19(9): 1102–1106.

CS263 Uribe Roca, M. C., F. Micheli, and R. Viotti. *Cannabis sativa* and dystonia secondary to Wilson's disease. **Mov Disord** 2004 Aug 10 (Epub ahead of print).

CS264 Stefanis, N. C., P. Delespaul, C. Henquet, C. Bakoula, C. N. Stefanis, and J. Van Os. Early adolescent cannabis exposure and positive and negative dimensions of psychosis. **Addiction** 2004; 99(10): 1333–1341.

CS265 Kalant, H. Adverse effects of cannabis on health: an update of the literature since 1996. **Prog Neuropsychopharmacol Biol Psychiatry** 2004; 28(5):849–863.

CS266 Shukla, P. C. and U. B. Moore. Marijuana-induced transient global amnesia. **South Med J** 2004; 97(8): 782–784.

CS267 Roy, B. and B. K. Dutta. In vitro lethal efficacy of leaf extract of *Cannabis sativa* Linn on the larvae of *Chironomous samoensis* Edward: an insect of public health concern. **Indian J Exp Biol** 2003; 41(11): 1338–1341.

CS268 Wade. D. T., P. Makela, P. Robson, H. House, and C. Bateman. Do cannabis-based medicinal extracts have general or specific effects on symptoms in multiple sclerosis? A double-blind, randomized, placebo-controlled study on 160 patients. **Mult Scler** 2004; 10(4): 434–441.

CS269 Brady, C. M., R. Das Gupta, C. Dalton, O. J. Wiseman, K. J. Berkley, and C. J. Fowler. An open-label pilot study of cannabis-based extracts for bladder dysfunction in advanced multiple sclerosis. **Mult Scler** 2004; 10(4): 425–433.

CS270 Vaney, C., M. Heinzel-Gutenbrunner, P. Jobin, et al. Efficacy, safety and tolerability of an orally administered cannabis extract in the treatment of spasticity in patients with multiple sclerosis: a randomized, double-blind, placebo-controlled, crossover study. **Mult Scler** 2004; 10(4): 417–424.

CS271 Finsterer, J., P. Christian, and K. Wolfgang. Occipital stroke shortly after cannabis consumption. **Clin Neurol Neurosurg** 2004; 106(4): 305–308.

CS272 Patel, S., B. F. Cravatt and C. J. Hillard. Synergistic Interactions between Cannabinoids and Environmental Stress in the Activation of the Central Amygdala. **Neuropsychopharmacology** 2004 Jul 28 (Epub ahead of print).

CS273 Velasco, G., I. Galve-Roperh, C. Sanchez, C. Blazquez, and M. Guzman. Hypothesis: cannabinoid therapy for the treatment of gliomas? **Neuropharmacology** 2004; 47(3): 315–323.

CS274 Burstein, S. H., M. Karst, U. Schneider, and R. B. Zurier. Ajulemic acid: A novel cannabinoid produces analgesia without a "high." **Life Sci** 2004; 75(12): 1513–1522.

CS275 Kogan, N. M., R. Rabinowitz, P. Levi, et al. Synthesis and antitumor activity of quinonoid derivatives of cannab-

inoids. **J Med Chem** 2004; 47(15): 3800–3806.

CS276 Kelleher, L. M., C. Stough, A. A. Sergejew, and T. Rolfe. The effects of cannabis on information-processing speed. **Addict Behav** 2004; 29(6): 1213–1219.

CS277 Verdoux, H. and M. Tournier. Cannabis use and risk of psychosis, an etiological link? **Presse Med** 2004; 33(8): 551–554.

CS278 Whalley, B. J., J. D. Wilkinson, E. M. Williamson, and A. Constanti. A novel component of cannabis extract potentiates excitatory synaptic transmission in rat olfactory cortex *in vitro*. **Neurosci Lett** 2004; 365(1): 58–63.

CS279 Kraft, B. and H. G. Kress. Cannabinoids and the immune system. Of men, mice and cells **Schmerz** 2004; 18(3): 203–210.

CS280 Solinas, M., A. Zangen, N. Thiriet, and S. R. Goldberg. Beta-endorphin elevations in the ventral tegmental area regulate the discriminative effects of Delta-9-tetrahydrocannabinol. **Eur J Neurosci**. 2004; 19(12): 3183–3192.

CS281 Kanayama, G., J. Rogowska, H. G. Pope, S. A. Gruber, and D. A. Yurgelun-Todd. Spatial working memory in heavy cannabis users: a functional magnetic resonance imaging study. **Psychopharmacology (Berl)** 2004; 176(3–4): 239–247.

CS282 Smith, A. M., P. A. Fried, M. J. Hogan, and I. Cameron. Effects of prenatal marijuana on response inhibition: an fMRI study of young adults. **Neurotoxicol Teratol** 2004; 26(4): 533–542.

CS283 Goldschmidt, L., G. A.Richardson, M. D. Cornelius, and N. L. Day. Prenatal marijuana and alcohol exposure and academic achievement at age 10. **Neurotoxicol Teratol** 2004; 26(4): 521–532.

CS284 Lozsadi, D. A., A. Forster, N. A. Fletcher. Cannabis-induced propriospinal myoclonus. **Mov Disord** 2004; 19(6): 708–709.

CS285 Hernandez-Avila, C. A., B. J. Rounsaville, and H. R. Kranzler. Opioid-, cannabis- and alcohol-dependent women show more rapid progression to substance abuse treatment. **Drug Alcohol Depend** 2004; 74(3): 265–272.

CS286 Russo, E. B., A. Merzouki, J. M. Mesa, K. A. Frey, and P. J. Bach. Cannabis improves night vision: a case study of dark adaptometry and scotopic sensitivity in kif smokers of the Rif mountains of northern Morocco. **J Ethnopharmacol** 2004; 93(1): 99–104.

CS287 D'Souza, D. C., E. Perry, L. MacDougall, et al. The psychotomimetic effects of intravenous delta-9-tetrahydrocannabinol in healthy individuals: implications for psychosis. **Neuropsychopharmacology** 2004; 29(8): 1558–1572.

CS288 Russo, E. B. Clinical endocannabinoid deficiency (CECD): can this concept explain therapeutic benefits of cannabis in migraine, fibromyalgia, irritable bowel syndrome, and other treatment-resistant conditions? **Neuro Endocrinol Lett** 2004; 25(1–2): 31–39.

CS289 Furler, M. D., T. R. Einarson, M. Millson, S. Walmsley, and R. Bendayan. Medicinal and recreational marijuana use by patients infected with HIV. **AIDS Patient Care STDS** 2004; 18(4): 215–228.

CS290 Nicholson, A. N., C. Turner, B. M. Stone, and P. J. Robson. Effect of Delta-9-tetrahydrocannabinol and cannabidiol on nocturnal sleep and early-morning behavior in young adults. **J Clin Psychopharmacol** 2004; 24(3): 305–313.

CS291 Rodriguez De Fonseca, F., M. A. Gorriti, A. Bilbao et al. Role of the endogenous cannabinoid system as a modulator of dopamine transmission: implications for Parkinson's disease and schizophrenia. **Neurotox Res** 2001; 3(1): 23–35.

CS292 Gadzicki, D., K. R. Muller-Vahl, D. Heller, et al. Tourette syndrome is not caused by mutations in the central cannabinoid receptor (CNR1) gene. **Am J Med Genet** 2004; 127B(1): 97–103.

CS293 Oliva, J. M., S. Ortiz, T. Palomo, and J. Manzanares. Spontaneous cannabinoid withdrawal produces a differential time-related responsiveness in cannabinoid CB1 receptor gene expression in the mouse brain. **J Psychopharmacol** 2004; 18(1): 59–65.

CS294 Notcutt, W., M. Price, R. Miller, et al. Initial experiences with medicinal extracts of cannabis for chronic pain: results from 34 'N of 1' studies. **Anaesthesia** 2004; 59(5): 440–452.

CS295 Gomez, M., M. Hernandez, B. Johansson, R. de Miguel, J. A. Ramos, and J. Fernandez-Ruiz. Prenatal cannabinoid and gene expression for neural adhesion molecule L1 in the fetal rat brain. **Brain Res Dev** 2003; 147(1–2): 201–207.

CS296 Amtmann, D., P. Weydt, K. L. Johnson, M. P. Jensen, and G. T. Carter. Survey of cannabis use in patients with amyotrophic lateral sclerosis. **Am J Hosp Palliat Care** 2004; 21(2): 95–104.

CS297 Contassot, E., M. Tenan, V. Schnuriger, M. F. Pelte, and P. Y. Dietrich. Arachidonyl ethanolamide induces apoptosis of uterine cervix cancer cells via aberrantly expressed vanilloid receptor-1. **Gynecol Oncol** 2004; 93(1): 182–188.

CS298 Iuvone, T., G. Esposito, R. Esposito, R. Santamaria, M. Di Rosa, and A. A. Izzo. Neuroprotective effect of cannabidiol, a non-psychoactive component from *Cannabis sativa*, on beta-amyloid-induced toxicity in PC12 cells. **J Neurochem** 2004; 89(1): 134–141.

CS299 Ng, R. S., D. A. Darko, and R. M. Hillson. Street drug use among young patients with Type 1 diabetes in the UK. **Diabet Med** 2004; 21(3): 295–296.

CS300 Dannon, P. N., K. Lowengrub, R. Amiaz, L. Grunhaus, and M. Kotler. Comorbid cannabis use and panic disorder: short term and long term follow-up study. **Hum Psychopharmacol** 2004; 19(2): 97,101.

CS301 Williams, L. J., A. Correa, and S. Rasmussen. Maternal lifestyle factors and risk for ventricular septal defects. **Birth Defects Res Part A Clin Mol Teratol** 2004; 70(2): 59–64.

CS302 Laure, P., T. Lecerf, A. Friser, and C. Binsinger. Drugs, recreational drug use and attitudes towards doping of high school athletes. **Int J Sports Med** 2004; 25(2): 133–138.

CS303 Costa, B., M. Colleoni, S. Conti, D. Parolaro, C. Franke, A. E. Trovato, and G. Giagnoni. Oral anti-inflammatory activity of cannabidiol, a non-psychoactive constituent of cannabis, in acute carrageenan-induced inflammation in the rat paw. **Naunyn Schmiedebergs Arch Pharmacol** 2004; 369(3): 294–299.

CS304 Jockers-Scherubl, M. C., U. Matthies, H. Danker-Hopfe, U. E. Lang, R. Mahlberg, and R. Hellweg. Chronic cannabis abuse raises nerve growth factor serum concentrations in drug-naive schizophrenic patients. J **Psychopharmacol** 2003; 17(4): 439–445.

CS305 Venance, L., R. Maldonado, and O. Manzoni. Endocannabinoids in the central nervous system **Med Sci (Paris)** 2004; 20(1): 45–53.

CS306 Stuyt, E. B. Hepatitis C in patients with co-occurring mental disorders and substance use disorders: is tobacco use a possible risk factor? **Am J Addict** 2004; 13(1): 46–52.

CS307 Tsai, J. C., S. Tsai, and W. C. Chang. Effect of ethanol extracts of three Chinese medicinal plants with laxative properties on ion transport of the rat intestinal epithelia. **Biol Pharm Bull** 2004; 27(2): 162–165.

CS308 Ducasse, E., J. Chevalier, D. Dasnoy, F. Speziale, P. Fiorani, and P. Puppinck. Popliteal artery entrapment associated with cannabis arteritis. **Eur J Vasc Endovasc Surg** 2004; 27(3): 327–332.

CS309 Janczyk, P., C. W. Donaldson, and S. Gwaltney. Two hundred and thirteen cases of marijuana toxicoses in dogs. **Vet Hum Toxicol** 2004; 46(1): 19–21.

CS310 Llewellyn, C. D., K. Linklater, J. Bell, N. W. Johnson, and S. Warnakulasuriya. An analysis of risk factors for oral cancer in young people: a case-control study. **Oral Oncol** 2004; 40(3): 304–313.

CS311 Westfall, R. E. Use of anti-emetic herbs in pregnancy: women's choices, and the question of safety and efficacy. Complement **Ther Nurs Midwifery** 2004; 10(1): 30–36.

CS312 Wilkinson, J. D., B. J. Whalley, D. Baker, et al. Medicinal cannabis: is delta9-tetrahydrocannabinol necessary for all its effects? **J Pharm Pharmacol** 2003; 55(12): 1687–1694.

CS313 Grant, P. and P. A. Gandhi. A case of cannabis-induced pancreatitis. **JOP** 2004; 5(1): 41–43.

CS314 Akerman, S., H. Kaube, and P. J. Goadsby. Anandamide is able to inhibit trigeminal neurons using an in vivo model of trigeminovascular-mediated nociception. **J Pharmacol Exp Ther** 2004; 309(1): 56–63.

CS315 Prentiss, D., R. Power, G. Balmas, G. Tzuang, and D. M. Israelski. Patterns of marijuana use among patients with HIV/AIDS followed in a public health care setting. **J Acquir Immune Defic Syndr** 2004; 35(1): 38–45.

CS316 Park, B., J. M. McPartland, and M. Glass. Cannabis, cannabinoids and reproduction. **Prostaglandins Leukot Essent Fatty Acids** 2004; 70(2): 189–197.

CS317 Singh, A. B. and P. Kumar. Aeroallergens in clinical practice of allergy in India. An overview. **Ann Agric Environ Med** 2003; 10(2): 131–136.

CS318 Jones, S. and J. Howl. Cannabinoid receptor systems: therapeutic targets for tumour intervention. **Expert Opin Ther Targets** 2003; 7(6): 749–758.

CS319 Chiriboga, C. A. Fetal alcohol and drug effects. **Neurologist** 2003; 9(6): 267–279.

CS320 Luo, J., J. H. Yin, H. Z. Wu, and Q. Wei. Extract from Fructus cannabis activating calcineurin improved learning and memory in mice with chemical drug-induced dysmnesia. **Acta Pharmacol Sin** 2003; 24(11): 1137–1142.

CS321 Degenhardt, L., W. Hall, and M. Lynskey. Exploring the association between cannabis use and depression. **Addiction** 2003; 98(11): 1493–1504.

CS322 Zajicek, J., P. Fox, H. Sanders, et al. Cannabinoids for treatment of spasticity and other symptoms related to multiple sclerosis (CAMS study): multicentre randomised placebo-controlled trial. **Lancet** 2003; 362(9395): 1517–1526.

CS323 Gaetani, S., V. Cuomo, and D. Piomelli. Anandamide hydrolysis: a new target for anti-anxiety drugs? **Trends Mol Med** 2003; 9(11): 474–478.

CS324 McCambridge, J., J. Strang, S. Platts, and J. Witton. Cannabis use and the

GP: brief motivational intervention increases clinical enquiry by GPs in a pilot study. **Br J Gen Pract** 2003; 53(493): 637–639.

CS325 Koenen, K. C., M. J. Lyons, J. Goldberg et al. Co-twin control study of relationships among combat exposure, combat-related PTSD, and other mental disorders. **J Trauma Stress** 2003; 16(5): 433–438.

CS326 Buggy, D. J., L. Toogood, S. Maric, P. Sharpe, D. G. Lambert, and D. L. Rowbotham. Lack of analgesic efficacy of oral delta-9-tetrahydrocannabinol in postoperative pain. **Pain** 2003; 106(1–2): 169–172.

CS327 Park, B., H. M. Gibbons, M. D. Mitchell, and M. Glass. Identification of the CB1 cannabinoid receptor and fatty acid amide hydrolase (FAAH) in the human placenta. **Placenta** 2003; 24(10): 990–995.

CS328 Guzman, M. Cannabinoids: potential anticancer agents. **Nat Rev Cancer** 2003; 3(10): 745–755.

CS329 Muller-Vahl, K. R. Cannabinoids reduce symptoms of Tourette's syndrome. **Expert Opin Pharmacother** 2003; 4(10): 1717–1725.

CS330 Naef, M., M. Curatolo, S. Petersen-Felix, L. Arendt-Nielsen, A. Zbinden, and R. Brenneisen. The analgesic effect of oral delta-9-tetrahydrocannabinol (THC), morphine, and a THC-morphine combination in healthy subjects under experimental pain conditions. **Pain** 2003; 105(1–2): 79–88.

CS331 Padley, J. R., Q. Li, P. M. Pilowsky, and A. K. Goodchild. Cannabinoid receptor activation in the rostral ventrolateral medulla oblongata evokes cardiorespiratory effects in anaesthetised rats. **Br J Pharmacol** 2003; 140(2): 384–394.

CS332 Semple, D. M., F. Ramsden, and A. M. McIntosh. Reduced binocular depth inversion in regular cannabis users. **Pharmacol Biochem Behav** 2003; 75(4): 789–793.

CS333 Sheweita, S. A. Narcotic drugs change the expression of cytochrome P450 2E1 and 2C6 and other activities of carcinogen-metabolizing enzymes in the liver of male mice. **Toxicology** 2003; 191(2–3): 133–142.

CS334 Luo, J., J. H. Yin, and Q. Wei. The effect of calcineurin activator, extracted from Chinese herbal medicine, on memory and immunity in mice. **Pharmacol Biochem Behav** 2003; 75(4): 749–754.

CS335 Clough, A. R., Z. Wang, R. S. Bailie, C. B. Burns, and B. J. Currie. Case-control study of the association between kava use and pneumonia in eastern Arnhem and Aboriginal communities (Northern Territory, Australia). **Epidemiol Infect** 2003; 131(1): 627–635.

CS336 Groger, A., A. Aslani, T. Wolter, E. M. Noah, and N. Pallua. A rare case of cannabis arteritis. **Vasa** 2003; 32(2): 95–97.

CS337 Grant, I., R. Gonzalez, C. L. Carey, L. Natarajan, and T. Wolfson. Non-acute (residual) neurocognitive effects of cannabis use: a meta-analytic study. **J Int Neuropsychol Soc** 2003; 9(5): 679–689.

CS338 Gilgun-Sherki, Y., E. Melamed, R. Mechoulam, and D. Offen. The CB1 cannabinoid receptor agonist, HU-210, reduces levodopa-induced rotations in 6-hydroxydopamine-lesioned rats. **Pharmacol Toxicol** 2003; 93(2): 66–70.

CS339 Pryce, G., Z. Ahmed, D. L. Hankey, et al. Cannabinoids inhibit neurodegeneration in models of multiple sclerosis. **Brain** 2003; 126(Pt. 10): 2191–2202.

CS340 Mathew, R. J., W. H. Wilson, and R. Davis. Postural syncope after marijuana: a transcranial Doppler study of the hemodynamics. **Pharmacol Biochem Behav** 2003; 75(2): 309–318.

CS341 Noland, J. S., L. T. Singer, S. K. Mehta, and D. M. Super. Prenatal cocaine/polydrug exposure and infant performance on an executive functioning task. **Dev Neuropsychol** 2003; 24(1): 499–517.

CS342 Taylor, D. R. and W. Hall. Respiratory health effects of cannabis: position statement of the Thoracic Society of Australia and New Zealand. **Intern Med J** 2003; 33(7): 310–313.

CS343 O'Leary, D. S., R. I. Block, B. M. Turner et al. Marijuana alters the human cerebellar clock. **Neuroreport** 2003; 14(8): 1145–1151.

CS344   Fried, P. A., B. Watkinson, and R. Gray. Differential effects on cognitive functioning in 13- to 16-year-olds prenatally exposed to cigarettes and marihuana. **Neurotoxicol Teratol** 2003; 25(4): 427–436.

CS345   Muller-Vahl, K. R., U. Schneider, H. Prevedel, et al. Delta 9-tetrahydrocannabinol (THC) is effective in the treatment of tics in Tourette syndrome: a 6-week randomized trial. **J Clin Psychiatry** 2003; 64(4): 459–465.

CS346   Verrico, C. D., J. D. Jentsch, and R. H. Roth. Persistent and anatomically selective reduction in prefrontal cortical dopamine metabolism after repeated, intermittent cannabinoid administration to rats. **Synapse** 2003; 49(1): 61–66.

CS347   Killestein, J., E. L. Hoogervorst, M. Reif, et al. Immunomodulatory effects of orally administered cannabinoids in multiple sclerosis. **J Neuroimmunol** 2003; 137(1–2): 140–143.

CS348   Daniels, I. R. and G. T. Layer. How should gynaecomastia be managed? **ANZ J Surg** 2003; 73(4): 213–216.

CS349   Cazalets, C., E. Laurat, B. Cador, et al. Grosbois. Cannabis arteritis: four new cases. **Rev Med Interne** 2003; 24(2): 127–130.

CS350   Saso, L. Effects of drug abuse on sexual response. **Ann Ist Super Sanita** 2002; 38(3): 289–296.

CS351   Ware, M. A., C. R. Doyle, R. Woods, M. E. Lynch, and A. J. Clark Cannabis use for chronic non-cancer pain: results of a prospective survey. **Pain** 2003;102(1–2): 211–216.

CS352   Cota, D., G. Marsicano, B. Lutz, et al. Endogenous cannabinoid system as a modulator of food intake. **Int J Obes Relat Metab Disord** 2003; 27(3): 289–301.

CS353   Croxford, J. L. Therapeutic potential of cannabinoids in CNS disease. **CNS Drugs** 2003; 17(3): 179–202.

CS354   Wade, D. T., P. Robson, H. House, P. Makela, and J. Aram. A preliminary controlled study to determine whether whole-plant cannabis extracts can improve intractable neurogenic symptoms. **Clin Rehabil** 2003; 17(1): 21–29.

CS355   Peters, F. T., H. H. Maurer, and P. Hellstern. Prevalence of illicit drug use in plasmapheresis donors. **Vox Sang** 2003; 84(2): 91–95.

CS356   Muller-Vahl, K. R., H. Prevedel, K. Theloe, H. Kolbe, H. M. Emrich, and U. Schneider. Treatment of Tourette syndrome with delta-9-tetrahydrocannabinol (delta 9-THC): no influence on neuropsychological performance. **Neuropsychopharmacology** 2003; 28(2): 384–388.

CS357   Ebrahim, S. H. and J. Gfroerer. Pregnancy-related substance use in the United States during 1996-1998. **Obstet Gynecol** 2003; 101(2): 374–379.

CS358   Zurier, R. B., R. G. Rossetti, S. H. Burstein, and B. Bidinger. Suppression of human monocyte interleukin-1beta production by ajulemic acid, a nonpsychoactive cannabinoid. **Biochem Pharmacol** 2003; 65(4): 649–655.

CS359   Flach, A. J. Delta-9-tetrahydrocannabinol (THC) in the treatment of end-stage open-angle glaucoma. **Trans Am Ophthalmol Soc** 2002; 100: 215–222; discussion 222–224.

CS360   Sarafian, T. A., S. Kouyoumjian, F. Khoshaghideh, D. P. Tashkin, and M. D. Roth. Delta 9-tetrahydrocannabinol disrupts mitochondrial function and cell energetics. **Am J Physiol Lung Cell Mol Physiol** 2003; 284(2): L298–L306

CS361   Clermont-Gnamien, S., S. Atlani, N. Attal, F. Le Mercier, F. Guirimand, and L. Brasseur. The therapeutic use of D9-tetrahydrocannabinol (dronabinol) in refractory neuropathic pain. **Presse Med** 2002; 31(39 Pt. 1): 1840–1845.

CS362   Jones, R. T. Cardiovascular system effects of marijuana. **J Clin Pharmacol** 2002; 42(11 Suppl): 58S–63S.

CS363   Brown, T. T. and A. S. Dobs. Endocrine effects of marijuana. **J Clin Pharmacol** 2002; 42(11 Suppl): 90S–96S.

CS364   Chowdhury, A. R. Effect of pharmacological agents on male reproduction. **Adv Contracept Deliv Syst** 1987; 3(4): 347–352.

CS365   Pardo, G., V. Legua, J. Remohi, and F. Bonilla-Musoles. Review and update: marijuana and reproduction. **Acta Ginecol (Madr)** 1985; 42(7): 420–429.

CS366 Williams, S. M., E. A. Mitchell, and B. J. Taylor. Are risk factors for sudden infant death syndrome different at night? **Arch Dis Child** 2002; 87(4): 274–278.

CS367 Mulheran, M., P. Middleton, and J. A. Henry. The acute effects of tetrahydrocannabinol on auditory threshold and frequency resolution in human subjects. **Hum Exp Toxicol** 2002; 21(6): 289–292.

CS368 Ware, M. A., A. Gamsa, J. Persson, and M. A. Fitzcharles. Cannabis for chronic pain: case series and implications for clinicians. **Pain Res Manag** 2002; 7(2): 95–99.

CS369 James, J. S. Marijuana safety study completed: weight gain, no safety problems. **AIDS Treat News** 2000; (348): 3–4.

CS370 Ciccocioppo, R., L. Antonelli, M. Biondini, M. Perfumi, P. Pompei, and M. Massi. Memory impairment following combined exposure to delta(9)-tetrahydrocannabinol and ethanol in rats. **Eur J Pharmacol** 2002; 449(3): 245–252.

CS371 Taylor, D. R., D. M. Fergusson, B. J. Milne, et al. A longitudinal study of the effects of tobacco and cannabis exposure on lung function in young adults. **Addiction** 2002; 97(8): 1055–1061.

CS372 Stock, S. L., E. Goldberg, S. Corbett, and D. K. Katzman. Substance use in female adolescents with eating disorders. **J Adolesc Health** 2002; 31(2): 176–182.

CS373 Sarafian, T. A., S. Kouyoumjian, D. Tashkin, and M. D. Roth. Synergistic cytotoxicity of Delta(9)-tetrahydrocannabinol and butylated hydroxyanisole. **Toxicol Lett** 2002; 133(2–3): 171–179.

CS374 Pistis, M., A. L. Muntoni, G. Pillolla, and G. L. Gessa. Cannabinoids inhibit excitatory inputs to neurons in the shell of the nucleus accumbens: an *in vivo* electrophysiological study. **Eur J Neurosci** 2002; 15(11): 1795–1802.

CS375 Dhawan, K., S. Kumar, and A. Sharma. Reversal of cannabinoids (delta9-THC) by the benzoflavone moiety from methanol extract of *Passiflora incarnata* Linneaus in mice: a possible therapy for cannabinoid addiction. **J Pharm Pharmacol** 2002; 54(6): 875–881.

CS376 Darling, M. R., G. M. Learmonth, and T. M. Arendorf. Oral cytology in cannabis smokers. **SADJ** 2002; 57(4): 132–135.

CS377 Brody, S. and R. Preut. Cannabis, tobacco, and caffeine use modify the blood pressure reactivity protection of ascorbic acid. **Pharmacol Biochem Behav** 2002; 72(4): 811–816.

CS378 Brophy. S. and A. Calin. Definition of disease flare in ankylosing spondylitis: the patients' perspective. **J Rheumatol** 2002; 29(5): 954–958.

CS379 Sauvanier, M., J. Constans, S. Skopinski et al. Lower limb occlusive arteriopathy: retrospective analysis of 73 patients with onset before the age of 50 years. **J Mal Vasc** 2002; 27(2): 69–76.

CS380 Boyce, S. H. and M. A. Quigley. Uvulitis and partial upper airway obstruction following cannabis inhalation. **Emerg Med (Fremantle)** 2002; 14(1): 106–108.

CS381 Gouzoulis-Mayfrank, E., S. Becker, S. Pelz, F. Tuchtenhagen, and J. Daumann. Neuroendocrine abnormalities in recreational ecstasy (MDMA) users: is it ecstasy or cannabis? **Biol Psychiatry** 2002; 51(9): 766–769.

CS382 Parker, L. A., R. Mechoulam, and C. Schlievert. Cannabidiol, a non-psychoactive component of cannabis and its synthetic dimethylheptyl homolog suppress nausea in an experimental model with rats. **Neuroreport** 2002; 13(5): 567–570.

CS383 Niveau, G. Cannabis-related flashback, a medico-legal case. **Encephale** 2002; 28(1): 77–79.

CS384 Muller-Vahl, K. R., U. Schneider, A. Koblenz, et al. Treatment of Tourette's syndrome with Delta 9-tetrahydrocannabinol (THC): a randomized crossover trial. **Pharmacopsychiatry** 2002; 35(2): 57–61.

CS385 Fried, P., B. Watkinson, D. James, and R. Gray. Current and former marijuana use: preliminary findings of a longitudinal study of effects on IQ in young adults. **CMAJ** 2002; 166(7): 887–891.

CS386   Alvaro, L. C., I. Iriondo, and F. J. Villaverde. Sexual headache and stroke in a heavy cannabis smoker. **Headache** 2002; 42(3): 224–226.

CS387   McLeod, A. L., C. J. McKenna, and D. B. Northridge. Myocardial infarction following the combined recreational use of Viagra and cannabis. **Clin Cardiol** 2002; 25(3): 133–134.

CS388   Solowij, N., R. S. Stephens, R. A. Roffman et al. Cognitive functioning of long-term heavy cannabis users seeking treatment. **JAMA** 2002; 287(9): 1123–1131.

CS389   Fergusson, D. M., L. J. Horwood, and K. Northstone. Maternal use of cannabis and pregnancy outcome. **BJOG** 2002; 109(1): 21–27.

CS390   Fox, S. H., M. Kellett, A. P. Moore, A. R. Crossman, and J. M. Brotchie. Randomised, double-blind, placebo-controlled trial to assess the potential of cannabinoid receptor stimulation in the treatment of dystonia. **Mov Disord** 2002; 17(1): 145–149.

CS391   Elsner, F., L. Radbruch, and R. Sabatowski. Tetrahydrocannabinol for treatment of chronic pain. **Schmerz** 2001; 15(3): 200–204.

CS392   Bachs, L. and H. Morland. Acute cardiovascular fatalities following cannabis use. **Forensic Sci Int** 2001; 124(2–3): 200–203.

CS393   Earleywine, M. Cannabis-induced Koro in Americans. **Addiction** 2001; 96(11): 1663–1666.

CS394   Kopelman, M. D., L. J. Reed, P. Marsden, et al. Amnesic syndrome and severe ataxia following the recreational use of 3,4-methylene-dioxy-methamphetamine (MDMA, 'ecstasy') and other substances. **Neurocase** 2001; 7(5): 423–432.

CS395   Bovasso, G. B. Cannabis abuse as a risk factor for depressive symptoms. **Am J Psychiatry** 2001; 158(12): 2033–2037.

CS396   Arnold, J. C., A. N. Topple, P. E. Mallet, G. E. Hunt, and I. S. McGregor. The distribution of cannabinoid-induced Fos expression in rat brain: differences between the Lewis and Wistar strain. **Brain Res** 2001; 921 (1–2): 240–255.

CS397   Lundqvist, T., S. Jonsson, and S. Warkentin. Frontal lobe dysfunction in long-term cannabis users. **Neurotoxicol Teratol** 2001; 23(5): 437–443.

CS398   Launay, D., V. Queyrel, P. Y. Hatron, U. Michon-Pasturel, E. Hachulla, and B. Devulder. Digital necrosis in a patient with anorexia nervosa. Association of vasculopathy and radial artery injury **Presse Med** 2000; 29(34): 1850–1852.

CS399   Voruganti, L. N., P. Slomka, P. Zabel, A. Mattar, and A. G. Awad. Cannabis induced dopamine release: an *in-vivo* SPECT study. **Psychiatry Res** 2001; 107(3): 173–177.

CS400   Tramer, M. R., D. Carroll, F. A. Campbell, D. J. Reynolds, R. A. Moore, and H. J. McQuay. Cannabinoids for control of chemotherapy induced nausea and vomiting: quantitative systematic review. **BMJ** 2001; 323(7303): 16–21.

CS401   Dowe, G., M. F. Smilkle, C. Thesiger, and E. M. Williams. Bloodborne sexually transmitted infections in patients presenting for substance abuse treatment in Jamaica. **Sex Transm Dis** 2001; 28(5): 266–269.

CS402   Fishwick, D., L. J. Allan, A. Wright, C. M. Barber, and A. D. Curran. Respiratory symptoms, lung function, and cell surface markers in a group of hemp fiber processors. **Am J Ind Med** 2001; 39(4): 419–425.

CS403   Scragg, R. K., E. A. Mitchell, R. P. Ford, J. M. Thompson, B. J. Taylor, and A. W. Stewart. Maternal cannabis use in the sudden death syndrome. **Acta Paediatr** 2001; 90(1): 57–60.

CS404   Flisher, A. J. and D. O. Chalton. Adolescent contraceptive non-use and covariation among risk behaviors. **J Adolesc Health** 2001; 28(3): 235–241.

CS405   Taylor, D. R., R. Poulton, T. E. Moffitt, P. Ramankutty, and M. R. Sears. The respiratory effects of cannabis dependence in young adults. **Addiction** 2000; 95(11): 1669–1677.

CS406   Disdier, P., B. Granel, J. Serratrice, et al. Cannabis arteritis revisited—ten new case reports. **Angiology** 2001; 52(1): 1–5.

CS407 Kosior, D. A., K. J. Filipiak, P. Stolarz, and G. Opolski. Paroxysmal atrial fibrillation in a young female patient following marijuana intoxication—a case report of possible association. **Med Sci Monit** 2000; 6(2): 386–389.

CS408 Mani, S. K., A. Mitchell, and B. W. O'Malley. Progesterone receptor and dopamine receptors are required in Delta 9-tetrahydrocannabinol modulation of sexual receptivity in female rats. **Proc Natl Acad Sci USA** 2001; 98(3): 1249–1254.

CS409 Schneider, F., N. Abdoucheli-Baudot, M. Tassart, F. Boudghene, and P. Gouny. Cannabis and tobacco: cofactors favoring juvenile obliterative arteriopathy. **J Mal Vasc** 2000; 25(5): 388–389.

CS410 Mackirdy, C. and D. Shepherd. Capgras syndrome: possibly more common among the Maori of New Zealand. **Aust NZ J Psychiatry** 2000; 34(5): 865–868.

CS411 Stokes, J. R., R. Hartel, L. B. Ford, and T. B. Casale. Cannabis (hemp) positive skin tests and respiratory symptoms. **Ann Allergy Asthma Immunol** 2000; 85(3): 238–240.

CS412 Hampson, A. J., M. Grimaldi, M. Lolic, D. Wink, R. Rosenthal, and J. Axelrod. Neuroprotective antioxidants from marijuana. **Ann N Y Acad Sci** 2000; 899: 274–282.

CS413 Goldschmidt, L., N. L. Day, and G. A. Richardson. Effects of prenatal marijuana exposure on child behavior problems at age 10. **Neurotoxicol Teratol** 2000; 22(3): 325–336.

CS414 Leweke, F. M., U. Schneider, M. Radwan, E. Schmidt, and H. M. Emrich. Different effects of nabilone and cannabidiol on binocular depth inversion in Man. **Pharmacol Biochem Behav** 2000; 66(1): 175–181.

CS415 Payne, H. C. Traumatic brain injury, depression and cannabis use—assessing their effects on a cognitive performance. **Brain Inj** 2000; 14(5): 479–489.

CS416 McDonald, A., N. D. Duncan, and D. I. Mitchell. Alcohol, cannabis and cocaine usage in patients with trauma injuries. **West Indian Med J** 1999; 48(4): 200–202.

CS417 Fried, P. A., B. Watkinson, and R. Gray. Growth from birth to early adolescence in offspring prenatally exposed to cigarettes and marijuana. **Neurotoxicol Teratol** 1999; 21(5): 513–525.

CS418 Balle, J., M. J. Olofsson, and J. Hilden. Cannabis and pregnancy. **Ugeskr Laeger** 1999; 161(36): 5024–5028.

CS419 Von Mandach, U., M. M. Rabner, J. Wisser, and A. Huch. LSD and cannabis abuse in early pregnancy with good perinatal outcome. Case report and review of the literature. **Gynakol Geburtshilfliche Rundsch** 1999; 39(3): 125–129.

CS420 Zenor, B. N., G. D. Weesner, and P. V. Malven. Endocrine and other responses to acute administration of cannabinoid compounds to non-stressed male calves. **Life Sci** 1999; 65(2): 125–133.

CS421 Okereke, U. N., B. E. Weber, and R. H. Israel. Spontaneous pneumomediastinum in an 18-year-old black Sudanese high school student. **J Natl Med Assoc** 1999; 91(6): 357–359.

CS422 Sherwood, R. A., J. Keating, V. Kavvadia, A. Greenough, and T. J. Peters. Substance misuse in early pregnancy and relationship to fetal outcome. **Eur J Pediatr** 1999; 158(6): 488–492.

CS423 Ameri, A. The effects of cannabinoids on the brain. **Prog Neurobiol** 1999; 58(4): 315–348.

CS424 Coghlan, D., M. Milner, T. Clarke, et al. Neonatal abstinence syndrome. **Ir Med J** 1999; 92(1): 232–233, 236.

CS425 Zimmer, A., A. M. Zimmer, A. G. Hohmann, M. Herkenham, and T. I. Bonner. Increased mortality, hypoactivity, and hypoalgesia in cannabinoid CB1 receptor knockout mice. **Proc Natl Acad Sci USA** 1999; 96(10): 5780–5785.

CS426 Lyketsos, C. G., E. Garrett, K. Y. Liang, and J. C. Anthony. Cannabis use and cognitive decline in persons under 65 years of age. **Am J Epidemiol** 1999; 149(9): 794–800.

CS427 Masset, D., J. H. Bourdon, J. Arditti-Djiane, and J. Jouglard. Impact of delta-9-tetrahydrocannabinol and its metabolites on the immune system. **Acta Clin Belg Suppl** 1999; 1: 39–43.

CS428 Ehrenreich, H., T. Rinn, H. J. Kunert, et al. Specific attentional dysfunction in adults following early start of cannabis use. **Psychopharmacology (Berl)** 1999; 142(3): 295–301.

CS429 Leech, S. L., G. A. Richardson, L. Goldschmidt, and N. L. Day. Prenatal substance exposure: effects on attention and impulsivity of 6-year-olds. **Neurotoxicol Teratol** 1999; 21(2): 109–118.

CS430 Disdier, P., L. Swiader, J. Jouglard, et al. Cannabis-induced arteritis vs. Buerger disease. Nosologic discussion apropos of two new cases. **Presse Med** 1999; 28(2): 71–74.

CS431 Gorriti, M. A., F. Rodriguez de Fonseca, M. Navarro, and T. Palomo. Chronic (-)-delta9-tetrahydrocannabinol treatment induces sensitization to the psychomotor effects of amphetamine in rats. **Eur J Pharmacol** 1999; 365(2–3): 133–142.

CS432 Ongradi, J., S. Specter, A. Horvath, and H. Friedman. Additive effect of marihuana and retrovirus in the anergy of natural killer cells in mice. **Orv Hetil** 1999; 140(2): 81–84.

CS433 Eames, S. L., J. Westermeyer, and R. D. Crosby. Substance use and abuse among patients with comorbid dysthymia and substance disorder. **Am J Drug Alcohol Abuse** 1998; 24(4): 541–550.

CS434 Jentsch, J. D., C. D. Verrico, D. Le, and R. H. Roth. Repeated exposure to delta 9-tetrahydrocannabinol reduces prefrontal cortical dopamine metabolism in the rat. **Neurosci Lett** 1998; 246(3): 169–172.

CS435 Matsunaga, T., K. Watanabe, H. Yoshimura, and I. Yamamoto. Quantitative analysis and pharmaco-toxicity of cannabinoids in commercially available cannabis seeds. **Yakugaku Zasshi** 1998; 118(9): 408–414.

CS436 Rubio, P., F. Rodriguez de Fonseca, J. L. Martin-Calderon, et al. Maternal exposure to low doses of delta9-tet-rahydrocannabinol facilitates morphine-induced place conditioning in adult male offspring. **Pharmacol Biochem Behav** 1998; 61(3): 229–238.

CS437 English, D. R., G. K. Hulse, E. Milne, C. D. Holman, and C. I. Bower. Maternal cannabis use and birth weight: a meta-analysis. **Addiction** 1997; 92(11): 1553–1560.

CS438 Block, R. I., W. J. Erwin, R. Farinpour, and K. Braverman. Sedative, stimulant, and other subjective effects of marijuana: relationships to smoking techniques. **Pharmacol Biochem Behav** 1998; 59(2): 405–412.

CS439 Daisley, H., A. Jones-Le Cointe, G. Hutchinson, and V. Simmons. Fatal cardiac toxicity temporally related to poly-drug abuse. **Vet Hum Toxicol** 1998; 40(1): 21–22.

CS440 Wang, M. Q., C. B. Collins, R. J. DiClemente, G. Wingood, and C. L. Kohler. Depressive symptoms as correlates of polydrug use for blacks in a high-risk community. **South Med J** 1997; 90(11): 1123–1128.

CS441 Westermeyer, J., S. Kopka, and S. Nugent. Course and severity of substance abuse among patients with comorbid major depression. **Am J Addict** 1997; 6(4): 284–292.

CS442 Schlicker, E., J. Timm, J. Zentner, and M. Gothert. Cannabinoid CB1 receptor-mediated inhibition of noradrenaline release in the human and guinea-pig hippocampus. **Naunyn Schmiedebergs Arch Pharmacol** 1997; 356(5): 583–589.

CS443 Middleman, A. B., L. M. Robertson, R. H. DuRant, V. Chiou, and S. J. Emans. Use of hormonal methods of birth control among sexually active adolescent girls. **J Pediatr Adolesc Gynecol** 1997; 10(4): 193–198.

CS444 Heishman, S. J., K. Arasteh, and M. L. Stitzer. Comparative effects of alcohol and marijuana on mood, memory, and performance. **Pharmacol Biochem Behav** 1997; 58(1): 93–101.

CS445 Ostrea, E. M. Jr., A. R. Ostrea, and P. M. Simpson. Mortality within the first 2 years in infants exposed to cocaine, opiate, or cannabinoid during gestation. **Pediatrics** 1997; 100(1): 79–83.

CS446 Durst, R. and P. Rebaudengo-Rosca. Attention deficit hyperactivity disorder, facilitating alcohol and drug abuse in an adult. **Harefuah** 1997; 132(9): 618–622, 680.

CS447 Holdcroft, A., M. Smith, A. Jacklin, et al. Pain relief with oral cannabinoids in familial Mediterranean fever. **Anaesthesia** 1997; 52(5): 483–486.

CS448 Elwan, O., A. A. Hassan, M. Abdel Naseer et al. Brain aging in a sample of normal Egyptians cognition, education, addiction and smoking. **J Neurol Sci** 1997; 148(1): 79–86.

CS449 Mirochnick, M., J. Meyer, D. A. Frank, H. Cabral, E. Z. Tronick, and B. Zuckerman. Elevated plasma norepinephrine after in utero exposure to cocaine and marijuana. **Pediatrics** 1997; 99(4): 555–559.

CS450 Meier, H. and H. J. Vonesch. Cannabis poisoning after eating salad. **Schweiz Med Wochenschr** 1997; 127(6): 214–218.

CS451 Sanudo-Pena, M. C., K. Tsou, E. R. Delay, A. G. Hohman, M. Force, and J. M. Walker. Endogenous cannabinoids as an aversive or counter-rewarding system in the rat. **Neurosci Lett** 1997; 223(2): 125–128.

CS452 Ruh, M. F., J. A. Taylor, A. C. Howlett, and W. V. Welshons. Failure of cannabinoid compounds to stimulate estrogen receptors. **Biochem Pharmacol** 1997; 53(1): 35–41.

CS453 Pope, H. G. Jr., A. Jacobs, J. P. Mialet, D. Yurgelun-Todd, and S. Gruber. Evidence for a sex-specific residual effect of cannabis on visuospatial memory. **Psychother Psychosom** 1997; 66(4): 179–184.

CS454 Lawson, T. M. and A. Rees. Stroke and transient ischaemic attacks in association with substance abuse in a young man. **Postgrad Med J** 1996; 72(853): 692–693.

CS455 Mallat, A., J. Roberson, and J. G. Brock-Utne. Preoperative marijuana inhalation—an airway concern. **Can J Anaesth** 1996; 43(7): 691–693.

CS456 Napiorkowski, B., B. M. Lester, M. C. Freier, et al. Effects of in utero substance exposure on infant neurobehavior. **Pediatrics** 1996; 98(1): 71–75.

CS457 Williams, J. H., N. A. Wellman, and J. N. Rawlins. Cannabis use correlates with schizotypy in healthy people. **Addiction** 1996; 91(6): 869–877.

CS458 Boros, C. A, D. W. Parsons, G. D. Zoanetti, D. Ketteridge, and D. Kennedy. Cannabis cookies: a cause of coma. **J Paediatr Child Health** 1996; 32(2): 194–195.

CS459 Navarro, M., R. de Miguel, F. Rodriguez de Fonseca, J. A. Ramos, and J. J. Fernandez-Ruiz. Perinatal cannabinoid exposure modifies the sociosexual approach behavior and the mesolimbic dopaminergic activity of adult male rats. **Behav Brain Res** 1996; 75(1–2): 91–98.

CS460 Richter, B., N. Marangos, A. Jeron, and S. Irscheid. 3 different malignancies of the aerodigestive tract after chronic abuse of cannabis products. **HNO** 1995; 43(12): 728–731.

CS461 Wiley, J. L., J. W. Huffman, R. L. Balster, and B. R. Martin. Pharmacological specificity of the discriminative stimulus effects of delta 9-tetrahydrocannabinol in rhesus monkeys. **Drug Alcohol Depend** 1995; 40(1): 81–86.

CS462 Navarro, M., P. Rubio, and F. R. de Fonseca. Behavioural consequences of maternal exposure to natural cannabinoids in rats. **Psychopharmacology (Berl)** 1995; 122(1): 1–14.

CS463 Romero, J., L. Garcia, J. J. Fernandez-Ruiz, M. Cebeira, and J. A. Ramos. Changes in rat brain cannabinoid binding sites after acute or chronic exposure to their endogenous agonist, anandamide, or to delta 9-tetrahydrocannabinol. **Pharmacol Biochem Behav** 1995; 51(4): 731–737.

CS464 Souilhac, J., M. Poncelet, M. Rinaldi-Carmona, G. Le Fur, and P. Soubrie. Intrastriatal injection of cannabinoid receptor agonists induced turning behavior in mice. **Pharmacol Biochem Behav** 1995; 51(1): 3–7.

CS465 Shiono, P. H., M. A. Klebanoff, R. P. Nugent, et al. The impact of cocaine and marijuana use on low birth weight and preterm birth: a multicenter study. **Am J Obstet Gynecol** 1995; 172(1 Pt. 1): 19–27.

CS466 Solowij, N., B. F. Grenyer, G. Chesher, and J. Lewis. Biopsychosocial changes associated with cessation of cannabis use: a single case study of acute and chronic cognitive effects, withdrawal and treatment. **Life Sci** 1995; 56(23–24): 2127–2134.

3 | Cocos nucifera

L.

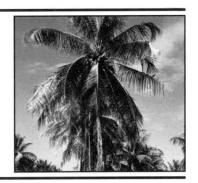

Common Names

Anaargeel	Iran	Kelapa	Malaysia
Arre kokosi	Albania	Khokhonate	South Africa
Bahia coconut palm	Brazil	Klapper	Netherlands
Boko	Philippines	Klapperboom	Netherlands
Cno coco	England	Kobari	India
Cno coco	Ireland	Kobbai	India
Cocco	Italy	Kobbai	Sri Lanka
Coco da Bahia	Brazil	Kobbera	India
Coco da India	Portugal	Kobbera	Sri Lanka
Coco fruto	Spain	Kok mak phao	Laos
Coco	Portugal	Kokas	Ethiopia
Coco	Spain	Kokkofoinika	Greece
Coconut	Guyana	Koko yashi	Japan
Cocotera	Spain	Koko	Spain
Cocotier	France	Kokonet	Ethiopia
Cocotier	Romania	Kokos orekonosnyi	Russia
Coqueiro da Bahia	Brazil	Kokos	Bulgaria
Coqueiro	Portugal	Kokos	Croatia
Cro bainney	The Isle of Man	Kokos	Czech Republic
Daab	India	Kokos	Germany
Dafu	Kenya	Kokos	Netherlands
Dafu	Mozambique	Kokos	Russia
Dafu	Tanzania	Kokos	Sweden
Dafu	Zaire	Kokos	Ukraine
Dua	Vietnam	Kokosa	Slovenia
Gawz el Hindi	Arabic countries	Kokoshneta	Iceland
Hentgagan engouz	Armenia	Kokosnoed	Denmark
Hindistancevizi	Turkey	Kokosnoot	Netherlands
I kokosit	Albania	Kokosnot	Sweden
Kafa	Turkey	Kokosnus	Israel
Karida	Greece	Kokosnuss	Germany
Karyda	Greece	Kokosnut	Netherlands
Ke ke ye zi	Taiwan	Kokosnut	Spain
Kelapa	Indonesia	Kokosov orah	Croatia

From: *Medicinal Plants of the World, vol. 3: Chemical Constituents, Traditional and Modern Medicinal Uses*
By: I. A. Ross © Humana Press Inc., Totowa, NJ

Kokosov orah	Serbia	Narial	India
Kokosov orech	Bulgaria	Narikela	India
Kokosov	Bulgaria	Narikol	India
Kokosova palma	Slovenia	Narival	Nepal
Kokosovaia pal'ma	Russia	Nariyal	India
Kokosovy orech	Czech Republic	Narkel	India
Kokosovy orech	Slovakia	Natsume yashi	Japan
Kokosovyj orech	Ukraine	Nazi	Mozambique
Kokosovyj orjekh	Russia	Nazi	Tanzania
Kokospalm	Netherlands	Nazi	Zaire
Kokospalm	Sweden	Niyog	Philippines
Kokospalme	Denmark	Niyok	Hawaii
Kokospalme	Germany	Niyok	Pacific Islands
Kokronoto	Surinam	Noce di cocco	Italy
Kokus	Israel	Noix de coco	France
Kokusnod	Faeroe Islands	Noz de coco	Portugal
Kokuszdio	Hungary	Nuca de cocos	Romania
Kookospahkina	Finland	Nuez de coco	Spain
Kookospalm	Estonia	Nyior	Malaysia
Kookospalmu	Finland	Palma de coco	Spain
Kronto	Surinam	Palma del cocco	Italy
Lag	Guyana	Palma kokosowa	Poland
Ma phra on	Thailand	Palmera de coco	Spain
Maak muu	Thailand	Polgaha	Sri Lanka
Mak un on	Myanmar	Qoqus	Israel
Maphrao	Thailand	T'ha'ari	Tahiti
Mar	India	Tenkaya	India
Mnazi	Mozambique	Tenkaya	Sri Lanka
Mnazi	Southeastern Africa	Tennai marama	India
Mnazi	Tanzania	Tennai marama	Sri Lanka
Mnazi	Zaire	Thenga	India
Naarakel	India	Thenga	Malaysia
Naariyal kaa per	India	Thenga	Sri Lanka
Naariyal kaa per	Pakistan	Thenginkai	India
Naariyal	India	Thengu	India
Naariyal	Pakistan	Thengu	Sri Lanka
Nadiya	India	Thenkaii	India
Nalikeran	Malaysia	Thenkaii	Sri Lanka
Nanivaara	India	Ungbin	Myanmar
Naral	India	Ye shu	China
Nargil	Arabic countries	Ye zi	China
Nargil	Iran		

BOTANICAL DESCRIPTION

Cocos nucifera is an unbranched monoecious plant of the PALMAE family. It grows to 30 m tall, with a crown of 25–35 paripinnate leaves, producing 12–16 new leaves per year. There is a central bud, which if cut off, leads to the death of tree. The trunk is straight or gently curved, with marked foliar scars, 30–50 cm in diameter, rises from a thickened base, and increases in height at a decreasing rate with age. The leaves are horizontal or somewhat hanging, 4–8 m in length and divided. Segments of leaves are numerous, linear-lanceolate, 0.5–1 m long and tapering. In the axil of each leaf is a spathe enclosing a long, stout, straw, or an orange-colored spadix. The spadix is composed of up to 40 branches, each bearing up to 300 small, fragrant, male flowers, and a few female, 2 cm long, globose flowers. The male and female flowers are produced separately in the leaf axils, usually on a long stalk. Approximately one-third of the female flowers develop into four to eight ripe fruits in 12–13 months, per inflorescence. The fruit is ovoid, three-angled drupe, up to 30 cm long, usually with thick, fibrous mesocarp (husk) and a hard, green-brown endocarp (shell) enclosing one seed. The seeds consist of 10 to 20 mm-thick white, fleshy endosperm (meat), covered by thin brown testa, surrounding a cavity party filled with a watery, sweet fluid (coconut water or milk). The latter is found mainly in immature fruits.

ORIGIN AND DISTRIBUTION

Evidence has been found that the place of origin is "submerged land to the north west of New Guinea." The major coconut areas lie between 20° N and 20° S of the equator. Although it is found beyond this region, 27° N and 27° S, cultivation has not been successful and the palm does not fruit. Many varieties are found in Melanesian region. It is most widely cultivated in the tropics: India, Ceylon, Malaysia, Indonesia, Philippines, South Sea Islands in the Pacific, East Africa, and Central and South Americas, up to 800 m above sea level, on humus-rich and porous soil or pure sand in coastal regions.

TRADITIONAL MEDICINAL USES

Admiralty Islands. The young root or leaves of the coconut plant are chewed for diarrhea[CN044].

Brazil. Decoction of the husk fiber is used to treat diarrhea and arthritis[CN070].

Cook Islands. Water extract of grated endosperm and *Citrus aurantium* juice is used to soak affected part in fractures and sprains[CN047]. Endosperm is taken orally for asthenia[CN051]. Oil, mixed with crushed

Phyllanthus virgatus, is rubbed around the ear for ear infections. Extract of different dried parts of the palm are taken orally for filariasis. A water solution of the crushed dried bark or husk and grated bark of *Hibiscus tiliaceus* is used externally to soak fractures and sprains. Crushed aerial root tips of *Ficus prolixa* are fried with coconut cream made of fresh endosperm, and the resulting oil is taken orally as a laxative in treating serious diseases[CN047].

Ecuador. Hot water extract of the plant is taken orally by females for sterility[CN055].

Fiji. Oil is used externally to prevent hair loss. The oil is warmed with crushed onion and garlic and applied aurally for earache[CN049]. Water of the unripe fruit is taken orally for kidney problems[CN049].

Ghana. Coconut milk is taken orally for diarrhea[CN098].

Guatemala. Hot water extract of the dried fruit is taken orally as a febrifuge and sudorific and for renal inflammation and scrofula. Hot water extract of the dried fruit is applied externally on wounds, ulcers, bruises, sores, skin infections, mucosa, dermatitis, inflammations, abscesses, and furuncles[CN056].

Haiti. Decoction of the dried pericarp is taken orally for amenorrhea. Fresh essential oil is applied externally on burns[CN051].

Hawaii. Water extract of the fruit is taken orally for asthma[CN024].

India. Infusion of the inflorescence is taken orally every morning for 3 days, coinciding with the menstrual cycle for leukorrhea and problems associated with the menstrual cycle[CN026]. A dose of 50 g daily of a mixture of *Cocos nucifera* fruit and *Ficus- benghalensis* latex is taken for 3 months to increase sexual potency in men[CN041]. Fruit is taken orally as a remedy for tapeworms[CN059].

Indonesia. Coconut oil is applied externally to treat wounds and injuries by the ethnic group of Ngada[CN159]. Shell is used as incense[CN057]. Hot water extract of the root is taken orally for fever, bloody diarrhea, and dysentery. Milk is taken orally by adults for poisoning[CN042]. Fruit milk is taken orally by females as a contraceptive[CN006]. Fruit juice is believed to diminish libido or fertility[CN008]. Seed oil with lemon juice and various tree roots is taken orally as an abortifacient[CN016]. Fruit ointment is applied externally for swollen legs. Fresh flowers, chewed with *Borassus flbellifer*, are used for gonorrhea[CN042].

Jamaica. Hot water extract of the dried shell is taken orally for diabetes[CN043]. Hot water extract of the root, with seven other plants, wine, and rum, is used as a tonic[CN060]. Extract of different parts are taken orally for diabetes[CN025].

Marquesas Islands. Fruit juice is mixed with *Cordia subcordata* and other plants and used for general menstrual disorders[CN003].

Mexico. A plaster made of fresh milk mixed with egg white is applied externally to prevent miscarriage[CN046].

Mozambique. Fruit is eaten by males as an aphrodisiac and used for relief of tumors[CN027].

Papua New Guinea. The fresh root of a young coconut is dug out and washed, then chewed and swallowed to relieve stomachache[CN022]. Fruit milk of *Cocos nucifera* is taken orally together with leaves of *Cleroden* sp., *Pouzolzia microhylla*, or *Macaranga tanarius* by pregnant women as an abortifacient agent[CN004].

Peru. Hot water extract of the fresh fruit is taken orally for blennorrhagia and asthma and as a diuretic, tenifuge, and galactagogue[CN054].

Thailand. Hot water extract of the fresh fruit juice is taken orally as a cardiotonic and neurotonic[CN062].

Tonga. Infusion of fresh kernel of coconut and Euodia hortensis are taken orally to treat retention of blood clots in the uterus after childbirth (locally called "toka-ala"). A mixture of *Cocos nucifera*, *Glochidion concolor*, *Vigna marina*, *Morinda citrifolia*, *Euodia hortensis*, and *Premna taitensis* with lemon juice is taken orally by pregnant women to treat severe bleeding during early pregnancy. Infusion of fresh kernel, taken twice daily with "tongan oil" prepared from *Aleurites moluccana* is used for dysuria caused by "kahi," a locally described syndrome affecting the gastrointestinal and genitourinary systems[CN045].

Trinidad. Hot water extract of the root is taken orally for amenorrhea[CN015].

Vanuatu. Hot water extract of the fruit, drunk in large quantities when very hot, is said to induce abortion[CN005]. Juice of the crushed root mixed with water is drank after delivery to restore strengh[CN023].

West Indies. Hot water extract of the root is taken orally for amenorrhea. Hot water extract of the mesocarp is taken orally by females for dysmenorrhea, amenorrhea, and menorrhagia[CN038].

CHEMICAL CONSTITUENTS

(ppm unless otherwise indicated)

14-O-(3-O-[β-D-galactopyranosyl-(1→2)-α-galactopyranosyl-(1→3)-α-L-arabinofuranosyl]-4-O-(α-L-arabino-furanosyl)-β-D- galactopyranosyl)-*trans*-zeatin-riboside: Milk[CN087]

Acetoin: Endosperm[CN030]
Alanine, phenyl: Lf[CN032]
Alanine: Endosperm[CN001]
Aluminium inorganic: Lf[CN011]
Amyrin, α: Sd oil[CN221]
Amyrin, β: Sd oil[CN221]
Arginine: Endosperm[CN001]
Aspartic acid: Endosperm[CN001]
Butane-2-3-diol: Endosperm[CN030]
Butane-2-3-dione: Endosperm[CN030]
Butyric acid, 2-methyl, methyl ester: Fr[CN220]
Butyroin: Fr[CN220]
Campesterol: Sd oil[CN221]
Caproic acid: Endosperm[CN030]
Catechins: Husk[CN066]
Cocamide diethanoloamide: Sd oil[CN082]
Cocamidopropyl betaine: Sd oil[CN214].
Cocos II protein: Pollen[CN114]
Cocos IIa protein: Pollen[CN114]
Cocos VI protein: Pollen[CN114]
Cocos VII protein: Pollen[CN114]
Cycloartenol, 24-methylene: Sd oil[CN221]
Cycloartenol: Sd oil[CN221]

Decalactone, δ: Endosperm[CN030]
Decanoic acid: Endosperm[CN030]
Docosane, N: Sd oil[CN221]
Dodecalactone, δ: Endosperm[CN030]
Dotriacontane, N: Sd oil[CN221]
Eicosane, N: Sd oil[CN221]
Ethyl lactate: Fr[CN220]
Fructose: Milk 2.22%[CN050], Rt[CN029]
Galactitol: Endosperm[CN028]
Gentisic acid: Lf[CN009]
Glucose: Milk 1.97%[CN050], Rt[CN029]
Glutamic acid: Endosperm[CN001], Lf[CN032]
Glycine: Endosperm[CN001], Lf[CN032]
Heneicosane, N: Sd oil[CN221]
Heptacosane, N: Sd oil[CN221]
Heptadecane, N: Sd oil[CN221]
Heptan-2-ol: Fr[CN220]
Hexacosane, N: Sd oil[CN221]
Histidine: Lf[CN032]
Lactose: Rt[CN029]
Lauric acid: Endosperm[CN030]
Leucine, iso: Endosperm[CN001], Lf[CN032]
Leucine: Lf[CN032]
Ligustrazine: Endosperm[CN030]
Limonene: Fr[CN220]
Linamarase: Endosperm[CN013]
Lysine: Endosperm[CN001], Lf[CN032]
Menthol: Fr[CN220]
Methionine: Endosperm[CN001], Lf[CN032]
Myristic acid: Sd oil[CN031]
Nonacosane, N: Sd oil[CN221]
Nonadecane, N: Sd oil[CN221]
Octacosane, N: Sd oil[CN221]
Octalactone, δ Endosperm[CN030]
Octanoic acid: Endosperm[CN030]
Pentacosane, N: Sd oil[CN221]
Phaseic acid, dihydro: Sap[CN040]
Phaseic acid, hydroxy: Sap[CN040]
Proline, hydroxy: Endosperm[CN001]
Proline: Lf[CN032]
Purin-6-one, 2-(3-methyl-but-2-enyl-amino): Milk[CN039]
Pyrasine, 2-3-5-trimethyl: Endosperm[CN030]
Raffinose: Rt[CN029]
Serine: Endosperm[CN001], Lf[CN032]
Sitosterol, β: Sd oil[CN221]
Sorbitol: Endosperm[CN028]
Squalene: Sd oil[CN221]
Stigmasterol: Sd oil[CN221]
Succinic acid: Rt[CN029]
Sucrose: Milk 0.43%[CN050]
Tannin (Cocos nucifera): Pl[CN061]

Terpineol, α: Fr[CN220]
Tetracosane, N: Sd oil[CN221]
Threonine: Lf[CN032]
Tocopherol, α: Sd oil[CN010]
Triacontane, N: Sd oil[CN221]
Triclosane, N: Sd oil[CN221]
Tyrosine: Lf[CN032]
Valine: Endosperm[CN001], Lf[CN032]

PHARMACOLOGICAL ACTIVITIES AND CLINICAL TRIALS

Acquired immunodeficiency syndrome activity. Coconut oil and "monolaurin"—a coconut oil byproduct—were administered to 12 women and 3 men who were in the early stage of human immunodeficiency virus infection. Ten patients took different doses of monolaurin, and five patients took coconut oil. It was believed that the treatment would lead to higher CD4 counts and a lower viral load. The trial was abandoned because it received only lukewarm approval from the government[CN155].

Allergenic activity. Dried fruit juice, administered intraperitoneally to guinea pigs at a dose of 10 mL/animal, was active. Dried fruit juice, administered intravenously to guinea pigs at a dose of 5 mL/animal, was active[CN036]. A patient with coconut anaphylaxis was confirmed by skin prick test. In vitro serum specific immunoglobulin E (IgE) was present[CN065]. Two patients with allergy manifested by life-threatening systemic reaction after consumption of coconut were investigated. Sera IgE from both patients indicated reduced coconut allergens with molecular weight of 35 and 36.5 kDa. IgE from 1 patient also bound a 55-kDa antigen. Preabsorption of sera with nut extracts suppressed IgE binding to coconut proteins. Preabsorption of sera with coconut produced a disappearance of IgE binding to protein bands at 35 and 36 kDa on a reduced immunoblot of walnut protein extract in one patient and suppression of IgE binding to a protein at 36 kDa in another patient[CN078]. Three cases of individuals allergic to cocamide diethanolamide were investigated. In two of the cases, multiple other cutaneous allergies were present. In both instances, cocamide diethanolamide was present in several personal care products used by the patients. In the third case, occupational exposure was suspected[CN082]. Coconut diethanolamide, administered to six patients with occupational contact dermatitis caused by coconut diethanolamide, produced sensitization from a barrier cream in two patients, hand-washing liquid in three, and one had been exposed to a hand-washing liquid and to a metalworking fluid containing coconut diethanolamide. Leave-on products (hand-protection foams) produced sensitization more rapidly (2–3 months) than rinse-off products (5–7 years). There was no contact allergy to another coconut-oil-derived sensitizer (cocamidopropyl betaine)[CN214]. Coconut diethanolamide, administered to a dentist, produced an occupational allergic contact dermatitis for hand-washing liquids[CN216]. Pollen extract, administered to 24 patients with allergy, asthma, and rhinitis produced positive skin prick test in all cases, and 19 of them were phadezym radioallergosorbent test-positive. Bronchial provocation test was positive in seven out of eight patients, and no late response or nonspecific reactions were observed[CN090]. An 8-month-old baby fed from birth with maternal milk was investigated. The first milk induced a severe gastrointestinal disorder, which disappeared when second milk was used. The third milk caused a relapse. The allergen was coconut, which was physicochemically modified in the second milk. It was confirmed by positive reintroduction test, positive skin test, and positive specific IgE test[CN091]. Pollen extract immunotherapy was studied in 96 allergic patients for 6–12 months. The clinical status measured by the symptom-medication scores demonstrated that the patients had significant clinical improvement after pollen extract immunotherapy. Serological study indicated a significant reduction of specific IgE and elevation of specific IgG in posttherapeutic patients' sera. There was no correlation between symptom-mediation scores and changes in specific serum IgE or IgG levels[CN097]. Proteins from fresh coconut and commercial extracts of coconut, administered to a patient with coconut anaphylaxis, produced a positive skin prick test. In vitro serum-specific IgE was present for coconut, hazelnut, Brazil nut, and cashew. Immunoblots demonstrated IgE binding to 35- and 50-kDa protein bands in the coconut and hazelnut extracts. Inhibition assays using coconut demonstrated complete inhibition of hazelnut specific IgE, but inhibition assays using hazelnut showed only partial inhibition of coconut-specific IgE[CN135]. A total of 100 patients (59 females and 41 males, aged 10–59 years, mean age 27.9 years) with allergic rhinitis underwent a skin prick test with 30 aeroallergens. Coconut produced 12% of positive results[CN194]. Oil, administered to β-lactoglobulin-treated brown Norway rats at a dose of 10% of diet supplemented with 0.5% curcumin for 3 weeks, lowered the circulatory release of rat chymase II in response to antigen[CN205]. The triethanolamine (TEA) salt of the condensation product of coconut fatty acids with a complex of polypeptides and amino acids derived from collagen (TEA-Coco-hydrolyzed protein), administered to a 21-year-old woman, produced a severe dermatitis of the face after using a proprietary skin cleanser. Patch testing revealed delayed hypersensitivity to TEA-Coco-hydrolyzed protein but not to other ingredients of the cleanser and positive results with other condensates of fatty acids and protein hydrolysates[CN218].

Aminopeptidase activity influence. Oil, administered to mice testis using acrylamides as substrates, produced no difference in soluble glutamyl-aminopeptidase (AP) angiotensin among the groups tested. Soluble aspartyl-AP and soluble pyroglutamyl-AP progressively decreased with the degree of saturation of the fatty acids used in the diet. Membrane-bound glutamyl-AP progressively increased with the degree of saturation of the fatty acids used in the diet. For membrane-bound aspartyl-AP activity, mice that were fed diets containing fish oil showed significantly higher levels than those fed sunflower oil, olive oil, and lard, but not those fed coconut oil[CN164].

Analgesic activity. Ethanol (50%) extract of the leaf, administered intraperitoneally to mice at a dose of 0.375 mg/kg, was inactive vs tail pressure method[CN036].

Anti-ancylostomiasis activity. Milk and meat of one nut eaten early in the morning by 22 adults on empty stomach was inactive[CN059].

Antibacterial activity. Ethanol (50%) extracts of the leaf, on agar plate at concentrations above 25 μg/mL, were inactive on *Bacillus subtilis*, *Escherichia coli*, *Salmonella typhosa*, and *Staphylococcus aureus*[CN058]. Tincture of the dried fruit (10 g plant material in 100 mL ethanol), on agar plate at a concentration of 30 μL/disc, was inactive on *Pseudomonas aeruginosa* and *Staphylococcus aureus* and produced weak activity on *Escherichia coli*[CN056]. Water extract of the husk fiber and fractions from adsorption chromatography were active on *Staphylococcus aureus*[CN070]. Hydrogenated oil, administered orally to Balb/c mice at a dose of 20% by weight for 4 wk and then infected with *Listeria monocytogenes* or treated with N-acetyl-L-cysteine (25 mg/mL intraperitoneally), produced no effect on survival. N-acetyl-L-cysteine reduced the recovery of *Listeria monocytogenes* from the spleen of the mice fed coconut oil diet[CN145]. There was a reduction in lymphocyte proliferation. An important increase in the production of reactive oxygen species was found after 12 h of the incubation with *Listeria monocyto-*

genes[CN166]. Hydrogenated oil, administered to *Listeria monocytogenes*-infected mice, produced a significant increase in peritoneal cells of coconut oil-fed mice and a reduction of bacterial recovery from the spleen[CN186]. Oil, administered to mice injected with a nonlethal dose of *Escherichia coli* at a dose of 20% by weight for 5 weeks, produced a decrease of peak plasma tumor necrosis factor (TNF)-α, interleukin (IL)-1 β, and IL-6 concentrations. Peak plasma IL-10 concentrations were higher in the coconut-fed group than in those fed the other diets, coconut oil diminished production of proinflammatory cytokines in vivo[CN187].

Anticarcinogenic effect. Coconut cake, administered to rat with 1,2-dimethylhydrazine-induced colon cancer at a dose of 25% of diet for 30 weeks, produced a significant decrease of the incidence and number of tumors, and β-glucuronidase and mucinase activities[CN134]. Hydrogenated oil, administered to Wistar female rats at doses of 8% and 24%, with or without a 24 mg/day/rat phytosterol supplement, produced no significant influence. Colonic glands were found in area of lymphoid follicles in all the groups but were more frequently in rats on high-fat diet[CN170].

Anticonvulsant activity. Ethanol (50%) extract of the leaf, administered intraperitoneally to mice at a dose 0.375 mg/mL, was inactive vs electroshock-induced convulsions[CN058].

Antidiarrheal activity. Water extract of coconut water, administered orally to adults, produced equivocal effect[CN019].

Antifungal activity. Ethanol (50%) extract of the leaf, on agar plate at a concentration of 25 μg/mL or more, was inactive on *Microsporum canis* and *Trichophyton mentagrophytes*[CN058]. Oil, on agar plate at a concentration of 05 mL/plate, was active on *Absidia corymbifera*, *Aspergillus flavus*, *Aspergillus niger*, and *Penicillium nigricans*[CN017]. Ethanol

(95%) extract of the dried shell, on agar plate at a concentration of 100 μg/mL, was active on *Microsporum audouini*, *Microsporum canis*, *Microsporum gypseum*, *Trichophyton mentagrophytes*, *Trichophyton rubrum*, *Trichophyton tonsurans*, *Trichophyton violaceum*, and *Epidermophyton floccosum*[CN033]. All fractions of the husk fiber, from adsorption chromatography, were inactive on *Candida albicans*, *Fonsecaea pedrosoi*, and *Cryptococcus neoformans*[CN070].

Antihypercholesterolemic activity. Oil was administered orally to male Wistar rats at doses of 12 or 24% of diet *ad libitum* for 4 weeks. Absorption of oleic acid in rats fed 24% oil was significantly greater than in controls during 0–8 hours but was not significantly different during 0–24 hours. There were no differences among groups in the distribution of cholesterol and oleic acid either in the lymph lipoproteins or in the lipid classes[CN097]. Oil was administered to 61 healthy males and 22 females aged 20–34 years, group I received a coconut–palm–coconut dietary sequence; group II, coconut–corn–coconut; group III, coconut oil during all three 5-week dietary periods. Compared with entry-level values, coconut oil raised the serum total cholesterol concentration greater than 10% in all three groups. The entry level of the ratio of low-density lipoprotein (LDL) to high-density lipoprotein (HDL) was not altered by coconut oil[CN107]. Oil was administered to 6-month-old ovariectomized rats with or without taurine for 28 days. Body mass gain, food intake, liver weight, and plasma apoliprotein (apo) A-1, apo B, LDL, and very low-density lipoprotein (VLDL) concentrations were not affected by the diet. Taurine lowered the plasma total cholesterol and increased liver total lipid and triglyceride in rats that were fed corn oil but not in those fed coconut oil. Taurine increased the 3-hydroxy-3-methylglutaryl coenzyme A (HMG-CoA) reductase messenger (m)RNA level in the liver of coconut-fed rats, but not in those fed corn oil[CN142]. Structured lipids (10%) synthesized from oil triglycerides, coconut oil, and coconut oil–safflower oil blends (1:0.7 w/w) were administered to rats for 60 days. The structured lipids lowered serum and liver cholesterol levels. Most of the decrease observed in serum was found in LDL fraction[CN143]. Oil, administered orally to male Wistar rats at a dose of 11% w/w for 6 months, produced a significant increase of serum total cholesterol (twofold), serum triglycerides (92.6%), LDL cholesterol (92.3%), and body weight gain (2.8-fold)[CN147].

Anti-inflammatory activity. Ethanol (50%) extract of the leaf, administered orally to male rats at a dose of 0.375 μg/kg, 1 hour before carrageenin injections, was inactive vs carrageenin-induced pedal edema[CN058].

Antilipidemic activity. Triglycerides structured lipids from coconut oil, administered to rats at a dose of 10% of diet for 60 days, produced a 15% decrease in total cholesterol and a 23% decrease in LDL cholesterol levels in the serum compared to coconut oil-fed rats. Total and free cholesterol levels in the liver of structured lipid-fed rats were lowered by 31 and 36%, respectively. The triglycerides in the serum and liver were decreased by 14 and 30%, respectively[CN140].

Anti-nociceptive activity. Aqueous extract of the husk fiber, administered orally to mice at doses of 200 or 400 mg/kg, produced an inhibition of the acetic acid-induced writhing response[CN063].

Antioxidant activity. Aqueous extract of the husk fiber, in cell culture, was active vs 2,2-diphenyl-1-picryl-hydrazyl-hydrate radicals[CN063]. Juice, in cell culture, was active vs 1,1-diphenyl-2-picrylhydrazyl, 2,2'-azino-bis(3-ethylbenz-thiazoline-6-sulfonic acid) and superoxide radicals but promoted the production of hydroxyl radicals and increased lipid peroxidation. The activity was most significant for fresh samples and diminished significantly when heated or treated with acid, alkali, or dialysis. Maturity of coconut drastically decreased the scavenging activity. Juice protected hemoglobin from nitrite-induced oxidation when added before the autocatalytic stage of the oxidation. Acid, alkali, or heat-treated or dialyzed juice showed a decreased ability in protecting hemoglobin from oxidation[CN069].

Antiparasitic activity. Polyphenolic-rich extract of the husk fiber, in cell culture at a concentration of 10 µg/mL, produced a reduction approx 44% of the association index between peritoneal mouse macrophages and *Leishmania amazonensis* promastigotes. It inhibited the growth of promastigote and amastigote developmental stages after 60 minutes. There was a concomitant increase of 182% in nitric oxide production by the infected macrophage in comparison to nontreated macrophages[CN064].

Antiproteinemic effect. Hydrogenated oil was administered orally to rats fed a protein-deficient diet at a dose of 200 g casein and 50 g coconut oil or 20 g casein and 50 g coconut oil for 28 days. The treatments produced a low concentration of protein and triacylglycerol (in serum VLDL, LDL–HDL 1 and 2–3), of cholesterol (in LDL–HDL1), and of phospholipids (in VLDL) in the protein-deficient groups. Relative amounts of linoleic and arachidonic acids in phospholipids of VLDL and HDL 2–3 were also lowered in the 20 g casein and 50 g coconut oil group[CN095]. Coconut fat, administered to rats, produced an increase in plasma esterase-1 activity[CN102]. Oil, administered to male Wistar rats at doses of 20% casein and 5% coconut oil or 2% casein and 5% coconut oil for 28 days, produced low concentration of protein, triacylglycerol, and VLDL in the plasma of 2% casein and 5% coconut oil group. Malondialdehyde content of the 2% casein and 5% coconut oil group was significantly higher than of control group. The lowest level of malondialdehyde was observed in the coconut oil group[CN103].

Antiviral activity. Crude extract of the husk fiber and one of the fractions from adsorption chromatography rich in catechin were active on acyclovir-resistant herpes-simplex virus type 1[CN070].

Anti-yeast activity. Tincture of the dried fruit, on agar plate at a concentration of 30 µL/disc, was inactive on *Candida albicans*. Extract of 10 g plant material in 100 mL ethanol was used[CN056]. Ethanol (50%) extract of the leaf, at a concentration of 25 µg/mL or more, was inactive on *Candida albicans* and *Cryptococcus neoformans*[CN058]. Seed oil, on agar plate at a concentration of 0.05 mL, was active on *Candida albicans*[CN017].

Apo B synthesis. Oil, administered to 1-month-old calves fed on a conventional milk replacer containing coconut oil, produced a twofold lower concentrations of total (^{35}S) proteins, (^{35}S) albumin, and (^{35}S) apo B in liver cells than in beef tallow-fed calves. The total amount of proteins secreted (including albumin) was similar in both groups. The amount of VLDL-(^{35}S) apo secreted was twofold lower in coconut oil-fed group[CN169]. Oil, administered to rabbits at a dose of 14% of the diet for 4 weeks, produced an increase in HDL-cholesterol (C) level from 170 to 250% over chow-fed control, with peak differences occurring at 1 week. Plasma apo A-I levels were also increased from 160 to 180%. After 4 weeks, there was no difference in plasma VLDL-C or LDL-C levels in the both groups. Hepatic level of apo A-I mRNA was increased in the coconut-fed groups. Treatment of cultured rabbit liver cells and sera with various saturated fatty acids did not alter apo A-I mRNA levels as observed in vivo[CN182].

Arrhythmogenic effect. Fruit juice, administered by intravenous infusion to dogs at a dose of 3 mL/minute, was active[CN036].

Atherosclerotic influence. Oil was administered orally to rabbits fed a semipurified, cholesterol-free atherogenic diet at a dose of 14% fat: coconut oil (CNO), corn oil (CO), palm kernel oil (PO), and cocoa butter (CB). Serum cholesterol levels (mg/dL) at 9 months were CO, 64; PO, 436; CB, 220; and CNO, 474. HDL cholesterol (%) was CO, 37; PO, 8.6; CB, 25; and CNO, 7. average artherosclerosis (arch + thoracic/2) was CO, 0.15; PO, 1.28; CB, 0.53; and CNO, 1.60[CN127]. Oil, administered to British Halflop rabbits at a dose of 3% of the diet, produced an increase of cholesterol, triacylglycerol, apo B, apo C-III, and apo E as compared to chow-fed rabbits. The apo A level did not differ from the chow-fed rabbits. There was a decrease in the low fractional catabolic rate of LDL-C[CN128]. Oil, administered with cholesterol (30 g/kg) to male golden Syrian hamsters at a dose of 150 g/kg of diet, developed lipid-rich lesions in the ascending aorta and aortic arch after 4 weeks. The lesions continued to progress throughout the next 8 weeks. Removal of cholesterol from the diet halted this progression. Oil, administered without supplemental cholesterol in the same dose for 16 weeks, doubled the size of lesions in the ascending aorta and decreased linearly the lesion size in the aortic arch[CN183].

Blood pressure effect. Fruit juice, administered intravenously by infusion to dogs at a dose of 3 mL/minute for 100 minutes, was active. Initial effect was a decrease in blood pressure[CN036]. Oil, administered to male weanling rats at a dose of 10% of diet for 5 weeks, produced significantly higher blood pressure than other groups. Systolic blood pressure was found related to the dietary intakes of saturated and unsaturated fatty acids. Prenatal exposure of the rats to a maternal low-protein diet abolished the hypertensive effect of the coconut oil diet[CN206].

Butyryl cholinesterase activity. Oil was administered to rats at different doses with or without clofibrate for 15 days. The hypolipidemic action of clofibrate was not influenced by the amount of fat. Clofibrate did not affect lower cholesterol concentration in rats fed the low fat diet, but it counteracted the rise in liver cholesterol seen in rats fed the high-fat diet. The high-fat diet produced slightly higher levels of butyryl cholinesterase in the small intestine but markedly raised intestinal esterase-1 activity[CN101].

Carcinogenic activity. Coconut oil acid diethanolamine condensate in ethanol was administered externally to 10 male and 10 female F344/N rats at doses of 25, 50, 100, 200, or 400 mg/kg body weight five times per week for 14 weeks. All of the rats survived the study. Final mean body weights and body weight gains of the 200 and 400 mg/kg males and females were significantly less than those of the controls. Clinical findings included irritation of the skin at the site of application in the 100, 200, and 400 mg/kg males and females. Cholesterol concentrations were significantly decreased in 200 and 400 mg/kg males. Histopathological lesions of the skin at the site of application included epidermal hyperplasia, sebaceous gland hyperplasia, chronic active inflammation, parakeratosis, and ulcer. The incidences and severities of skin lesions generally increased with increasing dose in males and females. The incidences of renal tube regeneration in the 100, 200, and 400 mg/kg females were significantly greater than the vehicle control incidence, and the severities in the 200 and 400 mg/kg females were increased. Coconut oil acid diethanolamine condensate in ethanol was administered externally to 10 male and 10 female B6C3F1 mice at doses of the 50, 100, 200, 400, or 800 mg /kg body weight five times per week for 14 weeks. All mice survived until the end of the study. Final mean body weights and body weight gains of dosed males and females were similar to those of the vehicle controls. The only treatment-related clinical finding was irritation of the skin at the site of application in males and females administered the 800 mg/kg dose. Weights of the liver and kidney of 800 mg/kg males and females, the liver of the 400 mg/kg females, and the lung of the 800 mg/kg females were significantly increased compared to the controls. Epididymal spermatozoal concentration was significantly increased in the 800-mg/kg males. Histopathological lesions of the skin at the site of application included epidermal hyperplasia, sebaceous gland hyperplasia, chronic active inflammation, parakeratosis, and ulcer. The incidences and severities of these skin lesions generally increased with increasing dose in males and females. Coconut oil acid diethanolamine condensate in ethanol was administered externally to 50 male and 50 female F344/N rats at doses of 50 or 100 mg/kg body weight five times a week for 104 weeks. The survival rates of treated male and female rats were similar to those of the vehicle controls. The mean body weights of dosed males and females were similar to those of the vehicle controls throughout most of the study. The only chemical-related clinical finding was irritation of the skin at the site of application in the 100-mg/kg females. There were marginal increases in the incidences of renal tubule adenoma or carcinoma (combined) in the 50-mg/kg females. The severity of nephropathy increased with increasing dose in the female rats. Nonneoplastic lesions of the skin at the site of application included epidermal hyperplasia, sebaceous gland hyperplasia, parakeratosis, and hyperkeratosis, and the incidences and severities of these lesions increased with increasing dose. The incidence of chronic active inflammation, epithelial hyperplasia, and epithelial ulcer of the forestomach increased with dose in female rats and the increases were significant in the 100-mg/kg group. Coconut oil acid diethanolamine condensate in ethanol was administered externally to 50 male and 50 female B6C3F1 mice at doses of 100 or 200 mg/kg body weight five times a week for 104 to 105 weeks. Survival of the mice was generally similar to that of the controls. Mean body weights of 100-mg/kg females from week 93 and 200-mg/kg females from week 77 were less than in the controls. The only clinical finding attributed to treatment was irritation of the skin at the site of application in males administered 200 mg/kg. The incidences of hepatic neoplasms (hepatocellular adenoma, hepatocellular carcinoma, and hepatoblastoma) were significantly increased in both sexes. Most of the incidences exceeded the historical control ranges. The incidences of eosinophilic foci in dosed groups of male mice were increased relative to that in controls. The incidences of renal tubule adenoma and renal tubule adenoma or carcinoma (combined) were significantly increased in the 200-mg/kg males. Several nonneoplastic lesions of the skin at the site of application were considered treatment related. Incidence of epidermal hyperplasia, sebaceous gland hyperplasia, and hyperkeratosis were greater in all dosed groups than in the controls. The incidence of ulcer in 200-mg/kg males and inflammation and parakeratosis in 200-mg/kg females were greater than in the controls. The incidence of thyroid gland follicular cell hyperplasia in all of the dosed groups was significantly greater than those in the control groups[CN148].

Cardiovascular effect. Coconut and coconut oil, administered to 32 coronary heart disease patients in 16 age- and sex-matched healthy controls with no difference in the fat, saturated fat, and cholesterol consumption, produced no effect[CN086]. Hydrogenated oil, administered to young male Wistar rats, at a dose of 10% of diet for 10 weeks, produced an increase in the risk of ventricular arrhythmias under conditions of both ischemia and reperfusion. The incidence of ventricular fibrillation was 67% in the oil-fed group. The time until the first occurrence of extrasystole, the incidence of ventricular tachycardia, and the incidence of reperfusion-induced ventricular fibrillation were influenced in a similar manner between groups. The fatty acid composition of myocardial tissue, the ratio of n-3 to n-6 fatty acids, and the double-bond index were significantly affected by the various diets[CN092]. Oil was administered by gastric intubation to male Sprague–Dawley rats at a dose of 86:14 w/w coconut oil/safflower oil for 10 days, containing either 0.8 mg Zn/kg or 111 mg Zn/kg. Zinc-deficient rats that were fed coconut oil had higher concentrations of triglycerides and total fatty acids in the heart than the control rats. The concentrations of phospholipids and total cholesterol were not different between zinc-deficient and control rats. Concentrations of lauric acid, myristic acid, palmitic acid, palmitoleic acid, and oleic acid were 65 to 192% higher in the hearts of zinc-deficient rats fed coconut diet than in the control rats. The level of arachidonic acid in phospholipids, which may represent desaturation activity, was not different in the zinc-deficient rats and control rats[CN093]. Oil was administered orally to rats fed a copper-deficient diet at doses of 10 g/100 g coconut oil or 10 g/100 g coconut oil with 1 g/100 g cholesterol. Rats fed the diet with coconut and cholesterol had left ventricular chamber volumes that were twofold larger than those of rats fed diet with coconut oil only. Copper deficiency reduced left ventricular chamber volume only in rats fed coconut oil and cholesterol. The results indicated that preload and contractility in the hearts of coconut oil-fed rats were greater than cardiac response to cholesterol addition to the coconut oil diet. Hearts in copper-deficient rats fed coconut oil and cholesterol exhibited eccentric hypertrophy and ventricular dysfunction[CN099]. Oil, administered orally to rats for 4 weeks, produced a significant

decrease in 5'-nucleotidase, phosphodiesterase I and p-nitrophenylphosphatase activity of cardiac sarcolemma. Sarcolemma from coconut-fed rats contained a significantly lower concentration of total polyunsaturated fatty acids (PUFAs) and a higher concentration of total monounsaturated fatty acids than that from safflower-fed rats. The fatty acid composition of the phosphatidylcholine exhibited the largest alterations because of coconut oil feeding. No dietary effect was observed in the sarcolemma content of cholesterol and phospholipids[CN122].

Cholestatic liver disease. Medium-chain fat from the oil, administered to bile duct-ligated rats, resulted in a decrease of consumption of the fat source compared to control rats; however, carbohydrate and protein intakes were not affected. Body weight gain was significantly greater in coconut-fed rats than in rats fed long-chain fat (Crisco vegetable shortening). Mortality was 44% in bile duct-ligated animals fed the long-chain fat and 0% in those fed medium-chain fat[CN118].

Cholesterol metabolism. Hydrogenated oil, administered orally to hamsters at a dose of 20% of diet for 4 weeks, induced hypercholesterolemia. Oil feeding had no effect on cholesterol synthesis but markedly inhibited cholesterol esterification in both the liver and the intestine. The diet-induced hypercholesterolemia was strongly correlated with an increase in acyl-CoA/cholesterol acyltransferase activity. The hypercholesterolemia increased aortic uptake of cholesterol and hence acyl-CoA/cholesterol acyltransferase activity[CN109]. Coconut fat, administered orally to rabbits with partial ileal bypass, produced a significant increase of serum total cholesterol and phospholipids concentrations. The effect on serum lipids of the type of fat was similar in control and partial ileal bypass rabbits[CN120]. Coconut—a main source of energy for two

Polynesian groups, Tokelauans and Puka-pukans—was investigated. Tokelauans obtained a much higher percentage of energy from coconut than the Pukapu-kans, 63% compared with 34%, so their intake of saturated fat is higher. The serum cholesterol levels are 35–40 mg higher in Tokelauans than in Pukapukans. Analysis of a variety of food samples and human fat biopsies showed a high lauric (12:0) and myristic (14:0) acids content. Vascular dis-ease is uncommon in both populations, and there is no evidence of the high saturated fat intake having a harmful effect in these populations[CN129]. Oil, administered orally to growing male Sprague–Dawley rats fed a diet containing unoxidized or oxidized cho-lesterol (5 g/kg) with coconut or salmon oil (100 g/kg) for 5 weeks, produced an effect independent of the dietary fat[CN132]. Hydro-genated coconut oil was administered to F(1)B Golden Syrian hamsters at a dose of 20 g/100 g for 10 weeks. The hamsters were ranked according to their plasma VLDL and LDL cholesterol as a low or medium group. Low-coconut oil group had significantly higher aortic total and esterified cholesterol concentrations than the low-cholesterol-fed group. Hamsters in the low-cholesterol-fed group had significantly higher aortic TNF-α concentrations than hamsters in the low-coconut oil group. Hamsters in the med-coconut oil group had significantly higher aortic IL-1-β concentrations than hamsters in the med-cholesterol group. Hamsters in both cholesterol fed groups had significantly lower plasma total cholesterol concentrations than hamsters in the low-coconut oil group[CN136].

Cholesterolemic effect. Oil, administered to phospholipids transfer protein knockout (PLTP0)-deficient mice, produced an increase of phospholipids and free choles-terol in the VLDL-LDL region of PLTP0 mice. Accumulation of phospholipids and free cholesterol was dramatically increased

in PLTP0/HL0 mice compared to PLTP0 mice. Turnover studies indicated that coco-nut oil was associated with delayed catabo-lism of phospholipids and phospholipids/ free cholesterol-rich particles. Incubation of these particles with hepatocytes of coconut-fed mice produced a reduced removal of phospholipids and free cholesterol by scav-enger receptor BI , even though scavenger receptor BI protein expression levels were unchanged[CN158].

Coagglutination activity. Oil was admin-istered to females at doses of a high-satu-rated fatty acids diet (HSAFA diet; 38.4% of energy from fat, polyunsaturated/satu-rated [P/S] fatty acid ratio 0.14) or low- satu-rated fatty acids diet (LSAFA; 19.7% of energy from fat, P/S ratio 0.17). The post-prandial plasma concentration of tissue plasminogen activator (t-PA) antigen was decreased in the HSAFA-fed group. Plasma t-PA antigen was correlated with plas-minogen activator inhibitor type 1 (PAI-1) activity when the participants consumed the HSAFA and LSAFA diet, although the diets did not affect the PAI-1 levels. There were no significant differences in postpran-dial variations in t-PA activity, factor VII coagulant activity, or fibrinogen levels as a result of the diets. Serum-fasting Lp(a) lev-els were lower in the HSAFA group and were lower in the LSAFA group. Serum Lp(a) concentrations did not differ when the women consumed the HSAFA and LSAFA diets[CN139].

Cytotoxic activity. Oil, in cell culture at a concentration of 300 µg/mL, was active on Ca-colon-HT29[CN034]. Coir fiber, adminis-tered intratracheally to guinea pigs, resolved the granulomas. Coir fiber and ash, in cell culture, produced a hemolytic activity and macrophage cytotoxicity more marked with ash compared with the fiber alone[CN126]. Extract of the husk fiber, in cell culture at a concentration of 10 µg/mL, inhibited the growth of promastigote and amastigote developmental stages of *Leishmania amazonensis* after 60 minutes[CN064]. Extract of the fiber husk (rich in catechins), in erythroleukemia cell line (K562) and normal human peripheral blood lymphocytes activated by phytohemagglutinin or phorbol ester, produced a dose-dependent effect. For phytohemagglutinin, this effect was irreversible, being already established on the first hours of culture[CN066]. Oil, administered to C57B16 mice at a dose of 21% fat by weight, produced a significant decrease in macrophage-mediated death of P815 cells by nitric oxide and did not alter the death of L929 cell by macrophages. Liposaccharide-stimulated TNF-α production by macrophages decreased with increasing unsaturated fatty acid content of the diet: fish oil < safflower oil < olive oil < coconut oil < low-fat diet[CN185].

Denture stomatitis. Coconut soap, associated with 05% sodium hypochlorite, used by patients for 15 days, significantly reduced clinical signs of denture stomatitis and was effective in controlling denture biofilm[CN131].

Desensitization effect. Saline extract of the dried pollen, administered subcutaneously to 96 allergic adults at variable doses, produced a clinical improvement and decreased IgE levels[CN020].

Dietary macronutrient distribution influence. Oil, administered to diet-induced overweight rats fed an energy-restricted diet with 60% of coconut oil, produced no difference between control and fat-fed group in weight loss and serum parameters. The coconut-fed group produced a greater reduction in the subcutaneous fat depot and of total body fat. Hepatic glycogen and glycogenic amino acid were altered in coconut-fed rats[CN163].

Diuretic activity. Decoction of the dried fruit, administered nasogastrically to rats at a dose 1 g/kg, was active[CN053]. Fruit juice, administered intravenously by infusion to dogs at a dose of 3 mL/minute for 100 minutes, produced weak activity[CN036]. Ethanol extract of the leaf, administered intraperitoneally to saline-loaded male rats at a dose of 0.185 mg/kg, was active. Urine was collected for 4 hours after treatment[CN058].

Epstein–Barr virus activation. Seed oil, in cell culture at a concentration of 50 µg/mL, was inactive on virus-transformed lymphoblasts[CN048].

Erythrocytic effect. Hydrogenated coconut oil, administered orally to healthy rats for 10 weeks, produced a significant effect on five of the six classes of erythrocytes identified. The proportion of cells in each class was dependent on the diet. There was no significant effect of diet on erythrocyte filterability index and no statistical correlation between erythrocyte filterability index and morphology[CN088].

Estrogenic effect. Seed oil, administered to female mice at a dose of 10% of diet, was active[CN007].

Exocrine pancreatic secretion. Oil, administered to piglets at a dose of 10 g/100 g of diet, did not affect the output of carboxylester hydrolase. Protein, chymotrypsin, carboxypeptidase A, elastase, and amylase outputs were not different among the dietary treatment groups. The outputs of trypsin and colipase were higher in the coconut-fed group[CN167]. Oil, administered to three barrows at a dose of 15 g fat/100 g diet, produced a significant increase of chymotrypsin secretion[CN207].

Fat digestibility. Fat, administered to male rats at a dose of 8% of diet for 2 weeks, produced no differential effect on growth. Glucose significantly depressed apparent lipid digestibility in coconut fat-fed rats[CN176].

Fatty acid composition influence. Oil was administered orally to mice bearing the L1210 murine leukemia cells at a dose of 16% of diet. A microsome-rich fraction prepared from the L1210 cells produced more monoenoic fatty acids (37% vs 12%) compared to mice fed the sunflower oil[CN124]. Oil, administered to chicken at concentrations of 10 and 20% of diet, produced changes in fatty acid composition of free fatty acid and triglyceride fractions of chick plasma parallel to that of the experimental diet. Plasma phospholipids incorporated low levels of 12:0 and 14:0 acids, whereas 18:0, the main saturated fatty acid of this fraction, increased after coconut oil feeding. The percentage of 18:2 acid significantly increased after coconut oil feeding[CN154]. Oil, administered to rats at a dose of 15% of diet for 4 weeks, produced an increase of total cholesterol in the liver and the decrease of total liver phospholipids[CN157]. Coconut/soy oil, administered by infusion into the duodenum of rats, produced the proportion of capric and lauric acids in the lymphatic triacylglycerol, reflecting the fatty acid composition in the diet. Results indicated that more than 50% of the capric and lauric acids could have been absorbed from the intestine as sn-monoacylglycerols[CN213]. Hydrogenated coconut oil was administered to rats at a dose of 7% of the diet (essential fatty acids deficient in both n-6 and n-3) for 28 weeks (1 week gestation, 3 weeks lactation, and 24 weeks thereafter). The fatty acid compositional changes indicative of an essential fatty acid deficiency, such as the decreases in the levels of 18:2 n-6 along with an accumulation of 20:3 n-9 were observed in all the salivary glands. In the submandibular glands, the proportions of 16:1, 18:1 n-9 and 18:1 n-7 were higher in hydrogenated coconut oil-fed group than in the other groups. Some differences in the fatty acid composition of the three glands were found[CN085].

Fatty acid metabolism. Oil was administered to preruminant Holstein Friesian male calves fed a conventional milk diet containing coconut oil for 19 days. Fatty acid oxidation was determined by measuring the production of CO_2 (total oxidation) and acid-soluble products (partial oxidation). Production of CO_2 was 1.7–3.6-fold lower and acid soluble products tend to be lower in liver slices of coconut oil-fed than beef-tallow-fed calves. Fatty acid esterification as neutral lipids was 2.6- to 3.1-fold higher in liver slices of coconut oil-fed group. The increase in neutral lipid production did not stimulate VLDL secretion by the hepatocytes, leading to a triacylglycerol accumulation in the cytosol of the calves fed coconut oil[CN178]. Oil, administered to preruminant calves fed a milk replacer containing coconut oil for 19 days, produced no significant difference in weight of the total body and tissue between the treated groups. Plasma glucose and insulin concentrations were lower in the coconut oil-fed group. Feeding on the coconut oil diet induced an 18-fold increase in the hepatic concentration of triacylglycerol. The perixomal oxidation rate of oleate was 1.5-fold higher in the hearts of calves fed coconut oil. The cytochrome C oxidase/citrate synthase activity ratio was lower in the liver of the coconut oil-fed animals[CN184]. Oil, administered as a ratio 7:1 w/w coconut oil/safflower oil by gastric intubation to zinc-deficient rats, reduced δ-desaturase activity in liver microsomes of rats fed coconut oil. Zinc-deficient rats on the coconut oil diet had unchanged δ-6-desaturase activity with linoleic acid as substrate and lowered activity with α-linolenic acid as substrate[CN197].

Food intake suppression. Oil, administered intragastrically to devazepide-treated rats at a dose of 1 g/4 mL 30 minutes before feeding, produced a decrease of devazepide effect[CN144].

Gastrin inhibition. Hydrogenated oil, administered to adult rats, produced a significant reduction in antral and plasma gastrin concentrations[CN171].

Gastrointestinal effect. Oil, administered to rats, induced the secretion of surfactant-like particles in the small intestine[CN160].

Genotoxic activity. Coconut oil acid diethanolamine condensate with or without S9 activation enzyme, in cell culture, produced no effect on *Salmonella typhimurium*. The treatment did not produce an increase in mutant L5178Y mouse lymphoma cell colonies, and no increased in the frequencies of sister chromatid exchanges or chromosomal aberrations in Chinese hamster ovary cells. In a peripheral blood micronucleus test in male and female mice from the 14-week test, positive results were obtained[CN148].

Genotype and diet effect. Coconut oil was administered to female Zucker rats throughout mating and lactation. Homozygous lean male and female rats, obese male, and lean heterozygous female rats were bred. Additional male rats were maintained on the same diet as their mothers until 11–12 days of age. Obese sucking rats had higher body weights than lean pups. Inguinal fat pad weights and pad-to-body weight ratios followed the pattern of obese greater than lean (FA/fa genes) pups that were greater than lean (FA/FA) pups. A similar relationship was found for adipose tissue lipogenic enzyme activities. At 11–12 weeks of age, measurements followed the general pattern of obese rats having greater value than lean rats (i.e., FA/fa = FA/FA). Coconut oil-fed fa/fa rats had lower hepatic lipogenic enzyme activities and lower fat cell numbers than safflower-fed fa/fa rats. High-fat diet did not result in a heterozygous effect in young adult lean male rats[CN079]. Hydrogenated coconut oil, corn oil, or menhaden oil were administered to diabetes-prone BHE/cdb and normal Sprague–Dawley rats. Both fat source and strain affected the temperature dependence of succinate-supported respiration. The transition temperature was greater in BHE/cdb rats than in the Sprague–Dawley rats. The efficiency of adenosine triphosphatase synthesis as reflected by the adenosine diphosphatase / O ratio was decreased in the BHE/cdb rats compared to Sprague–Dawley rats[CN084].

Glucose metabolism. Hydrogenated oil, administered to prediabetic weanling BHE rats fed a 6% fat and 64% sucrose diet, produced an increase of the fractional irreversible glucose turnover rates, fractional glucose carbon recycling, hepatic fatty acid synthesis rates, adipose fatty acid synthesis rate, lower muscle glycogen, and lower rates of incorporation of glucose into muscle glycogen than corn oil-fed rats. The diet had no effect on glucose mass and space, hepatic glycogen, or blood glucose levels[CN113]. Oil, administered to male Wistar rats at a dose of 25% by weight for 26 days, produced a significant increase in serum total cholesterol, LDLs, liver cholesterol, and liver weight. There was a decrease in serum HDLs, triacylglycerol levels, and abdominal fat weight; an increase in 3-hydroxy-3-methylglutaryl-CoA reductase activity in the liver; reduction in plasma lecithin-cholesterol acyltransferase activity; lower level of serum insulin; and liver glycogen in the coconut oil-fed rats. Glucose use was altered because lower glucose-6-phosphatase and increased glucokinase activities in the liver of coconut oil-fed rats were found[CN190]. Coconut palm wine was administered to rats at a dose of 24.5 mL/kg body weight/d for 15 days before conception and throughout gestation. On the 19th day of gestation, hypoglycemia was observed in both wine- and ethanol-treated groups. Synthesis of glycogen was elevated on exposure to ethanol/wine, but its degradation was enhanced only in ethanol-exposed rats. Key enzymes of the citric acid cycle and gluconcogenesis were inhibited on administration in both groups. The activities of glycolytic enzymes were increased[CN204]. Hydrogenated oil (6%), administered to BHE rats at a dose of 5% of diet, produced no influence on glucose. Hepatocytes isolated from rats fed coconut oil had a significantly lower affinity for insulin than menhaden oil-treated rats[CN104].

Glucose-6-phosphate dehydrogenase activity. Oil, administered to rats, reduced the G-6-PDH activity of lymphocytes by 16% and the activity of G-6-PDH in liver by 42%[CN192].

Glycemic index. The glycemic index of different commonly consumed products supplemented with increasing levels of coconut flour was determined in 10 normal and 10 diabetic subjects. The test food with 200–250 g coconut flour/kg had significantly low, gastrointestinal (GI) (< 60); with 150 g coconut flour/kg had GI ranging from 61.3 to 71.4. A very strong negative correlation (r –0.85, p < 0.005) was observed between the GI and dietary fiber content of food[CN067]. Oil, administered to lean Zucker rats at a dose of 5% of diet (87% saturated fatty acids) for 2 weeks, produced no differences in food intake, body weight, tissue level of glucagons-like peptide-1, plasma insulin, and glucagons levels in coconut oil- and olive oil-fed groups[CN174].

Hair damage prevention. Coconut oil application has a strong effect on hair as compared to sunflower and mineral oils. Among the three oils investigated, coconut oil was the only one that reduced the protein loss remarkably for both damaged and undamaged hair when used as a prewash and postwash grooming product[CN146].

Hemostatic effect. Coconut water, in citrated plasma of eight healthy volunteers, was observed. Replacement of up to 50% of diluted plasma by water did not influence initiation of coagulation. Replacing 50% of citrated plasma by coconut water reduced maximum amplitude of thrombelastography recording dose by 39%[CN072].

Hemotoxic activity. Fruit juice, administered by intravenous infusion to dogs at a dose of 5 mL/minute for 60 minutes, was active[CN036].

Hepatic activity. Hydrogenated oil, administered orally to male weanling rats at a dose of 10% of diet for 9 weeks, produced no significant alteration of hepatic 5-, 6-, and 9-desaturase activity. Addition of oil to the diet, simultaneously with lowering of the carbohydrate level, diminished the stimulatory effect of dietary sucrose vs glucose on 9-desaturase activity[CN121].

Hepatic lipid peroxidation. Oil, administered to apo E-deficient mice for 10 weeks, produced a significant increase in hepatic lipid peroxidation[CN172].

Hepatic mitochondrial effect. Oil, administered to chicken at a dose of 20% of the diet, produced a clear damage to the hepatic mitochondria accompanied by an accumulation of glycogen and lipid droplets in the hepatocyte cytoplasm. Pharmaceutical coconut oil induced a high percentage of cellular death when administered for 14 days. Fatty acid profiles in liver and hepatic mitochondria changed during 24 hours after pharmaceutical and cooking oils supplementation to the diet. The accumulation of shorter chain fatty acids (12:0) and (14:0) was higher after pharmaceutical than after cooking oil diet feeding. Mitochondrial ratios of saturated/unsaturated and saturated fatty acids (SUFAs)/PUFAs rapidly changed in parallel to these ratios in both diets. Most of the mitochondrial parameters measured recuperate to the control values when diets were supplied for 5–14 days. The maintenance of these ratios after 14 days pharmacological oil diet feeding was significantly higher than those in control[CN199].

Hydrogen peroxide release inhibition. Seed oil, administered to rats at a concentration of 8% of the diet, produced equivocal effect on macrophages. Capsaicin or curcumin enhanced the effect[CN021].

Hyperalphalipoproteinemic activity. Oil, administered orally to rabbits fed commercial chow or chow plus 14% w/w coconut oil, resulted in double increase the plasma levels of HDL cholesterol, phospholipids, and protein for up to 4 months without affecting HDL lipid and apoprotein composition. After 3 months also increased VLDL (107%) and LDL cholesterol (40%) levels, but the absolute increases in each of these lipoprotein fractions was less than half of that of HDL. Isotope kinetic studies of 125I-HDL protein indicated a double rate of production of HDL and no change in the efficiency of removal of HDL from plasma[CN115].

Hypercholesterolemic activity. Seed oil, administered by gastric intubation to dogs, was active. Seed oil, administered orally to adults, was active[CN037]. Oil, administered orally to rats at a dose of 79 g/day for 3 weeks, produced a significant increase of the final plasma cholesterol in groups that consumed yeast with coconut oil (91 mg/dL), in comparison to group consuming soybean protein with coconut oil (36 mg/dL)[CN089]. Coconut fat, administered to hyporesponsive and hyperresponsive inbred strains of rabbits with high or low response of plasma cholesterol to dietary SUFAs vs PUFAs, produced no influence on the efficiency of cholesterol absorption[CN106]. Fat, administered orally to young normolipidemic males at a dose of 30% of the diet with a polyunsaturated/saturated fat ratio of 4 or 0.25 for 8 weeks, produced a significant increase of total plasma cholesterol level[CN111]. Oil, administered to Mongolian gerbils, produced a hypercholesterolemia associated with elevations in VLDL, LDL, and HDL. The type of dietary fat did not influence lipoprotein composition and size[CN130]. Fresh and thermally oxidized oil, administered to rats at a dose of 20% of diet, produced an increase of total cholesterol, LDL and VLDL cholesterol, and triacylglycerol and phospholipids levels and a decrease in HDL cholesterol[CN149]. Oil, administered to 25 women at doses of 38.4% of energy from fat (HSAFA; PUFA/SUFA P/S ratio = 0.14) or 19.7% energy from fat (LSAFA; P/S ratio

0.17) for 3-week periods, produced no difference in serum total cholesterol, LDL cholesterol, and apo B concentrations between the diet periods. HDL cholesterol and apo A-I were 15% and 11%, respectively, higher during HSAFA diet period than during LSAFA diet period. The LDL/HDL-C and apo B/apo A-I ratios were higher during LSAFA diet period[CN152].

Hyperlipidemic activity. Palm wine was administered orally to female albino rats at a dose of 24.5 mL/kg body weight/day for 15 days before conception and during pregnancy. On days 13 and 19 of gestation, liver function and hyperlipidemia were seen in the fetuses. Hyperlipidemia was caused by increased biosynthesis since the incorporation of ^{14}C acetate into lipids and activity of HMG-CoA reductase and lipogenic enzymes were elevated[CN080]. Oil, administered to miniature pigs fed a pig chow supplemented with 17.1% of coconut oil for 30 d, produced a significant increase of cholesterol, triglyceride, HDL cholesterol and subfractions, LDL cholesterol and subfractions, and lipoprotein lipase activity in both genders. For cholesterol, triglyceride, HDL cholesterol (HDL-C and HDL[2]-C), LDL cholesterol (LDL-C, LDL[1 and 2]-C), and hepatic lipase, the female response to the diet was exaggerated compared to the male response[CN153].

Hyperthermic effect. Coconut oil, administered orally to rats with human recombinant TNF-α at a dose of 190 g/kg for 12 weeks, produced an antihypothermic effect and changes in serum albumin and Cu content 8 hours after treatment and in muscle and liver protein after 24 hours. The results indicated that changes in ecosanoid metabolism may be involved in the modulatory effect of the coconut oil-enriched diet[CN110].

Hypertriglyceridemic activity. Coconut oil, administered orally to rats at a dose of 14%:0.5% oil/cholesterol diet, produced an increase of lipids and apo B in the VLDL and intermediate-density lipoprotein fractions. The particle diameters of lipoproteins were similar in coconut oil- and olive oil-fed groups. The rates of triglyceride hydrolysis of both groups' VLDL by postheparin lipoprotein lipase in vitro were the same. The average fractional removal of apo B did not differ between diet groups[CN105]. Oil, administered to rabbits at a dose of 14%: 0.5% coconut oil/cholesterol of diet, produced an increase of plasma triglycerides 15 times higher than basal level. Postprandial triglyceride responses after the first high-fat/cholesterol meal were more prolonged in coconut-fed rabbits than in olive-fed group. Postprandial triglyceride responses after chronic coconut oil/cholesterol feeding were significantly greater compared to the olive oil-fed group. One coconut oil/cholesterol meal was associated with a 40% increase of postheparin plasma lipoprotein lipase activity and changed little in chronically fed coconut oil/cholesterol group[CN112].

Hypocholesterolemic activity. Kernel protein, administered orally to rats on a coconut oil diet, lowered the levels of cholesterol, phospholipids, and triglycerides in the serum and most tissues when compared to casein-fed animals. The increase of hepatic degradation of cholesterol to bile acids and hepatic cholesterol biosynthesis and the decrease of esterification of free cholesterol were noted. In the intestine, cholesterogenesis was decreased. The kernel proteins also decreased lipogenesis in the liver and intestine[CN077].

Hypoglycemic activity. Ethanol extract of the leaf, administered orally to rats at a dose of 250 mg/kg, produced less than a 30% drop in blood sugar level[CN058]. Fruit juice, administered intravenously by infusion to dogs at a dose of 3 mL/min for 100 min, was active[CN036]. Hot water extract of the dried shell, administered by gastric intubation to dogs at a dose of 200 mL/animal (20 g of air-dried plant material), produced weak activity[CN043]. The neutral detergent fiber from kernel, administered orally to rats at doses of 5%, 15%, and 30% of diet, resulted in significant decrease in the level of blood glucose and serum insulin, with increasing in the intake of fiber. The increase of fecal excretion of Cu, Cr, Mn, Mg, Zn, and Ca was present[CN075]. Neutral detergent fiber from coconut kernel, administered to rats at doses of 5, 15, and 30% of diet, produced an increase of fecal excretion of Cu, Cr, Mn, Mg, Zn, and Ca[CN180].

Hypolipidemic activity. Protein, administered orally to hypercholesterolemic rats, reduced total, LDL, and VLDL cholesterol; triglycerides; and phospholipids levels in the serum and increased the level of serum HDL cholesterol. The concentration of total cholesterol, triglycerides, and phospholipids in the tissues was lower than in the control group. There was increased activity of superoxide desmutase and catalase. An increase of hepatic cholesterogenesis, conversion of cholesterol to bile acids and fecal excretion of bile acids, and excretion of urinary nitrate and an decrease of malonaldehyde level in the heart were observed[CN071]. The neutral detergent fiber of kernel digested with cellulase and hemicellulase was administered orally to rats. Hemicellulose-rich fiber showed decreased concentration of total cholesterol and LDL and VLDL cholesterol and increased HDL cholesterol. Cellulose-rich fiber showed no significant alteration. There was increased HMG-CoA reductase activity and increased incorporation of labeled acetate into free cholesterol. Rats fed hemicellulose-rich fiber produced lower concentration of triglycerides and phospholipids and a lower release of lipoproteins into circulation. There were an increased concentration of hepatic bile acids and increased excretion of fecal sterols and bile acids[CN081].

Hypotensive activity. Fruit juice, administered by intravenous infusion to dogs at a dose of 10 mL/minute for 30 minutes, was active[CN036]. Water extract of the fresh leaf and stem, administered intravenously to dogs at a dose of 0.1 mL/kg, was active[CN002].

Hypothermic activity. Ethanol (50%) extract of the leaf, administered intraperitoneally to mice at a dose of 0.375 mg/kg, was inactive[CN058].

Ileal oleic acid uptake. Hydrogenated oil, administered to rats at a dose of 5 g/100 g of diet, produced saturable kinetics in ileal brush border membrane vesicles: V_{max} = 0.23 ± 03 µmol/mg protein/5 minutes and K_m = 196 ± 50.3 nmol for controls, and V_{max} = 04 ± 01 µmol/mg protein/5 minutes and K_m = 206 ± 85.3 nmol for coconut oil-fed group[CN198].

Immune function. Coconut oil, administered to rats fed a fat-rich diet (corn oil) or a diet poor in linoleate (coconut oil) at high and low concentrations, completely abolished the responses to *Escherichia coli* endotoxin[CN119].

Insulin secretion stimulation. Oil, administered orally to young suckling rabbits, quickened and strengthened the rise of immunoreactive serum insulin[CN123].

Intestinal brush border membrane. Oil, administered orally to rats at a dose of 10% for 5 weeks, produced an increase in level of saturated fatty acids in the brush border membrane from coconut oil-fed animals. Membrane fluidity was as follows: coconut oil less than commercial pellet diet less than corn oil less than fish oil. The membrane hexose content was high in the coconut-fed rats. Hexamines were elevated in coconut-treated rat brush borders. The activities of alkaline phosphatase, sucrase, and lactase were increased[CN209].

Intestinal esterase activity. Oil was administered to rats at different doses with or without clofibrate for 15 days. The hypolipidemic action of clofibrate was not influenced by the amount of fat. Clofibrate did not affect lower cholesterol concentration in rats fed the low-fat diet, but it counteracted the rise in liver cholesterol seen in rats fed the high-fat diet. The high-fat diet produced slightly higher levels of butyryl cholinesterase in the small intestine but markedly raised intestinal esterase-1 activity[CN101].

Intestinal neoplasia. Oil was administered to 8-week-old male Fischer rats divided into two groups of 60 each (sedentary and exposed to moderate exercise), at a dose of 21% of diet for 38 weeks. The exercising and sedentary rats fed coconut oil were significantly heavier than rats fed corn oil. In the rats fed coconut oil diet, nine carcinomas were recorded in the sedentary groups and five in the exercised rats, which developed significantly fewer neoplasms than corn oil-fed group[CN173].

Intestinal transport. Coconut water in different stages of maturation, administered to rats, produced a jejunal water absorption (17 ± 0.45 µL/minutes/cm), sodium excretion (–1694 ± 296 µEq/minutes/cm), and glucose absorption (5212.70 ± 2098.47 µg%/minutes/cm) in all the stages studied[CN137].

Intravenous hydration. The use of coconut water as a short-term intravenous hydration fluid for Solomon Island residents was investigated[CN076]. Fresh young coconut water, administered to eight healthy male volunteers in three doses in separate trials representing 50, 40, and 30% of the 120% fluid loss at 30 and 60 minutes of the 2-hour rehydration period. The percent of body weight loss than was regained (used as index of percent rehydration) was 75 ± 5%. The rehydration index, which provided an indication of how much of what was actually ingested and used for body weight restoration, was 1.56 ± 0.14. There was no difference at any time in serum Na⁺ and Cl⁻, serum osmolality, and net fluid balance among the trials. Coconut water was significantly sweeter, caused less nausea and more fullness and no stomach upset, and was easier to consume in a larger amount compared to carbohydrate-electrolyte beverage and plain water[CN161]. Water, administered to children with diarrhea, was inactive. The results indicated that coconut water composition, sodium and glucose concentrations, and osmolality values vary during maturation of the fruit. In no instance did the coconut water contain sodium and glucose concentrations of value as an oral rehydration solution[CN215].

Iron bioavailability. Oil, administered to suckling rats dosed with ^{59}Fe-labeled diet, produced a higher percentage of ^{59}Fe in the blood than those fed other fat sources. Administration to weanling rats produced a significantly higher percentage of ^{59}Fe retention than rats fed a formula-blend fat diet[CN168].

Jejunal oleic acid uptake. Hydrogenated oil, administered to rats at a dose of 5 g/100 g of diet, produced saturable kinetics in jejunal brush border membrane vesicles: V_{max} = 0.15 ± 01 μmol/mg protein/5 minutes, and K_m = 136 ± 29.1 nmol for controls, and V_{max} = 03 ± 01 μmol/mg protein/5 minutes and K_m = 124.5 ± 72.6 nmol for the coconut oil-fed group[CN198].

Juvenile hormone activity. Acetone extract of the dried stem produced weak activity on *Dysdercus cingulatus*[CN012].

Lauric acid incorporation. Lauric acid (50%) from the oil, administered to rats for 6 weeks, produced no significant difference between the experimental distribution of triacylglycerol types and the random distribution, calculated from the total fatty acid composition[CN116].

Lipid metabolism. Oil, administered orally to female C57BL/6 mice weaned at 21 d of age at a dose of 15% w/w for 6 weeks, increased the total lipids, triglycerides, LDL and VLDL cholesterol, and thiobarbituric acid-reactive substances (TBARS) and reduced glutathione concentrations, without changes in phospholipids or total cho-

lesterol concentrations compared to controls. The concentrations of total cholesterol, free and esterified cholesterol, triglycerides, and TBARS were increased in the macrophages of coconut-fed mice, whereas the content of total phospholipids did not change. The phospholipids composition showed an increase of phosphatidylcholine and a decrease of phosphatidylethanolamine. Incorporation of [^{3}H]-cholesterol into the macrophages and into the cholesterol ester fraction was increased. The coconut oil diet did not affect [^{3}H]-AA uptake, induced an increase in [^{3}H]-AA release, and enhanced AA mobilization induced by lipopolysaccharide[CN133]. Oil, administered to 28 persons with moderately elevated cholesterol level, decreased total cholesterol and LDL cholesterol (6.4 ± 0.8 and 4.2 ± 0.7 mmol/L), respectively, compared to butter diet (6.8 ± 0.9 and 4.5 ± 0.8 mmol/L). Apos A-1 and B were significantly higher on coconut oil and on butter than on safflower oil. In the group as a whole, HDL did not differ significantly in the three diets, whereas levels in women fed coconut oil were significantly higher than in the safflower oil group. Triacylglycerol level was lower in coconut oil group, but results were significant statistically only in women[CN212].

Lipid peroxide formation stimulation. Seed oil, administered to rats at a dose of 15% of diet for 6 weeks, was inactive on rat liver microsomes. Malondialdehyde concentration was unchanged among animals given different oils. Vitamin E level decreased among those fed soybean oil[CN018].

Lipogenetic effect. Kernel protein, administered orally to rats on a coconut oil diet, decreased lipogenesis in the liver and intestine. The kernel proteins also lowered the levels of cholesterol, phospholipids, and triglycerides in the serum and most tissues when compared to casein-fed animals. There was an increase in hepatic degradation of cholesterol to bile acids and hepatic cholesterol biosynthesis and a decrease in esterification of free cholesterol. In the intestine, cholesterogenesis was decreased[CN077].

Lipoprotein composition. Oil, administered to newborn chicken at a dose of 20% for 2 weeks, increased cholesterol concentration in all the lipoprotein fractions, whereas 10% coconut oil only increased cholesterol in LDL and HDL, an increase that was significant after 1 week of treatment. Similar results were obtained for triacylglycerol concentration after 2 weeks of treatment. Changes in phospholipids and total protein levels were less profound. Coconut oil decreased LDL and fluidity[CN208]. Oil, administered with or without 0.5% cholesterol to 36 young male Syrian hamsters for 6 weeks, produced higher plasma total triglyceride and total cholesterol in coconut oil without cholesterol supplementation-fed group than in the fish oil-fed group. With cholesterol supplementation, there was no significant difference in plasma total triglyceride level among the three dietary groups. The hepatic cholesteryl ester content was higher, and there was lower liver microsomal acyl-CoA/cholesterol acyltransferase activity in the cholesterol-supplemented coconut oil group compared to other groups. There was no significant difference in the excretion of fecal neutral and acidic sterols among the three dietary groups[CN211].

Lipoprotein lipase activity. Oil, administered to preruminant calves, produced no effect on palmitate oxidation rate by whole homogenates and induced higher palmitate oxidation by intermyofibrillar mitochondria. Carnitine palmitoyltransferase I activity did not significantly differ between the groups. Heart and longissimus thoracis muscle of calves fed coconut oil had higher lipoprotein lipase activity but produced no differences in fatty acid-binding protein content or activity of oxidative enzymes[CN181].

Liver function effect. Palm wine was administered orally to female albino rats at a dose of 24.5 mL/kg body weight/day) for 15 days before conception and during pregnancy. On days 13 and 19 of gestation, liver function and hyperlipidemia were seen in the fetuses. Altered liver function was evidenced by the increased activity of alcohol dehydrogenase, aldehyde dehydrogenase, glutamic oxaloacetic transaminase (GOT) (aspartate amino transferase), and glutamic pyruvic transaminase (GPT) (alanine amino transferase)[CN080].

Membrane fluidity and composition. Oil, administered to male weanling Wistar rats at a dose of 100 g fat/kg diet with 10% of the fat provided as corn oil, produced a 61.5% of lipid that were free to diffuse in the plasma membrane[CN203].

Myocardial infarction. Coconut oil, administered orally to rabbits with myocardial infarction induced by isoproterenol, produced a higher level of phospholipids in the heart and aorta. The concentrations of cholesterol and triglycerides were lower in the safflower oil fed group[CN108].

Nasal absorption. Sucrose ester of coconut fatty acid in aqueous ethanol solution (sucrose cocoate SL-40) administered intranasally to anesthetized male Sprague–Dawley rats at a dose of 0.5% sucrose cocoate with insulin, produced a rapid and significant increase in plasma insulin level with a concomitant decrease in blood glucose levels. Administration of a dose of 0.5% sucrose cocoate with calcitonin produced a rapid increase in plasma calcitonin levels and a concomitant decrease in plasma calcium levels[CN150].

Nephrotoxic activity. Fruit juice, administered by intravenous infusion to dogs at a dose of 3 mL/minute for 100 minutes, produced weak activity. Albuminuria was observed just before the end of infusion administration[CN036].

Neutrophil functions. Oil, administered to rats 21 days old at a dose of 15% final fat content of the diet for 6 weeks, produced a reduction in spontaneous and phorbol myristate acetate-stimulated H_2O_2 generation in glycogen-elicited peritoneal neutrophils relative to neutrophils from rats fed the control diet. The activity of superoxide desmutase, glutathione peroxidase, and catalase did not change in animals fed the fat-rich diets. The initial rate of O_2 generation in both resting neutrophils and phorbol myristate acetate-stimulated cells was significantly reduced when animals were fed coconut oil[CN188].

Ophthalmic absorption. Sucrose ester of coconut fatty acid in aqueous ethanol solution (sucrose cocoate SL-40), administered ophthalmically to anesthetized Sprague–Dawley male rats at a dose of 0.5% sucrose cocoate with insulin, produced an increase in plasma insulin level and a decrease in blood glucose levels[CN150].

Ornithine decarboxylase activity. Fixed oil (4.5%), *Clupeidae brevortia tyrannus* (4%), and *Zea mays* (1.5%); fixed oil (7.5%), *Clupeidae brevortia tyrannus* (1%), and *Zea mays* (1.5%); fixed oil (8.5%) and *Zea mays* (1.5%), administered orally to mice for 1 year, were active vs benzoyl peroxide-induced ornithine decarboxylase activity[CN035]. Oil, administered to 30 ultraviolet (UV)-irradiated Sencar and SKH-1 mice at doses of 1/14% (A diet), 7.9/7.1% (B diet), and 15/0% (C diet) corn oil/coconut oil for 6 weeks, produced no increase in enzyme activity. The level of ornithine decarboxylase activity in the UV-irradiated mice fed diet A was significantly higher than in mice fed the B or C diet. In the SKH-1 mice, ornithine decarboxylase activity was increased by 3 weeks and was significantly higher in mice fed diet C than in mice fed diet A. There was no significant effect of dietary fat on UV-induced skin tumor incidence[CN210].

Oxidative DNA damages. Oil, administered to Fischer F344 rats at a dose of 19.8% coconut oil and 2% corn oil for 12–15 weeks, produced an excretion of 8-oxo-7,8dihydro-2'-deoxyguanosine (8-oxodG)

in male group equal to 954 ± 367 pmol/kg/24 hours in the coconut oil fed group compared to 403 ± 150 pmol/kg/24 hours in the control. Calculated per whole animal, the excretion was 328 ± 128 pmol/24 hours in the coconut oil-fed rats and 137 ± 51 pmol/24 hours in the control[CN189].

Oxygen radical inhibition. Seed oil, administered to rats at a concentration of 8% of diet, produced equivocal effect on macrophages. Capsaicin or curcumin enhanced the effect[CN021].

Oxytocinase inhibition. Coconut oil, administered to mice, produced lower level of oxytocinase activity in the testis of mice compared to fish oil[CN162].

Pheromone (sex attractant). Ether extract of the stem, produced equivocal effect on *Aspiculuris tetraptera*, female and male *Dacus dorsalis*, male Mediterranean fruit flies, and male and female melon flies[CN014].

Pheromone (signaling). Ether extract of the stem, produced equivocal effect on *Aspiculuris tetraptera*, female and male *Dacus dorsalis*, male Mediterranean fruit flies, and male and female melon flies[CN014].

Phospholipidemic effect. Oil, administered to phospholipids transfer protein knockout (PLTP0)-deficient mice, produced an increase of phospholipids and free cholesterol in the VLDL–LDL region of PLTP0 mice. Accumulation of phospholipids and free cholesterol was dramatically increased in PLTP0/HL0 mice compared to PLTP0 mice. Turnover studies indicated that coconut oil was associated with delayed catabolism of phospholipids and phospholipids/free cholesterol-rich particles. Incubation of these particles with hepatocytes of coconut-fed mice produced a reduced removal of phospholipids and free cholesterol by SRBI, even though SRBI protein expression levels were unchanged[CN158].

Plasma fatty acids. Oil, administered to chicken at doses of 10% and 20% of the diet, produced an increase in the percentages of lauric and myristic acids in free fatty acid and triacylglycerol fractions in chick plasma, whereas these changes were less pronounced in phospholipids and cholesterol esters. The percentage of arachidonic acid was higher in plasma phospholipids than in the other fractions and was drastically decreased by coconut oil feeding. Linoleic acid, the main fatty acid of cholesterol esters, was increased[CN156]. Oil, administered to 37 children 1 year of age in the form of full vegetable-fat milk (3.5 g fat/dL, 100% vegetable fat from palm, coconut, and soybean oils), produced higher amounts of plasma linoleic acid and a plasma α-tocopherol concentrations than in the other milks tested[CN165]. Oil, administered to male Wistar rats at a dose of 40% of diet for 2 months, increased apo A-I concentration in plasma and did not change apo A-I mRNA level[CN175]. Oil, administered to 38 healthy children in a form of full vegetable-fat milk (3.5 g fat/dL, 100% vegetable fat from palm, coconut, and soybean oils), produced a significantly lower percentage of SUFAs in plasma triglycerides than in children fed standard-fat milk. Plasma PUFA levels were significantly higher than in children fed standard-fat milk[CN179]. Oil, administered to 41 healthy adults, produced a decrease of plasma lathosterol concentration, the ratio plasma lathosterol/cholesterol, LDL cholesterol, and apo B. Plasma total cholesterol, HDL cholesterol, and apo A levels were not significantly different between butter and coconut diets[CN193]. Oil, administered to male golden Syrian hamsters at a dose of 15% w/w for 4 weeks, produced the highest triglyceride levels of the diets studied[CN200]. Oil, administered to male golden Syrian hamsters at a dose of 4 g/kg of diet (12:0 and 14:0) for 7 weeks, produced the highest plasma cholesterol concentration compared to rapeseed and sunflower seed oil diets. Biliary lipids, lithogenic index, and bile acid profile of the gallbladder bile did not differ significantly among the six diets[CN201].

Platelets aggregation stimulation. Fruit juice, administered intravenously by infusion to dogs at a dose of 5 mL/min, was active. Total infusion was 300 mL[CN036]. Oil, administered orally to six New Zealand white rabbits fed a commercial diet supplemented with 60 g/kg of coconut oil low in all PUFA for 60 days, produced a platelets aggregation induced by both thrombin and collagen significantly lower with either fish or linseed oil (n-3 PUFA), than with corn oil (n-6 PUFA) or the low PUFA coconut oil[CN125].

Proinflammatory mediator production. Oil, administered to male C57B16 rats for 6 weeks, produced a decreased TNF-α level by resident macrophages (M phis) than in the fish oil-fed rats[CN177].

Prostaglandin outflow. Oil was administered to weanling male rats fed *ad libitum* a semisynthetic diet supplemented with 10% by weight of primrose oil, replaced partly or completely (25, 50, 75, or 100%) by hydrogenated coconut oil for 8 weeks. The release of prostanoids from the mesenteric vasculature was significantly reduced in the animals on the diet with the oil replaced by coconut oil[CN117].

Protective effect of vitamin A. Vitamin A, 240,000 IU, predissolved in 11.7 g of coconut oil and bolused directly into the rumen of mature wethers along with 4 g of chromic oxide or predissolved in 11.7, 23.4, or 35 g of coconut oil, produced significantly higher recoveries of vitamin A when dissolved in coconut oil (55.6%) compared to safflower oil (35.5%). Recoveries in abomasal digesta increased linearly with the amount of carrier coconut oil[CN195].

Pyretic activity. Fruit juice, administered intravenously to guinea pigs at a dose of 10 mL/kg four times at 1-hour intervals, was active[CN036].

Repellent activity. The lotions and creams containing coconut oil were efficient in protecting against *Simulium damnosum* bites[CN068].

Respiratory stimulant effect. Fruit juice, administered by intravenous infusion to dogs at a dose of 5 mL/minute for 60 minutes, was active[CN036].

Semen coagulation. Ethanol (50%) extract of the leaf, administered to rat semen at a concentration of 2%, was inactive[CN058].

Semen cryopreservation. Coconut water extender, administered with glycerol to the semen of six adult dogs at concentrations of 4, 6, and 8%, produced satisfactory effect. There was no difference among groups in motility and vigor. A smaller percentage of total and secondary abnormalities were observed using 6% glycerol[CN151].

Sensitization (skin). Fruit juice, administered subcutaneously to guinea pigs at a dose of 02 mg/animal, was active on skin. Edema occurred at the site of injection and recovered within 200 minutes. Fruit juice, administered subcutaneously to adults at a dose of 02 mg/person, was active on skin. Inflammation occurred at the site of injection and recovered within 90 minutes[CN036]. Aqueous extract of the husk fiber, administered externally to rabbits, produced no significant dermic or ocular irritation[CN063].

Shock prevention. Oil, administered to rats injected with *Escherichia coli* endotoxin, produced a significant effect[CN219].

Sickness behavior. Hydrogenated oil, administered to Swiss Webster mice at a dose of 17% w/w for 6 weeks, produced the bioactivity of plasma TNF-α equal to 32.6 ± 3.6 ng/mL in mice fed coconut oil diet compared to mice fed fish oil (98.2 ± 5.1 ng/mL)[CN202].

Spasmogenic activity. Ethanol (95%) extract of the fresh leaf and stem, administered to guinea pigs at a dose of 0.5 mL/L, was active on ileum. Water extract of the fresh leaf and stem, administered intraperitoneally to guinea pigs at a dose of 0.5 mL/L, was active on ileum[CN002].

Spermicidal effect. Ethanol (50%) extract of the leaf, administered to male rats, was inactive on sperm[CN058]. Fixed oil, administered to male adults at a concentration of 1:10, was inactive[CN052].

Subcellular membrane-bound enzymes activity. Oil, administered to male CFY weanling rats at a dose of 20% for 16 weeks, produced an increase of synaptosomal acetylcholinesterase activity in the coconut oil-fed group. The Mg^{2+}-adenosine triphosphate (ATPase) activity was similar among all groups in all the brain regions[CN196].

Superoxide production inhibition. Seed oil, administered to rats at a concentration of 8% of diet, produced equivocal effect on macrophages. Capsaicin or curcumin enhanced effect[CN021].

Tachycardiac activity. Fruit juice, administered by intravenous infusion to dogs at a dose of 5 mL/minute for 60 minutes, was active[CN036].

Toxicity assessment. Ethanol extract of the leaf, administered intraperitoneally to mice, was active, LD_{50} 0.75 g/kg[CN058]. Ethanol extract of the fresh leaf and stem, administered intraperitoneally to mice at the minimum toxic dose of 1 mL/animal, was active. Water extract of the fresh leaf and stem, administered intraperitoneally to mice at the minimum toxic dose of 1 mL/animal, was active[CN002]. Aqueous extract of the husk fiber, administered orally to mice, was active, LD_{50} 2.30 g/kg[CN063].

Tricarboxylate carrier influence. Oil, administered to rats at a dose of 15% of the diet for 3 weeks, produced a differential mitochondrial fatty acid composition and no appreciable change in phospholipids composition and cholesterol level. Compared with coconut oil-fed rats, the mitochondrial tricarboxylate carrier activity was markedly decreased in liver mitochondria from fish oil-fed rats. No difference in the Arrhenius plot between the two groups was observed[CN138].

Tumor prevention. The effect of kernel fiber on metabolic activity of intestinal and fecal β-glucuronidase activity during 1,2-dimethylhydrazine (DMH)-induced colon carcinogenesis was studied. Inclusion of fiber supported lower specific activity and less fecal output of β-glucuronidase than did the fiber-free diet[CN074]. Kernel, administered to animals treated with DMH, resulted in higher average weight. A decrease of cholesterol and increase of phospholipids and cholesterol/phospholipids ratio in most of tissues was found. HMG-CoA reductase activity was decreased in most of the tissues of the kernel and DMH, kernel and chili, and kernel, chili, and DMH groups. Histopathological studies showed that kernel-fed animals had fewer papillae, less infiltration into the submucosa, and fewer changes in the cytoplasm with decreased mitotic figures[CN083]. Oil, administered to rats for 4–8 weeks, produced a small but statistically insignificant reduction in TNF production. After 8 weeks, coconut oil suppressed production of the cytokine. Coconut oil produced no modulatory effect on the interleukin production[CN094]. Oil, administered orally at a dose of 20% of diet to virgin female Balb/c mice treated with 7,12-dimethylbenz[a]anthracene (DMBA), produced no effect on body weight, feed intake, or survival to 44 weeks of age and 36 weeks after the six DMBA doses. Mammary tumor incidence was the same in the coconut oil or menhaden oil but significantly higher in the corn oil group[CN100]. Oil was administered to female Wistar rats before mating and throughout pregnancy and gestation, and the male offspring were supplemented from weaning until 90 days of age. They were inoculated subcutaneously with Walker 256 tumor cells. Supplementation of the diet with coconut oil did not change cancer cachexia, except for a small decrease in serum triacylglycerol concentration[CN141].

Tumor-promoting effect. Fixed oil (4.5%) with 4% Clupeidae brevortia tyrannus and 1.5% Zea mays; 7.5% fixed oil, 1% Clupeidae

brevortia tyrannus, and 1.5% Zea mays; and 8.5% fixed and 1.5% Zea mays, administered to mice in the diet for 52 weeks, were active. Tumors were initiated with dimethylbenzanthracene and promoted with benzoyl peroxide for 52 weeks[CN035]. Oil, administered orally to female Sencar mice at doses of 5, 10, 15, and 20%, with addition of 5% corn oil for 1 week after initiation with 7,12-dimethylbenzanthracene and 3 weeks before the start of promotion with 12-O-tetradecanoylphorbol-13-acetate, produced no significant difference in latency or incidence of papillomas or carcinomas between the saturated fat diet groups[CN073]. Oil, administered to 30 Sencar and SKH-1 mice at doses of 1:14% (A diet); 7.9%:7.1% (B diet) and 15:0% (C diet) corn oil/coconut oil for 3 weeks before UV irradiation, produced tumor incidence that reached a maximum of 60, 60, and 53% for diets A, B, and C, respectively, with an average one to two tumors per Sencar mouse. For the SKH-1 mice, the diet groups reached 100% incidence by 29 weeks, with approx 12 tumors per mouse. No significant effect of dietary fat was found for tumor latency, incidence, or yield in either strain[CN210]. Oil (17%) with 3% of sunflower seed oil, administered to DMBA-treated female Sprague–Dawley rats in the diet, produced twice as many tumors as those fed 3% sunflower seed oil or 20% of either saturated fat alone. Tumor yields in the rats fed these mixed-fat diets were comparable to rats fed a 20% lard diet, which provided about the same amount of linoleic acid[CN217].

Uncoupling protein expression. Oil, administered to female Wistar rats fed ad libitum a high-fat diet with coconut oil for 7 weeks, promoted an increase in body fat content, body weight, and uncoupling protein levels. At the completion of experiment I, oil was administered to high-fat diet rats for 3 weeks. Adipose depots were strongly reduced in the rats fed the high fat diet enriched with coconut oil. Specific uncoupling protein was 3.4 times higher than in controls[CN191].

Vascular permeability increased. Fixed oil (4.5%), 4% *Clupeidae brevortia tyrannus*, and 1.5% *Zea mays*; 7.5% of fixed oil, 1% *Clupeidae brevortia tyrannus*, and 1.5% *Zea mays*; 8.5% fixed oil and 1.5% *Zea mays*, administered to mice in the diet for 52 weeks, was active vs vascular permeability induced by benzoyl peroxide[CN035].

REFERENCES

CN001 Atakeuchi, K. Amino acids in the endosperm of some Amazonian *Palmae*. **Chiba Daigaku Buuri Gakuba Kiyo Shizen Kagku** 1961; 3: 321–325.

CN002 Feng, P. C., L. J. Haynes, K. E. Magnus, J. R. Plimer, and H. S. A. Sherrat. Pharmacological screening of some West Indian medicinal plants. **J Pharm Pharmacol** 1962; 14: 556–561.

CN003 Suggs, R. C. Marquesan sexual behavior. Harcourt, Brace World, Inc, New York, 1966.

CN004 Haddon, A. C. Reports of the Cambridge anthropological expedition to Torres straits. Cambridge University Press, England 1908; 6: 107.

CN005 Deacon, A. B. Malekula, a vanishing people in the New Hebrides. George/Routledge and Sons, Ltd, London 1934; 233.

CN006 Brondegaard, V. J. Contraceptive plant drugs. **Planta Med** 1973; 23: 167–172.

CN007 Booth, A. N., E. M. Bickoff, and G. O. Kohler. Estrogen-like activity in vegetable oils and mill by-products. **Science** 1960; 131: 1807.

CN008 De Laszlo, H. and P. S. Henshaw. Plant materials used by primitive peoples to affect fertility. **Science** 1954; 119: 626–631.

CN009 Griffiths, L. A. On the distribution of gentisic acid in green plants. **J Exp Biol** 1959; 10: 43.

CN010 Mannan, A. and K. Ahmad. Studies on vitamine E in foods of East Pakistan. **Pak J Biol Agr Sci** 1966; 9: 13.

CN011 Lancaster, L. A. and B. Rajadurai. An automated procedure for the determination of aluminium in soil and plant digest. **J Sci Food Agr** 1974; 25: 381.

CN012 Gopakumar, B., B. Ambka, and V. K. K. Prabhu. Juvenomimetic activity in some South Indian plants and the probable cause of this activity in *Morus alba*. **Entomon** 1977; 2: 259–261.

CN013 Jansz, E. R., E. E. Jeya, N. Pieris, and D. J. Abeyratne. Cyanide liberation from linamarin. **J Natl Sci Counc Sri Lanka** 1974; 2: 57–65.

CN014 Keiser, I., E. J. Harris, D. H. Miyashita, M. Jacobson, and R. E. Perdue. Attraction of ethyl ether extracts of 232 botanicals to oriental fruit flies, melon flies, and Mediterranean fruit flies. **LLoydia** 195; 38(2): 141–152.

CN015 Wong, W. Some folk medicinal plants from Trinidad. **Econ Bot** 1976; 30: 103–142.

CN016 Devereux, G. A study of abortion in primitive societies. Julian, Inc, New York, 1976.

CN017 Jain, S. K. and S. C. Agrawal. Sporostatic effect of some oils against fungi causing otomycosis. **Indian J Med Sci** 1992; 46(1): 1–6.

CN018 Nardini, M., C. Scaccini, M. D'Aquino, P. Benedetti, M. A. Di Felice, and G. Tomassi. Lipid peroxidation in liver macrosomes of rats fed soybean, olive and coconut oil. **J Nutr Biochem** 1993; 4(1): 39–44.

CN019 Neto, U. F., L. Franco, K. Tabacow, and N. L. Machado. Negative findings for use of coconut water as an oral rehydration solution in childhood diarrhea. **J Amer Coll Nutr** 1993; 12(2): 190–193.

CN020 Karmakar, P. R., and B. P. Chatterjee. Placebo-controlled immunotherapy with *Cocos nucifera* pollen extract. **Int Arch Allergy Immunol** 1994; 103(2): 194–201.

CN021 Joe, B. and B. R. Lokesh. Role of capsaicin, curcumin and dietary N-3 fatty acids in lowering the generation of reactive oxygen species in rat peritoneal macrophages. **Biochem Biophys Acta** 1994; 1224(2): 255–263.

CN022 Holdsworth, D. Medicinal plants of the Gazelle peninsula, New Britain Island, Papua New Guinea, Part I. **Int J Pharmacog** 1992; 30(3): 185–190.

CN023 Bourdy, G. and A. Walter. Maternity and medicinal plants in Vanuatu I. The cycle of production. **J Ethnopharmacol** 1992; 37(3): 179–196.

CN024 Hope, B. E., D. G. Massey, and G. Fournier-Massey. Hawaiian *material medica* for asthma. **Hawaii Med J** 1993; 52(6): 160–166.

CN025 Morrison, E., and U. W. I. Jamaica. Local remedies....yeh or nay? **West Ind Med J Suppl** 1994; 2(43): 9.

CN026 Bhandary, M. J., K. R. Chandrashekar, and K. M. Kaveriappa. Medical ethnobotany of the Siddis of Uttara Kannada district, Karnataka, India. **J Ethnopharmacol** 1995; 47(3): 149–158.

CN027 Amico, A. Medicinal plants of southern Zambesia. **Fitoterapia** 1977; 48: 101–139.

CN028 Saittagaroon, S., S. Kawakishi, and M. Namiki. Generation of mannitol from copra meal. **J Food Sci** 1985; 50(3): 757–760.

CN029 Bopaiah, B. M., H. Shekara Shetty, and K. V. Nagaraja. Biochemical characterization of the root exudates of coconut palm. **Curr Sci** 1987; 56(16): 832–833.

CN030 Kinderlerer, J. L., and B. Kellard. Alkylpyrazines produced by bacterial spoilage of heat–treated and gamma-irradiated coconut. **Chem Ind (London)** 1987; 1987(16): 567–568.

CN031 Bibicheva, A. I., Z. P. Golovina, and L. A. Neofitova. Production of myristic acid from the waste of production of lauric aldehyde. **Maslo-Zhir Prom St** 1987; 4: 26.

CN032 Yeoh, H, H., Y. C. Wee, and L. Watson. Taxonomic variation in total leaf protein amino acid compositions of monocotyledonous plants. **Biochem Syst Ecol** 1986; 14(1): 91–96.

CN033 Venkataraman, S., T. R. Ramanujam, and V. S. Venkatasubbu. Antifungal activity of the alcoholic extract of coconut shell-*Cocos nucifera* Linn. **J Ethnopharmacol** 1980; 2(3): 291–293.

CN034 Salerno, J. W. and D. E. Smith. The use of sesame oil and other vegetable oils in the inhibition of human colon cancer growth *in vitro*. **Anticancer Res** 1991; 11(1): 209–215.

CN035 Locniskar, M., M. A. Belury, A. G. Cumberland, K. E. Patrick, and S. M. Fischer. The effect of dietary lipid on skin tumor promotion by benzoyl peroxide: comparison of fish, coconut and corn oil. **Carcinogenesis** 1991; 12(6): 1023–1028.

CN036 Ketusinh, O. Risks associate with intravenous infusion of coconut juice. **J Med Ass Thailand** 1954; 37(5): 249–271.

CN037 Chindavanig, A. Effect of vegetable oils on plasma cholesterol in man and dog. Master thesis, Department of Biochemistry, Faculty of Science, Mahidol University, Bangkok, Thailand, 1971; 58 pp.

CN038 Ayensu, E. S. Medicinal plants of the West Indies. Unpublished manuscript 1978; 110 pp.

CN039 Letham, D. S. A 6-oxypurine with growth promoting activity. **Plant Sci Lett** 1982; 26: 241–249.

CN040 Hoad, G. V. and P. Gaskin. Abscisic acid and related compounds in phloexudate of *Yucca flaccida* Haw, and coconut (*Cocos nucifera* L.). **Planta** 1980; 150: 347–348.

CN041 Lal, S. D. and B. K. Yadav. Folk medicine of Kurukshetra district (Haryana), India. **Econ Bot** 1983; 37(3): 299–305.

CN042 Hirschhorn, H. H. Botanical remedies of the former Dutch East Indies (Indonesia). I. *Eumycetes, Pteridophyta, Gymnospermae, Angiospermae* (Monocotyledons only). **J Ethnopharmacol** 1983; 7(2): 123–156.

CN043 Morrison, E. Y. S. A. and M. West. A preliminary study of the effects of some West Indian medicinal plants on blood sugar levels in the dog. **West Indian Med J** 1982; 31: 194–197.

CN044 Holdsworth, D. and B. Wamoi. Medicinal plants of the Admiralty Islands, Papua New Guinea. Part I. **Int J Crude Drug Res** 1982; 20(4): 169–181.

CN045 Singh, Y. N., T. Ikahihifo, M. Panuve, and C. Slatter. Folk medicine in Tonga. A study on the use of herbal medicines for obstetric and gynaecological conditions and disorders. **J Ethnopharmacol** 1984; 12(3): 305–329.

CN046 Cosminsky, S. Knowledge of body concepts of Guatemalan wives. **Anthropol Human Birth** 1982; 233–252.

CN047 Whistler, W. A. Traditional and herbal medicine in the Cook Islands.

J Ethnopharmacol 1985; 13(3): 239–280.

CN048 Ito, Y., S. Yanase, H. Tokuda, M. Kishishita, H. Ohigashi, M. Hirota, and K. Koshimizu. Epstein–Barr virus activation by tung oil, extracts of *Aleurite fordii* and its diterpene ester 12-o-hexadecanoyl-16-hydroxyphorbol-13-acetate. **Chem Lett** 1983; 1983(1): 87–95.

CN049 Singh, Y. N. Traditional medicine in Fiji: some herbal folk cures used by Fiji Indians. **J Ethnopharmacol** 1986; 15(1): 57–88.

CN050 Dan Hanh Khoi, Dao Trong Thang and Phung Thi Than. Chemical composition of coconut milk of varieties from southern Vietnam. **Rev Pharm** 1984; 27–36.

CN051 Weniger, B., M. Rouzier, R. Daugilh, D. Henrys, J. H. Henrys, and R. Anton. Popular medicine of the central plateau of Haiti. 2. Ethnopharmacological inventory. **J Ethnopharmacol** 1986; 17(1): 13–30.

CN052 Buch, J. G., R. K. Dikshit, and S. Mansuri. Effect of certain volatile oils on ejaculated human spermatozoa. **Indian J Med Res** 1988; 87(4): 361–363.

CN053 Caceres, A., L. M. Giron, and A. M. Martinez. Diuretic activity of plants used for the treatment of urinary aliments in Guatemala. **J Ethnopharmacol** 1987; 19(3): 233–245.

CN054 Ramirez, V. R., L. J. Mostacero, A. E. Garcia, et al. Vegetales empleados en medicina tradicional Norperuana. Banco Agrario del Peru & NACL Univ Trujillo, Trujillo, Peru, June 1988; 54 pp.

CN055 Gonzalez, F. and M. Silva. A survey of plants with antifertility properties described in the South American folk medicine. Abstr Princess Congress I Bangkok Thailand 1987; 20 pp.

CN056 Caceres, A., L. M. Giron, S. R. Alvarado and M. F. Torres. Screening of antimicrobial activity of plants popularly used in Guatemala for the treatment of dermatomucosal diseases. **J Ethopharmacol** 1987; 20(3): 223–237.

CN057 Sangat-Roemantyo, H. Ethnobotany of the Javanese medicine. **Econ Bot** 1990; 44(3): 413–416.

CN058 Dhawan, B. N., G. K. Patnaik, R. P. Rastogi, K. K. Singh, and J. S. Tandon. Screening of Indian plants for biological activity. VI. **Indian J Exp Biol** 1977; 15: 208–219.

CN059 Caius, J. F. and K. S. Mhaskar. The correlation between the chemical composition of anthelmintic and their therapeutic value in connection with the hook worm inquiry in the Madras presidency. XIX. Drugs allied to them. **Indian J Med Res** 1923; 11: 353.

CN060 Asprey, G. F., and P. Thornton. Medicinal plants of Jamaica. **West Indian Med J** 1955; 4: 69–82.

CN061 Wall, M. E., H. Taylor, L. Ambrosio, and K. Davis. Plant Antitumor agents III: a convenient separation of tannins from other plant constituents. **J Pharm Sci** 1969; 58: 839–841.

CN062 Wasuwat, S. A list of Thai medicinal plants, Asrct, Bangkok, Report no. 1 on Res Project 17. Research Report, A. S. R. C. T., No. 1 on Research Project 17 1967; 22 pp.

CN063 Alviano, D.S., K. F. Rodrigues, S. G. Leitao, et al. Antinociceptive and free radical scavenging activities of *Cocos nucifera* L. (*Palmae*) husk fiber aqueous extract. **J Ethnopharmacol** 2004; 92(2–3): 269–273.

CN064 Mendonca-Filho, R.R., I A. Rodrigues, D. S. Alviano, et al. Leishmanicidal activity of polyphenolic-rich extract from husk fiber of *Cocos nucifera* Linn. (*Palmae*). **Res Microbiol** 2004; 155(3): 136–143.

CN065 Nguyen, S. A., D. R. More, B. A. Whisman, and L. L. Hagan. Cross-reactivity between coconut and hazelnut proteins in a patient with coconut anaphylaxis. **Ann Allergy Asthma Immunol** 2004; 92(2): 281–284.

CN066 Kirszberg, C., D. Esquenazi, C. S. Alviano, and V. M. Rumjanek. The effect of a catechin-rich extract of *Cocos nucifera* on lymphocytes proliferation. **Phytother Res** 2003; 17: 1054–1058.

CN067 Trinidad, T.P., D. H. Valdez, A. S. Loyola, A. C. et al. Glycaemic index of different coconut (*Cocos nucifera*)-flour products in normal and diabetic subjects. **Br J Nutr** 2003; 90(3): 551–556.

CN068 Sylla, M., L. Konan, J. M. Doannio and S. Traore. Evaluation of the efficacity of coconut (*Cocos nucifera*), palm nut (*Eleais guineensis*) and gobi (*Carapa procera*) lotions and creams in indivirual protection against *Simulium damnosum* s.l. bites in Cote d'Ivoire. **Bull Soc Pathol Exot** 2003; 96(2): 104–109.

CN069 Mantena, S. K., Jagadish, S. R. Badduri, K. B. Siripurapu, and M.K. Unnikrishnan. *In vitro* evaluation of antioxidant properties of *Cocos nucifera* Linn. water. **Nahrung** 2003; 47(2): 126–131.

CN070 Esquenazi D., M. D. Wigg, M. M. Miranda, et al. Antimicrobial and antiviral activities of polyphenolics from *Cocos nucifera* Linn. (*Palmae*) husk fiber extract. **Res Microbiol** 2002; 153(10): 647–652.

CN071 Salil, G., and T. Rajamohan. Hypolipidemic and antiperoxidative effect of coconut protein in hypercholesterolemic rats. **Indian J Exp Biol** 2001; 39(10): 1028–1034.

CN072 Pummer, S., P. Heil, W. Maleck, and G. Petroianu. Influence of coconut water on hemostasis. **Am J Emerg Med** 2001; 19(4): 287–289.

CN073 Lo, H. H., M. F. Locniskar, D. Bechtel, and S. M. Fischer. Effects of type and amount of dietary fat on mouse skin tumor promotion. **Nutr Cancer** 1994; 22(1): 43–56.

CN074 Manoj, G., B. S. Thampi, S. Leelamma, and P. V. Menon. Effect of dietary fiber on the activity of intestinal and fecal beta-glucuronidase activity during 1,2-dimethylhydrazine induced colon carcinogenesis. **Plant Foods Hum Nutr** 2001; 56(1): 13–21.

CN075 Sindurani, J. A. and T. Rajamohan. Effects of different levels of coconut fiber on blood glucose, serum insulin and minerals in rats. **Indian J Physiol Pharmacol** 2000; 44(1): 97–100.

CN076 Campbell-Falck, D., T. Thomas, T. M. Falck, N. Tutuo, and K. Clem. The intravenous use of coconut water. **Am J Emerg Med** 2000; 18(1): 108–111.

CN077 Padmakumaran Nair, K. G., T. Rajamohan, and P. A. Kurup. Coconut kernel protein modifies the effect of coconut oil on serum lipids. **Plant Foods Hum Nutr** 1999; 53(2): 133–144.

CN078 Teuber, S.S. and W. R. Peterson. Systemic allergic reaction to coconut (*Cocos nucifera*) in 2 subjects with hypersensitivity to tree nut and demonstration of cross-reactivity to legumin-like seed storage proteins: new coconut and walnut food allergens. **J Allergy Clin Immunol** 1999; 103(6): 1180–1185.

CN079 Cleary, M. P., F. C. Phillips, and R. A. Morton. Genotype and diet effects in lean and obese Zucker rats fed either safflower or coconut oil diets. **Proc Soc Exp Biol Med** 1999; 220(3): 153–161.

CN080 Lal, J.J., C. V. Sreeranjit Kumar, M. V. Suresh, M. Indira, and P. L. Vijayammal. Effect of *in utero* exposure of Toddy (coconut palm wine) on liver function and lipid metabolism in rat fetuses. **Plant Foods Hum Nutr** 1998; 52(3): 209–219.

CN081 Sindhurani, J. A., and T. Rajamohan. Hypolipidemic effect of hemicellulose component of coconut fiber. **Indian J Exp Biol** 1998; 36(8): 786–789.

CN082 Fowler, J. F. Jr. Allergy to cocamide DEA. **Am J Contact Dermat** 1998; 9(1): 40–41.

CN083 Nalini, N., K. Sabitha, S. Chitra, P. Viswanathan, and V. P. Menon. Histopathological and lipid changes in experimental colon cancer: effect of coconut kernel (*Cocos nucifera* Linn.) and (*Capsicum annum* Linn.) red chilli powder. **Indian J Exp Biol** 1997; 35(9): 964–971.

CN084 Kim, M. J., and C. D. Berdanier. Nutrient–gene interactions determine mitochondrial function: effect of dietary fat. **FASEB J** 1998; 12(2): 243–248.

CN085 Alam, S. Q., and Y. Y. Shi. The effect of essential fatty acid deficiency on the fatty acid composition of different salivary glands and saliva in rats. **Arch Oral Biol** 1997; 42(10–11): 727–734.

CN086 Kumar, P. D. The role of coconut and coconut oil in coronary heart disease in Kerala, south India. **Trop Doct** 1997; 27(4): 215–217.

CN087 Kobayashi, H., N. Morisaki, Y. Tago, et al. Structural identification of a major cytokinin in coconut milk as 14-O-(3-O-[beta-D-galactopyranosyl-

(1→2)-alpha-D-galactopyranosyl-(1→3)-alpha-L-arabinofuranosyl]-4-O-(alpha-L-arabinofuranosyl)-beta-d-galactopyranosyl)-trans-zeatin riboside. **Chem Pharm Bull (Tokyo)** 1997; 45(2): 260–264.

CN088 Maccoll. A. J., K. A. James, and C. L. Booth. Erythrocyte morphology and filterability in rats fed on diets containing different fats and oils. **Br J Nutr** 1996; 76(1): 133–140.

CN089 Millan, N. and J. De Abreu. Effect of the type of dietary fat on cholesterolemia in rabbits fed brewer's yeast. **Arch Latinoam Nutr** 1996; 46(1): 71–74.

CN090 Karmakar, P. R. and B. P. Chatterjee. *Cocos nucifera* pollen inducing allergy: sensitivity test and immunological study. **Indian J Exp Biol** 1995; 33(7): 489–496.

CN091 Couturier. P., D. Basset-Stheme, N. Navette, and J. Sainte-Laudy. A case of coconut oil allergy in an infant: responsibility of "maternalized" infant formulas. **Allerg Immunol (Paris)** 1994; 26(10): 386–387.

CN092 Isensee, H. and R. Jacob. Differential effects of various oil diets on the risk of cardiac arrhythmias in rats. **J Cardiovasc Risk** 1994; 1(4): 353–359.

CN093 Eder, K. and M. Kirchgessner. The effect of zinc deficiency on heart and brain lipids in rats force–fed with coconut oil or fish oil diets. **Z Ernahrungswiss** 1994; 33(2): 136–145.

CN094 Tappia, P. S. and R. F. Grimble. Complex modulation of cytokine induction by endotoxin and tumour necrosis factor from peritoneal macrophages of rats by diets containing fats of different saturated, monounsaturated and polyunsaturated fatty acid composition. **Clin Sci (Lond)** 1994; 87(2): 173–178.

CN095 Bouziane, M., J. Prost, and J. Belleville. Changes in fatty acid compositions of total serum and lipoprotein particles, in growing rats given protein-deficient diets with either hydrogenated coconut or salmon oils as fat sources. **Br J Nutr** 1994; 71(3): 375–387.

CN096 Karmakar. P.R., A. Das, and B. P. Chatterjee. Placebo-controlled immunotherapy with *Cocos nucifera* pollen extract. **Int Arch Allergy Immunol** 1994; 103(2): 194–201.

CN097 Satchithanandam, S., M. Reicks, R. J. Calvert, M. M. Cassidy, and D. Kritchevsky. Coconut oil and sesame oil affect lymphatic absorption of cholesterol and fatty acids in rats. **J Nutr** 1993; 123(11): 1852–1858.

CN098 Yartey, J., E. K. Harisson, L. A. Brakohiapa, and F. K. Nkrumah. Carbohydrate and electrolyte content of some home-available fluids used for oral rehydration in Ghana. **J Trop Pediatr** 1993; 39(4): 234–237.

CN099 Jenkins, J. E. and D. M. Medeiros. Diets containing corn oil, coconut oil and cholesterol alter ventricular hypertrophy, dilatation and function in hearts of rats fed copper-deficient diets. **J Nutr** 1993; 123(6): 1150–1160.

CN100 Craig-Schmidt, M., M. T. White, P. Teer, J. Johnson, and H. W. Lane. Menhaden, coconut, and corn oils and mammary tumor incidence in BALB/c virgin female mice treated with DMBA. **Nutr Cancer** 1993; 20(2): 99–106.

CN101 Van Lith, H. A., M. Haller, G. Van Tintelen, A. G. Lemmens, L. F. Van Zutphen, and A. C. Beynen. Fat intake and clofibrate administration have interrelated effects on liver cholesterol concentration and serum butyryl cholinesterase activity in rats. **J Nutr** 1992; 122(11): 2283–2291.

CN102 Van Lith, H. A., G. W. Meijer, M. J. Van der Wouw, et al. Influence of amount of dietary fat and protein on esterase–1 (ES–1) activities of plasma and small intestine in rats. **Br J Nutr** 1992; 67(3): 379–390.

CN103 M'Fouara, J. C., M. N. Bouziane, J. Prost, and J. Belleville. Malondialdehyde production and erythrocyte membrane resistance to free radicals, in function of adequate or inadequate protein intake, associated with different oils (sunflower, soybean, coconut, salmon). **C R Seances Soc Biol Fil** 1992; 186(3): 263–277.

CN104 Pan, J. S., and C. D. Berdanier. Dietary fat saturation affects hepatocyte insulin binding and glucose metabolism in BHE rats. **J Nutr** 1991; 121(11): 1820–1826.

CN105 Van Heek, M. and D. B. Zilversmit. Mechanisms of hypertriglyceridemia in the coconut oil/cholesterol-fed rabbit. Increased secretion and decreased catabolism of very low density lipoprotein. **Arterioscler Thromb** 1991; 11(4):918–927.

CN106 Meijer, G. W., A. G. Lemmens, A. Versluis, L. F. Van Zutphen, and A. C. Beynen. The hypercholesterolemic effect of dietary coconut fat versus corn oil in hypo- or hyperresponsive rabbits is not exerted through influencing cholesterol absorption. **Lipids** 1991; 26(5): 340–344.

CN107 Ng, T. K., K. Hassan, J. B. Lim, M. S. Lye, and R. Ishak. Nonhypercholesterolemic effects of a palm-oil diet in Malaysian volunteers. **Am J Clin Nutr** 1991; 53(4 Suppl): 1015S–1020S.

CN108 Remla, A., P. V. Menon, and P. A. Kurup. Effect of coconut oil & safflower oil on lipids in isoproterenol induced myocardial infarction in rats. **Indian J Med Res** 1991; 94: 151–155.

CN109 Jackson, B., A. N. Gee, M. Martinez-Cayuela, and K. E. Suckling. The effects of feeding a saturated fat–rich diet on enzymes of cholesterol metabolism in the liver, intestine and aorta of the hamster. **Biochim Biophys Acta** 1990; 1045(1): 21–28.

CN110 Bibby, D. C. and R. F. Grimble. Dietary fat modifies some metabolic actions of human recombinant tumour necrosis factor alpha in rats. **Br J Nutr** 1990; 63(3): 653–668.

CN111 Mendis, S. and R. Kumarasunderam. The effect of daily consumption of coconut fat and soyabean fat on plasma lipids and lipoproteins of young normolipidaemic men. **Br J Nutr** 1990; 63(3): 547–552.

CN112 Van Heek, M. and D. B. Zilversmit. Postprandial lipemia and lipoprotein lipase in the rabbit are modified by olive and coconut oil. **Arteriosclerosis** 1990; 10(3): 421–429.

CN113 Kim, M. J., J. S. Pan, and C. D. Berdanier. Glucose turnover in BHE rats fed EFA deficient hydrogenated coconut oil. **Diabetes Res** 1990; 13(1): 43–47.

CN114 Jaggi, K. S., N. Arora, P. V. Niphadkar, and S. V. Gangal. Immunochemical characterization of *Cocos nucifera* pollen. **J Allergy Clin Immunol** 1989; 84(3): 378–385.

CN115 Quig, D. W., and D. B. Zilversmit. High-density lipoprotein metabolism in a rabbit model of hyperalphalipoproteinemia. **Atherosclerosis** 1989; 76(1): 9–19.

CN116 Bugaut, M. *In vivo* incorporation of lauric acid into rat adipose tissue triacylglycerols. **Lipids** 1989; 24(3): 193–203.

CN117 Huang, Y. S., B. A. Nassar, and D. F. Horrobin. The prostaglandin outflow from perfused mesenteric vasculature of rats fed different fats. **Prostaglandins Leukot Essent Fatty Acids** 1989; 35(2): 73–79.

CN118 Deems, R. O., and M. I. Friedman. Macronutrient selection in an animal model of cholestatic liver disease. **Appetite** 1988; 11(2): 73–80.

CN119 Wan, J. M., and R. F. Grimble. Effect of dietary linoleate content on the metabolic response of rats to *Escherichia coli* endotoxin. **Clin Sci (Lond)** 1987; 72(3): 383–385.

CN120 Schouten, J. A., A. C. Beynen, C. Mulder, and H. F. Hoitsma. The effect of dietary saturated fat versus polyunsaturated fat on serum cholesterol and phospholipid concentrations in rabbits with partial ileal bypass. **Z Ernahrungswiss** 1984; 23(2): 136–142.

CN121 De Schrijver, R. and O. S. Privett. Hepatic fatty acids and acyl desaturases in rats: effects of dietary carbohydrate and essential fatty acids. **J Nutr** 1983; 113(11):2217–2222.

CN122 Awad, T. B. and J. P. Chattopadhyay. Effect of dietary fats on the lipid composition and enzyme activities of rat cardiac sarcolemma. **J Nutr** 1983; 113(9):1878–1883.

CN123 Perret, J. P., N. Guiffray, and P. Mottaz. Stimulation of insulin secretion by medium-chain fatty acids in the diet of young rabbits. **Ann Nutr Metab** 1983; 27(2): 153–161.

CN124 Simon, I., C. P. Burns, and A. A. Spector. Electron spin resonance studies on intact cells and isolated lipid droplets from fatty acid-modified L1210 murine leukemia. **Cancer Res** 1982; 42(7): 2715–2721.

CN125 Vas Dias, F. W., M. J. Gibney, and T. G. Taylor. The effect of polyunsaturated fatty acids on the n–3 and n–6 series on platelet aggregation and platelet and aortic fatty acid composition in rabbits. **Atherosclerosis** 1982; 43(2–3): 245–257.

CN126 Saxena, R. P., R. K. Dogra, and J. W. Bhattacherjee. Coir fibre toxicity: *in vivo* and *in vitro* studies. **Toxicol Lett** 1982; 10(4): 359–365.

CN127 Kritchevsky, D., S. A. Tepper, G. Bises, and D. M. Klurfeld. Experimental atherosclerosis in rabbits fed cholesterol-free diets. **Atherosclerosis** 1982; 41(2–3): 279–284.

CN128 Olsson, G., A. M. Ostlund–Lindquist, G. Bondjers, O. Wiklund, and S. O. Olofsson. Quantification of plasma lipids and apolipoproteins in British Halflop rabbits. A comparison between normocholesterolemic rabbits, hypercholesterolemic rabbits (modified WHHL rabbits) and rabbits fed an atherogenic diet. **Atherosclerosis** 1988; 70(1–2): 81–94.

CN129 Prior, I. A., F. Davidson, C. E. Salmond, and Z. Czochanska. Cholesterol, coconuts, and diet on Polynesian atolls: a natural experiment: the Pukapuka and Tokelau island studies. **Am J Clin Nutr** 1981; 34(8): 1552–1561.

CN130 Nicolosi, R. J., J. A. Marlett, A. M. Morello, S. A. Flanagan, and D. M. Hegsted. Influence of dietary unsaturated and saturated fat on the plasma lipoproteins of Mongolian gerbils. **Atherosclerosis** 1981; 38(3–4): 359–371.

CN131 Barnabe, W., T. de Mendonca Neto, F. C. Pimenta, L. F. Pegoraro, and J. M. Scolaro. Efficacy of sodium hypochlorite and coconut soap used as disinfecting agents in the reduction of denture stomatitis, *Streptococcus mutans* and *Candida albicans*. **J Oral Rehabil** 2004; 31(5): 453–459.

CN132 Ringseis, R., and K. Eder. Dietary oxidized cholesterol increases expression and activity of antioxidative enzymes and reduces the concentration of glutathione in the liver of rats. **Int J Vitam Nutr Res** 2004; 74(1): 86–92.

CN133 Oliveros, L. B., A. M. Videla, and M. S. Gimenez. Effect of dietary fat saturation on lipid metabolism, arachidonic acid turnover, and peritoneal macrophage oxidative stress in mice. **Braz J Med Biol Res** 2004; 37(3): 311–320.

CN134 Nalini, N., V. Manju, and V.P. Menon. Effect of coconut cake on the bacterial enzyme activity in 1,2-dimethyl hydrazine induced colon cancer. **Clin Chim Acta** 2004; 342(1–2): 203–210.

CN135 Nguyen, S. A., D. R. More, B. A. Whisman, and L. L. Hagan. Cross-reactivity between coconut and hazelnut proteins in a patient with coconut anaphylaxis. **Ann Allergy Asthma Immunol** 2004; 92(2): 281–284.

CN136 Alexaki, A., T. A. Wilson, M. T. Atallah, G. Handelman, and R. J. Nicolosi. Hamsters fed diets high in saturated fat have increased cholesterol accumulation and cytokine production in the aortic arch compared with cholesterol-fed hamsters with moderately elevated plasma non-HDL cholesterol concentrations. **J Nutr** 2004; 134(2): 410–415.

CN137 Camargo, A. A. and U. Fagundes Neto. Intestinal transport of coconut water sodium and glucose in rats "*in vivo*". **J Pediatr (Rio J)** 1994; 70(2): 100–104.

CN138 Giudetti, A. M., S. Sabetta, R. di Summa, et al. Differential effects of coconut oil– and fish oil–enriched diets on tricarboxylate carrier in rat liver mitochondria. **J Lipid Res** 2003; 44(11): 2135–2141.

CN139 Muller, H., A. S. Lindman, A. Blomfeldt, I. Seljeflot, and J. I. Pedersen. A diet rich in coconut oil reduces diurnal postprandial variations in circulating tissue plasminogen activator antigen and fasting lipoprotein (a) compared with a diet rich in unsaturated fat in women. **J Nutr** 2003; 133(11): 3422–3427.

CN140 Rao, R., and B. R. Lokesh. TG containing stearic acid, synthesized from coconut oil, exhibit lipidemic effects in rats similar to those of cocoa butter. **Lipids** 2003; 38(9): 913–918.

CN141   Togni, V., C. C. Ota, A. Folador, et al. Cancer cachexia and tumor growth reduction in Walker 256 tumor-bearing rats supplemented with N-3 polyunsaturated fatty acids for one generation. **Nutr Cancer** 2003; 46(1): 52–58.

CN142   Kishida, T., S. Miyazato, H. Ogawa, and K. Ebihara.Taurine prevents hypercholesterolemia in ovariectomized rats fed corn oil but not in those fed coconut oil. **J Nutr** 2003; 133(8): 2616–2621.

CN143   Rao, R., and B. R. Lokesh. Nutritional evaluation of structured lipid containing omega 6 fatty acid synthesized from coconut oil in rats. **Mol Cell Biochem** 2003; 248(1–2): 25–33.

CN144   Bellissimo, N., and G. H. Anderson. Cholecystokinin-A receptors are involved in food intake suppression in rats after intake of all fats and carbohydrates tested. **J Nutr** 2003; 133(7): 2319–2325.

CN145   Puertollano, M. A., M. A. de Pablo, and G. Alvarez de Cienfuegos. Antioxidant properties of N-acetyl-L-cysteine do not improve the immune resistance of mice fed dietary lipids to *Listeria monocytogenes* infection. **Clin Nutr** 2003; 22(3): 313–319.

CN146   Rele, A. S., and R. B. Mohile. Effect of mineral oil, sunflower oil, and coconut oil on prevention of hair damage. **J Cosmet Sci** 2003; 54(2): 175–92.

CN147   Sethupathy, S., C. Elanchezhiyan, K. Vasudevan, and G. Rajagopal. Antiatherogenic effect of taurine in high fat diet fed rats. **Indian J Exp Biol** 2002; 40(10): 1169–1172.

CN148   National Toxicology Program. NTP Toxicology and Carcinogenesis Studies of Coconut Oil Acid Diethanolamine Condensate (CAS No. 68603-42-9) in F344/N Rats and B6C3F1 Mice (Dermal Studies). **Natl Toxicol Program Tech Rep Ser** 2001; 479: 1–226.

CN149   Srinivasan, K. N. and K. V. Pugalendi. Effect of excessive intake of thermally oxidized sesame oil on lipids, lipid peroxidation and antioxidants' status in rats. **Indian J Exp Biol** 2000; 38(8): 777–780.

CN150   Ahsan, F., J. J. Arnold, E. Meezan, and D. J. Pillion. Sucrose cocoate, a component of cosmetic preparations, enhances nasal and ocular peptide absorption. **Int J Pharm** 2003; 251(1–2): 195–203.

CN151   Cardoso Rde C., A. R. Silva, D. C. Uchoa, and L. D. da Silva. Cryopreservation of canine semen using a coconut water extender with egg yolk and three different glycerol concentrations. **Theriogenology** 2003; 59(3–4): 743–751.

CN152   Muller, H., A. S. Lindman, A. L. Brantsaeter, and J. I. Pedersen. The serum LDL/HDL cholesterol ratio is influenced more favorably by exchanging saturated with unsaturated fat than by reducing saturated fat in the diet of women. **J Nutr** 2003; 133(1): 78–83.

CN153   Thomas, T. R., J. Pellechia, R. S. Rector, G. Y. Sun, M. S. Sturek, and M. H. Laughlin. Exercise training does not reduce hyperlipidemia in pigs fed a high-fat diet. **Metabolism** 2002; 51(12): 1587–1595.

CN154   Garcia-Fuentes, E., A. Gil-Villarino, M. F. Zafra, and E. Garcia-Peregrin. Differential changes in the fatty acid composition of the main lipid classes of chick plasma induced by dietary coconut oil. **Comp Biochem Physiol B Biochem Mol Biol** 2002; 133(2): 269–275.

CN155   Anon. Clinical trials on AIDS start. **Reprowatch** 1999; 1–28: 6–11.

CN156   Garcia-Fuentes, E., A. Gil-Villarino, M. F. Zafra, and E. Garcia-Peregrin. Changes in plasma lipid composition induced by coconut oil. Effects of dipyridamole. **J Physiol Biochem** 2002; 58(1): 33–41.

CN157   Mohamed, A. I., A. S. Hussein, S. J. Bhathena, and Y. S. Hafez. The effect of dietary menhaden, olive, and coconut oil fed with three levels of vitamin E on plasma and liver lipids and plasma fatty acid composition in rats. **J Nutr Biochem** 2002; 13(7): 435–441.

CN158   Kawano, K., S. Qin S, C. Vieu, X. Collet, and X. C. Jiang. Role of hepatic lipase and scavenger receptor BI in clearing phospholipid/free cholesterol-rich lipoproteins in PLTP-deficient mice. **Biochim Biophys Acta** 2002; 1583(2): 133–140.

CN159 Sachs, M., J. von Eichel, and F. Asskali. Wound management with coconut oil in Indonesian folk medicine. **Chirurg** 2002; 73(4): 387–392.

CN160 Kalra, S., S. Mahmood, J. P. Nagpaul, and A. Mahmood. Changes in the chemical composition of surfactant–like particles secreted by rat small intestine in response to different dietary fats. **Lipids** 2002; 37(5): 463–468.

CN161 Saat, M., R. Singh, R. G. Sirisinghe, and M. Nawawi. Rehydration after exercise with fresh young coconut water, carbohydrate-electrolyte beverage and plain water. **J Physiol Anthropol Appl Human Sci** 2002; 21(2): 93–104.

CN162 Segarra, A. B., G. Arechaga, I. Prieto, et al. Effects of dietary supplementation with fish oil, lard, or coconut oil on oxytocinase activity in the testis of mice. **Arch Androl** 2002; 48(3): 233–236.

CN163 Simon, E., M. Del Puy Portillo, A. Fernandez-Quintela, M. A. Zulet, J. A. Martinez, and A. S. Del Barrio. Responses to dietary macronutrient distribution of overweight rats under restricted feeding. **Ann Nutr Metab** 2002; 46(1): 24–31.

CN164 Arechaga, G., I. Prieto, A. B. Segarra, et al. Dietary fatty acid composition affects aminopeptidase activities in the testes of mice. **Int J Androl** 2002; 25(2): 113–118.

CN165 Svahn, J. C., F. Feldl, N. C. Raiha, B. Koletzko, and I. E. Axelsson. Different quantities and quality of fat in milk products given to young children: effects on long chain polyunsaturated fatty acids and trans fatty acids in plasma. **Acta Paediatr** 2002; 91(1): 20–29.

CN166 Puertollano, M. A., M. A. de Pablo and G. Alvarez de Cienfuegos. Relevance of dietary lipids as modulators of immune functions in cells infected with *Listeria monocytogenes*. **Clin Diagn Lab Immunol** 2002; 9(2): 352–357.

CN167 Hedemann, M. S., A. R. Pedersen, and R. M. Engberg. Exocrine pancreatic secretion is stimulated in piglets fed fish oil compared with those fed coconut oil or lard. **J Nutr** 2001; 131(12): 3222–3226.

CN168 Pabon, M. L., and B. Lonnerdal. Effects of type of fat in the diet on iron bioavailability assessed in suckling and weanling rats. **J Trace Elem Med Biol** 2001; 15(1): 18–23.

CN169 Gruffat-Mouty, D., B. Graulet, D. Durand, M. E. Samson-Bouma, and D. Bauchart. Effects of dietary coconut oil on apolipoprotein B synthesis and VLDL secretion by calf liver slices. **Br J Nutr** 2001; 86(1): 13–19.

CN170 Quilliot, D., F. Boman, C. Creton, X. Pelletier, J. Floquet, and G. Debry. Phytosterols have an unfavourable effect on bacterial activity and no evident protective effect on colon carcinogenesis. **Eur J Cancer Prev** 2001; 10(3): 237–243.

CN171 Frank-Peterside, N. The effect of different dietary fats on gastrin levels in the pyloric antrum and plasma of weaner and adult Wistar rats. **Afr J Med Med Sci** 2000; 29(2): 135–139.

CN172 Ferre, N., J. Camps, A. Paul, et al. Effects of high-fat, low-cholesterol diets on hepatic lipid peroxidation and antioxidants in apolipoprotein E-deficient mice. **Mol Cell Biochem** 2001; 218(1–2): 165–169.

CN173 Thorling, E.B., N. O. Jacobsen, and K. Overvad. The effect of treadmill exercise on azoxymethane-induced intestinal neoplasia in the male Fischer rat on two different high-fat diets. **Nutr Cancer** 1994; 22(1): 31–41.

CN174 Rocca, A. S., J. LaGreca, J. Kalitsky, and P. L. Brubaker. Monounsaturated fatty acid diets improve glycemic tolerance through increased secretion of glucagon-like peptide-1. **Endocrinology** 2001; 142(3): 1148–1155.

CN175 Calleja, L., M. C. Trallero, C. Carrizosa, M. T. Mendez, E. Palacios-Alaiz, and J. Osada. Effects of dietary fat amount and saturation on the regulation of hepatic mRNA and plasma apolipoprotein A-I in rats. **Atherosclerosis** 2000; 152(1): 69–78.

CN176 Vissia, G. H., and A. C. Beynen. The lowering effect of dietary glucose versus starch on fat digestibility in rats is dependent on the type of fat in the diet. **Int J Vitam Nutr Res** 2000; 70(4): 191–194.

CN177 Wallace, F. A., E. A. Miles, and P. C. Calder. Activation state alters the effect of dietary fatty acids on pro-inflammatory mediator production by murine macrophages. **Cytokine** 2000; 12(9): 1374–1379.

CN178 Graulet, B., D. Gruffat-Mouty, D. Durand, and D. Bauchart. Effects of milk diets containing beef tallow or coconut oil on the fatty acid metabolism of liver slices from preruminant calves. **Br J Nutr** 2000; 84(3): 309–18.

CN179 Svahn, J. C., F. Feldl, N. C. Raiha, B. Koletzko, and I. E. Axelsson. Fatty acid content of plasma lipid fractions, blood lipids, and apolipoproteins in children fed milk products containing different quantity and quality of fat. **J Pediatr Gastroenterol Nutr** 2000; 31(2): 152–161.

CN180 Sindurani, J. A., and T. Rajamohan. Effects of different levels of coconut fiber on blood glucose, serum insulin, and minerals in rats. **Indian J Physiol Pharmacol** 2000; 44(1): 97–100.

CN181 Piot, C., J. Hocquette, P. Herpin, J. H. Veerkamp, and D. Bauchart. Dietary coconut oil affects more lipoprotein lipase activity than the mitochondria oxidative capacities in muscles of preruminant calves. **J Nutr Biochem** 2000; 11(4): 231–238.

CN182 Schwab, D. A., T. J. Rea, J. C. Hanselman, C. L. Bisgaier, B. R. Krause, and M. E. Pape. Elevated hepatic apolipoprotein A-I transcription is associated with diet-induced hyperalphalipoproteinemia in rabbits. **Life Sci** 2000; 66(18): 1683–1694.

CN183 Mangiapane, E. H., M. A. McAteer, G. M. Benson, D. A. White, and A. M. Salter. Modulation of the regression of atherosclerosis in the hamster by dietary lipids: comparison of coconut oil and olive oil. **Br J Nutr** 1999; 82(5): 401–409.

CN184 Piot. C., J. F. Hocquette, J. H. Veerkamp, D. Durand, and D. Bauchart. Effects of dietary coconut oil on fatty acid oxidation capacity of the liver, the heart and skeletal muscles in the preruminant calf. **Br J Nutr** 1999; 82(4): 299–308.

CN185 Wallace, F. A., S. J. Neely, E. A. Miles, and P. C. Calder. Dietary fats affect macrophage-mediated cytotoxicity towards tumour cells. **Immunol Cell Biol** 2000; 78(1): 40–48.

CN186 de Pablo, M. A., M. A. Puertollano, A. Galvez A, E. Ortega, J. J. Gaforio, and G. Alvarez de Cienfuegos. Determination of natural resistance of mice fed dietary lipids to experimental infection induced by *Listeria monocytogenes*. **FEMS Immunol Med Microbiol** 2000; 27(2): 127–133.

CN187 Sadeghi, S., F. A. Wallace, and P. C. Calder. Dietary lipids modify the cytokine response to bacterial lipopolysaccharide in mice. **Immunology** 1999; 96(3): 404–410.

CN188 Lopes, L. R., F. R. Laurindo, J. Mancini-Filho, R. Curi, and P. Sannomiya. NADPH-oxidase activity and lipid peroxidation in neutrophils from rats fed fat-rich diets. **Cell Biochem Funct** 1999; 17(1): 57–64.

CN189 Loft, S., E. B. Thorling, and H. E. Poulsen. High fat diet induced oxidative DNA damage estimated by 8-oxo-7, 8-dihydro-2-deoxyguanosine excretion in rats. **Free Radic Res** 1998; 29(6): 595–600.

CN190 Zulet, M. A., A. Barber, H. Garcin, P. Higueret, and J. A. Martinez. Alterations in carbohydrate and lipid metabolism induced by a diet rich in coconut oil and cholesterol in a rat model. **J Am Coll Nutr** 1999; 18(1): 36–42.

CN191 Portillo, M. P., F. Serra, E. Simon, A. S. del Barrio, and A. Palou. Energy restriction with high–fat diet enriched with coconut oil gives higher UCP1 and lower white fat in rats. **Int J Obes Relat Metab Disord** 1998; 22(10): 974–979.

CN192 Otton, R., F. Graziola , M. H. Hirata, R. Curi, and J. F. Williams. Dietary fats alter the activity and expression of glucose-6-phosphate dehydrogenase in rat lymphoid cells and tissues. **Biochem Mol Biol Int** 1998; 46(3): 529–536.

CN193 Cox, C., W. Sutherland, J. Mann, S. de Jong, A. Chisholm, and M. Skeaff.

Effects of dietary coconut oil, butter and safflower oil on plasma lipids, lipoproteins and lathosterol levels. **Eur J Clin Nutr** 1998; 52(9): 650–654.

CN194 Pumhirun, P., P. Towiwat, and P. Mahakit. Aeroallergen sensitivity of Thai patients with allergic rhinitis. **Asian Pac J Allergy Immunol** 1997; 15(4): 183–185.

CN195 Fichter, S. A., and G. E. Mitchell Jr. Coconut oil as a protective carrier of dietary vitamin A fed to ruminants. **Int J Vitam Nutr Res** 1997; 67(6): 403–406.

CN196 Srinivasarao, P., K. Narayanareddy, A. Vajreswari, M. Rupalatha, P. S. Prakash, and P. Rao. Influence of dietary fat on the activities of subcellular membrane-bound enzymes from different regions of rat brain. **Neurochem Int** 1997; 31(6): 789–794.

CN197 Eder, K., and M. Kirchgessner. Activities of liver microsomal fatty acid desaturases in zinc-deficient rats force-fed diets with a coconut oil/safflower oil mixture of linseed oil. **Biol Trace Elem Res** 1995; 48(3): 215–229.

CN198 Prieto, R. M., W. Stremmel, C. Sales, and J. A. Tur. Effect of dietary fatty acids on jejunal and ileal oleic acid uptake by rat brush border membrane vesicles. **Eur J Med Res** 1996; 1(7): 355–360.

CN199 Gil–Villarino, A., M. I. Torres, M. F. Zafra, and E. Garcia–Peregrin. Supplementation of coconut oil from different sources to the diet induces cellular damage and rapid changes in fatty acid composition of chick liver and hepatic mitochondria. **Comp Biochem Physiol C Pharmacol Toxicol Endocrinol** 1997; 117(3): 243–250.

CN200 Gonzalez, I., M. Escobar, and P. Olivera. Plasma lipids of golden Syrian hamsters fed dietary rose hip, sunflower, olive and coconut oils. **Rev Esp Fisiol** 1997; 53(2): 199–204.

CN201 Trautwein, E. A., A. Kunath-Rau, J. Dietrich, S. Drusch, and H. F. Erbersdobler. Effect of dietary fats rich in lauric, myristic, palmitic, oleic or linoleic acid on plasma, hepatic and biliary lipids in cholesterol-fed hamsters. **Br J Nutr** 1997; 77(4): 605–620.

CN202 Kozak, W., D. Soszynski, K. Rudolph, C. A. Conn, and M. J. Kluger. Dietary n-3 fatty acids differentially affect sickness behavior in mice during local and systemic inflammation. **Am J Physiol** 1997; 272(4 Pt. 2): 1298–1307.

CN203 Clamp, A. G., S. Ladha, D. C. Clark, R. F. Grimble, and E. K. Lund. The influence of dietary lipids on the composition and membrane fluidity of rat hepatocyte plasma membrane. **Lipids** 1997; 32(2): 179–184.

CN204 Lal, J. J., C. V. Kumar, M. V. Suresh, M. Indira, and P. L. Vijayammal. Effect of coconut palm wine (Toddy) on carbohydrate metabolism in pregnant rats and fetuses. **Plant Foods Hum Nutr** 1997; 50(1): 71–79.

CN205 Ju, H. R., H. Y. Wu, S. Nishizono, M. Sakono, I. Ikeda, M. Sugano, and K. Imaizumi. Effects of dietary fats and curcumin on IgE-mediated degranulation of intestinal mast cells in brown Norway rats. **Biosci Biotechnol Biochem** 1996; 60(11): 1856–1860.

CN206 Langley-Evans, S. C., A. G. Clamp, R. F. Grimble, and A. A. Jackson. Influence of dietary fats upon systolic blood pressure in the rat. **Int J Food Sci Nutr** 1996; 47(5): 417–425.

CN207 Gabert, V. M., M. S. Jensen, H. Jorgensen, R. M. Engberg, and S. K. Jensen. Exocrine pancreatic secretions in growing pigs fed diets containing fish oil, rapeseed oil or coconut oil. **J Nutr** 1996; 126(9): 2076–2082.

CN208 Castillo, M., J. H. Hortal, E. Garcia-Fuentes, M. F. Zafra, and E. Garcia-Peregrin. Coconut oil affects lipoprotein composition and structure of neonatal chicks. **J Biochem (Tokyo)** 1996; 119(4): 610–616.

CN209 Kaur, M., J. Kaur, S. Ojha, and A. Mahmood. Dietary fat effects on brush border membrane composition and enzyme activities in rat intestine. **Ann Nutr Metab** 1996; 40(5): 269–276.

CN210 Berton, T. R., S. M. Fischer, C. J. Conti, and M. F. Locniskar. Comparison of ultraviolet light-induced skin carcinogenesis and ornithine decarboxylase activity in sencar and hairless SKH-1 mice fed a constant level of dietary lipid varying in corn and coconut oil. **Nutr Cancer** 1996; 26(3): 353–363.

CN211   Lin, M. H., S. C. Lu, J. W. Hsieh, and P. C. Huang. Lipoprotein responses to fish, coconut and soybean oil diets with and without cholesterol in the Syrian hamster. **J Formos Med Assoc** 1995; 94(12): 724–731.

CN212   Cox, C., J. Mann, W. Sutherland, A. Chisholm, and M. Skeaff. Effects of coconut oil, butter, and safflower oil on lipids and lipoproteins in persons with moderately elevated cholesterol levels. **J Lipid Res** 1995; 36(8): 1787–1795.

CN213   Roche, M. E., and R. M. Clark. Lymphatic fatty acids from rats fed human milk and formula containing coconut oil. **Lipids.** 1994; 29(6): 437–439.

CN214   Pinola, A., T. Estlander, R. Jolanki, K. Tarvainen, and L. Kanerva. Occupational allergic contact dermatitis due to coconut diethanolamide (cocamide DEA). **Contact Dermatitis** 1993; 29(5): 262–265.

CN215   Fagundes Neto, U., L. Franco, K. Tabacow, and N. L. Machado. Negative findings for use of coconut water as an oral rehydration solution in childhood diarrhea. **J Am Coll Nutr** 1993; 12(2): 190–193.

CN216   Kanerva, L., R. Jolanki, and T. Estlander. Dentist's occupational aller- gic contact dermatitis caused by coco- nut diethanolamide, N-ethyl-4-toluene sulfonamide, and 4-tolyldiethanol- amine. **Acta Derm Venereol** 1993; 73(2): 126–129.

CN217   Hopkins, G. J., and K. K. Carroll. Relationship between amount and type of dietary fat in promotion of mammary carcinogenesis induced by 7,12-dimethylbenz[a]anthracene. **J Natl Cancer Inst** 1979; 62(4): 1009–1012.

CN218   Emmett, E. A., and R. C. Wright. Aller- gic contact dermatitis from TEA-Coco hydrolyzed protein. **Arch Dermatol** 1976; 112(7): 1008–1009.

CN219   Lim–Navarro, P. R. T., R. Escobar, M. Fabros, and C. S. Dayrit. Protection effect of coconut oil against *E. coli* endotoxin shock in rats. **Coconut Today** 1994; 11: 90–91.

CN220   Stalcup, A. M., K. H. Ekborg, M. P. Gasper, and D. W. Armstron. Enantio- meric separation of chiral components reported to be in coffee, tea and cocoa. **J Agr Food Chem** 1993; 41(10): 1684– 1689.

CN221   Mourafe, J. A., W. H. Brown, F. M. Whiting, and J. W. Stull. Unsaponi- fiable matter of crude and processed coconut oil. **J Sci Food Agr** 1975; 26: 523.

4 | Coffea arabica

L.

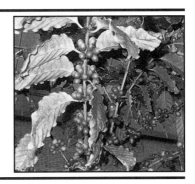

Common Names

Akeita	France	Kafa	Serbia
Araabia kohvipuu	Estonia	Kafe	Albania
Bunna	Ethiopia	Kafe	Bulgaria
Ca-fae	Thailand	Kafe	Czech Republic
Café	Africa	Kafe	Gambia
Café	Argentina	Kafe	Greece
Café	Bolivia	Kafe	Latin America
Café	Brazil	Kafe	Senegal
Café	Catalonia	Ka-fei	China
Café	Chile	Kaffe	Denmark
Café	Ecuador	Kaffe	Norway
Café	France	Kaffe	Sweden
Café	Peru	Kaffee	Germany
Café	Portugal	Kaffeeplante	Norway
Café	Spain	Kaffeestrauch	Germany
Café	Vietnam	Kaffi	Iceland
Cafea	Romania	Kafija	Latvia
Caffe	Finland	Kahawa	Africa
Caffe	Italy	Kahioa	Arabic countries
Caife	Ireland	Kahva	Bosnia
Chai	Georgia	Kahve	Turkey
Coffee	Guyana	Kahvi	Finland
Coffee	United Kingdom	Kape	Philippines
Coffee	United States	Kava	Croatia
Ga feh	China	Kava	Czech Republic
Gafae	Thailand	Kava	Lithuania
Ghah'veh	Iran	Kava	Slovakia
Ikhofi	Africa	Kava	Slovenia
Ikofu	South Africa	Kava	Ukraine
Ka'fe	Israel	Kave	Hungary
Kaafi	India	Kave	Israel
Kaapi	Central America	Kawa	Poland
Kaapi	Mexico	Kofe	Russia
Kaawa	Uganda	Koffee	India

From: *Medicinal Plants of the World, vol. 3: Chemical Constituents, Traditional and Modern Medicinal Uses*
By: I. A. Ross © Humana Press Inc., Totowa, NJ

Koffi	United Kingdom	Kope	Hawaii
Koffie	Netherlands	Kopi	Indonesia
Koffie	South Africa	Kopi	Malaysia
Koffieboom	Netherlands	Ko-pi	Sri Lanka
Kofi	Botswana	Ko-pyi	Korea
Kofi	South Africa	Lee-cah fee	United States
Kofii	India	Qahve	Azerbaijan
Kofje	Netherlands	Qahve	Yemen
Kohv	Estonia	Qahwah	Arabic countries
Koohii	Japan	Sourdj	Armenia

BOTANICAL DESCRIPTION

Coffee is a medium-size tree of RUBI-ACEAE family. The plants can live up to 25 years and grows to a height of 6–15 m; commercially are kept to the height of 175–185 cm. The leaf is developed from the axil and arranged in pairs. The leaves on the main trunk develop in pairs and spirally, whereas leaves from the branch develop in a fan-like manner. The size of the mature leaf of *Liberica* coffee is approx 15–30 cm × 5–15 cm, with 7–10 veins. The dorsal surface is smooth and shiny. The mature leaf of the *Robusta* coffee is about the same size, except that it has 8–13 veins, whereas the dorsal surface is shiny and wavy. The tree starts flowering at the age of 18–36 months. The flowers develop from the axil of the leaves in the form of several in a bunch. Coffee berries are green when immature and turn yellow and red at maturity and ripening. Usually, each berry will contain two cotyledon or beans. In the case of a single cotyledon, it is called peaberry. The time of maturity is approx 8–13 months for *Liberica* and 9–10 months for *Robusta*. Fruits and beans are round, 0.8–1.5 cm (*Robusta*) and 2–2.5 cm (*Liberica*), bean size 0.7–0.9 cm (*Robusta*) and 1.3–1.5 cm (*Liberica*).

ORIGIN AND DISTRIBUTION

Coffee originated from the tropical region of the African continent. In the first centuries, it was cultivated in Arabic countries: Aden and Yemen, later in Iran and India. At the end of the 17th century, the Dutch started to cultivate coffee on Jawa, Ceylon, and Surinam. In the 18th century, it was cultivated in Latin America and Brazil, then in Kenya, Tanzania, Malawa, and Uganda. Main producers currently are Brazil and Columbia.

TRADITIONAL MEDICINAL USES

Brazil. Decoction of the seed is taken orally for influenza[CA183].

Cuba. Hot water extract of the seed is taken orally by males as an anaphrodisiac[CA243].

Haiti. Decoction of the grilled fruit and leaf is taken orally for anemia, edema, asthenia, and rage. The fruit is taken orally for hepatitis and liver troubles. The soaked fruit is used externally for nervous shock. For headache, the leaf decoction is taken orally or the leaf is applied to the head[CA236].

Mexico. The leaves are made into a poultice and used to treat fever[CA168]. Hot water extract of the roasted seed is taken orally by nursing mothers to increase milk production[CA196].

Nicaragua. Leaves are used externally for headache, and the hot water extract is taken orally for stomach pain[CA181]. Decoction of the seed is taken orally for fever and used externally for cuts and hemorrhage[CA184].

Peru. Hot water extract of the dried fruit is taken orally as a stimulant for sleepiness and drunkenness[CA226]. Infusion of the leaf is taken orally to induce labor, and the hot water extract is taken orally as an antitussive in flu and lung ailments[CA200].

Thailand. Hot water extract of the dried seed is taken orally as a cardiotonic and neurotonic[CA245].

West Indies. Hot water extract of the seed is taken orally for asthma. Root juice is taken orally for scorpion sting[CA226].

CHEMICAL CONSTITUENTS

(*ppm unless otherwise indicated*)
Acetaldehyde, phenyl: Sd Hu[CA082]
Acetaldehyde: Sd[CA094]
Acetic acid: Sd[CA063]
Acetoin: Fr[CA087]
Acetol: Sd[CA131]
Acetone: Sd[CA063]
Acetophenone, 2-hydroxy-5-methyl: Sd Hu[CA082]
Acetophenone, 3'-4'-dihydroxy: Sd[CA095]
Acrylic acid, 2-3-dimethyl: Sd (roasted)[CA063]
Acrylic acid, 3-3-dimethyl: Sd (roasted)[CA063]
Adenine, 7-glucosyl: Pl[CA092]
Allantoic acid: Lf[CA135]
Allantoin: Lf[CA135]
Amine, dimethyl: Sd 4.0[CA129]
Amine, ethyl-methyl: Sd 1.0[CA129]
Amine, iso-butyl: Sd 1.0[CA129]
Amine, iso-pentyl: Sd 1.0[CA129]
Amine, N-pentyl: Sd 0.5-2.0[CA129]
Amine, N-propyl: Sd 0.5[CA129]
Arachidic acid: Sd[CA068]
Arbutin: Sd 0.1[CA096]
Atractyligenin, 2-O-(2-O-iso-valeryl-β-D-glucopyranosyl): Sd[CA250]
Atractyligenin, 2-O-(3-O-β-D-glucopyranosyl-2-iso-valeryl-β-D-glucopyranosyl): Sd[CA250]
Atractyligenin, 2-O-(3-O-β-D-glucosyl2-O-iso-valeroyl-β-D-glucosyl): Sd 0.024%[CA083]
Atractyligenin, 2-O-β-D-glucopyranosyl: Sd[CA250]
Atractyligenin, 3'-O-(β-D-glucosyl)-2'-(O-iso-valeroyl)-2-β-(2-deoxy), β-D-glucoside: Sd 170-460[CA117]
Atractyligenin: Sd 10 (free)-400 (total)[CA126]
Atractyligenin-2-O-(2-O-iso-valeryl-β-D-glucoside: Sd[CA116]
Atractyligenin-2-O-(β-D-glucoside): Sd 290-340[CA117]
Atractyligenin-2-O-β-D-glucoside: Sd 220[CA083]
Avenasterol, 5-dehydro: Sd[CA107]
Benzaldehyde, 3-4-dihydroxy: Sd[CA122]
Benzaldehyde: Sd Hu[CA082]
Benzofuran, 2-3-dihydro: Sd Hu[CA082]

Benzofuran, 2-methyl: Sd Hu[CA082]
Benzofuran: Sd Hu[CA082]
Benzoic acid, 2-4-dihydroxy: Sd[CA122]
Benzoic acid, 3-4-dihydroxy: Sd[CA122]
Benzothiazole: Sd Hu[CA075]
Benzoxazole, 2-4-dimethyl: Sd Hu[CA076]
Benzoxazole, 2-5-dimethyl: Sd Hu[CA076]
Benzoxazole, 2-6-dimethyl: Sd Hu[CA076]
Benzoxazole, 2-methyl: Sd Hu[CA076]
Benzoxazole, 4-methyl: Sd Hu[CA076]
Bifuryl, 2-2': Sd Hu[CA082]
But-2-en-1-4-olide, 2-3-4-trimethyl: Sd (roasted)[CA063]
But-2-en-1-4-olide, 2-3-dimethyl: Sd (roasted)[CA063]
But-2-en-1-4-olide, 3-4-dimethyl: Sd (roasted)[CA063]
But-2-en-1-al, 2-methyl: Sd (roasted)[CA063]
But-2-en-1-ol, 3-methyl: Sd (roasted)[CA063]
But-3-en-2-one, 4-(2'-furyl): Sd (roasted)[CA063]
Butan-1-al, 2-methyl: Sd (roasted)[CA063]
Butan-1-al, 3-methyl: Sd (roasted)[CA063]
Butan-1-al: Sd (roasted)[CA063]
Butan-2-3-dione, 1-(2'-furyl): Sd (roasted)[CA063]
Butan-2-one, 1-acetoxy: Sd (roasted)[CA063]
Butan-2-one, 4-(2'-furyl): Sd (roasted)[CA063]
Butan-2-one, 4-(2'-furyl-5'-methyl): Sd (roasted)[CA063]
Butan-2-one: Sd (roasted)[CA063]
Butan-3-one, 2-hydroxy: Sd (roasted)[CA063]
Butane-1-2-dione, 1-(2'-furyl): Sd (roasted)[CA063]
Butanedione: Sd (roasted)[CA063]
Butyric acid, 2-methyl: Fr[CA087]
Butyric acid, iso: Sd (roasted)[CA063]
Butyric acid, N: Sd (roasted)[CA063]
Butyrolactone, γ, α-methyl: Sd (roasted)[CA063]
Butyrolactone, γ: Sd (roasted)[CA063]
Cafesterol: Sd oil[CA062], Sd 0.3–5%[CA136, CA132]
Cafestol palmitate: Sd[CA130]
Cafestol, 16-methoxy: Sd[CA065]
Cafestol, 16-O-methyl: Sd 140[CA066], Lf[CA079]
Cafestol: Lf[CA079], Sd 1.2%[CA124]
Cafestol-2-one-11-O-(β-D-glucoside): Sd[CA118]
Caffeic acid: Sd 0.14–1.051%[CA064,CA078]
Caffeine: Sd 0.00004–3.98%[CA121,CA103], Pl[CA088], Call Tiss 0.9–1 mg/mL[CA099], Fr, Lf[CA077], Pc[CA111], Fr (unripe)[CA120]
Caffeoyl-quinic acid, 3: Sd[CA090]
Caffeoyl-quinic acid, 3-5-di-O: Sd[CA104]
Caffeoyl-quinic acid, 4: Sd[CA090]

Caffeoyl-quinic acid, 5: Sd[CA090]
Campesterol: Sd[CA107]
Candol B: Sd[CA070]
Carbon disulfide: Sd (roasted)[CA063]
Chlorogenic acid A, iso: Sd[CA112]
Chlorogenic acid B, iso: Sd[CA104]
Chlorogenic acid C, iso: Sd[CA112]
Chlorogenic acid, iso: Sd 0.05–1%[CA127]
Chlorogenic acid, neo: Sd 0.17–0.395%[CA127,CA064]
Chlorogenic acid: Sd 0.26–9.9%[CA134,CA114]
Chrysanthemin: Fr Pu[CA085]
Cinnamic acid, 3-4-dimethoxy: Sd 560[CA078]
Citric acid: Sd[CA081]
Cofaryloside: Sd 40[CA098]
Coffea arabica sterol (MP 128–130): Sd oil 2.7%[CA133]
Coffea arabica tryptamine derivative C-2: Fr (unripe) 0.1[CA120]
Coumaric acid, ortho: Sd 0.2%[CA078]
Coumaric acid, para: Sd 0.34%[CA078]
Cresol, meta: Sd Hu[CA082]
Cresol, ortho: Sd (roasted)[CA063]
Cresol, para: Sd Hu[CA082]
Crotonic acid, *cis*: Sd (roasted)[CA063]
Crotonic acid, *trans*: Sd (roasted)[CA063]
Cryptochlorogenic acid: Sd 0.4–2.63%[CA127]
Cyanidin-3-diglucoside: Fr Pu[CA085]
Cyclohex-2-en-1-one, 3-methyl: Sd Hu[CA082]
Cyclohexan-1-2-dione, 3-methyl: Sd (roasted)[CA063]
Cyclohexylmethylketone: Sd Hu[CA082]
Cyclopent-2-en-1-one, 2-3-dihydroxy: Sd[CA102]
Cyclopent-2-en-1-one, 2-3-dimethyl: Sd Hu[CA082]
Cyclopent-2-en-1-one, 2-hydroxy-3-methyl: Sd Hu[CA082]
Cyclopentan-1-2-dione, 3-5-dimethyl: Sd (roasted)[CA063]
Cyclopentan-1-2-dione, 3-methyl: Sd (roasted)[CA063]
Cyclopentane-1-2-dione, 3-ethyl: Sd (roasted)[CA063]
Cyclopentanone: Sd (roasted)[CA063]
Dimethyl disulfide: Sd Hu[CA082]
Dimethyl sulfide: Sd (roasted)[CA063]
Ethan-1-al: Sd (roasted)[CA063]
Ethanethiol: Sd (roasted)[CA063]
Ethanol: Sd (roasted)[CA063]
Ethyl acetate: Sd (roasted)[CA063]
Ethylamine: Sd 2[CA129]
Eugenol, iso: Sd Hu[CA082]

Ferulic acid: Sd 0.84%[CA078]
Feruloyl-quinic acid: Sd[CA090]
Formate, ethyl: Sd (roasted)[CA063]
Formate, methyl: Sd (roasted)[CA063]
Formic acid: Sd (roasted)[CA063]
Fucosterol: Sd[CA107]
Furan, 2-3-5-trimethyl: Sd Hu[CA082]
Furan, 2-5-dimethyl: Sd (roasted)[CA063]
Furan, 2-acetyl: Sd (roasted)[CA063]
Furan, 2-acetyl-5-methyl: Sd (roasted)[CA063]
Furan, 2-methyl: Sd (roasted)[CA063]
Furan, 2-methyl-5-(2'-furfuryl): Sd (roasted)[CA063]
Furan, 2-*N*-butyryl: Sd (roasted)[CA063]
Furan, 2-propionyl: Sd (roasted)[CA063]
Furan, 2-vinyl: Sd Hu[CA082]
Furan, 3-5-dimethyl-2-vinyl: Sd Hu[CA082]
Furan, 3-methyl-2-vinyl: Sd Hu[CA082]
Furan, 3-phenyl: Sd (roasted)[CA063]
Furan, 4-5-dimethyl-2-vinyl: Sd Hu[CA082]
Furan, 4-methyl-2-vinyl: Sd Hu[CA082]
Furan, 5-methyl-2-acetyl: Sd Hu[CA082]
Furan, 5-methyl-2-vinyl: Sd Hu[CA082]
Furan, tetrahydro, 2-methyl: Sd (roasted)[CA063]
Furan, tetrahydro: Sd (roasted)[CA063]
Furan: Sd (roasted)[CA063]
Furan-2-ethyl: Sd Hu[CA082]
Furan-2-iso-butenyl: Sd Hu[CA082]
Furan-2-iso-butyryl: Sd (roasted)[CA063]
Furan-2-iso-propyl: Sd Hu[CA082]
Furan-2-methyl-5-iso-propyl: Sd Hu[CA082]
Furan-2-methyl-5-*N*-propenyl: Sd Hu[CA082]
Furan-2-*N*-butyl: Sd Hu[CA082]
Furan-2-*N*-butyryl: Sd Hu[CA082]
Furan-2-*N*-pentyl: Sd Hu[CA082]
Furan-2-*N*-propenyl: Sd Hu[CA082]
Furan-2-*N*-propyl: Sd Hu[CA082]
Furan-2-propionyl: Sd Hu[CA082]
Furan-3-one, 2-(H), 2-5-dimethyl: Sd Hu[CA082]
Furan-3-one, tetrahydro, 2-methyl: Fr[CA087], Sd (roasted)[CA063]
Furfural, 5-methyl: Sd (roasted)[CA063]
Furfural: Sd (roasted)[CA063]
Furfuryl mercaptan: Sd Hu[CA082]
Furfuryl, 2, 2'-methyl-butyrate: Sd (roasted)[CA063]
Furfuryl, 2, acetate: Sd (roasted)[CA063]
Furfuryl, 2, alcohol: Sd (roasted)[CA063]
Furfuryl, 2, formate: Sd (roasted)[CA063]
Furfuryl, 2, methyl ether: Sd (roasted)[CA063]
Furfuryl, 2, methyl sulfide: Sd Hu[CA082]
Furfuryl, 2, propionate: Sd (roasted)[CA063]

Furfuryl, 2-2'-di: Sd (roasted)[CA063]
Furfuryl, 5-hydroxy-methyl: Sd Hu[CA082]
Furfuryl, 5-methyl: Sd Hu[CA082]
Furoate, ethyl: Sd Hu[CA082]
Furoate, methyl: Sd Hu[CA082]
Furyl, 2, (2'-methyl-5'-furyl-methane): Sd Hu[CA082]
Furyl, 2, acetone: Sd (roasted)[CA063]
Furyl, 2-2'-di, methane: Sd (roasted)[CA063]
Glycine: Sd[CA089]
Glycolic acid: Sd[CA105]
Glyoxal, methyl: Sd[CA131]
Glyoxal: Sd[CA131]
Guaiacol, 4-ethyl: Sd (roasted)[CA063]
Guaiacol, 4-vinyl: Sd (roasted)[CA063]
Guaiacol: Sd (roasted)[CA063]
Heptan-2-ol: Fr[CA087]
Heptan-3-ol: Fr[CA087]
Heptane-2-5-dione: Sd (roasted)[CA063]
Hexan-3-one: Sd (roasted)[CA063]
Hexane-2-3-dione: Sd (roasted)[CA063]
Hexane-2-5-dione: Sd (roasted)[CA063]
Histidine: Lf[CA135]
Hydrogen peroxide inorganic: Sd[CA089]
Hydrogen sulfide: Sd (roasted)[CA063]
Hydrolase, 7-methyl-*N*-nucleoside: Fr[CA119]
Hydrolase, nucleotide: Pl, Call Tiss[CA123]
Hydroquinone, 2-hydroxy: Sd[CA080]
Hydroquinone: Sd 2[CA096]
Indole, 2-methyl: Sd Hu[CA076]
Indole: Sd Hu[CA076]
Iso-amyl acetate: Sd[CA063]
Isoprene: Sd[CA063]
Isopropyl: Sd[CA063]
Kahweol eicosanoate: Sd[CA065]
Kahweol linoleate: Sd[CA065]
Kahweol oleate: Sd[CA065]
Kahweol palmitate: Sd[CA130]
Kahweol stearate: Sd[CA065]
Kahweol: Sd[CA110], Lf[CA079]
Kauren-18-oic acid, 16-17-dihydroxy: Sd[CA067]
Libertine, methyl: Sd[CA113]
Libertine: Sd[CA113]
Ligustrazine: Sd (roasted)[CA063]
Limonene: Fr[CA087]
Linalool, *cis*: Sd (roasted)[CA063]
Linalool, *trans*: Sd (roasted)[CA063]
Linalool: Sd (roasted)[CA063]
Linoleic acid: Sd[CA068]
Maleic anhydride, dimethyl: Sd (roasted)[CA063]
Maleic anhydride, methyl: Sd (roasted)[CA063]
Maltol: Sd Hu[CA082]

Mascaroside: Sd[CA097]
Mesityl: Sd Hu[CA082]
Methacrylic acid: Sd (roasted)[CA063]
Methanethiol: Sd (roasted)[CA063]
Methanol: Sd (roasted)[CA063]
Methyl acetate: Sd (roasted)[CA063]
Methylamine: Sd 27[CA129]
Myricetin: Fr 0.5[CA093]
Myristic acid: Sd[CA068]
NH$_3$ inorganic: Sd 820[CA129]
Nicotinic acid methyl ester: Sd (roasted)[CA063]
Nicotinic acid: Sd[L04511]
Oleic acid: Sd[CA068]
Oxazole, 2-4-5-trimethyl: Sd Hu[CA076]
Oxazole, 2-4-dimethyl: Sd Hu[CA076]
Oxazole, 2-4-dimethyl-5-acetyl: Sd Hu[CA076]
Oxazole, 2-4-dimethyl-5-ethyl: Sd Hu[CA076]
Oxazole, 2-5-dimethyl: Sd Hu[CA076]
Oxazole, 2-5-dimethyl-2-*N*-propyl: Sd Hu[CA076]
Oxazole, 2-5-dimethyl-4-ethyl: Sd Hu[CA076]
Oxazole, 2-5-dimethyl-4-*N*-butyl: Sd Hu[CA076]
Oxazole, 2-ethyl: Sd Hu[CA076]
Oxazole, 2-methyl-4-ethyl: Sd Hu[CA076]
Oxazole, 2-methyl-5-ethyl: Sd Hu[CA076]
Oxazole, 2-*N*-butyl: Sd Hu[CA076]
Oxazole, 2-phenyl: Sd Hu[CA076]
Oxazole, 4-5-dimethyl: Sd Hu[CA076]
Oxazole, 4-5-dimethyl-2-ethyl: Sd Hu[CA076]
Oxazole, 4-ethyl: Sd Hu[CA076]
Oxazole, 4-methyl-2-ethyl: Sd Hu[CA076]
Oxazole, 4-methyl-5-ethyl: Sd Hu[CA076]
Oxazole, 5-acetyl-2-methyl: Sd (roasted)[CA063]
Oxazole, 5-ethyl: Sd Hu[CA076]
Oxazole, 5-methyl-2-ethyl: Sd Hu[CA076]
Oxazole, 5-methyl-2-*N*-propyl: Sd Hu[CA076]
Oxazole, 5-methyl-4-ethyl: Sd Hu[CA076]
Oxindole, 3: Sd Hu[CA076]
Palmitic acid: Sd[CA068]
Pectic acid: Mesocarp, Epicarp[CA073]
Pectin: Mesocarp, Epicarp[CA071]
Pentan-1-al: Sd Hu[CA063]
Pentan-2-one, 1-acetoxy: Sd (roasted)[CA063]
Pentan-3-one, A-acetoxy: Sd (roasted)[CA063]
Pentane-2-3-dione: Sd (roasted)[CA063]
Pent-*trans*-2-en-4-one: Sd (roasted)[CA063]
Phenethyl alcohol: Sd Hu[CA076]
Phenethyl formate, β: Sd (roasted)[CA063]
Phenol, 2-6-dimethyl: Sd (roasted)[CA063]
Phenol: Sd (roasted)[CA063]
Phenylacetate, methyl: Sd (roasted)[CA063]
Phenylethanol, 4-methyl: Sd Hu[CA076]
Phosphoric acid inorganic: Sd[CA105]

Piceol: Sd (roasted)[CA063]
Pipecolic acid: Lf[CA077], Fr[CA077]
Piperidine: Sd 2[CA129]
Polysaccharide: Mesocarp, Epicarp[CA073]
Praline, hydroxyl: Lf, Fr[CA077]
Prop-2-en-1-al, 3-(2'-furyl): Sd (roasted)[CA063]
Propan-1-2-dione, 1-(2'-furyl): Sd (roasted)[CA063]
Propan-1-2-dione, 1-(2'-furyl-5'-methyl): Sd (roasted)[CA063]
Propan-1-al, 2-methyl: Sd (roasted)[CA063]
Propan-1-al, 3-(2'-furyl): Sd (roasted)[CA063]
Propan-1-al: Sd (roasted)[CA063]
Propan-1-ol: Sd (roasted)[CA063]
Propan-1-one, 1-(2'-furyl-5'-methyl): Sd (roasted)[CA063]
Propane, 1-hydroxy: Sd (roasted)[CA063]
Propanethiol: Sd (roasted)[CA063]
Propanone, 1-acetoxy: Sd (roasted)[CA063]
Propionate, methyl: Sd (roasted)[CA063]
Propionic acid: Sd (roasted)[CA063]
Protein: Sd Pu 11.9%[CA072]
Pyrazine, 2-3-5-trimethyl: Sd[CA069]
Pyrazine, 2-3-diethyl: Sd (roasted)[CA063]
Pyrazine, 2-3-diethyl-5-methyl: Sd (roasted)[CA063]
Pyrazine, 2-5-7-trimethyl: Sd[CA069]
Pyrazine, 2-5-dimethyl: Sd (roasted)[CA063]
Pyrazine, 2-6-dimethyl: Sd (roasted)[CA063]
Pyrazine, 2-acetyl: Sd Hu[CA076]
Pyrazine, 2-ethyl-3-5-6-methyl: Sd (roasted)[CA063]
Pyrazine, 2-ethyl-3-methyl: Sd (roasted)[CA063]
Pyrazine, 2-ethyl-5-methyl: Sd (roasted)[CA063]
Pyrazine, 2-ethyl-6-methyl: Sd (roasted)[CA063]
Pyrazine, 3-5-dimethyl-2-(2'-furyl): Sd Hu[CA076]
Pyrazine, 3-5-dimethyl-2-acetyl: Sd Hu[CA076]
Pyrazine, 3-6-dimethyl-2-(2'-furyl): Sd Hu[CA076]
Pyrazine, 3-6-dimethyl-2-acetyl: Sd Hu[CA076]
Pyrazine, 3-ethyl-2-5-dimethyl: Sd (roasted)[CA063]
Pyrazine, 3-ethyl-2-6-dimethyl: Sd (roasted)[CA063]
Pyrazine, 3-ethyl-2-methyl: Sd Hu[CA076]
Pyrazine, 3-methyl-2-(2'-furyl-4'-methyl): Sd Hu[CA076]
Pyrazine, 3-methyl-2-(2'-furyl-5'-methyl): Sd Hu[CA076]
Pyrazine, 3-methyl-2-acetyl: Sd Hu[CA076]
Pyrazine, 5-6-dimethyl-2-(2'-furyl): Sd Hu[CA076]
Pyrazine, 5-6-dimethyl-2-acetyl: Sd Hu[CA076]
Pyrazine, 5-7-dimethyl: Sd[CA069]

Pyrazine, 5-ethyl: Sd[CA069]
Pyrazine, 5-methyl-2-(2'-furyl-4'-5'-methyl): Sd Hu[CA076]
Pyrazine, 5-methyl-2-(2'-furyl-4'-5'-methyl): Sd Hu[CA076]
Pyrazine, 5-methyl-2-(2'-furyl-4'-methyl): Sd Hu[CA076]
Pyrazine, 5-methyl-2-(2'-furyl-5'-methyl): Sd Hu[CA076]
Pyrazine, 5-methyl-2-(2'-furyl-5'-methyl): Sd Hu[CA076]
Pyrazine, 5-methyl-2-acetyl: Sd Hu[CA076]
Pyrazine, 5-methyl-2-acetyl: Sd Hu[CA076]
Pyrazine, 6-methyl-2-(2'-furyl-4'-methyl): Sd Hu[CA076]
Pyrazine, 6-methyl-2-(2'-furyl-5'-methyl): Sd Hu[CA076]
Pyrazine, 6-methyl-2-acetyl: Sd Hu[CA076]
Pyrazine, diethyl-dimethyl: Sd Hu[CA076]
Pyrazine, methyl: Sd (roasted)[CA063]
Pyrazine, trimethyl: Sd (roasted)[CA063]
Pyrazine: Sd (roasted)[CA063]
Pyridine, 2-acetyl: Sd Hu[CA076]
Pyridine, 2-acetyl-methyl: Sd Hu[CA076]
Pyridine, 3-acetyl: Sd Hu[CA076]
Pyridine, 3-methyl: Sd (roasted)[CA063]
Pyridine: Sd (roasted)[CA063]
Pyroglutamic acid: Sd 0.05-0.15%[CA106]
Pyrrole, *N*-methyl: Sd (roasted)[CA063]
Pyrone, 3-hydroxy-2-methyl: Sd (roasted)[CA063]
Pyrrole, 1-5-dimethyl: Sd (roasted)[CA063]
Pyrrole, 1-ethyl: Sd (roasted)[CA063]
Pyrrole, 2, 5-methyl: Sd (roasted)[CA063]
Pyrrole, 2, *N*-methyl: Sd (roasted)[CA063]
Pyrrole, 2: Sd (roasted)[CA063]
Pyrrole, 2-4-dimethyl: Sd Hu[CA076]
Pyrrole, 2-4-dimethyl-3-ethyl: Sd Hu[CA076]
Pyrrole, 2-acetyl: Sd (roasted)[CA063]
Pyrrole, 2-acetyl-1-ethyl: Sd (roasted)[CA063]
Pyrrole, 2-acetyl-*N*-methyl: Sd (roasted)[CA063]
Pyrrole, 2-carboxaldehyde: Sd Hu[CA082]
Pyrrole, 2-ethyl: Sd Hu[CA082]
Pyrrole, 2-iso-butyl: Sd Hu[CA076]
Pyrrole, 2-methyl-*N*-acetyl: Sd Hu[CA082]
Pyrrole, 2-*N*-pentyl: Sd Hu[CA076]
Pyrrole, 2-propionyl: Sd Hu[CA082]
Pyrrole, 5-methyl-*N*-acetyl: Sd Hu[CA082]
Pyrrole, *N*-(2'-furfuryl), 2-carboxaldehyde: Sd Hu[CA082]
Pyrrole, *N*-(2'-furfuryl): Sd Hu[CA082]
Pyrrole, *N*-(2'-furfuryl-5'-methyl): Sd (roasted)[CA063]

Pyrrole, *N*-(3-methyl-butyl): Sd Hu[CA082]
Pyrrole, *N*-acetyl: Sd Hu[CA082]
Pyrrole, *N*-ethyl, 2-carboxaldehyde: Sd Hu[CA082]
Pyrrole, *N*-ethyl: Sd Hu[CA082]
Pyrrole, *N*-furfuryl-2-acetyl: Sd Hu[CA082]
Pyrrole, *N*-furfuryl-2-methyl: Sd Hu[CA082]
Pyrrole, *N*-methyl, 2-carboxaldehyde: Sd Hu[CA082]
Pyrrole, *N*-methyl: Sd Hu[CA082]
Pyrrole, *N*-methyl-2-acetyl: Sd Hu[CA082]
Pyrrole, *N*-*N*-pentyl: Sd Hu[CA082]
Pyrrole, *N*-propionyl: Sd Hu[CA082]
Pyrrole: Sd (roasted)[CA063]
Pyrrolidine: Sd 10[CA129]
Quercetin: Fr 0.5[CA093]
Quercetin-3-*O*-α-L-glucoside: Lf[CA100]
Quinic acid, 4-5-dicaffeoyl: Sd[CA104]
Quinic acid, 5-*O*-feruloyl: Sd[CA104]
Quinic acid, dicaffeoyl: Sd[CA090]
Quinic acid: Sd 0.55%[CA125], Sd (immature)[CA109], Sd[CA089]
Quinide: Sd (immature)[CA109]
Quinoline, 4-methyl: Sd Hu[CA076]
Quinoxaline, 2-3-dimethyl: Sd[CA069], Sd Hu[CA076]
Quinoxaline, 2-5-dimethyl: Sd Hu[CA076]
Quinoxaline, 2-ethyl: Sd[CA069]
Quinoxaline, 2-methyl: Sd Hu[CA076]
Quinoxaline, 5-methyl: Sd[CA069]
Quinoxaline: Sd Hu[CA076]
Salicylic acid methyl ester: Sd (roasted)[CA063]
Sitosterol, β: Sd oil 9.4%[CA133], Sd[CA107]
Stearic acid: Sd[CA068]
Stigmasterol: Sd[CA107]
Styrene, 3-4-dihydroxy: Sd[CA122]
Styrene, 3-4-dimethoxy: Sd Hu[CA082]
Styrene, 4-hydroxy-3-methoxy: Sd[CA122]
Succinimide, *N*-α-dimethyl: Sd (roasted)[CA063]
Sucrose: Sd[CA089]
Sulfide, 2-furfuryl-methyl: Sd (roasted)[CA063]
Sulfide, methyl-ethyl: Sd (roasted)[CA063]
Tannic acid: Sd[CA091]
Tannins: Aer[CA128]
Terpineol, α: Fr[CA087]
Theacrine: Sd[CA113]
Thenyl, 2-acetate: Sd (roasted)[CA063]
Thenyl, 2-alcohol: Sd (roasted)[CA063]
Theobromine: Pl[CA108], Sd, Pc[CA111]
Theophylline: Pc[CA111]
Thiazole, 2-4-5-trimethyl: Sd Hu[CA075]
Thiazole, 2-4-diethyl: Sd Hu[CA075]
Thiazole, 2-4-dimethyl: Sd Hu[CA075]

Thiazole, 2-4-dimethyl-5-ethyl: Sd Hu[CA075]
Thiazole, 2-5-diethyl: Sd Hu[CA075]
Thiazole, 2-5-dimethyl: Sd Hu[CA075]
Thiazole, 2-5-dimethyl-4-ethyl: Sd Hu[CA075]
Thiazole, 2-ethyl: Sd Hu[CA075]
Thiazole, 2-methyl: Sd Hu[CA076]
Thiazole, 2-methyl-4-ethyl: Sd Hu[CA075]
Thiazole, 2-methyl-5-ethyl: Sd Hu[CA075]
Thiazole, 2-*N*-butyl: Sd Hu[CA075]
Thiazole, 2-*N*-propyl: Sd Hu[CA076]
Thiazole, 4-5-dimethyl: Sd Hu[CA075]
Thiazole, 4-5-dimethyl-2-ethyl: Sd Hu[CA075]
Thiazole, 4-ethyl: Sd Hu[CA075]
Thiazole, 4-methyl: Sd Hu[CA075]
Thiazole, 4-methyl-2-acetyl: Sd Hu[CA075]
Thiazole, 4-methyl-2-ethyl: Sd Hu[CA075]
Thiazole, 4-methyl-5-ethyl: Sd Hu[CA075]
Thiazole, 5-ethyl: Sd Hu[CA075]
Thiazole, 5-ethyl-2-*N*-propyl: Sd Hu[CA076]
Thiazole, 5-methyl: Sd Hu[CA075]
Thiazole, 5-methyl-4-ethyl: Sd Hu[CA075]
Thiazole: Sd Hu[CA076]
Thiolan, 2-one: Sd (roasted)[CA063]
Thiophan-3-one, 2-methyl: Sd Hu[CA082]
Thiophene, 2-acetyl: Sd (roasted)[CA063]
Thiophene, 2-acetyl: Sd Hu[CA082]
Thiophene, 2-acetyl-3-methyl: Sd (roasted)[CA063]
Thiophene, 2-acetyl-4-methyl: Sd Hu[CA082]
Thiophene, 2-acetyl-5-methyl: Sd (roasted)[CA063]
Thiophene, 2-aldehyde: Sd (roasted)[CA063]
Thiophene, 2-methyl: Sd Hu[CA082]
Thiophene, 2-*N*-butyl: Sd Hu[CA082]
Thiophene, 2-*N*-propyl: Sd Hu[CA082]
Thiophene, 2-propionyl: Sd (roasted)[CA063]
Thiophene, 3-acetyl: Sd (roasted)[CA063]
Thiophene, 3-methyl, 2-carboxaldehyde: Sd Hu[CA082]
Thiophene, 3-methyl: Sd Hu[CA082]
Thiophene, 5-methyl, 2-acetyl: Sd Hu[CA082]
Thiophene, 5-methyl, 2-carboxaldehyde: Sd Hu[CA082]
Thiophene: Sd (roasted)[CA063]
Tocopherol: Sd oil 0.02-0.05%[CA133]
Toualdehyde, meta: Sd (roasted)[CA063]
Transferase, *N*-methyl: Pl, Call Tiss[CA123], Fr[CA119],
Trigonelline: Sd[CA101]
Tryptamide, 5-hydroxy: Sd[CA074]
Tryptamine, 5-hydroxy, *N*-β-(20-hydroxy-arachidoyl): Fr (unripe) 0.5[CA120]

Tryptamine, 5-hydroxy, N-β-(22-hydroxy-behenoyl): Fr (unripe) 0.5[CA120]

Tryptamine, 5-hydroxy, N-β-(arachidoyl): Fr (unripe)[CA120]

Tryptamine, 5-hydroxy, N-β-(behenoyl): Fr (unripe)[CA120]

Tryptamine, 5-hydroxy, N-β-(indoleoyl): Fr (unripe)[CA120]

Tryptamine, 5-hydroxy, N-β-(lignoceroyl): Fr (unripe)[CA120]

Tryptamine, 5-hydroxy: Wax[CA194], Sd[CA084]

Ursolic acid: Lf 0.05%[CA086]

Ut-2-en-1-4-olide, 2-3-4-trimethyl: Sd (roasted)[CA063]

Valeolactone, γ: Sd (roasted)[CA063]

Valeric acid, iso: Sd (roasted)[CA063]

Vitamin D: Sd oil[CA133]

Vitamin K-1: Sd 0.2[K18625]

Xanthine, 7-methyl: Pl[CA115]

Xanthine, para: Sd[CA113]

PHARMACOLOGICAL ACTIVITIES AND CLINICAL TRIALS

Abortifacient effect. In a population-based, case-controlled study of early spontaneous abortion in Sweden, 562 women who had spontaneous abortion at 6–12 weeks of gestation and 953 women who did not have abortion, indicated that the ingestion of caffeine may increase the risk of an early spontaneous abortion among nonsmoking women carrying fetus with normal karyotypes. Information on the ingestion of caffeine was obtained from in-person interviews. Plasma cotinine was measured as an indicator of cigarette smoking, and fetal karyotypes were determined from tissue samples. Multivariate analysis was used to estimate the relative risks associated with caffeine ingestion after adjustment for smoking and symptoms of pregnancy, such as nausea, vomiting, and tiredness. Among the nonsmokers, more spontaneous abortions occurred in women who ingested at least 100 mg of caffeine per day than in women who ingested less than100 mg/day, with the increase in risk related to the amount ingested; 100–299 mg/day: odds ratio, 1.3; 300–499 mg/day: odds ratio 1.4; 500 mg or more per day: odds ratio 2.2. Among smokers, caffeine ingestion was not associated with an excess risk of spontaneous abortion. When the analysis was stratified according to the results of karyotyping, the ingestion of moderate or high levels of caffeine was associated with an excess risk of spontaneous abortion when the fetus had a normal or unknown karyotype but not when the fetal karyotype was abnormal[CA021].

Alanine aminotransaminase level increase. Roasted seed powder, administered in unfiltered coffee to adults at a dose of 8 g/day, was active[CA172].

Allergenic activity. Ground coffee contains polyphenol haptens that activate the factor XII (Hageman factor)-dependent pathways of coagulation, fibrinolysis, and kinin generation in normal human plasma[CA006]. Extract of the dried aerial part, administered by inhalation to female adult who developed rhinitis and conjunctivitus on exposure to coffee plant, was active. A skin prick test and rhinoconjunctival provocation test to coffee leaf allergen extract were positive[CA201]. Seeds, administered by inhalation to adults at variable doses, were active. A 37-year-old worker in a coffee-roasting facility developed rhinoconjunctivis as a result of exposure to the dust of green, unroasted coffee bean[CA153]. Extract of the dried seed, administered by inhalation to female adults, was active. Extract of the fresh seed, administered by inhalation to females with rhinitis and conjunctivitus, produced a positive skin prick test and rhinoconjunctival provocation test to coffee leaf allergen extract[CA201].

α-Amylase inhibition. Powder of the dried seed, administered intragastrically to mice at a dose of 100 mg/kg, was active vs N-methyl-N'-nitro-N-nitroso-guanidine-induced mutagenesis[CA191].

Ambulatory blood pressure. The effect of regular coffee drinking on 24-hour ambulatory blood pressure in 22 men and women who were normotensive and 26 men and women who were hypertensive with a mean age of 72.1 years (range 54–89 years) was investigated. After 2 weeks of drinking caffeine-containing drinks or instant coffee (five cups/day, equivalent to 300 mg caffeine per day), changes in systolic blood pressure (SBP) and diastolic blood pressure (DBP) in the hypertensive group rise in mean SBP was greater by 4.8 (Standard error of the mean, 1.3) mmHg (p = 0.031) and increase in mean DBP was higher by 3 (1) mmHg (p = 0.010) in coffee drinkers than in abstainers. There were no significant differences between coffee drinkers and abstainers in the normotensive group[CA047]. In the group of 52 participants, the effect of coffee on blood pressure was estimated with the use of a random-effects model. In 11 trials, median duration was 56 days (range 14–79 days) and median dose of coffee was five cups per day. SBP and DBP increased by 2.4 (range 1–3.7) mmHg and 1.2 (range 0.4–2.1) mmHg, respectively, with coffee treatment compared to controls. Multiple linear regression analysis identified an independent, positive relationship between coffee consumption and changes in SBP. The effect on SBP and DBP was greater in trials with younger participants[CA050].

Anemia-producing activity. Hot water extract of the roasted coffee, administered orally to adults of both sexes, was inactive[CA167].

Anti-adhesive effect. Green and roasted coffee, used in a treatment mixture and as a pretreatment on beads, inhibited the *Streptococcus mutans*' sucrose-independent adsorption to saliva-coated hydroxyapatite beads. The inhibition of *Salmonella mutans* adsorption indicated that coffee-active molecules may adsorb to a host surface, preventing the tooth receptor from interacting with any bacterial adhesions. Among the known tested coffee components, trigonelline and nicotinic and chlorogenic acids are very active. Dialysis separation of roasted coffee components also showed that a coffee component fraction commonly considered as low-molecular weight coffee melanoidins may sensibly contribute to the roasted coffee's antiadhesive properties[CA001].

Anti-aging activity. Extract of the dried seed, administered externally to adults at a concentration of 0.5%, was active. The biological activity reported has been patented[CA151].

Antibacterial activity. Extract of the dried seed, on agar plate at a concentration of 0.1 mL/plate, was inactive on *Pseudomonas aeruginosa*, *Salmonella typhi*, *Salmonella typhimurium*, *Shigella dysenteriae*, *Shigella flexneri* 2A, *Vibrio mimicus*, *Yersinia enterolitica*, and *Escherichia coli*. Enteroinvasive, enterohemorrhagic, enteropathogenic and enterotoxic *Escherichia coli* was used[CA211]. Extract of the dried seed, on agar plate at a concentration of 0.1 mL/plate, produced weak activity on *Enterobacter cloacae*, *Aeromonas sobria*, *Clavibacter michiganense* ssp. *nebraskense*, *Staphylococcus aureus*, *Staphylococcus epidermidis*, *Vibro cholera* 0-1 V86 EL TOR, *Vibro cholerae* 0-1 569B classical strain, *Vibro cholera* non 0-1 strain, *Vibrio fluvialis*, and *Vibrio parahaemolyticus*. Extract of the dried seed, on agar plate at a concentration of 0.1 mL/plate, was active on *Plesiomonas shigelloides*[CA211]. Ethanol (95%) extract of the dried seed, on agar plate at a concentration of 1 mg/disc, was active on *Bacillus subtilis*[CA246]. EtOAc extract of the roasted seed, on agar plate at a concentration of 0.76 mg/mL, was active on *Streptococcus mutans*[CA204], and a concentration of 0.84 mg/mL was active on *Staphylococcus aureus*. Water extract of the roasted seed, on agar plate at a concentration of 12.7 mg/mL, was active on *Streptococcus mutans*, and a concentration of 13.5 mg/mL was active on *Staphylococcus aureus*. Infusion of the roasted seed, on agar plate at a concentration of 1.56 mg/mL, was active on

Streptococcus mutans and *Staphylococcus aureus*[CA204]. Decoction of the dark-roasted seed, on agar plate at concentrations of 3 and 6 mg/mL, was active on *Staphylococcus aureus*. Decoction of the medium-roasted seed, on agar plate at concentrations of 4, 6, 10, 11, and 34 mg/mL, were active on *Staphylococcus aureus*. Decoction of the light-roasted seed, on agar plate at concentrations of 6, 11, 12, 15, and 17 mg/mL, was active on *Staphylococcus aureus*[CA204].

Anticarcinogenic activity. The effects of coffee consumption on thyroid carcinomas and adenomas were investigated using a standard questionnaire is a case–control study in southwestern Germany, a know iodine-deficient area. The protective role of coffee drinking and the consumption of cruciferous vegetables, such as broccoli, were confirmed for both genders. Treatment for goiter and decaffeinated coffee consumption were associated with an increased risk for malignant tumors, but less so for adenomas[CA028].

Anticlastogenic activity. Powder of the roasted seed, administered intragastrically to mice and *Microtus montanus* at a dose of 100 mg/kg, was active vs N-methyl-N'-nitro-N-nitroso-guanidine-induced mutagenesis. β-carotene, curcumin, ellagic acid, and chlorogenic acid inhibited urethane-induced micronuclei formation. β-carotene, curcumin, and α-tocopherol inhibited micronuclei formation. Coffee potentiated the effect. A combination of curcumin, chlorogenic acid, eugenol, anethole, and α-tocopherol did not significantly inhibit micronuclei formation. Coffee did not alter the activity. A mixture of pure compounds was used[CA145].

Antifertility effect. Decoction of the dried seed, administered orally to female adults at a dose of 0.96 L/day, was active. Coffee intake delayed the time to conception and increased relative risk of failure to conceive[CA152]. Decoction of the dried seed,

administered orally to female adults at variable doses, was active. There was a correlation between heavy coffee drinking and difficulty in becoming pregnant in women in the United States[CA242]. Hot water extract of the roasted seed, administered in the drinking water of male rats at variable doses daily for 30 weeks, was inactive[CA228].

Antigen modification. Pig-to-rhesus monkey vein transplants were studied to identify the efficiency of green bean α-galactosidase in delaying hyperacute rejection. Biopsies were taken after occluding the grafts for light microscopy (hematoxylin and eosin), scanning electron microscopy, and immunostaining with *Griffonia simplicifolia* IB4 lectin, and for immunoglobulin (Ig) M, IgG, and IgC3. Galactosidase is effective in removing the terminal α-galactosidase and delays the onset of hyperacute rejection; however, its effect is temporary and it prolongs the survival of pig organs transplanted into primates[CA056].

Antihemolytic activity. Water extract of the dried seed, administered to rabbits' red blood cells at variable concentrations, was inactive vs *Staphylococcus aureus* α-toxin-induced hemolysis and produced weak activity vs *Vibrio parahaemolyticus*-induced hemolysis[CA213].

Anti-inflammatory activity. Extract of the green seed, administered externally to adult with skin inflammations by free radical inhibition at a concentration of 1%, was active[CA177].

Antimitogenic activity. Hot water extract of the fruit, administered orally to adults at variable doses, was active vs phytohemagglutinin-, concanavalin A-, and pokeweed mitogen-induced mitogenesis[CA241].

Antimutagenic activity. Extract of the seed, on agar plate at a concentration of 2.5 μg/mL, was active on *Salmonella typhimurium* TA100 and TA102 vs T-butyl peroxide-induced mutagenesis[CA169]. Hot water extract of the seed, on agar plate at a concentration of 3 mg/mL, was active on *Salmonella typhimurium* TA1535[CA223]. Infusion of the seed, on agar plate at a concentration of 100 µL/disc, was inactive on *Salmonella typhimurium* TA98 vs 2-amino-anthracene induced mutagenicity. Metabolic activation was required for activity[CA188]. Lyophilized extract of the seed, on agar plate at a concentration of 6.8 mg/mL, was active on *Salmonella typhimurium* TA1535 vs aflatoxin-2; 4-NQO-, MNNQ-, and ultraviolet light-induced mutagenicity[CA235]. Lyophilized extract of the seed, on agar plate at a concentration of 15 mg/mL, was active on *Salmonella typhimurium* TA100. Addition of catalase decreased the activity[CA230]. Decoction of the dried seed, at a concentration of 2% was active on *Drosophila melanogaster* vs cyclophosphamide-induced genotoxicity. A concentration of 5% was active vs urethane-induced genotoxicity. Methylene chloride/2-propanol (1:1) extract, at a concentration of 2%, was active on *Drosophila melanogaster* vs mitomycin C-induced genotoxicity[CA185]. Hot water extract of the roasted coffee, on agar plate at a concentration of 1%, was active on *Salmonella typhimurium* TA100 vs benzopyrene, AF-2, and 4NQO mutagenicity. Hot water extract of the roasted coffee, on agar plate at a concentration of 1%, was active on *Salmonella typhimurium* TA98 vs TRP-P-2, Glu-P-1, 2-acetylaminofluorene, and IQ mutagenicity. Hot water extract of the roasted coffee, on agar plate at a concentration of 1%, was inactive on *Salmonella typhimurium* TA100 vs β-propiolactone and glycidol mutagenicity. Hot water extract of the roasted coffee, on agar plate at a concentration of 1%, was inactive on *Salmonella typhimurium* TA100 vs acrolein mutagenicity[CA234].

Antioxidant activity. Green and roasted coffee beans were evaluated in relation to degree of roasting and species (*Coffea arabica* and *Coffea robusta*). The properties were evaluated by determining the reducing substances of coffee and its antioxidant activity in vitro and in vivo as protective activity against rat liver cell microsome lipid peroxidation measured as thiobarbituric acid-reacting substances. Reducing substances of *Robusta* samples were significantly higher when compared to those of *Arabica* samples ($p < 0.001$). Antioxidant activity for green coffee samples was slightly higher than for the corresponding roasted samples ($p < 0.001$). Extraction with three different organic solvents (ethyl acetate, ethyl ether, and dichloromethane) showed that the most protective compounds are extracted from acidified dark-roasted coffee solutions with ethyl acetate. Analysis of acidic extract by gel filtration chromatography produced five fractions. Higher molecular mass fractions showed protective activity. The small amounts of these acidic low-molecular-mass protective fractions isolated indicated that they contain strong protective agents[CA007]. Coffee and the sum of coffee and red wine on healthy subjects showed detectable capacity to scavenge radical cations in the colonic lumen, suggesting that antioxidant activity occurs in the colonic lumen. Fourteen subjects recorded their food intake three times for a period of 2–4 days, each time collecting all of the feces passed during the next 24 hours. Total antioxidant activity (6-hydroxy-2,5,7,8-tetramethulchroman-2-carboxylic acid) of fecal suspension was measured using the 2,2'-azinobis-(3-ethyl-benzothiazoline)-6-sulfonic acid radical cation decolorization assay. The average total antioxidant activity of feces was 26.6 mmol/kg wet feces. The total amount of antioxidant equivalents excreted over 24 hours, derived by multiplying the total antioxidant activity by the amount of feces passed during 24 hours, was 3.24 mmol, and this was significantly correlated with the average 24-hour intake of coffee and red wine, particularly to the sum of coffee and red wine[CA015]. Hot water extract of the seed, produced an inhibition of Fenton-catalyzed oxidation of 2'-deoxyguanosine[CA169].

Antispasmodic activity. Ethanol (50%) extract of the aerial parts was active on the guinea pig ileum vs acetylcholine - and histamine-induced spasms[CA139].

Anti-tumor activity. Water extract of the dried seed, administered intraperitoneally to mice, was active on CA-755 cells[CA171]. Hot water extract of the dried seed, administered in the drinking water of mice at a concentration of 0.5%, was active on spontaneous mammary tumors[CA180].

Antiviral activity. Hot water extract of the seed, in cell culture, produced weak activity on poliovirus 1[CA225].

Anti-yeast activity. Ethanol (100%) extract of the seed, on agar plate at a concentration of 18.7 mg/mL, was active on *Candida albicans*. Water extract of the seed, on agar plate was inactive on *Candida albicans*[CA205].

Arrhythmogenic effect. Hot water extract of the dried seed, administered orally to adults with cardiac abnormalities at a dose of 200 mg/person, produced equivocal effect[CA210].

Atherosclerotic effect. Hot water extract of the roasted coffee, administered orally to 85,747 female nurses, produced no correlation between coffee consumption and coronary heart disease[CA179].

Birth-weight effect. Caffeinated coffee alone had an adjusted odds ratio of 1.3 (95% confidence limits [CL] = 1.0, 1.7) for preterm delivery; mothers who consumed both caffeinated and decaffeinated coffee had an adjusted odds of 2.3 (95% CL = 1.3, 4), whereas those who consumed only decaffeinated coffee showed no increased odds of small-for-gestational age birth, low-birth-weight or preterm delivery. A reduction in mean birth-weight of –3 g per cup per week (95% CL = –5.9, –0.6) for caffeinated coffee and an increase of +0.4 g per cup per week (95% CL = 3.7, 4.5) for decaffeinated coffee was found[CA046].

Blood flow increase. Decoction of the seed, administered orally to adults, was active. Result was the same for both regular and decaffeinated coffee drinkers[CA164].

Bone mineral density. The association of caffeine consumption and bone mineral density has been investigated in 177 healthy women, age 19–26 years. Average caffeine intake was calculated from self-reports of the consumption of coffee, tea, colas, chocolate products, and selected medications during the previous 12 months. Mean caffeine intake was 99.9 mg/day. Bone mineral density at the femoral neck and the lumbar spine was measured by dual-energy X-ray absorptiometry. After adjusting for potential confounders, including height, body mass index, age and menarche, calcium intake, protein consumption, alcohol consumption, and tobacco use, caffeine consumption was not a significant predictor of bone mineral density. For every 100 mg of caffeine consumed, femoral neck bone mineral density decreased 6.9 mg/cm^2 and lumbar spine bone mineral density decreased 11.9 mg/cm^2. No single source of caffeine was significantly associated with a decrease in bone mineral density. Furthermore, the association between caffeine consumption and bone mineral density at either site did not differ significantly between those who consumed low levels of calcium (≤836 mg/day) and those who consumed high levels of calcium (>836 mg/day)[CA025]

Bone mineral effect. Coffee, taken by 258 healthy occupationally active men aged 40–63 years, significantly reduced the trabecular bone mineral content. The extent of alcohol intake did not differentiate bone mineral content values at the distal radius, whereas the significant detrimental effects of both smoking and coffee drinking on trabecular (but not cortical and total) bone mineral content were revealed. Simultaneously, smokers and ex-smokers, when compared to lifelong nonsmokers, had lower trabecular bone mineral content[CA014].

Brain metabolic response. Changes in brain lactate resulting from the combined effects of caffeine's stimulation of glycolysis and reduction of cerebral blood flow were determined by a rapid proton echoplanar spectroscopic imaging technique in a group of nine heavy caffeine users and nine caffeine-intolerant persons. They were studied at baseline and 1 hour after ingestion of caffeine citrate (10 mg/kg). Five of the caffeine users were restudied after a 1- to 2-month caffeine holiday. Significant increases in global and regionally specific brain lactate and psychological and physiological distress in response to caffeine ingestion were observed only among the caffeine-intolerant persons. Reexposure of the regular coffee drinkers to caffeine after a caffeine holiday resulted in little or no adverse clinical reaction but did result in significant rises in brain lactate, which were of a magnitude similar to that observed for the caffeine-intolerant group[CA051].

Caffeine intake, tolerance, and withdrawal. Caffeine in the form of brewed and instant coffee, tea, and caffeinated drinks was taken by 1934 individual twins from female–female pairs, including 486 monozygotic and 335 dizygotic pairs. The resemblance in twin pairs for total caffeine consumption, heavy caffeine use, caffeine intoxication, tolerance, and withdrawal was substantially greater in monozygotic than in dizygotic twin pairs and could be ascribed solely to genetic factors, with estimated broad heritabilities of between 35 and 77%[CA052].

Cancer-associated risk factor. Infusion of the seed, administered orally to adults, produced equivocal effect on urinary bladder cancer[CA156].

Carcinogenesis inhibition. Water-soluble fraction of the dried fruit, administered to female mice at a dose of 0.25% of diet, inhibited mammary tumor development in SHN virgin mice. Water-soluble fraction of the dried fruit, administered to female mice at a dose of 0.25% of diet, inhibited mammary glands in SHN virgin mice [CA202]. Decoction of the dried seed, administered in drinking water to rats at a concentration of 57.0 g/L, produced no effect on dimethylnitrosamine-induced glutathione S-transferase positive foci after subtotal hepatectomy[CA176]. Decoction of the dried seed, administered intragastrically to pregnant rhesuses at a dose of 10 mL/kg for 90 minutes before dosing with cyclophosphamide, N-nitrosodiethylamine, N-nitroso-N-ethylurea, or mitomycin, produced micronuclei and polychromatophilic nucleated erythrocytes in fetal liver, marrow, and blood[CA182]. Seeds, administered in ration of high mammary tumor strain of SHN/MEI virgin female mice, were active[CA175]. Hot water extract of the dried seed, administered in drinking water to rats at a dose of 6000 ppm, was active[CA158]. Hot water extract of the dried seed, administered orally to adults at variable doses, produced no effect on pancreatic cancer[CA207]. Hot water extract of the dried seed, administered orally to adults at variable doses, was inactive. Patients with newly diagnosed breast cancer ($n = 818$) were compared to surgical and neighborhood controls in a dietary case–control study of the relationship of dietary intake of coffee and total methylxanthine from coffee, tea, chocolate, and cocoa drinks. A nonsignificant negative association was found between methylxanthine consumption and breast cancer. This pattern was stronger in patients with high-fat diets after controlling several confounding hormonal factors. A diminished risk was found when consumption of methylxanthine of patients with breast cancer is compared to that of patients with benign disease[CA231]. Decoction of the dried seed, administered to male rats at a dose of 5% of diet, was active vs dimethylnitrosamine-induced carcinogenesis[CA218]. Lyophilized extract of the dried seed, administered intragastrically to mice at a dose of 50.0 g/kg of diet, was active. Animals were exposed to coffee *in utero*, as mother's diet was 1% instant coffee. After weaning, animals were given an instant coffee for 2 years. Incidence of neoplasms decreased from 70.6 to 34.8% in males and from 56.8 to 36.2% in females. The incidence of benign tumor was 2.72 vs 0% for controls[CA216]. Seed oil, administered to hamster at a concentration of 2.25% of diet, was active vs 7,12-dimethylbenz[a]anthracene (DMBA)-induced oral tumors. Seed, administered to hamsters at a concentration of 15% of diet, was active vs DMBA-induced oral tumors[CA173]. Seed, administered to rats at a concentration of 20% of diet, was active vs DMBA-induced carcinogenesis[CA143]. Decoction of the roasted coffee, administered orally to adults, was active on risk of colon or rectal cancer. Risk of colon cancer was reduced in drinkers of four or more cups of coffee per day. There was no effect on rectal cancer[CA147]. Methylene chloride/2-propanol (1:1) extract of the roasted coffee, administered in drinking water of male rats at a concentration of 10%, was inactive on urinary bladder[CA154]. Seed oil, administered to male rats at a dose of 0.10%, was active on the colon[CA170].

Carcinogenic activity. Decoction of the seed, administered orally to adults, was inactive. There was no association between colorectal adenomas and consumption of extract[CA189]. Roasted seed, administered to male rats at a dose of 6% of diet for 2 years, was inactive. Water extract of the roasted seed, administered to female rats at a dose of 6% of diet, was inactive. Regular and decaffeinated instant coffees were studied. Coffees with highest caffeine content showed lower tumor incidence[CA197]. Hot water extract of the roasted seed, administered orally to 18 rats at a dose of 2% for 120 days

of dosing with cycasin orally (150 mg/kg) on day 121, produced five tumors. Hot water extract of the roasted seed, administered orally to rats at a dose of 2%, was inactive[CA195].

Carcinogenic risk analysis. Pooled data of 564 cases and 2929 hospitals or population controls who had never smoked were enrolled in epidemiological studies to examine the association of coffee with an excess bladder cancer risk. The data were evaluated from 10 studies conducted in Denmark, Germany, Greece, France, Italy, and Spain. Information on coffee consumption and occupation was recoded following standard criteria. Unconditional logistic regression was applied adjusting for age, study center, occupation, and gender. Seventy nine percent of the study population reported having consumed coffee, and 2.4% were heavy drinkers, reporting having ingested on average 10 or more cups per day. There was no excess risk in coffee drinkers compared to nondrinkers. The risk did not increase monotonically with dose, but a statistically significant risk was seen for subjects having ingested 10 or more cups per day. This excess was seen in both males and females. There was no evidence of an association of the risk with duration or type of coffee consumption. Nonsmokers who are heavy coffee drinkers may have a small excess risk of bladder cancer. Although these results cannot be attributed to confounding by smoking, the possibility of bias in control selection cannot be discarded. On the basis of the data, only a small proportion of cancers of the bladder among nonsmokers could be attributed to coffee drinking[CA018].

Cardiac mechanoenergetics. Caffeine in a concentration higher than 0.05 mM, corresponding to the maximum blood concentration after a healthy human subject consumed a cup of coffee, depresses left ventricular systolic and diastolic functions and decreases a measure of total mechanical energy per beat in terms of SBP-volume area more severely in failing hearts at concentrations lower than those in normal hearts[CA060].

Cardioexcitatory activity. Hot water extract of the dried seed, administered orally to adults, produced weak activity. There was no change in electrocardiogram pattern, but some subjects showed sinus arrhythmia, sinus tachycardia, and incomplete right bundle branch block, premature ventricular contraction, and premature atrial contraction[CA224].

Cardiovascular effects. Caffeinated coffee was taken by 72 males and 72 females with a mean age of 21 years. Ingestion of caffeine had no effect on initial mood or working memory, but it improved encoding of new information, counteracted the fatigue, and increased blood pressure and pulse rate[CA044].

Cerebral blood flow. The possibility of caffeine-mediated changes in blood flow velocity in the middle cerebral artery induced by tests of cerebrovascular responsiveness was examined by transcranial doppler sonography. Velocity in the middle cerebral artery measures were obtained as healthy college students hypoventilated, hyperventilated, and performed cognitive activities (short-term remembering, generating an autobiographical image, and solving problems), each in 31-second tests. The measures were obtained from the same persons, in separate testing sessions, when they were noncaffeinated and under two levels of caffeine (45 mg/12 oz and 117 mg/8 oz). Compared with the no-caffeine control condition, a smaller amount of caffeine had no significant effects on global velocity in the middle cerebral artery but a larger amount suppressed the velocity by 5.8%. Time course analyses indicated that the velocity followed a triphasic pattern to increase over baselines during hypoventilation, regardless of caffeine condition; slowed below baselines during hyperventilation (with the degree of slowing attenu-ated under caffeine); and increased over baselines during all cognitive activities (ranges 3.8–6.9%)[CA042].

Chemopreventive effect. Chlorogenic acid had a regressive effect on induced aberrant crypt foci, as well as on development of aberrant crypt foci in azoxymethane-induced colorectal carcinogenesis in rats. Rice germs and γ-aminobutyric acid-enriched defatted rice germ inhibited azoxymethane-induced aberrant crypt foci formation and colorectal carcinogenesis in rats. Ferulic acid, also known to be contained in coffee beans and rice, prevented azoxymethane aberrant crypt foci formation and intestinal carcinogenesis in rats[CA017].

Cholesteryl ester transfer protein activity. French press or filtered coffee, consumed by 46 healthy normolipidemic subjects for 24 weeks, produced a long-term increase in cholesteryl ester transfer protein, as well as phospholipid transfer protein activity; the increase in cholesteryl ester transfer protein activity may contribute to the rise in low-density lipoprotein (LDL) cholesterol. Relative to the baseline values, French-press coffee significantly increased average cholesteryl ester transfer protein activity by 12% after 2 weeks, by 18% after 12 weeks, and by 9% after 24 weeks. Phospholipid transfer protein activity was significantly increased by 6% after 2 weeks and by 10% after 12 weeks. Lecithin/cholesterol acyltransferase activity was significantly decreased by 6% after 12 weeks and by 7% after 24 weeks. The increase in cholesteryl ester transfer protein clearly preceded the increase in LDL cholesterol, but not the increase in total triglycerides (TGs). However, consumption of French-press coffee produced a persistent rise in cholesteryl ester transfer protein activity, whereas the rise in serum TGs was transient[CA032].

Water extract of the green seed, administered intravenously to male rats at a dose of 70 mg/kg, was inactive. Water extract of the roasted seed, administered intravenously to male rats at a dose of 0.84 mg/kg, was active[CA155].

Chromosome aberration induced. Lyophilized extract of the roasted seed, in cell culture at a concentration of 3.9 mg/mL, was active on human lymphocytes. Caffeinated and decaffeinated coffees without S9 mix was tested. The extract produced weak activity with S9 mix[CA233]. Extract of the roasted seed, in cell culture at variable concentrations, was active on human lymphocytes. Metabolic activation reduced the effect[CA239].

Central nervous system effects. Ethanol (60%) extract of the dried seed, administered orally to adults at a dose of 30 mL/person, increased acuteness of hearing[CA244]. Water extract of the roasted seed, administered orally to adults, produced an increase in work performance[CA141].

Cognitive and psychomotor performance. Coffee and tea, consumed four times during the day by 30 healthy volunteers, maintained aspects of cognitive and psychomotor performance throughout the day and evening when caffeinated beverages were administered repeatedly. Tea, coffee, or water was administered in a randomized five-way crossover design. A psychometric battery consisting of critical flicker fusion, choice reaction time, and subjective sedation tests was administered predose and at frequent time points postdose. The Leeds sleep evaluation questionnaire was completed each morning, and a wrist Actigraph was worn for the duration of the study. Caffeinated beverages maintained critical flicker fusion threshold throughout the whole day, independent of caffeine dose or beverage type. During the acute phase of the beverage ingestion, caffeine significantly sustained performance compared with water after the first beverage of critical flicker fusion and subjective sedation and after the second beverage for the recogni-

tion component of the choice reaction time task. There were significant differences between tea and coffee at 75 mg caffeine dose after the first drink. Compared to coffee, tea produced a significant increase in critical flicker fusion threshold between 30 and 90 minutes postconsumption. After the second beverage, caffeinated coffee at 75 mg dose significantly improved reaction time, compared with tea at the same dose, for the recognition component of the choice reaction time task. Caffeinated beverages had a dose-dependent negative effect on sleep onset, time, and quality. Day-long tea consumption produced similar alert effects as coffee, despite lower caffeine levels, but it is less likely to disrupt sleep[CA036].

Colonic cancer risk. French-press coffee, consumed by men and women with mean age of 43 ± 11 years, did not influence the colorectal mucosal proliferation rate but may increase the detoxification capacity and antimutagenic properties in the colorectal mucosa through an increase in glutathione concentration[CA033].

Comutagenic activity. Hot water extract of the roasted seed with methylglyoxal, DL-glyceraldehyde, dihydroxyacetone, and autoxidized linoleic acid, on agar plate at a concentration of 1%, were active on *Salmonella typhimurium* TA100[CA234].

Coronary heart disease. In a study of 20 randomly selected groups of 179 Finnish men and women aged 30–59 years, it was determined that coffee drinking did not increase the risk of coronary heart disease or death. In men, the effects of smoking and a high serum cholesterol level largely explain slightly increased mortality from coronary heart disease and all causes in heavy coffee drinkers. Habitual coffee drinking, health behavior, major known coronary heart disease risk factors, and medical history were assessed at the baseline examination. Each subject was followed up 10 years after the survey using the national hospital discharge and death registers. Multivariate analyses were performed using the Cox proportional hazards model. In men, the risk of nonfatal myocardial infarction was not associated with coffee drinking. The highest coronary heart disease mortality was found among those who did not drink coffee at all. Also, in women, all-cause mortality decreased by increasing coffee drinking. The prevalence of smoking and the mean level of serum cholesterol increased with increasing coffee drinking. Non-coffee drinkers more often reported a history of various diseases and symptoms, and they were also more frequently users of several drugs compared with coffee drinkers[CA023]. A risk of coronary events (death, nonfatal infarction, or coronary artery surgery) was estimated in a group of more than 11,000 men and women aged 40–59 years by approx 7.7 years of study. Coffee and tea consumption showed a strong inverse relation. Coffee showed a weak but beneficial gradient with increasing consumption, associated with beneficial effects for mortality and coronary morbidity, although there was a residual benefit of coffee consumption in avoiding heart disease among men[CA058]. Decoction of the dried seed, administered to adults of both sexes at variable doses, produced equivocal effect. In a 12-year cohort study on the influence of coffee intake on coronary heart disease in 38,500 subjects it was indicated that during the first 6 years a strong correlation between high coffee intake and coronary death was found. After the first 6 years, the correlation was significantly decreased[CA140].

Cytotoxic activity. Ethanol (50%) extract of the aerial parts, in cell culture, was inactive on CA-9KB, effective dose$_{50}$ greater than 20.0 µg/mL[CA139].

Dermatitis-producing effect. Hot water extract and powder of the dried seed, administered externally to adults, were active[CA212].

Down syndrome effect. Data from a case–control study of 997 live-born infants or fetuses with Down syndrome and 1007 live-born controls with a birth defect indicated that among nonsmoking mothers, high coffee consumption is more likely to reduce the viability of a Down syndrome conceptus than that of a normal conceptus[CA020].

Embryotoxic effect. Hot water extract of the Folger's instant coffee, administered by gastric intubation to pregnant mice at a dose of 1.28 mg/animal, was inactive[CA229]. Hot water extract of the roasted seed, administered in drinking water of pregnant rats at variable doses daily for 30 weeks, was inactive[CA228].

Estrogenic effect. Unsaponifiable fraction of the seed oil, administered subcutaneously to immature female rats at a dose of 117 mg/animal, was inactive[CA138]. Subcutaneous administration to ovariectomized female guinea pigs was active[CA248].

Fatalities. Extract of the roasted seed, administered rectally to a 37-year-old woman with breast cancer after radical mastectomy and chemotherapy at a dose of 0.95 L/person four times daily, was active. Death was attributed to fluid and electrolyte imbalance. Sodium and chloride could not be detected. Extract of the roasted seed, administered rectally to a 46-year-old woman at a dose of 10–12 coffee enemas, three to four an hour, produced convulsive seizures and eventually death[CA219]. Decoction of the dark-roasted seed, on agar plate, was active on *Staphylococcus aureus*, with lethal dose$_{50}$ of 16 mg/mL. Concentrations of 23, 35, and 40 mg/mL, were active on *Escherichia coli*. Decoction of the medium-roasted seed at concentrations of 29, 41, 50, and 52 mg/mL, were active on *Escherichia coli*. Decoction of the light-roasted seed at concentrations of 40, 46, 50, and 57 mg/mL, were active on *Escherichia coli*. Decoction of the roasted seed, on agar plate at concentrations of 28 and 41 mg/mL, was active on *Escherichia coli*. Decoction of the medium-roasted seed, on agar plate at a concentration of 4 mg/mL, was active on *Sarcina lutea*[CA178].

Fertilization inhibition. Hot water extract of the roasted seed, administered in the drinking water of female rats at variable doses daily for 30 weeks, was inactive[CA228].

Fibrinogen level increase. Hot water extract of the dried seed, administered to adults at a dose of five cups/day, produced weak activity[CA150].

Fungal activity. Coffee leaves, fruits, and soil were cultured and inoculated into mice. A fungus isolated from the liver of a mouse inoculated with soil showed temperature-dependent dimorphism and in vitro mycelium and yeast phases characteristic of *Paracoccidioides brasiliensis*. Yeast cells of the fungus produced disseminated infection after intraperitoneal inoculation in Wistar rats from which the fungus was reisolated. An antigen reacting with sera from patients with paracoccidioidomycosis was obtained from this *Paracoccidioides brasiliensis* strain; antigen identity with strain 339 and with four other *Paracoccidioides brasiliensis* strains was detected by gel immunodiffusion. However, when the exoantigen was submitted to sodium dodecyl sulfate-polyacrylamide gel electrophoresis, a low gp43 expression in the new strain, which was called Ibia[CA002], was observed.

Gallbladder diseases. The relation of ultrasound-documented gallbladder disease with coffee drinking in 13,938 adult participants was examined between 1988 and 1994. The prevalence of total gallbladder disease was unrelated to coffee consumption in either men or women. However, among women, a decreased prevalence of previously diagnosed gallbladder disease was found with increased coffee drinking. These findings do not support a protective effect of coffee consumption on total gallbladder disease, although coffee may decrease the risk of symptomatic gallstones in women[CA022].

γ-Glutamyltransferase effect. In a cross-sectional study involving 1353 males aged 35–59 years, it was concluded that coffee consumption is inversely related to serum γ-glutamyltransferase and that coffee may inhibit the inducing effects of aging and possibly of smoking on serum γ-glutamyltransferase in the liver[CA030].

Gastroesophageal reflux effect. Coffee, a known lower esophageal sphincter relaxant, was tested in 185 and 258 cases of esophageal adenocarcinoma and gastric adenocarcinoma, respectively, and 815 controls. There was no association between lower esophageal sphincter-relaxing foods and symptoms of chronic reflux. There was no association between dietary factors known to cause lower esophageal relaxation and the risk of adenocarcinoma of the esophagus or gastric cardia. The results indicated that dietary factors associated with lower esophageal sphincter relaxation and transient gastroesophageal reflux are not associated with any important risk of esophageal malignancy[CA012].

Gastrointestinal effect. It was demonstrated that coffee promotes gastroesophageal reflux. It stimulated gastrin release and gastric acid secretion, but studies on the effect on lower esophageal sphincter pressure yielded conflicting results. Coffee also prolonged the adaptive relaxation of the proximal stomach, suggesting that it might slow gastric emptying. However, other studies indicated that coffee does not affect gastric emptying or small bowel transit. It induced cholecystokinin release and gallbladder contraction, which may explain why patients with symptomatic gallstones often avoid drinking coffee. Coffee increased rectosigmoid motor activity within 4 minutes after ingestion in some people. Their effects on the colon were comparable to those of a 1000-kcal meal. Because coffee contains no calories and its effects on the gastrointestinal tract cannot be ascribed to its volume load, acidity, or osmolality; it must have pharmacological effects. Caffeine alone could not account for these gastrointestinal effects[CA009].

Genotoxicity inhibition. Hot water extract of the fruit, administered intragastrically to mice at a dose of 500 mg/kg, was active vs adriamycin-, cyclophosphamine-, procarbazine-, and mitomycin-induced genotoxicity. Genotoxicity was measured by the presence of micronucleated polychromatic erythrocytes in bone marrow[CA240].

Glutathione-S-transferase induction. Seed oil, administered to hamsters at a concentration of 2.25% of diet, was active[CA173]. The seed, administered in ration of female mice, was active[CA221].

Hialuronidase inhibition. Hot water extract of the seed, at a concentration of 0.01%, produced 53% inhibition, probably resulting from tannins[CA137].

Homocysteine effects. Elevated homocysteine concentration is considered an independent risk factor for cardiovascular diseases and has been associated with neural tube defects. In a study of 290 young women aged 25–30 years and in 288 older women aged 60–65 years total homocysteine concentrations were measured. All of the participants completed questionnaires about factors, including lifestyle, health, and use of vitamin supplements. Smoking status, coffee consumption, SBP, and body mass index were positively associated, and estrogen replacement therapy and tea consumption were inversely associated with total homocysteine in some of the models. According to the criteria used, between 1 and 36% of the women had suboptimal folate intake. Folic acid is a strong predictor of total homocysteine concentration; however, several dietary and other lifestyle factors are important as well[CA026]. Coffee, consumed by 26 volunteers (18–53 years of age) at a dose of 1 L/day for 4 weeks, raised plasma concentrations of total homocys-

teine in healthy individuals. Coffee increased homocysteine concentrations in 24 of 26 individuals. Circulating concentrations of vitamin B_6, vitamin B_{12}, and folate were unaffected[CA027]. Infusion of the seed oil, administered orally to more than 15,000 adults of both sexes at variable doses, was active on plasma[CA190].

Hypercholesterolemic effect. Triacylglycerols has been determined to be the major lipid constituents of the coffee oil, along with sterol esters, sterols/triterpene alcohol, hydrocarbons, and the hydrolyzed products of triacylglycerols as the minor components. Fatty acid composition of total oil, neutral lipids, polar lipids, and pure triacylglycerols showed the presence of fatty acids of C14, C16, C18, and C20 carbon chains. Palmitic and linoleic acids were the major fatty acids and comprise approx 38.7% and 35.9%, respectively. Pancreatic lipase hydrolysis revealed that the linoleoyl and palmityl moieties are preferentially esterified at the Sn-2 and Sn-1,3 positions of triacylglycerols, respectively. The presence of high amounts of palmitic acid at Sn-1,3 position in coffee oil may be partly responsible for its hypercholesterolemic effects[CA004]. Coffee oil was administered orally to 11 healthy normolipemic volunteers at a dose of 2 g/day for 3 weeks. After a 2-week washout period, the reverse treatments were applied for another 3 weeks. Six subjects received oil supplying 72 mg/day of cafestol and 53 mg/day of kahweol, and five received oil that provided 40 mg of cafestol, 19 mg of 16-O-methyl-cafestol, and 2 mg of kahweol/day. The average cholesterol level increased by 0.65 mmol/L (13%) on coffee oil. The TG level increased by 0.49 mmol/L (61%). No effects on serum lipids or lipoprotein cholesterol levels were significantly different between variety *Arabica* or *Robusta* oils. The treatments elevated serum lipid levels; therefore, cafestol must be involved and kahweol cannot be the sole cholesterol-raising diterpene[CA005]. Coffee total lipids, coffee nonsaponifiable matter, and coffee diterpene alcohols have been examined in adult Syrian hamsters. The animals were fed either a commercial laboratory chow diet containing 5% fat and low in saturated fat (1.46 g/100 g diet) and cholesterol (0.03 g/100 g diet) or a semisynthetic diet set in gelatin, containing 10% fat and high in saturated fat (4 g/100 g diet) and cholesterol (90.5 g/100 g diet). The coffee lipid extracts were dissolved in olive oil (concentration either 5 mg of total lipid, 0.5 mg nonsaponifiable matter or 0.5 mg diterpene alcohols for 250 µL olive oil) in study 1 and in coconut oil (concentrations either 20 mg total lipid, 2 mg nonsaponifiable matter, or 2 mg diterpene alcohols per 250 µL) in study 2. A dose of 250 µL of these solutions was administered daily by gavage. Control animals received 250 µL vehicle only. For serum lipid analysis, blood samples were obtained on days 0, 7, and 14 in study 1 and on days 0, 7, 14, and 21 in study 2. The results indicated a tendency of serum total cholesterol (TC) and high-density lipoprotein (HDL) cholesterol to increase with administration of coffee total lipid, nonsaponifiable, and diterpene alcohols. In contrast, in study 2 there were no significant differences in serum lipids between control and coffee lipid-treated groups across time. The results support the concept that coffee lipids may be hypercholesterolemic and indicate that diterpene could be the lipid component responsible for such an effect. However, it appears that this hypercholesterolemic effect is apparent only when the background diet is low in saturated fat and cholesterol. A high-saturated fat/high-cholesterol diet may mask the hypercholesterolemic effect of coffee lipid[CA010]. Hot water extract of the dried kernel, administered intragastrically to male hamsters, was active vs feeding high-fat diet[CA160]. Hot water extract of the boiled seed, adminis-

tered in drinking water of hamster and rats at a concentration of 0.5 g/mL, was inactive[CA187]. Decoction of the dried seed, administered orally to adults, produced equivocal results[CA157,CA163]. Decoction of the roasted coffee, administered orally to 20 healthy volunteers at a dose of 600 mL/day for 4 weeks, produced a significant increase of LDL and TG levels, and LDL–HDL ratio. Decoction of the boiled coffee passed through a conventional paper filter, administered orally to 20 healthy volunteers at a dose of 600 mL/day for 4 weeks, produced no change in LDL and TG levels and LDL–HDL ratio. Filtering removed more than 80% of the lipid-soluble substances present in boiled coffee[CA161]. Heartwood, administered orally to adults for 24 hours, produced an increase of cholesterol level[CA238]. Hot water extract of the seed, administered orally to 1629 middle-aged adults, produced an increase of serum cholesterol level and intake of fat. Hot water extract of the seed, administered orally to 1625 middle-aged adults, produced equivocal effect. Consumers of filtered coffee had no significant change in serum cholesterol level[K12893]. Powder of the seed, administered orally to adults at a dose of 8 g/day dosed daily in unfiltered coffee, was active[CA172]. Hexane-diethyl ether extract of the roasted seed, administered intragastrically to hamsters at a dose of 2 mg/animal, was active. Lipid fraction of the roasted seed, administered to hamsters at a dose of 20 mg/animal, was active. Nonsaponifiable fraction of the roasted seed, administered to hamsters at a dose of 2 mg/animal, was active. The effect was found only in diet low in saturated fat and cholesterol[CA174]. Decoction of the dried seed, administered orally to adults of both sexes at variable doses, decreased the level of cholesterol. Decoction of the dried seed, administered orally to adults at a dose of five cups per day, produced weak activity, and when administered to new coffee drinkers of both sexes at variable doses, decreased cholesterol level[CA247].

Hypertiglyceridemic activity. Hot water extract of the boiled seed, administered in drinking water of hamster and rats at a concentration of 0.5 g/mL, was inactive[CA187].

Hypoglycemic activity. Flower, green seed, and leaf, administered by gastric intubation to mice, were active[CA208].

Immunostimulant activity. Hot water extract of fruit, in the drinking water of mice at a concentration of 0.5%, increased the percentage of thymocytes expressing mature CD4 or CD8 markers and increased the proportion of peripheral lymphocytes expressing CD25, a marker of activation[CA186]. Hot water extract of the fruit, administered orally to adults at variable doses, was active on lymphocytes vs suppressor T-cells and natural-killer cells and inactive vs helper T-cells[CA241]. Methanol extract of the dried pericarp, administered in drinking water of mice at a concentration of 0.5%, was active on lymphocytes B. The extract enhanced lipopolysaccharide-induced activation[CA148]. Extract of the dried seed, administered intramuscularly to adult calves at a concentration of 10 mL/animal, was active[CA203].

Insecticidal activity. Ethanol (50%) extract of the aerial parts, at a concentration of 1%, was inactive on *Musca domestica* and *Tribolium castaneum*[CA128].

K-*ras* gene mutagenesis. The relationship between consumption of coffee and mutations in the K-*ras* gene in exocrine pancreatic cancer was investigated in 185 patients, 121 for whom tissue was available. Mutations in codon 12 of K-*ras* were detected by the artificial restriction fragment-length polymorphism technique. Mutations were found in tumors from 94 of 121 patients (77.7%) and were more common among regular coffee drinkers than among non-regular coffee drinkers (82% vs 55.6%, p = 0.018, n = 107). The weekly intake of coffee was significantly higher among patients with a mutated tumor (mean of 14.5 cup/week vs 8.8 among patients with a wild-type tumor, p < 0.05). Regarding non-regular drinkers, the odds ratio of a mutated tumor adjusted by age, sex, smoking, and alcohol drinking was 3.26 for drinkers of 2–7 cups/week, 5.77 for drinkers of 8–14 cups/week, and 9.99 for drinkers of more than 15 cups/week (p = 0.01)[CA057].

Leukocytosis activity. Hot water extract of the seed, administered orally to adults at a dose of five cups per day, produced weak activity[CA150].

Lipid profile alteration. Hot water extract of the seed, administered orally to adults at a dose of five cups per day, produced weak activity on apolipoprotein (apo) B HDL-C and apo A-1[CA150].

Lipoprotein modification. Decoction of the seed, administered orally to 22 adults at a dose of five to six strong cups for 1 day, was active. Consumption of cafestol and kahweol resulted in decreased lipoprotein A levels. Filtering coffee removed the diterpenes[CA146]. Decoction of the dried stem bark, administered orally to 150 healthy adults of both sexes who consumed five or more cups of boiled coffee and 159 filter coffee consumers at a dose of 1.2 L/day, was active on human serum. Median level of serum lipoprotein was higher in the boiled coffee drinkers[CA144].

Liver dysfunction. In a 4-year study in 1221 liver dysfunction-free (serum aspartate aminotransferase [AST] and alanine aminotransferase [ALT] <39 IU/L and no medical care for or no past history of liver disease) males aged 35–56 years, was investigated for the association of coffee consumption with the development of increased serum AST and/or ALT activities. From the analysis using the Kaplan-Meier method, the estimated incidence of serum AST and/or ALT ≥ 40 IU/L, ≥ 50 IU/L, and ≥ 60 IU/L decreased with an increase in coffee consumption. From the Cox proportional hazards model, coffee drinking was independently inversely associated with the development of serum AST and/or ALT $\geq$ 40 IU/L, $\geq$ 50 IU/L, and $\geq$ 60 IU/L, controlling for age, body mass index, alcohol intake, and cigarette smoking[CA041].

Maternal risks. Three-hundred six mothers who gave birth to babies with cleft lip, or palate, or both were matched with 306 mothers who gave birth to healthy babies in the same area during the same period. Significantly more babies in the cleft palate group had a family history of clefts (48/306 compared with 7/306) in the cases studied; combined cleft lip and palate was significantly more common among boys (82/157 compared with 57/149) and cleft palate alone among girls (48/149 compared with 22/157). There was no difference between the groups regarding dietary preferences, but during pregnancy the mothers who gave birth to babies with defects tended to drink less alcohol and less coffee[CA038].

Mean platelet volume increase. Hot water extract of the seed, administered orally to adults at a dose of five cups per day, produced weak activity[CA150].

Metabolism. Decoction of the seed, administered orally to adults at variable doses, was active. Volunteers consumed food containing hydroquinone or glycopyranoside derivative (arbutin). Blood and urine levels of the compounds and conjugates were assayed[CA150].

Miscellaneous effects. Decoction of the dried seed, administered orally to 171 healthy nonsmoking adults of both sexes over the age of 50 years, indicated that coffee may decrease postprandial falls in SBP and can increase DBP in untreated hypertensives[CA192].

Mitogenic activity. Hot water extract of the fruit, administered orally to adults at variable doses, was inactive on lymphocytes vs T-lymphocyte proliferation. Hot water extract of the fruit, administered orally to adults at variable doses, was inactive on lymphocytes B vs B-cell proliferation[CA241].

Molluscicidal activity. Water extract of the roasted seed, was inactive on *Biomphalaria pfeifferi*[CA237].

Mood effects. In a full crossover design study, the effect of coffee and tea on acute physiological responses and mood indicated that caffeinated beverages acutely stimulate the autonomic nervous system and increase alertness. In the study, caffeine levels in tea were 37.5 and 75 mg and in coffee 75 and 150 mg in one group. In another group caffeine, level was manipulated. SBP, DBP, heart rate, skin temperature, skin conductance, and mood were monitored over each 3-hour study session. Tea and coffee produced mild autonomic stimulation and an elevation on mood. There were no effects of tea vs coffee or caffeine dose, despite a fourfold variation in the latter. In one study, increasing beverage strength was associated with greater increases in DBP and energetic arousal. In the other, caffeinated beverages increased DBP, SBP, and skin conductance and lower heart rate and skin temperature compared to water. Significant dose–response relationships to caffeine were seen only for SBP, heart rate, and skin temperature. There were significant effects of caffeine on energetic arousal but no consistent dose–response effects[CA035].

Mutagenic activity. Freeze-dried roasted and instant coffee, at a dose of 20 mg/plate, induced between 6 and 10 times the revertants found in negative controls of *Salmonella typhimurium*. Green coffee beans had no mutagenic activity. Mutagenicity increased with roasting time to 4 minutes, the time normally used roast coffee. The genotoxic compounds were quickly formed at temperature of 220°C. Mutagenic activity was independent of the roasting procedure[CA011]. Water extract of the dried fruit, in cell culture at a concentration of 2 mg/mL, was active on hamster lung cells without microsomal activation[CA206]. Hot water extract of the seed, on agar plate at concentration of 40 mg/plate, was active on *Salmonella typhimurium* TA102 and inactive on *Salmonella typhimurium* TA100 [CA169]. Hot water extract of the seed, on agar plate at concentration of 50 mg/plate, was active on *Salmonella typhimurium* TA100 and inactive on *Salmonella typhimurium* TA1535, TA1537, TA1538, and TA98[CA165]. Hot water extract of the seed, administered intragastrically to mice at a dose of 6 g/animal, was inactive on *Escherichia coli* K12 and *Salmonella typhimurium* TA1530. The effect was assayed on bacteria injected intravenously coincidentally with extract administration and harvested 1.5 hours later[CA165]. Ethanol (95%) and hot water extracts of the solid residue of brewed coffee, on agar plate at a concentration of 12.5 mg/plate, were inactive on *Salmonella typhimurium* TA100 and TA98. Hot water extract of the distillates of brewed coffee overheated to 150°C, on agar plate at a concentration of 5 mg/plate, was inactive on *Salmonella typhimurium* TA100. Metabolic activation had no effect on the results. MeCl$_2$ extract of distillates of brewed coffee overheated to 300°C, on agar plate at a concentration of 100 μg/plate, was inactive on *Salmonella typhimurium* TA100 and TA98. Extract was toxic at higher doses. MeCl$_2$ extract of distillates of brewed coffee overheated to 300°C, on agar plate at a concentration of 300 μg/plate, was active on *Salmonella typhimurium* TA98. Metabolic activation was required for activity. MeCl$_2$ extracts of distillates and solid residue of brewed coffee, on agar plate at a concentration of 5 mg/plate, were inactive on *Salmonella typhimurium* TA100 and TA98. MeCl$_2$ extract of distillates of brewed coffee overheated to 150°C, on agar plate at a concentration of 750 μg/plate, was active on *Salmonella typhimurium* TA98. Metabolic activation was required for activity[CA232]. Hot water extract of the seed, on agar plate at a concentration of 10 g/L, was active on *Salmonella typhimurium* TA98[CA166]. Hot water extract of the roasted seed, on agar plate at a concentration of 14 mg, was active on *Salmonella typhimurium* TA100. The activity shown was the result of caffeine[CA227].

Myocardial infarction. A group of 340 of age-, sex-, and community-matched individuals drinking caffeinated and decaffeinated coffee was investigated. The odds ratio for drinking four or more cups per day of caffeinated coffee was 0.84 (95 % confidence interval [CI], 0.49–1.42) compared with drinking one cup or less per week, after adjustment for coronary risk factors. The odds ratio for drinking more than one cup per day of decaffeinated coffee vs nondrinkers was 1.25 (95% CI, 0.76–2.04)[CA053].

Neuron-sprouting stimulation. Chromatographic fraction of the dried seed, in cell culture at a concentration of 1 μg/mL, was active on SK-N-SH cells[CA249].

Nuclear aberration reduction. Decoction of the seed, administered intragastrically with methylurea and sodium nitrite to mice at a dose of 1 g/animal, was active. Decoction of the seed, administered intragastrically with methylurea and sodium nitrite to mice at a dose of 600 mg/animal, was active on colon[CA214].

Occupational respiratory allergy. There was a significant correlation between sensitization to green coffee bean and work-related symptoms (asthma and/or rhinitis) ($p < 0.01$), common allergic symptoms ($p < 0.05$), and atopy by prick test ($p < 0.01$)[CA061].

Ovarian cancer risk. In a study of 549 women with newly diagnosed epithelial ovarian cancer and 516 control women, it was concluded that coffee and caffeine consumption may increase the risk of ovarian cancer among premenopausal women. Coffee and alcohol consumption was assessed through a semiquantitative food-frequency questionnaire, and information on tobacco smoking was collected through personal interview. There was no risk for ovarian cancer overall associated with tobacco or alcohol use in either premenopausal or postmenopausal women. Association of borderline significance for tobacco and invasive serous cancers and alcohol and mucinous cancers were observed but reduced after adjustment for coffee consumption[CA029].

Ovulation inhibition effect. Hot water extract of the roasted seed, administered in drinking water of female rats at variable doses daily for 30 weeks, was inactive[CA228].

Pancreatic cancer risk. In a study of 583 individuals with histologically confirmed pancreatic cancer and 4813 controls, it was determined that consumption of total alcohol, wine, liquor, beer, and coffee was not associated with pancreatic cancer[CA039].

Parkinson's disease. The association of smoking, alcohol, and coffee consumption with Parkinson's disease was investigated in 196 subjects who developed Parkinson's disease from 1976 to 1995. Each incident case was matched by age ($\pm$ 1 year) and sex to a general population control subject. The findings suggest an inverse association between coffee drinking and Parkinson's disease; however, this association did not imply that coffee has a direct protective effect against Parkinson's disease[CA024]. In a study of 8004 Japanese-American men aged 45–60 years, it was indicated that higher coffee intake is associated with a significantly lower incidence of Parkinson's disease. Data were analyzed from 30 years of follow-up. During the follow-up, 102 men were identified as having Parkinson's disease. Age-adjusted incidence of Parkinson's disease declined consistently with increased amounts of coffee intake from 10.4 per 10,000 person-years in men who drank coffee to 1.9 per 10,000 person-years in men who drank at least 450 g/day. Similar relationships were observed with total caffeine intake and for caffeine from noncoffee sources. Consumption of in-

creasing amounts of coffee was also associated with lower risk of Parkinson's disease in men who were never, past, and current smokers at baseline. Other nutrients in coffee, including niacin, were unrelated to Parkinson's disease incidence. The relationship between caffeine and Parkinson's disease was unaltered by intake of milk and sugar[CA037].

Peroxide formation stimulation. Hot water extract of the seed was active. Polyphenolics catalyzed the oxidation of O_2 to H_2O_2[CA169].

Pharmacokinetic interactions. The most serious coffee (caffeine)-related central nervous system (CNS) effects include seizures and delirium. Other symptoms affecting the cardiovascular system range from moderate increases in heart rate to more severe cardiac arrhythmia. Although tolerance develops to many of the pharmacological effects of caffeine, tolerance may be overwhelmed by the nonlinear accumulation of caffeine when its metabolism becomes saturated. This might occur with high levels of consumption or as the result of pharmacokinetic interaction between caffeine and medications. The polycyclic aromatic hydrocarbon-inducible cytochrome P450 IA2 participated in the metabolism of caffeine, as well as of several clinically important drugs. A number of drugs, including certain selective serotonin reuptake inhibitors (particularly fluvoxamine), antiarrhythmics (mexiletine), antipsychotics (clozapine), psoralens, idrocilamine and phenylpropanolamine, bronchodilators (furafylline and theophylline), and quinolones (enoxacin), have been reported to be potent inhibitors of this isoenzyme. Thus, pharmacokinetic interactions at the cytochrome P450 IA2 enzyme level may cause toxic effects during concomitant administration of caffeine and certain drugs used for cardiovascular, CNS, gastrointestinal, infectious, and respiratory and skin disorders[CA031]. Decoction of the dried seed was administered orally to nine healthy patients of both sexes with ileostomies at a dose of 720 mL (one, two, or three cups of French-press coffee with a standardized breakfast) for three separate days in random order. Ileostomy effluent was collected for 14 hours and urine for 24 hours. Stability of cafestol and kahweol was assessed under simulated gastrointestinal tract conditions. Corrected mean absorption of diterpenes expressed as percentages of the amount consumed and the amount entering the duodenum were 67% and 88%, respectively, for cafestol and 72% and 93%, respectively, for kahweol. There was a loss of diterpenes during incubation in vitro with gastric juice (cafestol 24% and kahweol 32%), during storage with ileostomy effluent (cafestol 18% and kahweol 12%), and during freeze-drying (cafestol 26% and kahweol 32%). Mean excretion of glucuronidated plus sulphated conjugates in urine was 1.2% of the ingested amount for cafestol and 0.4% of the ingested amount for kahweol. Approximately 70% of the ingested cafestol and kahweol was absorbed in ileostomy volunteers. Only a small part of the diterpenes was excreted as a conjugate of glucuronic acid or sulphate in urine[CA199].

Pheromone. Ether extract of the stem was active on *Aspiculuris tetraptera* and male Mediterranean fruit flies. Ether extract of the stem produced equivocal effect on *Dacus dorsalis* and melon flies of both sexes[CA142].

Prophylactic effect. The therapeutic effect of a 30% extract from coffee beans has been investigated in newborn calves in herds that endemically showed a high proportion of infections within the gastroenteric and/or respiratory system in calves. Fifty newborn calves were given a subcutaneous injection of 10 mL of the extract on the first and third days of life. Another 50 calves received physiological saline as control. On the first 2 days of life, the group treated with the extract had fewer animals

with body temperature below physiological values; during the first period of diarrhea (between days 4 and 6), there was a significantly lower tendency of diarrhea, and after the second period of diarrhea (day 9), a better and quicker recovery and a lower tendency of exsiccation as the control calves. The average duration of illness was shorter (4.7 instead of 7 days), and the average number of therapeutical interventions were less (3.1 instead of 4.5) than in control calves. Within the four herds endemically showing a high number of cases of diarrhea in newborn calves, the morbidity could be dropped by 35% by the administration of one to three subcutaneous injections of 10 mL of the extract[CA008].

Prostaglandin inhibition. Water extract of the dried seed, administered in drinking water of rats at a dose of 5%, was active. Prostaglandin I-2 synthesis in the rat thoracic aorta was assayed[CA217].

Psychomotor performance. Coffee, taken by 17 introverts and 19 extroverts at doses of 2 and 4 mg caffeine/kg during the morning and evening, did not support the hypothesis that caffeine differentially affects extroverts and introverts. In this randomized, double-blind, crossover study, the subjects drank coffee during the mornings and evenings. At 30-minute intervals for 180 minutes after drinking coffee, the participants completed the Profile of Mood States, a battery of self-report visual analog scales, and the Digital Symbol Substitution Test. Caffeine affects on mood and task performance did not significantly interact with extroversion, except for nonsignificant trends for caffeine to increase happiness and vigor more among extroverts than introverts. No three-way interactions of group, time, and dose were found on any scales or on the Digital Symbol Substitution Test[CA043].

Renin–angiotensin–aldosterone system activity. Plasma renin activity and enzyme-converting angiotensin I to angiotensin II activity, serum concentration of aldosterone, and catecholamines in patients with hypertension and patients with low or normal plasma renin activity, drinking one cup of coffee were measured by radioimmunoassay, and blood pressure was measured by ambulatory monitoring. Drinking one cup of coffee produced, after 1–2 hours, elevated SBP and after 1 hour DBP in patients with low renin–angiotensin–aldosterone system activity who habitually drink coffee. Patients with normal renin–angiotensin–aldosterone system activity had elevations only in DBP from 1 to 2 hours after drinking. Plasma catecholamines, aldosterone con-centrations, blood renin activity, and enzyme-converting angiotensin I to angiotensin II activities were not elevated[CA055].

Respiratory effect. Respiratory consequences of work in coffee processing were studied in 764 female workers exposed to dusts associated with the processing of green and roasted coffee. A group of 387 females not exposed to respiratory irritants served as controls for the prevalence of acute and chronic respiratory symptoms. A greater prevalence of all acute and chronic respiratory symptoms was consistently found among exposed workers than among control workers. The highest prevalence of chronic respiratory symptoms was recorded for chronic cough (40%), followed by acute symptoms of dry cough (58.7%). Mean acute reductions of lung function throughout the work shift were recorded in all of the studied groups; the mean across-shift decrease as a percentage of preshift values was particularly marked in forced expiratory flow at 75% ([FEF25]; –26.7%), forced expiratory flow at 50% ([FEF50]; –20.6%), followed by forced expiratory volume in 1 second (–9.9) and forced vital capacity (–3.7%). The preshift (baseline) values of ventilatory capacity were decreased in comparison to the predicted ones, and were low-

est for FEF50 and FEF25. Disodium cromoglycate significantly diminished across-shift reductions for FEF50 and FEF25 in a subgroup of the examined workers[CA013].

Rheumatoid arthritis risk. Coffee, consumed by 6809 subjects with no clinical arthritis, indicated that the amount of coffee consumed was directly proportional to the prevalence of rheumatoid factor positivity. The consumption of coffee was first studied for its association with rheumatoid factor (sensitized sheep cell agglutination titer) in a cross-sectional survey and second for its prediction of rheumatoid in a cohort of 18,981 men and women who had neither arthritis nor a history of it at the baseline examination. In the cross-sectional survey, the amount of coffee consumes was directly proportional to the prevalence of rheumatoid factor. Adjusted for age and sex, this association was significant, but after further adjustment for smoking, the linear trend declined below significance. In the cohort study, there was an association between coffee consumption and the risk of rheumatoid factor-positive rheumatoid arthritis that did not result from age, sex, level of education, smoking, alcohol intake, body mass index, or serum cholesterol. After adjusting for these potential confounders, the users of four or more cups a day still have a relative risk of 2.2 (95% CI at 1.13–4.27) for developing rheumatoid factor-positive rheumatoid arthritis compared with those drinking less. Coffee consumption did not predict the development of rheumatoid factor-negative rheumatoid arthritis[CA034].

RNA (messenger) polymerase inhibition. Petroleum ether extract of the green seed, administered in ration of female mice at variable doses for 12 days, produced strong activity[CA220]. The seed, administered in ration of female mice at variable concentrations for 12 days, was active[CA220].

Serum homocysteine concentration. The influence of nutritional factors associated with total homocysteine in 260 school teachers, 151 women, and 109 men with a median age of 64 years was performed by observational analyses of baseline and 2–4 months follow-up tests that designed to test the feasibility of conducting a large-scale clinical trial of vitamin supplements. In multivariable linear regression and generalized linear models, there was a positive, significant dose–response relationship between coffee consumption and total homocysteine ($p = 0.01$)[CA048].

Serum lipids and lipoproteins. Serum concentrations of TC, TGs, and HDL cholesterol were measured in a group of 4587 males aged 48–56 years, drinking instant and brewed coffee. LDL cholesterol levels were calculated from the values of TC, TG, and HDL cholesterol. The consumption of brewed coffee was unrelated to any parameter, and instant coffee consumption showed a highly significant positive association with serum LDL cholesterol levels and an inverse association with serum TG levels. For each cup of instant coffee a day, LDL cholesterol levels were 0.82 mg/dL (95% CI, 0.29–1.35) higher, and TG levels in a natural log-scale were 0.014 mg/dL (95% CI, 0.006–0.022) lower. A tendency for positive association between instant coffee intake and serum TC levels ($p = 0.09$) was observed. HDL cholesterol levels were unrelated to instant coffee consumption[CA049].

Sex hormone-binding globulin level increase. Water extract of the seed, administered to 50 premenopausal women at variable doses daily, was active. Blood samples were obtained from each woman on days 11 and 22 of her menstrual cycle. High intakes of caffeinated coffee, green tea, and total caffeine were commonly correlated with increasing sex hormone-binding globulin on days 11 and 22 of the cycle after controlling for potential confounders. Green tea but not caffeinated coffee intake was inversely correlated with estradiol on day 11 of the cycle.

Although the effect of caffeine cannot be distinguished from the effects of coffee and green tea, consumption of caffeine-containing beverages favorably altered hormone levels associated with the risk of developing breast cancer[CA149].

Sister chromatid exchange stimulation. Lyophilized extract of the essential oil, administered by gastric intubation to mice at a dose of 50 mL/kg in two doses, was inactive[CA209]. Lyophilized extract of the dried seed, administered by gastric intubation to hamsters at a dose of 2.5 g/kg, was inactive[CA209].

Skin depigmentation effect. Extract of the dried seed, administered externally to adults at a dose of 5%, was active. Skin-lightening cosmetics contained extract of *Coffea arabica* seeds (containing chlorogenic acid) as melanin-formation inhibitors. The extract has been incorporated into cosmetics for skin-aging prevention or into hair preparations for hair protection. Biological activity reported has been patented[CA193].

Smooth muscle relaxant activity. The aqueous extracts of green and roasted coffees were assayed on isolated guinea pig tracheal spirals. Contractile and relaxant activities were compared with histamine and theophylline, respectively. Green coffee extracts induced concentration dependent contraction, but the maximal tension never exceeded 76.3% ± 5.2 of a maximal histamine contraction (0.69 ± 0.07 g/mm² vs 0.52 ± 0.05 g/mm²; $p = 0.01$). One gram of green coffee dust had a biological activity equivalent to 1.23 ± 0.1 mg of histamine. The pD2 value of histamine was −5.17 ± 0.05. The potency of green coffee was unaffected by mepyramine maleate (1 μg/mL, final bath concentration), whereas that of histamine was reduced 500-fold. Tissues contracted with histamine were not significantly relaxed by green coffee extracts. By contrast, roasted coffee extracts induced concentration-dependent relaxation of uncontracted and histamine contracted tissues. Tissues contracted with green coffee extracts were also completely relaxed by roasted coffee extracts. The pD2 value of theophylline was -4.10 ± 0.03. The relaxant activity of 1 g of roasted coffee was equivalent to 1.95 ± 0.16 mg of theophylline. The potency of these extracts was significantly reduced after propranolol (1 µg/L; dose ratio 1.56)[CA159].

Stress relief. A survey of 261 house staff, nurses, and medical oncologists in a cancer research hospital and oncologists in outside clinical practices was carried out to measure burnout, physiological distress, and physical symptoms. Each participant completed a questionnaire that quantified life stressors, personality attributes, burnout, psychological distress, physical symptoms, coping strategies, and social support. The results indicated that house staff experienced the greatest burnout. They also reported greater emotional exhaustion, a feeling of emotional distance from patients, and a poorer sense of personal accomplishment. Nurses reported more physical symptoms than house staff and oncologists. However, they were less emotionally distant from patients. Women reported a lower sense of accomplishment and greater distress. The four most frequent methods of relaxing were talking to friends, using humor, drinking coffee or eating, and watching television[CA019].

Suicidal risk. Data from 36,689 adult men and women (25–64 years of age) who participated in a population survey between 1972 and 1992 indicated that clustering of the heavy use of alcohol, cigarettes, and coffee could serve as a new marker for increased risk of suicide. The mortality of the cohort was monitored for a mean of 14.4 years, which yielded 169 suicides. Criteria for heavy use of each psychoactive substance were defined as: alcohol more than 120 g/week, cigarettes more than 21/day, and coffee more than 7 cups/day. Approximately

50% of the men and 80% of the women did not use any of the psychoactive substances heavily. Every third man and every fifth woman used one substance heavily. The prevalence for those who exceeded criteria for joint heavy use of two substances was 9% for men and 1% for women. Joint-heavy use of all three substances was rare. The adjusted risk of suicide increased linearly with increasing level of joint heavy use of alcohol, cigarette, and coffee. Among subjects with heavy use of one substance, the risk was 1.55, with joint-heavy use of two substances 2.22, and with joint-heavy use of all three substances 3.99 compared with no heavy use[CA016].

Sunscreen effect. Seed oil, administered externally to adults at a concentration of 30%, was active. Biological activity reported has been patented[CA222].

Symptomatic gallstone disease. In a 10-year study, 46,008 men aged 40–75 years without history of gall stone disease were investigated for the association of coffee and caffeinated drink consumption with symptomatic gallstone disease or cholecystectomy, diagnosed by ultrasonography or X-ray. After adjusting for other known or suspected risk factors, compared with men who did not consume regular coffee, the adjusted relative risk (RR) for those who consistently drank two to three cups of regular coffee per day was 0.60 (95% CI, 0.42–0.86); four or more cups per day the RR was 0.55 (95% CI, 0.33–0.92). The risk of gall stone disease declined with increasing caffeine intake. RR for men in the highest category of caffeine intake (>800 mg/day) compared with men in the lowest category (≤25 mg/day) was 0.55 (95% CI, 0.35–0.87). Decaffeinated coffee was not associated with a decreased risk[CA045]. The effect of coffee drinking in relation to alcohol drinking, smoking, and obesity was investigated in the population of 7637 males, aged 48–59 years; 1360 men with a possible pathologic condition influencing liver enzyme levels, and 182 former alcohol drinkers; the effect of coffee on serum γ-glutamyltransferase (GGT) was examined by a multiple linear regression model and analysis of variance adjusting for alcohol drinking, smoking and body mass index. The adjusted percentage of difference in serum GGT was –4.3 (95% CI, –5 to –3.5) per cup. The inverse coffee–GGT relationship was most prominent among men drinking 30 mL or more of ethanol and smoking 15 or more cigarettes/day, and positive associations of alcohol and smoking with GGT were attenuated by coffee drinking, more clearly among men with body mass index of 25 kg/m^2 or greater. Adjusted percentages of difference in serum GGT were –2.6% (p = 0.0003) per cup of brewed coffee and –5.1% (p = 0.0001) per cup of instant coffee[CA054].

Thymidylate synthetase inhibition. Hot water extract of the dried seed, administered in drinking water of mice at a concentration of 0.5%, was active[CA180].

Thyroid effect. Coffee oil, administered orally to 11 healthy normolipemic volunteers at a dose of 2 g/day for 3 weeks, produced no effect on serum total and free thyroxine, triiodothyronine, and thyroid-stimulating hormone [CA005].

Toxicity. Atractyloside, a diterpenoid glycoside that occurs naturally in plants, may be present at levels as high as 600 mg/kg of dried plant material. Consumption of plants containing atractyloside or carboxyatractyloside has caused fatal renal proximal tubule necrosis and/or centrilobular hepatic necrosis in man and farm animals. Although pure atractyloside and crude plant extracts disrupt carbohydrate homeostasis and induce similar pathophysiological lesions in the kidney and liver, it is also possible that the toxicity of atractyloside may be confounded by the presence of other natural constituents in plants. Atractyloside competitively inhibits the adenine nucleoside

carrier in isolated mitochondria and thus blocks oxidative phosphorylation. This has been assumed to explain changes in carbohydrate metabolism and the toxic effects in liver and kidney. In vitro proximal tubular cells are selectively sensitive to atractyloside, whereas other renal cell types are quite resistant. There are also differences in the response of liver and renal tissue to atractyloside. Thus, not all of the clinical, biochemical, and morphological changes caused by atractyloside can simply be explained on the basis of mitochondrial phosphorylation. The relevance to a wider human risk is shown by the presence of atractyloside analogues in dried roasted coffee beans (17.5–32 mg/kg)[CA003]. Ethanol (50%) extract of the aerial parts, administered intraperitoneally to mice, was active, lethal dose$_{50}$ of 1 g/kg[CA139]. Water extract of the roasted seed, administered to female rats at a dose of 6% of diet for 2 years, was inactive. Both regular and decaffeinated instant coffees were tested[CA198].

Urinary diterpenes excretion. Absorption and excretion of the cholesterol-raising coffee diterpenes cafestol and kahweol were observed in nine healthy patients with ileostomies. Ileostomy effluent was collected for 14 hours, and urine was collected for 24 hours. Approximately 70% of the ingested cafestol and kahweol was absorbed. Only small part of the diterpene was excreted as a conjugate of glucuronic acid or sulphate in urine, mean excretion was 1.2% of the ingested amount for cafesterol and 0.4% for kahweol[CA059].

Urinary hydrogen peroxide. Instant coffee, taken by healthy human volunteers, indicated that coffee drinking is rapidly and reproducibly followed by increased levels of hydrogen peroxide detectable in the urine for up to 2 hours after drinking coffee. The levels of hydrogen peroxide indicated that exposure of human tissues to hydrogen peroxide might be greater than is commonly supposed. It is possible that hydrogen peroxide in urine could act as an antibacterial agent and that hydrogen peroxide is involved in the regulation of glomerular function[CA040].

White blood cell-macrophage stimulant. Water extract of the freeze-dried fruit, at a concentration of 2 mg/mL, was inactive on macrophages. Nitrate formation was used as an index of the macrophage stimulating activity to screen effective foods[CA215].

Weight-gain inhibition. Lyophilized extract of the dried seed, administered intragastrically to mice at a dose of 50 g/kg of diet, was active. Animals were exposed to coffee in utero, as mother's diet was 1% instant coffee. After weaning, animals were given instant coffee in diet for 2 years. Increase in energy expenditure was shown by increase in caloric intake and depressed growth[CA216].

REFERENCES

CA001 Dagla, M., R. Tarsi, A. Papetti, P. Grisoli, C. Daccaro, C. Pruzzo, and G. Gazzani. Antiadhesive effect of green and roasted coffee on *Streptococcus mutans'* adhesive properties on saliva-coated hydroxyapatite beads. **J Agr Food Chem** 2002; 50(5): 1225–1229.

CA002 Silva-Vergara, M. L., R. Martinez, A. Chadu, M. Madeira, G. Freitas-Silva, and C. M. Leite-Maffei. Isolatioon of *Paracoccidioides brasiliensis* strain from the soil of a coffee plantation in Ibia, State of Minas Gerais, Brasil. **Med Mycol** 1998; 36(1): 37–42.

CA003 Obatomi, D. K. and P. H. Bach. Biochemistry and toxicology of the diterpenoid glycoside atractyloside. **Food Chem Toxicol** 1998; 36(3): 35–46.

CA004 Kanhal, M. A. Lipid analysis of *Coffea arabica* Linn. beans and their possible hypercholesterolemic effects. **J Food Sci Nutr** 1997; 48(2): 135–139.

CA005 Mensink, R. P., W. J. Lebink, I. E. Lobbezoo, M. P. Weusten-Van der Wouw, P. L. Zock, and M. B. Katan. Diterpene composition of oils from Arabica and Robusta coffee beans and their effects on serum lipids in man. **J Int Med** 1995; 237(6): 543–550.

CA006 Becker, C. G., N. Van Hamont, and M. Wagner. Tobacco, cocoa, coffee and ragweed: cross-reacting allergens that activate factor-XII-dependent pathways. **Blood** 1981; 58(5): 861–867.

CA007 Daglia, M., A. Papetti, C. Gregotti, F. Berte, and G. Gazzani. *In vitro* antioxidant and *ex vivo* protective activities of green and roasted coffee. **J Agr Food Chem** 2000; 48(5): 1449–1454.

CA008 Ponepal, V., U. Spielberger, G. Riedel-Caspari and F. W. Schmidt. Use of *Coffea arabica* tosta extract for the prevention and therapy of polyfactorial infectious diseases in newborn calves. **Deutsche Tierarztliche Wochenschrift** 1996; 103(10): 390–394.

CA009 Boekema, P. J., M. Samsom, G. P. van Berge Henegouven,, and A. J. Smout. Coffee, and gastrointestinal function: facts, and fiction. A review. **Scand J Gastroenterol Suppl** 1999; 230: 35–39.

CA010 Ratnayake, W. M., G. Pelletier, R. Hollywood, S. Malcolm, and B. Stavric. Investigations of the effect of coffee lipids on serum cholesterol in hamsers. **Food Chem Toxicol** 1995; 33(3): 195–201.

CA011 Albertini, S., U. Friederich, C. Schlatter, and F. E. Wurgler. The influence of roasting procedure on the formation of mutagenic compounds in coffee. **Food Chem Toxicol** 1985; 23(6): 593–597.

CA012 Terry, P., J. Lagergren, A. Wolk, and O. Nyren. Reflux-inducing dietary factors, and risk of adenocarcinoma of the esophagus, and gastric cardia. **Nutr Cancer** 2000; 38(2): 186–191.

CA013 Zuskin, E., J. Mustajbegovic, E. N. Schachter, J. Kern, D. Ivankovic, and S. Heimer. Respiratory function in female workers occupationally exposed to organic dusts in food processing industries. **Acta Med Croat** 2000; 54(4–5): 183–191.

CA014 Medra, S. M., E. A. Janowska, and E. Rogucka. The effect of smoking tobacco, and drinking of alcohol, and coffee on bone mineral density of healthy men 40 years of age. **Polskie Archiwum Medycyny Wewnetrznej** 2000; 103(3–4): 187–193.

CA015 Garsetti, M., N. Pellegrini, C. Baggio, and F. Brighenti. Antioxidant activity in human faeces. **Br J Nutr** 2000; 84(5): 705–710.

CA016 Tanskanene, A., J. Tuomilehto, H. Viinamaki, E. Vartiainen, J. Lehtonen, and P. Puska. Joint heavy use of alcohol, cigarettes, and coffee, and the risk of suicide. **Addiction** 2000; 95(11): 1699–1704.

CA017 Mori, H., K. Kawabata, K. Matsunaga, et al. Chemopreventive effects of coffee bean, and rice constituents on colorectal carcinogenesis. **Biofactors** 2000; 12(1–4): 101–105.

CA018 Sala, M., S. Cordier, J. Chang-Claude, et al. Coffee consumption, and bladder cancer in nonsmokers: a poled analysis of case-control studies in European countries. **Cancer Causes Control** 2000; 11(10): 925–931.

CA019 Kash, K. M., J. C. Holland, W. Breitbart, et al. Stress, and burnout in oncology. **Oncology (Huntington)** 2000; 14(11): 1621–1633.

CA020 Torfs, C. P. and R. E. Christianson. Effect of maternal smoking, and coffee consumption on the risk of having a recognized Down syndrome pregnancy. **Am J Epidem** 2000; 152(12): 1185–1191.

CA021 Cnatingius, S., L. B. Signorello, G. Anneren, et al. Caffeine intake and the risk of first-trimester spontaneous abortion. **N Engl J Med** 2000; 343(25): 1839–1845.

CA022 Ruhl, C. E., and J. E. Everhart. Association of coffee consumption with gallbladder disease. **Am J Epidemiol** 2000; 152(11): 1034–1038.

CA023 Kleemola, P., P. Jousilahti, P. Pietinen, E. Vartiainen, and J. Tuomilehto. Coffee consumption and the risk of coronary heart disease, and death. **Arch Intern Med** 2000; 160(22): 3393–3400.

CA024 Benedetti, M. D., J. H. Bower, D. M. Maraganore, S. K. MacDonnell, B. J. Peterson, J. E. Ahlskog, D. J. Schaid, and W. A. Rocca. Smoking, alcohol, and coffee consumption preceding Parkinson's disease: a case-control study. **Neurology** 2000; 55(9): 1350–1358.

CA025 Conlisk, A. J., and D. A. Galuska. Is caffeine associated with bone mineral density in young adult women? **Prevent Med** 2000; 31(5): 562–568.

CA026 Rasmussen, L. B., L. Ovesen, I. Bulow, N. Knudsen, P. Laurberg, and H. Perrild. Folate intake, lifestyle factors, and homocysteine concentrations in younger, and older women. **Am J Clin Nutr** 2000; 72(5): 1156–1163.

CA027 Urgert, R., T. van Vliet, P. L. Zock, and M. B. Katan. Heavy coffee consumption, and plasma homocysteine: a randomised controlled trial in healthy volunteers. **Am J Clin Nutr** 2000; 72(5): 1107–1110.

CA028 Frentzel-Beyme, R. and U. Helmert. Association between malignant tumors of the thyroid gland and exposure to environmental protectiveand risk factors. **Rev Environm Health** 2000; 15(3): 337–358.

CA029 Kuper, H., L. Titus-Ernstoff, B. L. Harlow, and D. W. Cramer. Population based study of coffee, alcohol and tobacco use and risk of ovarian cancer. **Int J Canc** 2000; 88(2): 313–318.

CA030 Nakanishi, N., K. Nakamura, K. Nakajima, K. Suzuki, and K. Tatara. Coffee consumption and decreased serum gamma-glutamyltransferase: a study of middle–aged Japanese men. **Eur J Epidemiol** 2000; 16(5): 419–423.

CA031 Carillo, J. A. and J. Benitez. Clinically significant pharmacokinetic interactions between dietary caffeine and medications. **Clin Pharmacokinetics** 2000; 39(2): 127–153.

CA032 De Roos, B., A. Van Tol, R. Urgenr, et al. Consumption of French-press coffee raises cholesteryl ester transfer protein activity levels before LDL cholesterol in normolipidemic subjects. **J Intern Med** 2000; 248(3): 211–216.

CA033 Grubben, M. J., C. C. Van Den Braak, R. Broekhuizen, et al. The effect of unfiltered coffee on potential biomarkers for colonic cancer risk in healthy volunteers: a randomized trial. **Alim Pharm Therap** 2000; 14(9): 1181–1190.

CA034 Heliovaara, M., K. Alio, P. Knekt, O. Impivaara, A. Reunanen, and A. Aromaa. Coffee consumption, rheumatoid factor and the risk of rheumatoid arthritis. **Ann Rheum Dis** 2000; 59(8): 631–635.

CA035 Quinlan, P. T., J. Lane, K. L. Moore, J. Aspen, J. A. Rycroft, and D. C. O'Brien. The acute physiological and mood effects of tea and coffee: the role of caffeine level. **Pharm Biochem Behav** 2000; 66(1): 19–28.

CA036 Hindmarch, I., U. Rigney, N. Stanley, P. Quinlan, J. Rycroft, and J. Lane. A naturalistic investigation of the effects of day-long consumption of tea, coffee and water on alertness, sleep onset and sleep quality. **Psychopharmacology** 2000; 149(3): 203–216.

CA037 Ross, G. W., R. D. Abbott, H. Petrovitch, et al. Association of coffee and caffeine intake with the risk of Parkinson disease. **JAMA** 2000; 283(20): 2674–2679.

CA038 Koren, G. Caffeine during pregnancy? In moderation. **Can Family Phys** 2000; 46(4): 801–803

CA039 Villneuve, P. J., K. C. Johnson, A. J. Hanley, and Y. Mao. Alcohol, tobacco and coffee consumption and the risk of pancreatic cancer: results from Canadian Enhanced Surveillance System case-control project. Canadian Cancer Registries Epidemiology Research Group. **Eur J Cancer Prev** 2000; 9(1): 49–58.

CA040 Long, L. H. and B. Halliwell. Coffee drinking increases levels of urinary hydrogen peroxide detected in healthy human volunteers. **Free Radical Res** 2000; 32(5): 463–467.

CA041 Nakanishi, N., K. Nakamura, K. Suzuki, and K. Tatara. Effects of coffee consumption against the development of liver dysfunction: a 4-year follow up study of middle-aged Japanese male office workers. **Industrial Health** 2000; 38(1): 99–102.

CA042 Perod, A. L., A. E. Roberts, and W. M. McKinney. Caffeine can affect velocity in the middle cerebral artery during hyperventilation, hypoventilation,, and thinking: a transcranial Doppler study. **J Neuroimaging** 2000; 10(1): 33–38.

CA043 Liguori, A., J. A. Grass, and J. R. Hughes. Subjective effects of caffeine among introverts and extraverts in the morning and evening. **Exp Clin Psychopharmacol** 1999; 7(3): 244–249.

CA044 Smith, A. P., R. Clark, and J. Gallagher. Breakfast cereal and caffeinated coffee: effects on working memory, attention, mood and cardiovascular function. **Phys Behav** 1000; 67(1): 9–17.

CA045 Leitzmann, M. F., W. C. Willett, E. B. Rimm, et al. A prospective study of coffee consumption, and the risk of symptomatic gallstone disease in men. **JAMA** 1999; 281(22): 2106–2112.

CA046 Eskenazi, B., A. L. Stapleton, M. Kharazzi, and W. Y. Chee. Association between maternal decaffeinated and caffeinated coffee consumption and fetal growth and gestational duration. **Epidemiology** 1999; 10(3): 242–240.

CA047 Rakic, V., V. Burke and L. J. Beilin. Effects of coffee on ambulatory blood pressure in older men and women: a randomized controlled trial. **Hypertension** 1999; 33(3): 869–893.

CA048 Stolzenberg-Solomon, R. Z., E. R. Miller 3rd, M. G. Maguire, J. Selhub, and L. J. Appel. Association of dietary protein intake and coffee consumption with serum homocysteine concentrations in an older population. **Am J Clin Nutr** 1999; 69(3): 467–475.

CA049 Miyake, Y., S. Kono, M. Nishiwaki, et al. Relationship of coffee consumption with serum lipids and lipoproteinds in Japanese men. **Ann Epidemiol** 1999; 9(2): 121–126.

CA050 Jee, S. H., P. K. Whelton, I. Suh, and M. J. Klag. The effect of chronic coffee drinking on blood pressure: a meta-analysis of controlled clinical trials. **Hypertension** 1999; 33(2): 647–652.

CA051 Dager, S. R., M. E. Layton, W. Strauss, et al. Human brain metabolic response to caffeine and the effects of tolerance. **Am J Psychiatry** 1999; 156(2): 229–237.

CA052 Kendler, K. S. and C. A. Prescott. Caffeine intake, tolerance, and withdrawal in women: a population-based twin study. **Am J Psychiatry** 1999; 156(2): 223–228.

CA053 Sesso, H. D., J. M. Gaziano, J. E. Buring, and C. H. Hennekens. Coffee and tea intake and the risk of myocardial infarction. **Am J Epidemiol** 1999; 149(2): 162–167.

CA054   Honjo, S., S. Kono, M. P. Coleman, et al. Coffee drinking and serum gamma-glutamyltransferase: an extended study of Self-Defence Officials of Japan. **Ann Epidemiol** 1999; 9(5): 325–331.

CA055   Mazurek, W. and M. Negrusz-Kawecka. Effect of coffee on blood pressure and activity rennin-angiotensin-aldosterone system and catecholamines concentration in patients with essential hypertension. **Polski Merkuriusz Lekarski** 1999; 7(40): 159–163.

CA056   Luo, Y., J. Wen, C. Luo, R. D. Cummings, and D. K. Cooper. Pig xenogeneic antigen modification with green coffee bean alpha-galactosidase. **Xenotransplantation** 1999; 6(4): 238–248.

CA057   Porta, M., N. Malats, L. Guarner, et al. Association between coffee drinking and K-ras mutations in exocrine pancreatic cancer. PANKRAS II Study Group. **J Epidemiol Comm Health** 1999; 53(11): 702–709.

CA058   Woodward, M., and H. Tunstall-Pedoe. Coffee and tea consumption in the Scottish Heart Health Study follow up: conflicting relations with coronary risk factors, coronary disease, and all cause mortality. **J Epidemiol Comm Health** 1999; 53(8): 481–487.

CA059   De Roos, B., S. Meyboom, T. G. Kosmeijer-Schiul, and M. B. Katan. Absorption and urinary excretion of the coffee diterpenes cafestol and kahweol in healthy ileostomy volunteers. **J Intern Med** 1998; 244(6): 451–460.

CA060   Fujii, W, M. Takaki, A. Yoshida, H. Ishidate, H. Ito, and H. Suga. Effects of intracoronary caffeine on left ventricular mechanoenergetics in Ca^{2+} overload failing rat hearts. **Japanese J Phys** 1998; 48(5): 373–381.

CA061   Larese, F., A. Fiorito, F. Casasola, et al. Sensitization to green coffee beans, and work-related allergic symptoms in coffee workers. **Am J Indust Med** 1998; 34(6): 623–627.

CA062   Hauptmann, H., and J. Franca. Cafesterol. II. **J Amer Chem Soc** 1943; 65: 81.

CA063   Stoffelsma, J., G. Sipma, D. K. Kettenes, and J. Pypker. New volatile components of roasted coffee. **J Agr Food Chem** 1968; 16(6): 1000.

CA064   Sondheimer, E. On the distribution of caffeic acid and the chlorogenic acid isomers in plants. **Arch Biochem Biophys** 1958; 74: 131–138.

CA065   Pettitt Jr, B. C. Identification of the diterpene esters in *arabica* and *canephora* coffees. **J Agr Food Chem** 1987; 35(4): 549–551.

CA066   Speer, K. 16-O-methylcafestrol, a new diterpene in coffee. Food Chem Consum Proc Eur Conf Food Chem 5th 1989; 1989(1): 302–306.

CA067   Obermann, H. and G. Spiteller. 16,17-dihydroxy-9-kauren-18-oic acid. A compound of roasted coffee. **Chem Ber** 1975; 108: 1093.

CA068   Haggag, M. Y. A study of the lipid content of *Coffea arabica* seeds. **Pharmazie** 1975; 30: 409.

CA069   Vitzthum, O. G. and P. Werkhoff. Cycloalkapyrazines in coffee aroma. **J Agr Food Chem** 1975; 23(3): 510.

CA070   Wahlberg, I., C. R. Enzell, and J. W. Rowe. Ent-16-kauren-19-ol from coffee. **Phytochemistry** 1975; 14: 1677.

CA071   Correa, J. B. C., S. Adebrecht, and J. D. Fontana. Polysaccharides from the epicarp and mesocarp of coffee beans. II. Fractionation and partial acid hydrolysis of water-soluble pectin. **An Acad Brasil Cienc** 1974; 46: 349.

CA072   Molina, M. R., G. De La Fuente, M. A. Batten, and R. Bressani. Decaffeination. A process to detoxify coffee pulp. **J Agr Food Chem** 1974; 22(6): 1055.

CA073   Correa, J. B. C., E. O. Coelho, and J. D. Fontana. Polysaccharide from the epicarp and the mesocarp of coffee beans. III. Structural features of pectic acid. **An Acad Brasil Cienc** 1974; 46: 357.

CA074   Buegin, E. Lowering the carboxylic acid-5-hydroxy-tryptamide content of unroasted coffee beans. Patent-Ger Offen-2,429,233 1975.

CA075   Vitzthum, O. G. and P. Werkhoff. Oxazoles and thiazoles in coffee aroma. **J Food Sci** 1974; 39: 1210.

CA076   Vitzthum, O. G. and P. Werkhoff. Newly discovered nitrogen-containing heterocycles in coffee aroma. **Z Lebensm-Unters Forsch** 1974; 156: 300.

CA077 Higuchi, K., T. Suzuki, and H. Ashihara. Pipecolic acid from the developing fruits (pericarp and seeds) of *Coffea arabica* and *Camellia sinensis*. **Colloq Sci Int Café [C.R.]** 1995; 16: 389–395.

CA078 Andrade, P. B., R. Leitao, R. M. Seabra, M. B. Oliveira, and M. A. Ferreira. Development of an HPLC/diode-array detector method for simultaneous determination of seven hydroxyl-cinnamic acids in green coffee. **J Liq Chrom Rel Technol** 1997; 20(13): 2023–2030.

CA079 Kolling-Speer, I. and K. Speer. Diterpenes in coffee leaves. **Colloq Sci Int Café 1997; 17(15): 1–154.**

CA080 Hiramoto, K., X. G. Li, M. Makimoto, T. Kato, and K. Kikugawa. Identification of hydroxyhydroquinone in coffee as a generator of reactive oxygen species that break DNA single strands. **Mutat Res** 1998; 419(1/2/3): 43–51.

CA081 Spiro, M. Coffee, tea and chemistry. **Chem Rev** 1997; 6(5): 11–15.

CA082 Vitzthum, O. G. and P. Werkhoff. Steam volatile aroma constituents of roasted coffee-neutral fraction. **Z Lebensm-Unters Forsch** 1976; 160: 277.

CA083 Obermann, H. and G. Spiteller. The structures of the "coffee atractylosides". **Chem Ber** 1976; 109: 3450.

CA084 Gal, S. and E. Jenny. Extraction of the irritating substances from crude coffee. Patent-Swiss-568,719 1975.

CA085 Barboza, C. A., and J. R. Ramirez-Martinez. Anthocyanins in pulp of the coffee cultivar Bourbon Rojo. **Colloq Sci Int Café [C.R.]** 1992; 14: 272–276.

CA086 Waller, G. R., M. Jurzyste, T. K. B. Karns, and P. W. Geno. Isolation and characterization of ursolic acid from *Coffea arabica* L. (coffee) leaves. **Colloq Sci Int Café [C.R.]** 1991; 14: 245–247.

CA087 Stalcup, A. M., K. H. Ekborg, M. P. Gasper, and D. W. Armstron. Enantiomeric separation of chiral components reported to be in coffee, tea or cocoa. **J Agr Food Chem** 1993; 41(10): 1684–1689.

CA088 Koge, K., Y. Orihara, and T. Furuya. Caffeine production by polyurethane foam-immobilized coffee (*Coffea arabica* L.) cells. **Biochem Eng 2001 Proc Asia Pac Biochem Eng Conf** 1992; 299–301.

CA089 Tsuji, S., T. Shibata, K. Ohara, N. Okada, and Y. Ito. Factors affecting the formation of hydrogen peroxide in coffee. **Shokuhin Eiseigaku Zasshi** 1991; 32(6): 504–512.

CA090 Correia, A. M. N. G. Effect of roasting on the evolution of chlorogenic acids in coffee. **Gov Rep Announce Index (US)** 1991; 91(19): 309 pp.

CA091 Savolainen, H. Tannin content of tea, and coffee. **J Appl Toxicol** 1992; 12(3): 191–192.

CA092 Schulthess, B. H., P. Ruedi, and T. W. Baumann. 7-glucosyladenine, a new adenine metabolite in coffee cell suspension cultures. **Colloq Sci Int Café [C. R.]** 1993; 15(2): 770–772.

CA093 Hertog, M. G. L., P. C. H. Hollman, and B. Van Der Putte. Content of potentially anticarcinogenic flavonoids of tea infusions, wines, and fruit juices. **J Agr Food Chem** 1993; 41(8): 1242–1246.

CA094 Miyake, T. and T. Shibamoto. Quantitative analysis of acetaldehyde in foods and beverages. **J Agr Food Chem** 1994; 41(11): 1968–1970.

CA095 Nishina, A., F. Kajishima, M. Matsunaga, H. Tezuka, H. Inatomi, and T. Osawa. Antimicrobial substance, 3',4'-dihydroxyacetophenone, in coffee residue. **Biosci Biotech Biochem** 1994; 58(2): 293–296.

CA096 Deisinger, P. J., T. S. Hills, and J. C. English. Human exposure to naturally occurring hydroquinone. **J Toxicol Environ Health** 1996; 47(1): 31–46.

CA097 Ducruix, A., C. Pascard, M. Hammoniere, and J. Poisson. The crystal and molecular structure of mascaroside, a new bitter glycoside from coffee beans. **Acta Crystallogr Ser B** 1977; 33: 2846.

CA098 Richter, R., H. Obermann, and G. Spiteller. A new kauran-18-oic acid ester from green coffee beans. **Chem Ber 1977; 110: 1963.**

CA099 Frischknecht, P. M., T. W. Baumann, and H. Wanner. Tissue culture of *Coffea arabica*-growthand caffeine formation. Planta Med 1977; 31: 344.

CA100 Gonzalez, J., R. Noriega, and R. Sandoval. Contribution to the study of flavonoids of coffee tree (*Coffea*) leaves. **Rev Colomb Quim** 1975; 5: 85.

CA101 Tohda, C., N. Nakamura, K. Komatsu, and M. Hattori. Trigonelline-induced neurite outgrowth in human neuroblastoma SK-N-SH cells. **Biol Pharm Bull** 1999; 22(7): 679–682.

CA102 Tillack, B. and H. G. Maier. Reducing agents in roasted coffee. **Lebensmittelchemie** 1999; 53(6): 159–160.

CA103 Huang, C. T., C. F. Chen, and T. H. Tsai. Determination of the caffeine content in the tea and coffee. **J Chin Med** 1999; 10(2): 135–141.

CA104 Trugo, L. C. and R. Macrae. Chlorogenic acid composition of instant coffees. **Analyst (London)** 1984; 109(3): 263–266.

CA105 Scholze, A. and H. G. Maier. Acids of coffee. VIII. Glycolic and phosphoric acid. **Z Lebensm-Unters Forsch** 1984; 178(1): 5–8.

CA106 Engelhardt, U., K. Peters, and H. G. Maier. Pyroglutamic acid in bean coffee. **Z Lebensm-Unters Forsch** 1984; 178(4): 288.

CA107 Duplatre, A., C. Tisse, and J. Estienne. Identification of Arabica and Robusta (coffee) species by studying the sterol fraction. **Ann Falsif Expert Chim Toxicol** 1984; 77(828): 259–270.

CA108 Frischknecht, P. M. and T. W. Baumann. Stress induced formation of purine alkaloids in plant tissue culture of *Coffea arabica*. **Phytochemistry** 1985; 24(10): 2255–2257.

CA109 Hucke, J., and H. G. Maier. Quinic acid lactone in coffee. **Z Lebensm-Unters Forsch** 1985; 180(6): 479–484.

CA110 Lam, L. K. T. and L. W. Wattenberg. Preparation of the palmitates of kahweol and cafestrol. **Org Prep Proc Int** 1985; 17(4/5): 264–267.

CA111 Suzuki, T. and G. R. Waller. Purine alkaloids of the fruits of *Camellia sinensis* L. and *Coffea arabica* L. during fruit development. **Ann Bot (London)** 1985; 56(4): 537–542.

CA112 Okuda, T., T. Hatano, I. Agata, S. Nishibe, and K. Kimura. Tannins in *Artemisia montana*, *A. princeps*, and

CA113 Kappeler, A. W., and T. W. Baumann. Purine alkaloid pattern in coffee beans. **Colloq Sci Int Café [C.R.]** 1985; 11: 273–279.

CA114 Trugo, L. C., C. A. B. de Maria, and C. C. Werneck. Simultaneous determination of total chlorogenic acid and caffeine in coffee by high performance gel filtration chromatography. **Food Chem** 1991; 42(1): 81–87.

CA115 Baumann, T. W., T. W. Koetz, and R. Morah. N-methyltransferase activities in suspension cultures of *Coffea arabica*. **Plant Cell Rep** 1983; 2(1): 33–35.

CA116 Richter, H. and G. Spiteller. A new atractyligenin glycoside from green coffee beans. **Chem Ber** 1978; 111: 3506.

CA117 Maier, H. G. and H. Wewetzer. Determination of diterpene glycosides in coffee. **Z Lebensm-Unters Forsch** 1978; 167: 105.

CA118 Richter, H. and G. Spiteller. A new furokaurane glycoside from green coffee-bean. **Chem Ber 1979; 112: 1088.**

CA119 Waller, G. R. and M. F. Roberts. N-methyltransferases and 7-methyl-N-nucleoside hydrolase activity *in vitro* of *Coffea arabica* fruits, and the biosynthesis of caffeine:, and the *in vivo* metabolism of caffeine. **Proc IUPAC 11th International Symp Chem Nat Prod** 1978; 4(2): 55–71.

CA120 Folstar, P., F. A. Schols, H. C. Van Der Plas, W. Pilnik, C. A. Landheer, and A. Van Veldhuizen. New tryptamine derivatives isolated from wax of green coffee beans. **J Agr Food Chem 1980; 28(4): 872–874.**

CA121 Waller, G. R. and C. F. Cumberland. High production of caffeine by sterile tissue cultures of *Coffea arabica*. **Colloq Sci Int Café [C.R.]** 1980; 9: 611–618.

CA122 Koenig, W. A., W. Rahn, and R. Vetter. Identify and quantify emetic active constituents in roast coffee. **Colloq Sci Int Café [C.R.]** 1980; 9: 145–149.

CA123 Waller, G. R., T. Suzuki, and M. F. Roberts. Cell-free metabolism of caffeine in *Coffea arabica*. **Colloq Sci Int Café [C.R.]** 1980; 9: 627–635.

CA124 Hirsbrunner, P. and R. Bertholet. Saponification treatment of spent coffee grounds. Patent-US-4,293,581 1981.

CA125 Kampmann, B and H. G. Maier. Acids of coffee. I. Quinic acid. Z Lebensm-Unters Forsch 1982; 175(5): 333–336.

CA126 Aeschach, R., A. Kusy, and H. G. Maier. Diterpenes of coffee. I. Atactyligenin. **Z Lebensm-Unters Forsch** 1982; 175(5): 337–341.

CA127 Walkowski, A. and W. Meissner. Changes in the content of chlorogenic acids in row coffee beans during accelerated aging. **Zesz Nauk Akad Ekon Poznaniu Ser** 1981; 1(88): 94–97.

CA128 Atal, C. K., J. B. Srivasava, B. K. Wali, R. B. Chakravarty, B. N. Bhawan, and R. P. Rastogi. Screening of Indian plants for biological activity. Part VIII. **Indian J Exp Biol** 1978; 16: 330–349.

CA129 Neurath, G. B., M. Dunger, F. G. Pein, D. Ambrosius, and O. Schreiber. Primary and secondary amines in the human environment. **Food Cosmet Toxicol** 1977; 15: 275–282.

CA130 Pezzuto, J. M., N. P. D. Nanayakkara, C. M. Compadre, et al. Characterization of bacterial mutagenicity mediated by 13-hydroxy-ent-kaurenoic acid (steviol) and several structurally related derivatives and evaluation of potential to induce glutathione-S-transferase in mice. **Mutat Res** 1986; 169: 93–103.

CA131 Kasai, H., K. Kumeno, Z. Yamaizumi, et al. Mutagenicity of methylgyoxal in coffee. **Jap J Cancer Res (Gann)** 1982; 73: 681–683.

CA132 Wettsten, A., H. Fritzsche, F. Hunziker, and K. Miescher. Steroids. XXXII. The constitution of cafesterol. **Helv Chim Acta** 1941; 24: 332E.

CA133 De Paula, R. D. Investigation of coffee oil. **Anais Assoc Brasil Quim** 1943; 2: 57.

CA134 Shiroya, M. and S. Hattori. Studies on the browning and blackening of plant tissues. III. Occurrence in the leaves of *Dahlia* and several other plants of chlorogenic acid as the principal browning agent. **Physiol Plant** 1955; 8: 358–369.

CA135 Hoffman, E., D. Schlee, and H. Reinbothe. On the occurrence and dis-

tribution of allantoin in *Boraginaceae*. **Flora Abt A Physiol Biochem (Jena)** 1969; 159: 510–518.

CA136 Slotta, K. H. and K. Neisser. On the chemistry of coffee. III. Determination of cafesterol and other compounds in coffee oil. **Ber Deutsch Hem Ges** 1938; 71: 19991–1994.

CA137 Vincent, D., G. Segonzae, and R. Issandou-Carles. Action of purine alkaloids and caffeine-containing drugs on hyauronidase. **C R Seances Soc Biol Ses Fil** 1954; 148: 1075.

CA138 Hauptmann, H, J. Franca, and L. Bruck-Lacerda. Cafestol. III. The supposed estrogenic activity of cafestrol. **J Amer Chem Soc** 1943; 65: 993.

CA139 Bhakuni, D. S., M. L. Dhar, M. M. Dhar, B. N. Dhawan, B. Gupta, and R. . Srimali. Screening of Indian plants for biological activity. **Part III. Indian J Exp Biol** 1971; 9: 91.

CA140 Stensvold, I., A. Tverdal, and B. K. Jacobsen. Cohort study of coffee intake and death from coronary heart disease over 12 years. **Br Med J** 1996; 544–545.

CA141 Koley, J., B. N. Coley, and S. R.Maitra. Effect of drinking tea, coffee and caffeine on work performance. **Indian J Physiol Allied Sci** 1973; 27: 96.

CA142 Keiser, I., E. J. Harris, D. H. Miyashita, M. Jacobson, and R. E. Perdue. Attraction of ethyl ether extracts of 232 botanicals to oriental fruit flies, melon flies, and Mediterranean fruit flies. **Loydia** 1975; 38(2): 141–152.

CA143 Schwaireb, M. H., M. M. El-Mofty, A. M. Rizk, A. M. Abdel-Galil, and H. H. Hrasani. Effects of green coffee and green tea on induce mammary gland tumorigenesis in rats. **J Herbs Spices Med Plants** 1995; 3(4): 59–69.

CA144 Urgert, R., M. P. M. E. W. Van Der Wouw, R. Hovenier, P. G. Lund-Larsen, and M. B. Katan. Chronic consumers of boiled coffee have elevated serum levels of lipoprotein (A). **J Intern Med** 1996; 240(6): 367–371.

CA145 Abraham, S. K. Anti-genotoxic effects in mice after the interaction between coffee and dietary constituents. **Food Chem Toxicol** 1996; 3(1): 15–20.

CA146 Urgert, R., M. P. M. E. Weusten-Van Der Wouw, R. Hovenier, S. Meyboom,

A. C. Beynen, and M. B. Catan. Diterpenes from coffee beans decrease serum levels of lipoprotein (A) in humans: results from four randomized controlled trials. **Eur J Clin Nutr** 1997; 51(7): 431–436.

CA147 Tavani, A., A. Pregnolato, C. La Vecchia, E. Negri, R. Talamini, and S. Franceschi. Coffee and tea intake and risk of cancers of the colon and rectum: a study of 3,530 cases and 7,057 controls. **Int J Cancer** 1997; 73(2): 193–197.

CA148 Kobayashi, T., M. Yasuda, K. Iijima, K. Toriizuka, J. C. Cyong, and H. Nagasawa. Effect of coffee cherry on the activation of splenic lymphocytes in mice. **Anticancer Res** 1997; 17(2A): 913–916.

CA149 Nagata, C., M. Kabuto, and H. Shimizu. Association of coffee, green tea,, and caffeine intakes with serum concentrations of estradiol and sex hormone-binding globulin in premenopausal Japanese women. **Nutr Cancer** 1998; 30(1): 21–24.

CA150 Burr, M. L., E. S. Limb, P. M. Sweetnam, A. M. Fehily, L. Amarah, and A. Hutchings. Instant coffee, and cholesterol: a randomized controlled trial. **Eur J Clin Nutr** 1995; 49(10): 779–784.

CA151 Myazaki, H. and T. Yamada. Skin cosmetics containing coffee bean extracts. Patent-Japan Kokai Tokkyo Koho-08 301,722 1996.

CA152 Wiliams, M. A., R. R. Monson, M. B. Goldman, and R. Mittendorf. Coffee and delayed conception. **Lancet** 1990; 335(8705): 1603.

CA153 Glauser, T., A. Bircher, and B. Wuthrich. Allergic rhinoconjunctivis by handling green coffee beans. **Schweiz Med Wochenschr** 1992; 122(35): 1279–1281.

CA154 Lina, B. A., A. A. Rutten, , and R. A. Woutersen. Effect of coffee drinking on cell proliferation in rat urinary bladder epithelium. **Food Chem Toxicol** 1993; 31(12): 947–951.

CA155 Tse, S. Y. H. Coffee contains cholinomimetic compound distinct from caffeine. I: purification and chromatographic analysis. **J Pharm Sci** 1991; 80(7): 665–669.

CA156 Anon. Coffee, tea, and mate. **Lancet** 1991; 338(8769): 752.

CA157 Anon. Regular or decaf/ Coffee consumption and serum lipoproteins. **Nutr Rev** 1992; 50(6): 175–178.

CA158 Hasegawa, R. and N. Ito. Liver medium-term bioassay in rats for screening of carcinogens and modifying factors in hepatocarcingenesis. **Food Chem Toxicol** 1992; 30(11): 979–992.

CA159 Zuskin, E., P. G. Duncan, and J. S. Douglas. Pharmacological characterization of extracts of coffee dusts. **Br J Int Med** 1983; 40: 193–198.

CA160 Sanders, T. A. B., and S. Sandaradura. The cholesterol-raising effect of coffee in the Syrian hamster. **Biol Reprod** 1992; 68(2): 431–434.

CA161 Ahola, I., M. Jauhiainen, and A. Aro. The hypercholesterolemic factor in boiled coffee is retained by a paper filter. **J Intern Med** 1991; 230(4): 293–297.

CA162 Lindahl, B., I. Johansson, F. Huhtasaari, G Hallmanns, and K. Asplund. Coffee drinking and blood cholesterol. Effects of brewing method, food intake and life style. **J Internal Med** 1991; 230(4): 299–305.

CA163 El Shabrawy, M., and F. M. Felimban. A study of the impact of Arabic coffee consumption on serum cholesterol. **J Roy Soc J Health** 1993; 113(6): 288–291.

CA164 Van Den Brink, G., J. E. Brinkman, Y. L. Kan, H. S. Lau, and S. J. Troost. Influence of caffeine from coffee on heart rate and blood pressure of pharmacy students. **Pharm Week Bull** 1992; 127(12): 308–310.

CA165 Aeschbachter, H. L. and H. P. Wurzner. An evaluation of instant and regular coffee in the Ames mutagenicity test. **Toxicol Lett** 1979; 5: 139–145.

CA166 Kato, T., K. Hiramoto, and K. Kikugawa. Possible occurrence of new mutagens with the DNA breaking activity in coffee. **Mutat Res** 1994; 306(1): 9–17.

CA167 Mehta, S. W., M. E. Pritchard, and C. Stegman. Contribution of coffee and tea to anemia among NANNES. II.

Participants. **Nutr Res** 1992; 12(2): 209–222.

CA168   Zamora-Martinez, M. C., and C. N. P. Pola. Medicinal plants used in some rural populations of Oaxaca, Puebla and Veracuz, Mexico. **J Ethnopharmacol** 1992; 35(3): 229–257.

CA169   Stadler, R. H., R. J. Turesky, O. Muller, J. Markovic, and P. M. Leong-Morgenthaler. The inhibitory effects of coffee on radical-mediated oxidation and mutagenicity. **Mutat Res** 1994; 308(2): 177–190.

CA170   Gershbein, L. L. Action of dietary trypsin, pressed coffee oil, silymarin and iron salt on 1,2-dimethylhydrazine tumorigenesis by gavage. **Anticancer Res** 1994; 14(3A): 1113–1116.

CA171   Schroeder, E. Preliminary study of Chinese anticancer drugs. **An Paul Med Cir** 1978; 105(1): 67–94.

CA172   Urgert, R., A. G. M. Schulz, and M. B. Katan. Effects of cafestol and kahweol from coffee grounds on serum lipids and serum lipids and serum liver enzymes in humans. **Am J Clin Nutr** 1995; 61(1): 149–154.

CA173   Miller, E. G., A. P. Gonzales-Sanders, A. M. Couvillon, et al. Inhibition of oral carcinogenesis by green coffee beans and limonoid glucosides. **ACS Symp Ser** 1994; 546: 220–229.

CA174   Ratnayake, W. M. N., and G. Pelletier. Investigation of the effect of coffee lipids on serum cholesterol in hamsters. **Food Chem Toxicol** 1995; 33(3): 195–201.

CA175   Nagasawa, H., M. Yasuda, S. Sakamoto, and H. Inatomi. Protection by coffee cherry against spontaneous mammary tumor development in mice. **Anticancer Res** 1995; 15(1): 141–146.

CA176   Hasegawa, R., T. Ogiso, K. Imaida, T. Shirai, and N. Ito. Analysis of the potential carcinogenicity of coffee and its related compounds in a medium-term liver bioassay of rats. **Food Chem Toxicol** 1995; 33(1): 15–20.

CA177   Brin, A. J. and N. Goutelard. Cosmetic or pharmaceutical composition for topical application active free radicals. Patent-Eur. Pat. Appl.-629,397 1994; 16 pp.

CA178   Daglia, M., M. T. Cuzzoni, and C. Dacarro. Anibacterial activity of coffee. **J Agr Food Chem** 1994; 42(10): 2270–2272.

CA179   Willett, W. C., M. J. Stampfer, J. E. Manson, et al. Coffee consumption and coronary heart disease in women. **J Am Med Ass** 1996; 275(6): 458–462.

CA180   Nagasawa, H., M. Yasuda, S. Sakamoto, and H. Inatomi. Suppression in coffee cherry of the growth of spontaneous mammary tumors in SHN mice. **Anticancer Res** 1996; 16(1): 151–153.

CA181   Barrett, B. Medicinal plants of Nicaragua's Atlantic coast. **Econ Bot** 1994; 48(1): 8–20.

CA182   Abraham, S. K. Inhibitory effects of coffee on transplacental genotoxicity in mice. **Mutat Res** 1995; 347(1): 45–52.

CA183   Stehmann, J. R. and M. G. L. Brandao. Medicinal plants of Lavras Novas (Minas Gerais, Brazil). Fitoterapia 1995; 56(6): 515–520.

CA184   Coee, F. G. and G. J. Anderson. Ethnobotany of the Garifuna of eastern Nicaragua. **Econ Bot** 1996; 50(1): 71–107.

CA185   Abraham, S. K. and U. Graf. Protection by coffee against somatic genotoxicity in *Drosophila*: role of bioactivation capacity. **Food Chem Toxicol** 1996; 34(1): 1–14.

CA186   Kobayashi, T., M. Yasuda, K. Iijima, K. Toriizuka, J. C. Cyong, and H. Nagasawa. Effects of coffee cherry on the immune system in SHN mice. Anticancer Res 1996; 16(4A): 1827–1830.

CA187   Beynen, A. C., M. P. M. E. Van Der Wouw, B. De Roos, and M. B. Katan. Boiled coffee fails to raise serum cholesterol in hamsters and rats. **Br J Nutr** 1996; 76(5): 755–764.

CA188   Badria, F. A. Is man helpless against cancer? An environmental approach: antimutagenic agents from Egyptian food, and medicinal preparations. **Cancer Lett** 1994; 84(1): 1–5.

CA189   Baron, J. A., E. R. Greenberg, R. Haile, J. Mandel, R. S. Sandler, and L. Mott. Coffee and tea and the risk of recurrent colorectal adenomas. **Cancer Epidemiol Biomark Prevent** 1997; 6(1): 7–10.

CA190   Nhgard, O., H. Refsum, P. M. Ueland, et al. Coffee consumption and plasma total homocysteine: the hordaland and homocysteine study. **Am J Clin Nutr** 1997; 65(1): 136–143.

CA191 Abraham, S. K. Anti-enotoxic effects in mice after the interaction between coffee and dietary constituents. **Food Chem Toxicol** 1996; 34(1): 15–20.

CA192 Rakic, V., L. J. Beilin, and V. Burke. Effect of coffee and tea drinking on postprandial hypotension in older men and women. **Clin Exp Pharmacol Physiol** 1996; 23(6–7): 559–563.

CA193 Nishibe, Y., N. Tomono, H. Hirasawa, and T. Okada. Skin-lightening cosmetics containing extracts of *Coffea arabica* seeds. Patent-Japan Kokai Tokkyo Koho-08 92,057 1996; 12 pp.

CA194 Hirsbrunner, P. and E. Brambilla. Separation of serotonin from coffee wax. Patent-Ger Offen-2,532,308 1976; 14 pp.

CA195 Mori, H. and I. Hirono. Effect of coffee on carcinogenicity of cycasin. **Br J Cancer** 1977; 35: 369.

CA196 Latorre, D. L. and F. A. Latorre. Plants used by the Mexican Kickapoo Indians. Econ Bot 1977; 31: 340–357.

CA197 Wurzner, H. P., E. Lindstrom, L. Vuataz, and H. Luginbuhl. A 2-year feeding study of instant coffees in rats. II. Incidence and types of neoplasms. **Food Cosmet Toxicol** 1977; 15: 289.

CA198 Wurzner, H. P., E. Lindstrom, L. Vuataz, and H. Luginbuhl. A 2-year feeding study of instant coffees in rats. I. Body weight, food consumption, hematological parameters and plasma chemistry. **Food Cosmet Toxicol** 1977; 15: 7.

CA199 De Ross, B., S. Meyboom, T. G. Kosmeijer-Schuil, and M. B. Katan. Absorption and urinary excretion of the coffee diterpenes cafestola and kahweol in healthy ileostomy volunteers. **J Intern Med** 1998; 244(6): 451–460.

CA200 Duke, J. A. and V. R. Martinez. Amazonian ethnobotanical dictionary. CRC Press, Boca Raton, FL, 1994: 181.

CA201 Axelsson, I. G. K. Allergy to the coffee plant. **Allergy** 1994; 49(10): 885–887.

CA202 Nagasawa, H., M. Yasuda, and H. Inatomi. Further study on the effects of coffee cherry on spontaneous mammary tumourigenesis in mice: effects of

methanol extract. **Anticancer Res** 1996; 16(6B): 3507–3513.

CA203 Ponepal, V., U. Spielberger, G. Riedel-Caspari, and F. W. Schmidt. Use of *Coffea-arabica-toasta* extract in propylaxis and therapy of multifactorial infectious diseases in newborn calves. **Dtsch Tieraerztl Wochenschr** 1996; 103(10): 390–394.

CA204 Daglia, M., A. Papetti, C. Dacarro, and G. Gazzani. Isolation of an antibacterial component from roasted coffee. **J Pharm Biomed Anal** 1998; 18(1/2): 219–225.

CA205 Vaijayanthimala, J., C. Anandi, V. Udhaya, and K. V. Pugalendi. Anticandidal activity of certain South Indian medicinal plants. **Phytother Res** 2000; 14(3): 207–209.

CA206 Nakasato, F., M. Nakayasu, Y. Fujita, M. Nagao, M. Terada, and T. Sugimura. Mutagenicity of instant coffee on cultured Chinese hamster lung cells. **Mutat Res** 1984; 141(2): 109–112.

CA207 Kinlen, L. J. and K. McPherson. Pancreas cancer and coffee and tea consumption: a case-control study. **Br J Cancer** 1984; 49(1): 93–96.

CA208 Sampaio, E. D., F. D. Furtado, M. J. Furtado, M. N. Cavalcante, and O. D. Riedel. Hypoglycemic effect of raw coffee beans (*Coffea arabica* L. *Rubiaceae*). **Rev Med Univ Fed Ceara** 1979; 19(1/2): 49–53.

CA209 Aeschbacher, H. U., H. Meier, E. Ruch, and H. P. Wurzner. Investigation of coffee in sister chromatid exchange and micronucleus tests *in vivo*. **Food Chem Toxicol** 1984; 22(10): 803–807.

CA210 Dobmeyer, D. J., R. A. Stine, C. V. Leier, R. Greenberg, and S. F. Schaal. The arrhythmogenic effects of caffeine in human beings. **N Engl J Med** 1983; 308(14): 814–816.

CA211 Toda, M., S. Okubo, R. Hiyoshi, and T. Shimamura. The bactericidal activity of tea and coffee. **Lett Appl Microbiol** 1989; 8(4): 123–125.

CA212 Piraccini, B. M., F. Bardazzi, C. Vincenzi, and M. P. Tardio. Occupational contact dermatitis due to coffee. **Contact Dermatitis** 1990; 23(2): 114.

CA213 Okubo, S., H. Ikigai, M. Toda, and T. Shimamura. The anti-haemolysin activity of tea and coffee. **Lett Appl Microbiol** 1989; 9(2): 65–66.

CA214 Aeschbacher, H. U. and E. Jaccaud. Inhibition by coffee on nitrosourea-mediated DNA damage in mice. **Food Chem Toxicol** 1990; 28(9): 633–637.

CA215 Miwa, M., Z. L. Kong, K. Shinohara, and M. Watanabe. Macrophage stimulating activity of foods. **Agr Biol Chem** 1990; 54(7): 1863–1866.

CA216 Stalder, R., A. Bexter, H. P. Wurzner, and H. Luginbuhl. A carcinogenicity study of instant coffee in Swiss mice. **Ed Chem Toxicol** 1990; 28(12): 829–837.

CA217 El Tahir, K. E. H., E. A. Hamad, A. M. Ageel, M. A. Abu Nasif, and E. A. Gadkarim. Influence of tea, and coffee beverages on prostacyclin synthesis by the rat aorta. Prostaglandins **Leukotrienes Essent Fatty Acids** 1990; 40(1): 63–66.

CA218 Li, Y., R. Q. Yan, G. Z. Tan, X. X. Duan, and L. L. Tan. Comparative study on the inhibitory effect of green tea, coffee,, and levamisole on the hepatocacinogenetic action of dimethylnitrosamine. **Chung-Hua Chung Liu Tsa Chin** 1991; 13(3): 193–195.

CA219 Eisele, J. W. and D. T. Reay. Death related to coffee enemas. **JAMA** 1980; 244: 1608–1609.

CA220 Lam, L. K. T., V. L. Sparnins, and L. W. Wattenberg. Isolation and identification of kahweol palmitate and cafestol palmitate as active constituents of green coffee beans that enhance glutathione S-transferase activity in the mouse. **Cancer Res** 1982; 42: 1193–1198.

CA221 Lam, L. K. T., V. L. Sparnins, and L. W. Wattenberg. Isolation and identification of kahweol palmitate and cafestol palmitate as active constituents of green coffee beans that enhance glutathione (GSH) S-transferase activity. **Proc Am Ass Cancer Res** 1982; 23: 88.

CA222 Grollier, J. F. and S. Pessis. Use of coffee oil as a solar radiation filter on the skin. Patent-Fr Demande-2,479,688 1981; 3 pp.

CA223 Stich, H. F., M. P. Rosin and L. Bryson. Inhibition of the mutagenicity of a model nitrosation reaction by natu-rally occurring phenolics, coffee and tea. **Mutat Res** 1982; 95: 119–128.

CA224 Lilahut, N. and S. Tancharoen. Studies of the effect of coffee on EKG of non-coffee drinker. Undergraduate Special Project Report 19878; 22 pp.

CA225 Konowalchuk, J. and J. I. Speirs. Antiviral effect of commercial juices and beverages. **Appl Environ Microbiol** 1978; 35: 1219.

CA226 Ayensu, E. S. Medicinal plants of the West Indies. Unpublished Manuscript 1978; 110 pp.

CA227 Nagao, M., Y. Takahashi, H. Yamanaka, and T. Sugimura. Mutagens in coffee and tea. **Mutat Res** 1979; 68: 101–106.

CA228 Nolen, G. A. The effect of brewed and instant coffee in reproduction and teratogenesis in the rats. **Toxicol Appl Pharmacol** 1981; 58: 171–183.

CA229 Murphy, S. J. and C. P. Benzamin. The effects of coffee on mouse development. **Microbiol Lett** 1981; 17: 91–99.

CA230 Fujita, F. Y., K. Wakabayashi, M. Nagao, and T. Sugimura. Characteristics of major mutagenicity of instant coffee. **Mutat Res** 1985; 142(4): 145–148.

CA231 Lubin, F., E. Ron, Y. Wax, and B. Modan. Coffee and methylxanthines and breast cancer: a case-control study. **J Nat Cancer Inst** 1985; 74(3): 569–573.

CA232 Blair, C. A. and T. Shibamoto. Ames mutagenicity tests of overheated brewed coffee. **Food Chem Toxicol** 1984; 22(12): 971–975.

CA233 Aeschbacher, H. U., E. Ruch, H. Meier, H. P. Wurzner, and R. Munoz-Box. Instant and brewed coffees in the in vitro human lymphocyte mutagenicity test. **Food Chem Toxicol** 1985; 23(8): 747–752.

CA234 Yamaguchi, T. and M. Iki. Inhibitory effect of coffee extract against some mutagens. **Agr Biol Chem** 1986; 50(12): 2983–2988.

CA235 Obana, H., S. I. Nakamura, and R. I. Tanaka. Suppressive effects of coffee on the SOS responses induced by UV and chemical mutagens. **Mutat Res** 1986; 175; 47–50.

CA236 Weniger, B., M. Rouzier, R. Daguilh, D. Henrys, J. H. Henrys, and R. Anton. Popular medicine of the central plateau of Haiti. 2. Ethnopharmacological inventory. **J Ethnopharmacol** 1986; 17(1): 13–30.

CA237 Kloos, H., F. W. Thiongo, J. H. Ouma, and A. E. Buttersworth. Preliminary evaluation of some wild and cultivated plants for snail control in Machakos district, Kenya. **J Trop Med Hyg** 1987; 90(4): 197–204.

CA238 Kark, J. D., Y. Friedlander, N. A. Kaufmann, and Y. Stein. Coffee, tea, and plasma cholesterol: the Jerusalem lipid research clinic prevalence study. **Br Med J** 1985; 291(6497): 699–701.

CA239 Aeschbacher, H. U., E. Ruch, H. Meier, H. P. Wurzner, and R. Munoz-Box. Instant and brewed coffees in the *in vitro* human lymphocyte mutagenicity test. **Food Cosmet Toxicol** 1985; 23(8): 747–752.

CA240 Abraham, S. K. Inhibition of the *in vivo* genotoxicity by coffee. **Food Chem Toxicol** 1989; 27(12): 787–792.

CA241 Melamed, I., J. D. Kark, and Z. Spirer. Coffee and the immune system. **Int J Immunopharmacol** 1990; 12(1): 129–134.

CA242 Christianson, R. E., F. W. Oechsli, and B. J. Van Dert Berg. Caffeinated beverages and decreased fertility. **Lancet** 1989; 1989(8634): 378.

CA243 Roig Y Mesa, J. T. Plantas medicinales, aromaticas o venenosas de Cuba, Ministerion de Agricultura, Republica de Cuba, Havana. 1945; 872 pp.

CA244 Coleman, D. E. S. The effect of certain homeopathic remedies upon the hearing. **J Am Inst Homeopathy** 1922; 15: 279–281.

CA245 Wasuwat, S. A list of Thai medicinal plants, ASRCT, Bangkok. Report no. 1 on Res. Project 17. Research Report, A. S. R. C.T., No. 1 on Research Project 17, 1967; 22 pp.

CA246 Nishina, A., F. Kajishima, M. Matsunaga, H. Tezuka, H. Inatomi, and T. Osawa. Antimicrobial substance, 3',4'-dihydroxyacetophenone, in coffee residue. **Biosci Biotech Biochem** 1994; 58(2): 293–296.

CA247 Wei, M., C. A. Macera, C. A. Horning, and S. N. Blair. The impact of changes in coffee consumption on serum cholesterol. **J Clin Epidemiol** 1995; 48(10): 1189–1196.

CA248 De G Paula, R. D. Investigation of coffee oil. **Anail Assoc Brasil Quim** 1943; 2: 57.

CA249 Tohda, C., N. Nakamura, K. Komatsu, and M. Hattori. Trigonelline-induced neurite outgrowth in human neuroblastoma SK-N-SH cells. Biol Pharm Bull 1999; 22(7): 679–682.

CA250 Fontana, G., G. Mantia, P. Vetri, F. Venturella, V. Hopps, and G. Cascio. Effects on the carbohydrate metabolism of "coffee atractylosides". **Fitoterapia** 1994; 65(1): 29–33.

CA251 Booth, S.L., H.T. Madabushi, K.W. Davidson, and J.A. Sadowski. Tea and coffee brews are not dietary sources of vitamin K-1 (phylloquinone). **JAMA** 1995; 95(1): 82–83.

5 | Daucus carota

L.

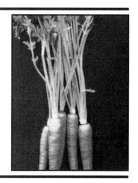

Common Names

Boktel	Malaysia	Gazar baladi	India
Bokti	Indonesia	Gazar	India
Bortol	Sudan	Gazur	India
Cairead	Ireland	Gelbe Rube	Germany
Caretysen	Cornwall	Gele peen	Netherlands
Carot	Cambodia	Gele Wortel	Netherlands
Carot	Vietnam	Gujjur	India
Carota	Italy	Gujjur-jo-beej	India
Carota salvatica	Italy	Gularot	Faeroe Islands
Carote	Italy	Gulerod	Denmark
Carotola	Germany	Gullerodder	Denmark
Carotte sauvage	Mauritius	Gulrot	Norway
Carotte	France	Have-gulerod	Denmark
Carradje	The Isle of Man (Manx)	Havijk	Iran
Carrot sauvage	Belgium	Havuc	Turkey
Carrot sauvage	Canada	Hong cai tou	China
Carrot sauvage	France	Hong da gen	China
Carrot sauvage	Tunisia	Hong lu fai	China
Carrot	Guyana	Hong luo bo	China
Carrot	United Kingdom	Hu lu fai	China
Carrot	United States	Hu luo bo	China
Cenoura brava	Portugal	Huang luo bo	China
Cenoura selvagem	Brazil	Hu-lo-po-tze	China
Cenoura	Portugal	Ikherothi	Africa
Curral	Scotland	Ilikherothi	Africa
Curran	Scotland	Jazar barri	Iraq
Dauco marino	Italy	Kaareti	New Zealand
Daucus carotte	France	Karot	Australia
Gaajara	India	Karot	Cambodia
Gahzar	India	Karot	Netherlands Antilles
Gaiweruam	Germany	Karot	Philippines
Gajar	India	Karote	Albania
Gajjarakkilangu	India	Karote	Hawaii
Gajor	India	Karoti	Samoa

From: *Medicinal Plants of the World, vol. 3: Chemical Constituents, Traditional and Modern Medicinal Uses*
By: I. A. Ross © Humana Press Inc., Totowa, NJ

Karoto	Greece	Ruokaporkana	Finland
Karotte	Germany	Sargarepa	Croatia
Karotten	Germany	Sargarepa	Hungary
Karotter	Denmark	Sargarepa	Serbia
Karuvathu kelengu	India	Segwere	South Africa
Kdyuir	Turkmenistan	Speisemohre	Germany
Khaerot	Thailand	Speisemohren	Germany
Lobak merah	Malaysia	Spisegulerod	Denmark
Marchew	Poland	Vild gulerod	Benin
Meacan dearg	Ireland	Vild gulerod	Denmark
Mohre	Germany	Viljelty porkkana	Finland
Mohrrube	Germany	Vill gulrot	Norway
Morkov	Bulgaria	Wild carrot	Canada
Morkov	Macedonia	Wild carrot	England
Morkov	Romania	Wild carrot	New Zealand
Morkov	Russia	Wild gulerod	Denmark
Morkva	Ukraine	Wilde mohre	Germany
Moronen	Wales	Wilde peen	Belgium
Morot	Sweden	Wilde peen	Netherlands
Mrkva	Yugoslavia	Wilde wortel	Belgium
Niistsikapa's	United States	Wildmorot	Sweden
Nora-ninjij	Japan	Wortel	Indonesia
Pahari gajar	India	Wortel	Netherlands
Pastanaga	Spain	Wortel	South Africa
Pastenade	France	Yang hua luo bo	China
Pastenaga	France	Ye hu luo bo	China
Pastinaca selvatica	Italy	Zanahoria Silvestre	Dominican Republic
Peen	Netherlands	Zanahoria silvestre	Chile
Phakchi-daeng	Thailand	Zanahoria silvestre	Peru
Pitta gajur	India	Zanahoria silvestre	Spain
Porkkana	Finland	Zanahoria silvestre	Venezuela
Queen Anne's lace	Canada	Zanahoria	Puerto Rico
Risch melna	Switzerland	Zanahoria	Spain

BOTANICAL DESCRIPTION

Carrot is an erect (30–120 cm high) annual or biennial herb of the UMBELLIFERAE family with branched stem arising from a large, succulent, thick, fleshy 5–30 cm long tap root. The color of the root in the cultivated varieties ranges from white, yellow, orange, light purple, or deep red to deep violet. The shape varies from short stumps to tapering cones. Leaves are finely dissected, twice or thrice-pinnate, segments are linear to lanceolate, 0.5–3 cm long. Upper leaves are reduced, with a sheathing petiole. Stem is striate or ridged, glabrous to hispid, up to 1 m tall. Flowers are borne in compound, more or less globose, to 7-cm-in-diameter umbels. Rays are numerous, bracts 1–2 pinnated, lobes linear, 7–10 bracteoles similar to bracts. Flowers are white or yellowish; the outer are usually the largest. Sepals are minute or absent, there are five petals and stamens, ovary inferior with two cells and one ovule per cell, two styles. Fruits are oblong, with bristly hairs along ribs, 2–4 mm long.

ORIGIN AND DISTRIBUTION

Cultivated carrot originated in Afghanistan then spread to China in the 13–14th century and reached England in the 15th century. It was introduced to North America by settlers and is grown widely in temperate and tropical regions of the world.

TRADITIONAL MEDICINAL USES

Algeria. Hot water extract of the seed, mixed with *Euphorbia* species and a beetle, is taken orally to facilitate childbirth[DC010].

Arabic countries. The dried seeds are used as an abortifacient in the form of a pessary in Unani medicine[DC191].

Belgium. Dried root is taken orally for diabetes[DC088].

Brazil. Water extract of the dried root is taken orally as a nerve tonic and stimulant[DC089].

Canary Islands. Infusion of the dried aerial parts is taken orally for cystitis[DC208].

China. Decoction of the seed is taken orally as an emmenagogue[DC108]. Root juice is taken orally for cancer of the stomach, bowel, and uterus, and for ulcers[DC108].

Egypt. Hot water extract of the fruit is taken orally to facilitate pregnancy and as an emmenagogue, aphrodisiac, diuretic, and antispasmodic[DC151]. Hot water extract of the dried fruit is taken orally as a diuretic and for urinary colic[DC174].

England. Hot water extract of the root and seed are taken orally to induce the menstrual cycle[DC017].

Europe. Decoction of the dried leaf is taken orally for diabetes mellitus[DC140]. Hot water extract of the root is taken orally as an emmenagogue[DC019] and anthelmintic[DC237]. Hot water extract of the seed is taken orally to induce menstruation[DC011].

Fiji. Fresh leaf juice is used as a nose drop for headache. Fresh root is taken orally for heart diseases[DC207].

France. Hot water extract of the fruit is taken orally as an emmenagogue[DC227].

Greece. Infusion of the dried flowers is taken orally as a tonic and to relieve sluggishness[DC083].

India. Decoction of the fresh root is taken orally for jaundice and inflammation, as an anthelmintic, and externally for leprosy[DC118].

Dried seeds are mixed with crude sugar and eaten to terminate early pregnancy[DC188]. Hot water extract of the dried root is taken orally as a tonic, expectorant, diuretic, stomachic, and liver cleanser[DC219]. Hot water extract of the leaf is taken orally as a uterine stimulant during parturition[DC020]. Hot water extract of the seed is taken orally as an abortifacient, emmenagogue, and aphrodisiac[DC008]. The dried seeds are used as a powerful abortifacient[DC239]. The root is taken orally as a hypotensive medication[DC098].

Iran. Water extract of the fruit is taken orally as an emmenagogue[DC014].

Italy. Decoction of the root is used as a gargle for loss of speech[DC072]. Root juice is taken orally as an anthelmintic and cicatrizing agent, for leukorrhea, and to improve sight[DC224]. The fresh root is used externally for dermatitis and burns. The fresh root juice is taken orally for loss of voice and persistent coughs, and the decoction is taken orally for diuresis[DC222]. The root is taken orally as a diuretic and a digestive and to treat uricemia and constipation[DC102].

Kuwait. The seeds are taken orally as an emmenagogue[DC113].

Madeira. Infusion of the entire plant is taken orally for jaundice[DC101].

Mexico. Hot water extract of the fresh root is taken orally as a cardiotonic[DC173]. The flowers or root, boiled together with *Cassia fistula* and "Rosa de Castilla," are taken orally before breakfast to induce abortion. To correct delayed menstruation, the liquid is taken daily for 40 days[DC234].

Morocco. The fruit is taken orally for urinary tract infections[DC253].

New Caledonia. Infusion of the fruit is taken orally as an emmenagogue[DC009].

Pakistan. Hot water extracts of the leaf and seed are taken orally as stimulants of the uterus during parturition[DC003].

Peru. Hot water extracts of the dried root and dried aerial parts are taken orally as a carminative, emmenagogue, and vermifuge[DC218].

Philippines. Hot water extract of the leaf is taken orally as a stimulant of the uterus during parturition[DC001].

Rodrigues Islands. Decoction of the entire plant is taken orally for gout, jaundice, and mouth ulcers[DC100].

South Korea. Hot water extract of the dried fruit is taken orally as an abortifacient and emmenagogue[DC206].

Tunisia. Dried leaf is used externally for chilblains[DC254].

Turkey. The seed, ground with the seeds of *Brassica rapa* and *Raphanus sativus*, is taken orally as a tonic[DC099].

United States. Hot water extract of the fruit is taken orally to stimulate menstruation[DC012]. Hot water extract of the seed is taken orally as an emmenagogue[DC021]. Seeds are taken orally as an emmenagogue, diuretic, and abortifacient[DC182]. The fresh root is taken orally for general nervousness, and the hot water extract is taken orally as a diuretic in dropsy and as a tonic[DC250]. Hot water extract of the dried root and seed is taken orally as a carminative, diuretic, and stimulant[DC249].

CHEMICAL CONSTITUENTS

(ppm unless otherwise indicated)
Aesculetin coumarin: Lf, Rt[DC248]
Alanine(DL): Bd[DC236]
Alanine: Sd[DC065], Rt[DC126,DC200]
Alcanols (C22–C30): Lf 305[DC172]
Aldolase: Call Tiss[DC036]
Alkanes (C13–C58): Rt[DC126]
Alkanes (C15–C39): Lf 0.033[DC172]
Amine, ethyl-methyl: Rt 7[DC199]
Ammonia-lyase: Pl[DC194]
Amylase: Call Tiss[DC036]
Amyrin, α: Aer[DC198]
Amyrin, β: Aer[DC198]
Aniline, *N*-methyl: Rt 0.8[DC199]
Aniline: Rt 30.9[DC199]
Anthocyanins: Call Tiss[DC233], Pl[DC085]
Apigenin: Lf[DC087]
Apigenin-4'-O-β-D-glucoside: Sd[DC177], Fr[DC170]
Apigenin-7-galactomannoside: Sd[DC177]
Arabinoside: Rt[DC200]
Arachic acid: Fr fixed oil 0.31%[DC134]

Arginine: Pl[DC161]
Asaraldehyde: Sd EO[DC023]
Asarone, *cis*: Fr EO 4.10%[DC090]
Asarone, *trans*: Fr EO 40.325[DC090]
Asarone: Sd EO[DC023], Fr EO 6.08%[DC090]
Ascorbic acid, dehydro: Rt[DC244]
Ascorbic acid: Rt[DC093]
Aspartic acid: Pl[DC161]
Astragalin: Sd[DC177]
Avenasterol, 7-dehydro: Fr EO[DC134]
Benzene, 4-methyl-iso-propenyl: Sd[DC149]
Benzoic acid, 4-hydroxy: Rt[DC246]
Benzylamine, *N*-methyl: Rt 16.50[DC199]
Benzylamine: Rt 2.80[DC199]
Bergapten: Rt 0.3[DC175], Call Tiss 115[DC076], Fr[DC142]
Betaine: Sh 0.3 μmol/g[DC181]
Bisabolene, β: Sd EO[DC171], Fr EO 20.13%[DC090], Sd EO 1.5%[DC029]
Bisabolene, γ, *trans*: Rt[DC144]
Bisabolene, γ: Rt[DC067]
Bisabolene: Sd EO[DC023], Rt[DC064]
Borneol acetate: Rt[DC064]
Caffeic acid: Aer, Rt[DC245], Lf[DC248], Call Tiss[DC246]
Caffeoylquinic acid: Rt[DC111]
Calcium inorganic: Rt[DC153]
Campesterol: Lf[DC172], Aer, Rt[DC198]
Capric acid: Fr fixed oil 1.56%[DC134]
Car-3-ene monoterpene: Fr EO 1.27%[DC090]
Carota-1-4-β-oxide sesquiterpene: Sd EO 66[DC131]
Carotene, α, all-*trans*: Rt[DC106]
Carotene, α: Rt[DC157], Lf[DC030]
Carotene, β, 9-*cis*: Rt[DC135]
Carotene, β, all-*trans*: Rt[DC135]
Carotene, β: Rt[DC078]
Carotene, ε: Rt[DC022]
Carotene, γ: Lf[DC030], Rt[DC157]
Carotene: Rt[DC243]
Carotol: EO[DC042], Sd[DC146], Sd EO[DC033]
Caryophyllene, β: Rt[DC144]
Caryophyllene: Rt[DC067]
Chlorogenic acid, iso: Rt[DC159], Lf[DC248]
Chlorogenic acid, *trans*: Aer[DC129]
Chlorogenic acid: Rt[DC031], Aer[DC245], Call Tiss[DC060], Lf[DC248]
Chlorophyll: Fr Ju 0.2[DC197]
Chloroplasts: Rt[DC143], Call Tiss[DC063], Lf[DC030]
Cholesterol: Lf[DC172]
Choline, phosphatidyl: Pl[DC120]
Choline: Sd[DC018]

Chromone, 5-7-dihydroxy-2-methyl: Rt[DC024]
Chrysanthemin: Call Tiss[DC184]
Chrysin: Fr[DC170]
Chrysoeriol: Lf[DC087]
Cinnamic acid, *trans*; Pl[DC194]
Cinnamic acid: Call Tiss[DC060]
Citric acid, iso: Rt[DC240]
Citric acid: Rt[DC240]
Coenzyme Q-10: Pl[DC058]
Cosmosiin: Fr[DC170]
Coumaric acid, para: Rt[DC040], Call Tiss[DC246]
Coumarin, iso, 3-4-dihydro-8-hydroxy-6-mehoxy-3-methyl: Rt[DC041], Call Tiss[DC037]
Coumarin, iso: Rt[DC159]
Cpsmosiin: Lf[DC170]
Cryptoxanthin, β: Rt[DC122]
Cyanidin diglycoside: Rt[DC247]
Cyanidin-3-(sinapoyl-xylosyl-glucosyl-galactoside): Pl, Lf[DC125]
Cyanidin-3-0-galactoside: Call Tiss[DC184]
Cyanidin-3-5-digalactoside: Call Tiss[DC184]
Cyanidin-3-glucogalactoside: Call Tiss[DC184]
Cymen-8-ol, para: Sd 0.9[DC149]
Cynaroside: Fr[DC170], Aer[DC129], Lf[DC170]
Cysteine: Pl[DC161]
Dauca-4-8-diene sesquiterpene: Sd EO 4.1%[DC029]
Daucarin: Sd[DC189]
Daucic acid: Rt[DC039]
Daucol, dehydroxy: Sd EO[DC033]
Daucol: Sd EO[DC033]
Daucosterol: Lf[DC087]
Dauc-*trans*-8-en-4-β-ol sesquiterpene: Sd EO 4.1%[DC029]
Daucus carota agglutinin: Rt[DC180]
Daucus carota alkaloid 2: Sd[DC018]
Daucus carota exopolygalacturonase: Rt[DC027]
Daucus carota protein (75 kDa): Pl[DC028]
Daucus carota tertiary alkaloid: Sd[DC166]
Dehydrogenase, glutamic acid: Pl[DC168]
Diosgenin: Call Tiss 0.6%[DC121]
Elemicin: Sd 0.2%[DC149]
Esterase, pectin: Rt[DC119]
Ethanolamine, phosphatidyl: Pl[DC196]
Ethylamine: Rt 1[DC199]
Eugenin: Call Tiss[DC037], Rt[DC156]
Eugenol methyl ether phenylpropanoid: Fr EO 1.23%[DC090]
Eugenol phenylpropanoid: 0.70%[DC149], Fr EO 1.72%[DC090]
Extensil: Rt[DC055]
Falcarindiol monoacetate: Rt[DC057]

Falcarindiol-1-acetate: Rt[DC069]
Falcarinol: Rt 10[DC069]
Farnesene, β, *trans*: Sd EO 2.5%[DC029]
Ferulic acid: Rt[DC040], Call Tiss[DC060], Lf[DC248]
Fructokinase, phospho: Rt[DC150]
Fructose: Rt[DC228]
Fumarase: Call Tiss[DC036]
Fumaric acid: Rt[DC240]
Galactose: Rt[DC200]
Galactosidase, β: Pl[DC161]
Galacturonanase, exo-D: Rt[DC112]
Gentisic acid: Call Tiss[DC246]
Geraniol: Sd 300[DC149]
Geranyl-2-methyl-butyrate: 0.05%[DC149]
Glucose: Rt[DC228], Bd[DC236]
Glucosidase, α: Pl[DC161]
Glucosidase, β: Pl[DC161]
Glucuronidase, β: Pl[DC161]
Glutamic acid: Pl[DC161], Rt[DC200]
Glycerol, phosphatidyl: Pl[DC120]
Glycine: Sd[DC065], Pl[DC161], Rt[DC126], Bd[DC236]
Guaiacol, para-vinyl: Sd 0.4%[DC149]
Hentraicontane, N: Sd[DC032]
Heptacosane, N: Bd[DC236], Sd[DC032]
Heptadeca-2-9-diene-4-6-diyn-8-ol-acetoxy: Rt[DC069]
Heraclenin: Rt, Aer[DC178]
Histidine: Pl[DC161], Rt[DC200]
Hydroxylase, cinnamic acid-4: Pl[DC168]
Indole, acetic acid: Call Tiss[DC155]
Inosidol, phosphatidyl: Pl[DC196]
Invertase: Pl[DC231]
Ionone, β: Sd 0.03%[DC149]
Kaempherol: Rt[DC075], Fr[DC170]
Lauric acid: Fr Fixed oil 2.08%[DC134]
Leucine, iso: Pl[DC161], Rt[DC200]
Leucine: Rt[DC126], Bd[DC236], Pl[DC161], Sd[DC065]
Lignin: Pl[DC034]
Limonene: Rt[DC064]
Linoleic acid: Sd 12.2%[DC195]
Linolenic acid: Sd oil[DC148]
Lupeol: Rt[DC198]
Lutein: Rt 2.8[DC068]
Luteolin: Fr[DC170], Rt 1.4[DC073]
Luteolin-7-O-(6''-O-malonyl)-β-D glucoside: Aer[DC129]
Luteolin-7-O-β-D-glucoronide: Aer[DC129]
Lyase, phenylalanine-ammonia: Call Tiss[DC109], Pl[DC168]
Lycopene: Lf[DC030], Call Tiss[DC063], Rt[DC157]
Lysine: Pl[DC154], Rt[DC200]
Malic acid: Rt[DC240]

Malvidin-3-5-diglucoside: Rt[DC032]
Mannose: Rt[DC200]
Melatonin: Rt 55.3 pg/g[DC084]
Mellein, 6-hydroxy, (-): Rt[DC024]
Mellein, 6-methoxy, (-): Rt[DC024]
Mellein, 6-methoxy: Pl[DC124], Rt[DC193]
Methionine: Pl[DC154]
Methylamine: Rt 3.80[DC199]
Mevalonic acid: Rt 4[DC232]
Myrcene: Rt[DC144]
Myricetin: Rt 1[DC073]
Myristic acid: Sd oil[DC148]
Myristicin: Rt 34.4[DC179]
Nerol acetate: EO 2.51%[DC107]
Nerol: Fr EO 0.30%[DC107]
Neurosporene: Rt[DC157]
NH$_3$ inorganic: Rt 3970[DC199]
Nonacosane, N: Bd[DC236], Sd[DC032]
Nucleotidase, 3': Pl[DC165]
Octacosane, N: Sd[DC032]
Oleic acid: Sd oil[DC136], Sd 11.6%[DC195], Fr
    Fixed oil 76.25%[DC134]
Paeonol: Fr EO 1.33%[DC090]
Palmitic acid: Sd oil[DC148], Fr fixed oil
    3.25%[DC134]
Palmitoleic acid: Rt[DC114], Fr fixed oil
    0.31%[DC134]
Peroxidase: Rt[DC032]
Petroselinic acid: Sd oil[DC145], Sd 71.2%[DC195]
Phellandrene, α: Rt[DC144]
Phenethylamine, N-methyl: Rt 2[DC199]
Phenetrhylamine: Rt 2[DC199]
Phenylalanine: Rt[DC200]
Phosphatase, acid: Pl[DC161]
Phytofluene: Rt[DC157]
PIK-A49: Pl[DC080]
Pimpinellin, iso: Call Tiss[DC095]
Pinene, α: Sd[DC146], Rt[DC064], Sd EO 0.9%[DC029]
Pinene, β: Rt[DC064]
Polysaccharides: Pl[DC077]
Proline, 4-hydroxy: Rt[DC200]
Proline: Rt[DC126], Pl[DC161], Sh 0.1 μmol/g[DC181]
Protein: Pl[DC038], Sd 30%[DC229]
Psoralen, 5-methoxy: Pl, Cr[DC123], Fr[DC082]
Psoralen: Rt 0.3[DC175,DC142]
Putrescine: Call Tiss[DC152]
Pyrazine, 2-methoxy-3-sec-butyl: Rt[DC064]
Qercitrin: Fr[DC170]
Quercetin: Rt[DC075], Fr[DC170]
Quinic acid: Rt[DC240]
Rhamnose: Rt[DC200]
Ribonuclease, deoxy: Pl[DC165]

Ribonuclease: Pl[DC165]
RNase: Call Tiss[DC036]
Rutin: Rt[DC075]
Scopoletin: Rt[DC024], Lf[DC248]
Serine: Sd[DC065], Bd[DC236], Rt[DC200]
Shikimic acid: Rt[DC240]
Sitosterol, β: Sd[DC035], Rt[DC057], Bd[DC236], Lf[DC172],
    Aer[DC198]
Sterase: Pl[DC161]
Stigmasterol: Lf[DC172], Aer, Lf[DC198]
Suberin: Rt[DC046]
Succinic acid: Rt[DC240]
Sucrose: Rt[DC228]
Syringic acid: Rt[DC246]
Taraxasterol: Aer, Rt[DC198]
Tartaric acid: Rt[DC240]
Terpinen-4-ol: Rt[DC064]
Terpinene, α: Rt[DC144]
Terpinene, γ: Rt[DC064]
Terpineol, α: Pl[DC257]
Terpinolene: Rt[DC144]
Threonine: Rt[DC200]
Tiglic acid: Sd EO[DC023]
Toluidine: Rt 7.20[DC199]
Transaminase, glutamate-oxalacetate: Call
    Tiss[DC036]
Transaminase, glutamate-pyruvate: Call
    Tiss[DC036]
Tryptophan: Rt[DC126], Pl[DC154]
Tyrosine: Bd[DC236], Sd[DC065], Pl[DC161], Rt[DC200]
Ubiquinone 10: Call Tiss 0.125[DC062], Pl
    160[DC061]
Umbelliferone: Lf[DC241]
Uronic acid: Rt[DC200]
Valine: Rt[DC126], Bd[DC236], Sd[DC065], Pl[DC161]
Vanillic acid: Call Tiss[DC246]
Xanthotoxin: Pl, Cr[DC123], Rt 0.3[DC175], Call
    Tiss[DC095], Fr[DC082]
Xylitol: Rt[DC110]
Xylose: Rt[DC200]
Zeatin, cis: Call Tiss[DC160] Zeatin: Call
    Tiss[DC160]

PHARMACOLOGICAL ACTIVITIES AND CLINICAL TRIALS

Abortifacient effect. Ethanol (95%) extract of the dried seed, administered by gastric intubation to pregnant mice at doses of 30 mg/animal and 40 mg/kg on days 4–6, was inactive[DC238]. Petroleum ether extract of the dried seed, administered subcutaneously to pregnant rats beginning on day 7 of pregnancy, was active[DC127]. Petroleum ether extract of the dried seed, administered subcutaneously to pregnant rats at a dose of 2 mL/kg, was active. The effect was blocked by progesterone given on days 7–19 of pregnancy[DC205]. Seed essential oil, administered to pregnant mice at a dose of 5 mg/kg, was active[DC171]. Acetone extract of the fresh root, at a concentration of 1 μg/mL, produced weak activity and the propanol extract was inactive on *Salmonella typhimurium* TA98 vs 2-amino-3-methylimidazo (4,5-F) quinoline-induced mutagenicity[DC053]. Fresh fruit juice, administered by gastric intubation to male mice at a dose of 0.5 mL/animal, was active on *Schizosaccharomyces pombe*. The animals were treated with the juice and nitrosation precursors, then yeast cells were injected into the venous plexus of the orbit. Four hours later, the animals were sacrificed and the livers removed, plated with yeast and examined. Results were significant at $p < 0.001$ level[DC197]. Infusion of the stem, on agar plate at a concentration of 100 μL/disc, produced strong activity on *Salmonella typhimurium* TA98 vs 2-amino-anthracene-induced mutagenicity. Metabolic activation was not required for activity. Weak activity was produced on *Salmonella typhimurium* TA100 vs ethyl methanesulfonate-induced mutagenicity. Metabolic activation was not required for activity[DC255]. Methanol extract of the dried root, on agar plate at a concentration of 50 μL/disc, was inactive on *Bacillus subtilis* NIG-1125 His Met and *Escherichia coli* B/R-WP2-TRP[DC203]. Root juice, on agar plate at a concentration of 500.0 μL/plate produced weak activity on *Salmonella typhimurium* TA98 vs 2-nitrofluorine- and 1-nitropyrene-induced mutagenesis[DC056]. Water extract of the fresh root, on agar plate plus S9 mix at a dose of 0.4 mL/plate, was active on *Salmonella typhimurium* TA 100 vs TRP-P-2 mutagenicity[DC215]. Water extract of the fresh root, on agar plate at a concentration of 500 μg/plate, produced weak activity on *Salmonella typhimurium* TA100 vs N-nitrosoamine-induced mutagenicity[DC115].

Agglutinin activity. Water extract of the fresh root at variable concentrations was active on *Streptococcus mutans*[DC180].

AIDS therapeutic effects. Water extract of the dried rhizome taken orally by adults was active. A pharmaceutical solution containing fruit bodies of *Tremella fuciformis*, *Daucus carota* rhizome, *Astragalus mongholicus* root, and *Zizyphus jujuba* fruits, honey, vitamin A palmitate, zinc sulfate, and vitamin C was useful for controlling acquired immunodifficiency syndrome (AIDS), cancer, and infections[DC139].

Anti-allergenic activity. Water extract of the fresh root, in cell culture at a concentration of 100 μL/mL, was inactive on Leuk-RBL 2H3 vs biotinylated anti-deoxyriboneucleoprotein immunoglobulin E /avidin-induced β-hexosaminidase release[DC086].

Anti-amoebic activity. Essential oil, in broth culture at a concentration of 0.5 μL/mL, was active on *Entamoeba histolytica*[DC091].

Antibacterial activity. Essential oil, on agar plate at a concentration of 0.43 mg/mL, produced weak activity on *Streptococcus-β hemolytic* and *Staphylococcus aureus*, equivocal on *Escherichia coli*, minimal inhibitory concentration (MIC) 1.74 mg/mL and inactive on *Proteus mirabilis*, MIC 17.4 mg/mL. Fruit essential oil on agar plate was active on *Staphylococcus aureus*, MIC 0.12 mg/mL, and *Streptococcus-β hemolytic*, MIC 0.23 mg/mL, inactive on *Proteus mirabilis*, MIC 18.5 mg/mL, and equivocal on *Escherichia coli*, MIC 9.25 mg/mL[DC107]. Ethanol (70%) extract of the fruit, on agar plate, was active on *Bacillus megaterium*, *Staphylococcus albus*, *Staphylococcus aureus*, and *Bacillus cereus*[DC190]. Ethanol (95%) and water extracts of the entire plant, on agar plate, were inactive on *Escherichia coli* and *Staphylococcus aureus*[DC026]. Fresh root, macerated, in pieces and shredded, was active on *Listeria monocytogenes*[DC137]. Fresh shredded root dipped in chlorine and packaged under an atmosphere containing 3% oxygen and 97% nitrogen, was active on *Listeria monocytogenes*. Bacterial growth was inhibited on shredded carrots more than on whole carrots. There was no inhibition on cooked carrots[DC132]. The root, on agar plate, was active on *Streptococcus mutans*[DC048].

Anticlastogenic activity. Plant juice, administered intragastrically to male mice at a dose of 1 mL/kg, produced weak activity on reticulocyte vs γ-ray irradiation[DC047].

Anticytotoxic activity. Ethanol (95%) extract of the fresh root, at a concentration of 80 mg/mL in cell culture, was active on Vero cells vs *N*-nitrosopiperidine, *N*-nitrosodibutylamine, and *N*-nitrosodimethylamine cytotoxicity. A dose of 20 mg/mL was inactive vs *N*-nitrosopiperidine, nitrosodimethylamine, *N*-nitrosopyrrolidine, and *N*-nitrosodibutylamine cytotoxicity[DC104].

Anti-edema activity. Methanol extract of the root, applied externally to mice at a dose of 2 mg/ear, produced inhibition ratio of 37[DC071].

Anti-estrogenic effect. Ethanol (95%) extract of the dried seed, administered by gastric intubation of ovariectomized mice at a dose of 40 mg/kg daily for 3 days, produced weak activity[DC238]. Petroleum ether extract of the dried seed, at a dose of 10 mg/kg, was active[DC117].

Antifertility effect. Hot water extract of the dried seed, administered by gastric intubation to female rats, was active[DC201].

Antifungal activity. Acetone, water, and ethanol (95%) extracts of the dried fruit, on agar plate at a concentration of 50%, were inactive on *Neurospora crassa*[DC252]. The essential oil, at a concentration of 1000 ppm on agar plate, produced weak activity on *Aspergillus flavus*[DC068]. Ethanol (50%) extract of the dried root, on agar plate at a concentration of 500 mg/mL, was active on *Botrytis cinerea* and inactive on *Aspergillus fumigatus*, *Aspergillus niger*, *Fusarium oxysporum*, *Penicil-*

lium digitatum, *Rhizopus nigrans*, and *Trichophyton mentagrophytes*[DC212]. Seed essential oil, in broth culture at variable concentrations, was active on *Cladosporium werneckii*[DC192]. The root, on agar plate, was active on *Porphyromonas gingivalis*[DC048].

Antigen expression inhibition. Fresh plant juice, in the ration of female mice, was active vs IgE antibody expression in ovalbumin-sensitized mice[DC116].

Antihalitosis effect. Dried root ingested by adults was active. The biological activity has been patented[DC050].

Antihepatotoxic activity. Water extract of the fresh root, administered intragastrically to male rats at a dose of 20 mL/kg, was active vs lindane-induced hepatotoxicty[DC118]. Supernatant of the fresh root, administered intragastrically to male mice at a dose of 50 mL/kg, decreased serum bilirubin, urea, lactic dehydrogenase, serum glutamic pyruvic transaminase, and serum glutamic oxaloacetic transaminase levels vs carbon tetrachloride (CCl_4)-induced hepatotoxicity[DC092].

Antihyperglycemic activity. Decoction, ethanol (80%),[DC088] and water[DC103] extracts of the dried root, administered intragastrically to mice at a dose of 25 g/kg, were active vs glucose-induced hyperglycemia. Dried leaf, administered to male mice at a concentration of 6.25% of the diet for 28 days, was inactive vs streptozotocin-induced hyperglycemia[DC140]. Fresh root, taken orally by 15 adults of both sexes with type II diabetes at a dose of 280 g/person, was active[DC133].

Anti-implantation effect. Chloroform–methanol (9:1) fraction of ethanol (95%) extract, a chloroform-soluble fraction and an ethyl acetate-soluble fraction of a water extract, methanol-soluble fraction of a petroleum ether extract and chloroform soluble fraction of petroleum ether extract of the seed, administered orally to female rats at a dose of 50 mg/kg, were active vs foot shock[DC230]. Water and petroleum ether extracts of the seed, administered orally to female rats at doses of 100 and 20 mg/kg, respectively, were active[DC006]. Petroleum ether extract of the seed, administered orally to female rats at a dose of 500 mg/kg, was inactive[DC044]. Ethanol (50%) extract of the dried seed, administered orally to female rats at a dose of 500 mg/kg, was inactive[DC167]. Ethanol (95%) extract of the dried fruit, administered orally to pregnant rats at a dose of 500 mg/kg, produced 60% inhibition of implantation[DC169]. Petroleum ether extract of the dried seed, administered subcutaneously to pregnant rats at a dose of 6 mL/kg, was inactive[DC187]. Seed essential oil, administered to pregnant mice at a dose of 5 mg/kg, was active[DC171].

Antimycobacterial activity. Ethanol (95%) and water extracts of the entire plant, on agar plate, were inactive on *Mycobacterium tuberculosis*[DC026]. Leaf juice, on agar plate, produced weak activity on *Mycobacterium tuberculosis*, MIC less than 1:20[DC007].

Anti-nematodal activity. Methanol extract of the fruit, at a concentration of 1 mg/mL, was active, and the water extract, at a concentration of 10 mg/mL, produced weak activity on *Toxacara canis*[DC147].

Antioxidant activity. Plant juice, at a dose of 100 μL/kg, produced weak activity vs Fenton's reagent-induced lipid peroxidation[DC047]. The root, at a concentration of 1%, produced weak activity at 120° F[DC096]. Water extract of the fresh root, at a concentration of 10 μM trolox equivalent per gram, produced weak activity vs oxygen radical absorption capacity assay with hydroxyl and peroxyl radical generators, and Cu^{2+} (reactive species) activity[DC052]. Fresh root homogenate produced 31.8% inhibition of lipid peroxidation[DC093].

Antioxytocic effect. Methanol extract of the dried seed, at a concentration of 0.5 mg/mL, was equivocal vs oxytocin-induced contractions[DC221].

Antiprogesterone effect. Petroleum ether extract of the dried seed, administered subcutaneously to pregnant rats at doses of 2 mL/kg and 0.6 mL/animal, were active[DC205].

Petroleum ether extract of the seed, administered subcutaneously to pregnant rats at a dose of 0.6 mL/animal, was active[DC223].

Antispasmodic activity. Petroleum ether fraction chromatographed and fraction eluted with chloroform, at a concentration of 0.50 mg/mL, was active on the guinea pigileum vs histamine-induced contractions[DC226]. Tertiary alkaloid fraction of the dried seeds produced weak activity on the dog trachea vs acetylcholine (ACh)- and KCl-induced contractions, and active on the guinea pig ileum. A concentration of 25 μg/mL was active on the rat uterus vs ACh- and oxytocin-induced contractions, results significant at $p < 0.02$ level[DC166]. Methanol extract of the dried seed, at a concentration of 0.1 mg/mL, was active on the guinea pig ileum vs histamine-induced contractions[DC221].

Anti-thyroid activity. Boiled root, taken orally by adults at a dose of 554 g/person, produced weak activity on iodine uptake by the thyroid. The root, taken orally by adults, at a dose of 352 g/person, produced slight to high iodine uptake by the thyroid[DC251].

Anti-tumor activity. Petroleum ether extract of the dried seed, administered intraperitoneally to male mice at a concentration of 3 mg/kg, was active on Chinese hamster cells-V79[DC059]. The root, administered in the ration of female rats for 1 month before 7,12-dimethybenz[a]anthracene treatment, reduced tumor size[DC045]. Water extract of the aerial parts, administered intraperitoneally to mice at a dose of 400 mg/kg, was inactive on Leuk (Friend Virus-Solid) and Leuk-L1210. A dose of 500 mg/kg was inactive on Sarcoma 180 (ASC)[DC235]. Water extract of the dried root taken orally by adults was active. A pharmaceutical solution containing fruit bodies of *Tremella fuciformis*, *Daucus carota* root, *Astragalus mongholicus* root, and *Zizyphus jujuba* fruits, honey, vitamin A palmitate, zinc sulfate, and vitamin C was useful for controlling AIDS, cancer, and infections[DC139]. Hot water extracts of the fresh leaf and fresh root, in cell culture, produced strong activity on Raji cells vs phorbol myristate acetate-promoting expression of Epstein-Barr virus (EBV) early antigen[DC070]. Methanol extract of the fresh root, at a concentration of 200 mg/mL, was inactive on Raji cells vs EBV activation induced by 12-O-hexadecanoylphorbol (40 ng/mL)[DC097].

Anti-yeast activity. Ethanol (50%) extract of the dried root, on agar plate at a concentration of 500 mg/mL, was inactive on *Candida albicans* and *Saccharomyces pastorianus*[DC212].

Cardiotonic activity. Petroleum ether fraction chromatographed and fraction eluted with chloroform, administered by perfusion at a concentration of 0.20 mg/mL, was inactive on the guinea pig heart[DC226].

Catalase inhibition. Water extract of the fresh root, administered intragastrically to infant mice at a dose of 50 mL/kg, was active. The treatment was administered for seven successive days, followed by a single dose of 20% v/v CCl_4 in olive oil subcutaneously at 1 mL/kg on the last day 1 hour after the administration of the carrot extract[DC074]. Chloroform–methanol (9:1) fraction of the ethanol (95%) extract, ethyl acetate fraction of the water extract, and chloroform-soluble fraction of the water extract of the seed were active on the nonpregnant rat uterus[DC225].

Central nervous system (CNS) depressant activity. Ethanol (95%) extract of the seed, administered orally to mice and rats at a dose of 50 mg/kg, was inactive[DC020].

CNS stimulant activity. Ethanol (95%) extract of the seed, administered orally to mice and rats at a dose of 50 mg/kg, was inactive[DC020].

Conditioned taste aversion. Frozen leaf and stem, administered intragastrically to rats at a dose of 562 mg/kg, was inactive. The test substance was temporarily paired with the introduction of sodium saccharin solution. Consumption of the saccharin solution 2 days after the test was used to estimate aversiveness of the test substance[DC216].

Cytotoxic activity. Ethanol (50%) extract of the root, in cell culture, was inactive on CA-9KB, effective dose $(ED)_{50}$ greater than 20 µg/mL[DC013]. Methanol extract of the fresh root, in cell culture at a concentration of 200 µg/mL, was inactive on macrophage cell line RAW 264.7[DC054]. Water extract of the aerial parts, in cell culture, was inactive on CA-9KB, ED_{50} greater than 0.1 mg/mL[DC235].

Dermatitis-producing effect. Ether extract of the fresh entire plant, applied by patch at a concentration of 1%, was active[DC130]. Fresh root, in a mixture containing *Apium graveolens*, *Aromatica rusticana*, *Solanum tuberosum*, and *Petroselinum crispum*, was active[DC220].

Desmutagenic activity. Fresh plant juice, on agar plate at a concentration of 0.5 mL/disc, was inactive on *Salmonella typhimurium* TA98[DC213]. Homogenate of the fresh root, at a concentration of 100 µL/disc on agar plate, was active on *Salmonella typhimurium* TA98 and TA100 vs 1,4-dinitro-2-methyl pyrrole mutagenesis[DC211].

Diuretic activity. Ethanol (70%) extract of the dried fruit, administered intravenously to dogs at a dose of 150 mg/kg, increased diuresis 1.7-fold[DC141]. Ethanol (95%) extract of the seed, administered orally to rats at a dose of 100 mg/kg, was inactive[DC020]. Seed essential oil, administered intravenously to dogs at a concentration of 4 µL/kg, produced 2.4-fold increase in urine flow and an increase in K^+, Na^+, and Cl^- excretion. Ethanol (70%) extract of the seed essential oil, administered intravenously to dogs at a dose of 20 mg/kg, produced 1.6-fold increase in urine flow[DC141].

Embryotoxic effect. Ethanol (95%) extract of the dried seed, administered by gastric intubation to pregnant rats at a dose of 40 mg/animal on days 4–6, was inactive[DC238]. A dose of 0.10 g/kg, administered by gastric intubation to pregnant rats on days 1–10, was inactive, and a dose of 0.25 mg/kg on days 1–10 was equivocal. Six of 10 animals were pregnant vs 10 of 10 in the control group[DC209]. Ethanol (50%) extract of the dried seed, administered by gastric intubation to pregnant rats at a dose 200 mg/kg, was equivocal[T05679]. The water extract, at a dose of 0.5 g/kg on days 1–10, was inactive[DC209]. Petroleum ether extract, administered subcutaneously to pregnant rats at a dose of 1 mL/kg, was inactive and a dose of 2 mL/kg was active. Results were significant at $p < 0.05$ level[DC187]. Powdered dried seed, administered by gastric intubation to pregnant rats at doses of 2–4.5 g/kg on days 1–10, was inactive[DC209]. Petroleum ether extract of the seed chromatographed and fraction eluted with chloroform, administered orally to female rats at a dose of 20 mg/kg, was active[DC256]. Ethanol (95%) extract of the seed, administered orally to female rats at a dose of 50 mg/kg, was inactive. Chloroform-soluble and ethyl acetate-soluble fractions of a water extract of the seed, administered orally to female rats at a dose of 50 mg/kg, were active vs foot shock. Chloroform- and methanol-soluble fractions of the petroleum ether extract of the seed, administered orally to female rats at a dose of 50 mg/kg, was inactive[DC230]. Petroleum ether extract of the seed, administered subcutaneously to pregnant rats at a dose of 0.6 mL/animal, was active[DC223]. Seed essential oil, administered subcutaneously to pregnant rats on days 1, 2, 7, and 8, was active[DC206].

Estrogenic effect. Ethanol (95%) extract of the dried seed, administered by gastric intubation to infant female mice at doses of 20 and 40 mg/animal daily for 3 days, produced weak activity[DC238]. Doses of 50, 100, and 500 mg/kg, administered subcutaneously to ovariectomized rats, produced weak activity[DC214]. Petroleum ether extract of the dried seed, administered subcutaneously to ovariectomized rats at doses of 2 and 6 mL/kg, was active, results significant at $p < 0.01$ level[DC185]. Ethanol (95%) extract of the root, administered subcutaneously to female infant mice, was active [DC015,DC016]. Ethanol (95%) extract of the root, administered subcutaneously to female infant mice, was inactive[DC004]. The seed essential oil was inactive[DC171]. Root, in the ration of female infant mice, produced activity equivalent to 2 μg stilbestrol in 100 g carrot (dry weight)[DC002].

Estrous cycle disruption effect. Petroleum ether extract of the dried seed, administered subcutaneously to rats at a dose of 2 mL/kg, was active. Results were significant at $p < 0.001$ level[DC186].

Glutathione formation induction. Water extract of the fresh root, administered intragastrically to infant mice at a dose of 25 mL/kg, was active. The treatment was administered for seven successive days followed by a single dose of 20% v/v CCl_4 in olive subcutaneously at 1 mL/kg on the last day, 1 hour after the administration of the carrot extract[DC074].

Glutathione peroxidase inhibition. Water extract of the fresh root, administered intragastrically to infant mice at a dose of 50 mL/kg, was active. The treatment was administered for seven successive days followed by a single dose of 20% v/v CCl_4 in olive subcutaneously at 1 mL/kg on the last day, 1 hour after the administration of the carrot extract[DC074].

Glutathione reductase stimulation. Water extract of the fresh root, administered intragastrically to infant mice at a dose of 25 mL/kg, was active. The treatment was administered for seven successive days followed by a single dose of 20% v/v CCl_4 in olive subcutaneously at 1 mL/kg on the last day, 1 hour after the administration of the carrot extract[DC074].

Glutathione S-transferase induction. Fresh leaf was inactive on *Spodoptera frugiperda*[DC210].

Glutathione S-transferase inhibition. Water extract of the fresh root, administered intragastrically to infant mice at a dose of 50 mL/kg, was active. The treatment was administered for 7 successive days followed by a single dose of 20% v/v CCl$_4$ in olive subcutaneously at 1 mL/kg on the last day, 1 hour after the administration of the carrot extract[DC074].

Goitrogenic activity. Fresh root, in the ration of rats at a dose of 9 g/day for 26 days, was active[DC204].

Hemagglutinin activity. Saline extract of the dried seed, at a concentration of 10%, was active on the human red blood cells[DC202].

Hypocholestrolemic activity. Fresh root, taken orally by human adults at a dose of 200 g/person, was active. Daily ingestion at breakfast for 3 weeks decreased cholesterol in serum by 11%, increased fecal bile acid and fat excretion by 50%, and increased stool weight by 25%[DC163].

Hypoglycemic activity. Dried leaf, in the ration of male mice at a concentration of 6.25% of the diet for 28 days, was inactive vs streptozotocin-induced hyperglycemia[DC140]. Ether extract of the fresh root, administered subcutaneously to dogs, rabbits, and human adults, was active[DC025].

Hypotensive activity. Essential oil, administered intravenously to dogs at a dose of 3 µL/kg, was active. The ethanol (70%) extract, administered intravenously to dogs at a dose of 75 mg/kg, was active. There was a dip followed by rise in blood pressure[DC141]. Ethanol (80%) extract of the aerial parts, at a dose of 10 mg/kg, was not blocked by atropine. The extract did not inhibit pressor response of norepinephrine either[DC081]. Ethanol (95%) extract of the seed, administered intravenously to dogs at a dose of 10 mg/kg, produced a transient effect that was blocked by atropine[DC020]. Petroleum ether fraction chromatographed and fraction eluted with chloroform, administered intravenously to rabbits at a dose of 0.80 mg/kg, was inactive[DC226]. Methanol extract, administered intravenously to dogs and rabbits at a

dose of 2–5 mg/kg, was inactive[DC221]. Seed essential oil, administered intravenously to dogs at a concentration of 4 µL/kg, was active[DC141].

Immunostimulant activity. Fresh plant juice, in the ration of female mice, was active in ovalbumin-sensitized mice[DC116]. Water extract of the dried root, taken orally by human adults, was active. A pharmaceutical solution containing fruit bodies of *Tremella fuciformis, Daucus carota* root, *Astragalus mongholicus* root and *Zizyphus jujuba* fruits, honey, vitamin A palmitate, zinc sulfate, and vitamin C is claimed useful as an immunostimulant for controlling AIDS, cancer, and infections[DC139].

Inotropic effect (negative). Ethanol (80%) extract of the aerial parts, at a concentration of 0.3 mg/mL, was active on the guinea pig atrium[DC081].

Inotropic effect (positive). Ethanol (95%) extract of the seed, at a concentration of 4 mg/mL, was active on the perfused frog heart[DC020].

Insecticidal activity. Water extract of the dried root, at variable concentrations, was inactive on *Blatella germanica* and *Oncopeltus fasciatus,* and a dose of 40 mg/kg, administered intravenously, was inactive on *Periplaneta americana*[DC242].

Interferon induction stimulation. Fresh plant juice, in cell culture, was active on mice splenocytes[DC116].

Interleukin-4 release inhibition. Fresh plant juice, in cell culture, was active on mice splenocytes[DC116].

Lipid peroxidase inhibition. Water extract of the fresh root, administered intragastrically to infant mice at a dose of 50 mL/kg, was active. The treatment was administered for 7 successive days followed by a single dose of 20% v/v CCl$_4$ in olive subcutaneously at 1 mL/kg on the last day, 1 hour after the administration of the carrot extract[DC074].

Lipid peroxide formation inhibition. Fresh fruit juice, taken orally by human adults at a dose of 16 mg of β carotene/person, was active[DC094]. Hot water extract of the fresh leaf produced strong activity vs *t*-butyl hydroperoxide/heme-induced luminol-enhanced chemiluminescence[DC070]. Hot water extract of the fresh root produced weak activity vs *t*-butylhydroperoxide/heme-induced luminol-enhanced chemiluminescence[DC070].

Liver regeneration stimulation. Seed essential oil, administered subcutaneously to partially hepatectomized male rats at a dose of 100 mg/animal daily for 7 days, was inactive[DC176].

Luteal suppressant effect. Petroleum ether extract of the dried seed, administered subcutaneously to female rats at a dose of 0.6 mL/animal, was active[DC164].

Mutagenic activity. Methanol extract of the fresh root, on agar plate, was inactive on *Salmonella typhimurium* TA98 and TA100[DC162]. Root juice, on agar plate at a dose of 200 μL/mL, produced weak activity on *Salmonella typhimurium* TA100 and a dose of 400 μL/mL was inactive on *Salmonella typhimurium* TA98[DC051].

Nematocidal activity. Water extract of the dried fruit, in cell culture at a concentration of 10 mg/mL, and methanol extract at a concentration of 1 mg/mL, were active on *Toxacara canis*[DC105].

Oviposition stimulation. Ethanol (95%) extract of the aerial parts was active on black swallowtail butterfly[DC129].

Ovulation inhibition effect. Water, ethanol (95%), and petroleum ether extracts of the seed, administered orally to rabbits at a dose of 100 mg/kg, were inactive[DC005].

Pheromone effect (sex attractant). Water extract of the root was active on *Costelytra zealandica*[DC043].

Progesterone synthesis inhibition. Fresh root, on the perfused ovaries of rabbits fed a carrot-rich diet, was active[DC049].

Pro-oxidant activity. The root, at a concentration of 1%, was active at 120° F on peanut oil[DC096].

Protein synthesis inhibition. Buffer of the fresh root produced weak activity, IC_{50} 158 μg protein/mL[DC086].

Quinone reductase induction. Acetonitrile extract of the dried root, in cell culture at a concentration of 7.9 mg/g, was active on Hematoma-Mouse-ICIC7. The sample was assayed for the induction of detoxifying enzymes that may have anticarcinogenic activity[DC079].

Sister chromatid exchange inhibition. Fresh root juice, in the drinking water of rats at a dose of 300 mL animal, was active on Chinese hamster ovary cells. The plasma from the rats treated with carrot juice and cyclophoshamide reduced sister chromatid exchange in DNA-repair-deficient and in normal human lymphocytes in the Chinese hamster ovary cells when compared to cyclophoshamide treated only[DC128].

Skeletal muscle relaxant activity. Petroleum ether fraction chromatographed and fraction eluted with chloroform, at a concentration of 0.50 mg/mL, was inactive on the frog rectus abdominus muscle vs ACh-induced contractions[DC226].

Skeletal muscle stimulant activity. Ethanol (95%) extract of the seed, at a concentration of 10 mg/mL, was inactive on frog rectus abdominus muscle[DC020].

Smooth muscle relaxant activity. Alkaloid fraction (tertiary) of the dried seed, at a concentration of 25 μg/mL was active on the rabbit and rat ileum[DC166].

Spasmogenic activity. Ethanol (95%) extract of the seed, at a concentration of 1.5 mg/mL, was active on the dog tracheal chain. The extract, at a concentration of 1 mg/mL, was active on the guinea pig, rabbit, and rat ileum. The activity was equal to approx 0.1 μg/mL of acetylcholine. The action was blocked by atropine[DC020].

Spasmolytic activity. Ethanol (80%) extract of the aerial parts, at a concentration of 3 mg/mL, was active on the rabbit aorta vs K+-induced contractions[DC081].

Toxicity assessment. Ethanol (50%) extract of the root, administered intraperitoneally to mice, produced LD$_{50}$ 500 mg/kg[DC013].

Tumor promotion inhibition. Methanol extract of the dried leaf, in cell culture at a concentration of 200 μg/disc, was inactive on EBV vs 12-O-hexadecanoylphorbol-13-acetate-induced EBV activation[DC217].

Uterine relaxation effect. Alkaloid fraction of the dried seed, at a concentration of 25 μg/mL, was active on the rat uterus[DC166]. Methanol extract of the dried seed, at a concentration of 0.5 mg/mL, was equivocal[DC221]. Petroleum ether fraction of the seed, chromatographed and fraction eluted with chloroform, at a concentration of 0.50 mg/mL, was active on the nonpregnant rat uterus vs oxytocin-induced contractions[DC226].

Uterine stimulant effect. Petroleum ether fraction of the seed, chromatographed and fraction eluted with chloroform, at a concentration of 0.5 mg/mL, was active on the nonpregnant rat uterus vs oxytocin-induced contractions[DC226]. Ethanol (95%) extract of the seed, at a concentration of 1 mg/mL, was inactive on the rat uterus. The amplitude was diminished but not the tone[DC020].

Vasodilator activity. Alkaloid fraction (tertiary) of the dried seed, administered to frog by perfusion at a dose of 2.5 mg/kg, was active vs barium chloride-induced vasoconstriction[DC166].

White blood cell stimulant. Root juice, administered intraperitoneally to mice at a dose of 0.2 mL/animal, increased neutrophil accumulation by 71%[DC066].

White blood cell-macrophage stimulant. Water extract of the freeze-dried root, at a concentration of 2 μg/mL, was inactive. Nitrite formation was used as an index of the macrophage stimulating activity[DC138].

REFERENCES

DC001 Quisumbing, E. Medicinal plants of the Philippines. Department of Agriculture and Natural Resources Tech Bull 16, Manila; 1951.

DC002 Ferrando, R., M. M. Guilleux, and A. Guerrillot-Venet. Oestrogen content of plants as a function of conditions of culture. **Nature** 1961; 192: 1205.

DC003 Ahmad, Y. S. A note of the plants of the medicinal value found in Pakistan. Govt of Pakistan Press, Karachi 1957.

DC004 Walker, B. S., and J. C. Janney. Estrogenic substances. II. An analysis of plant sources. **Endocrinology** 1930; 389.

DC005 Kapoor, M., S. K. Garg, and V. S. Mathur. Antiovulatory activity of five indigenous plants in rabbits. **Indian J Med Res** 1974; 62: 1225–1227.

DC006 Garg, S. K., and V. S. Mathur. Effects of chromatographic fractions of *Daucus carota* (seeds) on fertility in female albino rats. **J Reprod Fertil** 1972; 31: 143.

DC007 Fitzpatrick, F. K. Plant substances active against *Mycobacterium tuberculosis*. **Antibiot Chemother** 1954; 4: 528.

DC008 Saha, J. C., E. C. Savini, and S. Kasinathan. Ecbolic properties of Indian medicinal plants. Part I. **Indian J Med Res** 1961; 49: 130–151.

DC009 Rageau, J. Les plantes medicinales de la Nouvelle Caledonie. Trav & Doc de Lorstom No 23, Paris 1973.

DC010 Hilton-Simpson, M. W. Arab medicine and surgery. Oxford Univ Press, Humphrey Milford, London, 1922.

DC011 Jochle, W. Menses-inducing drugs: their role in Antique, Medieval and Rennaissance gynecology and birth control. **Contraception** 1974; 10: 425–439.

DC012 Krochmal, A., and C. Krochmal. Medicinal plants of the United States. Quadrangle, the New York Times Book Co., New York 1973.

DC013 Bhakuni, D. S., M. L. Dhar, B. N. Dhawan, B. Gupta, and R. C. Srimali. Screening of Indian plants for biological activity. Part III. **Indian J Exp Biol** 1971; 9: 91.

DC014 Hooper, D., and H. Field. Useful plants and drugs of Iran and Iraq. **Field Mus Hist Publ Bot Ser** 1937; 9(3): 73.

DC015 Ferrando, R., M. M. Guilleux, and A. Guerillot-Vinet. Estrogen content of wheat, carrots and grass hay. **C R Seances Soc Biol Ses Fil** 1963; 157: 1024.

DC016 Ferrando, R., M. M. Guilleux, and A. Guerillot-Vinet. Influence of manures in the soil on the estrogen content of plants (wheat and carrot). **Bull Acad Nat Med (Paris)** 1961; 145: 598.

DC017 Culpeper, N. Culpeper's complete herbal. W. Fulsham + Co., Ltd., London 1650.

DC018 Gambhir, S. S., A. K. Sanyal, S. P. Sen, and P. K. Das. Studies on *Daucus carota*. Part II. Cholinergic activity of the quaternary base isolated from water-soluble fraction of alcoholic extract of seeds. **Indian J Med Res** 1966; 54: 1053.

DC019 Watt, J. M., and M. G. Breyer-Brandwijk. The medicinal and poisonous plants of southern and eastern Africa. 2nd ed, E. + S. Livingstone, Ltd., London 1962.

DC020 Gambhir, S. S., A. K. Sanyal, S. P. Sen, and P. K. Das. Studies on *Daucus carota*. Part I. Pharmacological studies with the water-soluble fraction of the alcoholic extract of the seeds: a preliminary report. **Indian J Med Res** 1966; 54: 178.

DC021 Burlage, H. M. Index of the plants of Texas with reputed medicinal and poisonous properties. Published by author 1968.

DC022 Rao, C. N. True Vitamin A Value of Some Vegetables. **J Nutr Diet** 1967; 4: 10.

DC023 Chu, J. H., and T. C. Lee. The constituents of Chinese drug, hu-lo-po-tze the seeds of *Daucus carrota* L. **Yao Hsueh Hsuehh Pao** 1953; 1: 75–77.

DC024 Coxon, D. T., R. F. Curtis, K. R. Price, and G. Levett. Abnormal metabolites produced by *Daucus carota* roots stored under conditions of stress. **Phytochemistry** 1973; 12: 1881–1885.

DC025 Franke, M., S. Malczynski, B. Giedosz, and J. Onysymow. Hypoglycemic action of a carrot extract. **C R Soc Biol** 1934; 115: 1363–1366.

DC026 Gottshall, R. Y., E. H. Lucas, A. Lickfeldt, and J. M. Roberts. The occurrence of antibacterial substances active against *Mycobacterium tuberculosis* in seed plants. **J Clin Invest** 1949; 28: 920–923.

DC027 Suzuki, Y. Purification, and properties of carrot exo-polygalacturonase. Abstr 3rd Congress of the Federation of Asian and Oceanian Biochemists; POS02-005, Bangkok, Thailand, 1983.

DC028 Thuleau, P., A. Graziana, R. Ranjeva, and J. I. Schroeder. Solubilized proteins from carrot (*Daucus carota* L.) membranes bind calcium channel blockers and form calcium-permeable ion channels. **Proc Nat Acad Sci (USA)** 1993; 90: 765–769.

DC029 Mazzoni, V., F. Tomi, and J. Casanova. A daucane-type sesquiterpene from *Daucus carota* seed oil. **Flavour Franrance** 1999; 14(5): 268–272.

DC030 Rhodes, B. B., and C. V. Hall. Effects of CPTA 2-(4-chlorophenyltio)-triethylamine hydrochloride, temperature, and genotype on carotene synthesis in carrot leaves. **Hortscience** 1975; 10: 22.

DC031 Knypl, J. S., K. M. Chylinska, and M. W. Brzeski. Increased level of chlorogenic acid and inhibitors of indole-3-acetic acid oxidase in roots of carrot infested with the northern root-knot nematode. **Physiol Plant Pathol** 1975; 6: 51.

DC032 Brown, S. O., Hamilton, R. J., and S. Shaw. Hydrocarbons from seeds. **Phytochemistry** 1975; 14: 2726.

DC033 Cheema, A. S., R. S. Dhillon, B. C. Gupta, B. R. Chhabra, and P. S. Kalsi. Chemical investigation of the terpenoids from *Daucus carota*. **Riechst Aromen Koerperpflegem** 1975; 25: 138.

DC034 Sugano, T., T. Tanaka, E. Yamamoto, and A. Nishi. Behaviour of phenylalanine ammonia-lyase in carrot cells in suspension cultures. **Phytochemistry** 1975; 14: 2435–2436.

DC035 Behari, M., and C. K. Andhival. Chemical investigation of the seeds of *Daucus carota*. **Indian J Chemist** 1975; 13: 639A.

DC036 Neuman, K. H., A. Schafer, and J. Blaschke. Investigation on differentiation and enzyme activity of carrot tissue cultures. **Planta Med Suppl** 1975; 188.

DC037 Sarkar, S. K., and Phan Chon Ton. Biosynthesis of 6-hdroxy-8-methoxy-3-methyl-3,4-dihydroisocoumarin and 5-hydroxy-7-methoxy-2-methylchromone in carrot root tissues treated with ethylene. **Physiol Plant** 1975; 33: 108.

DC038 Okamura, S., K. Sueki, and A. Nishi. Physiological changes of carrot cells in suspension culture during growth and senescence. **Physiol Plant** 1975; 33: 251.

DC039 Barton, D. H. R., B. D. Brown, D. D. Ridley, D. A. Widdowson, A. J. Keys, and C. J. Leaver. The structure of daucic acid. **J Chem Soc Perkin Trans I** 1975; 2069.

DC040 Sarkar, S., and C. T. Phan. Some hydroxy-cinnamic acids of the carrot root. **Plant Sci Lett** 1974; 2: 41.

DC041 Ton, P. C., and S. K. Sarkar. Biosynthesis of isocoumarins in carrot roots tissues. Induction by substances other that ethylene and effects of metabolic inhibitors. **Rev Can Biol** 1975; 34: 23.

DC042 Kulesza, J., J. Kula, and W. Kwiatkowski. Oil of carrot seed as the source of the carotol for the synthesis of the new odoriferous compounds. **An Acad Brasil Cienc** 1972; 448: 412.

DC043 Osborne, G. O., and J. F. Boyd. Chemical antractans for larvae of Costelytra zealandica (Coleoptera, Scarabaeidae). **N Z J Zool** 1974; 1: 371.

DC044 Garg, S. K. Antifertility effect of oil from few indigenous plants on female albino rats. **Planta Med** 1974; 26: 391–393.

DC045 Dorogokuplya, A. G., S. F. Postol'nikov, E. G. Troitskaya, and L. K. Adil'gireeva. Role of carotene-containing foods in the occurrence of experimental tumors. **Alma-At Gos Med Inst Alma Ata** 1975; 153.

DC046 Kolattukudy, P. E., K. Kronman, and A. J. Poulose. Determination of structure and composition of suberin from the roots of carrot, parsnip, rutabaga, turnip, red beet and sweet potato by combined gas-liquid chromatography and mass spectrometry. **Plant Physiol** 1975; 55: 567.

DC047 Shimoi, K., S. Masuda, B. Shen, M. Furugori, and N. Kinae. Radioprotective effects of antioxidative plant flavanoids in mice. **Mutat Res** 1996; 350(1): 153–161.

DC048 Tokida, F., and Y. Yamazaki. Dentifrice containing caryophyllene and plant extracts. Patent-Japan Kokai Tokyo Koho-08 231,361 1996; 7 pp.

DC049 Keenan, D. L., A. M. Dharmarajan, and H. A. Zacur. Dietary carrot results in diminished ovarian progesterone secretion, whereas a metabolite, retinoic acid, stimulates progesterone secretion in the in vitro perfused rabbit ovary. **Fertil Steril** 1997; 68(2): 358–363.

DC050 Sakamoto, Y. Compositions containing parsley and carrot extracts and vegetable oils for controlling bad breath. Patent-Japan Kokai Tokyo Koho-09-59,138 1997; 4 pp.

DC051 Kassie, F., W. Parzefall, S. Musk, et al. Genotoxic effects of crude juice from Brassica vegetables and juices and extracts from phytopharmaceutical preparations and spices of cruciferous plants origin in bacterial and mammalian cells. **Chem Biol Interact** 1996; 102(1): 1–16.

DC052 Cao, G. H., E. Sofic, and R. L. Prior. Antioxidant capacity of tea and common vegetables. **J Agr Food Chem** 1996; 44(11): 3426–3431.

DC053 Rauscher, R., R. Edenharder, and K. L. Platt. In vitro antimutagenic and in vivo anticlastogenic effects of carotenoids and solvent extracts from fruits and vegetables rich in carotenoids. **Mutat Res** 1998; 413(2): 129–142.

DC054 Kim, O. K., A. Murakami, Y. Nakamura, and H. Okigashi. Screening of edible Japanese plants for nitric oxide generation inhibitory activities in raw 264.7 cells. **Cancer Lett** 1998; 125(1/2): 199–207.

DC055 Sudarshanakrishna, K. R., K. R. Viswanathan, H. K. Sreenath, and K. Santhanam. Extraction and assay of extensin in some vegetables. **J Food Sci Technol** 1998; 35(1): 87–89.

DC056 Tang, X., and R. Edenharder. Inhibitions of mutagenicity of 2-nitrofluorene, 3-nitrofluaranthene and 1-nitropyrene by vitamins, porphyrins and related compounds, and vegetable and fruit juices and solvent extract. **Food Chem Toxicol** 1997; 35(3/4): 373–378.

DC057 Maki, A., J. Kitajima, F. Abe, G. A Stewart, and M. F. Ryan. Isolation, identification and bioassay of chemicals affecting nonpreference carrot-root resistance to carrot-fly larva. **J Chem Ecol** 1989; 15(6): 1883–1897.

DC058 Aragozzini, F., R. Gualandris, E. Maconi, and R. Craveri. Coenzyme Q-10 in plant cell cultures. **Ann Microbiol Enzimol** 1984; 34(1): 75–81.

DC059 Majumder, P. K., and M. Gupta. Effect of the seed extract of carrot (*Daucus carota* Linn.) on the growth of Ehrlich ascites tumor in mice. **Phytoter Res** 1998: 12(8): 584–585.

DC060 Braun, G., and U. Seitz. Accumulation of caffeic, ferulic, and chlorogenic acid in relation to the accumulation of cyanidin in two lines of *Daucus carota*. **Biochem Physiol Pflanz** 1975; 168: 93.

DC061 Ikeda, T., T. Matsuoto, and M. Noguchi. Culture conditions on higher plant cells in suspension culture. Part 7. Formation of ubiquinone by tobacco plant cells in suspension culture. **Phytochemistry** 1976; 15: 568–569.

DC062 Noguchi, M., T. Matsumoto, K. Okunishi, and T. Ikeda. Production of ubiquinone 10 from callus. Patent-Japan Kokai-76 32,788 1976.

DC063 Mok, M. C., W. H. Gabelman, and F. Skoog. Carotenoid synthesis in tissue cultures of *Daucus carota*. **J Amer Soc Hort Sci** 1976; 101: 442.

DC064 Cronin, D. A., and P. Stanton. 2-methoxy-3-sec-butylpyrazine-an important contributor to carrot aroma. **J Sci Food Agr** 1976; 27: 145.

DC065 Behari, M., and C. K. Andhiwal. Amino acids in certain medicinal plants. **Acta Cienc Indica** 1976; 2(3): 229–230.

DC066 Yamazaki, M., and T. Nishimura. Induction of neutrophil accumulation by vegetable juice. **Biosci Biotech Biochem** 1992; 56(1): 150–151.

DC067 Lund, E. D., and J. H. Bruemmer. Sesquiterpene hydrocarbons in processed stored carrot sticks. **Food Chem** 1992; 43(5): 331–335.

DC068 Granado, F., B. Olmedilla, I. Blanco and E. Rojas-Hidalgo. Carotenoid composition in raw and cooked Spanish vegetables. **J Agr Food Chem** 1992; 40(11): 2135–2140.

DC068 Dwivedi, S. K., and N. K. Dubey. Potential use of the essential oil of *Trachyspermum ammi* against seed-borne fungi of guar (*Cyamopsis tetragonoloba* L. (Taub.)). **Mycopathologia** 1993; 121(2): 101–104.

DC069 Lund, E. D. Polyacetylenic carbonyl compounds in carrots. **Phytochemistry** 1992; 31(10): 3621–3623.

DC070 Maeda, H., T. Katsuki, T. Akaike, and R. Yasutake. High correlation between lipid peroxide radical and tumor-promoter effect: suspension of tumor promotion in the Epstein-Barr virus/B-lymphocyte system and scavenging of alkyl peroxide radicals by various vegetable extracts. **Jap J Cancer Res (Gann)** 1992; 83(9): 923–928.

DC071 Yasukawa, K., A. Yamaguchi, J. Arita, S. Sakurai, A. Ikeda, and M. Takido. Inhibitory effect of edible plant extracts on 12-o-tetradecanoylphorbol-13-acetate-induced ear oedema in mice. **Phytother Res** 1993; 7(2): 185–189.

DC072 De Feo, V., and F. Senatore. Medicinal plants and phytotherapy in the amalfital coast, Salerno province, Campania, southern Italy. **J Ethnofarmacol** 1993; 39(1): 39–51.

DC073 Hertog, M. G. L., P. C. H. Hollman, and M. B. Katani. Content of potentially anticarcinogenic flavanoids of 28 vegetables and 9 fruits commonly consumed in the Netherlands. **J Agr Food Chem** 1992; 40(12): 2379–2383.

DC074 Bishayee, A., and M. Chatterjee. Carrot aqueous extract protection against hepatic oxidative stress and lipid peroxidation induced by acute carbon tetrachloride intoxication in mice. **Fitoterapia** 1993; 64(3): 261–265.

DC075 Bel Rhlid, R., S. Chabot, Y. Piche, and R. Chenevert. Isolation and identification of flavanoids from RI t-DNA-transformed roots (*Daucus carota*) and their significance in vascular-arbuscular mycorrhiza. **Phytochemistry** 1993; 33(6): 1369–1371.

DC076 Zobel, A. M., and S. A. Brown. Furanocoumarins on the surface of callus cultures from species of the *Rutaceae* and *Umbelliferae*. **Can J Bot** 1993; 71(7): 966–969.

DC077 Konno, H., Y. Yamasaki, and K. Katoh. Extracellular polysaccharides from the culture medium of cell suspension cultures of carrot. **Okayama Daigaku Shigen Seibutsu, Kagaku Kenkyusho Hokoku** 1993; 1(2): 91–103.

DC078 Sato, M. Solubility and extraction of beta-carotene from carrot. **Kenkyu Kiyo Kagoshima Diagaku Kyoikugakubu Shizen Kagakuhen** 1992; 44: 103–108.

DC079 Prochaska, H. J., A. B. Santamaria, and P. Talalay. Rapid detection of inducers of enzymes that protect against carcinogens. **Proc Nat Acad Sci USA** 19923; 89: 2394–2398.

DC080 Yang, W. N., and W. Boss. Regulation of phosphatidylinositol 4-kinase by the protein activator PIK-A49. **J Biol Chem** 1994; 269(5): 3852–3857.

DC081 Gilani, A. H., F. Shaheen, and S. A. Saeed. Cardiovascular actions of *Daucus carota*. **Arch Pharm Res** 1994; 17(3): 150–153.

DC082 Ceska, O., S. K. Chaudhary, P. J. Warrington, and M. J. Ashwood-Smith. Phytoactive furocoumarins in fruit of some Umbelifers. **Phytochemistry** 1987; 26(1): 165–169.

DC083 Malamas, M., and M. Marselos. The tradition of medicinal plants in Zagori, Epirus (northwestern Greece). **J Ethnofarmacol** 1992; 37(3): 197–203.

DC084 Hattori, A., H. Migitaka, M. Ilgo, et al. Identification of melatonin in plants and its effects on plasma melatonin levels and binding to melatonin receptors in the verterbrates **Biochem Mol Biol Int** 1995; 35(3): 627–634.

DC085 Han, A., K. P. Zanewich, S. B. Rood, and D. K. Dougall. Gibberellic acid decreases anthocyanin accumulation in wild carrot cell suspension cultures but does not alter 3' nucleosidase activity. **Physiol Plant** 1994; 92(1): 47–52.

DC086 Tanaka, Y., M. Kataoka, Y. Konishi, T. Nishimune, and Y. Takagaki. Effects of vegetable foods on beta-hexosaminidase release from rat basophilic leukemia cells (RBL-2H3). **Jap J Toxicol Environ Health** 1992; 38(5): 418–424.

DC087 Shaaban, E. G., M. Abou-Karam, N. S. El-Shaer, E. D. Seif, and A. Ahmed. Flavanoids from cultivated *Daucus carota*. **Alexandria J Pharm Sci** 1994; 8(1): 5–7.

DC088 Neef, H., P. Declercq, and G. Laekeman. Hypoglycaemic activity of selected European plants. **Phytother Res** 1995; 9(1): 45–48.

DC089 Elisabetsky, E., W. Figueiredo, and G. Oliveria. Traditional Amazonian nerve tonics as antidepressant agents: *Chaunochiton kappleri*: a case study. **J Herbs Spices Med Plants** 1992; 1(1/2): 125–162.

DC090 Kameoka, H., K. Sarara, and M. Miyazawa. Components of essential oils of kakushitsu (*Daucus carota* L., and *Carpesium abrotanoides* L.). **Nippon Nogei Kagaku Kaishi** 1989; 63(2): 185–188.

DC091 De Blasi, V., S. Debrot, P. A. Menoud, L. Gendre, and J. Schowing. Amoebicidal effect of essential oils *in vitro*. **J Toxicol Clin Exp** 1990; 10(6): 361–373.

DC092 Bishayee, A., A. Sarkar ,and M. Chaterjee. Hepatoprotective activity of carrot (*Daucus carota* L.) against carbon tetrachloride intoxication in mouse liver. **J Ethnopharmacol** 1995; 47(2): 69–74.

DC093 Al-Saikhan, M. S., L. R. Howard, and J. C. Miller Jr. Antioxidant activity and total phenolics in different genotypes of potato (*Solanum tuberosum* L.). **J Etnopharmacol** 1995; 70(1): 69–74.

DC094 Abbey, M., M. Noakes, and P. J. Nestel. Dietary supplementation with orange and carrot juice in cigarette smokers lowers oxidation products in copper-oxidized low-density lipoproteins. **J Amer Diet Ass** 1995; 95(6): 671–675.

DC095 Zobel, A. M., and S. A. Brown. Furanocoumarins on the surface of callus cultures from species of the *Rutaceae* and *Umbeliferae*. **Can J Bot** 1993; 71(7): 966–969.

DC096 Gazzani, G. Anti- and pro-oxidant activity of some vegetables in the Mediterranean diet. **Riv Sci Aliment** 1994; 23(3): 413–420.

DC097 Murakami, A., S. Jiwanjiinda, K. Koshimizu, and H. Ohigashi. Screening for *in vitro* anti-tumor promoting activities of edible plants from Thailand. **Cancer Lett** 1995; 95(1/2): 137–146.

DC098 Sharma, M. P., J. Ahmad, A. Hussain, and S. Khan. Folklore medicinal plants of Mewat (Gurgaon district), Haryana, India. **Int J Pharmacog** 1992; 30(2): 135–137.

DC099 Yesilada, E., G. Honda, E. Sezik, M. Tabata, T. Fujita, T. Tanaka, Y. Takeda and Y. Takaishi. Traditional medicine in Turkey. V. Folk medicine in the inner Taurus mountain. **J Ethnopharmacol** 1995; 46(3): 133–152.

DC100 Gurib-Fakim, A., M. D. Sweraj, J. Gueho, and E. Dulloo. Medicinal plants of the Rodrigues. **Int J Pharmacol** 1996; 34(1): 133–152.

DC101 Rivera, D., and C. Obon. The ethnopharmacology of Madeira and Porto Santo Islands, a review. **J Ethnopharmacol** 1995; 46(2): 2–14.

DC102 De Feo, V., R. Aquino, A. Menghini, E. Ramundo, and F. Senatoare. Traditional phytotherapy in the Peninsula sorrentina, Campania, Southern Italy. **J Ethnopharmacol** 1992; 36(2): 113–125.

DC103 Neef, H., P. De Clercq, and G. Laekeman. Hypoglycemic activity of selected European plants. **Pharm World Sci** 1993; 15(6): H11-.

DC104 Martinez, A., I. Cambero, Y. Ikken, M. L. Marin, A. I. Haza, and P. Moralez. Protective effect of broccoli, onion, carrot, and licorice extracts against cytotoxity of N-nitrosamines evaluated by 3-(4, 5-dimethylthiazol-2-yl)-2,5-diphenyltetrazolium bromide assay. **J Agr Food Chem** 1998; 46(2): 585–589.

DC105 Kiuchi, F. Studies on the nematocidal constituents of natural medicines. **Nat Med** 1995; 49(4): 364–372.

DC106 Van Breemen, R. B. Innovations in carotenoid analysis using LC/MS. **Anal Chem** 1996; 68(9): 299–304.

DC107 Kilibarda, V., N. Nanusevic, N. Dogovic, R. Ivanic, and K. Savin. Content of the essential oil of the carrot and its antibacterial activity. **Pharmazie** 1996; 51(10): 777–7778.

DC108 Duke, J. A., and E. S. Ayensu. Medicinal plants of China. Reference Publications, Inc. Algonac, Michigan1985; 1(4): 52–361.

DC109 Heinzmann, U., and U. Seitz. Synthesis of phenylalanine ammonia-lyase in anthocyanin-containing and anthocyanin-free callus cells of *Daucus carota*. **Planta** 1977; 135: 63.

DC110 Counsell, J. N., and D. J. Roberton. Xylitol- a sweetener which is kind to the teeth. **Food Process Ind** 1976; 45(54): 24–26.

DC111 Skorikova, Y. G., and E. A. Isagulyan. Polyphenols of carrots and cucumbers. **Konservn Ovoshchesush Prom-St** 1977; 1977(2): 14.

DC112 Heinrichova, H. Isolation, characterization, and mode of action of exo-D-galacturonanase form carrot. **Collect Czech Chem Commun** 1977; 42: 3214.

DC113 Alami, R., A. Macksad, and A. R. El-Gindy. Medicinal plants in Kuwait. Al-Assiriya Printing Press, Kuwait 1976.

DC114 Gregor, H. D. Lipid composition of *Daucus carota* roots. **Phytochemistry** 1977, 16: 953–955.

DC115 Ikken, Y., I. Cambero, M. L. Marin, A. Martinez, A. I. Haza, and P. Morales. Antimutagenic effect of fruit and vegetable aqueous extracts against N-nitrosamines evaluated by the Ames test. **J Agr Food Chem** 1998; 46(12): 5194–5200.

DC116 Akiyama, H., K. Hoshino, M. Tokuzumi, R. Teshima, H. Mori, T. Inakuma, Y. Ishiguro, Y. Goda, J. I. Sawada, and M. Toyoda. The effect of feeding carrots on immunoglobulin E production and anaphylactic response in mice. **Biol Pharm Bull** 1999; 22(6): 551–555.

DC117 Majumder, P. K., S. Dasgupta, R. K. Mukhopadhaya, U. K. Mazumdar, and M. Gupta. Anti-steroidogenic activity of the petroleum ether extract and fraction 5 (fatty acids) of carrot (*Daucus carota* L.) seeds in mouse ovary. **J Ethnopharmacol** 1997; 57(3): 209–212.

DC118 Balasubramaniam, P., L. Pari, and V. P. Menon. Protective effect of carrot (*Daucus carota* L.) against lindane-induced hepatotoxicity in rats. **Phytother Res** 1998; 12(6): 434–436.

DC119 Markovic, O. Pectinusterase from carrot (*Daucus carota*). **Experientia** 1978; 34: 561.

DC120 Gregor, H. D. Lipids of *Daucus carota* cell suspension culture. **Chem Phys Lipids** 1977; 20: 77.

DC121 Khanna, P., R. Khanna, M. Sogani, and S. K. Manot. *Daucus carota* seedling callus a new source of diosgenin. **Indian J Exp Biol** 1977; 15: 586.

DC122   Bureau, J. L., and R. J. Bushway. HPLC determination of carotenoids in fruits and vegetables in the United States. **J Food Sci** 1986; 51(1): 128–130.

DC123   Ceska, O., S. K. Chaudhary, P. J. Warrington, and M. J. Ashwood-Smith. Furocoumarins in the cultivated carrot, *Daucus carota*. **Phytochemistry** 1986; 25(1): 81–83.

DC124   Kurosaki, F., K. Matsui, and A. Nishi. Production and metabolism of 6-methoxymellein in cultured carrot cells. **Physiol Plant Pathol** 1984; 25(3): 313–322.

DC125   Harborne, J. B., A. M. Mayer, and N. Bar-Nun. Identification of the major anthocyanin of carrot cells in tissue culture as cyanidin 3-(sinapoylxylosylglucosylgalactoside). **Z Naturforsch Ser** 1983; C38(11/12): 1055–1056.

DC126   Adhiwal, C. K., and K. Kishore. Some chemical constituents of the roots of *Daucus carota*, Nantes. **Indian Drugs** 1985; 22(6): 334–335.

DC127   Kaliwal, B. B., A. R. Nazeer, and A. M. Rao. Dose on temporal effect of carrot seed (*Daucus carota*) extract on pregnancy in albino rats. **Comp Physiol Ecol** 1984; 9(3): 173–177.

DC128   Darroudi, F., H. Targa, and A. T. Natarajan. Influence of dietary carrot on cytostatic drug activity of cyclophosphamine and its main directly acting metabolite: induction of sister-chromatide exchanges in normal human lymphocytes, Chinese hamster ovary cells, and their DNA repair–deficient. **Mutat Res** 1988; 198(2): 327–335.

DC129   Feeny, P., K. Sachdev, L. Rosenberry, and M. Carter. Luteolin-7-O-(6"-O-malonyl)-beta-D-glucoside and trans-chlorogenic acid: oviposition stimulants for the black swallowtail butterfly. **Phytochemistry** 1988; 27(11): 3439–3448.

DC130   Munoz, D., I. Urrutia, I. Leanizbarrutia, and L. Fernandez de Corres. Contact dermatitis from plants in a geriatric nurse. **Contact Dermatitis** 1989; 20(3): 227–228.

DC131   Dhillon, R. S., V. K. Gautam, P. S. Kalsi, and B. R. Chhabra. Carota-1,4-beta-oxide, a sesquiterpene from *Daucus carota*. **Phytochemistry** 1989; 28(2): 639–640.

DC132   Beuchat, L. R., and R. E. Brackett. Inhibitory effects of raw carrots on *Listeria monocytogenes*. **Appl Environ Microbiol** 1990; 56(6): 1734–1742.

DC133   Philippides, P., N. Katsilambros, A. Galanopulous, et al. Glycaemic response to carrot in type II diabetic patients. **Diabetes Nutr Metal Clin Exp** 1988; 1(4): 363–364.

DC134   Kilibarda, V., R. Ivanic, K. Savin, and M. Miric. Fatty oil from the fruit of wild (*Daucus carota* L. ssp. *caroto*) and cultivated carrot (*Daucus carota* L. ssp. *sativa* (Hoffm.) Arcang.). **Pharmazie** 1989; 44(2): 166–167.

DC135   Ben-Amotz, A., A. Lers, and M. Avron. Stereoisomers of beta-carotene and phytoene in the *Alga dunaliella bardawil*. **Plant Physiol** 1990; 86(4): 1286–1291.

DC136   Mallet, J. F., E. M. Gaydou, and A. Archavlis. Determination of petroselinic acid in *Umbeliferae* seed oils by combined GC and NMR spectroscopy analysis. **J Amer Oil Chem Soc** 1990; 67(10): 607–610.

DC137   Nguyan-The, C., and B. M. Lund. The lethal effect of carrot on *Listeria* species. **J Appl Bacteriol** 1991; 70(6): 479–488.

DC138   Miwa, M., Z. L. Kong, K. Shinohara, and M. Watanabe. Macrophage stimulation activity of foods. **Agr Biol Chem** 1990; 54(7): 1863–1866.

DC139   Xu, W.G. Oral immunostimulants containing vitamins and medicinal plants for controlling AIDS, cancer and infections. Patent-faming Zhuanli Shenquing Gongkai Shuomingshu CN-1, 033,939 1989; 13 pp.

DC140   Swanston-Flatt, S. K., C. Day, P. R. Flatt, B. J. Gould, and C.J. Bailey. Glycaemic effects of traditional European plant treatments for diabetes studies in normal and streptozotocin diabetic mice. **Diabetes Res** 1989; 10(2): 69–73.

DC141   Mahran, G. H., H. A. Kadry, Z. G. Isaac, C. K. Thabet, M. M. Al-Aziziz, and M. M. El-Olemy. Investigation of diuretic drug plants. 1. Phytochemical screening and pharmacological evaluation of *Anethum graveolens* L., *Apium graveolens* L., *Daucus carota* L., and *Eruca sativa*.Mill. **Phytother Res** 1991; 5(4): 169–172.

DC142 Zobel, A. M., and S. A. Brown. Psoralens on the surface of seeds of *Rutaceae* and fruits of *Umbelliferae* and *Leguminosae*. **Can J Bot** 1991; 69(3): 485–488.

DC143 Koch, L., F. Madl, P. Schlick, S., et al. Beta-carotene concentrate from carrot. Patent-Hung Teljes-55,752 1991; 12 pp.

DC144 Senalik, D., and P. W. Simon. Quantifying intra-plant variation of volatile terpenoids in carrot. **Phytochemistry** 1987; 26(7): 1975–1979.

DC145 Gunstone, F. D. The carbon-13 NMR spectra of six oils containing petroselinic acid and of aquilegia oil and meadowfoam oil which contain delta 5 acids. **Chem Phys Lipids** 1991; 58(1/2): 159–167.

DC146 Cu, J. Q., F. Perineau, M. Dealmas, and A. Gaset. Comparison of the chemical composition of carrot seed essential oil extracted by different solvents. **Flavour Fragrance J** 1989; 4(4): 225–231.

DC147 Kiuchi, F., N. Nakamura, N. Miyashita, S. Nishizawa, Y. Tsuda, and K. Kondo. Nematocidal activity of some anthelmintics, traditional medicines, and spices by a new assay method using larvae of *Toxocara canis*. **Shoyakugaku Zasshi** 1989; 43(4): 279–287.

DC148 Zaka, S., B. Asghar, and S. A. Khan. The fatty acid composition of seed oils of the Pakistani *Umbelliferae*. Part VI. *Seseli libanotis* and *Daucus carota* seed oils. **Sci Int (Lahore)** 1990; 2(4): 313–315.

DC149 Buttery, R. G., D. R. Black, W. F. Addon, L. C. Ling, and R. Teranishi. Identification of additional volatile constituents of carrot roots. **J Agr Food Chem** 1979; 27(1): 1.

DC150 Caldwekll, R. A., and J. F. Turner. Phosphofructokinase of carrot roots. **Phytochemistry** 1979; 18: 318–320.

DC151 Hilal, S. H., A. M. El Shamy, and M. Y. Haggag. A study of the volatile and fixed oils of the fruits of *Daucus carota* var. *boissieri*. **Egypt J Pharm Sci** 1975; 16: 509.

DC152 Montague, M. J., W. Koppenbrink, and E. G. Jaworski. Polyamine metabo-lism in embryogenic cells of *Daucus carota*. I. Changes in intracellular content and rates of synthesis. **Plant Physiol** 1978, 62: 430–433.

DC153 Speck, P., F. Escher, and J. Solms. Effect of salt pretreatment on quality and storage stability of air-dried carrots. **Lebensm Wiss Technol** 1977; 10: 308.

DC154 Widholm, J. Selection and characterization of a *Daucus carota* cell line resistant to four amino acid analogs. **J Exp Bot** 1978; 29: 1111.

DC155 Bender, L., and K. H. Neumann. Investigation on the indole-3-acetic acid metabolism of carrot tissue cultures (*Daucus carota*). **Z Pflanzenphysiol** 1978; 88: 209.

DC156 Stoessl, A., and J. B. Stothers. Carbon-13 NMR studies. Part 79. Postinfectional inhibitors from plants. Part XXXII. A carbon-13 biosynthetic study of stress metabolites from carrot roots: eugenin and 6 methoxymellein. **Can J Bot** 1978; 56: 2589.

DC157 Buishand, J. G., and W. H. Gabelman. Investigation on the inheritance of root color and carotenoid content in carrot, *Daucus carota*. **Diss Abstr Int B** 1978; 39: 2656.

DC158 Schaefer, A., J. R. Blaschke, and K. H. Neumann. On DNA metabolism of carrot tissue cultures. **Planta** 1978; 139: 97.

DC159 Sarkar, S. K., and C. T. Phan. Naturally-occuring and ethylene-induced phenolic compounds in the carrot root. **J Food Prot** 1979; 42: 526–534.

DC160 Salem, S., D. Linstedt, and J. Reinert. The cytokinins of cultured carrot cells. **Protoplasma** 1979; 101: 526–534.

DC161 Sasse, F., D. Backs-Husemann, and W. Barz. Isolation and characterization of vacuoles from cell suspension cultures of *Daucus carota*. **Z Naturforsch** 1979; Ser C 34: 103–109.

DC162 Takahashi, Y., M. Nagao, T. Fujino, Z. Yamaizumi, and T. Sugimura. Mutagens in Japanese pickle identified as flavanoids. **Mutat Res** 1979; 68: 117–123.

DC163 Robertson, J., W. G.Brydon, K. Tadesse, P. Wenham, A. Walls, and M. A. Eastwood. The effect of raw carrot on serum lipids and colon function. **Amer J Clin Nutr** 1979; 1889–1892.

DC164 Kaliwal, B. B., and M. A. Rao. Inhibition of implantation by carrot seed extract and its rectification by progesterone in albino rats. **J Karnatak Univ** 1977; 12: 167–172.

DC165 Misawa, M. Production of natural substances by plant cell cultures described in Japanese patents. Plant Tissue Culture its Bio-technol Appl Int Congr 1st 1977; 17–26.

DC166 Gambhir, S. S., S. P. Sen, A. K. Sanyal, and P. K. Das. Antispasmodic activity of the tertiary base of *Daucus carota* Linn. seeds. **Indian J Physiol Pharmacol** 1979; 23: 225–228.

DC167 Anon. Antifertility agents. **Ann Rep Central Drug Res Inst, Lucknow, India** 1978; 1–10.

DC168 Sugano, N., K. Koide, Y. Ogawa, Y. Moriya, and A. Nishi. Increase in enzyme levels during the formation of phenolic acids in carrot cell cultures. **Phytochemistry** 1978; 17: 1235–1237.

DC169 Chaudhury, R. R. Controversies in the clinical evaluation of antifertility plants. Clinical Pharmacology &Therapeutics, P. Turner (ed.), Macmillan, New York, 1980; pp. 474–482.

DC170 El-Moghazi, A. M., S. A. Ross, A. F. Halim, and A. Abou-Rayya. Flavanoids of *Daucus carota*. **Planta Med** 1980; 40: 382–383.

DC171 Dung, J. Y., L. C. Hsu, S. W. Zhu, and Y. Zhou. Studies on the anti-fertility constituents in carrot seeds (*Daucus carota* L.). **Chung Ts'ao Yao** 1981; 12(2): 13.

DC172 Andhiwal, C. K., K. Kishore, and J. A. Ballantine. Hydrocarbons, alcohol and phytosterols from the leaves of *Daucus carota*, Nantes. **J Indian Chem Soc** 1980; 57: 1044–1045.

DC173 Lozoya, X. Mexican medicinal plants used for treatment of cardiovascular diseases. **Amer J Chinese Med** 1980; 8: 86–95.

DC174 Khafagy, S. M., Sabri, N. N., and A. H. A. Donia. Chemical characterization and preliminary pharmacological screening of the bitter principle isolated from *Daucus carota* L. *var. boissieri* Schweinf. growing in Egypt. **J Drug Res (Egypt)** 1979; 11; 115–120.

DC175 Ivie, G. W., D. L. Holt, and M. C. Ivey. Natural toxicants in human foods: psoralens in raw and cooked parsnip root. **Science** 1981; 213: 909–910.

DC176 Gershbein, L. L. Regeneration of rat liver in the presence of essential oils and their components. **Food Cosmet Toxicol** 1977; 15: 173–182.

DC177 Gupta, K. R., and G. S. Nintanjan. A new flawone glycoside from seeds of *Daucus carota*. **Planta Med** 1982; 46: 240–241.

DC178 Ivie, G. W., R. C. Beier, and D. L. Holt. Analysis of the garden carrot (*Daucus carota* L.) for linear furocoumarins (psoralens) at the sub parts per million level. **J Agr Food Chem** 1982; 30(3): 413–416.

DC179 Yates, S. G., and R. E. England. Isolation and analysis of carrot constituents: myristicin, falcarinol, and falcarindiol. **J Agr Food Chem** 1982; 30(2): 317–320.

DC180 Ramstorpa, M., P. Carlsson, D. Bratthall, and B. Mattiasson. Isolation and partial characterization of a substance from carrots, *Daucus carota* with ability to agglutinate cells of *Streptococcus* mutants. **Caries Res** 1982; 16: 423–427.

DC181 Storey, R., and R. G. Wyn Jones. Quaternary ammonium compounds in plants in relation to salt resistance. **Phytochemistry** 1977; 16: 447–453.

DC182 Krag, K. J. Plants used as contraceptives by the North American Indians. An ethnobotanic study. **Thesis-by-Harvard University** 1976; 117 pp.

DC183 Duehrssen, E., and K. H. Neumann. Characterization of satellite DNA of *Daucus carota* L. **Z Pflanzenphysiol** 1980; 100: 447–454.

DC184 Hemingson, J. C., and R. P. Collins. Anthocyanins present in cell cultures of *Daucus carota*. **J Nat Prod** 1982; 45(4): 385–389.

DC185 Kaliwal, B. B., and M. A. Rao. Effect of carrot seed (*Daucus carota*) extract on estrous cycle as compared with that of estradiol-17-beta in albino rats. **Comp Physiol Ecol** 1983; 8(2): 101–104.

DC186 Kaliwal, B. B., and M. A. Rao. Inhibition of ovarian compensatory hypertrophy by carrot seed (*Daucus carota*) extract of estradiol-17beta in hemicastrated albino rats. **Indian J Exp Biol** 1981; 19: 1058–1060.

DC187   Kaliwal, B. B., and M. A. Rao. Dose and durational effect of carrot seed extract (*Daucus carota*) on implantation in albino rats. **Comp Physiol Ecol** 1979; 4: 92–97.

DC188   Lal, S. D., and B. K. Yadav. Folk medicine of Kurukshetra district (Haryana), India. **Econ Bot** 1983; 37(3): 299–305.

DC189   Makaranko, P. N., and E. P. Komissarenko. Daukarin. Patent-USSR-1,012, 910 1983.

DC190   Ross, S. A., S. E. Megalla, D. W. Bishay, and A. H. Awad. Studies for determining antibiotic substances in some Egyptian plants. Part I. Screening for antimicrobial activity. **Fitoterapia** 1980; 51: 303–308.

DC191   Razzack, H. M. A. The concept of birth control in Unani medical literature. Unpublished manuscript of author. 1980; 64 pp.

DC192   Batt, C., M. Solberg, and M. Ceponis. Effect of volatile components of carrot seed oil on growth and aflatoxin production by *Aspergillus parasiticus*. **J Food Sci** 1983; 48(3): 762–764.

DC193   Kurosaki, F., and A. Nishi. Isolation and antimicrobial activity of the phytoalexin 6-methoxymellein from cultured carrot cells. **Phytochemistry** 1983; 22(3): 669–672.

DC194   Noe, W., and H. U. Seitz. Studies on the regulatory role of trans-cinnamic acid on the activity of the phenylalanine ammonia-lyase(pal)in suspension cultures of *Daucus carota* L. **Z Naturforsch Ser C** 1983; 38(5/6): 408–412.

DC195   Kleiman, F., and G. F. Spencer. Search for new industrial oils: 16. *Umbelliflorae*-seed oils rich in petroselinic acid. **J Amer Oil Chem Soc** 1982; 59: 29–32.

DC196   Kleinig, H., and C. Kopp. Lipids, lipid turnover, and phospholipase D in plant suspension culture cells (*Daucus carota*). **Planta** 1978; 139(1): 61–65.

DC197   Barale, R., D. Zucconi, R. Bertani, and N. Loprieno. Vegetables inhibit, *in vivo*, the mutagenicity of nitrite combined with nitrosable compounds. **Mutat Res** 1983; 120(2/3): 145–150.

DC198   Hooper, S. N., and R. F. Chandler. Herbal remedies of the maritime Indians: phytosterols and triterpenes of 67 plants. **J Ethnopharmacol** 1984; 10(2): 181–194.

DC199   Neurath, G. B., M. Dunger, F. G. Pein, D. Ambrosius, and O. Schreiber. Primary and secondary amines in the human environment. **Food Cosmet Toxicol** 1977; 15: 275–282.

DC200   Stevens, B. J. H., and R. R. Selvendran. Structural features of cell-wall polysaccharides of the carrot *Daucus carota*. **Carbohydr Res** 1984; 128(2): 321–333.

DC201   Prakash, A. O. Biological evaluation of some medicinal plant extracts for contraceptive efficacy. **Contraceptive Delivery Systems** 1984; 5(3): 9–10.

DC202   Hardman, J. T. M. L. Beck, and C. E. Owensby. Range form lectins. **Transfusion** 1983; 23(6): 519–522.

DC203   Ishii, R., K. Yoshikawa, H. Minakata, H. Komura, and T. Kada. Specifities of bio-antimutagens in plant kingdom. **Agr Biol Chem** 1984; 48(10): 2587–2591.

DC204   Sarkar, S. R., L. R. Singh, B. P. Uniyal, S. K. Mukherjee, and K. K. Nagpal. Effect of common vegetables on thyroid funtions in rats-a preliminary study. **Def Sci J** 1983; 33(4): 317–321.

DC205   Kaliwal, B. B., R. Nazeer Ahamed, and M. Appaswamy Rao. Abortifacient effect of carrot seed (*Daucus carota*) extract and its reversal by progesterone in albino rats. **Comp Physiol Ecol** 1984; 9(1): 70–74.

DC206   Woo, W. S., E. B. Lee, K. H. Shin, S. S. Kang, and H. J. Chi. A review of research on plants for fertility regulation in Korea. **Korean J Pharmacog** 1981; 12(3): 153–157.

DC207   Singh, Y. N. Traditional medicine in Fiji: some herbal folk cures used by Fiji Indians. **J Ethnopharmacol** 1986; 15(1):57–88.

DC208   Darias, V., L. Bravo, E. Barquin, D. M. Herrera, and C. Fraile. Contributions to the ethnopharmacological study on the Canary Islands. **J Ethnopharmacol** 1986; 15(2): 169–193.

DC209   Lal, R., M. Gandhi, A. Sankaranarayanan, V. S. Mathur, and P. L. Pharma. Antifertility effect of *Daucus carota* seeds in female albino rats. **Fitoterapia** 1986; 67(4): 243–246.

DC210   Yu, S.J. Interactions of allelochemicals with detoxication enzymes of insecticide-susceptible and resistant fall armyworms. **Pestic Biochem Physiol** 1984; 22: 60–68.

DC211 Osawa, T., H. Ishibashi, M. Namiki, T. Kada, and K. Tsuji. Desmutagenic action of food components on mutagens formed by the sorbic acid nitrite reaction. **Agr Biol Chem** 1986; 50(8): 1971–1977.

DC212 Guerin, J. C., and H. P. Reveillere. Antifungal activity of plant extracts used in therapy. II. Study of a 40 plant extracts against 9 fungi species. **Ann Pharm Fr** 1985; 43(1): 77–81.

DC213 Yamaguchi, T., Y. Yamashita, and T. Abe. Desmutagenic activity of peroxidase on autoxidised linolenic acid. **Agr Biol Chem** 1980; 44(4): 959–961.

DC214 Kant, A., D. Jacob, and N. K. Lohiya. The estrogenic efficacy of carrot (*Daucus carrota*) seeds. **J Adv Zool** 1986; 7(1): 36–41.

DC215 Shinohara, K., S. Kuroki, M. Miwa, Z. L. Kong, and H. Hosoda. Antimutagenicity of dialyzates of vegetables and fruits. **Agr Biol Chem** 1988; 52(6): 1369–1375.

DC216 Yokel, R. A., and C. D. Ogzewalla. Effects of plant ingestion in rats determined by the conditioned taste aversion procedure. **Toxicon** 1981; 19(2): 223–232.

DC217 Koshimizu, K., H. Ohigashi, H. Tokuda, A. Kondo, and K. Yamaguchi. Screening of edible plants against possible anti-tumor promoting activity. **Cancer Lett** 1988; 39(3): 247–257.

DC218 Ramirez, V. R., L. J. Mostacero, A. E. Garcia, C. F. Mejia, P. F. Pelaez, C. D. Medina, and C. H. Miranda. Vegetales empleados en medicina tradicional norperuana. Banco Agrario del Peru & Nacl Univ Trujillo, Trujillo, Peru, June 1988; 54 pp.

DC219 Singh, V. P., S. K. Sharma, and V. S. Khare. Medicinal plants from Ujjain district Madhya Pradesh- part II. **Indian Drugs Pharm Ind** 1980; 1980(5): 7–12.

DC220 Ratka, P., and T. Sloboda. Phototoxic reaction from vegetables. **Contact Dermatitis** 1986; 15(1): 39–40.

DC221 Dhar, V.J. Studies on *Daucus carota* seeds. **Fitoterapia** 61(3): 255–258.

DC222 Antonone, R., F. de Simone, P. Morrica, and E. Ramundo. Traditional phytotherapy in the Roccamonfina volcanic group, Campania, southern Italy. **J Ethnopharmacol** 1988; 22(3): 295–306.

DC223 Kaliwal, B. B. Efficacy of carrot seed (*Daucus carota*) extract in inhibiting implantation and its reversal as compared with estradiol-17-beta in albino rats. **J Curr Biosci** 1989; 6(3): 77–82.

DC224 Lokar, L. C., and L. Poldini. Herbal remedies in the traditional medicine of the Venezia Giulia region (north east Italy). **J Ethnopharmacol** 1988; 22(3): 231–239.

DC225 Dhar, V. J. S. K. Garg, and V. S. Mathur. Studies on the new indigenous antifertility agents. **Bull P. G. I.** 1974; 8: 72–73.

DC226 Dhar, V. J. V. S. Mathur, and S. K. Garg. Pharmacological studies on *Daucus carota*. Part I. **Planta Med** 1975; 28: 12–15.

DC227 Perrot, E., and R. R. Paris. Les plantes medicinales. Part I. Presses Universitaires dex France, Paris, France 1971.

DC228 Gawadi, A. G. The sugars of the roots of *Daucus carota*. **Plant Physiol** 1947; 22: 438.

DC229 Earle, F. R., C. A. Glass, G. C. Geisinger, I. A. Wolff, and Q. Jones. Search for new industrial oils. IV. **J Amer Oil Chem Soc** 1960; 37: 440.

DC230 Garg, S. K. Antfertility effect of some chromatographic fractions of *Daucus carota*. **Indian J Pharmacol** 1975; 7: 40–42.

DC231 Ueda, Y., H. Ishiyama, M. Fukui, and A. Nishi. Invertase in cultured *Daucus carota* cells. **Phytochemistry** 1974; 13: 383.

DC232 Wills, R. B. H., and E. V. Scurr. Mevalonic acid concentrations in fruit and vegetable tissues. **Phytochemistry** 1975; 14: 1643.

DC233 Alfermann, A. W., D. Merz, and E. Rheinhard. Induction of anthyocyanin biosynthesis in tissue cultures of *Daucus carota*. **Planta Med Suppl** 1975; 70.

DC234 Kelly, I. Folk practices in North Mexico, birth customs, folk medicine, and spiritualism in the Laguna zone.

Institute of Latin American Studies, University of Texas Press, Austin, Texas 1965; 1–166.

DC235 Abbott, B. J. J. Leiter, J. L. Hartwell, et al. Screening data from the cancer chemotherapy national service center screening laboratories. XXXIV. Plant extracts. **Cancer Res** 1966; 26: 761–935.

DC236 Behari, M., and C. K., Andhiwal. Chemical investigation of the seeds of *Daucus carota* nantes. **Indian J Chem** 1975; 13A: 639.

DC237 Dragendorff, G. Die heilpflanzen der verschiedenen volker und zeiten. F. Enke, Stuttgart 1898; 885 pp.

DC238 Sharma, M. M., G. Lal, and D. Jacob. Estrogenic and pregnancy interceptory effects of carrot, *Daucus carota* seeds. **Indian J Exp Biol** 1976; 506–508.

DC239 Nayar, S.L. Poisonous seeds of India. Part I. **J Bombay Nat Hist Soc** 1954; 52(1): 1–18.

DC240 Schramm, R. Paper chromatography of organic acids in storage roots of some *Umbelliferae*. **Acta Soc Bot Pol** 1961; 30: 285–292.

DC241 Crowden, R. K., J. B. Harborne, and V. H. Heywood. Chemosystematics of the *Umbelliferae* - a general survey. **Phytochemistry** 1969; 8: 1963–1984.

DC242 Heal, R. E., E. F. Rogers, R. T. Wallace, and O. Starnes. A survey of plants for insecticidal activity. **Lloydia** 1950; 13(1): 89–162.

DC243 Pospisilova, J., V. Toul, and R. Dupal. Rapid modification of the method of determining provitamin A in plants. **Sbornik Ceskoslov Akad Zemedel Ved** 1959; 5: 583–594.

DC244 Tipson, R. S. A qualitative test for dehydroascorbic acid. **J Amer Pharm Ass** 1945; 34: 190–192.

DC245 Herrmann, K. On the occurrence of caffeic acid and chlorogenic acid in fruits and vegetables. **Naturwissenschaften** 1956; 43: 109.

DC246 Netien, G., and J. Combet. Phenolic acids present in *in vitro* plant tissue cultures compared to the original plant. **C R Acad Sci Ser D** 1971; 272: 2491–2494.

DC247 Krishnamoorthy, V., and T. R. Seshadri. Survey of anthocyanins from Indian sources: Part III. **J Sci Ind Res-B** 1962; 21: 591–593.

DC248 Herrmann, K. Oxidative enzymes and phenolic substrate in vegetables and fruit. I. Hydroxycinnamic acids. **Z Lebensm-Unters Forsch** 1957; 106: 341–348.

DC249 Anon. The Herbalist. Hammond Book Company, Hammond Indiana 1931; 400 pp.

DC250 Liebstein, A. M. Therapeutic effects of various food articles. **Amer Med** 1927; 33: 33–38.

DC251 Greer, M. A., and E. B. Astwood. The antithyroid effect of certain foods in man as determined with radioactive iodine. **Endocrinology** 1948; 43: 105–119.

DC252 Kubas, J. Investigations on known or potential antitumoral plants by means of microbiological tests. Part III. Biological activity of some cultivated plant species in *Neurospora crassa* test. **Acta Biol Cracov Ser Bot** 1972; 15: 87–100.

DC253 Bellakhdar, J., R. Claisse, J. Fleurentin, and C. Younos. Repertory of standard herbal drugs in the Moroccan Pharmacopoea. **J Ethnopharmacol** 1991; 35(2): 123–143.

DC254 Boukef, K., H. R. Souissi, and G. Balansard. Contribution to the study on plants used in traditional medicine in Tunisia. **Plant Med Phytother** 1982; 16(4): 260–278.

DC255 Badria, F. A. Is man helpless against cancer? An environmental approach: Antimutagenic agents from Egyptian food and medicinal preparations. **Cancer Lett** 1994; 84(1): 1–5.

DC256 Garg, S. K., V. S. Mathur, and R. R. Chaudhury. Screening of Indian plants for antifertility activity. **Indian J Exp Biol** 1978; (16): 1077–1079.

DC257 Burbott, A. J., R. Croteau, W. E. Shine, and W. D. Loomis. Biosynthesis of cyclic monoterpenes by cell freee extracts of *Mentha piperita*. Int Congr Essent Oils (PAP) 6th Allured Publ Corp Oak Park, Ill 1974; 17: 1.

6 | Ferula assafoetida

L.

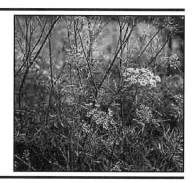

Common Names

Anjadana	Pakistan	Hing	Bangladesh
Asafetida	England	Hing	India
Asafetida	Croatia	Hingu	India
Asafetida	Finland	Ingu	India
Asafetida	Germany	Inguva	India
Asafetida	Guyana	Kama I anguza	Afghanistan
Asafetida	Iceland	Kama I anguza	Pakistan
Asafetida	Lithuania	Kayam	India
Asafetida	Netherlands	Ma ha hing	Laos
Asafetida	Poland	Merde du diable	France
Asafetida	Russia	Mvuje	Mozambique
Asafetida	Spain	Mvuje	Tanzania
Asafetida	Sweden	Mvuje	Zaire
Asafetida	United States	Ordoggyoker	Hungary
Asafetide	France	Perungayam	India
Asafootida	Estonia	Perunkaya	India
Asafotida	Germany	Perunkayan	Sri Lanka
Asant	Germany	Pirunpaska	Finland
Assa Foetida	France	Pirunpihka	Finland
Assafetida	Italy	Raamathan	India
A-wei	China	Rechina fena	Iran
Aza	Greece	Sagapeen	Netherlands
Devil's dung	United States	Setan bokosu	Turkey
Djoflatao	Iceland	Seytan tersi	Turkey
Driveldrikis	Latvia	Sheingho	Myanmar
Duivelsdrek	Netherlands	Shing-kun	Tibet
Dyvelsdrak	Denmark	Stinkasant	Germany
Dyvelsdrekk	Norway	Stinking gum	United States
Dyvelstrack	Sweden	Teufelsdreck	Germany
Ferule persique	France	Velna suds	Latvia
Godenvoedsel	Netherlands	Zapaliczka cuchnaca	Poland
Hajupihka	Finland	Zaz	Iran
Hengu	India		

From: *Medicinal Plants of the World, vol. 3: Chemical Constituents, Traditional and Modern Medicinal Uses*
By: I. A. Ross © Humana Press Inc., Totowa, NJ

BOTANICAL DESCRIPTION

Ferula assafoetida is an herbaceous, mono-ecious, perennial plant of the UMBEL-LIFERAE family. It grows to 2 m high with a circular mass of leaves. Flowering stems are 2.5–3 m high and 10 cm thick, with a number of schizogenous ducts in the cortex containing the resinous gum. Stem leaves have wide sheathing petioles. Compound large umbels arise from large sheaths. Flowers are pale greenish yellow. Fruits are oval, flat, thin, reddish brown and have a milky juice. Roots are thick, massive, and pulpy. It yields a resin similar to that of the stems. All parts of the plant have the distinctive fetid smell.

ORIGIN AND DISTRIBUTION

Asafoetida is native to central Asia, eastern Iran to Afghanistan, where it grows from 600 to 1200 m above the sea level. Although not native to India, it has been used in Indian medicine and cookery for ages. Today it is grown chiefly in Iran and Afghanistan, from where it is exported to the rest of the world.

TRADITIONAL MEDICINAL USES

Afghanistan. Hot water extract of the dried gum is taken orally for hysteria and whooping cough and to treat ulcers[FA071].

Brazil. Hot water extract of the dried leaf and stem is taken orally by males as an aphrodisiac. Extract is taken orally as nerve and general tonics[FA035]. Oleoresin powder, crushed with the fingertips, is used as a condiment[FA041].

China. Decoction of the plant is taken orally as a vermifuge[FA038].

Egypt. Dried gum is applied vaginally as a contraceptive before or after coitus. Fifty-two percent of the women interviewed practiced this method, and 48% of them depended on indigenous methods and/or prolonged lactation[FA064]. Hot water extract of the dried root is taken orally as an antis-pasmodic, a diuretic, a vermifuge, and an analgesic[FA072].

Fiji. Paste made from the dried resin is applied to the chest for whooping cough. Fried *Ferula* is taken with *Allium sativum* and sugar to cleanse the new mother. Fried *Ferula*, *Piper nigrum*, and *Cinnamonum camphora* is taken orally for headache and toothache. Hot water extract of the dried resin is taken orally for upset stomach[FA056].

India. Extract of dried *Ferula assafoetida* with *Brassica alba* and rock salt is diluted with vinegar and taken orally as an abortifacient[FA057]. Hot water extract of the dried gum is taken orally as a carminative, an antispasmodic, and an expectorant in chronic bronchitis. Mixed with cayenne pepper and sweet flag, it is used as a remedy for cholera[FA070]. Exudate of the dried gum resin is eaten to prevent guinea worm disease[FA046]. Gum resin with salt and the bark juice of *Moringa pterygosperma* is used externally for stomachaches[FA052]. A dry *Lampyris noctiluca* without head is mixed with 200–300 mg of *Ferula* and taken mornings and evenings for gallstones and kidney stones. For old stones, potassium nitrate is added to the mixture[FA054]. Hot water extract of the dried resin is taken orally as an emmenagogue[FA061].

Malaysia. Gum is chewed by females for amenorrhea[FA028].

Morocco. Gum is chewed as an antiepileptic[FA037].

Nepal. Water extract of the resin is taken orally as an anthelmintic[FA036].

Saudi Arabia. Dried gum is used medicinally for whooping cough, asthma, and bronchitis[FA068].

United States. Fluid extract of the resin is taken orally as an emmenagogue, a stimulating expectorant, an anthelmintic, an aphrodisiac, and a stimulant to the brain and nerves. It is claimed to be a powerful antispasmodic[FA029].

CHEMICAL CONSTITUENTS

(*ppm unless otherwise indicated*)

(E)-3-Methylsulfinyl-2-propenyl sec-butyl disulfide: Pl[FA077]

(E)-3-Methylsulfinyloxy-2-propenyl sec-butyl disulfide: Pl[FA077]

(Z)-3-Methylsulfinyloxy-2-propenyl sec-butyl disulfide: Pl[FA077]

2,3-Dihydro-7-hydroxy-2R*,3R*-dimethyl-2-[4,8-dimethyl-3(E),7-nonadienyl]-furo[3,2-C]coumarin: Rt[FA080]

2,3-Dihydro-7-hydroxy-2R*,3R*-dimethyl-2-[4-methyl-5- (4-methyl-2-furyl)-3(E)-pentenyl]-furo[3,2-C]coumarin: Rt[FA080]

2,3-Dihydro-7-hydroxy-2R*,3R*-dimethyl-2-[4-methyl-5-(4-methyl-2-furyl)-3(E),7-pentenyl]-furo[2,3-B]chromone: Rt[FA078]

2,3-Dihydro-7-hydroxy-2R*,3R*-dimethyl-3-[4,8-dimethyl-3(E),7-nonadie nyl]-furo[3,2-C]coumarin: Rt[FA082]

2,3-Dihydro-7-hydroxy-2S*,3R*-dimethyl-2-[4,8-dimethyl-3(E),7-nonadien-6-onyl]-furo[3,2-C]coumarin: Rt[FA080]

2,3-Dihydro-7-hydroxy-2S*,3R*-dimethyl-2-[4,8-dimethyl-3(E),7-nonadienyl]-furo[2,3-B]chromone: Rt[FA078]

2,3-Dihydro-7-hydroxy-2S*,3R*-dimethyl-2-[4-methyl-5-(4-methyl-2-furyl)-3(E)-pentenyl]-furo[3,2-C]coumarin: Rt[FA080]

2,3-Dihydro-7-hydroxy-2S*,3R*-dimethyl-2-[4-methyl-5-(4-methyl-2-furyl)-3(E),7-pentenyl]-furo[2,3-B]chromone: Rt[FA078]

2,3-Dihydro-7-hydroxy-2S*,3R*-dimethyl-3-[4,8-dimethyl-3(E),7-nonadie nyl]-furo[3,2-C]coumarin: Rt[FA082]

2,3-Dihydro-7-hydroxy-2S*,3R*-dimethyl-3-[4-methyl-5-(4-methyl-2-furyl)- 3(E)-pentenyl]-furo[3,2-C]coumarin: Rt[FA082]

2,3-Dihydro-7-methoxy-2R*,3R*-dimethyl-2-[4,8-dimethyl-3(E),7-nonadienyl]-furo[3,2-C]coumarin: Rt[FA0780]

2,3-Dihydro-7-methoxy-2S*,3R*-dimethyl-2-[4,8-dimethyl-3(E),7-nonadienyl]-furo[3,2-C]coumarin: Rt[FA080]

2,3-Dihydro-7-methoxy-2S*,3R*-dimethyl-2-[4,8-dimethyl-3(E),7-nonadien-6-onyl]-furo-[3,2-C]coumarin: Rt[FA080]

2,3-Dihydro-7-methoxy-2S*,3R*-dimethyl-2-[4-methyl-5-(4-methyl-2-furyl)-3(E)-pentenyl]-furo[3,2-C]coumarin: Rt[FA080]

2,3-Dihydro-7-methoxy-2S*,3R*-dimethyl-3-[4,8-dimethyl-3(E),7-nonadie nyl]-furo]3,2-c]coumarin: Rt[FA082]

3,4,5-Trimethyl-2-(methylsulfinyloxymethyl)thiophene: Pl[FA077]

3,4,5-Trimethyl-2-thiophenecarboxylic acid: Pl[FA077]

Arabinose, L: Gum resin[FA024]

Arabinose: Gum[FA008]

Asacoumarin A: Resin 29.6[FA002]

Asacoumarin B: Resin 61.6[FA002]

Asadisulphide: Resin 46.7[FA024]

Assafoetidnol A: Rt[FA079]

Assafoetidnol B: Rt[FA079]

Asaresinotannoid A: Gum resin[FA024]

Asaresinotannoid B: Gum resin[FA024]

Asaresinotannol A: Gum[FA008]

Asaresinotannol B: Gum[FA008]

Assafoetidin: Gum resin[FA001]

Badrakemin acetate: Gum resin 1500[FA019]

Badrakemin: Gum resin 1750[FA019]

Bis(3-methylthio-2E-propenyl) disulfide: Pl[FA077]

Borneol acetate: Sd EO 9.33%[FA013]

Butyl-propenyl-disulfide, secondary: Sd EO 35.12%[FA013]

Coladonin: Gum resin 1250[FA019]

Conferol: Rt 10[FA005]

Cynaroside: Fr[FA006]

Diallyl disulfide: EO[FA010]

Diallyl sulfate: EO[FA010]

Diallyl sulfide: EO[FA010]

Dimethyl trisulfide: EO[FA015]

Disulfide, 1-(1-methyl-thio-propyl)-1-propenyl: Gum[FA016]

Disulfide, 2-butyl-3-methyl-thio-allyl: Gum[FA016]

Disulfide, 2-butyl-methyl: EO[FA015]

Disulfide, 2-butyl-propenyl: Gum[FA016]

Disulfide, di-2-butyl: EO[FA015]

Farnesiferol A: Gum resin[FA022]

Farnesiferol B: Rt 19.2[FA009], Gum resin[FA022]

Farnesiferol BC: Rt 200[FA009], Gum resin[FA023], Gum 1.67%[FA004]

Ferocolicin: Gum resin[FA001]

Feruginin: Rh 90[FA011]

Ferula assafoetida polysaccharide: Gum resin[FA020]

Ferulic acid: Gum resin[FA024], Gum[FA008], EO[FA010]

Foetidin: Rt 500[FA018], Pl[FA017]

Foetisulfide A: Pl[FA077]
Foetisulfide B: Pl[FA077]
Foetisulfide C: Pl[FA077]
Foetisulfide D: Pl[FA077]
Foetithiophene A: Pl[FA077]
Foetithiophene B: Pl[FA077]
Foliferidin: Gum resin 500[FA019]
Galactose: Gum[FA008], Gum resin[FA024]
Galbanic acid: Gum 2.06%[FA004]
Geraniol acetate: EO[FA010], Sd EO 7.71%[FA013]
Glucose: Gum[FA008,FA024]
Glucuronic acid: Gum resin[FA024]
Gummosin: Gum resin 1500[FA019],
    Rt 769.2[FA005]
Jaeschkeanadiol, 5-α-(3-4-diacetoxy-benzoyl-
    9-β-angeloxy: Rh 190[FA011]
Jaeschkeanadiol, 5-α-(3-methoxy-4-hydroxy-
    benzoyl): Rh 1200[FA011]
Jaeschkeanadiol, 5-α-(4-hydroxy-benzoyl)-9-
    β-angeloxy: Rh 260[FA011]
Jaeschkeanadiol, 5-α-(para-hydroxy-benzoyl):
    Rh 1500[FA011]
Jaeschkeanadiol, 9-β-hydroxy: Rh 470[FA011]
Jaeschkeanadiol: Rh 6100[FA011]
Kamolonol: Gum resin[FA003]
Karatavicinol: Gum resin 3000[FA019]
Linoleic acid: Sd 12.8%[FA014]
Lucuronic acid: Gum[FA008]
Luteolin: Fr[FA006]
Mogoltadone: Gum resin[FA003]
Myristic acid: Sd EO 21.23%[FA013]
Oleic acid: Sd 5.3%[FA014]
Petroselinic acid: Sd 76.5%[FA013]
Phellandrene, α: EO[FA010]
Phellandrene: Sd EO 5.48%[FA013], Gum EO
    6.4%[FA012]
Pinene, α: EO[FA010]
Pinene, β: EO[FA010]
Polyanthin: Gum resin[FA003]
Polyanthinin: Gum resin[FA003]
Prop-cis-2-enyl, 2-butyl, disulfide (R): EO[FA007]
Propenyl disulfide, sec-butyl: Gum EO
    51.9%[FA012]
Prop-trans-2-enyl, 2-butyl, disulfide: EO[FA007]
Rhamnose: Gum[FA008,FA024]
Samarcandin acetate: Gum resin 4000[FA019]
Samarcandin, epi: Rt 9.2[FA005]
Sodium ferulate: Pl[FA073]
Terpineol, α: Sd EO 12.71%[FA013]
Tetrasulfide, di-2-butyl: EO[FA015]
Trisulfide, 2-butyl-methyl: EO[FA015]
Trisulfide, di-2-butyl: EO[FA015]

Umbelliferone: Gum resin[FA021], Gum[FA008],
    EO[FA010]
Umbelliprenin, 5-hydroxy: Gum 362.5[FA004]
Umbelliprenin: Rt 23[FA005]
Umbelliprenin8-acetoxy-5-hydroxy: Gum
    175[FA004]
Umbelliprenin8-hydroxy: Gum 1550[FA004]
Umbelliprenin9-hydroxy: Gum 387.5[FA004]
Undecyl sufonyl acetic acid: Gum EO
    18.8%[FA012]

PHARMACOLOGICAL ACTIVITIES AND CLINICAL TRIALS

Allergenic activity. Oleoresin powder, administered externally to adults, was active. Reactions to patch test occurred most commonly in patients who were regularly exposed to the substance, or who already had dermatitis on the fingertips. Previously unexposed patients had few reactions (i.e., no irritant reactions)[FA041].

Antibacterial activity. Dried gum resin, on agar plate, was active on *Clostridium perfringens* and *Clostridium sporogenes*[FA030].

Anticarcinogenic activity. Dried resin, administered orally to Sprague–Dawley rats at doses of 1.25 and 2.5% w/w of the diet, produced a significant reduction in the multiplicity and size of palpable N-methyl-N-nitrosourea-induced mammary tumors, and a delay in mean latency period of tumor appearance[FA076]. Oral administration to mice increased the percentage of life span by 52.9%. Intraperitoneal administration did not produce any significant reduction in tumor growth. The extract also inhibited a two-stage chemical carcinogenesis induced by 7,12-dimethylbenzathracene and croton oil on mice skin with significant reduction in papilloma formation[FA085].

Anticholesterolemic activity. Resin, administered to rats fed an atherogenic diet, at a dose of 1.5%, failed to reduce the serum cholesterol levels[FA092].

Anticoagulant activity. Water extract of the gum, administered intravenously to dogs and rats at variable doses, was active[FA065].

Antifertility effect. A mixture of *Embella ribes* fruit, *Piper longum* fruit, borax, *Ferula* dried gum, *Piper betle*, *Polianthes tuberosa*, and *Abrus precatorius*, administered orally to female adults at a dose of 0.28 g/person starting from the second day of menstruation twice daily for 20 days, without sexual intercourse during the dosing period, produced the effect for 4 months. The biological activity reported has been patented[FA049]. Gum, administered by gastric intubation to male mice at a dose of 5 mg/kg for 32 days, was active[FA069]. Methanol extract of the resin, administered orally to Sprague–Dawley rats at a dose of 400 mg/kg daily for 10 days, prevented pregnancy in 80% of the rats. When administered as a polyvinylpyrrolidone 1:2 complex, 100% pregnancy inhibition was observed at this dose. Lower doses of the extract produced a marked reduction in the mean number of implantations. Significant activity was observed in the hexane and chloroform eluents of sulfur-containing extract in an immature rat bioassay, the methanol extract was devoid of any estrogenic activity[FA093].

Antifungal activity. Ethanol (95%) extract of the dried gum on agar plate was active[FA039]. Essential oil of rhizome, on agar plate at a concentration of 400 ppm, was active on *Microsporum gypseum* and *Trichophyton rubrum*, and produced weak activity on *Trichophyton equinum*[FA055]. Extract of asafetida, on agar plate at concentrations of 5–10 mg/mL, inhibited *Aspergillus parasiticus* aflatoxin production[FA083].

Antihepatotoxic activity. A mixture of the methanol-insoluble fraction of the dried resin, fresh garlic, curcumin, ellagic acid, butylated hydroxytoluene, and butylated hydroxyanisole, administered by gastric intubation to ducklings at a dose of 10 mg/animal, was active vs aflatoxin B1-induced hepatotoxicity[FA034].

Antihypercholesterolemic activity. Gum, administered to female rats at a concentra-

tion of 1% of diet, was inactive[FA050]. A hot mixture of *Nigella sativa*, *Commiphora myrrha*, *Ferula assafoetida*, *Aloe vera*, and *Boswellia serrata*, administered by gastric intubation to rats at a dose of 0.5 g/kg for 7 days, was active vs streptozotocin-induced hyperglycemia[FA042].

Antihyperglycemic activity. Hot water extract of the dried gum, *Nigella sativa*, *Myrrhis odorata*, and *Aloe* sp. in equal parts, administered by gastric intubation to rats at a dose of 10 mL/kg for 7 days, was active vs streptozotocin-induced hyperglycemia. Results were significant at $p < 0.05$ level[FA058]. Hot water extract of the dried gum, administered by gastric intubation to rats at a dose of 10 mL/kg for 7 days, was inactive[FA047]. A hot mixture of *Nigella sativa*, *Commiphora myrrha*, *Ferula assafoetida*, *Aloe vera*, and *Boswellia serrata*, administered by gastric intubation to rats at a dose of 0.5 g/kg for 7 days, was active vs streptozotocin-induced hyperglycemia[FA042].

Antihypertensive effect. Water extract of the dried gum resin, administered intravenously to dogs at variable doses, was active[FA067].

Anti-implantation effect. A powdered mixture of *Ferula assafoetida*, *Piper longum*, *Embella ribes*, and borax, administered orally to female adults, was active. Biological activity reported has been patented[FA027].

Anti-inflammatory effect. Ethanol (95%) extract of the resin, administered orally to two groups of 50 patients with irritable colon, was active. Results were significant at $p < 0.001$ level[FA048].

Antimutagenic activity. Water extract of the dried gum, on agar plate at a concentration of 2 mg/plate, was inactive on *Salmonella typhimurium* TA100 vs aflatoxin B1-induced mutagenesis and a concentration of 10 mg/plate, was inactive on *Salmonella typhimurium* TA98[FA032]. Asafoetida, on agar plate at a dose of 0.5 µg/plate was active on *Salmonella typhimurium* TA98 and

TA100 vs aflatoxin B1-induced mutagenesis[FA088]. Asafoetida, on agar plate, was active on *Salmonella typhimurium* TA100 and TA1535 microsomal activation-dependent mutagenicity of 2-acetamidofluorene[FA090].

Antioxidant activity. Asafetida, administered orally to Sprague–Dawley rats at doses of 1.25% and 2.5% w/w, significantly restored the level of antioxidant system, depleted by N-methyl-N-nitrosourea treatment. There was a significant inhibition in lipid peroxidation as measured by thiobarbituric acid-reactive substances in the liver of rats[FA076].

Antiparasitic activity. Oleo-gum resin from roots and stems was active on *Trichomonas vaginalis*[FA074].

Antispasmodic activity. Gum extract, administered to isolated guinea pig ileum at a dose of 3 mg/mL, produced a decrease of spontaneous contraction to $54 \pm 7\%$ of control. Exposure of precontracted ileum by acetylcholine, histamine, and KCl to *Ferula* gum extract produced a concentration-dependent relaxation. Preincubation with indomethacin, propanolol, atropine, and chlorpheniramine before exposure to the gum, did not produce any relaxation[FA075].

Antitumor activity. Water extract of the dried oleoresin, administered by gastric intubation to mice at a dose of 50 mg/animal daily for 5 days, was active on CA-Ehrlich ascites, 53% increase in life span (ILS)[FA044]. Water extract administered intraperitoneally was inactive on Dalton's lymphoma, 4.8% ILS, and CA-Ehrlich ascites, 5.5% ILS[FA044].

Antiulcerogenic activity. Colloidal solution, administered orally to rats at a dose of 50 mg/kg, 60 minutes before experiment, produced significant protection against gastric ulcers induced by 2 hours cold restraint stress, aspirin, and 4 hours pylorus ligation[FA081].

Apoptosis effect. Sodium ferulate, administered to human lymphocytes cell culture, induced apoptosis[FA073].

Carcinogenesis inhibition. Gum, administered to mice at a dose of 40 mg/g of diet, was active. The dose was inactive vs 3'-methyl-4-dimethylaminoazobenzene-induced carcinogenesis[FA033].

Cardiac depressant activity. Tincture of the gland, administered by perfusion to rabbits, produced weak activity on the heart[FA025].

Chemomodulatory influence. Asafetida, administered orally to Sprague–Dawley rats at doses of 1.25% and 2.5% w/w in diet, produced an increase in the development and differentiation of ducts/ductules and lobules and a decrease in terminal end buds as compared to both normal and N-methyl-N-nitrosourea-treated control animals. Asafetida treatment significantly reduced the levels of cytochrome P450 and b5. There was an enhancement in the activities of glutathione-S-transferase, deoxythymidine-diaphorase, superoxide desmutase, catalase, and reduced glutathione[FA076].

Central nervous (CNS) effects. Ethanol extract of the dried gum, administered orally to adults at a dose of 20 mL/person, was active[FA066].

Cytotoxic activity. Ethanol (90%) extract of the dried plant, in cell culture administered at a concentration 0.25 mg/mL, was active on human lymphocytes. The extract was active on Vero cells, effective dose (ED_{50} 0.15 mg/mL; Chinese hamster ovary (CHO) cells, ED_{50} 0.575 mg/mL; and Dalton's lymphoma, ED_{50} 0.6 mg/mL[FA040]. Water extract of the dried gum, in cell culture at a concentration of 500 µg/mL, produced weak activity on CA-mammary-microalveolar cells[FA045].

Digestive enzyme inhibition. Asafoetida, administered orally to rats at a dose of 2500 mg% for 8 weeks, decreased the levels of phosphatases and sucrase in the small intestine[FA089].

DNA synthesis inhibition. Ethanol (90%) extract of the dried entire plant at a concentration of 0.25 mg/mL, was active[FA040].

Fibrinolytic activity. Ether extracts of the dried gum and gum resin, administered orally to 10 healthy subjects fed 100 g of butter to produce alimentary hyperlipemia, were active[FA031].

Gastric mucosal exfoliant activity. Powder of the dried entire plant, administered by gastric intubation to adults at a dose of 0.2 g for 1 hour, was active[FA059].

Hepatic mixed function oxidase inhibition. Oleoresin, administered to rats at a dose of 250 mg%, was active[FA043].

Hypocholesterolemic activity. A hot mixture of *Nigella sativa*, *Commiphora myrrha*, *Ferula assafoetida*, *Aloe vera*, and *Boswellia serrata*, administered by gastric intubation to rats at a dose of 0.5 g/kg for 7 days, was active vs streptozotocin-induced hyperglycemia[FA042].

Hypoglycemic activity. Hot water extract of the dried gum, *Nigella sativa*, *Myrrhis odorata*, and *Aloe* sp. in equal parts, administered by gastric intubation to rats at a dose of 10 mL/kg for 7 days, was active. Results were significant at $p < 0.001$ level[FA058]. Hot water extract of the dried gum, administered by gastric intubation to rats at a dose of 10 mL/kg for 7 days, was inactive[FA047]. A hot mixture of *Nigella sativa*, *Commiphora myrrha*, *Ferula assafoetida*, *Aloe vera*, and *Boswellia serrata*, administered by gastric intubation to rats at a dose of 0.5 g/kg for 7 days, was active vs streptozotocin-induced hyperglycemia[FA042].

Hypolipemic activity. A hot mixture of *Nigella sativa*, *Commiphora myrrha*, *Ferula assafoetida*, *Aloe vera* and *Boswellia serrata*, administered by gastric intubation to rats at a dose of 0.5 g/kg for 7 days, was active vs streptozotocin-induced hyperglycemia[FA042].

Hypotensive activity. Tincture of the gland, administered intravenously to rabbits, was active[FA025]. Water extract of the dried gum resin, administered intravenously to dogs at variable doses, was active[FA067]. Gum extract, administered to anaesthetized rats at doses of 0.3–2.2 mg/100 g body weight, significantly reduced the mean arterial blood pressure[FA075].

Mutagenic activity. Ethanol (95%) extract of the dried resin, on agar plate at a concentration of 15 mg/plate, produced weak activity on streptomycin-dependent strains of *Salmonella typhimurium* TA98. Metabolic activation has no effect on the result[FA060]. Resin, on agar plate at a concentration of 200 µg/plate, was active on *Salmonella typhimurium* TA1537 and inactive on *Salmonella typhimurium* TA1538 and *Salmonella typhimurium* TA98[FA062].

Olfactory status influence. Asafoetida extract, administered to allergic (group I) and nonallergic rhinitis (group II) patients at a dose of 10% aqueous solution, produced an elevation of olfactory thresholds by 55.8% in group I and 66.8% for both groups[FA086].

Pancreatic digestive enzymes effect. Asafetida, administered orally to albino rats at a dose of 250 mg% for 8 weeks, enhanced pancreatic lipase activity, stimulated pancreatic amylase and chymotrypsin. The stimulatory influence was not observed when their intake was restricted to a single oral dose[FA087].

Protein digestibility. Asafetida did not affect the digestibility of protein in sorghum[FA084].

Sister chromatid exchange stimulation. Gum, administered by gastric intubation to mice at a dose of 1 g/kg, was active. The results were significant at p less than 0.01 level. A dose of 0.5 g/kg, produced weak activity[FA051]. Asafoetida, administered orally to mice, produced weak activity in spermatogonia[FA091].

Smooth muscle relaxant activity. Tincture of the gland, administered to rabbits, was active on the bladder and intestine[FA025].

Toxic effect. Gum, administered orally to adults, was active. A case of methemoglobinemia occurred in a 5-week-old male infant, after administration of asafetida preparation to alleviate colic. Treatment was with intravenous methylene blue and the infant recovered[FA053].

Tumor-promoting activity. Water extract of the dried oleoresin, administered externally to mice at a dose of 200 μL/animal, was active vs 7,12-dimethylbenz[a]anthracene and croton oil treatment[FA044].

Uterine stimulant effect. Hot water extract of the plant, administered to female rats, was inactive on estrogen of uterus. Extract administered to pregnant rats, was inactive on uterus[FA026].

Vasodilator activity. Water extract of the dried gum resin, administered to frogs, was active on the vein[FA067].

REFERENCES

FA001 Banerji, A., B. Mallick, A. Chatterjee, H. Budzikiewicz, and M. Breuer. Assafoetidin and ferocolicin, two sesquiterpenoid coumarins from *Ferula assafoetida* Regel. **Tetrahedron** 1988; 29(13): 1557–1560.

FA002 Kajimoto, T., K. Yahiro, and T. Nohara. Sesquiterpenoid and disulphide derivatives from *Ferula assafoetida*. **Phytochemistry** 189; 28(6): 1761–1763.

FA003 Hofer, O., M. Widhalm, and H. Greger. Circular dichroism of sesquiterpene-umbelliferone ethers and structure elucidation of a new derivative isolated from the gum resin 'asafetida'. **Monatsh Chem** 1984; 115(10): 1207–1218.

FA004 Appendino, G., S. Taglipietra, G. M. Nano, and J. Jakupovic. Sesquiterpene coumarin ethers from asafetida. **Phytochemistry** 1994; 35(1): 183–186.

FA005 Nassar, M. I., E. A. Abu-Mustafa, and A. A. Ahmed. Sesquiterpene coumarins from *Ferula assafoetida* L. **Pharmazie** 1995; 50(11): 766–767.

FA006 Pangarova, T. T., and G. G. Zapesochnaya. Flavonoids of *Ferula assafoetida*. **Chem Nat Comp** 1973; 9(6): 768.

FA007 Kjaer, A., M. Sponholtz, K. O. Abraham, M. L. Shankaranarayana, M. L. Raghavan, and C. P. Natarajan. 2-butyl propenyl disulfides from asafetida: separation, characterization and absolute configuration. **Acta Chem Scand Ser B** 1976; 30: 137.

FA008 Mahram, G. H., T. S. M. A. El-Alfy, and H. A. Ansary. A phytochemical study of the gum and resin of Afghanian assafoetida. **Bull Fac Pharm Cairo Univ** 1975; 12: 119.

FA009 Nassar, M. I. Spectral study of farnesiferol B from *Ferula assafoetida* L. **Pharmazie** 1994; 49(7): 542–543.

FA010 Mahran, G. H., T. S. M. A. El Alfy, and S. M. A. Ansari. A phytochemical study of volatile oil of Afghanian asafoetida. **Bull Fac Pharm Cairo Univ** 1973; 12(2): 101–117.

FA011 Singh, M. M., A. Agnihotri, S. N. Garg, S. Agarwal, D. N. Gupta, G. Keshri, and V. P. Kamboj. Antifertility and hormonal properties of certain carotene sesquiterpenes of *Ferula jaeschkeana*. **Planta Med** 1988; 54(6): 492–494.

FA012 Ashraf, M., R. Ahmad, S. Mahood, and M. K. Bhatty. Studies of the essential oils of the Pakistani species of the family *Umbelliferae*. XLV. *Ferula assafoetida*, Linn (Herra Hing) gum oil. **Pak J Sci Ind Res** 1980; 23: 68–69.

FA013 Ashraf, M., R. Ahmad, S. Mahood, and M. K. Bhatty. Studies of the essential oils of the Pakistani species of the family *Umbelliferae*. Part XXXV. *Ferula assafoetida*, Linn (Hing) seed oil. **Pak J Sci Ind Res** 1979; 22(6): 308–310.

FA014 Kleiman, R., and G. F. Spencer. Search for new industrial oils: 16. *Umbelliflorae*-seed oils rich in petroselinic acid. **J Amer Oil Chem Soc** 1982; 59: 29–32.

FA015 Rajanikanth, B., B. Ravindranath, and M. L. Shankaranarayana. Volatile polysulphides of asafetida. **Phytochemistry** 1984; 23(4): 899–900.

FA016 Shankaranarayana, M. L., B. Raghavan, and C. P. Natarajan. Odorous compounds of asafetida. VII. Isolation and identification. **Indian Food Pack** 1982; 36(5): 65–76.

FA017 Abu-Mustafa, E. A., A. Khattab, S. Meshaal, et al. Foetidin, a new sesquiterpenoid coumarin from *Ferula assafoetida*. **Abstr Internat Res Congr Nat Prod Coll Pharm Univ N Carolina Chapel Hill NC July 7-12** 1985; 1985: Abstr-42.

FA018 Buddrus, J., H. Bauer, E. A. Abu-Mustafa, A. Khattab, S. Meshaal, E. A. M. El-Khrisy, J., and M. Lincheid. Foetidin, a sesquiterpenoid coumarin from *Ferula assa-foetida*. **Phytochemistry** 1985; 24(4): 869–870.

FA019 Hofer, O., M. Widhalm, and H. Greger. Circular dichroism of sesquiterpene-umbelliferone ethers and structure elucidation of a new derivative isolated from the gum resin "asa foetida." **Monatsh Chem** 1984; 115(10): 1207–1218.

FA020 Guarnieri, A., and M. Amorosa. The structure of gum polysaccharide from gum-resin ammoniac. II. Smith degradation. **Ann Chim (Rome)** 1970; 60(2): 108–115.

FA021 Fujita, M., T. Furuya, and H. Itokawa. Crude drugs containing coumarins and their derivatives. III. Chromatographic separation and determination of umbelliferone and its homologs. **Yakugaku Zasshi** 1958; 78: 395–398.

FA022 Caglioti, L., H. Naef, D. Arigoni, and O. Jeger. Sesquiterpenes and azulenes. CXXVII. The constituents of asafetida. II. Farnesiferol B and C. **Helv Chim Acta** 1959; 42: 2557–2570.

FA023 Caglioti, L., H. Naef, D. Arigoni, and O. Jeger. Sesquiterpenes and azulenes.126. The constituents of asafoetida. I. Farnesiferol A**. Helv Chim Acta** 1958; 41: 2278–2292.

FA024 Mahran, G. H., T. S. M. A. El-Alfy, and H. A. Ansary. A phytochemical study of the gum and resin of Afghanian asafoetida. **Bull Fac Pharm** 1975; 12(2): 119–132.

FA025 Boyd, L. J. The pharmacology of the homeopathic drugs. I. **J Amer Inst Homeopathy** 1928; 21: 7.

FA026 Misra, M. B., S. S. Mishra, and R. K. Misra. Screening of a few indigenous abortifacients. **J Indian Med Ass** 1969; 52: 535.

FA027 Das, P. C. Oral contraceptive. Patent-Brit-1,025,372 1966.

FA028 Gimlette, J. D. A dictionary of Malayan medicine, Oxford University Press, New York, USA, 1939.

FA029 Anon. Lilly's handbook of pharmacy and therapeutics, 5th rev, Eli Lilly and Co, Indianapolis 1898.

FA030 Garg, D. K., A. C. Banerjea, and J. Verma. The role of intestinal *Clostridia* and the effect of asafetida (Hing) and alcohol in flatulence. **Indian J Microbiol** 1980; 20(3): 194–197.

FA031 Bordia, A., and S. K. Arora. The effect of essential oil (active principle) of asafetida on alimentary lipemia. **Indian J Med Res** 1975; 63(5): 707–711.

FA032 Soni, K. B., M. Lahiri, P. Chakcradeo, S. V. Bhide, and R. Kuttan. Protective effect of food additives on aflatoxin-induced mutagenicity and hepatocarcinogenicity. **Chem Lett** 1997; 115(2): 129–133.

FA033 Aruna, K., and V. M. Sivaramakrishnan. Anticarcinogenic effect of some Indian plant products. **Food Chem Toxicol** 1992; 30(11): 953–956.

FA034 Soni, K. B., A. Rajan, and R. Kuttan. Inhibition of aflatoxin-induced liver damage in ducklings by food additives. **Mycotoxin Res** 1993; 9(1): 22–27.

FA035 Elisabetsky, E., W. Figueiredo, and G. Oliveria. Traditional Amazonian nerve tonics as antidepressant agents: *Chaunochiton kappleri*: a case study. **J Herbs Spices Med Plants** 1992; 1(1/2): 125–162.

FA036 Bhattarai, N. K. Folk Anthelmintic drugs of central Nepal. **Int J Pharmacol** 1992; 30(2): 145–150.

FA037 Bellakhdar, J., R. Claisse, J. Fleuretin, and C. Younos. Repertory of standard herbal drugs in the Moroccan Pharmacopoeia. **J Ethnopharmacol** 1991; 35(2): 123–143.

FA038 Duke, J. A., and E. S. Ayensu. Medicinal plants of China. Reference publications, Inc. Algonac, Michigan 1985 1(4): 52–361.

FA039 Thyagaraja, N., and A. Hosono. Effect of spice extract on fungal inhibition. **Food Sci Technol (London)** 1996; 29(3): 286–288.

FA040 Unnikrishn, M. C., and R. Kuttan. Cytotoxicity of extracts of spices to cultured cells. **Nutr Cancer** 1988; 11(4): 251–257.

FA041 Seetharam, K. A., and J. S. Pasricha. Condiments and contact dermatitis of the finger-tips. **Indian J Dermatol Venerol Leprol** 1987; 53(6): 325–328.

FA042 Al-Awadi, F., and M. Shoukry. The lipid lowering effect of an anti-diabetic plant extract. **Acta Diabetol** 1988; 25(1): 1–5.

FA043 Sambaiah, K., and K. Srinivasan. Influence of spices and spice principles on hepatic mixed function oxygenase system in rats. **Indian J Biochem Biophys** 1989; 26(4): 254–258.

FA044 Unnikrishn, M. C., and R. Kuttan. Tumour reducing and anticarcinogenic activity of selected spices. **Cancer Lett** 1990; 51(1): 85–89.

FA045 Sato, A. Studies on anti-tumor activity of crude drugs. I. The effects of aqueous extracts of some crude drugs in short-term screening test. **Yakugaku Zasshi** 1989; 109(6): 407–423.

FA046 Joshi, P. Herbal drugs used in Guinea worm disease by the tribals of southern Rajasthan (India). **Int J Pharmacog** 1991; 29(1): 33–38.

FA047 Al-Awadi, F. M., and K. A. Gumaa. Studies on the activity of individual plants of an antidiabetic plant mixture. **Acta Dabetol** 1987; 24(1): 37–41.

FA048 Rahlfs, V. W., and P. Mossinger. Asa foetida in the treatment of the irritable colon. A double blind study. **Dtsch Med Wochenschr** 1979; 104: 140–143.

FA049 Das, P. C. Oral contraceptive (long-acting). Patent-Brit-1,445,599 1976; 11 pp.

FA050 Kamanna, V. S., and N. Chandrasekhara. Effect of garlic (*Allium sativum* Linn.) on serum lipoproteins and lipoprotein cholesterol levels in albino rats rendered hypercholesterolemic by feeding cholesterol. **Lipids** 1982; 17(7): 483–488.

FA051 Abraham, S. K., and P. C. Kesavan. Genotoxicity of garlic, turmeric and asafetida in mice. **Mutat Res** 1984; 136(1): 85–88.

FA052 John, D. One hundred useful raw drugs of the Kani tribes of Trivandrum forest division, Kerala, India. **Int J Crude Drug Res** 1984; 22(1): 17–39.

FA053 Kelly, K. J., J. Nue, B. M. Camitta, and G. R. Honig. Methemoglobinemia in an infant treated with the folk remedy glycerited asafetida. **Pediatrics** 1984; 73(5): 717–719.

FA054 Tiwar, K. C., R. Majumder, and S. Bhattacharjee. Folklore medicines from Assam and Arunachal Pradesh (district Tirap). **Int J Crude Drug Res** 1979; 17(2): 61–67.

FA055 Dikshi, A., and A. Husain. Antifungal action of some essential oils against animal pathogens. **Fitoterapia** 1984; 55(3): 171–176.

FA056 Singh, Y. N. Traditional medicine in Fiji: some herbal folk cures used by Fiji Indians. **J Ethnopharmacol** 1986; 15(1): 57–88.

FA057 Venkataraghavan, S., and T. P. Sundareesan. A short note on contraceptive in Ayurveda. **J Sci Res Pl Med** 1981; 2(1/2): 39.

FA058 Al-Awadi, F. M., M. A. Khattar, and K. A. Gumaa. On the mechanism of the hypoglycaemic effect of a plant extract. **Diabetologia** 1985; 28(7): 432–434.

FA059 Desai, H. G., and R. H. Kalro. Effect of black pepper & asafetida on the DNA content of gastric aspirates. **Indian J Med Res** 1985; 81: 325–329.

FA060 Shashikanth, K. N., and A. Hosono. *In vitro* mutagenicity of tropical spices to streptomycin dependent strains of *Salmonella typhimurium* TA98. **Agr Biol Chem** 1986; 50(11): 2947–2948.

FA061 Kamboj, V. P. A review of Indian medicinal plants with interceptive activity. **Indian J Med Res** 1988; 1988(4): 336–355.

FA062 Siwaswamy, S. N., B. Balachandran, S. Balanehru, and V. M. Sivaramakrishnan. Mutagenic activity of south Indian food items. **Indian J Exp Biol** 1991; 29(8): 730–737.

FA063 Self, P. A., F. D. Horowitz, and L. Y. Paden. Olfactions in newborn infants. **Dev Psychol** 1972; 7(3): 349–363.

FA064 El-Dean Mahmoud, A. A. G. Study of indigenous (folk ways) birth control methods in Alexandria. Thesis-University of Alexandria-Higher Institute of Nursing 1972.

FA065 Mansurov, M. M. Effect of *Ferula asafetida* on the blood coagulability. **Med Zh Uzb** 1967; 1967(6): 46–49.

FA066 Coleman, D. E. S. The effect of certain homeopathic remedies upon the hearing. **J Amer Inst Homeopathy** 1922; 15: 279–281.

FA067 Sarkis'yan, R. G. Effect of *Ferula* on arterial pressure. **Med Zh Uzb** 1969; 1969(9): 23–24.

FA068 Seabrook, W. B. Adventures in Arabia among the Bedouins, Druses, whirling dervishes & Yezidee devil worshipers. Blue Ribbon Book, New York 1927; 99–105.

FA069 Walia, K. Effects of asafetida (7-hydroxycoumarin) on mouse spermatocytes. **Cytologia** 1973; 38: 19–724.

FA070 Subrahmanyan, V., L. V. L. Sastry, and M. Srinivasan. Asafoetida. **J Sci Ind Res B** 1954; 13: 382–386.

FA071 Mahran, G. H., T. S. M. A. El Alfy, and S. M. A. Ansari. A phytochemical study of volatile oil of Afghanian asafetida. **Bull Fac Pharm Cairo Univ** 1973; 12(2): 101–107.

FA072 Buddrus, J., H. Bauer, E. Abu-Mustafa, A. Khattab, S. Mishaal, E. A. M. El-Khrisy, and M. Linscheid. Foetidin, a sesquiterpenoid coumarin from *Ferula assa-foetida*. **Phytochemistry** 1985; 24(4): 869–870.

FA073 Lu, Y., C. Xu, Y. Yang, and H. Pan. The effect of antioxidant sodium ferulate on human lymphocytes apoptosis induced by H_2O_2. **Zhongguo Yi Xue Ke Xue Yuan Xue Bao** 1998; 20(1): 44–48.

FA074 Ramadan, N.I., and F. M. Al Khadrawy. The *in vitro* effect of Assafoetida on *Trichomonas vaginalis*. **J Egypt Soc Parasitol** 2003; 33(2): 615–630.

FA075 Fatehi, M., F. Farifteh, and Z. Fatehi-Hassanabad. Antispasmodic and hypotensive effects of *Ferula asafoetida* gum extract. **J Ethnopharmacol** 2004; 91(2–3): 321–324.

FA076 Mallikarjuna, G.U., S. Dhanalakshmi, S. Raisuddin, and A. R. Rao. Chemomodulatory influence of *Ferula asafoetida* on mammary epithelial differentiation, hepatic drug metabolizing enzymes, antioxidant profiles and N-methyl-N-nitrosourea-induced mammary carcinogenesis in rats. **Breast Cancer Res Treat** 2003; 81(1): 1–10.

FA077 Duan, H., Y. Takaishi, M. Tori, S. Takaoka, G. Honda, M. Ito, Y. Takeda, O. K. Kodzhimatov, K. Kodzhimatov, and O. Ashurmetov. Polysulfide derivatives from *Ferula foetida*. **J Nat Prod** 2002; 65(11): 1667–1669.

FA078 Nagatsu, A., K. Isaka, K. Kojima, et al. New sesquiterpenes from *Ferula ferulaeoides* (Steud.) Korovin. VI. Isolation and identification of three new dihydrofuro[2,3-B]chromones. **Chem Pharm Bull (Tokyo)** 2002; 50(5): 675–677.

FA079 Abd El-Razek, M.H., S. Ohta, A. A. Ahmed, and T. Hirata. Sesquiterpene coumarins from the roots of *Ferula assa-foetida*. **Phytochemistry** 2001; 58(8): 1289–1295.

FA080 Isaka, K., A. Nagatsu, P. Ondognii, O. Zevgeegiin, P. Gombosurengyin, K. Davgiin, K. Kojima, and Y. Ogihara. Sesquiterpenoid derivatives from *Ferula ferulaeoides*. V. **Chem Pharm Bull (Tokyo)** 2001; 49(9): 1072–1076.

FA081 Agrawal, A.K., C. V. Rao, K. Sairam, V. K. Joshi, and R. K. Goel. Effect of *Piper longum* Linn, *Zingiber officinalis* Linn and *Ferula* species on gastric ulceration and secretion in rats. **Indian J Exp Biol** 2000; 38(10): 994–998.

FA082 Kojima, K., K. Isaka, P. Ondognii, Oet al. Sesquiterpenoid derivatives from *Ferula ferulaeoides*. IV. **Chem Pharm Bull (Tokyo)** 2000; 48(3): 353–356.

FA083 Soni, K.B., A. Rajan, and R. Kuttan. Reversal of aflatoxin induced liver damage by turmeric and curcumin. **Cancer Lett** 1992; 66(2): 115–121.

FA084 Pradeep, K.U., P. Geervani, and B. O. Eggum. Influence of spices on utilization of sorghum and chickpea protein. **Plant Foods Hum Nutr** 199; 41(3): 269–276.

FA085 Unnikrishnan, M.C., and R. Kuttan. Tumour reducing and anticarcinogenic activity of selected spices. **Cancer Lett** 1990; 51(1): 85–89.

FA086 Mann, S.S., S. Maini, K. S. Nageswari, H. Mohan, and A. Handa. Assessment of olfactory status in allergic and non-allergic rhinitis patients. **Indian J Physiol Pharmacol** 2002; 46(2): 186–194.

FA087   Platel, K., and K. Srinivasan. Influence of dietary spices and their active principles on pancreatic digestive enzymes in albino rats. **Nahrung** 2000; 44(1): 42–46.

FA088   Soni, K. B., M. Lahiri, P. Chackradeo, S. V. Bhide, and R. Kuttan. Protective effect of food additives on aflatoxin-induced mutagenicity and hepatocarcinogenicity. **Cancer Lett** 1997; 115(2): 129–133.

FA089   Platel, K., and K. Srinivasan. Influence of dietary spices or their active principles on digestive enzymes of small intestinal mucosa in rats. **Int J Food Sci Nutr** 1996; 47(1): 55–59.

FA090   Soudamini, K. K., M. C. Unnikrishnan, K. Sukumaran, and R. Kuttan. Mutagenicity and anti-mutagenicity of selected spices. **Indian J Physiol Pharmacol** 1995; 39(4): 347–353.

FA091   Abraham, S. K., and P. C. Kesavan. Genotoxicity of garlic, turmeric and asafoetida in mice. **Mutat Res** 1984; 136(1): 85–88.

FA092   Kamanna, V.S., and N. Chandrasekhara. Effect of garlic (*Allium sativum* Linn) on serum lipoproteins and lipoprotein cholesterol levels in albino rats rendered hypercholesteremic by feeding cholesterol. **Lipids** 1982; 17(7): 483–488.

FA093   Keshri, G., V. Lakshmi, M. M. Singh, and V. P. Kamboj. Post-coital antifertility actiivty of *Ferula assafoetida* extract in female rats. **Pharmac Biol** 1999; 37(4): 273–278.

7 | Hordeum vulgare

L.

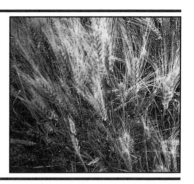

Common Names

Almindelig	Denmark	Jecam	Serbia
Arlysen	Cornwall	Jeczmien	Poland
Arpa	Hungary	Jeemen	Czech Republic
Arpa	Turkey	Koarn	Netherlands
Arpa	Turkmenistan	Korn	Sweden
Barley	Guyana	Mach'ca	Ecuador
Barley	United Kingdom	Mehrzeilige Gerste	Germany
Barley	United States	Mitmerealine oder	Estonia
Barlysyn	Wales	Monitahoohra	Finland
Byg	Denmark	Oarn	The Isle of Man (Manx)
Bygg	Faeroe Islands	Ohra	Finland
Bygg	Iceland	Orge	France
Bygg	Norway	Orz	Romania
Cebada	Spain	Orzo	Italy
Cevada	Portugal	Paare(i)	New Zealand
Echemik	Bulgaria	Saat-Gerste	Germany
Elb	Albania	Sechszeilige Gerste	Gemany
Eorna	Scotland	Sibada	Hawaii
Garase	South Africa	Sibada	Pacific Islands
Gerst	Netherlands	Too moo	China
Gerste	Germany	Usurp	China
Gewone gerst	Netherlands	Yachmen	Russia
Haidd	Wales	Yachmin	Ukraine
Jecam	Croatia		

BOTANICAL DESCRIPTION

Hordeum vulgare is grass that may be either a winter or a spring annual of the POACEAE (GRAMINAE) family. It forms a rosette type of growth in fall and winter, developing elongated stems and flower heads in early summer. Winter varieties form branched stems or tillers at the base, so several stems rise from a single plant. The stems of both winter and spring varieties may vary in length from 30 to 120 cm, depending on variety and growing conditions.

From: *Medicinal Plants of the World, vol. 3: Chemical Constituents, Traditional and Modern Medicinal Uses*
By: I. A. Ross © Humana Press Inc., Totowa, NJ

Stems are round, hollow between nodes, and develop five to seven nodes below the head. At each node, a clasping leaf develops. In most varieties, the leaves are coated with a waxy chalk-like deposit. Shape and size of leaves vary with variety, growing conditions, and position on the plant. The spike contains the flowers and consists of spikelets attached to the central stem or rachis. Stem intervals between spikelets are 2 mm or less in dense-headed varieties and up to 4–5 mm in lax or open-headed kinds. Three spikelets develop at each node on the rachis. *Hordeum vulgare* is six-row variety, where all three of the spikelets at each node develop a seed. Each spikelet has two linear to lanceolate glumes rising from near the base and flat and terminates in an awn. The glumes, minus the awn, are approximately half the length of the kernel in most varieties, but this varies from less than half to equal to the kernel in length. Glumes may be covered with hairs, weakly haired, or hairless. The awns on the glumes may be shorter than the gume, equal in length, or longer. The barley kernel consists of the caryopsis, or internal seed, the lemma, and palea. In most barley varieties, the lemma and palea adhere to the caryopsis and are a part of the grain following threshing. The lemmas in barley are usually awned. Awns vary in length from very short up to as much as 12 in. Edges of awns may be rough or "barbed" (bearded) or nearly smooth. Awnless varieties are also known. In six-row barley, awns are usually more developed on the central spikelets than on the lateral ones. The barley kernel is generally spindle shaped. In commercial varieties, the length ranges from 7 to 12 mm.

ORIGIN AND DISTRIBUTION

Grains found in pits and pyramids in Egypt indicated that barley was cultivated there more than 5000 years ago. The most ancient glyph or pictograph found for barley is dated approx 3000 BC. References to barley and beer are found in the earliest Egyptian and Sumerian writings. The origin of barley is still not known. There are differing views among researchers regarding whether the original wild forms were indigenous to Eastern Asia, particularly Tibet, or to the Near East, Eastern Mediterranean area, or both. Varieties are constantly changing as new ones are developed and tested while others pass out of cultivation.

TRADITIONAL MEDICINAL USES

Afghanistan. Flowers are taken orally by females for contraception[HV127].

Argentina. Decoction of the dried fruit is taken orally for diarrhea and to treat respiratory and urinary tract infections[HV063].

China. Decoction of the dried fruit is taken orally for diabetes[HV033].

Egypt. Dried fruits are smoked as a treatment for schistosomiasis[HV109]. The fruit is used intravaginally as a contraceptive before and after coitus. Fifty-three percent of 1200 puerperal women interviewed practiced this method, of whom 47% depended on indigenous method and/or prolonged lactation[HV130].

Guatemala. Hot water extract of the dried seed is taken orally for renal inflammation and kidney disease[HV120]. Hot water extract of the dried seed is used externally for dermatitis, inflammations, erysipelas, and skin eruptions[HV122].

India. Powdered flowers of *Calotropis procera*, fruits of *Piper nigrum*, seed ash of *Hordeum vulgare*, and rose water are taken orally for cholera[HV115].

Iran. Flour is used as a food. A decoction of the dried seed is used externally as an emollient and applied on hemorrhoids and infected ulcers. A decoction of the dried seed is taken orally as a diuretic and antipyretic and used for hepatitis, diarrhea, scorbutism, nephritis, bladder inflammation, gout, enema, and its tonic effect. Decoction of the dried seed is applied to the nose to reduce internasal inflammation[HV019].

Italy. Seeds are eaten as a urinary antiseptic[HV049]. Compresses of boiled seeds are used to soothe rheumatic and joint pains[HV123]. Infusion of the dried seed is used as a galactogogue[HV039].

Korea. Hot water extract of the dried entire plant is taken orally for beriberi, coughs, influenza, measles, syphilis, nephritis, jaundice, dysentery, and ancylostomiasis; for thrush in infants; and as a diuretic. Extract of the dried entire plant is used externally for prickly heat[HV113].

Peru. Hot water extract of dried fruits is used externally for measles and as an emollient and taken orally as a diuretic[HV121].

South Korea. Hot water extracts of the fruit and dried seeds are taken orally by pregnant women to induce abortion[HV126,HV116]. Hot water extracts of the fruits taken orally by females as a contraceptive[HV126].

Turkey. Decoction of the fruit is taken orally for common colds[HV074].

United States. Infusion of the dried seed is taken orally for dysentery, diarrhea, and colic and for digestive and gastrointestinal disorders[HV099].

CHEMICAL CONSTITUENTS

(ppm unless otherwise indicated)
Abscisic acid: Sd[HV034]
Aconitic acid: Rt[HV026]
Aesculetin: Protoplast[HV091]
Aesculin: Protoplast[HV091]
Agmatine, para-coumaroyl: Sh 2.5[HV002]
Alkyl resorcinol (C17:0): Sd[HV103]
Alkyl resorcinol (C19:0): Sd[HV103]
Alkyl resorcinol (C19:1): Sd[HV103]
Alkyl resorcinol (C21:0): Sd[HV103]
Alkyl resorcinol (C23:0): Sd[HV103]
Alkyl resorcinol (C25:0): Sd[HV103]
Amine, diethyl: Sd 5.7[HV111]
Amine, dimethyl: Sd 1.6[HV111]
AMP, cyclic: Sd, Seedling[HV022]
Apigenin-7-O-β-D-diglucoside: Lf[HV107]
Arabinitol, 2-carboxy: Lf 814 nmol/g[HV071]
Azidoalanine: Pl[HV205]
Barwin: Sd 6[HV011]
Benzaldehyde, 2-5-dihydroxy: Lf[HV078]
Benzene-1-3-diol, 5-pentadecyl: Lf[HV078]

Benzoquinone, 1-4: Call Tiss, Rt, Lf[HV023]
Benzoxazin-3(4H)-one, 1-4, (2H), 2-4-dihydroxy: Seedling[HV036]
Benzoxazin-3-one, 1-4, 2-4-dihydroxy-7-methoxy: Aer[HV101]
Benzoxazolinone, 6-methoxy: Seedling[HV036]
Betaine: Sh 15 μmol/g, Rt 2 μmol/g[HV110]
Butyronitrile, 3-β-D-glucopyranosyloxy-3-methyl: Epidermis[HV013]
Butyronitrile, 4-β-D-glucopyranosyloxy-3-hydroxy-methyl: Epidermis[HV013]
Caffeic acid: Fr[HV029]
Calmodulin: Sh[HV105], Cotyledon[HV081]
Carnitine: Lf 0.83–3.6 nmol/g[HV125]
Catechin-(4-α-8)-catechin-(4-α-8)-catechin: Fr[HV054]
Catechin-(4-α-8)-gallocatechin-(4-α-8)-catechin: Fr[HV054]
Catechin, (+): Sd[HV106]
Chlorogenic acid: Fr[HV029]
Chlorophyll, proto: Lf[HV021]
Choline: Sd 1.08 mg/g[HV004]
Chrysoeriol-7-galactoside: Lf[HV107]
Chrysoeriol-7-O-β-D-glucoside: Lf[HV107]
Corydine, (+): Rt[HV001]
Coumaric acid, para, *cis*: Cell wall[HV088]
Coumaric acid, para, *trans*: Cell wall[HV088]
Coumaric acid, para: Fr[HV029]
Cramine: Lf 0.04–1.18%[HV060]
Cryptopine, allo, α: Rt[HV001]
Cyclohexanamine, *N*-cyclohexyl: Lf[HV078]
Cynaroside: Lf[HV107]
Cystathionine: Seedling 0.07[HV132]
Delphinidin, pro: Fr[HV054]
Dicentrine: Rt[HV001]
Docos-1-ene: Lf[HV078]
Eicos-*trans*-3-ene: Lf[HV078]
Eicos-*trans*-5-ene: Lf[HV078]
Eicos-*trans*-9-ene: Lf[HV078]
Ethanolamine, phosphatidyl: Lf[HV124]
Ethylamine: Sd 3.4[HV111]
Ferulic acid, *trans*, 5-hydroxy: Cell wall[HV088]
Ferulic acid, *trans*: Cell wall[HV088]
Ferulic acid: Sd[HV037]
Flavone, 5-7-dihydroxy-3'-4'-5'-trimethoxy: St/Lf[HV087]
Fucosterol, 28-iso: Em[HV025]
Fusariotoxin T-2: Pl[HV160]
Gallocatechin-(4-α-8)-catechin-(4-α-8)-catechin: Fr[HV054]
Gallocatechin-(4-α-8)-gallocatechin-(4-α-8)-catechin: Fr[HV054]

Gallocatechin-(4-α-8)-gallocatechin-(4-α-8)-catechin: Fr[HV054]

Gallocatechin-(4-α-8)-gallocatechin-(4-α-8)-gallocatechin: Fr[HV054]

Gallocatechin, (+):Fr[HV054]

γ-3 hordein: Sd[HV180]

Gibberellin A-1: Seedling[HV027]

Gibberellin A-3: Seedling[HV027]

Gibberellin: Sd[HV034]

Glaucentrine: Rt[HV001]

Glaucine, (+): Rt[HV001]

Glucan, β: Sd[HV057,HV190]

Glycine-betaine: Lf[HV031]

Glycoprotein D-1-G-1: Lf[HV119]

Gramine: Seedling[HV024], Aer[HV055], Protoplast, Lf[HV090], Rt[HV067]

Heptadecane, N: Lf[HV078]

Heterodendrin, epi: Epidermis[HV013]

Hexadecanoic acid methyl ester: Lf[HV078]

Hor v 9: Pl[HV164]

Hordein B: Caryopsis[HV035]

Hordenine: Rt[HV067], Seedling 63[HV094]

Hordeum protein 26kDa: Sd 80[HV095]

Hordeum protein 30kDa: Sd 80[HV095]

Hordeum protein 32kDa: Sd 3.0[HV095]

Hordeum thaumatin-like protein R: Sd[HV009]

Hordeum thaumatin-like protein S: Sd[HV009]

Hordeum vulgare protease inhibitor: Fr[HV008]

Hordeum vulgare protein MW 28000: Sd w/o seedcoat[HV085]

Hordeum vulgare protein MW 30000: Sd w/o seedcoat[HV085]

Hordeumin: Sd[HV072]

Hordothionin, ω: Sd[HV015]

Hydroxamic acid: Lf, Protoplast[HV090]

Indole: Lf[HV078]

Indole-3-acetic acid: Kernel[HV043]

Indole-3-carboxylic acid: Seedling[HV006]

Jasmonic acid: Sh, Fr[HV082]

Linoleic acid, 15(R)-hydroxy: Sd <1.0[HV016]

Linoleic acid: Lf[HV083]

Linolenic acid: Lf[HV083]

Lipid transfer protein 1: Sd[HV179]

Lipid transfer protein CW-18: Lf[HV012]

Lipid transfer protein CW-21: Lf[HV012]

Lunasin: Pl[HV163]

Lutonarin: Sh[HV053]

Lutonarin-3'-methyl ether: Sh[HV053]

Mannitol: Rt[HV007]

Melatonin: Sd 378.1 pg/g[HV069]

Methylamine: Sd 4.5[HV111]

Methyl-D-glucopyranoside: Lf[HV078]

Mugineic acid, 2'-deoxy: Rt[HV133]

Mugineic acid, 3-hydroxy: Rt[HV133]

Mugineic acid: Rt[HV133]

Naphthal-2-en-amine, N-phenyl: Lf[HV078]

NH$_3$ inorganic: Sd[HV111]

Nucellain: Endosperm[HV018]

Octadec-1-ene: Lf[HV078]

Octadeca-cis-9-cis-12-cis-15-trienoic acid methyl ester: Lf[HV078]

Octadeca-cis-9-cis-15-dienoic acid methyl ester: Lf[HV078]

Oleic acid: Lf[HV083]

Orientin, iso, 3'-methyl ether: Lf[HV107]

Orientin, iso, 7-(ferulyl-glucoside): Lf[HV107]

Orientin, iso, 7-arabinosyl-glucoside: Lf[HV107]

Orientin, iso, 7-O-β-D-glucoside: Lf[HV107]

Orientin, iso, 7-rhamnoglucoside: Lf[HV107]

Orientin, iso: Lf[HV107]

Palmitic acid: Lf[HV083]

Palmitoleic acid: Lf[HV083]

Phytic acid: Sd[HV057]

Phytol, iso: Lf[HV078]

Phytol: Lf[HV078]

Piperidine, 2-2-6-6-tetramethyl: Lf[HV078]

Piperidine: Sd 1[HV111]

Plastohydroquinone 9: Call Tiss, Rt, Lf[HV023]

Plastoquinone 9: Call Tiss, Rt, Lf[HV023], Seedling[HV129]

Polysaccharide (*Hordeum vulgare*): Sd[HV089]

Procyanidin B-3: Sd[HV106]

Prodelphinidin B-3 dimer: Sd[HV106]

Prodelphinidin B-3: Sd[HV106]

Prodelphinidin T-1: Sd[HV188]

Prodelphinidin T-2: Sd[HV188]

Prodelphinidin T-3: Sd[HV188]

Proline: Sh 0.4 μmol/g, Rt 1.9 Œ°mol/g[HV110]

Propane, diamino: Seedling[HV086]

Propelargonidin dimer: Sd[HV106]

Propene, 1-cyano-3-β-D-glucopyranosyl-oxy-2-methyl: Epidermis[HV013]

Protein Z(4): Sd[HV179]

Protein: Rt, Lf[HV028]

Putrescine: Seedling[HV086]

Pyrazine, 2-5-diethyl: Lf[HV078]

Pyrrolidine: Sd 0.9[HV111]

Pyrrolinium, 1-(3-amino-propyl): Seedling[HV086]

Quinic acid, feruloyl: Lf[HV097]

Roquefortine C: Sd[HV102]

Salazosulfapyridine: Pl[HV140]

Salicylic acid: Sh 1[HV066]

Salipurposide, iso: Lf[HV032]

Saponarin, 6''-feruloyl: Lf 11[HV017]

Saponarin, 6''-sinapoyl, 4'-glucoside: Lf 6[HV017]

Saponarin, 6″-sinapoyl: Lf 22[HV017]
Saponarin: Sh[HV053]
Satiomem: Sd[HV014]
Scopoletin: Protoplast[HV091]
Shikimic acid, feruloyl: Lf[HV097]
Sinapic acid, *trans*: Cell wall[HV088]
Sitosterol, β: Em[HV025]
Starch: Sd[HV020]
Stearic acid: Lf[HV083]
Stigmasterol: Em[HV025]
Sutherlandin: Epidermis[HV013]
Tocopherol, α: Seedling[HV129], Call Tiss, Rt, Lf[HV023]
Tocoquinone, α: Call Tiss, Rt, Lf[HV023]
Trichothecene: Pl[HV160]
Tricin: Lf/St[HV087]
Tricin-7-O-β-D-glucoside: Lf[HV107]
Trigonelline: Sd 8.9[HV118]
Tryptamine: Lf 3[HV065]
Tryptophan: Seedling[HV006]
Tyramine, *N*-methyl: Fr[HV048], Seedling 48[HV094], Rt[HV001]
Tyramine: Seedling 26[HV094]
Umbelliferone: Fr[HV029]
Vanillic acid: Fr[HV029]
Vitamin B-1: Sd 4.47[HV005]
Vitamin B-2: Sd 1.28[HV005]
Vitamin K-1: Call Tiss, Rt, Lf[HV023]
Vitexin-7-O-β-D-diglucoside: Lf[HV107]
Vitexin, iso, 2″ (3″)-O-glucosyl: Lf 590.9[HV010]
Vitexin, iso, 2″-O-diglucoside: Lf[HV080]
Vitexin, iso, 2″-O-glucoside: Lf[HV041]
Vitexin, iso, 2″-O-glucosyl: Lf[HV064]
Vitexin, iso, 4′-7-diglucoside: Lf 7[HV017]
Vitexin, iso, 7-diglucoside: Lf[HV107]
Vitexin, iso, 7-O-β-D-diglucoside: Lf[HV107]
Vitexin, iso, 7-rhamnosyl-glucoside: Lf 13[HV017]
Vitexin, iso: 2″-O-glucosyl: Lf[HV040]
Vitexin, iso: Lf[HV058]
Vitexin-7-rhamnoglucoside: Lf[HV107]

PHARMACOLOGICAL ACTIVITIES AND CLINICAL TRIALS

5-Hydroxytryptamine inhibition. Ethanol (80%) extract of the dried stem bark, in cell culture at a dose of 10 μg/mL, inhibited the uptake of serotonin (5HT) in rat brainstem neurons[HV046].

Acquired immune deficiency syndrome therapeutic effect. Hot water extract of the dried fruit, administered orally to patients with acquired immuodeficiency syn-

drome (AIDS) four to five doses/week for a year for the purpose of in clearing heat and detoxifying the blood, produced an improvement in the patient's health[HV093].

Allergenic activity. Extract of the dried seed, administered externally to male adults at a concentration of 10%, was active[HV044]. Allergens, administered by ingestion or inhalation to 40 children aged 3–6 months who suffered from diarrhea, vomiting, eczema, or weight loss after the introduction of the cereal in the diet and to 18 food-allergic adults and eight patients with Baker's asthma, produced strong effect in children[HV172]. Protein Z(4), administered to four patients with beer allergy, provoked weak positive response to skin testing in two of the patients and was recognized by the four individual sera tested. Lipid transfer protein 1 showed reactivity with three of four individual sera and induced strong positive skin prick test responses in all four of the patients tested[HV179]. Two cases of severe systemic reactions resulted from beer ingestion: one case of anaphylaxis requiring emergency care and one of generalized urticaria and angioedema were reported. Barley was recognized as the specific ingredient responsible for the observed allergic reaction[HV183]. Beer and malt allergens were found in three patients with urticaria. Urticaria from beer was an immunoglobulin E (IgE)-mediated hypersensitivity reaction induced by a protein component of approx 10 kDa deriving from barley[HV184]. A 50-year-old man, who developed bronchial asthma after exposure to barley flour, was confirmed by skin prick test and serum-specific IgE. Bronchial challenge test with every allergen showed no response, except for an immediate response to barley flour. The most relevant clinical feature was an immediate asthmatic response developed after oral provocation with either barley-made beer or barley flour itself that indicated IgE-mediated food-induced bronchial asthma[HV195]. A 32-year-old storeman developed occupational asthma resulting from barley grain dust in the packaging of flour, barley, and peanuts. He developed immediate symptoms of sneezing, cough, and dyspnea on exposure to barley only. Bronchial provocation test to the barley confirmed the diagnosis[HV197].

Ameliatory effect. Decoction of the grain, at a dose of 250 mL, produced a decrease in the passage time of whole blood with a microchannel array flow analyzer[HV173].

Anti-allergenic activity. Alcohol-soluble prolamines, administered to patients with gluten-sensitive enteropathy and dermatitis herpetiformis, produced monoclonal antibodies and serum reaction[HV165].

Anti-amoebic activity. Ethanol (50%) extract of the seed, in broth culture at a concentration of 125 µg/mL, was active on *Entamoeba histolytica*[HV001].

Anti-atherogenic activity. β-Glucan in barley cellulose, administered to Syrian golden F(1)B hamsters at doses of 2, 4, or 8 g/100 g in a semipurified hypercholesterolemic diet of 0.15 g/g cholesterol, 20 g/100 g of hydrogenated coconut oil and 15 g/100 g of cellulose, produced cholesterol-lowering effect. Compared with control hamsters, dose-dependent decreases that were similar in magnitude in plasma total and low-density lipoprotein (LDL) cholesterol concentrations were observed in hamsters fed the β-glucan diet at weeks 3, 6, and 9. Liver cholesterol concentrations were also reduced significantly in hamsters consuming 8 g/100 g β-glucan[HV210].

Antibacterial activity. Decoction of the dried fruit, on agar plate, was inactive on *Pseudomonas aeruginosa*[HV063]. Ethanol (95%) and water extracts of the dried fruit, on agar plate at a concentration of 50 µL/plate, were inactive on *Staphylococcus aureus*[HV073]. Water extract of the dried fruit, on agar plate, at a concentration of 1 mg/mL, was inactive on *Salmonella typhi*[HV030]. Hot water extract of the dried fruit, on agar plate at a concentration of 62.5 mg/mL, was inactive on *Escherichia coli* and *Staphylococcus aureus*[HV056].

Tincture of the dried seed, on agar plate at a concentration of 30 µL/disc, was inactive on *Escherichia coli*, *Pseudomonas aeruginosa*, and *Staphylococcus aureus*. Extract of 10 g plant material in 100 mL ethanol was used[HV122].

Anticoagulation activity. Serpin BSZx (an inhibitor of trypsin and chemotrypsin) inhibited thrombin, plasma kallikrein, factor VIIa/tissue factor, and factor Xa at heparin-independent association rates. Only factor Xa turned a significant fraction of BSZx over as substrate. Activated protein C and leukocyte elastase were slowly inhibited by BSZx, whereas factor XIIa, urokinase and tissue type plasminogen activator, plasmin and pancreas kallikrein, and elastase were not or only weakly affected. Trypsin from *Fusarium* was not inhibited, while interaction with subtilisin Carlsberg and Novo was rapid, but most BSZx was cleaved as a substrate[HV192].

Antidiabetic activity. The plant, administered to diabetic rats, produced a decrease of blood glucose concentration, water consumption, and weight loss. No differences were found in healthy animals[HV157].

Antidiarrheal activity. Extract of the germinating seeds, administered in the ration of male rats, was active vs cecocolectomy-induced diarrhea[HV045]. Germinated barley and scutellum fraction of germinated barley, administered to rats, prevented diarrhea caused by cecocolectomy and increased the protein content and sucrose activity of small intestinal mucosa[HV150]. The aleurone and scutellum fractions of barley grains before and after germination, administered to rats with diarrhea, were active. The addition of fractions of germinated barley and not barley collected before germination increased the fecal output and jejunal mucosal protein content. The effect of malted barley was similar to that of germinated barley foodstuff[HV151].

Antifungal activity. Dried stem, on agar plate, was active on *Sphacelia segetum*[HV131]. Hot water extract of the dried fruit, on agar plate at a concentration of 62.5 mg/mL, was inactive on *Aspergillus niger*[HV056]. Water extract of the seed, on agar plate at a concentration of 5 mg/mL, was inactive on *Helicobacter pylori*[HV076]. Protein fraction of the seed without seed coat, on agar plate at a concentration of 2 μg/disc, was active on *Neurospora crassa* and *Trichoderma* sp.[HV085]. Protein fraction of the seed without seed coat, on agar plate at a concentration of 2 μg/disc, was active on *Neurospora crassa*[HV085].

Antihepatotoxic activity. Methanol extract of the dried fruit, administered by gastric intubation to rabbits at a dose of 0.5 g/kg, was active vs CCl_4-induced hepatotoxicity. A mixture of *Machilus* sp., *Alisma* sp., *Amomum xanthioides*, *Bulboschoenus maritimus*, *Artemisia iwaymogis*, *Atractylodes japonica*, *Crataegus cuneata*, *Hordeum vulgare*, *Citrus sinensis*, *Polyporus umbellatus*, *Agastache rugosa*, *Raphanus sativus*, *Poncirus trifoliatus*, *Curcuma zeodaria*, *Citrus aurantium*, *Saussurea lappa*, *Glycyrrhiza glabra*, and *Zingiber officinale* was used[HV112].

Antihypercholesterolemic activity. Dried bran, administered in ration of male rats, was active[HV068]. Methanol extract of the dried fruit, administered by gastric intubation to rabbits at a dose of 500 mg/kg, was active vs CCl_4-induced hepatotoxicity. A mixture of *Machilus* sp., *Alisma* sp., *Amomum xanthioides*, *Bulboschoenus maritimus*, *Artemisia iwaymogis*, *Atractylodes japonica*, *C. cuneata*, *Hordeum vulgare*, *Citrus sinensis*, *Polyporus umbellatus*, *Agastache rugosa*, *Raphanus sativus*, *Poncirus trifoliatus*, *Curcuma zeodaria*, *Citrus aurantium*, *Saussurea lappa*, *Glycyrrhiza glabra*, and *Zingiber officinale* was used. Results were significant at $p < 0.01$ level[HV112]. Gum, administered orally to male rats for 4 weeks, was active. Biological activity reported had been patented[HV104]. Chromatographic fraction of the green leaf juice, administered to rats at a dose of 1% of diet, was active vs cholesterol-loaded animals. The results were significant at $p < 0.005$ level[HV117]. Seeds,

administered to 20 men with hypercholesterolemia aged 41 ± 5 years, resulted in significant fall in serum total cholesterol, LDL cholesterol, and phospholipids, and LDL and very low-density lipoprotein (VLDL). A dose of 50/50 w/w mix with rice, administered to seven women with mild hypercholesterolemia aged 56 ± 7 years twice daily for 2–4 weeks, produced a significant improvement of serum lipid profiles. In the normolipemic subjects, serum lipids were unaffected[HV193]. Bran flour and oil extract, administered to 79 patients with hypercholesterolemia, aged 48.2 years at a dose of 3 g oil extract or 30 g flour for 30 days, significantly decreased total serum cholesterol. LDL cholesterol was decreased 6.5% with addition of bran flour and 9.2% with oil. High-density lipoprotein (HDL) cholesterol decreased significantly in the bran flour group but not in the oil group[HV059]. Fiber (nonstarch polysaccharides), administered to 21 men with mild hypercholesterolemia aged 30–59 years for 4 weeks, produced a significant fall in plasma total cholesterol and LDL cholesterol. The triglyceride and glucose concentrations did not change significantly[HV204].

Antihyperglycemic activity. Dried seeds, administered orally to six patients with noninsulin-dependent diabetes mellitus at a dose of 50 g/person, was active. A single dose resulted in a glycemic index of 53.4[HV047]. Water extract of the dried fruit, administered intragastrically to rats at a dose of 150 mg/kg, produced weak activity on blood vs streptozotocin-induced hyperglycemia[HV033]. Dried seeds, administered orally to eight adults with normal glucose tolerance at a dose of 50 g/person, were active[HV052]. Flour, administered in the ration of male rats, was active vs streptozotocin-induced hyperglycemia[HV062]. Barley gum, administered to 4-week-old male Sprague–Dawley rats as a 2% dietary supplement for 14 days, lowered serum cholesterol concentration and suppressed the elevation of serum and liver triglyceride concentrations[HV154]. Thick and thin rolled oat made from raw or preheated kernel, administered to healthy subjects, produced high glucose, insulin, and metabolic responses[HV181]. Barley flour naturally high in β-glucan and β-glucan-enriched flour, administered to 11 healthy men, resulted in a decrease of the insulin response. Plasma glucose and insulin concentrations increased significantly. Cholesterol concentration dropped below the fasting concentration 4 hours after the meal and was significantly lower than after low-fiber meal. The cholecystokinin remained elevated for a long time after the barley-containing meals[HV185]. Boiled intact and milled kernels with different amylase-amylopectin ratios, administered to healthy subjects, produced lower metabolic responses and higher satiety scores when compared to white wheat bread. The boiled flours produced higher glucose and insulin responses than did the corresponding boiled kernels. The impact of amylase to amylopectin on the metabolic responses was marginal[HV198]. The intact kernels, administered to healthy subjects at concentrations of 40 and 80% (SCB-40 and SCB-80), produced the glycemic and insulinemic indices 39 and 33 for SCB-80, compared to pumpernickel bread 69 and 61, respectively. The glycemic index for SCB-40 was 66[HV199].

Anti-inflammatory activity. Germinated barley foodstuff, administered to mice with DSS-induced colitis, prevented disease activity and loss of body weight after induction of colitis. Serum interleukin (IL)-6 level, mucosal STAT3 expression, necrosis factor-κB activity, and mucosal damages were decreased and cecal butyrate content increased. The germinated barley foodstuff-fed mice had lower bile acid concentration than the control group[HV161]. Green barley extract, in LPS-activated human monocytes cell line culture (THP-1), was active[HV178].

Antimutagenic activity. Methanol extract of the dried fruit and leaf, on agar plate at a concentration of 50 μL/disc, was inactive on *Bacillus subtilis* NIG-1125 HIS MET and *Escherichia coli* B/R-WP2-TRP[HV114].

Antioxidant activity. Water extract of the roasted seed, at a concentration of 1 mg/mL, produced strong activity vs a liposome model system. A concentration of 25 mg/mL was active vs 2,2-diphenyl-1-picryl-hydrazyl-hydrate-induced radical. A concentration of 5 mg/mL was inactive vs linoleic acid system[HV079]. Ethanol (80%) extract of the freeze-dried leaf, at a concentration of 60 μg/mL, was active vs oxidation of ethyl linoleate by Fenton's reagent[HV010]. Young leaf extract, administered orally to 36 patients with type 2 diabetes at a dose of 15 g daily for 4 weeks, enhanced the scavenging of oxygen free radicals, saved the LDL-vitamin E content, and inhibited LDL oxidation[HV177]. Purified green barley extract, in human mononuclear culture of cells isolated from perithelial blood and synovial fluid of patients with rheumatoid arthritis, was active[HV178]. Leaf essence, administered to atherosclerotic New Zealand White male rabbits at a dose of 1% of diet, produced a decrease of plasma total cholesterol, triacylglycerol, lucigenin-chemiluminescence, and luminal-chemiluminescence levels. The value of T_{50} of red blood cell hemolysis and the lag phase of LDL oxidation increased in barley-treated group compared with the control. Ninety percent of the intimal surface of the thoracic aorta was covered with atherosclerotic lesions in the control group, but only 60% of the surface was covered in the barley group. This inhibition was associated with a decrease in plasma lipids and an increase in antioxidative abilities[HV003].

Anti-tumor activity. Commercial barley bran (13% dietary fiber) from the aleurone/subaleurone layer; outer-layer barley bran, including the germ (25.5% dietary fiber); and spent barley grain bran (product of the brewery including the hull) (47.7% dietary fiber) were administered to male Sprague–Dawley rats as a 5% dietary supplement for

7 months. Commercial barley bran was most effective in reducing tumor incidence and burden. Tumor burden and tumor mass index were reduced significantly by outer-layer barley bran and spent barley grain bran. Commercial barley bran and spent barley grain bran, administered to rats with 1,2-dimethylhydrazine-induced intestinal tumor, produced a higher incidence and burden of tumor[HV153]. Fiber was administered to 4-week-old male Sprague–Dawley rats with dimethylhydrazine-induced tumors at a dose of 5% of diet. The insoluble fiber-rich fraction (spent barley grain) was significantly more effective at preventing induced tumors than the soluble commercial barley bran. The incidence of rats affected, tumor mass index, and plasma cholesterol concentration were reduced by spent barley grain. Outer-layer barley bran was moderately effective in cancer prevention[HV155]. The crude and partially purified lunasin, in stably *ras*-transfected mouse fibroblast cell culture, suppressed colony formation induced with isopropylthiogalactoside. This fraction also inhibited histone acetylation in mouse fibroblast (NIH 3T3) and human breast (MCF-7) cells in the presence of the histone deacetylase inhibitor sodium butyrate[HV163].

Anti-ulcer activity. Water extract of the green leaf juice, administered by gastric intubation to rats at a dose of 500 mg/kg, was active vs stress-induced (restraint) ulcers. The results were significant at $p < 0.001$ level. Water extract was active vs acetic acid-induced and aspirin-induced ulcers. The results were significant at $p < 0.01$ and $p < 0.005$ levels, respectively. Water extract was inactive vs pylorus ligation-induced ulcers[HV116]. Extract of the dried seedling, administered orally to adults at a dose of 30 g/person, was active[HV077]. Germinated barley foodstuff, administered orally to male Sprague–Dawley rats on day 6 after initiation of colitis, was active vs dextran sodium sulfate-induced colitis. Germinated barley foodstuff treatment reduced colonic inflam-

mation with an increase in cecal butyrate levels[HV139]. Fiber and protein factions of germinated barley foodstuff, administered to dextran sodium sulfate-induced colitis Sprague–Dawley rats, significantly attenuated the clinical signs of colitis and decreased serum α1-acid glycoprotein levels, with an increase in cecal butyrate production, whereas germinated barley foodstuff-protein did not. Germinated barley foodstuff with or without salazosulfapyridine, administered to rats after the onset of colitis, accelerated colonic epithelial repair and improved clinical signs[HV140]. Germinated barley foodstuff, administered orally to patients with mild to moderate active ulcerative colitis at a dose of 30 g/person daily for 4 weeks, produced a significant clinical and endoscopic improvement independent of disease extent. The improvement was associated with an increase in stool butyrate concentrations and in luminal *Bifidobacterium* and *Eubacterium* levels. After the end of treatment, the patients had an exacerbation of the disease[HV141]. Germinated barley foodstuff with or without *Clostridium butyricum*, administered to 3% dextran sodium sulfate-induced colitis in Sprague–Dawley rats for 8 days, prevented bloody diarrhea and mucosal damage and increased the fecal short-chain fatty acid levels[HV143]. Germinated barley foodstuff, administered to Sprague–Dawley rats for 5 days, prevented bloody diarrhea and mucosal damage, elevated fecal acetic acid and *N*-butyric acid levels, and tended to increase the number of *Eubacteria* and *Bifidobacteria*. The number of *Enterobacteriaceae*, the total number of aerobes and *Bacteroidaceae*, were lowered by germinated barley foodstuff treatment[HV144]. Germinated barley foodstuff, administered to HLA-B27 transgenic rats for 13 weeks, produced an increase of bacterial butyrate production and the decrease of cecal occult blood, colonic mucosal hyperplasia, colonic mucosal necrosis factor-κB-DNA binding activity, and the production of IL-8[HV145]. Butyrate from germinated barley foodstuff, administered orally or intracecally to Sprague–Dawley rats, produced reduction of mucosal damage only by intrathecal administration. Bacterial butyrate production and reduction of mucosal damage depended on the dose of germinated barley foodstuff in the diet[HV146]. Germinated barley foodstuff and scutellum fraction of germinated barley, administered to Sprague–Dawley rats with colitis induced by 3% dextran sodium sulfate, prevented bloody diarrhea and mucosal damage in colitis. The germinated samples did not produce a protective effect. Germinated barley foodstuff increased mucosal protein and RNA content in the colitis model[HV149]. Germinated barley foodstuff, administered to 18 patients with mildly to moderately active ulcerative colitis at a dose of 20–30 g germinated barley foodstuff daily for 4 weeks, produced a significant decrease in clinical activity index scores compared to the control group. No side effects related to germinated barley foodstuff were observed. Germinated barley foodstuff therapy increased fecal concentrations of *Bifidobacterium* and *Eubacterium limosum*[HV170]. Germinated barley foodstuff, administered to patients with mild to moderate active ulcerative colitis, irresponsible to or intolerant of standard treatment at a dose of 20–30 g germinated barley foodstuff daily for 4 weeks, resulted in a significant clinical and endoscopic improvement associated with an increase in stool butyrate concentrations[HV174].

Antiviral activity. Ethanol (50%) extract of the seed, in cell culture at a concentration of 50 µg/mL, produced weak activity on Ranikhet virus[HV001]. Decoction of the dried seed, in cell culture, produced weak activity on WA-rotavirus[HV042]. Protein fraction of the seed without seed coat, on agar plate at a concentration of 2 µg/disc, was active on CA-Ehrlich ascites[HV085].

Anti-yeast activity. Tincture of the dried seed, on agar plate at a concentration of 30 µL/disc, was inactive on *Candida albicans*.

Extract of 10 g plant material in 100 mL ethanol was used[HV122].

Cardiovascular activity. β-glucan, administered to 18 men with mild hypercholesterolemia with a mean body weight index of 27.4 ± 4.6 at a dose of 8.1–11.9 g β-glucan per day, produced no significant change in total, LDL and HDL cholesterol, triacylglycerol, fasting glucose, and postprandial glucose[HV169].

Cholesterol biosynthesis inhibition. The inhibitor I from oily nonpolar fraction of flour, administered to chicken at a dose of 2.5–20 ppm, produced a significant decrease in hepatic cholesterogenesis and serum total and LDL cholesterol and an increase in lipogenic activity[HV158].

Cholesterol-7-α-hydroxylase inhibition. Petroleum ether extract of the fresh fruit, administered to pigs at a concentration of 3.5 g/kg of diet for 29 days, produced 40% inhibition of the hepatic enzyme activity[HV092].

Citrate lyase inhibition. Petroleum ether extract of the fresh fruit, administered to pigs at a concentration of 3.5 g/kg of diet for 29 days, was active on the hepatic enzymes[HV092].

Cyclo-oxygenase inhibition. Methanol extract of the ether-insoluble fraction of the fresh seed, administered to rats at a dose of 100 µg/mL, inhibited platelets by 46%. Methanol extract of ether-soluble fraction inhibited platelets by 29%[HV051].

Cytotoxic activity. Water extract of the dried fruit, in cell culture at a concentration of 500 µg/mL, produced weak activity on CA-mammary-microalveolar[HV098]. Ethanol (50%) extract of the seed, in cell culture, was inactive on CA-9KB, ED_{50} greater than 20 µg/mL[HV001]. Methanol extract of the dried seed, in cell culture, was inactive on SNU-1 human cells, IC_{50} greater than 0.3 mg/mL, and on SNU-C4 human cells, IC_{50} greater than 0.3 mg/mL[HV061]. Protein fraction of the seed without seed coat, in cell culture at a concentration of 2 µg/disc, was active on

CA-Ehrlich ascites[HV085]. Methanol extract of the aerial parts, in cell culture at a concentration of 50 mg/mL, was equivocal on CA-9KB[HV075].

Diuretic activity. Decoction of the dried seed, administered nasogastrically to rats at a dose of 1 g/kg, produced strong activity[HV120].

Estrogenic effect. Ethanol (95%) extract of the aerial parts, administered subcutaneously to infant mice, was active[HV128].

Fatty acid synthase inhibition. Petroleum ether extract of the fresh fruit, administered to pigs at a concentration of 3.5 g/kg of diet for 29 days, was active on hepatic enzymes[HV092].

Gastrointestinal activity. Water extract of the green leaf juice, administered by gastric intubation to rats at a dose of 500 mg/kg, was inactive vs pylorus ligation-induced ulcers[HV116]. Fiber, administered orally to young male Wistar rats at a dose of 500 g extrudates/kg of diet for 6 weeks, produced a higher concentration of neutral sterols in the intestinal content of the barley-fed group than in the control group ($p < 0.005$) and affected indirectly the amount of formed secondary bile acids[HV134]. Fiber, administered orally to young male Wistar rats at a dose of 50 g/100 g extrudates or mixtures for 6 weeks, produced greater food intake in the last 2 weeks and increased ceca and colon masses, cecal and colon contents, concentration of resistant starch in cecal, most of colon contents, and β-glucan level in the small intestine, cecum, and colon. The numbers of coliforms and *Bacteroides* were lower and those of *Lactobacillus* were higher than in the control group. The dose increased weight gain in the sixth week. Short-chain fatty acids were higher in the cecal, colon, and feces content of the test group. The proportion of secondary bile acids was lower and the amount of neutral sterol was higher in feces of fiber-treated animals. The concentrations of excreted bile acids increased up to 30% during the

feeding period[HV138]. Germinated barley foodstuff, administered to Sprague–Dawley rats fed on various diets with the same protein and dietary fiber levels, produced an increase fecal output compared with commercial water-soluble and insoluble dietary fibers. The dietary fiber from germinated barley foodstuff increased the fecal output and mucosal protein content. The protein fraction of germinated barley foodstuff degraded to the peptide form did not increase the fecal output or mucosal protein content[HV152]. Germinated barley foodstuff from aleurone and scutellum fractions of germinated barley, administrated to healthy volunteers at a dose of 9 g daily for 14 days, significantly increased fecal butyrate content and fecal *Bifidobacterium* and *Eubacterium*. Ten anaerobic microorganisms selected from intestinal microflora were cultured in vitro in germinated barley foodstuff medium. After 3 days of incubation, seven strains (*Bifidobacterium breve, Bifidobacterium longum, Lactobacillus acidophilus, Lactobacillus casei* ssp. *casei, Bacteroides ovatus, Clostridium butyricum,* and *Eubacterium limosum*) lowered the medium pH producing short-chain fatty acid. Germinated barley foodstuff changed the intestinal microflora and increased probiotics such as *Bifidobacterium*. Butyrate was produced by the mutual action of *Eubacterium* and *Bifidobacterium*[HV186]. Germinated barley foodstuff from aleurone layer, scutellum, and germ, administered to 10 healthy volunteers at a dose of 30 g/day/person for 28 days, produced an increased fecal butyrate content, fecal weight, and water content. There were no significant changes in body weight and major abnormalities in hematologic and urinary analysis[HV187]. Fiber, administered to nine patients with ileostomies at a dose of 35 g/day, increased the ileal excretion of starch[HV191]. Flaked and finely milled barley, eaten by patients with ileostomies, showed that only 2 ± 1% of starch remained undigested after the consumption of finely milled barley and $17 \pm 1\%$ resisted digestion, partly as oligosaccharides but largely as intact unpitted starch granules bound by intact cell walls. The energy excretion from the stoma was three times higher after flaked that after milled barley. Nonstarch polysaccharide, starch, and fat made almost equal contributions to the higher energy excretion[HV196]. Bran flour, administered to 44 volunteers at a dose of 30 g/day, decreased the transit time by 8.02 hours from baseline and increased daily fecal weight by 48.6 g[HV201]. Groats were administered to volunteers at a dose of 1 g carbohydrate/kg body weight, three times or at three different doses of 0.75, 1, and 1.5 g carbohydrate/kg body weight. After consumption of 1 g carbohydrate/kg body weight, produced a mean mouth to cecum transit time of 8.4 ± 0.4 hour. After consumption of the high dose, a mean mouth-to-cecum transit time of 9.0 ± 0.5 hours was produced. Particle size did not significantly affect the mouth-to-caecum transit time[HV206]. Germinated barley foodstuff, administered to Sprague–Dawley rats, prevented diarrhea and mucosal damages; increased mucosal protein, DNA, and RNA content; and depressed bacterial translocation and elevation of myeloperoxidase activity induced by methotrexate[HV147]. β-glucan-rich barley fraction, administered to ileostomy subjects at a dose of 13.0 g β-glucan/day for 2 days, increased the cholesterol excretion higher than with the oat bran with β-glucanase and wheat flour diets. Bile acid excretion was 755 (133–1187) mg/day[HV194]. Carbohydrates, administered to healthy subjects at a dose of 90 g for dinner in random order 1 week apart, significantly increased the breath hydrogen and improved glucose tolerance. No difference in the rates of glucose disappearance or gut glucose absorption was observed. Serum-free fatty acid concentrations were significantly reduced the morning after the barley meal[HV202]. Germinated barley foodstuff, administered to Sprague–Dawley rats with constipation induced by loperamide, produced an increase of bowel movements, fecal water content, and concentration of short-chain fatty acids in cecal content, especially butyrate[HV148].

Glucose tolerance effect. Fiber, administered orally to type 2 diabetic Goto–Kakizaki male rats for 9 months, improved the area under the plasma glucose concentration time curves, lowered the fasting plasma glucose and glycosylated hemoglobin levels, and decreased plasma total cholesterol, triglycerides, and free fatty acid levels[HV135]. Fiber, administered orally to 8-week-old male Goto–Kakizaki strain rats, at a dose of 1.79 g/day/rat for 3 months, improved glucose tolerance and lowered the plasma cholesterol and triglyceride levels. The fasting plasma glucose level was significantly lower in comparison to rice and corn starch-fed rats[HV136]. High barley (high-fiber diet), administered to 10 women (20.4 ± 1.3 year-old, 19.2 ± 2 kg/m^2) for 4 weeks with a 1-month interval, resulted in lowering plasma total and LDL cholesterol concentrations and reduced plasma triacylglycerol concentration. The barley diet increased stool volume. There was no significant difference in glucose tolerance between diet regimens[HV168]. Barley bread containing lactic acid and reference barley bread, administered in the morning to 10 healthy men and women, produced a significant lowering of the incremental glycemic area and of the glucose response at 95 minutes after ingestion of the bread with lactic acid. At 45 minutes after the meal, the insulin level was significantly lower after the lactic acid bread, compared with reference barley bread[HV176].

Glucose-6-phosphate dehydrogenase inhibition. Petroleum ether extract of the fresh fruit, administered to pigs at a concentration of 3.5 g/kg of diet for 29 days, was active on hepatic enzymes[HV092].

Glutamate–oxaloacetate–transaminase inhibition. Methanol extract of the dried fruit, administered by gastric intubation to rabbits at a dose of 500 mg/kg, was active vs CCl_4-induced hepatotoxicity. A mixture of *Machilus* sp., *Alisma* sp., *Amomum xanthioides*, *Bulboschoenus maritimus*, *Artemisia iwaymogis*, *Atractylodes japonica*, *Crataegus cuneata*, *Hordeum vulgare*, *Citrus sinensis*, *Polyporus umbellatus*, *Agastache rugosa*, *Raphanus sativus*, *Poncirus trifoliatus*, *Curcuma zeodaria*, *Citrus aurantium*, *Saussurea lappa*, *Glycyrrhiza glabra*, and *Zingiber officinale* was used. Results were significant at $p < 0.01$ level[HV112].

Glutamate–pyruvate–transaminase inhibition. Methanol extract of the dried fruit, administered by gastric intubation to rabbits at a dose of 500 mg/kg, was active vs carbon tetrachloride (CCl_4)-induced hepatotoxicity. A mixture of *Machilus* sp., *Alisma* sp., *Amomum xanthioides*, *Bulboschoenus maritimus*, *Artemisia iwaymogis*, *Atractylodes japonica*, *Crataegus cuneata*, *Hordeum vulgare*, *Citrus sinensis*, *Polyporus umbellatus*, *Agastache rugosa*, *Raphanus sativus*, *Poncirus trifoliatus*, *Curcuma zeodaria*, *Citrus aurantium*, *Saussurea lappa*, *Glycyrrhiza glabra*, and *Zingiber officinale* was used. Result was significant at $p < 0.01$ level[HV112].

Growth inhibition. Germinated barley foodstuff, administered orally to 4-week-old female ICR mice at a dose of 10% for 24 weeks, produced no effect on the growth rate of mice[HV142].

Hair growth influence. Purified procyanidin B-3, in hair epithelial cell culture, produced high hair-growing activity and in vivo anagen-inducing activity. (+)-Catechin produced no hair-growing activity[HV162].

3-Hydroxy-3-methylglutaryl coenzyme A reductase inhibition. Petroleum ether extract of the fresh fruit, administered to pigs at a concentration of 3.5 g/kg of diet for 29 days, produced 40% inhibition of the hepatic enzyme activity[HV092].

Hypocholesterolemic activity. Fixed oil of the bran, administered orally to adults of both sexes at a dose of 30 mg/day, was active. Flour bran, administered orally to adults at a dose of 3 g/day, was active[HV059]. Dried bran, administered in the ration of male rats, was active[HV068]. Petroleum ether extract of the fresh fruit, administered to pigs at a concentration of 3.5 g/kg of diet, produced a decrease of serum total cholesterol, LDL cholesterol, and HDL cholesterol after 29 days of feeding[HV092]. Flour, administered orally to adults with hypercholesterolemia at a dose of 44 g/day, produced a decrease of total and LDL cholesterol levels[HV100].

Hypoglycemic activity. Water extract of the fermented root, administered intravenously to rabbits, was active[HV007]. The dried seed, administered orally to eight healthy volunteers at a dose of 50 g/person, was active. A single dose resulted in a glycemic index of 68.7 and an insulinemic index of 71.1[HV047].

Hypolipemic activity. Fiber, administered orally to nine adults with ileostomies at a dose of 13 g/day, increased the excretion of cholesterol[HV072]. Petroleum ether extract of the fresh fruit, administered to pigs at a concentration of 3.5 g/kg of diet, was inactive[HV092]. Purified green barley extract, in human mononuclear culture of cells isolated from perithelial blood and synovial fluid of patients with rheumatoid arthritis, was active[HV178]. Leaf essence, administered to atherosclerotic New Zealand White male rabbits at a dose of 1% of diet, produced a decrease of plasma total cholesterol, triacylglycerol, lucigenin–chemiluminescence, and luminal–chemiluminescence levels. The value of T_{50} of red blood cell hemolysis and the lag phase of LDL oxidation increased in barley-treated group compared with the control. Ninety percent of the intimal surface of the thoracic aorta was covered with atherosclerotic lesions in the control group, but only 60% of the surface was covered in the barley group. This inhibition was associated with a decrease in plasma lipids and an increase in antioxidative abilities[HV003].

Hypotriglyceridemic activity. Fixed oil of the bran, administered orally to adults of both sexes at a dose of 30 mg/day, was active. Flour bran, administered orally to adults at a dose of 3 g/day, was inactive[HV059].

Laxative effect. Powdered dried bran, administered orally to 44 adults at a dose of 30 g/person, was active on gastrointestinal motility. Transit time decreased by 8 hours, and fecal mass increased by 48.6 g/day[HV050].

Lipid metabolism. Fiber, administered orally to male type 2 diabetic Goto–Kakizaki rats for 9 months, improved the area under the plasma glucose concentration time curves, lowered the fasting plasma glucose and glycosylated hemoglobin levels, and decreased plasma total cholesterol, triglycerides and free fatty acid levels[HV135].

Lipolytic effect. Ethanol (95%) extract of the dried entire plant in combination with *Rhizoma zingiberis*, *Ligustrum chuanxiong*, *Lilium brownii*, *Nephelium longa*, and *Polygonum multiflorum*, administered in drinking water to C57BL/6J obese mice at a concentration of 5%, was active[HV070].

Lipoxygenase inhibition. Methanol extract of ether-insoluble and ether-soluble fractions of the fresh seed, administered to rats at a dose of 100 µg/mL, was inactive on platelets[HV051].

Lung function. Exposure of six men to barley dust for 2 days decreased ventilatory capacity. Five volunteers not previously exposed to barley dust, when exposed to the dust for 2 hours, decreased the ventilatory capacity ranging from 200 mL to 800 mL, with recovery taking up to 72 hours. All of the subjects had decreases in flow at 50% vital capacity but little or no change in flow at 75% vital capacity. In three subjects, there was a drop in specific conductance

that lasted for less than 24 hours[HV209]. Sixty-nine of 80 dockworkers handling grains reported evening feverish episodes/ symptoms not related to smoking or atopic status. No gross deficits in lung function were detected[HV200].

Malic enzyme inhibition. Petroleum ether extract of the fresh fruit, administered to pigs at a concentration of 3.5 g/kg of diet for 29 days, was active on hepatic enzymes[HV092].

Mineral utilization. Germinated barley foodstuff, administered orally to 5-week-old Sprague–Dawley rats for 14 days, promoted the absorption of calcium (Ca) and magnesium (Mg) by the gastrointestinal tract. The absorption of iron and potassium was not attenuated and mineral absorption was not inhibited[HV142]. Barley husk, administered to 5- and 9-week-old rats at different doses, produced a lowering of zinc (Zn) and Ca absorption already at dose 20 g dietary fiber/ kg dry matter and had a small negative effect on potassium absorption. Phytate did not appear as a major factor affecting mineral absorption in barley husk. All of the diets containing barley husk had very low molar ratios (phytate:Zn was 4)[HV159]. Processed or unprocessed barley was administered to healthy subjects in two single meals containing porridge or breakfast (60 g) cereals for 2 months. Zn absorption from hydrothermally-treated barley porridge was significantly higher than from the control porridge; Ca absorption did not differ. Zn absorption from breakfast cereals of malted barley with phytase activity was significantly higher than from flakes of barley without phytase activity; Ca absorption was not significantly different[HV167]. Standard barley and β-glucan-enriched barley dehulled grains was administered to 10 healthy hydrogen-producing adults at a dose of 35 g. The percentage of the ^{13}C dose oxidized was greater after standard barley than after enriched barley consumption. The area under the curve for H_2 was greater after enriched barley intake. There was no difference in CO_2 production[HV171]. Hull fiber extract, in Caco-2 cell culture, produced no effect on the rate of transepithelial ^{45}Ca transport across Caco-2 cell monolayers and the uptake of ^{45}Ca into Caco-2 cells[HV182]. A low-phytate barley-fiber concentrate was administered to young women at a dose of 15 g barley fiber (high-fiber, high-protein diet) and 15 g barley fiber (high-fiber, low-protein diet). The mean daily intake of the cations was 25.4 and 22.9 mmol Ca, 10.1 and 10 mmol Mg, 166.8 and 119.3 μmol Zn, and 186.2 and 154 μmol Fe, respectively. Mean balances were 1.9 and –0.8 mmol Ca, –0.2 and –0.5 mmol Mg, –4.6, and –18.4 μmol Zn, respectively. The mean apparent iron absorption was 5.4 and –23.2 μmol[HV203].

Monocytic differentiation. Prodelphinidin B-3, T1, T2, and T3 from bran polyphenol extract, in HL60 human myeloid leukemia cell culture, induced 26–40% nitro blue tetrazolium positive cells and 22–32% α-naphthyl-butyrate esterase-positive cells. Proanthocyanidins potentiated all-*trans*-retinoic acid-induced granulocytic and sodium butyrate-induced monocytic differentiation in HL60 cells[HV188].

Mutagenic activity. Ethanol (70%) extract of the dried seed, on agar plate at a concentration of 50 mg/mL, was inactive on *Escherichia coli* PQ 37. The water and chloroform extracts of the ethanol (70%) extract were inactive. Metabolic activation had no effect on the results[HV096].

Oxidative effect. Ethanol (95%) extract of the dried entire plant, administered in drinking water to C57BL/6J obese mice at a concentration of 5%, increased glucose oxidation in epididymal fat pads. Extract of mixture of following plants: *Hordeum vulgare*, *Rhizoma zingiberis*, *Ligustrum chuanxiong*, *Lilium brownii*, *Nephelium longa*, and *Polygonum multiflorum* was used[HV070].

Pepsin inhibition. Water extract of the green leaf juice, administered by gastric

intubation to rats at a dose of 500 mg/kg, was inactive vs pylorus ligation-induced ulcers[HV116].

Periodontal effect. Fiber, administered to male Alpk:APfSD rats for 107 weeks with sacrifices at 26, 53, and 77 weeks, produced oronasal fistulation and severe periodontitis[HV156].

Phosphogluconate dehydrogenase inhibition. Petroleum ether extract of the fresh fruit, administered to pigs at a concentration of 3.5 g/kg of diet for 29 days, was active on hepatic enzymes[HV092].

Protein synthesis inhibition. Chromatographic fraction of the dried seed, in cell culture, was active on reticulocyte lysate of rabbits, inhibitory concentration$_{50}$ 15.25 ng/mL[HV084].

Proteinemic effect. Methanol extract of the dried fruit, administered by gastric intubation to rabbits at a dose of 500 mg/kg, produced an increase in serum albumin and protein content vs CCl_4-induced hepatotoxicity. A mixture of *Machilus* sp., *Alisma* sp., *Amomum xanthioides*, *Bulboschoenus maritimus*, *Artemisia iwaymogis*, *Atractylodes japonica*, *Crataegus cuneata*, *Hordeum vulgare*, *Citrus sinensis*, *Polyporus umbellatus*, *Agastache rugosa*, *Raphanus sativus*, *Poncirus trifoliatus*, *Curcuma zeodaria*, *Citrus aurantium*, *Saussurea lappa*, *Glycyrrhiza glabra*, and *Zingiber officinale* was used. Results were significant at $p < 0.01$ level[HV112].

Respiratory effect. Barley ear inhaled by a 2.5-year-old child produced fever, dyspnea, right paracardiac infiltrate with pleural reaction on X-rays, and normal bronchoscopy after 8 days. On day 11, extensive right pneumothorax, and on day 20, right axillary inflammatory lesion were observed. On day 28, the ear of barley was expulsed and there was complete recovery[HV207]. Barley spike, inhaled into the tracheobronchial tree of 18 children under the age of 5 years, produced coughing and choking in 14 of the children. The spikes were removed by laryngoscopy in 12 patients and by rigid bronchoscopy in two. Four patients with history of cough, dyspnea, fever, and serious respiratory diseases, such as pneumothorax, lobar pneumonia, and pleural empyema, required surgical intervention. All of the children made satisfactory recoveries[HV189]. Dust extract of barley, in cell culture on nonsensitized guinea pig tracheal smooth muscle pretreated with drugs, produced constrictor effect that was significantly inhibited by atropine indicating an interaction of the extracts with parasympathetic nerves. Inhibition of contraction of other mediators was less effective and varied with the dust extract[HV208].

Toxic effect. β-glucan-enriched soluble barley fiber, administered orally to Wistar rats at concentrations of 0.7, 3.5, and 7.0% β-glucan for 28 days, increased the number of circulating lymphocytes in males. The increase was not dose-dependent and was not observed in females. A dose-dependent increase in full and empty cecum weight was observed. There were no adverse effects on general condition and behavior, growth, feed and water consumption, feed conversion efficiency, red blood cell and clotting potential parameters, clinical chemistry values, and organ weight. Necropsy and histopathology findings revealed no treatment-related changes in any organ evaluated[HV137]. β-glucan (64%) preparation (barley β-fiber), administered to CD-1 mice at concentrations of 1, 5, or 10% of diet (0.7, 3.5, and 7% β-glucan) for 28 days, produced no adverse effect in hematological or clinical chemistry measurements, in organ weights and immunopathology in either sex after treatment or after the recovery period[HV166]. Azidoalanine and the azide-treated extracts, in Chinese hamster and normal human skin fibroblast cell cultures, significantly increased the frequency of sister chromatid exchanges observed in both cultures. This increase was approximately twofold, as compared with the control[HV205].

Toxicity assessment. Ethanol (50%) extract of the seed, administered intraperitoneally to mice, produced a maximum tolerated dose of 1 g/kg[HV001]. Hexane extract of the green leaf juice, administered in ration of rats, produced lethal dose$_{50}$ greater than 10 g/kg[HV117].

Tyrosinase inhibition. Methanol (80%) extract of the dried seedling, in cell culture at a concentration of 100 μg/mL, was inactive[HV038].

Urease inhibition. Water extract of the seed, in cell culture at a concentration of 0.3 mg/mL, was inactive[HV076].

Weight gain inhibition. Ethanol (95%) extract of the dried entire plant, administered in drinking water to C57BL/6J obese mice at a concentration of 5%, was active. The extract also contained Rhizoma zingiberis, Ligustrum chuangxiong, Lilium brownii, Nephelium longa, and Polygonum multiflorum[HV070].

REFERENCES

HV001 Dhar, M. L., M. M. Dhar, B. N. Dhawan, B. N. Mehrotha, and C. Ray. Screening of Indian plants for biological activity. Part I. **Indian J Exp Biol** 1968; 6: 232–247.

HV002 Stoessl, A. The antifungal factors in barley—3. Isolation of P-coumaroylagmatine. **Phytochemistry** 1965; 4: 973–976.

HV003 Yu Y. M., C. H. Wu, Y. H. Tseng, C. E. Tsai, and W. C. Chang. Antioxidative and hypolipidemic effects of barley leaf essence in a rabbit model of atherosclerosis. **Jpn J Pharmacol** 2002; 89(2): 142–148.

HV004 McElroy, L. W., H. A. Rigney, and H. H. Draper. Choline content of live stock feeds used in Western Canada. **Sci Agr** 1948; 28: 268–271.

HV005 Spencer, E. V., A. D. Robinson, L. W. McElroy, and J. Kastelic. Collaborative analysis of wheat, oats and barley for their thiamine and riboflavin. **Can J Res Ser F** 1949; 27: 194–198.

HV006 Mendez, J. Indole auxins in barley seedlings. **Phytochemistry** 1967; 6: 313–315.

HV007 Donard, E., and H. Labbe. The coexistence in barley rootlets of hyperglycemic and hypoglycemic substances. **Comp Rend** 1933; 196: 1047–1050.

HV008 Cheunsoontorn, S., and N. Udompon-sanontha. Nutritional value of ant larvae (*Oecophylla smaragdina* Hym.). **Abstr 3rd Congress of the Federation of Asian and Oceanian Biochemists Bangkok Thailand** 1983.

HV009 Hejgaard, J., S. Jacobsen, and I. Svendsen. Two antifungal thaumatin-like proteins from barley grain. **FEBS Lett** 1991; 291(1): 127–131.

HV010 Osawa, T., H. Katsuzaki, Y. Hagiwara, H. Hagiwara, and T. Shibamoto. AS novel antioxidant isolated from young green barley leaves. **J Agr Food Chem** 1992; 40(7): 1135–1138.

HV011 Svensson, B., I. B. Svendsen, P. Hojrup, P. Roepstorff, S. Ludvigsen, and F. M. Poulsen. Primary structure of barwin: a barley seed protein closely related to the C-terminal domain of proteins encoded by wound-induced plant genes. **Biochemistry** 1992; 31(37): 8767–8770.

HV012 Molina, A., A. Segura, and F. Garcia-Olmedo. Lipid transfer proteins (NSLTPS) from barley and maize leaves are potent inhibitors of bacterial and fungal plant pathogens. **FEBS Lett** 1993; 316(2): 119–122.

HV013 Purmohseni, H., W. D. Ibenthal, R. Machinek, G. Remberg, and V. Wray. Cyanoglucosides in the epidermis of *Hordeum vulgare*. **Phytochemistry** 1993; 33(2): 295–297.

HV014 Upreti, R. K., S. Ahmad, S. Shukla, and A. M. Kidwai. Experimental anorexigenic effect of a membrane proteoglycan isolated from plants. **J Ethnopharmacol** 1994; 42(1): 53–61.

HV015 Mendez, E., A. Rocher, M. Calero, T. Girbes, L. Citores, and F. Soriano. Primary structure of omega-hordothionin, a member of a novel family of thionins from barley endosperm, and its inhibition of protein synthesis in eucaryotic and procaryotic cell-free system. **Eur J Biochem** 1996; 239(1): 67–73.

HV016 Hamberg, M., and G. Hamberg. 14(R)-hydroxylinoleic acid, an oxylipid from oat seeds. **Phytochemistry** 1996; 42(3): 729–732.

HV017 Ohikawa, M., J. Kinjo, Y. Hagiwara, et al. Three new anti-oxidative saponarin analogs from young green barley leaves. **Chem Pharm Bull** 1998; 46(12): 1887–1890.

HV018 Linnestad, C., D. N. P. Doan, R. C. Brown, et al. Nucellain, a barley homolog of the dicot vacuolar-processing protease, is localized in nuclear cell walls. **Plant Physiol** 1998; 118(4): 1169–1180.

HV019 Zagari, A. Medicinal plants. Vol 4, 5th ed., Tehran University Publications, No 1810/4, Tehran, Iran 1992; 969 pp.

HV020 Stalay, A. E. Starch granulation. Patent-Neth Appl-73 10,688 1975.

HV021 Savchenko, G. E. Effect of chloramphenicol on the accumulation and transformation of protochlorophyll in barley leaves. **Biol Nauch-Tekhn Progress** 1974: 60.

HV022 Bonnafous, J. C., J. L. Olive, J. L. Borgna, and M. Mousseron-Canet. Cyclic AMP in barley seeds and seedlings, and the bacterial or fungal contamination. **Biochimie** 1975; 57: 661.

HV023 Lichtenthaler, H. K., and V. Straub. The formation of lipoquinones in tissue cultures. **Planta Med Sauppl** 1975; 198.

HV024 Gross, D., H. Lehmann, and H. R. Shutte. Biosynthesis of *Graminae*. **Biochem Physiol Pflanz** 1974; 166: 281.

HV025 Lenton, J. R., L. J. Goad, and T. W. Goodwin. Sitosterol biosynthesis in *Hordeum vulgare*. **Phytochemistry** 1975; 14: 1523–1528.

HV026 Zimlyanukhin, L. A. Dynamics of aconitic acid formation in corn and barley roots. **Fiziol I Fiz-Khim Mekhanizmy Regulyatsii Obmen Protsessov Organizma** 1974; 1974(3): 18.

HV027 Faull, K. R., B. G. Coombe, and L. G. Paleg. Extraction and characterization of gibberellins from *Hordeum vulgare* seedlings. **Aust J Plant Physiol** 1974; 1: 183.

HV028 Vassilev, G. N., and N. P. Mashev. Synthesis, chemical structure and cytokinin-like activity of some derivatives of N-Phenyl-N'-alk-yl or arylt thiourea and their influence on the nitrogen metabolism in barley seedlings. **Biochem Physiol Pflanz** 1974; 165: 467.

HV029 Solomakhina, V. A., N. V. Novotel'-nov, and M. T. Golovkina. Extraction of phenolic compounds from barley and their determination. **Ezv Vyssh Uchebn Zaved Pishch Tekhnol** 1975; 1975(3): 183.

HV030 Perez, C., and C. Anesini. *In vitro* antibacterial activity of Argentine folk medicinal plants against *Salmonella typhi*. **J Ethnopharmacol** 1994; 44(1): 41–46.

HV031 Nakamura, T. H., M. B. Ishitani, P. Harinasut, M. Nomura, T. H. Takabe, and T. T. Takabe. Distribution of glycinebetaine in old and young leaf blades of salt-stressed barley plants. **Plant Cell Physiol** 1996; 37(6): 873–877.

HV032 Reuber, S., B. Jende-Strid, V. Wray, and G. Weissenbock. Accumulation of the chalcone isosalipurposide in primary leaves of barley flavonoid mutants indicates a defective chalcone isomerase. **Physiol Plant** 1997; 101(4): 827–832.

HV033 Park, J, H., B. K. Kim, M. K. Park, et al. Anti-diabetic activity of herbal drugs. **Korean J Pharmacog** 1997; 28(2): 72–74.

HV034 Kobayashi, M., M. Gomi, J. Agematsu, T. Asami, S. Yoshida, and A. Sakurai. Fluctuation of endogenous gibberelin and abscisic acid levels in germinating seeds of barley. **Biosci Biotech Biochem** 1995; 59(10): 1969–1970.

HV035 Davies, J. T., P. R. Shewry, and N. Harris. Spatial and temporal patterns of B hordein synthesis in developing barley (*Hordeum vulgare* L.) caryopses. **Cell Biol Int** 1993; 17(2): 195–203.

HV036 Mayoral, A. M., C. Gutierrez, M. L. Ruiz, and P. Castanera. A high performance liquid chromatography method for quantification of diboa, dimboa and mboa from aqueous extracts of corn and winter cereal plants. **J Liq Chromatogr** 1994; 17(12): 2651–2665.

HV037 Zupfer, J. M., K. E. Churchil, D. C. Rasmusson, and R. G. Fulcher. Variation in ferulic acid concentration among diverse barley cultivars measured by HPLC and microspectrophotometry. **J Agr Food Chem** 1998; 46(4): 1350–1354.

HV038 Shin, N. H., K. S. Lee, S. H. Kang, K. R. Min, S. H. Lee, and Y. S. Kim. Inhibitory effects of herbal extracts on dopa oxidase activity of tyrosinase. **Nat Prod Sci** 1997; 3(2): 111–121.

HV039 Bruckner, C. The use of plant galactagogues in middle Europe. **Gleditschia** 1989; 17(2): 189–201

HV040 Shibamoto, T., Y. Hagiwara, H. Hagiwara, and T. Osawa. Flavonoid with strong antioxidative activity isolated from young barley leaves. **ACS Symp Ser** 1994; 547: 154–163.

HV041 Nakajima, S., Y. Hagiwara, H. Hagiwara, and T. Shibamoto. Effect of the antioxidant 2'-O-glycosylisovitexin from young green barley leaves on acetaldehyde formation in beer stored at 50C for 90 days. **J Agr Food Chem** 1998; 46(4): 1529–1531.

HV042 Song, M. J., and D. H. Kim. Inhibitory effect of herbal medicines on rotavirus infection. **Korean J Pharmacog** 1998; 292): 125–128.

HV043 Dundelova, M., and S. Prochazka. The level of indolyl-3-acetic acid in kernels of winter wheat (*Triticum aestivum* L.) and spring barley (*Hordeum vulgare* L.). **Rostl Vyroba** 1989; 35(4): 381–389.

HV044 Periera, F., M. Rafael, and M. H. Lacerda. Contact dermatitis from barley. **Contact Dermatitis** 1998; 39(5): 261.

HV045 Kanauchi, O., T. Nakamura, K. Agata, T. Fushiki, and H. Hara. Effects of germinated barley foodstuff in preventing diarrhea and forming normal feces in ceco-colectomized rats. **Biosci Biotech Biochem** 1998; 62(2): 366–368.

HV046 Cho, H. M., J. S. Jung, T. H. Lee, et al. Inhibitory effects of extracts from traditional herbal drugs on 5-hydroxytryptamine uptake in primary cultured rats brainstem neurons. **Korean J Pharmacog** 1995; 26(4): 349–354.

HV047 Shukla, K., J. P. Narain, P. Puri, et al. Glycemic response to maize, bajra and barley. **Indian J Physiol Pharmacol** 1991; 35(4): 249–254.

HV048 Poocharoen, B., J. F. Barbour, L. M. Libbey, and R. A. Scanlan. Precursors of N-nitrosodimethylamine in malted barley. 1. Determination of hordenine and gramine. **J Agr Food Chem** 1992; 40 (11): 2216–2221.

HV049 De Feo, V., and F. Senatore. Medicinal plants and phytotherapy in the Amafitan Coast, Salerno province, Campania, Southern Italy. **J Ethnopharmacol** 1993; 39(1): 39–51.

HV050 Luptn, J. R., J. L. Morn, and M. Robinson. Barley bran flour accelerates gastrointestinal transit time. **J Amer Diet Ass** 1993; 93(8): 881–885.

HV051 Sekiya, K., T. Fushimi, T. Kanamori, et al. Regulation of arachidonic acid metabolism in platelets by vegetables. **Biosci Biotech Biochem** 1993; 57(4): 670–671.

HV052 Miller, J. B., E. Pang, and L. Bramall. Rice: a high or low glycemic index food? **Amer J Clin Nutr** 1992; 56(6): 1034–1036.

HV053 Poplavskaya, R. S. Flavonoid accumulation of leaves of spring barley during development. **Vestsi Akad Navuk BSSR Biyal Navuk** 1991; 1991(5): 17–20.

HV054 Brandon, M. J., L. Y. Foo, L. J. Porter, and P. Meredith. Proanthocyanidins of barley and sorghum: composition as a function of maturity of barley ears. **Phytochemistry** 1982; 21(12): 2953–2957.

HV055 Rustamani, M. A., K. Kanehisa, H. Tsumuki, and T. Shiraga. Additional observations on *Aphid* densities and gramine contents in barley lines. **Appl Entomol Zool** 1992; 27(1): 151–153.

HV056 Anesini, C., and C. Perez. Screening of plants used in argentine folk medicine for antimicrobial activity. **J Ethnopharmacol** 1993; 39(2): 119–128.

HV057 Sasatamoinen, M., S. Plaami, J. Kumpulainen, and O. Rantanen. Concentrations of water soluble and insoluble beta-glucan and phytic acid in 6 row and 2-row barley. **Cereal Res Commun** 1991; 19(4): 391–397.

HV058 Hagiwara, Y., and H. Hagiwara. Isovitexin derivative from plant leaves as a xanthine oxidase inhibitor. Patent-Japan Kokai Tokkyo Koho-05,238,943 1993; 10 pp.

HV059 Lupton, J. R., M. C. Robinson, and J. L. Morin. Cholesterol-lowering effect of barley bran flour and oil. **J Amer Diet Ass** 1994; 94(1): 65–70.

HV060 Toshida, H., H. Tsumuki, K. Kanehisa, and L. J. Corcuera. Release of gramine from the surface of barley leaves. **Phytochemistry** 1993; 34(4): 1011–1013.

HV061 Hyun, J. W., K. H. Lim, J. E. Shin, et al. Antineoplastic effect of extracts from traditional medicinal plants and various plants. **Korean J Pharmacol** 1994; 25(2): 171–177.

HV062 Mahdi, G. S., D. J. Naismith, R. G. Price, S. A. Taylor, J. Risteli, and L. Risteli. Modulating influence of barley on the altered metabolism of glucose and of basement membranes in the diabetic rat. **Ann Nutr Metab** 1994; 38(2): 61–67.

HV063 Perez, C., and C. Anesini. Inhibition of *Pseudomonas aeruginosa* by Argentinean medicinal plants. **Fitoterapia** 1994; 65(2): 169–172.

HV064 Nishiyam, T., Y. Hagiwara, H. Hagiwara, and T. Shibamoto. Inhibition of malonaldehyde foration from lipids by an isoflavonoid isolated from young green barley leaves. **J Amer Oil Chem Soc** 1993; 70(8): 811–813.

HV065 Miyagawa, H., H. Toda, T. Tsurushima, T. Ueno, and J. Shishiyama. Accumulation of tryptamine in barley leaves irradiated with UV light. **Biosci Biotech Biochem** 1994; 58(9): 1723–1724.

HV066 Scott, I. M., and H. Yamamoto. Mass spectrometric quantification f salicylic acid in plant tissues. **Phytochemistry** 1994; 37(2): 336.

HV067 Liu, D. L., and J. L. Lovett. Biologically active secondary metabolites of barley. II. Phytotoxicity of barley allelochemicals. **J Chem Ecol** 1993; 19(10): 2231–2244.

HV068 Jackson, K. A., D. A. I. Suter, and D. L. Topping. Oat bran, barley and malted barley lower plasma cholesterol relative to wheat bran but differ in their effects on liver cholesterol in rats fed diet with and without cholesterol. **J Nutr** 1994; 124(9): 1678–1684.

HV069 Hattori, A., H. Migitaka, M. Iigo, et al. Identification of melatonin in plants and its effects on plasma melatonin levels and binding to melatonin receptors in vertebrates. **Biochem Mol Biol Int** 1995; 35(3): 527–634.

HV070 Wijaya, E., Z. M. Wu, and F. Ng. Effect of 'Slimax', a Chinese herbal mixture, on obesity. **Int J Pharmacog** 1995; 33(1): 41–46.

HV071 Moore, B. D., E. Isidoro, and J. R. Seemann. Distribution of 2-carboxy-arabibitol among plants. **Phytochemistry** 1993; 34(3): 703–707.

HV072 Ohba, R., S. Kitaoka, S. Ohda, and S. Ueda. Storage stability and thermal stability of hordeumin, an anthocyanin pigment from barley. **Biosci Biotech Biochem** 1995; 59(4): 746–748.

HV072 Lia, A., G. Hallmans, A. S. Sandberg, B. Sundberg, P. Aman, and H. Andersson. Oat beta-glucan increases bile acid excretion and a fiber-rich barley fraction increases cholesterol excretion in ileostomy subjects. **Amer J Clin Nutr** 1995; 62(6): 1245–1251.

HV073 Perez, C., and C. Anesini. Antibacterial activity of alimentary plants against *Staphylococcus aureus* growth. **Amer J Chinese Med** 1994; 22(2): 169–174.

HV074 Fujita, T., E. Sezik, M. Tabata, E. Yesilada, G. Honda, Y. Takeda, T. Taanka, and Y. Takaishi. Traditional medicine in Turkey. VII. Folk medicine in middle and west Black Sea regions. **Econ Bot** 1995; 49(4): 406–422.

HV075 Arisawa, M. Cell growth inhibition of KB cells by plant extracts. **Nat Med** 1994; 48(4): 338–347.

HV076 Bae, E. A., M. J. Han, N. J. Kim, and D. H. Kim. Anti-*Helicobacter pylori* activity of herbal medicines. **Boil Pharm Bull** 1998; 21(9): 990–992.

HV077 Mitsuyama, K., T. Saiki, O. Kanauchi, et al. Treatment of ulcerative colitis with germinated barley foodstuff feeding: a pilot study. **Aliment Pharmacol Ther** 1998; 12(12): 1225–1230.

HV078 Munoz, O., V. H. Argandona, and L. J. Corcuera. Chemical constituents from shoots of *Hordeum vulgare* infected by the *Aphid schizapsis graminum*. **Z Naturforsch Ser C** 1998; 53C(9/10): 811–817.

HV079 Duh, P. D., and G. C. Yen. Antioxidative activity of three herbal water extracts. **Food Chem** 1997; 60(4): 639–645.

HV080 Miyake, T., and T. Shibamoto. Inhibition of malonaldehyde and acetaldehyde formation from blood plasma oxidation by naturally occurring antioxidants. **J Agr Food Chem** 1998; 46(9): 3694–3697.

HV081 Lukas, T. J., D. B. Iverson, M. Schleicher, and D. M. Watterson. Structural characterization of a higher plant calmodulin. **Plant Physiol** 1984; 75(3): 788–795.

HV082 Meyer, A., O. Miersch, C. Buttner, W. Dathe, and G. Sembdner. Occurrence of the plant growth regulator jasmonic acid in plants. **J Plant Growth Regul** 1984; 3: 1–8.

HV083 Dorne, A. J, G. Cadel, and R. Douce. Polar lipid composition of leaves from nine typical alpine species. **Phytochemistry** 1986; 25(1): 65–68.

HV084 Asano, K., B. Svensson, and F. M. Polsen. Isolation and characterization of inhibitors of animal cell-free protein synthesis from barley seeds. **Carlsberg Res Commun** 1984; 49(7): 619–626.

HV085 Roberts, W. K., and C. P. Selitrennikoff. Isolation and partial characterization of two antifungal proteins from barley. **Biochim Biophys Acta** 1986; 880: 161–170.

HV086 Smith, T. A., S. J. Croker, and R. S. T. Loeffler. Occurrence in higher plants of 1-(3-aminopropyl)-pyrrolinium and pyrroline: products of polyamine oxidation. **Phytochemistry** 1986; 25(3): 683–689.

HV087 Kaneta, M., and N. Sugiyama. Identification of flavone compounds in eighteen *Gramineae* species. **Agr Biol Chem** 1973; 37: 2663–2665.

HV088 Oashi, H., E. Yamamoto, N. G. Lewis, and G. H. N. Towers. 5-Hydroxyferulic acid in *Zea mays* and *Hordeum vulgare* cell walls. **Phytochemistry** 1987; 26(7): 1915–1916.

HV089 Lehtonen, M., and R. Aikasalo. Betaglucan in two-and six-rowed barley. **Cereal Chem** 1987; 64(3): 191–193.

HV090 Argandona, V. H., G. E. Zuniga, and L. J. Corcuera. Distribution of gramine and hydroxamic acids and wheat leaves. **Phytochemistry** 1987; 26(7): 1917–1918.

HV091 Werner, C., and P. Matile. Accumulation of coumarylglucosides in vacuoles of barley protoplasts. **J Plant Physiol** 1985; 118(3): 237–249.

HV092 Quewshi, A.A., T. D. Crenshaw, N. Abuirmeileh, D. M. Peterson, and C.

E. Elson. Influence of minor plant constituents on porcine hepatic lipid metabolism. **Atherosclerosis** 1987; 64(2/3): 109–115.

HV093 Yu, J., and K. J. Chen. Clinical observations of AIDS treated with herbal formulas. **Int J Orient Med** 1989; 14(4): 189–193.

HV094 Johansson, I. M., and B. Schubert. Separation of hordenine and N-methyl derivatives from germinating barley by liquid chromatography with dual-electrode coulometric detection. **J Chromatogr** 1990; 498(1): 241–247.

HV095 Leah, R., H. Tommerup, I. Svendsen, and J. Mundy. Biochemical and molecular characterization of three barley seed proteins with antifungal properties. **J Biol Chem** 1991; 266(3): 1564–1573.

HV096 Pang, H. A., Y. W. Lee, N. J. Suh, and I. M. Chang. Toxicological study on Korean tea materials: screening of potential mutagenic activities by using SOS-chromotest. **Korean J Pharmacog** 1990; 21(1): 83–87.

HV097 Laman, M. A., and R. S. Poplavskaya. Hydroxycinnamine acid derivatives in spring barley. **Vestsi Akad Navuk BSSR Ser Biyal Navuk** 1990; 1990(2): 37–39.

HV098 Sato, A. Studies on anti-tumor activity of crude drugs. I. The effects of aqueous extracts of some crude drugs in shortterm screening test. **Yakugaku Zasshi** 1989; 109(6): 407–423.

HV099 Giordano, J., and P. J. Levine. Botanical preparations used in Italian folk medicine: possible pharmacological and chemical basis of effect. **Social Pharmacol** 1989; 3(1/2): 83–110.

HV100 Newman, R.K., S. E. Lewis, C. W. Newman, R. J. Boik, and R. T. Ramage. Hypocholesterolemic effect of barley foods on healthy men. **Nutr Rep Int** 1989; 39(4): 749–760.

HV101 Barria, B. N., S. V. Cpaj, and H. M. Niemeyer. Occurrence of Diboa in wild Hordeum species and its relation to Aphid resistance. **Phytochemistry** 1992; 31(1): 89–91.

HV102 Haggblom, P. Isolation o-froquefortine C from feed grain. **Appl Environ Microbiol** 1990; 56(9): 2924–2926.

HV103 Hengtrakul, P., K. Lorenz, and M. Mathias. Alkylresorcinol homologs in cereal grains. **J Food Compos Anal** 1991; 4(1): 52–57.

HV104 Hyldon, R. G., and J. S. O'Mahony. Treating hypercholesterolemia. Patent-US-4,175,124 1979; 3 pp.

HV105 Grand, R. J. A., A. C. Nairn, and S. V. Perry. The preparation of calmodulins from barley (Hordeum sp) and Basidiomycete fungi. **Biochem J** 1980; 185: 755–760.

HV106 Mc Murrough, I. High-performance liquid chromatography of flavonoids in barley and hops. **J Chromatogr** 1981; 218: 683–693.

HV107 Frost, S., J. B. Harborne, and L. King. Identification of the flavonoids in five chemical races of cultivated barley. **Hereditas** 1977; 85: 163–168.

HV108 Banerjee, M., and A. K. Sharma. Variations in DNA content. **Experientia** 1979; 35: 2–43.

HV109 Kloos, H., W. Sidrak, A. A. M. Michael, E. W. Mohareb, and G. I. Higashi. Disease concepts and treatment practices relating to Schistosomiasis haematobium in upper Egypt. **J Trop Med Hyg** 1982; 85(3): 99–117.

HV110 Storey, H., and R. G. Wyn Jones. Quaternary ammonium compounds in plants in relation to salt resistance. **Phytochemistry** 1977; 16: 447–453.

HV111 Neurath, G. B., M. Dunger, F. G. Pein, D. Ambrosius, and O. Schreiber. Primary and secondary amines in the human environment. **Food Cosmet Toxicol** 1977; 15: 275–282.

HV112 Hong, N. D., J. W. Kim, B. W. Kim, and J. G. Shon. Studies on the efficacy of the combined preparation of crude drugs. 6. Effect of "Saengkankunbitang" on activities of the liver enzyme, protein contents and the excretory action of bile juice in the serum of CCL4-intoxicated rabbits. **Korean J Pharmacog** 1982; 13: 33–38.

HV113 Han, D. S., S. J. Lee, and H. K. Lee. Ethnobotanical survey in Korea. Proc Fifth Asian Symposium on Medical Plants and Spices Seoul Korea August 20-24 1984 PH Han DS Han Yn Han, and WS Woo (eds) 1984; 5: 125–144.

HV114 Ishii, R., K. Yoshikawa, H. Minakata, H. Komura, and T. Kada. Specifities of bio-antimutagens in plant kingdom. **Agr Biol Chem** 1984; 48(10): 2587–2591.

HV115 Sahu, T. R., Less known uses of weeds as medicinal plants. **Ancient Sci Life** 1984; 3(4): 245–249.

HV116 Ohtake, H., H. Yuasa, C. Komura, T. Miyauchi, Y. Hagiwara, and K. Kubota. Studies on the constituents of green juice from young barley leaves. Antiulcer activity of fractions from barley juice. **Yakugaku Zasshi** 1985; 105(11): 1046–1051.

HV116 Woo, W. S., E. B. Lee, K. H. Shin, S. S. Kang, and H. J. Chi. A review of research on plants for fertility regulation in Korea. **Korean J Pharmacog** 1981; 12(3): 153–170.

HV117 Ohtake, H., S. Nonaka, Y. Sawada, Y. Hagiwara, H. Hagiwara, and K. Kubota. Studies on the constituents of green juice from young barley leaves. Effect on dietary induced hypercholesterolemia in rats. **Yakugaku Zasshi** 1985; 105(11): 1052–1057.

HV118 Evans, L. S., and W. A. Tramontano. Trigonelline and promotion of cell arrest in G2 of various legumes. **Phytochemistry** 1984; 23(9): 1837–1840.

HV119 Matsuoka, Y., H. Seki, K. Kubota, H. Ohtake, and Y. Hagiwara. Anti-inflammatory effect of glycoprotein, D 1-G1, isolated from barley leaves. **Ensho** 1983; 3(4): 602–604.

HV120 Caceres, A., L. M. Giron, and A. M. Martinez. Diuretic activity of plants used for the treatment of urinary ailments in Guatemala. **J Ethnopharmacol** 1987; 19(3): 233–245.

HV121 Ramiez, V. R., L. J. Mostacero, A. E. Garcia, et al. Vegetales empleados en medicina traditional Norperuana. Banco Agrario Del Peru & NACL Univ Trujillo, Trujillo, Peru, June, 1988; 54 pp.

HV122 Caceres, A., L. M. Giron, S. R. Alvarado, and M. F. Torres. Screening of antimicrobial activity of plants popularly used in Guatemala for the treatment of dermatomucosal diseases. **J Ethnopharmacol** 1987; 20(3): 223–237.

HV123 Leporatti, M. L., and A. Pavesi. New or uncommon uses of several medicinal plants in some areas of central Italy. **J Ethnopharmacol** 1990; 29(2): 213–223.

HV124 Chetal, S., D. S. Wagle, and H. S. Nainawatee. Phosphatidylethanolamine in wheat and barley leaves under water stress. **Phytochemistry** 1982; 21(6): 1432–1433.

HV125 Ariffin, A., P. H. Mc Neil, R. J. Cooke, C. Wood, and D. R. Thomas. Carnitine content of greening barley leaves. **Phytochemistry** 1982; 21(6): 1431–1432.

HV126 Lee, E. B., H. S. Yun, and W. S. Woo. Plants and animals used for fertility regulation in Korea. **Korean J Pharmacog** 1977; 8: 81–87.

HV127 Hunte, P., M. Safi, A. Macey, and G. B. Kerr. Indigenous methods of voluntary fertility regulation in Afghanistan. **Natl Demographic Family Guidance Survey of Settled Population Afghanistan** 1975; 4: 1.

HV128 Kapoor, P. D., and A. K. Pal. Estrogenic activity of pasture plants used as cattle feed. **Indian J Exp Biol** 1965; 3: 61–63.

HV129 Peake, I. R., P. J. Dunphy, and J. F. Pennock. The chemical diversity of the plastochromanols. **Phytochemistry** 1970; 9: 1345.

HV130 El-Dean Mahmoud, A. A. G. Study of indigenous (folk ways) birth control methods in Alexandria. **Thesis-MS-University of Alexandria-Higher Institute of Nursing** 1972.

HV131 Celayeta, F. D. Action of the tissues of various plants on the growth of *Sphacelia segetum*. **Farmacognosia (Madrid)** 1960; 20: 91–101.

HV132 Datko, A. H., S. H. Mudd, and J. Giovaneli. A sensitive and specific assay for cystathione: cystathione content of several plant tissues. **Ann Biochem** 1974; 62(2): 531–545.

HV133 Kawai, S., Y. Sato, S. I. Takagi, and K. Nomoto. Separation and determination of mugineic acid and its analogues by high-performance liquid chromatography. **J Chromatogr** 1987; 391: 325–327.

HV134 Dongowski G, M. Huth, and E. Gebhardt. Steroids in the intestinal tract of rats are affected by dietary-fibre-rich barley-based diets. **Br J Nutr** 2003; 90(5): 895–906.

HV135 Li J., T. Kaneko, L. Q. Qin, J. Wang, Y. Wang, and A. Sato. Long-term effects of high dietary fiber intake on glucose tolerance and lipid metabolism in GK rats: comparison among barley, rice, and cornstarch. **Metabolism** 2003; 52(9): 1206–1210.

HV136 Li J., T. Kaneko, Y. Wang, L. Q. Qin, and A. Sato. Effects of dietary fiber on the glucose tolerance in spontaneously diabetic rats–comparison among barley, rice, and corn starch. **Nippon Eiseigaku Zasshi** 2003; 58(2): 281–286.

HV137 Delaney B., T. Carlson, S. Frazer, et al. Evaluation of the toxicity of concentrated barley beta-glucan in a 28-day feeding study in Wistar rats. **Food Chem Toxicol** 2003; 41(4): 477–487.

HV138 Dongowski G., M. Huth, E. Gebhardt, and W. Flamme. Dietary fiber-rich barley products beneficially affect the intestinal tract of rats. **J Nutr** 2002; 132(12): 3704–3714.

HV139 Fukuda M., O. Kanauchi, Y. Araki, et al. Prebiotic treatment of experimental colitis with germinated barley foodstuff: a comparison with probiotic or antibiotic treatment. **Int J Mol Med** 2002; 9(1): 65–70.

HV140 Kanauchi O., T. Iwanaga, A. Andoh, et al. Dietary fiber fraction of germinated barley foodstuff attenuated mucosal damage and diarrhea, and accelerated the repair of the colonic mucosa in an experimental colitis. **J Gastroenteol Hepatol** 2001; 16(2): 160–168.

HV141 Kanauchi O, T. Iwanaga, and K. Mitsuyama. Germinated barley foodstuff feeding. A novel neutraceutical therapeutic strategy for ulcerative colitis. **Digestion** 2001; 63 Suppl 1: 60–67.

HV142 Kanauchi O., Y. Araki, A. Andoh, et al. Effect of germinated barley foodstuff administration on mineral utilization in rodents. **J Gastroenterol** 2000; 35(3): 188–194.

HV143 Araki Y., Y. Fujiyama, A. Andoh, S. Koyama, O. Kanauchi, and T. Bamba. The dietary combination of germinated barley foodstuff plus *Clostridium butyricum* suppresses the dextran sulfate sodium-induced experimental colitis in rats. **Scand J Gastroenterol** 2000; 35(10): 1060–1067.

HV144 Araki Y., A. Andoh, S. Koyama, Y. Fujiyama, O. Kanauchi, and T. Bamba.

Effects of germinated barley foodstuff on microflora and short chain fatty acid production in dextran sulfate sodium-induced colitis in rats. **Biosci Biotechnol Biochem** 2000; 64(9): 1794–1800.

HV145 Kanauchi O., A. Andoh, T. Iwanaga, et al. Germinated barley foodstuffs attenuate colonic mucosal damage and mucosal nuclear factor kappa B activity in a spontaneous colitis model. **J Gastroenterol Hepatol** 1999; 14(12): 1173–1179.

HV146 Kanauchi O., T. Iwanaga, K. Mitsuyama, et al. Butyrate from bacterial fermentation of germinated barley foodstuff preserves intestinal barrier function in experimental colitis in the rat model. **J Gastroenterol Hepatol** 1999; 14(9): 880–888.

HV147 Kanauchi O., K. Mitsuyama, T. Saiki, K. Agata, T. Nakamura, and T. Iwanaga. Preventive effects of germinated barley foodstuff on methotrexate-induced enteritis in rats. **Int J Mol Med** 1998; 1(6): 961–966.

HV148 Kanauchi O., Y. Hitomi, K. Agata, T. Nakamura, and T. Fushiki. Germinated barley foodstuff improves constipation induced by loperamide in rats. **Biosci Biotechnol Biochem** 1998; 62(9): 1788–1790.

HV149 Kanauchi O., K. Mitsuyama, T. Saiki, K. Agata, T. Nakamura, and T. Iwanaga. Effects of germinated barley foodstuff on dextran sulfate sodium-induced colitis in rats. **J Gastroenterol** 1998; 33(2): 179–188.

HV150 Kanauchi O., T. Nakamura, K. Agata, T. Fushiki, and H. Hara. Effects of germinated barley foodstuff in preventing diarrhea and forming normal feces in ceco-colectomized rats. **Biosci Biotechnol Biochem** 1998; 62(2): 366–368.

HV151 Kanauchi O., T. Nakamura, K. Agata, and T. Fushiki. Preventive effect of germinated barley foodstuff on diarrhea induced by water-soluble dietary fiber in rats. **Biosci Biotechnol Biochem** 1997; 61(3): 449–354.

HV152 Kanauchi O., T. K. Agata, and T. Fushiki. Mechanism for the increased defecation and jejunum mucosal protein content in rats by feeding germinated barley foodstuff. **Biosci**

Biotechnol Biochem 1997; 61(3): 443–448.

HV153   McIntosh G. H., R. K. Le Leu, P. J. Royle, and G. P. Young. A comparative study of the influence of differing barley brans on DMH-induced intestinal tumours in male Sprague-Dawley rats. **J Gastroenterol Hepatol** 1996; 11(2): 113–119.

HV154   Oda T, S. Aoe, S. Imanishi, Y. Kanazawa, H. Sanada and Y. Ayano. Effects of dietary oat, barley, and guar gums on serum and liver lipid concentrations in diet-induced hypertriglyceridemic rats. **J Nutr Sci Vitaminol (Tokyo)** 1994; 40(2): 213–217.

HV155   McIntosh G. H., L. Jorgensen, and P. Royle. The potential of an insoluble dietary fiber-rich source from barley to protect from DMH-induced intestinal tumors in rats. **Nutr Cancer** 1993; 19(2): 213–221.

HV156   Robinson M., D. Hart, and G. H. Pigott.The effects of diet on the incidence of periodontitis in rats. **Lab Anim** 1991; 25(3): 247–253.

HV157   Naismith D. J., G. S. Mahdi, and N. N. Shakir. Therapeutic value of barley in the management of diabetes. **Ann Nutr Metab** 1991; 35(2): 61–64.

HV158   Qureshi A. A., W. C. Burger, D. M. Peterson, and C. E. Elson. The structure of an inhibitor of cholesterol biosynthesis isolated from barley. **J Biol Chem** 1986; 261(23): 10544–10550.

HV159   Donangelo C. M., and B. O. Eggum. Comparative effects of wheat bran and barley husk on nutrient utilization in rats. 2. Zinc, calcium and phosphorus. **Br J Nutr** 1986; 56(1): 269–280.

HV160   Puls R., and J. A. Greenway. Fusariotoxicosis from barley in British Columbia. II. Analysis and toxicity of syspected barley. **Can J Comp Med** 1976; 40(1): 16–19.

HV161   Kanauchi O., I. Serizawa, Y. Araki, et al. Germinated barley foodstuff, a prebiotic product, ameliorates inflammation of colitis through modulation of the enteric environment. **J Gastroenterol** 2003; 38(2): 134–141.

HV162   Kamimura A., and T. Takahashi. Procyanidin B-3, isolated from barley and identified as a hair-growth stimulant, has the potential to counteract inhibitory regulation by TGF-beta1. **Exp Dermatol** 2002;11(6): 532–541.

HV163   Jeong H. J., Y. Lam, and B. O. de Lumen. Barley lunasin suppresses ras-induced colony formation and inhibits core histone acetylation in mammalian cells. **J Agric Food Chem** 2002; 50(21): 5903–5908.

HV164   Astwood J.D., and R. D. Hill. Molecular characterization of Hor v 9. Conservation of a T-cell epitope among group IX pollen allergens and human VCAM and CD2. **Adv Exp Med Biol** 1996; 409: 269–277.

HV165   Vainio E., and E. Varjonen. Antibody response against wheat, rye, barley, oats and corn: comparison between gluten-sensitive patients and monoclonal antigliadin antibodies. **Int Arch Allergy Immunol** 1995; 106(2): 134–138.

HV166   Delaney B., T. Carlson, G. H. Zheng, et al. Repeated dose oral toxicological evaluation of concentrated barley beta-glucan in CD-1 mice including a recovery phase. **Food Chem Toxicol** 2003 ; 41(8): 1089–1102.

HV167   Fredlund K., E. L. Bergman, L. Rossander-Hulthen, M. Isaksson, A. Almgren, and A. S. Sandberg. Hydrothermal treatment and malting of barley improved zinc absorption but not calcium absorption in humans. **Eur J Clin Nutr** 2003; 57(12): 1507–1513.

HV168   Li J., T. Kaneko, L. Q. Qin, J. Wang, and Y. Wang. Effects of barley intake on glucose tolerance, lipid metabolism, and bowel function in women. **Nutrition** 2003; 19(11-12): 926–929.

HV169   Keogh G. F., G. J. Cooper, T. B. Mulvey, et al. Randomized controlled crossover study of the effect of a highly beta-glucan-enriched barley on cardiovascular disease risk factors in mildly hypercholesterolemic men. **Am J Clin Nutr** 2003; 78(4): 711–718.

HV170   Kanauchi O., T. Suga, M. Tochihara, et al. Treatment of ulcerative colitis by feeding with germinated barley foodstuff: first report of a multicenter open control trial. **J Gastroenterol** 2002; 37 Suppl 14: 67–72.

HV171   Lifschitz C. H., M. A. Grusak, and N. F. Butte. Carbohydrate digestion in humans from a beta-glucan-enriched barley is reduced. **J Nutr** 2002; 132(9): 2593–2596.

HV172 Armentia A., R. Rodriguez, A. Callejo, et al. Allergy after ingestion or inhalation of cereals involves similar allergens in different ages. **Clin Exp Allergy** 2002; 32(8): 1216–1222.

HV173 Suganuma H., T. Inakuma, and Y. Kikuchi. Amelioratory effect of barley tea drinking on blood fluidity. **J Nutr Sci Vitaminol (Tokyo)** 2002; 48(2): 165–168.

HV174 Bamba T., O. Kanauchi, A. Andoh, and Y. Fujiyama. A new prebiotic from germinated barley for nutraceutical treatment of ulcerative colitis. J **Gastroenterol Hepatol** 2002; 17(8): 818–824.

HV175 Kaplan R.J., and C. E. Greenwood. Influence of dietary carbohydrates and glycaemic response on subjective appetite and food intake in healthy elderly persons. **Int J Food Sci Nutr** 2002; 53(4): 305–316.

HV176 Ostman E. M., H. G. Liljeberg Elmstahl, and I. M. Bjorck. Barley bread containing lactic acid improves glucose tolerance at a subsequent meal in healthy men and women. **J Nutr** 2002; 132(6): 1173–1175.

HV177 Yu Y. M., W. C. Chang, C. T. Chang, C. L. Hsieh, and C. E. Tsai. Effects of young barley leaf extract and antioxidative vitamins on LDL oxidation and free radical scavenging activities in type 2 diabetes. **Diabetes Metab** 2002; 28(2): 107–114.

HV178 Cremer L., A. Herold, D. Avram, and G. Szegli. A purified green barley extract with modulatory properties upon TNF alpha and ROS released by human specialised cells isolated from RA patients. **Roum Arch Microbiol Immunol** 1998; 57(3–4): 231–242.

HV179 Garcia-Casado G., J. F. Crespo, J. Rodriguez, and G. Salcedo. Isolation and characterization of barley lipid transfer protein and protein Z as beer allergens. **J Allergy Clin Immunol** 2001; 108(4): 647–649.

HV180 Palosuo K., H. Alenius, E. Varjonen, N. Kalkkinen, and T. Reunala. Rye gamma-70 and gamma-35 secalins and barley gamma-3 hordein cross-react with omega-5 gliadin, a major allergen in wheat-dependent, exercise-induced anaphylaxis. **Clin Exp Allergy** 2001; 31(3): 466–473.

HV181 Granfeldt Y., A. C. Eliasson, and L. Bjorck. An examination of the possibility of lowering the glycemic index of oat and barley flakes by minimal processing. **J Nutr** 2000; 130(9): 2207–2214.

HV182 Kennefick S., and K. D. Cashman. Inhibitory effect of wheat fibre extract on calcium absorption in Caco-2 cells: evidence for a role of associated phytate rather than fibre per se. **Eur J Nutr** 2000; 39(1): 12–17.

HV183 Bonadonna P., M. Crivellaro, A. Dama, G. E. Senna, G. Mistrello, and G. Passalacqua. Beer-induced anaphylaxis due to barley sensitization: two case reports. **J Invest Allerg Clin Immunol** 1999; 9(4): 268–270.

HV184 Curioni A., B. Santucci, A. Cristaudo, et al. Urticaria from beer: an immediate hypersensitivity reaction due to a 10-kDa protein derived from barley. **Clin Exp Allergy** 1999; 29(3): 407–413.

HV185 Bourdon I., W. Yokoyama, P. Davis, et al. Postprandial lipid, glucose, insulin, and cholecystokinin responses in men fed barley pasta enriched with beta-glucan. **Am J Clin Nutr** 1999; 69(1): 55–63.

HV186 Kanauchi O., Y. Fujiyama, K. Mitsuyama, et al. Increased growth of *Bifidobacterium* and *Eubacterium* by germinated barley foodstuff, accompanied by enhanced butyrate production in healthy volunteers. **Int J Mol Med** 1999; 3(2): 175–179.

HV187 Kanauchi O., K. Mitsuyama, T. Saiki, T. Fushikia, and T. Iwanaga. Germinated barley foodstuff increases fecal volume and butyrate production in humans. **Int J Mol Med** 1998; 1(6): 937–941.

HV188 Tamagawa K., S. Fukushima, M. Kobori, H. Shinmoto, and T. Tsushida. Proanthocyanidins from barley bran potentiate retinoic acid-induced granulocytic and sodium butyrate-induced monocytic differentiation of

HL60 cells. **Biosci Biotechnol Biochem** 1998; 62(8): 1483-1487.

HV189   Ammari, F. F., K. T. Faris, and T. M. Mahafza. Inhalation of wild barley into the airways: two different outcomes. **Saudi Med J** 2000; 21(5): 468–470.

HV190   Robertson J. A., G. Majsak-Newman, and S. G. Ring. Release of mixed linkage (1→3),(1→4) beta-D-glucans from barley by protease activity and effects on ileal effluent. **Int J Biol Macromol** 1997; 21(1–2): 57–60.

HV191   Lia A., B. Sundberg, P. Aman, A. S. Sandberg, G. Hallmans, and H Andersson. Substrates available for colonic fermentation from oat, barley and wheat bread diets. A study in ileostomy subjects. **Br J Nutr** 1996; 76(6): 797–808.

HV192   Dahl S. W., S. K. Rasmussen, L. C. Petersen, and J. Hejgaard. Inhibition of coagulation factors by recombinant barley serpin BSZx. **FEBS Lett** 1996; 394(2): 165–168.

HV193   Ikegami S., M. Tomita, S. Honda, et al. Effect of boiled barley-rice-feeding in hypercholesterolemic and normolipemic subjects. **Plant Foods Hum Nutr** 1996; 49(4): 317–328.

HV194   Lia A., G. Hallmans, A. S. Sandberg, B. Sundberg, P. Aman, and H. Andersson. Oat beta-glucan increases bile acid excretion and a fiber-rich barley fraction increases cholesterol excretion in ileostomy subjects. **Am J Clin Nutr** 1995; 62(6): 1245–1251.

HV195   Vidal C., and A. Gonzalez-Quintela. Food-induced and occupational asthma due to barley flour. **Ann Allergy Asthma Immunol** 1995; 75(2): 121–124.

HV196   Livesey G., J. A. Wilkinson, M. Roe, et al. Influence of the physical form of barley grain on the digestion of its starch in the human small intestine and implications for health. **Am J Clin Nutr** 1995; 61(1): 75–81.

HV197   Yap J.C., C. C. Chan, Y. T. Wang, S. C. Poh, H. S. Lee, and K. T. Tan. A case of occupational asthma due to barley grain dust. **Ann Acad Med Singapore** 1994; 23(5): 734–736

HV198   Granfeldt Y., H. Liljeberg, A. Drews, R. Newman, and I. Bjorck. Glucose and insulin responses to barley products: influence of food structure and amylose-amylopectin ratio. **Am J Clin Nutr** 1994; 59(5): 1075–1082.

HV199   Liljeberg H., and I. Bjorck. Bioavailability of starch in bread products. Postprandial glucose and insulin responses in healthy subjects and *in vitro* resistant starch content. **Eur J Clin Nutr** 1994; 48(3): 151–163.

HV200   Cockcroft A. E., M. McDermott, J. H. Edwards, and P. McCarthy. Grain exposure—symptoms and lung function. **Eur J Respir Dis** 1983; 64(3): 189–196.

HV201   Lupton J. R., J. L. Morin, and M. C. Robinson. Barley bran flour accelerates gastrointestinal transit time. **J Am Diet Assoc** 1993; 93(8): 881–885.

HV202   Thorburn A., J. Muir J, and J. Proietto. Carbohydrate fermentation decreases hepatic glucose output in healthy subjects. **Metabolism** 1993; 42(6): 780–785.

HV203   Wisker E, R. Nagel, T. K. Tanudjaja, and W. Feldheim. Calcium, magnesium, zinc, and iron balances in young women: effects of a low-phytate barley-fiber concentrate. **Am J Clin Nutr** 1991; 54(3): 553–559.

HV204   McIntosh G. H., J. Whyte, R. McArthur, and P. J. Nestel. Barley and wheat foods: influence on plasma cholesterol concentrations in hypercholesterolemic men. **Am J Clin Nutr** 1991; 53(5): 1205–1209.

HV205   Arenaz P., and L. Hallberg. Genotoxicity of azidoalanine in mammalian cells. **Environ Mol Mutagen** 1989; 13(3): 263–270.

HV206   De Vries J. J., T. Collin, C. M. Bijleveld, J. H. Kleibeuker, and R. J. Vonk. The use of complex carbohydrates in barley groats for determination of the mouth-to-caecum transit time. **Scand J Gastroenterol** 1988; 23(8): 905–912.

HV207   Paillard S., P. Cochat, and L. David. A migrating ear of barley: a curious story of an intrabronchial foreign body. **Pediatrie** 1987; 42(6): 447–449.

HV208   Zuskin E., J. Mustajbegovic, and V. Sitar-Srebocan. Pharmacologic study of the effects of the components of beer *in vitro*. **Lijec Vjesn** 1997; 119(3-4): 103–105.

HV209 McCarthy P. E., A. E. Cockcroft, and M. McDermott. Lung function after exposure to barley dust. **Br J Ind Med** 1985; 42(2): 106–110.

HV210 Delaney, B., R. J. Nicolosi, T. A. Wilson, T. Carlson, S. Frazer, G. H. Zheng, R. Hess, K. Ostergren, J. Haworth and N. Knutson. Beta-glucan franctions from barley and oats are similarly antiatherogenic in hypercholesterolemic Syrian golden hamsters. **J Nutr** 2003; 133(2): 468–475.

8 | Larrea tridentata

(D. C.) Cov.

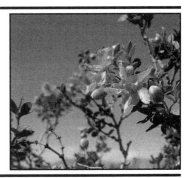

Common Names

Black bush	United States	Gobernadora	United States
Chaparral	England	Grease bush	United States
Chaparral	United States	Greasewood	United States
Creosote bush	England	Guamis	Spain
Creosote bush	United States	Hediondilla	Spain
Creosotum	United States	Jarilla	Spain
Dwarf Evergreen Oak	United States	Kreosotestrauch	Germany
Gobernadora	England	Paloondo	Spain
Gobernadora	Spain		

BOTANICAL DESCRIPTION

Larrea tridentata is a member of the caltrop family ZYGOPHYLLACEAE. It is a native, drought-tolerant, evergreen shrub slowly growing to 2–4 m tall and 1.8 m wide, with numerous flexible stems projecting at an angle from its base. The bush is a group of four to 12 plants that shoot up from one plant in all directions. The root system consists of a shallow taproot and several lateral secondary roots, each approx 3 m in length and 20–35 cm deep. The taproot extends to a depth of approx 80 cm. The leaves are thick, waxy, resinous, 12–25 mm long, alternate leaves with two leaflets, pointed, yellow-green in color, covered with a varnish; darker and aromatic after rainfall. These leaves grow directly from the branches of the bush. The bush may lose some of leaves during extreme drought. Yellow flowers are solitary and axillary, numerous, up to 2 cm wide, mostly bloom from February to August, some individuals maintain flowers year-round. Fruits are small, reddish-white, globose, consisting of five united, indehiscent, one-seeded carpels that may or may not break apart after maturing. Each carpel is densely covered by long, gray or white trichomes.

ORIGIN AND DISTRIBUTION

Larrea tridentata occurs throughout the Mojave, Sonoran, and Chihuahuan Deserts. Its distribution extends from southern California northeast through southern Nevada to the southwest corner of Utah and southeast through southern Arizona and New Mexico to western Texas and north-central Mexico. It is known to attain ages of several thou-

From: *Medicinal Plants of the World, vol. 3: Chemical Constituents, Traditional and Modern Medicinal Uses*
By: I. A. Ross © Humana Press Inc., Totowa, NJ

sand years; some clones may be the earth's oldest living organisms. The age of the largest clone in Johnson Valley, California, is estimated at 9400 years; one estimated the average longevity to be 1250 years at a study site in Dateland, CA, and 625 years at a San Luis site. *Larrea tridentata* commonly grows on gentle well-drained slopes, plains, valley floors, and sand dunes and in arroyos at elevations up to 1515 m and occurs on calcareous, sandy, and alluvial soils with a layer of caliche. It can survive without any added water. Often the most abundant shrub, even forming pure stands.

TRADITIONAL MEDICINAL USES

Mexico. Decoction of the bark and dried branches is taken orally as an abortive and for diabetes. Decoction of the dried root is taken orally by pregnant humans as an abortive and for diabetes[LT034]. Infusion of the shade-dried entire plant is taken orally to treat infectious diseases[LT011]. Decoction of the dried leaf is taken orally for treatment of diabetes. Hot water extract of the dried leaf is taken orally as a blood purifier; to treat kidney problems, urinary tract infections, and frigidity; for gallstones, rheumatism and arthritis, diabetes, wounds, and skin injuries, displacement of the womb, and paralysis; and to dissolve tumors[LT032].

United States. Hot water extract of the dried leaf is taken orally as a stimulating expectorant and tonic, for tuberculosis, and is drank by Indians of the Southwest for bowel cramps, as a diuretic, and for venereal disease. Hot water extract of the dried leaf is used externally for wound healing[LT038]. Hot water extract of the dried plant is taken orally for cancer. Effects described are from multicomponent reaction[LT029].

CHEMICAL CONSTITUENTS

(ppm unless otherwise indicated)
(−)-3,3'-Didemethoxyverucosin: Pl[LT048]
(−)-8'-Epi-larreatricin: Pl [LT048]
(−)-Larreatricin: Pl[LT048]

(+)-3,3'-Didemethoxyverucosin: Pl[LT048]
Acetophenone: EO[LT027]
Agarofuran, α: EO[LT027]
Anisic acid methyl ester, ortho: EO[LT027]
Ayanin: Lf[LT027]
Benzaldehyde: EO[LT027]
Benzoic acid ethyl ester: EO[LT027]
Benzoic acid hex-3-enyl ester: EO[LT027]
Benzoic acid N-hexyl ester: EO[LT027]
Benzyl acetate: EO[LT027]
Bergamotene, α: EO[LT027]
Borneol acetate: EO[LT027]
Borneol: EO[LT027]
Butan-1-al, 3-methyl: EO[LT027]
Butanoic acid benzyl ester: EO[LT027]
Butanoic acid, 2-methyl: EO[LT027]
Butyric acid, iso: EO[LT027]
Calamenene: EO[LT027]
Camphene: EO[LT027]
Camphor: EO[LT027]
Car-3-ene: EO[LT027]
Chrysoeriol-6-8-di-C-β-D-glucoside: Lf[LT023]
Cineol 1-8: EO[LT027]
Cinnamic acid ethyl ester, hydro: EO[LT027]
Copanene: EO[LT027]
Curcumene, α: EO[LT027]
Cymene, para: EO[LT027]
Edulane: EO[LT027]
Erythrodiol, 3-β-(3-4-dihydroxy-cinnamoyl): St 0.073–8[LT035, LT028]
Eudesmol, β: EO[LT027]
Eudesmol, γ: EO[LT027]
Farnesol: EO[LT027]
Fenchene, α: EO[LT027]
Furan, tetrahydro, 3-4-dimethyl: EO[LT027]
Gossypetin, 3-3'-7-tri-O-methyl: Lf[05600]
Gossypetin, 3-7-di-O-methyl: Lf[LT008]
Gossypetin-3-3'-7-8-tetramethyl ether: Lf[LT030]
Guaiacin, didehydro, 3'-3'-demethoxy-6-O-demethyl: Lf/Tw 2.8[LT005]
Guaiacin, iso, nor, 3'-demethoxy, triacetate: Lf/Tw[LT025]
Guaiacin, iso, nor, 3'-demethoxy: Pl[LT031], Lf/Tw 53, St 1.49[LT035]
Guaiacin, iso, nor: St 1.4[LT035]
Guaiacin, iso: 3'-6-di-O-demethyl: Lf/Tw 32.6[LT005]
Guaiacin, iso: 3'-demethoxy-6-O-demethyl: St 0.2[LT006], Lf/Tw 3.5[LT005]
Guaiacin, iso: St 0.2[LT006]
Guaiaretic acid, nor-dihydro, 3'-O-methyl: Pl[LT018], Lf[LT007]

Guaiaretic acid, nor-dihydro, 4-O-methyl: Lf[LT012]

Guaiaretic acid, nor-dihydro: Lf/Tw[LT003], Lf[LT012], Pl[15279], Lf & St[LT038], Oleoresin[LT024], Aer 0.696%[LT049], St 26.9[LT035]

Guaiazulene: EO[LT027]

Hept-1-en3-one: EO[LT027]

Heptan-2-one: EO[LT027]

Herbacetin, 3-7-di-O-methyl: Lf[LT009]

Herbacetin-3-7-8-trimethyl ether: Lf[LT030]

Hex-1-en-3-one: EO[LT027]

Hex-3-enyl acetate: EO[LT027]

Hexan-1-al: EO[LT027]

Hexan-3-ol: EO[LT027]

Hexan-3-one: EO[LT027]

Larrea divaricata flavonoid: Lf, St[LT038]

Larrea divaricata sterol (MP126-128): Lf, St[LT038]

Larrea lignan 1-B: Lf[LT007]

Larrea lignan 1-C: Lf[LT007]

Larrea lignan 1-D: Lf[LT007]

Larrea lignan 1-E: Lf[LT007]

Larrea lignan 1-F: Lf[LT007]

Larrea lignan 1-H: Lf[LT007]

Larrea lignan 1-I: Lf[LT007]

Larrea lignan 2-D: Lf[LT007]

Larreantin: Rt[LT033]

Larreatricin, 3-3''-dimethoxy: St 1.9[LT006]

Larreatricin, 3-4-dehydro: St 0.087–1.2[LT035,LT006]

Larreatricin, 4-epi, 3''-hydroxy: Lf & Tw 7.4[LT006]

Larreatricin, 4-epi: St, Lf & Tw 3[LT006]

Larreatricin: St 9.6[LT006]

Larreatridenticin: St 0.8[LT035,LT006]

Limonene: EO[LT027]

Linalool, *cis*, oxide: EO[LT027]

Linalool, *trans*, oxide: EO[LT027]

Linalool: EO[LT027]

Meso-3,3'-didemethoxynectandrin B: Pl[LT048]

Muurolene, α: EO[LT027]

Myrcene: EO[LT027]

Naphthalene, 1-2-dihydro, 1-5-5-trimethyl: EO[LT027]

Naphthalene, methyl: EO[LT027]

Nonan-2-one: EO[LT027]

Nordihydroguaiaretic acid: Lf, Tw[LT040]

Ocimene, β: EO[LT027]

Oct-1-en-3-one: EO[LT027]

Palmitic acid ethyl ester: EO[LT027]

Pentadecan-2-one: EO[LT027]

Pentadecanoic acid ethyl ester: EO[LT027]

Pinene, α: EO[LT027]

Pinene, β: EO[LT027]

Pyran-5-ol, tetrahydro, 2-6-6-trimethyl-2-vinyl, *cis*: EO[LT027]

Rossal-2-ene: EO[LT027]

Rossalene, 2: EO[LT027]

Santalene, β: EO[LT027]

Sitosterol, β: St 2-3.5[LT028,LT035]

Sucrose: Lf/Tw[LT003], Lf & St[LT038]

Terpineol, α: EO[LT027]

Tetradecan-2-one: EO[LT027]

Tetradecane, N: EO[LT027]

Tricosane, N: EO[LT027]

Tridecan-2-one: EO[LT027]

Tridecane, N: EO[LT027]

Undecan-2-one: EO[LT027]

Vicenin 2: Lf[LT023]

PHARMACOLOGICAL ACTIVITIES AND CLINICAL TRIALS

Alkaline phosphatase stimulation. Extract of the leaf, administered orally to adults, was active. Patients with subacute hepatic necrosis had negative workup, except for consumption of 15 tablets of the herbal extract per day for 4 months[LT017].

Anthelmintic activity. Water and petroleum ether extracts of the dried oleoresin were active on *Eimeria tenella* in chicken[LT024].

Anti-amoebic activity. The resin of *Larrea* produced inhibitory activity at a concentration of 1 ppm on *Entamoeba invadens* PZ axenic cultures. The nordihydroguaiaretic acid activity was observed at 10^{-6} to 10^{-8} concentrations[LT047].

Antibacterial activity. Methylene chloride extract of the dried aerial parts of the plants, on agar plate at a concentration of 1 g/mL, was active on *Bacillus subtilis*[LT016]. Methanol extract of the shade-dried plant, on agar plate at a concentration of 0.6 mg/mL, was inactive on *Staphylococcus aureus*. A concentration of 10 mg/mL was inactive on *Escherichia coli* and *Pseudomonas aureuginosa*[LT011].

Antidiabetic activity. Masoprocol, a compound derived from *Larrea*, administered orally to streptozotocin-induced diabetic rats at a dose of 0.83 mmol/kg body weight twice daily for 4 days, lowered glucose concentrations an average of 35% compared with vehicle (14.2 ± 1.1 vs 21.7 ± 1.0 mmol/L, $p < 0.001$). The animals were fed a 20% fat diet for 2 weeks before iv injection with streptozotocin (STZ, 0.19 mmol/kg). Diabetic animals (glucose 16–33 mmol/L) were treated with vehicle, metformin (0.83 mmol/kg), or masoprocol. Masoprocol decreased triglyceride level 80% compared with vehicle; nonesterified fatty acids and glycerol concentration by approx 65%, in comparison to vehicle. Adipocytes isolated from normal animals, treated with masoprocol (30 μmol/L) had higher basal and insulin-stimulated glucose clearance than adipocytes treated with vehicle ($p < 0.05$)[LT045]. Oral administration of masoprocol to two mouse models for type 2 diabetes reduced plasma glucose concentration approx 8 mmol/L in male C57BL/ks-db/db or C57BL/6J-ob/ob mice. The decline in plasma glucose concentration after masoprocol treatment in the mice was achieved without any change in plasma insulin concentration. Oral glucose tolerance improved, and the ability of insulin to lower plasma glucose concentrations was accentuated in masoprocol-treated db/db mice[LT013].

Antifungal activity. Ethanol and methanol (41.5–100%) extracts prepared from 6 g of dried leaf and stem powders were active on *Aspergillus flavus*, *Aspergillus niger*, *Penicillium chrysogenum*, *Penicillium expansum*, *Fusarium poae*, and *Fusarium moniliforme*[LT039].

Antihypertriglyceridemic activity. Masoprocol (nordihydroguaiaretic acid), administered orally to rodent models of type 2 diabetes at a dose range of 10 to 80 mg/kg twice daily for 4 to 8 days, decreased serum glucose and triglyceride levels. Masoprocol, at a dose of 40 or 80 mg/kg twice daily, significantly reduced hepatic triglyceride secretion ($p < 0.01$) and liver triglyceride content ($p < 0.001$), whereas lower doses of masoprocol decreased serum triglyceride without an apparent reduction in hepatic triglyceride secretion. The adipose tissue hormone-sensitive lipase was decreased, while adipose tissue lipoprotein lipase activity was increased in masoprocol-treated rats[LT044].

Anti-implantation effect. Chloroform extracts of the dried leaf, twig, and stem, administered intragastrically to pregnant rats at a dose of 0.58 g/kg for 10 days, were active. The phenolic fraction, at a dose of 0.52 g/kg and methanol extract at a dose of 0.70 g/kg, were active. Water extract, at a dose of 1 g/kg and petroleum ether extract at a dose of 0.38 g/kg, were inactive[LT035].

Anti-tumor activity. Water extract of the dried root, administered intraperitoneally to mice at a dose of 400 mg/kg, was inactive on Leuk (friend virus-solid) and Leuk-L1210. A dose of 500 mg/kg was inactive on sarcoma 180(ASC)[LT036].

Antiviral activity. Chloroform/methanol extract (1:1) of the dried leaf, in cell culture, was active on HIV-1 virus. TAT transactivation was inhibited[LT007]. Ethanol acetate soluble fraction of the dried leaf, in cell culture at a concentration of 0.75 μg/mL, was active on HIV virus vs HIV cytopathic effect[LT022].

Anti-yeast activity. Methanol extract of the shade-dried plant, on agar plate at a concentration of 1.25 mg/mL, was inactive on *Candida albicans*[LT011].

Cytotoxic activity. Water extract of the dried root, in cell culture, was inactive on CA-9KB, ED_{50} greater than 0.1 μg/mL[LT036]. The methanol extract was active on Leuk-P388, ED_{50} 0.57 μg/mL[LT004].

Detoxification activity. Phenolic resin, in increasing levels, was mixed with alfalfa pellets and fed to wood rats. Three detoxification pathways and urine pH, which are related to detoxification of allelochemicals, were measured. The excretion rate of two-phase II detoxification conjugates, glucuronides, and sulfides increased with increasing resin intake, whereas excretion of hippuric acid was independent of resin intake. Urine pH declined with increasing resin ingestion. The results indicated that a wood rat's tolerance to resin intake is related to the capacity for amination, sulfation, or pH regulation[LT042].

Gene expression inhibition. Chloroform/methanol extract (1:1) of the dried leaf, in cell culture, was active on hepatoma-Cos-7, IC_{50} 600.0 μg/mL vs TAT-dependent activation of HIV promoter bioassay[LT022].

Hepatotoxic activity. The leaf, taken orally by a female adult, was active[LT021]. A patient consumed 15 tablets of the leaf per day for 4 months. Approximately 1 year after stopping consumption, liver enzymes returned to normal and fatigue was no longer a complaint[LT017]. Infusion of the dried leaf, taken orally by a female adult at variable doses, was active. The 60-year-old woman who took Larrea tridentata for 10 months developed severe hepatitis for which no other cause could be found. Despite aggressive supportive therapy, the patient's condition deteriorated and required orthotropic liver transplantation[LT019]. Dried leaves, administered orally to adults at variable doses, were active. A public warning has been issued by the US Centers for Disease Control based on reports of liver toxicity after use of Larrea tridentata tea[LT015]. Dried leaves, administered orally to adults of both sexes at variable doses, were active[LT010]. The plant, administered orally to adults at variable doses, was active[LT020]. Dried leaves, administered orally to adults at variable doses, were active. One case of hepatotoxicity induced by Larrea tridentata taken as a nutritional supplement was reported[LT014]. Thirteen patients were identified for whom Larrea tridentata tincture for internal use was prescribed. Additionally, 20 female and three male patients were identified from whom an extract of Larrea tridentata in castor oil for topical use was prescribed. None of the patients had history of liver disease. In all of the cases, Larrea tridentata was given as either part of a complex herbal formula individualized for each patient containing less than 10% Larrea tridentata tincture or an extract in castor oil for topical use. The four patients with complete before and after blood chemistry panels and complete blood counts had no indication of liver damage from use of Larrea tridentata. This included one patient who was taking medications with significant potential for hepatotoxicity. No patient showed any sign of organ damage during the follow-up period[LT043]. Nordihydroguaiaretic acid is a lignan found in high amounts (up to 10% by dry weight) in the leaves and twigs of Larrea tridentata. It has been shown to reduce cystic nephropathy in the rats, but no reports have been made concerning the hepatotoxic potential of the compound. Larrea-containing medications induce hepatotoxicity and nephrotoxicity in humans. Intraperitoneal administration of nordihydroguaiaretic acid produced LD_{50} 75 mg/kg. Administration is associated with a time- and dose-dependent increase in serum alanine aminotransferase levels, which suggest liver damage. Freshly isolated mouse hepatocytes are more sensitive to nordihydroguaiaretic acid than human melanoma cells. Glucuronidation was identified as a potential detoxification mechanism for nordihydroguaiaretic acid[LT040].

Insecticide activity. Acetone extracts of the dried leaf, dried root, and dried stem, at a low concentration, were inactive on Culex quinquefasciatus[LT002]. Water extract of the dried leaf, administered intravenously, produced weak activity on Periplaneta americana[LT037].

Pigmented cholelithiasis prophylaxis. Powdered hydroalcoholic extract of the leaf was administered to Syrian golden hamster (ChCM). The extract was added to the lithogenic diet (basic diet plus 25 000 IU of vitamin A) at the 4% level for 70 days. The results indicated that the *Larrea*-fed group did not develop pigment cholelithiasis, whereas the group that received the lithogenic diet alone developed cholelithiasis in 63% of the cases. It is suggested that the active principle present in the leaves of *Larrea*, are responsible for the prevention is nordihydroguaiaretic acid, a potent antioxidant. However, the hamsters that received the diet containing *Larrea* showed serious signs of toxicity and pathological changes, such as marked reduction of growth, pronounced irritability and aggressiveness, and a marked hypoplasia of testicular and accessory sex glands[LT046].

Plant growth inhibitor. Water extract of the aerial parts, administered externally, was toxic to tomato plant seedlings[LT001].

Prothrombin time increased. Extract of the leaf, administered orally to adults, was active. Patients with subacute hepatic necrosis had negative workups, except for their consumption of 15 tablets of the herbal extract daily for 4 months[LT017].

Skin cancer chemoprevention. Topically applied nordihydroguaiaretic acid prevented phorbol ester promotion of tumors in mouse skin, indicating that nordihydroguaiaretic acid may be a candidate drug for the chemoprevention of skin cancer. Nordihydroguaiaretic acid, investigated as a potential inhibitory agent for ultraviolet-B (UVB)-induced signaling pathways in the human keratinocyte cell line HaCaT, significantly inhibited UVB-induced c-fos and activator protein-1 transactivation. It also inhibited the activity of phosphatidylinositol 3-kinase, a UVB-inducible enzyme that contributes c-fos expression and activator protein-1 transactivation by inhibiting the phosphatidylinositol 3-kinase signaling pathway[LT041].

REFERENCES

LT001   Bennett, E. L., and J. Nbonner. Isolation of plant growth inhibitors from *Thamnosma montana*. **Amer J Bot** 1953; 40: 29.

LT002   Hartzell, A., and F. Wilcoxon. A survey of plant products for insecticidal properties. **Contrib Boyce Thompson Inst** 1941; 12: 127–141.

LT003   Waller, C. W., and O. Gisvold. A phytochemical investigation of *Larrea divaricata* Cav. **J Amer Pharm Ass** 1945; 34: 78–81.

LT004   Luo, Z. Y., D. Meksuriyen, C. A. J. Erdelmeier, H. H. S. Fong, and G. A. Cordell. Larreantin, a novel, cytotoxic naphthoquinone from *Larrea tridentata*. **J Org Chem** 1988; 53(10): 2183–2185.

LT005   Konno, C., H. Z. Xue, Z. Z. Lu, et al. 1-ARYL tetralin lignans from *Larrea tridentata*. **J Nat Prod** 1989; 52(5): 1113–1117.

LT006   Konno, C., Z. Z. Lu, H. Z. Xue, et al. Furanoid lignans from *Larrea tridentata*. **J Nat Prod** 1990; 53(2): 396–406.

LT007   Gnabre, J., R. Chih, C. Huang, et al. Characterization of anti-HIV lignans from *Larrea tridentata*. **Tetrahedron** 1995; 51(45): 12203–12210.

LT008   Sakakibara, M., and T. J. Mabry. A new 8-hydroxyflavonol from *Larrea tridentata*. **Phytochemistry** 1975; 14: 2097–2098.

LT009   Sakakibara, M., B. N. Timmermann, N. Nakatani, H. Waldrum, and T. J. Mabry. New 8-hydroxyflavonol from *Larrea tridentata*. **Phytochemistry** 1975; 14: 849–851.

LT010   Sheikh, N. M., R. M. Philen, and L. A. Love. Chaparral-associated hepatotoxicity. **Arch Inter Med** 1997; 157(8): 813–919.

LT011   Navarro, V., M. L. Villarreal, G. Rojas, and X. Lozoy. Antimicrobial evaluation of some plants used in Mexican traditional medicine for the treatment of infectious diseases. **J Ethnopharmacol** 1996; 53(3): 143–147.

LT012   Ma, Y., L. Qi, J. N. Gnabre, R. C. C. Huang, F. E. Chou, and Y. Ito. Purification of anti-HIV lignans from *Larrea tridentata* by pH-zone-refining countercurrent chromatography. **J Liq Chromatogr** 1998; 21(1/2): 171–181.

LT013 Luo, J., T. Chuang, J. Cheung, et al. Masoprocol (nordihydroguaiaretic acid): a new antihyperglycemic agent isolated from the creosote bush (*Larrea tridentata*). **Eur J Pharmacol** 1998; 346(1): 77–79.

LT014 Clark, F., and D. R. Reed. Chaparral-induced toxic hepatitis. California and Texas, 1992. **MMWR Morbid Mortal Wkly Rep** 1992; 41(43): 812–814.

LT015 Anon. From the Food and Drug Administration. Public Warning about herbal product "Chaparral". **J Amer Med Ass** 1993; 269(3): 328.

LT016 Dentali, S. J., and J. J. Hoffmann. Potential anti-infective agents from *Eriodictyon angustifolium* and *Salvia apiana*. **Int J Pharmacog** 1992; 30(3): 223–231.

LT017 Katz, M., and F. Saibil. Herbal hepatitis: Subacute hepatitis necrosis secondary to Chaparral leaf. **J Clin Gastroenterol** 1990; 12(2): 203–206.

LT018 Gnabre, J. N., J. N. Brady, D. J. Clanton, et al. Inhibition of human immunodeficiency virus type 1 transcription and replication by DNA sequence-selective plant lignans. **Proc Natl Acad Sci** 1995; 92(24): 11239–11243.

LT019 Gordon, D. W., G. Rosental, J. Hart, R. Sirota, and A. L. Baker. The broadening spectrum of liver injury caused by herbal medication. **JAMA** 1995; 273(5): 489–501.

LT020 Koff, R. S. Herbal hepatotoxicity revisiting a dangerous alternative. **JAMA** 1995; 273(5): 502.

LT021 Smith, B. C., and P. V. Desmond. Acute hepatitis induced by ingestion of the herbal medication Chaparral. **Aust N Z J Med** 1993; 23(5): 526.

LT022 Gnabre, J. N., Y. Ito, Y. Ma, and R. C. Huang. Isolation of anti-HIV-1 lignans from *Larrea tridentata* by counter-current chromatography. **J Chromatogr A** 1996; 719(2): 353–364.

LT023 Sakakibara, M., T. J. Mabry, M. L. Bouillant, and J. Chopin. 6,8-Di-C-glucosylflavones from *Larrea tridentata* (*Zygophyllaceae*). **Phytochemistry** 1977; 16: 1113–1114.

LT024 Zamora, J. M., and E. C. Mora. Cytotoxic, antimicrobial and phytochemical properties of *Larrea tridentata* Cav. **Diss Abstr Int B** 1985; 45(12): 3809–3810.

LT025 Fronczek, F. R., P. Caballero, N. H. Fischer, S. Fernandez, E. Hernandez, and L. M. Hurtado. The molecular structure of 3'-demethoxynorisoguaiacin triacetate from creosote bush (*Larrea tridentata*). **J Nat Prod** 1987; 50(3): 497–499.

LT026 Gonzalez-Coloma, A., C. S. Wisdom, and P. W. Rundel. Ozone impact on the antioxidant nordihydroguaiaretic acid content in the external leaf resin of *Larrea tridentata*. **Biochem Syst Ecol** 1988; 16(1): 59–64.

LT027 Bohnstedt, C. F., and T. J. Mabry. The volatile constituents of the genus *Larrea* (*Zygophyllaceae*). **Rev Latino-amer Quim** 1979; 10: 128–131.

LT028 Xue, H. Z., Z. Z. Lu, C. Konno, et al. 3-Beta-(3,4-dihydroxycinnamoyl) erythrodiol and 3-beta-(-4-hydroxycinnamoyl) erythrodiol from *Larrea tridentata*. **Phytochemistry** 1988; 27(1): 233–235.

LT029 Nebelkopf, E. Herbs and cancer. Part II. **Herbalist** 1981; 6(1): 26–39.

LT030 Bernhard, H. O., and K. Thiele. Additional flavonoids from the leaves of *Larrea tridentata*. **Planta Med** 1981; 41: 100–103.

LT031 Nuzzo, N. A., A. M. Martin, C. Konno, C. D. Fakroddin, H. H. S. Fong, and D. P. Waller. Effect of nor-3'-demethoxyisoguaiacin (NDI) on fertility in female rats. **Biol Reprod** 1987; 36(1): Abstr-301.

LT032 Winkelman, M. Frequently used medicinal plants in Baja California Norte. **J Ethnopharmacol** 1986; 18(2): 109–131.

LT033 Luo, Z. Y., D. Meksuriyen, C. A. J. Erdelmeier, H. H. S. Fong, and G. A. Cordell. Larreantin, a novel, cytotoxic naphthoquinone from *Larrea tridentata*. Abstr International Congress on Natural Products, Research Park City, UT. July 17-21 1988; 1988: Abstr-013.

LT034   Dimayuga, R. E., R. F. Murillo, and M. L. Pantoja. Traditional medicine of Baja California sur Mexico II. **J Ethnopharmacol** 1987; 20(3): 209–222.

LT035   Konno, C., A. M. Martin, B. X. Ma, et al. Search for fertility regulating agents from *Larrea tridentata*. Proc First Princess Chulabhorn Science Congress Bangkok 1989; 1989: 328–337.

LT036   Abbott, B. J., J. Leiter, J. L. Hartwell, et al. Screening data from the cancer chemotherapy National Service Center Screening Laboratories. XXXIV. Plant extracts. **Cancer Res** 1966; 26: 761–935.

LT037   Jacobson, M. Insecticides from plants. A review of the literature, 1941-1953. Agr Handbook No.154, USDA 1958: 299 pp.

LT038   Waller, C. W., and O. Gisvold. A phytochemical investigation of *Larrea divaricata* Cav. **J Amer Pharm Ass Sci Ed** 1945; 34: 78–81.

LT039   Tequila-Meneses, M., M. Cortez-Rocha, E. E. Rosas-Burgos, S. Lopez-Sandoval, and C. Corrales-Maldonado. Effect of alcoholic extracts of wild plants on the inhibition of growth of *Aspergillus flavus, Aspergillus niger, Penicillium chrysogenum, Penicillium expansum, Fusarium moniliforme* and *Fusarium poae* moulds. **Rev Iberoam Microl** 2002; 19(2): 84–88.

LT040   Lambert, J. D., D. Zhao, R. O. Meyers, R. K. Kuester, B. N. Timmermann, and R. T. Dorr. Nordihydroguaiaretic acid: hepatotoxicity and detoxification in the mouse. **Toxicon** 2002; 40(12): 1701–1708.

LT041   Gonzalles, M., and G. T. Bowden. Nordihydroguaiaretic acid-mediated inhibition of ultraviolet B-induced activator protein-1 activation in human keratinocytes. **Mol Carcin** 2002; 34(2): 102–111.

LT042   Mangione, A. M., D. Dearing, and W. Karasow. Detoxification in relation to toxin tolerance in desert woodrats eating creosote bush. **J Chem Ecol** 2001; 27(12): 559–2578.

LT043   Heosn, S., and E. Yarnell. The safety of low-dose *Larrea tridentata* (DC) Coville (creosote bush or chaparral): A retrospective clinical study. **J Alt Complement Med** 2001; 7(2): 175–185.

LT044   Scribner, K. A., T. M. Gadbois, M. Gowri, S. Azhar, and G. M. Reaven. Masoprocol decreases serum triglyceride concentrations in rats with fructose-induced hypertriglyceridemia. **Metabolism** 2000; 49(9): 1106–1110.

LT045   Reed, M.J., K. Meszaros, L. J. Entes, et al. Effect of masoprocol on carbohydrate and lipid metabolism in a rat model of type II diabetes. **Diabetologia** 1999; 42(1): 102–106.

LT046   Granados, H., and R. Cardenas. Biliary calculi in the golden hamster. XXXVII. The prophylactic action of the creosote bush (*Larrea tridentata*) in pigmented cholelithiasis produced by vitamin A. **Rev Gastroenterol Mex** 1994; 59(1): 31–35.

LT047   Segura, J. J. Effects of nordihydroguaiaretic acid and ethanol on the growth of *Entamoeba invadens*. **Arch Invest Med (Mex)** 1978; 1: 157–162.

LT048   Moinuddin, S. G., S. Hishiyama, M. H. Cho, L. B. Davin, and N. G. Lewis. Synthesis and chiral HPLC analysis of the dibenzyltetrahydrofuran lignans, larreatricins, 8'-epi-larreatricins, 3,3'-didemethoxyverrucosins and meso-3,3'-didemethoxynectandrin B in the creosote bush (*Larrea tridentata*): evidence for regiospecific control of coupling. **Org Biomol Chem** 2003; 1(13): 2307–2313.

LT049   Page. J. O. Determination of nordhydroxyguaiaretic acid in creosote bush. **Anal Chem** 1955; 27: 1266–1268.

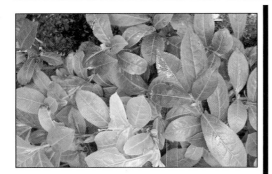

Plate 1. *Camellia sinensis* (*see* full discussion in Chapter 1).

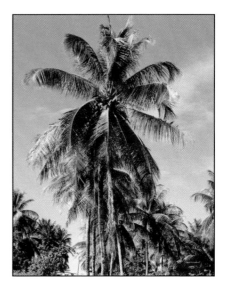

Plate 3. *Cocos nucifera* (*see* full discussion in Chapter 3).

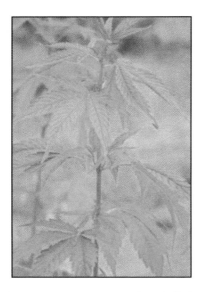

Plate 2. *Cannabis sativa* (*see* full discussion in Chapter 2).

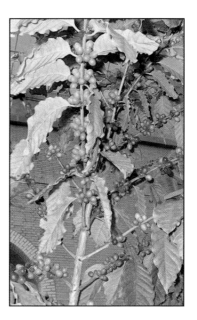

Plate 4. *Coffea arabica* (*see* full discussion in Chapter 4).

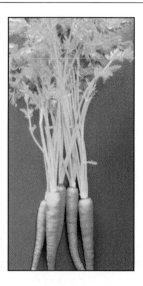

Plate 5. *Daucus carota* (*see* full discussion in Chapter 5).

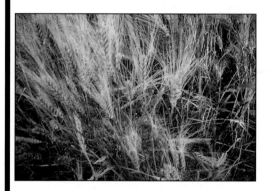

Plate 7. *Hordeum vulgare* (*see* full discussion in Chapter 7).

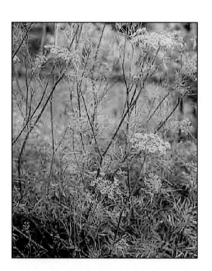

Plate 6. *Ferula assafoetida* (*see* full discussion in Chapter 6).

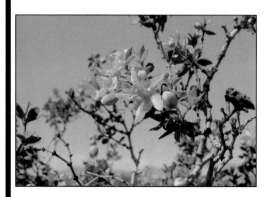

Plate 8. *Larrea tridentata* (*see* full discussion in Chapter 8).

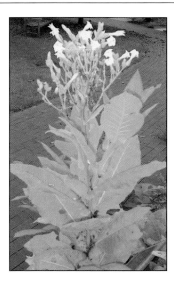

Plate 9. *Nicotiana tabacum* (*see* full discussion in Chapter 9).

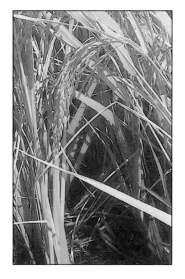

Plate 11. *Oryza sativa* (*see* full discussion in Chapter 11).

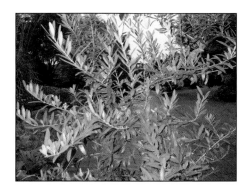

Plate 10. *Olea europaea* (*see* full discussion in Chapter 10).

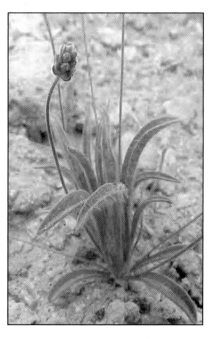

Plate 12. *Plantago ovata* (*see* full discussion in Chapter 12).

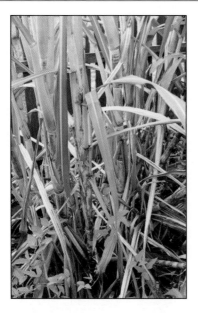

Plate 13. *Saccharum officinarum* (*see* full discussion in Chapter 13).

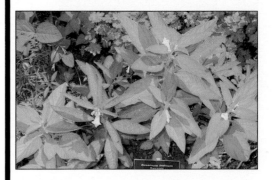

Plate 15. *Sesamum indicum* (*see* full discussion in Chapter 15).

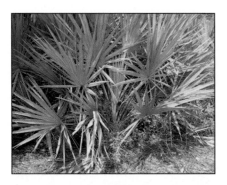

Plate 14. *Serenoa repens* (*see* full discussion in Chapter 14).

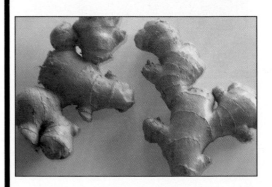

Plate 16. *Zingiber officinale* (*see* full discussion in Chapter 16).

9 | Nicotiana tabacum

L.

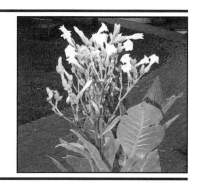

Common Names

A´-li	Colombia	Tabacco Virginia	Italy
Aco	Wales	Tabacni izdelki	Slovenia
Baco	Wales	Tabaco	Brazil
Dé-oo-wé	Colombia	Tabaco	Mexico
Dohány	Hungary	Tabaco	Portugal
Duhan	Albania	Tabaco	Spain
Duhan	Croatia	Tabaco	Venezuela
Duvan	Serbia	Tabák	Czech Republic
Duvn	Serbia	Tabak	Germany
Dybaco	Wales	Tabak	Netherlands
E´-li	Colombia	Tabak	South Africa
Echter tabak	Germany	Tabak	Russia
Faco	Wales	Tabaka	Surinam
Fyglys	Wales	Tabako	France
Grand tabac	France	Tabako	Netherlands Antilles
Hogesoppu	India	Tabako	Philippines
Kanvoc	Greece	Tabako	Spain
Kapva	Greece	Tabaku	Netherlands Antilles
Kherm´-ba	Ecuador	Tabat	France
Lukux-ri	Colombia	Tamaku	India
Maco	Wales	Tambaku	India
Mahora	Romania	Tamrakatu	India
Mu-lu´	Colombia	Tembakau	Indonesia
Myglys	Wales	Tembakau	Malaysia
Navadni tobak	Slovenia	Temmdki	Turkmenistan
Nhybaco	Wales	Thybaco	Wales
Nicotiane	France	Tobac	Ireland
Pagári-mulé	Colombia	Tobacco	Australia
Petun	Brazil	Tobacco	Guyana
Pogaku	India	Tobacco	Iceland
Pokala	India	Tobacco	Italy
Pugaiyilai	India	Tobacco	Kenya
Tabac	France	Tobacco	New Zealand
Tabac	Spain	Tobacco	United Kingdom

From: *Medicinal Plants of the World, vol. 3: Chemical Constituents, Traditional and Modern Medicinal Uses*
By: I. A. Ross © Humana Press Inc., Totowa, NJ

Tobacco	United States	Tütün	Turkey
Tobacco	West Indies	Twak	South Africa
Tobak	Denmark	Tybaco	Wales
Tobak	Sweden	Tyton szlachetny	Poland
Tobaken	Sweden	Tyutyun	Bulgaria
Tobakk	Norway	Tyutyun	Ukraine
Tobakken	Denmark	Ugwayi	Botswana
Tombaca	Scotland	Ugwayi	South Africa
Tombagey	The Isle of Man (Manx)	Vaaristubukas	Estonia
Toombak	Sudan	Virginiantupakka	Finland
Tubbak	Faeroe Islands	Virginiatobak	Sweden
Tumbako	Mozambique	Virginiatobakk	Norway
Tumbako	Tanzania	Virginischer tabak	Germany
Tumbako	Zaire	Virginsk tobak	Denmark
Tupakka	Finland	Ye´-ma	Brazil
Tutun	Romania		

BOTANICAL DESCRIPTION

Nicotiana tabacum is a stout annual of the TOMENTOSAE family, approx 1–3 m high. The stem is erect with few branches. Leaves are ovate, elliptic, or lanceolate, up to 100 cm or more in length, usually sessile or sometimes petiolate with frilled wing or auricle. The inflorescence is a panicle with distinct rachis and several compounds branches. Flowers are light red, light pink, or white. The fruit is a capsule approx 15–20 mm long, narrowly elliptic ovoid or orbicular. Seeds spherical or broadly elliptic, 0.5 mm long, brown, with fluted ridges.

ORIGIN AND DISTRIBUTION

Nicotiana tabacum originated from the borders of Argentina and Bolivia. It has been cultivated in pre-Columbian times in the West Indies, Mexico, Central America, and the northern region of South America. It is now found worldwide as a cultivated crop.

TRADITIONAL MEDICINAL USES

Argentina. Leaves are smoked by adults in ayahuasca mixture during healing rituals[NT481].

Brazil. Dried leaf is used as an insecticide[NT609]. Leaves are heated and the juice is squeezed out, mixed with ash from bark of *Theobroma subircanum* or other *Theobroma* species to make an intoxicating snuff. Snuff is not a hallucinogenic, but it does produce inebriation[NT617]. The Tukanoan peoples of the Vaupes rub a decoction of the leaf briskly over sprains and bruises. The leaf juice is taken orally to induce vomiting and narcosis[NT619].

Colombia. The Witotos and Boras used the fresh leaf as poultice over boils and infected wounds. The Tikuna men mix the crushed leaves with oil from palms and used as a hair treatment to prevent baldness. The juice is taken orally by the Tukanos to induce vomiting and narcosis[NT619].

Cuba. Extract of the leaf is taken orally to treat dysmenorrhea[NT614].

East Africa. Dried leaves of *Nicotiana tabacum* and *Securinega virosa* are mixed in a paste and used externally to destroy worms in sores[NT592].

Ecuador. The Jivaros use the leaf juice for indisposition, chills, and snake bites and to treat pulmonary ailments. The Aguarunas apply leaf juice by clyster, alone or mixed with ayahuasca, to induce vomiting before tobacco-ayahuasca enema. The Kulina customarily smoke all night when taking ayahuasca[NT619].

Fiji. Fresh root is taken orally for asthma and indigestion. Fresh root juice is applied ophthalmically as drops for bloodshot eyes and other problems. Seed is taken orally for rheumatism and to treat hoarseness[NT594].

Guatemala. Leaves are applied externally by adults for myasis, headache, and wounds[NT464]. A mixture of the leaf with menthol VapoRub is applied externally for children for cough[NT470]. Hot water extract of the dried leaf is applied externally for ringworms, fungal diseases of the skin[NT516], wounds, ulcers, bruises, sores, mouth lesions, stomatitis, and mucosa[NT607]. The leaf is taken orally for kidney diseases[NT605].

Haiti. Decoction of the dried leaf is taken orally for bronchitis and pneumonia[NT598].

India. Juice of *Securinega leucopyrus* is mixed with the dried leaf and applied externally for parasites[NT517]. Fresh leaf is mixed with corncob or *Amorphophallus paeonifolium* to treat asthma[NT467].

Iran. Infusion of the dried leaf is applied externally as an insect repellent. Ointments made from crushed leaves are used for baldness, dermatitis, and infectious ulcerations and as a pediculicide. Juice is applied externally as an insect repellent[NT358]. Leaf is added to the betel quid and used as a mild stimulant[NT329].

Kenya. Water extract of the dried leaf is applied ophthalmically for corneal opacities and conjunctivitis[NT466].

Malaysia. Infusion of the dried leaf is taken orally as a sedative[NT414].

Mexico. Extract of the plant, massaged on the abdomen with saliva, is used to facilitate expulsion of placenta[NT438]. Exudate from the leaf and stem is used as a dentifrice for gum inflammation[NT469].

Nepal. Leaf juice is applied externally to treat scabies[NT463].

Nicaragua. Leaves are chewed for toothache[NT465] and applied externally for aches, pains, bites, stings, and skin rashes[NT468].

Nigeria. Hot water extract of the fresh leaf is taken orally as a sedative[NT580].

Papua New Guinea. Dried plant, mixed with the bark of *Galbulima belgraveana* and *Zingiber officinale* is taken orally for head lice[NT611]. Young leaf tip is chewed to relieve stomachache. Decoction of the young leaf is taken orally to treat gonorrhea[NT455].

Paraguay. Extract of the plant is administered orally to cows as an insecticide and insect repellent[NT456]. Smoked or chewed dried leaf will spoil the milk of nursing mothers. Dried resin accumulated in the stem of a smoking pipe is applied externally against botfly larvae and severe pediculosis[NT600].

Peru. Decoction of the leaf with ayahuasca beverage (*Banisteriopsis caapi* and *Psychotria viridis*) is taken orally for hallucinating effect during shamanic training. A diet of cooked plantain and smoked fish follows each use[NT585]. Hot water extract of the dried flower and leaf is used externally for snake and spider bites[NT606]. The Witotos and Boras used the fresh leaves as poultice over boils and infected wounds. The Tikuna men mix the crushed leaves with oil from palms as a hair dressing to prevent baldness. The Jivaros use the tobacco juice for indisposition, cold, chills, and snake bites and to treat pulmonary ailments[NT619]

Sierra Leone. Leaf is chewed and rubbed on area to dress umbilical stump[NT586].

Tanzania. Leaves are placed in the vagina to stimulate labor[NT618].

Turkey. Powdered leaf is applied externally for wounds[NT459].

United States. Extract of the plant is taken orally to treat tiredness, ward off diseases, and quiet fear[NT364].

CHEMICAL CONSTITUENTS

(ppm unless otherwise indicated)
2,3,6-Trimethyl-1,4-naphthoquinone: Pl[NT037]
2-Methylquinone: Lf smoke[NT160]
2-Naphthylamine: Lf[NT038]
3-(Nitrosomethyloamino)propionic acid: Pl[NT107]

3-Hydroxypyridine: Lf smoke[NT188]

3-Hydroxypyridine: Lf smoke[NT188]

4-(Methylnitrosamino)-1-(3-pirydyl)-1-butanol: Lf[NT011]

4-(Methylnitrosamino)-1-(3-pirydyl)-1-butanone: Lf[NT005]

4-(Methylnitrosamino)-4-(3-pyridyl)butyric acid: Lf[NT087]

4-(Nitrosomethyloamino)-1-(3-pirydyl)butyric acid: Pl[NT106]

4-(Nitrosomethyloamino)butyric acid: Pl[NT107]

4-(N-nitrosomethyloamino)-4-(3-pirydyl)butyric acid: Pl 0.01-0.95[NT107]

4-Aminobiphenyl: Lf smoke[NT160]

6-Methyl-3-hydroxypyridine: Lf smoke[NT188]

Abienol, cis: Pl[NT424]

Abscisic acid, β-D-glucopyraoside: Stigma[NT596]

Abscisic acid, cis-2-trans-4: Petiole[NT581]

Abscisic acid, methyl ester: Stigma[NT596]

Abscisic acid: Petal, Cy, Ovary, Style, Stamen, An, Stigma[NT596]

Acetaldehyde: Lf[NT599]

Acetamide: Lf[NT543]

Acetic acid: An[NT391], Lf[NT440]

Acetonitrile: St[NT376]

Acetophenone, 3-4-dimethoxy: Lf, Rt, St, Bk, Tw[NT428]

Acetophenone: Lf, Rt, St, Bk, Tw[NT428]

Acrolein: Lf[NT599]

Acrylonitrile: Lf[NT022]

Actinidiolide, dihydro: Lf, Rt, St, Bk, Tw[NT428]

Actinidol, 3-oxo: Lf, Rt, St, Bk, Tw[NT428]

Adenine, 6-benzyl: Call Tiss[NT518]

Aesculetin: Lf[NT448]

Agropine: St 7%[NT538]

Alainine: Sd[NT515]

Alanine, phenyl: Sd[NT515]

Albumin: cured Lf[NT359]

Alkyl-2-cyclopenten-2-ol-1-one: Lf smoke[NT188]

Alkyl-2-hydroxy-2-cyclopenten-1-one: Lf smoke[NT171]

Amine, N-nitroso-diethanol: Lf[NT599]

Amine, N-nitroso-dimethyl: Lf[NT599]

Amyrin, β: Lf[NT540], Sd oil[NT491], Sd[NT480]

Anabasine, N'-formyl: Lf 4.3–8.6[NT565]

Anabasine, N'-methyl, (2'S): Pl[NT562]

Anabasine, N'-nitroso: Lf[NT599]

Anabasine, N-methyl: Lf[NT472]

Anabasine, N-nitroso: Lf[NT599]

Anabasine: An[NT391], Lf, Pl[NT437], Cx, Rt[NT508]

Anatabine, N'-formyl: Lf[NT506]

Anatabine, N'-methyl: Lf 1[NT565]

Anatabine: An[NT391], Lf[N5T01], Pl[NT437], Lf[NT543], Rt[NT508]

Anatalline: Rt 10.4[NT321], Pl[NT562]

Anethole: Lf, Rt, St, Bk, Tw[NT428]

Aniline-HCl: Lf smoke[NT160]

Antheraxanthin: Lf[NT363]

Anthralin: Smoke[NT183]

Arachidic acid: Lf[NT544]

Areginine: Sd[NT515]

Arginine: Pl[NT562]

Aristolochene, 5-epi: Pl[NT510]

Aspartic acid: Sd[NT515]

ATP: St[NT397]

Avenasterol, 7-dehydro: Sd[NT515]

Azetidine-2-carboxylic acid: Pl[NT377]

Basm-4-en-6-one, 7-8-epoxy: Lf[NT561]

Basman-6-one, 1(R)-3(R)-3(R)-epoxy-4(S)-8(S)-dihydroxy, (2S-8S-11R-12S): Fl[NT356]

Basman-6-one, 1(R)-3(R)-epoxy-4(S)-8(R)-dihydroxy, (2S-7R-11S-12S): Fl[NT356]

Benzaldehyde, 3-4-dimethoxy: Lf, Rt, St, Bk, Tw[NT428]

Benzaldehyde: Lf, Rt, St, Bk, Tw[NT428]

Benzene, 1-2-4-trihydroxy: Lf[NT448]

Benzene, allyl: Lx (St)[NT376]

Benzene, N-propyl: Lx (St)[NT376]

Benzene, tert-butyl: Lx (St)[NT376]

Benzo-(A)-anthracene: Lf 2.6 μg/100 Cig[NT434]

Benzo-(A)-fluorene: Lf 4.9 μg/100 Cig[NT434]

Benzo-(A)-pyrene: Lf 1.7 μg/100 Cig[NT434]

Benzo-(F)-fluoranthene: Lf 2.1 μg/100 Cig[NT434]

Benzo-(G-H-I)-perylene: Lf 0.3 μg/100 Cig[NT434]

Benzo-(K)-fluoranthene: Lf 1.2 μg/100 Cig[NT434]

Benzo[e]pyrene: Smoke[NT183]

Benzofuran, octahydro, 6-hydroxy-4-4-7-(A)-trimethyl: Lf, Rt, St, Bk, Tw[NT428]

Benzoic acid: Lf 36[NT498]

Benzonitrile: Lf[NT472]

Benzopyrene: Lf[NT599]

Benzoquinone, 1-4: Call Tiss, Rt, Lf[NT379]

Benzyl acetate: Lf, Rt, St, Bk, Tw[NT428]

Benzyl alcohol: Lf, Rt, St, Bk, Tw[NT428]

Bicycle-(4-4-O)-decan-9-one, 1-3-7-7-tetramethyl-2-oxa: Lf, Rt, St, Bk, Tw[NT428]

Bicyclo-(4-4-O)-dec-5-en-9-oe, 1-3-7-7-tetramethyl-2-oxa: Lf, Rt, St, Bk, Tw[NT428]

Bicyclo(5.4.0)-undecan-3-one, 4-oxa-7(R)-11-11-trimethyl, (1S): Lf 0.016[NT349]

Bicyclodamascenone A: Lf EO[NT430]
Bicyclodamascenone B: Lf EO[NT430]
Biphenyl methane: Lf, Rt, St, Bk, Tw[NT428]
Bipyridine, 2-3': Pl[NT562]
Bipyridyl, 2-3', 5-methyl: Lf 0.9[NT565]
Bipyridyl, 2-3': Lf[NT506]
Bipyridyl, 2-3'-5-methyl: Lf 11[NT565]
Blumenol A β-D-glucopyranoside: Lf[NT548]
Blumenol C: Lf 0.23[NT572]
Brassicasterol: Sd[NT515]
But-2-en-4-olide, 3-(4-methyl-1-pentyl):
    Lf 0.002[NT349]
But-3-en-2-one, 3-methyl: Lx (St)[NT376]
Butan-1-ol, 4-(methyl-nitrosamino)-4-(3-
    pyridyl): Lf[NT599]
Butan-1-one, 4-(N-methyl-N-nitrosamino)-1-
    (3-pyridyl): Lf[NT599]
Butan-4-olide, 4-ethyl: Lf, Rt, St, Bk, Tw[NT428]
Butane-2-3-dione: Lx (St)[NT376]
Buten-2-al: Lx (St)[NT376]
But-trans-2-en-1-one, 1-(2-3-6-trimethyl-
    phenyl): Lf[NT535]
Butyraldehyde: Lf[NT022]
Butyric acid, N, caffeoyl-4-amino: Pl[NT350]
Butyric acid, N, N-caffeoyl-4-amino: Bd[NT350]
Butyric acid: Lf[NT440], An[NT391]
Butyronitrile, 1: Lx (St)[NT376]
Cadinene, Δ: Lf[NT565]
Cadinenol: Lf, Rt, St, Bk, Tw[NT428]
Caffeic acid: Lf[NT591], Sd oil[NT491]
Calamanene: Lf, Rt, St, Bk, Tw[NT428]
Campest-7-en-ol: Sd[NT515]
Campestanol: Sd[NT515]
Campesterol acyl glycoside: Lf[NT368]
Campesterol ester: Lf[NT368]
Campesterol glycoside: Lf[NT368]
Camphor: Lf, Rt, St, Bk, Tw[NT428]
Capnos-11-ene-2-10-dione, 4-6-8-trihydroxy:
    Fl[NT345]
Capnos-12(20)-en-2-one, 8(R)-11(S)-epoxy-
    4(S)-6(R)-dihydroxy, (1S-3R-7R): Fl[NT356]
Capnos-12(20)-ene, 4(S)-6(R)-diol, 2(R)-
    11(R), 8(R)-11(R)-diepoxy, (1S-3S):
    Fl[NT356]
Capric acid: Lf[NT413]
Caproic acid: Lf[NT440]
Capronic acid, iso: An[NT391]
Capsidiol: Pl[NT454]
Capsidol: Rt[NT457]
Carboxylase, ribulose-diphosphate: Pl[NT371]
Cardinene, γ: Lf[NT565]
Carotene, β: Call Tiss[NT411]

Carotene: Lf[NT363]
Carvone: Lf, Rt, St, Bk, Tw[NT428]
Caryophyllene, β: Lf, Rt, St, Bk, Tw[NT428]
Catechol: Lf[NT022]
Cedrene, α: Lf, Rt, St, Bk, Tw[NT428]
Cedrol: Lf, Rt, St, Bk, Tw[NT428]
Cembr-2-en-12-one, 4-6-dihydroxy-7-8-epoxy-
    20-nor, (1S-2-trans-4S-6R-7R-8R): Fl[NT335]
Cembra-2-6-12-(20)-triene-4-8-diol, 11-
    hydroperoxy: Lf 0.1[NT330]
Cembra-2-7-11-trien-6-one, 4(R)-hydroxy,
    (1S-2-trans-4R-6R-7-trans-11-trans): Fl[NT451]
Cembra-2-7-11-trien-6-one, 4(S)-hydroxy,
    (1S-2-trans-4S-6R-7-trans-11-trans): Fl[NT451]
Cembra-2-7-11-triene-4-6-diol, (1S-2-trans-
    4R-6R-7-trans-11-trans): Fl[NT451]
Cembra-2-7-11-triene-4-6-diol, (1S-2-trans-
    4S-6R-7-trans-11-trans): Fl[NT451]
Cembra-2-7-11-triene-4-6-diol, α: Lf[NT460]
Cembra-2-7-12 (20-triene-4-6-11-triol),
    (1S-2-trans-4S-6R-7-trans): Fl[NT451]
Cembra-2-7-dien-12-one, 4-6-dihydroxy-20-
    nor, (1S-2-trans-4S-6R-7-trans): Fl[NT335]
Cembra-2-7-diene-4-6-diol, 11-12-epoxy,
    (1S-2-trans-4R-6R-7-trans-11-trans): Fl[NT451]
Cembra-2-7-diene-4-6-diol, 11-12-epoxy,
    (1S-2-trans-4S-6R-7-trans-11-trans): Fl[NT451]
Cembra-3-7-11-15-tetraen-6-ol: Gum[NT567]
Cembra-trans-2-12(20)-dien-6-one, 4(S)-8(R)-
    11(S)-trihydroxy, 1(S): Fl[NT341]
Cembra-trans-2-12(20)-dien-6-one, 4(S)-8(S)-
    11(S)-trihydroxy, 1(S): Fl[NT341]
Cembra-trans-2-12(20)-dien-6-one, 8(R)-
    11(S)-epoxy-4(S)-hydroxy, 1(S): Fl[NT328]
Cembra-trans-2-12(20)-diene-4(S)-6(R)-7(S)-
    triol, 8(R)-11(S)-epi-dioxy: Fl[NT337]
Cembra-trans-2-12(20)-diene-4(S)-6(R)-7(S)-
    triol, 8(R)-11(S)-epoxy, (1S): Fl[NT337]
Cembra-trans-2-8(19)-12(20)-triene-4(S)-
    6(R)-7(R)-11(S)-tetraol, (1S): Fl[NT341]
Cembra-trans-2-8(19)-12(20)-triene-4(S)-
    6(R)-7(S)-11(S)-tetraol, (1S): Fl[NT341]
Cembra-trans-2-en-6-one, 8(R)-11(S)-epoxy-
    4(S)-12(R)-dihydroxy, 1(S): Fl[NT328]
Cembra-trans-2-trans-11-diene-4-(S)-6(R)-
    diol, 7(R)-8(R)-epoxy. 1(S): Lf[NT333]
Cembra-trans-2-trans-11-diene-4(S)-6(R)-diol,
    7(S)-8(S)-epoxy, 1(S): Fl[NT333]
Cembra-trans-2-trans-12-dien-6-one, 8(R)-
    11(S)-epoxy-4(S)-hydroxy, 1(S): Fl[NT328]
Cembra-trans-2-trans-6-12(20)-trien-4-ol,
    8-11-epoxy, (1S-4R-11S): Lf 0.05[NT546]

Cembra-*trans*-2-*trans*-6-12(20)-triene-4(R)-8(S)-11(S)-triol, (1S): Fl 14.5[NT575]

Cembra-*trans*-2-*trans*-6-12(20)-triene-4(S)-8(S)-11(S)-triol, (1S): Fl[NT342]

Cembra-*trans*-2-*trans*-6-diene-4-12-diol, 8-11-epoxy, (1S-4S-8S-11R12S): Lf 0.01[NT552]

Cembra-*trans*-2-*trans*-6-*trans*-10-triene-4(R)-8(S)-12(R)-triol, (1S): Fl[NT342]

Cembra-*trans*-2-*trans*-6-*trans*-10-triene-4(R)-8(S)-12(S)-triol, (1S): Fl[NT342]

Cembra-*trans*-2-*trans*-6-*trans*-10-triene-4(S)-8(S)-12(R)-triol, (1S): Fl[NT342]

Cembra-*trans*-2-*trans*-6-*trans*-10-triene-4(S)-8(S)-12(S)-triol, (1S): Fl[NT342]

Cembra-*trans*-2-*trans*-6-*trans*-11-triene-4-6-diol, 4-O-methyl, (1S-4R): Lf[NT570]

Cembra-*trans*-2-*trans*-6-*trans*-12-trien-4-ol, 8-11-epoxy, (1-2-4-R-8R-11S): Lf 0.03[NT546]

Cembra-*trans*-2-*trans*-6-*trans*-12-trien-4-ol, 8-11-epoxy, (1S-4S-8R-11S): Lf 0.2[NT546]

Cembra-*trans*-2-*trans*-6-*trans*-12-triene-4-6-diol, 12-hydroperoxy, (1S-4R-6R-12S): Lf[NT570]

Cembra-*trans*-2-*trans*-7-*trans*-10-triene-4-6-diol, 12-hydroperoxy, (1S-4S-6R-12R): Fl[NT569]

Cembra-*trans*-2-*trans*-7-*trans*-10-triene-4-6-diol, 12-hydroperoxy, (1S-4S-6R-12S): Fl[NT569]

Cembra-*trans*-2-*trans*-7-*trans*-11-triene, 4(S)-10(S)-dihydroxy, (1S): Fl[NT347]

Cembra-*trans*-2-*trans*-7-*trans*-11-triene-10-one, (1S): Fl[NT347]

Cembra-*trans*-2-*trans*-7-*trans*-11-triene-10-one, 4(R)-6(R)-dihydroxy, (1S): Fl[NT347]

Cembra-*trans*-2-*trans*-7-*trans*-11-triene-4(R)-6(R)-10(R)-triol, (1S): Fl[NT347]

Cembra-*trans*-2-*trans*-7-*trans*-11-triene-4(R)-6(R)-10(S)-triol, (1S): Fl[NT347]

Cembra-*trans*-2-*trans*-7-*trans*-11-triene-4(R)-6(R)-13(R)-triol, (1S): Fl[NT346]

Cembra-*trans*-2-*trans*-7-*trans*-11-triene-4(S)-6(R)-10(R)-triol, (1S): Fl[NT347]

Cembra-*trans*-2-*trans*-7-*trans*-11-triene-4(S)-6(R)-10(S)-triol, (1S): Fl[NT347]

Cembra-*trans*-2-*trans*-7-12(20)-triene-4(R)-6(R)-11(S)-triol, (1S): Fl 36.1[NT575]

Cembra-*trans*-2-*trans*-7-12(20)-triene-4(S)-6(R)-11(R)-triol, (1S): Fl 9[NT575]

Cembra-*trans*-2-*trans*-7-12(20)-triene-4(S)-6(R)-11(S)-triol: Lf[NT553]

Cembra-*trans*-2-*trans*-7-12(20)-triene-4(S)-6(R)-diol, 10(R)-11(R)-epoxy, (1S): Fl[NT344]

Cembra-*trans*-2-*trans*-7-12(20)-triene-4(S)-6(R)-diol, 10(S)-11(S)-epoxy, (1S): Fl[NT344]

Cembra-*trans*-2-*trans*-7-12(20)-triene-4-6-diol, 11-hydroperoxy, (1S-4R-6R-11S): Fl[NT569]

Cembra-*trans*-2-*trans*-7-12(20)-triene-4-6-diol, 11-hydroperoxy, (1S-4S-6R-11S): Fl[NT569]

Cembra-*trans*-2-*trans*-7-*cis*-11-triene-4(R)-6(R)-10(S)-triol, (1S): Fl[NT347]

Cembra-*trans*-2-*trans*-7-*cis*-11-triene-4(S)-6(R)-20-triol, (1S): Fl[NT346]

Cembra-*trans*-2-*trans*-7-dien-6-one, 11(S)-12(S)-epoxy-4(S)-hydroxy, 1(S): Fl[NT328]

Cembra-*trans*-2-*trans*-7-diene-4(R)-6(R)-diol, 11(R)-12(R)-epoxy, 2(S): Fl[NT344]

Cembra-*trans*-2-*trans*-7-diene-4(S)-6(R)-11(S)-12(R)-tetraol, (1S): Fl[NT341]

Cembra-*trans*-2-*trans*-7-diene-4(S)-6(R)-diol, 11(R)-12(R)-epoxy, 1(S): Fl[NT344]

Cembra-*trans*-2-*trans*-7-diene-4(S)-6(R)-diol, 11(S)-12(S)-epoxy: Lf[NT553]

Cembra-*trans*-2-*trans*-7-diene-4-6-diol, 11-12-epoxy, (1S-4R-11S-12S): Lf 0.09[NT546]

Cembra-*trans*-2-*trans*-7-*trans*-10-*trans*-6-one, 4(S)-12(S)-dihydroxy, 1(S): Fl[NT328]

Cembra-*trans*-2-*trans*-7-*trans*-10-triene-4(R)-6(R)-12(R)-triol, (1S): Fl 13.3[NT575]

Cembra-*trans*-2-*trans*-7-*trans*-10-triene-4(R)-6(R)-12(S)-triol, (1S): Fl 21.7[NT575]

Cembra-*trans*-2-*trans*-7-*trans*-10-triene-4(S)-6(R)-12(R)-triol, (1S): Fl 20.5[NT575]

Cembra-*trans*-2-*trans*-7-*trans*-10-triene-4(S)-6(R)-12(S)-triol: Lf[NT553]

Cembra-*trans*-2-*trans*-7-*trans*-11-triene-4(R)-6(R)-diol: Lf[NT553]

Cembra-*trans*-2-*trans*-7-*trans*-11-triene-4(S)-6(R)-diol: Lf[NT553]

Cembra-*trans*-2-*trans*-7-*trans*-11-triene-4-6-diol, 4-O-methyl, (1S-4R-6R): Lf[NT570]

Cembra-*trans*-2-*trans*-7-*trans*-11-triene-4-8-diol, 4-8-di-O-methyl: Lf[NT570]

Cembratriendiol, α: Lf[NT509]

Cembratriendiol, β: Lf[NT509]

Cembrene: Lf 0.031[NT541]

Cembrenodienol, α: Lf[NT507]

Cembrenodienol, β: Lf[NT507]

Cerotic acid: Sd[NT515]

Cerotic acid: Sd[NT515]

Chlorogenic acid: Lf[NT365]

Chlorophyll A: Call Tiss[NT411]
Chlorophyll B: Call Tiss[NT411]
Cholest-7-enol, 4-α-methyl: Sd oil[NT491]
Cholest-7-enol: Sd oil[NT491]
Cholesta-7-24-dien-3-β-ol, 4-α-24-dimethyl: Sd[NT490]
Cholesta-7-24-dien-3-β-ol, 4-α-methyl-24-ethyl: Sd[NT490]
Cholesta-8-24-dien-3-β-ol, 4-α-14-α-24-trimethyl: Sd[NT490]
Cholestanol: Sd[NT515]
Cholesterol acyl glycoside: Lf[NT368]
Cholesterol ester: Lf[NT368]
Cholesterol glycoside: Lf[NT368]
Cholesterol, 24-methylene: Sd oil[NT491]
Cholesterol: Sd oil[NT491], Lf[NT540]
Choline, phosphatidyl: Pl[NT577]
Choline: Pl[NT562]
Chrysene: Lf smoke 5.1 μg/100 Cig[NT434]
Cineol, 1–8: Lf, Rt, St, Bk, Tw[NT428]
Cinnamonitrile, dihydro: Cured Lf[NT472]
Cinnamyl alcohol: Lf, Rt, St, Bk, Tw[NT428]
Citric acid: Lf[NT388], cured Lf[NT544]
Citronellol: Lf, Rt, St, Bk, Tw[NT428]
Citrostadienol: Sd oil[NT491]
Clerosterol: Sd[NT515]
Coenzyme Q-10: Pl[NT417]
Collidine, γ: Lf[NT472]
Coniferyl alcohol: Lf smoke[NT171]
Cotinine: Lf 95.9[NT565]
Cotinine: Lf[NT506]
Coumarin: Lf, Rt, St, Bk, Tw[NT428]
Cresol, *m*-: Lf[NT327]
Cresol, ortho: Lf[NT327]
Cresol, para: Lf[NT327]
Crotonaldehyde: Lf[NT599]
Cupalene: Lf, Rt, St, Bk, Tw[NT428]
Cupalene: Lf, Rt, St, Bk, Tw[NT428]
Curcumene, α: Lf, Rt, St, Bk, Tw[NT428]
Cycloartanol, 24-methylene: Lf[NT540], Sd[NT480]
Cycloartanol, 31-nor: Sd[NT490]
Cycloartanol: Sd oil[NT491], Sd[NT480]
Cycloartenol, 24-methylene: Sd oil[NT491]
Cycloartenol, 31-nor: Sd oil[NT491]
Cycloartenol: Lf[NT540], Sd[NT480]
Cycloeucalenol: Sd oil[NT491]
Cyclohex-2-en-1-4-dione, 2-6-6-trimethyl-4-methylene: Lf, Rt, St, Bk, Tw[NT428]
Cyclohexanone, 4-hydroxy-2-2-6-trimethyl: Lf, Rt, St, Bk, Tw[NT428]
Cyclohexanone, 4-hydroxy-3-3-5-trimethyl: Lf, Rt, St, Bk, Tw[NT428]

Cyclopent-1-ene, 2-methyl-5-iso-propyl, 1-carboxylic acid: Lf[NT533]
Cyclopent-2-en-1-one, 2-3-dimethyl: Lf, Rt, St, Bk, Tw[NT428]
Cyclopropane-1-carboxylic acid-1-amino: Call Tiss[NT564]
Cyperone, α, 2-keto: Lf[NT565]
Cysteine: Sd[NT515]
Damascene, β, 3-hydroxy: Lf EO[NT559]
Damascene, β, 3-hydroxy: Lf, Rt, St, Bk, Tw[NT428]
Damascene, β, 4-hydroxy: Lf EO[NT559]
Damascene, β, 8-9-dihydro, 3-hydroxy: Lf EO[NT559]
Damascene, β: Lf, Rt, St, Bk, Tw[NT428]
Damascenone, β: Lf, Rt, St, Bk, Tw[NT428]
Damascenone: Lf, Rt, St, Bk, Tw[NT428]
Daucosterol: Lf[NT320]
Debneyol, 1-β-hydroxy, 12-O-β-D-glucoside: Lf 7.4[NT343]
Debneyol, 1-hydroxy: Pl 3[NT602]
Debneyol, 7-epi: Pl 1.1[NT602]
Debneyol, 8-hydroxy: Pl 3[NT602]
Debneyol: Pl[NT510]
Deca-*cis*-2-*trans*-4-dienoic acid, 6-iso-propyl-3-methyl-9-oxo: cured Lf[NT431]
Decane: Smoke[NT183]
Deca-*trans*-2-*trans*-4-dienoate, 9-oxo-6-iso-propyl-3-methyl, methyl: Lf[NT530]
Deca-*trans*-2-*trans*-4-dienoic acid, 6-iso-propyl-3-methyl-9-oxo, (−): Lf[NT622]
Deca-*trans*-2-*trans*-7-dienoic acid, 6-iso-propyl-3-methyl-9-oxo: cured Lf[NT431]
Deca-*trans*-4-9-dienoic acid, 3-hydroxy-6-iso-propyl-3-methyl-9-(5-oxo-tetrahydrofuran-2-yl): Lf[NT348]
Dec-*trans*-4-en-9-one, 1-3-dihydroxy-6-iso-propyl-3-methyl, (3-ε-6-ε): 0.009[NT549]
Dec-*trans*-4-enoic acid, 3-ε-hydroxy-9-oxo-3-ε-methyl-6-(S)-iso-propyl: Cured Lf[NT420]
Dec-*trans*-4-enoic acid, 3-hydroxy-6-iso-propyl-3-methyl-9-oxo, (6S): Lf 0.037[NT514]
Dec-*trans*-4-enoic acid, 3-hydroxy-6-iso-propyl-3-methyl-9-oxo: Lf 0.008[NT514]
Dehydratase, Δ-amino-levulinic acid: Call Tiss[NT386]
Dehydrogenase, NADP-linked-glyceraldehyde: Pl[NT371]
Docosan-1-ol: Lf[NT540]
Dodeca-*trans*-6-*trans*-9-dienoic acid, 3-psi-hydrohy-4-psi-9-dimethyl: Cured Lf[NT473]

Dotriacontanoic acid: Sd[NT515]

Drim-8-en-11-ol: Lf[NT535]

Drim-8-en-7-one: Lf[NT367]

Driman-8-9-(R)-diol, 11-nor: 0.006[NT623]

Driman-8-ol, 11-nor, (DL): 0.007[NT623]

Duva-3-9-(17)-13-trien-1-ol, 5-8-oxido: Lf, Rt, St, Bk, Tw[NT428]

Duva-4-8-13-triene-1-3-diol: Lf[NT361]

Duvatienediol, α: Trichome[NT444], Pl[NT445]

Duvatienediol, β: Trichome[NT444], Pl[NT445]

Duvatriene-1-3-diol, β-4-8-13: Lf[NT405]

Elem: Lf, Rt, St, Bk, Tw[NT428]

Esculin: Smoke[NT183]

Estragole: Lf[NT579]

Ethanol, (4-hydroxy-3-methoxy-phenyl)-2: Lf 19[NT498]

Ethanol, 2-phenoxy: Lf, Rt, St, Bk, Tw[NT428]

Ethanolamine, phosphatidyl: Pl[NT577]

Eugenol: Lf[NT327]

Eugenol: Smoke[NT183]

Fanesyl-acetone: Lf, Rt, St, Bk, Tw[NT428]

Fatty acid: Lf smoke[NT171]

Fluoranthene: Smoke[NT183]

Formaldehyde: Lf[NT599]

Formic acid: Lf[NT440]

Fructose: Sd[NT515]

Fucosterol, 28-iso: Sd oil[NT491]

Fumaric acid: cured Lf[NT544]

Furfural, 5-methoxy-methyl: Cured Lf[NT544]

Furfuryl alcohol: Cured Lf[NT413]

Geraniol: Lf, Rt, St, Bk, Tw[NT428]

Geranyl-geraniadiene: Lf 720[NT557]

Geranyl-linalool, 20-hydroxy, 3-O-[α-L-rhamnopyranosyl(1-4)]-β-D-glucopyrano-side-20-[β-D-glucopyranosyl(1-2)]-[α-L-rhamnopyranosyl(1-6)]-β-D-glucopyrano-side (trans-6-trans-10-cis-14): Lf[NT353]

Geranyl-linalool, 20-hydroxy, 3-O-[α-L-rhamnopyranosyl(1-4)]-β-D-glucopyranoside-20-O-[α-L-rhamno-pyranosyl(1-4)]-[α-L-rhamnopyranosyl(1-6)]-β-D-glucopyranoside (trans-6-trans-10-cis-14): Lf[NT353]

Gibberellin A-1: Call Tiss[NT432]

Globulin: Cured Lf[NT359]

Glucose: Sd[NT515]

Glutamic acid: Sd[NT515]

Glutamyl, γ-L, L-glutamic acid: Pl[NT385]

Glutathione: Pl 0.15–0.20 mM[NT419]

Glutelin: Cured Lf[NT359]

Glutinosone: Lf[NT608]

Glycerol, phosphatidyl: Pl[NT577]

Glycine: Sd[NT515]

Glycine-betaine: Lf 2.8 mM[NT461]

Glycoprotein: Call Tiss[NT396]

Gramisterol: Sd oil[NT491]

Guaiacol, 4-ethyl: Lf[NT327]

Guaiacol, 4-methyl: Lf[NT327]

Guaiacol, 4-propyl: Lf[NT327]

Guaiacol, 4-vinyl: Lf[NT327]

Guaiacol, methyl: Cured Lf[NT413]

Guaiacol: Lf[NT327]

Harman indole: Lf[NT323]

Harman, nor: Lf[NT323]

Hentriacontane-10-12-dione: Stigma[NT522]

Hept-2-enoate, 6-oxo-3-iso-propyl, methyl: Lf[NT530]

Hept-5-en-2-one, 6-methyl: Lf, Rt, St, Bk, Tw[NT428]

Hept-6-en-2-ol, (E)-5-iso-propyl-7-(2-methy-tetrahydro-fur-2-yl): Lf[NT372]

Hept-6-en-2-one, (E)-5-iso-propyl-7-(2-methyl-tetrahydro-fur-2-yl): Lf[NT372]

Hepta-4-(E)-6-dienoic acid, 3-iso-propyl-6-methyl, methyl ester: Cured Lf 0.075[NT398]

Hepta-4-6-dien-1-ol, 3-iso-propyl-6-methyl, (E): Lf[NT406]

Heptacosane-10-12-dione: Stigma[NT522]

Heptacosanoic acid: Sd[NT515]

Heptadeca-8-cis-11-cis dienal: Lf EO[NT505]

Heptadeca-8-cis-11-cis-14 cis trienal: Lf EO[NT505]

Heptadecanoic acid: Cured Lf[NT544]

Heptadecenoic acid: Cured Lf[NT544]

Heptanoic acid: Cured Lf[NT413]

Hept-trans-2-ene-1-6-diol, 3-iso-propyl, (6-ε): Lf 0.01[NT549]

Hept-trans-2-enoate, 6-oxo-3-iso-propyl, me-thyl: Lf[NT530]

Hept-trans-3-en-2-one, 5-hydroxy-5-iso-propyl, (−): Lf[NT442]

Hept-trans-3-en-2-one, 5-hydroxy-5-iso-pro-pyl: Lf 0.021[NT514]

Hex-5-en-2-one: Lx (St)[NT376]

Hexadecane: Smoke[NT183]

Hexan-4-olide, 5-methyl: Lf 0.006[NT349]

Hexane-1-5-dio, 2-iso-propyl, (2-S-5-ε): Lf 0.02[NT549]

Hexanoate, 5-oxo-2-(S)-iso-propyl: Lf[NT530]

Hexatriacontanon-2-6-10-14-18-22-26-30-33-aen-1-35-diol, 3-7-11-15-19-23-27-31-35-nonamethyl: Cured Lf 4.5[NT435]

Hexatriaconta-octa-2-6-10-14-18-22-26-30-en-1-34-diol, 3-7-11-15-19-23-27-31-octamethyl-35-methylene: Cured Lf 39[NT435]

Histidine: Sd[NT515]

Histones: Call Tiss[NT395]

Humulene, α: Lf, Rt, St, Bk, Tw[NT428]

Hydrazine sulfate: Lf smoke[NT160]

Hydrocyanic acid inorganic: Cured Lf[NT423]

Hydroquinone, 2-iso-propyl: Lf[NT448]

Hydroquinone: Lf smoke[NT171]

Hydroquinone: Lf[NT022]

Hydroxyacetophenone: Lf smoke[NT171]

Hydroxyphenyl alcohol: Lf smoke[NT171]

Indole: Cured Lf[NT472]

Indole-3-acetic acid: Call Tiss[NT421], Pl[NT433]

Inositol, phosphatidyl: Pl[NT577]

Ionol, α, 3-oxo: Lf 0.47[NT572]

Ionol, β, 3-hydroxy: Lf, Rt, St, Bk, Tw[NT428]

Ionol, β, 3-hydroxy-5-6-epoxy: Lf 0.046[NT534]

Ionol, β, 7-8-dihydro-3-hydroxy: Lf[NT374], Rt, St, Bk, Tw[NT428]

Ionone, β, 3-hydroxy, (R)-(-): Lf[NT393]

Ionone, β, 3-hydroxy: Lf, Rt, St, Bk, Tw[NT428]

Ionone, β, 4-oxo: Lf, Rt, St, Bk, Tw[NT428]

Ionone, β: Lf, Rt, St, Bk, Tw[NT428]

Ionyl, β, 3-hydroxy-5-6-epoxy, β-D-glucopyranoside: Cured Lf[NT548]

Iso-amyl acetate: Lf, Rt, St, Bk, Tw[NT428]

Isoperoxidase (A-A): Pl[NT389]

Isoperoxidase (A-B): Pl[NT389]

Isoperoxidase (A-D): Pl[NT389]

Isoperoxidase (A-E): Pl[NT389]

Isoperoxidase (C-N): Pl[NT389]

Isophorone: Lf, Rt, St, Bk, Tw[NT428]

Isoprene: Lf[NT022]

Kaempferol-3-rhamnoglucoside: Lf 0.02%[NT484]

Kaepferol: Lf 50[NT484]

Kynurenic acid, 6-hydroxy: Pl[NT562]

Labd-13-en-15-ol, 8-12-epoxy, 12(R)-13-*trans*: Fl[NT338]

Labd-13-en-15-ol, 8-12-epoxy, 12(S)-13-*trans*: Fl[NT338]

Labd-13-ene- 8-12-15-triol, 12(S)-13-*trans*: Fl[NT338]

Labd-14-ene, 13-η-hydroxy-8-α-12-η-epoxy: Lf[NT373]

Labd-8(17)-en-12-al, 13-14-15-16-tetra-nor: Lf[NT535]

Labd-8(17)-en-13-one, 15-16-dinor: Lf[NT535]

Labd-8-en-12 al, 13-14-15-16-tetra-nor: Lf[NT535]

Labd-8-en-13-one, 15-16-di-nor: Lf[NT535]

Labd-8-ene-7-13-dione, 14-15-di-nor: Fl[NT338]

Labdan-13-one, 11-12-epoxy-8-hydroxy-14-15-di-nor, 11(S)-12(R): Fl[NT338]

Labdane, 15-16-di-nor, 8-13-epoxy: Lf[NT535]

Labdane, 15-16-di-nor, 8-α-13, 9-α-13-diepoxy: Lf[NT535]

Lanos-8-en-3-β-ol, 24-methylene: Sd oil[NT491]

Lanost-8-en-3-β-ol, 31-nor: Sd oil[NT491]

Lanost-9(11)-en-3-β-ol, 31-nor, 24-methyl: Sd[NT490]

Lanost-9(11)-en-3-β-ol, 31-nor: Sd[NT490]

Lanosterol, 24-dihydro: Sd oil[NT491]

Lanosterol, 31-nor: Sd oil[NT491]

Lanosterol: Sd oil[NT491]

Laurc acid: Cured Lf[NT413]

Leucine, D: Call Tiss[NT392]

Leucine, iso: Sd[NT515]

Leucine, L: Call Tiss[NT392]

Leucine: Sd[NT515]

Leucinopine lactam: Crown Gall Tumor Tiss[NT583]

Leucinopine: Crown Gall Tumor Tiss[NT583]

Levulinic acid: Cured Lf[NT544]

Ligase, leucine-tRNA: Pl[NT571]

Limonene: Smoke[NT183]

Linalool: Lf, Rt, St, Bk, Tw[NT428]

Linoleic acid: Sd oil[NT400], Cured Lf[NT544]

Linolenic acid: Sd oil[NT400], Cured Lf[NT544]

Loliolide, dehydro: Lf 0.027[NT547]

Loliolide-β-D-glucopyranoside: Lf 8.3[NT558]

Lophenol, 24-(R)-ethyl: Sd[NT490]

Lophenol, 24-methyl: Sd[NT490]

Lophenol: Sd oil[NT491]

Lubimin: Lf[NT446]

Lupein: Lf[NT363]

Lupeol: Sd oil[NT491]

Lutidine, 2-3: Lf[NT322]

Lutidine, 2-4: Lf[NT322]

Lutidine, 2-5: Lf[NT322]

Lutidine, 2-6: Lf[NT322], Cured Lf[NT543]

Lutidine, 3: Cured Lf[NT543]

Lutidine, 3-5: Cured Lf[NT472]

Lyase, L-phenylalanine ammonia: Pl[NT624]

Lysine: Sd[NT515]

Magestigma-4-*trans*-7-diene-3(S)-9(R)-diol, 6(R): Lf[NT503]

Maleimide, methyl-ethyl: Lf, Rt, St, Bk, Tw[NT428]

Malic acid: Cured Lf[NT544]

Malonic acid: Cured Lf[NT544]

Megastigma-4-*trans*-7-diene-3(S)-9(S)-diol, 6(R): Lf[NT503]

Megastigma-5(13)-(E)-dien-6-9-diol: Cured Lf[NT479]

Megastigma-5-*trans*-8-dien-4-one: Lf[NT529]

Megastigmastrienone, 8-9-dihydro, 8-9-dihydroxy: Lf[NT500]

Megastigmastrienone, iso, 8-9-dihydro, 8-9-dihydroxy: Lf[NT500]

Megastigmastrienone: Lf, Rt, St, Bk, Tw[NT428]

Megastigum-7-ene-5-6-9-triol, (5R-6S-7-trans-9S): Lf[NT597]

Melissic acid: Sd[NT515]

Methionine: Sd[NT515]

Mikimopine: Rt 480[NT339]

Morpholine, N-nitroso: Lf[NT599]

Myosmine: Lf[NT322], Cured Lf[NT543]

Myristic acid: Cured Lf[NT544]

N1-nitrosonornicotine: Lf[NT072]

Naphthalene, 1-2-dihydro, 3-iso-propenyl-5-methyl: Lf[NT487]

Naphthalene, 2-methoxy: Lf, Rt, St, Bk, Tw[NT428]

Naphthalene, methyl: Lf, Rt, St, Bk, Tw[NT428]

Naphthalene: Lf, Rt, Stem, Bk, Tw[NT428]

Naphthalene-1-ol, 1-2-3-4-tetrahydro, cis-2-iso-propenyl-8-methyl: Lf[NT487]

Naphthoquinone, 1-4, 2-3-6-trimethyl: Lf[NT326]

Nectarin I: Fl[NT357]

Neophytadiene: Lf[NT540]

Neoxanthin: Lf[NT363]

NH_3 inorganic: Lf Ju[NT425]

Nicotanoside A: Sd 0.13%[NT351]

Nicotanoside B: Sd 0.29%[NT351]

Nicotanoside C: Sd 0.71%[NT352]

Nicotanoside E: Sd 0.16%[NT351]

Nicotanoside F: Sd 1.155%[NT352]

Nicotelline: Pl[NT562]

Nicotiana tabacum diterpene I: Fl[NT336]

Nicotiana tabacum glycoprotein: Lf, Lf smoke Condensate, Lf Tar[NT603]

Nicotiana tabacum heptaacyl glyceride 3: Stigma[NT563]

Nicotiana tabacum heptaacyl glyceride: Stigma[NT563]

Nicotiana tabacum pentaacyl glyceride 2: Stigma[NT563]

Nicotiana tabacum tetraacyl glyceride: Stigma[NT563]

Nicotiana tabacum virus inhibitor: Lf, St[NT527]

Nicotianamine: Lf 0.05% μM[NT439]

Nicotianine: Lf[NT324]

Nicotine, nor, 1'-(6-hydroxy-octanoyl): Lf 1.6[NT565]

Nicotine, nor, 1'-(7-hydroxy-octanoyl): Lf[NT550]

Nicotine, nor, 1'-(hydroxy-octanoyl): Lf 1.1[NT565]

Nicotine, nor, 1'-acetyl: Lf[NT550]

Nicotine, nor, 1'-hexanoyl: Lf[NT550]

Nicotine, nor, 1'-octanoyl: Lf[NT550]

Nicotine, nor, 1'-propionyl: Lf[NT550]

Nicotine, nor, N-(4-dimethyl-amino-butanoyl): Lf 0.83[NT531]

Nicotine, nor, N'-acetyl: Lf[NT506]

Nicotine, nor, N'-butanoyl: Lf[NT506]

Nicotine, nor, N'-carboethoxy: Lf 4[NT531]

Nicotine, nor, N'-formyl: Lf[NT506]

Nicotine, nor, N'-hexanoyl: Lf[NT506]

Nicotine, nor, N'-iso-propyl: Pl[NT562]

Nicotine, nor, N'-nitroso: Lf[NT378], Cured Lf 1.1–1.8[NT407], Pl[NT562]

Nicotine, nor, N'-octanoyl: Lf[NT506]

Nicotine, nor: An[NT391], Call Tiss[NT499], Lf[NT526], Pl[NT437], Rt, Cx[NT508]

Nicotine: Lf[NT360], Cured Lf[NT408], Aer[NT436], Pl[NT562], Call Tiss 11.46 mg/5.05 g[NT576] Cured Lf smoke[NT543], Rt, Stigma/Style, Stamen, Ovary, Petal, Cx, Sd (immature), Sd, Ovule, Fl[NT508]

Nicotine-N'-oxide: Cured Lf smoke[NT543]

Nicotinic acid, 6-hydroxy: Pl[NT562]

Nicotinic acid, methyl ester: Lf, Rt, St, Bk, Tw[NT428]

Nicotinic acid, N-glucoside: Pl[NT562]

Nicotinic acid: Pl[NT562]

Nicotinoyl-1-O-β-D-glucopyranose: Pl[NT354]

Nicotyrine: An[N06589], Lf[NT440], Cured Lf smoke[NT543]

N'-nitrosoanabasine: Lf[NT087]

N'-nitrosoanatabine: Lf[NT166]

N'-nitrosonornicotine: Lf[NT087]

N-nitrosoproline: Pl[NT107]

N-nitrosopyrrolidine: Lf[NT087]

N-nitrososarcosine: Pl[NT107]

N-N-octanoylnornicotine: Lf[NT294]

Non-3-en-8-one, 2-5-diepoxy-2(R)-hydroxy-5(R)-iso-propyl: Lf[NT348]

Non-3-en-8-one,1-5-epi-dioxy-2(S)-hydroxy-5-iso-propyl: Lf[NT348]

Non-3-ene-2-8-diol, 5-iso-propyl, (E): Lf[NT406]

Non-6-en-2-one, 5-iso-propyl-8-hydroxy, (E): Lf[NT406]

Non-6-en-2-one, 5-iso-propyl-8-hydroxy-8-methyl, (E): Lf[NT406]

Non-8-en-4-olide, 3(R)-7(R)-epoxy-4(R)-8-dimethyl: Lf 0.002[NT349]

Nonacosane-8-10-dione: Stigma[NT522]

Nonan-2-ol, 3-3-5-trimethyl-8-iso-propyl-4-9-dioxa-bicyclo-(3.3.1): Lf[NT406]

Nonan-2-one, 5-iso-propyl-6-7-epoxy-8-hydroxy-8-methyl, (E): Lf[NT406]

Nonane-2-8-diol, 3-4-epoxy-5-iso-propyl, (2-ε-3-5-4-S-5-S-8-ε): Lf 0.001[NT549]

Nonane-2-8-diol, 3-4-epoxy-5-iso-propyl-2-metyl, (3-R-4-S-5-S-8-ε): Lf 0.006[NT549]

Nona-*trans*-2-en-8-ol, 3-methyl-4-oxo: Lf[NT476]

Nona-*trans*-2-*trans*-6-dienal, 5-iso-propyl-2-methyl-8-oxo: Lf 0.004[NT514]

Non-*cis*-6-en-4-olide: Lf 0.36[NT349]

Non-*trans*-2-en-4-one, 3-methyl: Lf[NT535]

Non-*trans*-3-en-8-one, 1-2-dihydrohy5-iso-propyl-2-methyl, (5-S): Lf 0.03[NT549]

Non-*trans*-3-en-8-one, 1-2-dihydrohy5-iso-propyl-2-methyl, 2-epi, (S-5): Lf 0.4[NT549]

Non-*trans*-5-en-4-olide, 2(R)-7-iso-propyl-4(S)-methyl: Lf[NT348]

Nonvolatile acids: Lf[NT493]

Nuclease: Pl[NT422]

Nucleotidase, 3': Pl[NT576]

Obtusifoliol: Sd oil[NT491]

Occidenol: Lf[NT608]

Occidentalol: Lf[NT608]

Occidol: Lf[NT565]

Oct-2-en-4-olide, 3-methyl-7-oxo: Lf 0.003[NT349]

Octa-5-*trans*-7-dienoic acid, 4-iso-propyl-7-methyl, methyl ester: cured Lf 0.75[NT398]

Octacosanoic acid: Sd[NT515]

Octadec-*trans*-9-en-18-olide: Lf[NT535]

Octan-2-one, 7-hydroxy-3-3-dimethyl: Cured Lf[NT478]

Octanoic acid: Lf[NT440]

Octa-*trans*-2-7-diene-1-6-(S)-iol, 2-6-dim-ethyl: Lf 0.03[NT532]

Oct-*trans*-2-enoic acid, Y-iso-propyl-7-oxo: Cured Lf[NT431]

Oct-*trans*-5-en-4-olide, 4-iso-propyl-7-oxo: Lf 0.016[NT514]

Oleic acid: Sd oil[NT400], Cured Lf[NT544]

Oleic acid: Smoke[NT183]

Oxalic acid: Cured Lf[NT544]

Oxidase, β-indolyl-acetic acid: Call Tiss[NT390]

Oxidase, indole-acetic acid: Stem pith[NT384]

Palmitic acid, methyl ester: Lf, Rt, St, Bk, Tw[NT428]

Palmitic acid: Sd oil[NT400], Lf[NT540], Cured Lf[NT544]

Palmitin, mono: Pl[NT416]

Pantolactone: Lf, Rt, St, Bk, Tw[NT428]

Pent-2-4-dienen-5-olide, 3-iso-propyl: Lf 0.005[NT349]

Pent-2-en-4-olide, 3-ethyl-4-methyl: Lf 0.005[NT349]

Pent-2-en-4-olide, 3-iso-propyl: Lf 0.008[NT349]

Pent-2-en-4-olide, 4-methyl-3-(3-oxo-1-butyl): Lf 0.005[NT349]

Pent-2-en-5-olide, 5-propyl: Lf, Rt, St, Bk, Tw[NT428]

Pentacosane-8-10-dione: Stigma[NT522]

Pentadeca-4-9-dien-14-on-1-al, 6-8-dihydroxy-11-iso-propyl-4-8-dimethyl: Lf[NT494]

Pentadecan-15-olide: Lf[NT535]

Pentadecan-2-one, 6-10-14-trimethyl: Lf, Rt, St, Bk, Tw[NT428]

Pentadecanal, 6-10-14-trimethyl, *trans*-2-ethylidene: Lf[NT535]

Pentadecanal: Lf EO[NT500]

Pentadecanoic acid: Cured Lf[NT413]

Pentadeca-*trans*-3-*trans*-8-*cis*-12-14-tetraen-2-one, 5-iso-propyl-8-12-dimethyl: Lf smoke[NT554]

Pentadeca-*trans*-3-*trans*-8-12-14-tetraen-2-one, 5-iso-propyl-8-12-dimethyl: Lf smoke[NT554]

Pentadeca-*trans*-4-*trans*-9-dienoic acid, 6(R)-8(R)-dihydroxy-4-8-dimethyl-11(S)-iso-propyl-14-oxo: Lf[NT332]

Pentadeca-*trans*-4-*trans*-9-dienoic acid, 6(R)-8(S)-dihydroxy-4-8-dimethyl-11(S)-iso-propyl-14-oxo: Fl, Lf[NT332]

Pentan-2-one: Lx (St)[NT376]

Pentan-4-olide, 3(R)-methyl, 4(R): Lf 0.002[NT349]

Pentan-4-olide, 3(R)-methyl, 4(S): Lf 0.002[NT349]

Pentan-4-olide, 4(5-methyl-2-furyl): Lf 0.022[NT349]

Pentan-5-olide, 3-iso-propyl: Lf, Rt, St, Bk, Tw[NT428]

Pentan-5-olide, 5-pentyl: Lf, Rt, St, Bk, Tw[NT428]

Pentan-5-olide, 5-propyl: Lf, Rt, St, Bk, Tw[NT428]

Peroxidase, iso, A-1: Pl[NT370]

Peroxidase, iso, A-2: Pl[NT370]

Peroxidase: Call Tiss[NT383], Cy[NT387], Lf[NT409]

Phenol, 2-6-dimethoxy: Lf[NT327]

Phenol, *m*-ethyl: Lf[NT327]

Phenol, *m*-methoxy: Lf[NT327]

Phenol, ortho-tert-butyl: Cured Lf[NT413]

Phenol, para-ethyl: Lf[NT327]

Phenol, para-methoxy: Lf[NT327]

Phenol: Lf[NT327]

Phenol: Smoke[NT183]

Phenolic cyano compound: Lf smoke[NT171]

Phenyl acetate, methyl: Lf, Rt, St, Bk, Tw[NT428]
Phenylacetic acid: Lf 46[NT498]
Phenylethanol, 2: Lf, Rt, St, Bk, Tw[NT428]
Phenylethyl, 2-iso-valerate: Lf[NT535]
Phorbol myristate acetate: Smoke[NT183]
Phosphatase, acid: Lf[NT409]
Phosphatidic acid: Pl[NT577]
Phthadiene, neo: Lf[NT399]
Phthalate, dibutyl: Lf, Rt, St, Bk, Tw[NT428]
Phthalate, diethyl: Lf, Rt, St, Bk, Tw[NT428]
Phytofuran: Lf[NT399], Rt, St, Bk, Tw[NT428]
Phytol: Lf[NT540]
Phytuberin: Lf[NT446]
Phytuberol, dihydro, 2-α-methoxy: Pl[NT539]
Phytuberol, dihydro, 2-β-methoxy: Pl[NT539]
Phytuberol: Pl[NT539]
Picoline, 2: Cured Lf smoke[NT412]
Picoline, 3: Cured Lf smoke[NT412]
Picoline, α: Lf[NT322]
Picoline, β: Lf[NT322]
Picoline, γ: Lf[NT322]
Piperidin-2-one, N-methyl: Cured Lf smoke[NT543]
Piperidin-2-one: Cured Lf smoke[NT543]
Piperonal: Lf, Rt, St, Bk, Tw[NT428]
Plastohydroquinone 9: Call Tiss[NT411], Rt, Lf[NT379]
Plastoquinone 9: Call Tiss[NT411], Rt, Lf[NT379]
Polysaccharide(pectic): Pl 0.078%[NT504]
Proline: Call Tiss[NT392]
Propan-2-ol, 2-(1-methyl-4-iso-propyl-7-8-dioxa-bicyclo-(3.2.1)-oct-6-yl), endo: Lf[NT406]
Propionaldehyde: Lf[NT022]
Propionamide: Cured Lf smoke[NT543]
Propionic acid: Lf[NT440], An[NT391]
Propionitrile: Lx (St)[NT376]
Protein (fraction I): Lf[NT545]
Protein (*Nicotiana tabacum*): Pl[NT474]
Protein PR-R: Lf[NT523]
Protein: Stem pith[NT384], Call Tiss[NT394]
Putrescine, caffeoyl: Pl[NT562]
Putrescine, feruloyl: Pl[NT562]
Putrescine, N-methyl: Pl[NT562]
Putrescine, para-coumaroyl: Pl[NT562]
Putrescine: Pl[NT562]
Pyrazine, 2-3-dimethyl: Cured Lf[NT472]
Pyrazine, 2-5-dimethyl: Cured Lf[NT472]
Pyrazine, 2-ethyl-6-methyl: Cured Lf[NT472]
Pyrazine, 2-methyl: Cured Lf smoke[NT412]
Pyrazine, butyl: Cured Lf smoke[NT543]
Pyrazine, ethyl: Cured Lf smoke[NT543]
Pyrazine, methyl: Cured Lf[NT472]
Pyrazine, pentyl: Cured Lf smoke[NT543]

Pyrazine, propyl: Cured Lf smoke[NT543]
Pyrazine, triethyl: Cured Lf[NT472]
Pyrene: Lf smoke 6.8 mg/100 Cig[NT434]
Pyrene: Smoke[NT183]
Pyrid-2-(1-H)-one, 5-6-dihydro: cured Lf[NT472]
Pyridine, 2(14), 5-6-dihydro: Lf 37[NT498]
Pyridine, 2-acetyl: Cured Lf smoke[NT543]
Pyridine, 2-ethyl: Cured Lf[NT472]
Pyridine, 3-(dimethyl-pyrryl): Cured Lf[NT472]
Pyridine, 3-acetyl: Cured Lf smoke[NT543]
Pyridine, 3-aldehyde: Cured Lf[NT472]
Pyridine, 3-cyano: Cured Lf smoke[NT543]
Pyridine, 3-cyano: Cured Lf[NT472]
Pyridine, 3-ethyl: Lf[NT322]
Pyridine, 3-hydroxy: Cured Lf[NT472]
Pyridine, 3-vinyl: Lf[NT322], Cured Lf smoke[NT543]
Pyridine, butenyl: Cured Lf smoke[NT543]
Pyridine, phenyl-3: Cured Lf[NT472]
Pyridine, propenyl: Cured Lf smoke[NT543]
Pyridine: Lf[NT322], Cured Lf[NT412], Cured Lf smoke[NT543]
Pyridyl, 2-3'-bi: Cured Lf smoke[NT543]
Pyridyl, 2-3'-di: Lf[NT322]
Pyridyl, 2-4'-di: Lf[NT502]
Pyridyl, 3-3'-di: Lf[NT502]
Pyridyl, 4-4'-di: Lf[NT502]
Pyrindin-7-one, 3-6-6-trimethyl-5-6-dihydro-7-(H)-2: Lf[NT369]
Pyrogallol: Smoke[NT183]
Pyrrole, 1-acetic acid, 2-formyl-5-ethoxy-methyl): Lf 36[NT498]
Pyrrole, 1-methyl: Lx (St)[NT376]
Pyrrole, 2-acetyl: Cured Lf[NT472]
Pyrrole, N-methyl-2-acetyl: Lf, Rt, St, Bk, Tw[NT428]
Pyrrole: Cured Lf[NT472]
Pyrrolid-2-one, N-methyl: Cured Lf smoke[NT543]
Pyrrolid-2-one: Cured Lf smoke[NT543]
Pyrrolidine, N-nitroso: Lf[NT599]
Pyrrolidinyl-β-D-fructopyranose, 1-deoxy-1-(S)-2-(3-pyridyl)-1: Lf[NT555]
Quercetin: Lf[NT591]
Quercetin: Smoke[NT183]
Quercitrin, iso: Cured Lf[NT410], Lf 50[NT484]
Quinolin-9-one, iso, 1-3-6-6-tetramethyl-5-6-7-8-tetrahydro: Lf[NT369]
Quinoline, iso: Cured Lf[NT472]
Quinoline: Cured Lf[NT472]
Raffinose: Sd[NT515]
Resorcinol: Smoke[NT183]

Ribonuclease, deoxy: Pl[NT576]
Ribonuclease: Pl[NT576]
Rishitin: Lf[NT565]
Rishitin-3-O-(α-L-rhamnopyranosyl(1-4)-β-D-glucopyranosyl(1-4)-β-D-glucopyranoside): Lf 2.2[NT625]
Rishitin-β-sophoroside: Lf[NT573]
Rutin: Lf 25-9700[NT484, NT615]
Saccharopine, L: Lf 0.67[NT489]
Salicylate, iso-amyl: Lf, Rt, St, Bk, Tw[NT428]
Scopoletin: Lf[NT401]
Scopolin: Lf[NT401], Pl[NT562]
Serine, O-acetyl: Pl[NT471]
Serine: Sd[NT515]
Sitosterol acyl glycoside: Lf[NT368]
Sitosterol ester: Lf[NT368]
Sitosterol glycoside: Lf[NT368]
Sitosterol, β: Lf[NT368], Pl[NT424], Sd oil[NT491]
Skatole: Cured Lf[NT472]
Solanadione, nor: Lf, Rt, St, Bk, Tw[NT428]
Solanascone, 10-β-hydroxy, β-D-glucoside: Lf 6.8[NT340]
Solanascone, 13-hydroxy, β-D-glucopyranoside: Lf 0.6[NT331]
Solanascone, 15-hydroxy, β-D-glucopyranoside: Lf 0.4[NT331]
Solanascone, 15-hydroxy, β-D-glucoside: Lf 12.3[NT462]
Solanascone, 2-3-dehydro: Lf[NT565]
Solanascone, 3-hydroxy, β-sophoroside: Lf 5.7[NT496]
Solanascone, 3-hydroxy-β-sophoside: Lf[NT568]
Solanascone, 9-β-D-glucoside: Lf 1.2[NT340]
Solanascone: Lf[NT528]
Solanascone: Lf[NT565]
Solanascone-3-O-β-sophoroside: Lf 10[NT625]
Solanesol: Cured Lf[NT475], Lf 0.74%[NT560]
Solanofuran: Lf, Rt, St, Bk, Tw[NT428]
Solanol: Lf, Rt, St, Bk, Tw[NT428]
Solanone: Lf, Rt, St, Bk, Tw[NT428]
Solanoquinone: Lf[NT626]
Solavetinon-3-O-β-D-glucoside: Lf 9.3[NT625]
Solavetinone, (−): Cured Lf[NT477]
Solavetinone, 13-hydroxy: Cured Lf[NT477]
Solavetinone, 3-hydroxy: Lf[NT568]
Solavetinone, 9-β-hydroxy: Cured Lf[NT477]
Solavetinone: Cured Lf[NT488], Lf[N1657]
Solavetinone: Lf 0.03[NT488]
Solavetivone: Cured Lf[NT488]
Spiloxabovolide: Lf, Rt, St, Bk, Tw[NT428]
Squalene: Lf[NT540]
Squalene: Smoke[NT183]

Squalene-2-3-oxide: Seedling, Lf[NT325]
Stachyose: Sd[NT515]
Starch: Call Tiss[NT394]
Stearic acid: Sd oil[NT400], Lf[NT540], Cured Lf[NT544]
Stigmast-7-en-3-β-ol: Sd[NT515]
Stigmastal-2-3-dien-ol: Sd[NT515]
Stigmastenol, δ-7: Sd[NT515]
Stigmasterol acyl glycoside: Lf[NT368]
Stigmasterol ester: Lf[NT368]
Stigmasterol glycoside: Lf[NT368]
Stigmasterol: Lf[NT368], Pl[NT424], Call Tiss[NT382], Sd oil[NT491], Lf[NT540]
Styrene: Lx (St)[NT376]
Succinamopine antibiotic: Crown Gall Tumor Tiss[NT492]
Succinic acid: Cured Lf[NT544]
Succinimide, *trans*-2-ethylidene-3-methyl: Lf 5[NT498]
Sucrose, 6-O-acetyl-2-3-4-tri-O-(3S-methyl-pentanoyl): Fl[NT501]
Sucrose: Sd[NT515]
Sulfurylase, ATP: Pl[NT418]
Syringone, aceto, α-hydroxy: Rt[NT519]
Syringone, aceto: Rt[NT519]
Terpineol, α: Lf, Rt, St, Bk, Tw[NT428]
Tetradecane: Smoke[NT183]
Theaspirone, 8-9-dehydro: Lf EO[NT556]
Threonine: Sd[NT515]
Thunberga-*trans*-2-*trans*-6-diene-4-11-diol, 8-12-epoxy, (1S-4S-8R-11S-12R): Cured Lf[NT429]
Thunberga-*trans*-2-*trans*-6-diene-4-12-diol, 8-11-epoxy, (1S-4R-8R-11S-12R): Lf 0.016[NT536]
Thunberga-*trans*-2-*trans*-6-diene-4-12-diol, 8-11-epoxy, (1S-4S-6R-11S-12R): Lf[NT536]
Thymol: Lf, Rt, St, Bk, Tw[NT428]
Tobacco F-1 protein: Lf[NT542]
Tobacco glycoprotein: Cured Lf[NT163]
Tobacco saponin A: Sd[NT610]
Tobacco saponin B: Sd[NT610]
Tocopherol, α: Lf[NT540], Call Tiss[NT411], Rt[NT379]
Tocoquinone, α: Call Tiss[NT411], Lf, Rt[NT379]
Toluene: Lx (St)[NT376]
Transferase, amino, alanine: Call Tiss[NT366]
Trichodiene, 15-hydroxy: Pl 0.2[NT355]
Trideca-5-10-12-trien-2-one, (E)-6-12-dim-ethyl-9-iso-propyl: Lf[NT372]
Tridecan-2-one: Lf[NT535]
Trideca-*trans*-3-*trans*-7-diene-2-12-dione, 6-hydroxy-9-iso-propyl-6-methyl: Fl 0.04[NT514]

Tyramine: Lf[NT520]
Tyrosine: Sd[NT515]
Ubelliferone: Pl[NT627]
Ubiquinone 10: Call Tiss 0.0075[NT427], Pl 360[NT426]
Undec-5-en-4-olide, (E)-4-methyl-7-iso-pro-pyl-10-oxo: Lf[NT372]
Undeca-2-one, 6-10-dimethyl: Lf, Rt, St, Bk, Tw[NT428]
Undeca-3-*trans*-6-dien-2-ol, 2-6-dimethyl-10-oxo: Lf[NT476]
Undeca-5-9-dien-2-one, 6-19-dimethyl: Lf, Rt, St, Bk, Tw[NT428]
Undecane: Smoke[NT183]
Undecen-4-olide, 5-(E), 7(S)-10-oxo-4: Lf[NT375]
Undec-*trans*-5-en-10-one, 1-4-epoxy-2(R)-hydroxy-7-iso-propyl-4(R)-methyl: Lf[NT348]
Undec-*trans*-5-en-10-one, 1-4-epoxy-2(R)-hydroxy-7-iso-propyl-4(S)-methyl: Lf[NT348]
Undec-*trans*-5-en-4-olide, 2(R)-hydroxy-7(S)-iso-propyl-4(S)-methyl-10-oxo: Lf[NT348]
Undec-*trans*-5-ene, 2-10-dihydroxy-1-4-epoxy-7-iso-propyl-4-methyl: Lf[NT537]
Undec-*trans*-5-ene, 2-10-dione, 4-hydroxy-7-iso-propyl-4-methyl: Lf 0.005[NT514]
Undec-*trans*-5-ene, epi, 2-10-dihydroxy-1-4-epoxy-7-iso-propyl-4-methyl: Lf[NT537]
Valeric acid, β-methyl: Lf[NT440]
Valeric acid, iso: Lf[NT440]
Valeric acid: Lf[NT440], An[NT391]
Valine: Sd[NT515]
Vanillin: Lf 1.51[NT450]
Vetivone, β, 11-12-dihydroxy: Cured Lf[NT477]
Violaxanthin: Lf[NT363]
Virg-3-ene, 18-oxo: Fl[NT334]
Vitamin K-1: Call Tiss[NT411], Rt, Lf[NT379]
Xylenol, 2-3: Lf[NT327]
Xylenol, 2-4: Lf[NT327]
Xylenol, 2-5: Lf[NT327]
Xylenol, 2-6: Lf[NT327]
Xylenol, 3-5: Lf[NT327]
Zeaxanthin: Lf[NT363]

PHARMACOLOGICAL ACTIVITIES AND CLINICAL TRIALS

8-Oxodeoxyguanosine level increase.
Nitrosamine 4-(methylnitrosamino)-1-(3-pyridyl)-1-butanone, administered intragastrically to A/J mice at doses 0.25 or 0.5 mg/mouse, three times a week for 3 weeks, produced a significant elevation of 8-oxodeoxyguanosine in lung DNA 2 hours after the last administration. A single-dose treatment (4 mg/mouse) produced an insignificant increase of lesion in the lung DNA. In the liver, the increase was only significant by multiple doses of the higher dose. At 4 and 24 hours after treatment, the 8-oxodeoxyguanosine levels declined to the basal levels in both liver and lung. Administration of a single dose (20 mg/animal) to F344 rats, produced a significant increase of 8-oxodeoxyguanosine in rat lung DNA and an insignificant increase in liver DNA. The 8-oxodeoxyguanosine level in rat kidney, a nontarget tissue, was inert to nitrosamine treatment[NT090].

Abortifacient effect.
The smoke of the dried leaf by pregnant women was active[NT486].

Acetylhydrolase activity.
Smoke extract, administered to rats at a dose of 0.5 cigarettes/kg for 5 days, did not alter plasma platelet-activating factor acetylhydrolase activity during the treatment. Combination of smoke extract and 17-α-ethynylestradiol decreased plasma platelet-activating factor acetylhydrolase activity by 90%. The effect of medroxyprogesterone on plasma platelet-activating factor acetylhydrolase activity was not influenced by smoke extract[NT267]. Administration of an increasing concentrations of extract to confluent cultures of collagen-producing mouse fibroblasts or primary osteoblasts from chick embryo calvarias, produced no effect on glycolysis and DNA synthesis. There was no influence on cell proliferation in fibroblasts, but it was inhibited at the highest extract concentration in osteoblasts. Adenosine triphosphatase (ATPase) activity was not detectable in fibroblast medium but was decreased in osteoblast medium. At the highest concentration, [³H]hydroxyproline and [³H]proline contents in the cell layers were decreased to the following respective values:

fibroblasts 56% and 45% and osteoblasts 50% and 29%, respectively. When incubation with smokeless tobacco (STE) was discontinued for 1 day, recovery did not occur[NT094].

Age-related alterations. Smoke, administered to old CBA/CA mice, produced spontaneous death more frequently than in the control animals. Prevalence of hepatocellular carcinoma was higher and body weight was lower in the smoke-treated mice than in controls. There were differences in organ indices. The reactivity against sheep erythrocytes antigen was lower in mice kept in smoke than in controls. The ratio of normal reactivity (against sheep erythrocytes) and autoreactivity (against mouse erythrocytes) showed a decrease in the smoke-treated mice[NT108].

Airspace permeability increase. Cigarette smoke condensate in rat lungs produced a 59.7% increase in epithelial permeability over control values, peaking 6 hours after instillation and returning to control values by 24 hours. Instillation of human recombinant tumor necrosis factor (TNF)-α produced an increase in epithelial permeability in the rat lung. Only a vestigial amount of TNF-α was detected in bronchoalveolar lavage fluid in vivo or in culture medium from bronchoalveolar lavage leucocytes from smoke-treated animals. Anti-TNF antibody did not abolish the increased epithelial permeability produced by cigarette smoke condensate. One hour after instillation of cigarette smoke condensate there was a marked decrease in the reduced glutathione content in the lung in association with increased oxidized glutathione levels. Reduced glutathione levels in bronchoalveolar lavage fluid decreased following cigarette smoke condensate[NT264].

Aldosterone synthesis inhibition. Nicotine, anabasine, and cotinine, in freshly isolated rat adrenal cells at concentrations up to 100 mM, did not inhibit stimulated corticosterone production but inhibited aldosterone production in a dose-dependent manner. The relative inhibitory potency was: cotinine > anabasine > nicotine. Cotinine, anabasine, and nicotine, at a concentration of 100 mM, inhibited adrenocorticotropic hormone (ACTH)-stimulated aldosterone synthesis by 75, 44, and 21%, respectively. Angiotensin (ANG)-II-stimulated aldosterone synthesis was inhibited by 92, 78, and 62%, respectively. The plasma cotinine concentration range attained in tobacco smokers was between 1 and 10 mM. When tested with [^{3}H]corticosterone and [^{3}H]progesterone as exogenous substrates, 1–10 mM cotinine produced a significant dose-dependent inhibition of ACTH- and ANG-II-stimulated aldosterone synthesis[NT276].

Allergenic activity. Cigarette smoke condensate, in cell culture at concentrations of 6.6–20 μg/mL, produced an inhibition of cell surface antigen-presenting major histocompatibility complex class I expression and immunoglobulin (Ig) synthesis. Intraperitoneal administration to C57BL/6 mice before challenge with ovalbumin antigen produced a decrease of antiovalbumin-specific antibody response. This inhibition affected Ig protein synthesis then membrane bound major histocompatibility complex class I expression. Supplementation with selenium significantly reduced the inhibitory effects[NT004]. IgE antibodies against crude tobacco leaf were present in smokers, nonsmokers, and ex-smokers, and the atopic individuals were far more likely to show such responses than nonatopic individuals. It has also been established that IgE antibodies can be detected against at least three specific tobacco leaf allergens, namely crossed immunoelectrophoresis (CIE) antigens 19, 23, and 30, but these IgE antibodies did not correlate with any type of clinical smoke sensitivity. There is no concrete evidence for the presence of IgE antibodies in man against smoke extract. There is preliminary evidence that smoke challenge under controlled conditions in an environmental chamber does not induce significant decreases in forced expiratory volume in 1 second (FEV1) or peak flow in smoke-sensitive subjects, even though they complain of symptoms. Tobacco leaf was immunogenic in rabbits, but it is not known if any tobacco incineration products *per se* are immunogenic in man[NT143]. Tobacco glycoprotein from the cured leaf, administered intradermally by three injections to mice, produced a long-lasting IgE antibody response. No hemagglutinating antibodies were produced[NT163]. Smoke from Kentucky Reference IRI cigarettes, administered in a Prototype Mark II Walton Horizontal Smoke Exposure Machine to Balb/c mice within 24 hours after birth for up to 10 weeks, produced no difference in the magnitude of the splenic plaque-forming cells response in smoke-exposed and untreated control animals immunized with sheep red blood cells on sequential days up to day 9 postpartum. On day 10, the plaque-forming cells' response of smoke-exposed mice was reduced by 33%, on day 14, there was a 60% reduction, whereas animals exposed to smoke from 4 to 10 weeks showed a 90% reduction of the splenic plaque-forming cells response[NT175]. Tobacco smoke, administered to normal CFW mice, produced a significantly increased susceptibility to the lethal effects of histamine. The lethal dose $(LD)_{50}$ for mice subjected to smoke was 45 mg/kg of histamine, whereas in normal CFW mice the LD_{50} was 1.1 g/kg. The histamine susceptibility of smoked mice was markedly diminished by injecting the animals with isoproterenol. Normal CFW mice and sham control mice exhibited an epinephrine-induced hyperglycemia, whereas the blood glucose values for smoked mice given epinephrine were similar to those for sham mice given only saline. Results indicated that tobacco smoke can contain a

component that causes an autonomic imbalance, hence rendering the mice more susceptible to histamine[NT185]. Tobacco leaf extract, administered to CFW female mice with developed type 1 skin and mast cell sensitivities, produced IgG1- and IgE-tobacco-mast-cell-sensitizing antibodies detected by 2 and 48 hours after immunization[NT186].

Alveolar macrophages fluorescence. Cigarette smoke, administered to rats at a dose of two cigarettes for 1 or 5 days, produced an increased fluorescence after 1 day of exposure and enhanced after 5 consecutive days. Larger and more granular/complex alveolar macrophages were more fluorescent than smaller and less granular/complex cells. Smoke-exposed rats (5 days of exposure) lavaged immediately after the exposure had less cells in their bronchoalveolar lavage fluid than control animals. Rats lavaged 3 smoke-free days after the exposure, produced an increase in cell recovery, probably resulting from to less airway obstruction[NT283].

Analgesic activity. Nicotine or tobacco smoke, administered to male Sprague–Dawley rats, produced analgesia measured by tail-flick latencies. A second treatment, 24 hours after the first, failed to produce analgesia, thereby demonstrating the rapid development of tolerance. The restraint, which was a necessary part of the tobacco smoke exposure, also produced analgesia, although of a more transient nature and lesser magnitude than that resulting from tobacco smoke exposure. Tolerance also developed to restraint stress-induced analgesia. The long-term (43 weeks) daily exposure of rats to tobacco smoke or restraint stress resulted in the development of cross-tolerance. Long-term tobacco smoke exposure resulted in increased tail-flick latency when the animals had been withdrawn from tobacco smoke for 24 hours[NT298].

Anesthetic activity. Nicotine, administered to mice, increased the latent time of biting the clip in the tail press test ($p <$

0.001) and retarded tail withdrawal latency in the tail immersion test ($p < 0.01$), compared to controls[NT081].

Angiogenesis inhibition. Cigarette smoke or smoke extract, administered to ulcerated rats once daily for 3 days, produced concomitant and dose-dependent reduction of angiogenesis and constitutive nitric oxide synthase activity[NT232].

Antibacterial activity. Tincture of the dried leaf (10 g plant material in 100 mL ethanol), on agar plate at a concentration of 30.0 µL/disc, was inactive on *Escherichia coli*, *Pseudomonas aeruginosa*, and *Staphylococcus aureus*[NT607]. Methanol extract of the dried leaf, on agar plate at a concentration of 25 mg/mL, was active on *Bacillus subtilis*, *Corynebacterium pyogenes*, *Pseudomonas aeruginosa*, *Serratia marcescens*, *Shigella dysenteriae*, and *Staphylococcus aureus* and inactive on *Escherichia coli*, *Klebsiella pneumoniae*, and *Proteus vulgaris*[NT482]. Smoke condensate, in murine alveolar macrophage cell line (MH-S) cells, significantly enhanced the replication of *Legionella pneumophila* in macrophages and selectively downregulated the production of interleukin (IL)-6 and TNF-α induced by bacterial infection[NT027].

Anti-convulsant activity. Methanol (50%) extract of the dried leaf, administered to mice, was active vs leptazol-induced convulsions[NT591]. Ethanol (70%) extract of the fresh leaf, administered intraperitoneally to mice of both sexes at variable doses, was active vs metrazole- and strychnine-induced convulsions[NT580].

Anti-estrogenic effect. Aqueous extract of the dried leaf smoke, administered to female adults at a concentration of 25.0 µL/plate, was active on granulosa cells. Results significant at $p < 0.001$ level[NT595].

Antifungal activity. Hot water extract of the dried leaf, in broth culture, was inactive on *Epidermophyton floccosum*, *Microsporum canis*, *Trichophyton mentagrophytes* var. *algondonosa*, and *Trichophyton mentagro-phytes* var. *granulare*[NT516]. Undiluted methanol extract of the fresh leaf, on agar plate, was active on *Aspergillus fumigatus*[NT604]. Saponin solution of the fresh seed, administered to infected plants, was active on *Puccinia recondita*[NT610].

Antiglaucomic activity. Water extract of the callus tissue, administered intravenously to rabbits at a dose of 250 µg/animal, produced a 55% drop in intraocular pressure[NT443].

Antioxidant activity. Smoke, administered by inhalation to mice for 10 weeks, produced an increase of catalase, glutathione peroxidase and glutathione reductase activity. The activity of superoxide dismutase was unaltered[NT019]. Administration to DBA/2, C57BL/6J, and ICR mice at a dose of 3 cigarettes/day 5 days/week for 7 months, produced a decrease in the antioxidant defense of bronchoalveolar lavage fluids in the DBA/2 and C57BL/6J strains and an increase in ICR mice. Lung elastin content was significantly decreased in DBA/2 and C57BL/6J mice but not in ICR mice. Emphysema was present in DBA/2 and C57BL/6J but not in ICR mice. When administered to pallid mice with a severe serum α(1)-proteinase inhibitor (α[1]-PI) deficiency for 4 months, there was an acceleration of the development of the spontaneous emphysema assessed with morphometrical and biochemical (lung elastin content) methods[NT034]. Rutin and chlorogenic acid from STE leaf extract, in murine mast cell culture, reduced reactive oxygen species levels and inhibited histamine release in antigen-IgE-activated cells. They augmented the inducible cytokine messages, i.e., IL-10, IL-13, interferon (IFN)-γ, IL-6, and TNF-α in IgE-sensitized mast cells after antigen challenge. Results indicated that tobacco polyphenolic antioxidants differentially affected two effector functions of antigen-IgE-activated mast cells[NT042]. Cigarette smoke, administered to Sprague–Dawley rats for 2 hours/day for 4 weeks, enhanced N-methyl-

D-aspartate receptor (NMDAR) subunits 2A and 2B concentrations in the hippocampus. Lipid peroxidation and antioxidant enzyme activities did not show any change. The results indicated that cigarette smoke induces NMDAR 2A and 2B expression in the hippocampus not because of an increased lipid peroxidation but because cigarette smoke has no effect on lipid peroxidation and antioxidant enzyme activities in the hippocampus[NT199]. Tobacco smoke, administered to rats for 2 days or 8 weeks (6 hours/day, 3 days/week), significantly increased the number of cells recovered by bronchoalveolar lavage (BAL). Manganese(III)meso-tetrakis(N,N'-diethyl-1,3-imidazolium-2-yl) porphyrin 10150 significantly decreased BAL cell number in tobacco smoke-treated rats. Squamous cell metaplasia, following 8 weeks of tobacco smoke exposure, was 12% of the total airway epithelial area in animals exposed to tobacco smoke without AEOL 10150, compared with 2% in animals exposed to tobacco smoke, but treated with AEOL 10150 ($p < 0.05$)[NT201]. Cigarette smoke, administered to albino rats for 30 minutes/day for 30 days, increased the lipid peroxide levels in liver, lung, and kidney of smoke-treated rats. No changes were found in the brain and heart. The activity of the antioxidant enzymes was also elevated in the livers, lungs, and kidneys of the test animals. Brain and heart did not show any change in the activities of all of these antioxidant enzymes, except an increase of glutathione-S-transferase in brain. The level of reduced glutathione was lowered in the livers, lungs, and kidneys of the test animals when compared to controls. There were no significant changes in brain and heart[NT220]. Whole cigarette smoke, administered to rats daily for 1, 2, 7, or 14 days, increased expression of manganese superoxide dismutase, glutathione peroxidase, and metallothionein. Copper–zinc superoxide dismutase and catalase expression did not change from control levels. The distribution of manganese superoxide dismutase expression was similar in control and smoke-exposed animals. Catalase, copper–zinc superoxide dismutase, glutathione peroxidase, and metallothionein showed widespread expression in the lung by in situ hybridization. Copper–zinc superoxide dismutase, glutathione peroxidase, and metallothionein were highly expressed in bronchial epithelium. Catalase expression levels were similar in all cell types. Results indicated that most of these antioxidant enzymes and scavengers showed prominent bronchial expression but that manganese superoxide dismutase showed a unique pattern, with intense hot spots in the epithelium of the small airways[NT249]. Water-soluble substances in cigarette smoke in nerve terminals prepared from the rat cerebral cortex, significantly reduced the spontaneous increase in thiobarbituric acid-reactive substances in synaptosomes in a dilution factor-dependent manner. The aqueous extract also inhibited the elevation of lipid peroxidation induced by 2,2'-azobis (2-amidinopropane) dihydrochloride, a peroxyl radical generator. Smoke substances scavenged superoxide radicals generated from stimulated human leukocytes and from the xanthine/xanthine oxidase system. These effects were not mimicked by nicotine. The antioxidant effects of smoke substances were preserved for several days at 5°C or –80°C[NT252]. Cigarette smoke, administered to rats for 3 months, decreased activities of glutathione reductase, catalase, and brush-border enzyme γ-glutamyl transpeptidase and the levels of glutathione in the kidney. The activities of glutathione peroxidase and lipid peroxide levels were increased. Urinary excretion of γ-glutamyl transpeptidase, glutathione, and lipid peroxide were also higher[NT263].

Antistress effect. Smoke of the dried leaf, administered to rats at variable doses, produced equivocal activity. Smoke, administered to C57B1/6 and Balb/c mice, and MNRA and MR rats in a chamber for 19 days, produced no emotional-stress reaction. A difference in the free preference of space containing tobacco smoke was observed among inbred animals with active and passive emotional-stress reaction phenotypes[NT043].

Antiviral activity. Leaf, on agar plate at a concentration of 2%, was active on herpes simplex 1 virus and reduced plague formation in monkey kidney cells. Undiluted leaves produced strong activity on Coxsackie B5 virus, herpes simplex 1 virus, and measles virus. Viral reproduction was inhibited[NT574]

Anti-yeast activity. Tincture of the dried leaf (10 g plant material in 100 mL ethanol), on agar plate at a concentration of 30 μL/disc, was inactive on *Candida albicans*[NT607].

Apoptosis. Smoke extract, in rat lung alveolar L2 cells, induced apoptotic cell death. A concentration of 0.25% resulted in a 50% increase of caspase-3 and matrix metalloproteinase activities[NT191]. Chloroform extract of the cigarette smoke, in a human gastric epithelial cell line (AGS) for 5 hours, induced apoptosis in a dose- and time-dependent manner in AGS cells and a decrease of bcl-2 and an increase of caspase-3 activity. Pretreatment with Z-DEVD-FMK (specific inhibitor of caspase-3) dose-dependently blocked the DNA fragmentation induced by the chloroform extract. Chloroform extract time- and dose-dependently increased the level of cytochrome C in the cytoplasm, which might activate caspase-3. The ethanol extract was not active[NT197]. Mainstream cigarette smoke, administered to Sprague–Dawley rats for 18 or 100 days, produced a significant and time-dependent increase in the proportion of apoptotic cells in the bronchial and bronchiolar epithelium. Oral *N*-acetylcysteine did not affect the background frequency of apoptosis but significantly decreased smoke-induced apoptosis. A mixture of sidestream and mainstream smoke, administered to Sprague–Dawley rats for 28 days, produced a more than 10-fold increase in the frequency of pulmonary alveolar macrophages undergoing apoptosis. Exposure to smoke produced an acute increase of cells positive for proliferating cell nuclear antigen[NT213]. Cigarette smoke, administered to rats at concentrations of 2 and 4% for 1 hour daily for 1, 3, 6, and 9 days, produced a time- and concentration-dependent increase in apoptosis in the rat gastric mucosa. The effect was accompanied by an increase in xanthine oxidase activity. The increased apoptosis and xanthine oxidase activity could be detected after even a single exposure. In contrast, the p53 level was elevated only in the later stage of cigarette smoke exposure. The apoptotic effect could be blocked by pretreatment with xanthine oxidase inhibitor (allopurinol, 20 mg/kg intraperitoneally) or a hydroxyl free radical scavenger (dimethyl sulfoxide [DMSO], 0.2%, 1 mL/kg intravenously). Neither of these treatments had any effect on the p53 level of the mucosa[NT221].

Aromatase inhibition. Aqueous extract of cigarette smoke, administered to female adults at a concentration of 25 μL/plate, was active on granulosa cells[NT595]. Synthesis and testing of a series of acylated nornicotines and anabasines for their ability to inhibit aromatase showed an interesting correlation of activity with the length of the acyl carbon chain, with maximum activity at C-11. The acylated derivatives showed activity, which was significantly greater than that of nicotine and anabasine. In vivo studies in rats indicated that administration of this inhibitor delayed the onset of nitrosomethyurea (NMU)-induced breast carcinoma and altered the estrous cycle by suppression of the aromatase enzyme system. Toxicity studies indicated relatively low toxicity with LD_{50} for *N-N*-octanoylnornicotine at 367 mg/kg body weight[NT294].

Arrhythmogenic effect. Water extract of the dried leaf, administered intravenously to cats at doses of 10–20 mg/kg, produced weak activity[NT588].

Arterial endothelial injury. Environmental smoke, administered to ovariectomized rats treated with subcutaneous placebo or 17-β-estradiol pellets for 6 weeks, produced a more than fourfold increase of carotid artery low-density lipoprotein (LDL) accumulation compared with filtered air exposure. The effect was largely mediated by increased permeability. No protective effect of estradiol was observed. Acute smoke exposure of a buffer solution containing LDL produced a more than sixfold increase in the highly reactive carbonyl glyoxal. Perfusion of this solution through carotid arteries produced 105% increase in permeability. Perfusion of glyoxal alone produced a 50% increase in carotid artery permeability[NT202].

Aryl hydrocarbon hydroxylase induction. Smoke of cured leaf, administered by inhalation to mice and rats at an undiluted concentration, produced an induction in lungs and kidneys. There was no induction in bowels and liver[NT403].

Atherogenic effect. Smoke, administered by inhalation to mice for 10 weeks, produced an increase of lipid peroxidation and a decrease of reduced glutathione level in the heart. Levels of total cholesterol, LDL cholesterol, and triglycerides were increased. The high-density lipoprotein (HDL) cholesterol levels decreased in serum[NT019].

Bacterial colonization of lower respiratory tract. Cigarette smoke, administered for 3 days before and after intratracheal instillation of bacterial suspension containing six bacterial species (*Staphylococcus aureus*, *Staphylococcus epidermidis*, *Streptococcus pneumonia*, *Proteus mirabilis*, *Haemophilus influenza*, *Peptostreptococcus* spp.) to male Wistar albino rats with or without vitamin E supplements (100 mg/kg/day), significantly increased the colony numbers of all isolated bacteria species in smoke-treated rats than in the control group and in the smoke- and vitamin E-supplemented rats ($p < 0.05$). Only *Staphylococcus aureus* and *Staphylococcus epidermidis* were isolated from vitamin E-supplemented rats[NT234].

Behavioral changes. Nicotine, administered to rats for 7 days, significantly increased rat locomotion activity. This sensitization to nicotine was blocked by mecamylamine (1 mg/kg) and by the administration of 6 mg/kg of the following cembranoids: eunicin, eupalmerin acetate (EUAC), and (4R)-2,7,11-cembratriene-4-6-diol (4R). None of these compounds modified locomotor activity of nonsensitized rats[NT210]. Nicotine, administered by continuous infusion to adolescent rats on postnatal days 30 to 47.5, using a dosage regimen that maintains plasma levels similar to those found in smokers or in users of the transdermal nicotine patch, produced a decrease of grooming in female rats on 44 day of administration, an effect not seen in males. This effect is opposite to the effects of nicotine in adult rats. Two weeks after cessation of nicotine administration, females showed deficits in locomotor activity and rearing. The males again were unaffected. The behavioral deficits appeared at the same age at which gender-selective brain cell damage emerges. Nicotine exposure enhanced passive avoidance, with the effect intensifying and persisting throughout the posttreatment period[NT216]. Smokeless tobacco extract (STD), administered by gavage to pregnant Sprague–Dawley rats on gestational days 6–20 at doses equivalent to 1.33 (STD-1), 4 (STD-2), and 6 mg nicotine/kg (STD-3) three times daily, reduced maternal weight gain at the 2 higher doses. During the preweaning period, significant pup weight reductions were noted in the STD-2 pups until postnatal day 6 and in the STD-3 group until postnatal day 15. In the

STD-1 group, no statistically significant weight reduction was noted. The incidence of deaths was increased in a dose-related manner. No significant differences were noted for pinna detachment and incisor eruption. Smoke treatment significantly affected earlier eye opening and vaginal patency. No significant effects were seen on negative geotaxis, but for surface righting, a decreased success rate was noted. Open field activity increased from the preweaning to postweaning periods. During the preweaning period, the STD-3 offsprings were more active, and during postweaning, the STD-1 offsprings were more active. No difference was noted in vertical activity or in the number of stereotypical movements. No treatment-related difference was noted in the active avoidance shuttle box[NT277].

Benzo(a)pyrene hydroxylase induction. Masheri, a pyrolyzed tobacco product, administered orally to Swiss mice, Sprague–Dawley rats, and Syrian golden hamsters at a dose of 10% diet for 20 months, produced a significant induction of cytochrome P450 and benzo(a)pyrene hydroxylase in proximal and distal parts of the three species[NT100].

Benzopyrene hydroxylase induction. Methyl chloride extract of the leaf, administered intragastrically to rats at a dose of 3 mg/animal daily for 21 months in DMSO solvent, was active. The rats were divided into two groups. One was fed a vitamin A diet, and the other was fed a vitamin A-deficient diet. Treatment with the extract increased pulmonary and hepatic benzopyrene hydroxylase level over controls in both groups. The vitamin A-deficient group had significantly higher hepatic and lower pulmonary levels when compared to the vitamin-fed group[NT519].

Benzphetamine demethylase stimulation. Methyl chloride extract of the leaf, administered intragastrically to rats at a dose of 3 mg/animal daily for 21 months in DMSO solvent, was active. The rats were divided into two groups. One was fed a vitamin A diet, and the other was fed a vitamin A-deficient diet. In the vitamin-deficient group, treatment with the extract increased benzphetamine demethylase level vs control[NT519].

Biochemical effect. Tobacco smoke was administered by inhalation in Hamburg II machine to senescence accelerated SAM-P/8 and SAM-R/1 mice 10 minutes/day, 5 days/week for 5 weeks. The treatment increased lung weight and the ratio of albumin to total protein in the bronchoalveolar lavage fluid, a decrease elastase inhibitory capacity/trypsin inhibitory capacity in bronchoalveolar lavage fluid, and a decrease in the glutathione (GSH) content and the GSH/sulfhydryl (SH) ratio of the lung, compared with those not exposed. There was focal infiltration of macrophages into alveoli with hyaline membrane and thickened alveolar wall in SAM-P/8 with tobacco exposure[NT110].

Birth-weight effect. Cigarette smoke, administered to pregnant rats daily for a 2-hour period throughout gestation, significantly decreased the average birth-weight of pups compared with both pair-fed and *ad libitum* control groups. The body weights of the pups exposed to smoke were no longer significantly different from those in the pair-fed and *ad libitum* control groups at weeks 1 and 2 after birth, respectively. The study indicated that fetal growth retardation caused by exposure to cigarette smoke during pregnancy does not persist after birth[NT273].

Blood pressure effect (biphasic). Water extract of the dried leaf, administered intravenously to cats and rats at doses of 0.1 and 5–20 mg/kg, produced an initial hypotensive effect followed by hypertension[NT588].

Breathing inhibition. Cigarette smoke from low-nicotine research cigarettes and gas phase smoke obtained by passing the smoke through a glass-fiber Cambridge filter was administered to anesthetized Sprague–

Dawley rats at a dose of 6, 50%. Inhalation of gas phase smoke alone evoked a transient inhibitory effect on breathing, prolonging expiratory time (Te) to a peak of 159 ± 6% of the base line. The response was similar to that triggered by inhaling the unfiltered smoke (Te = 177 ± 12%). The bradypnea started within 1–4 breaths after the onset of smoke inhalation, lasted for three to five breaths and was completely abolished by vagotomy. This inhibitory effect of gas phase smoke on breathing was also largely prevented after a pretreatment with either intravenous infusion or aerosol inhalation of a hydroxyl radical scavenger, dimethylthiourea[NT292].

Bronchoconstrictor activity. Inhalation of cured leaf, administered to adults as an undiluted concentration, was active on asthma[NT381].

Bupivacaine kinetics. Smoke, administered by Hamburg II smoking machine to mice for 4 or 8 days, produced no effect after 4 days and a significant increase of metabolism and elimination of bupivacaine in the treated group. The smoke acted at different levels, i.e., metabolism, elimination and binding of bupivacaine, increased the permeability of the cell membranes, and facilitates the penetration of bupivacaine and desbutylbupivacaine in erythrocytes[NT067].

Cadmium-induced alterations. Mainstream smoke generated from University of Kentucky 2R1 reference cigarettes, administered to cadmium-treated young female Long–Evans rats at a dose of 10 puffs daily for 12 weeks, produced no significant changes in lung function or morphometry[NT285].

Carboxyhemoglobin effect. Cigarette smoke was administered by inhalation with a modified Walton horizontal smoke exposure machine to mice at intermittent doses. During the first 30 seconds of each 1-minute cycle, the subjects were exposed to smoke diluted either 1:10 or 1:5 with air. This treatment produced carboxyhemoglobin values significantly higher than those in marijuana smoke-treated mice. Mice exposed to six or eight puffs of tobacco smoke had mean carboxyhemoglobin values of 24.6 and 28.5% saturation, respectively. No acute lethal effects were observed in mice receiving multiple daily episodes of eight puffs per episode of marijuana smoke, whereas mice exposed to a single eight-puff episode of tobacco smoke suffered approx 50% acute lethal effects[NT135].

Carcinogenic activity. Methyl chloride extract of the leaf, administered intragastrically to rats at a dose of 3 mg/animal daily for 21 months in DMSO solvent, was active. The rats were divided into two groups. One was fed a vitamin A diet, and the other was fed a vitamin A-deficient diet. Cumulative tumor incidence in vitamin-deficient rats was significantly greater than that in vitamin-fed rats. Vitamin-deficient rats had a preponderance of pituitary adenomas, whereas vitamin-fed rats showed lung and forestomach tumors[NT519]. Smoke and snuff of the dried leaf, administered to adults at variable doses, were active[NT329]. Forty-one users of STE and 38 cigarette smokers, produced a decrease of total [4-(methylnitrosamino)-1-3-pirydyl)-1-butanone and its glucuronide] in users of STE and smokers. The 1-hydroxypyrene level was unchanged in tobacco smokers and reduced in smokers who used medicinal nicotine (nicotine patch). The overall mean total [4-(methylnitrosamino)-1-3-pirydyl)-1-butanone and its glucuronide] levels among smokers who used the nicotine patch was significantly lower than among smokers who used the OMNI cigarette[NT001]. A mixture of sidestream and mainstream smoke, administered to male A/J mice at concentrations of 99, 120, and 176 mg/m³ of total suspended particulate material for 5 months, produced significantly more lung tumors by the highest smoke concentrations, although response to the high dose was slightly less than response from the medium dose. Lung tumor incidences were in all three groups significantly higher than in controls. Lung displacement volume and plasma cotinine level were increased in a dose-dependent manner[NT006]. Tobacco specific nitrosamines were administered to a line of human papillomavirus-immortalized bronchial epithelial cells at concentrations of 100 or 400 μg/mL for 7 days. The transformed cells produced progressively growing subcutaneous tumors on inoculation into nude mice. Immunofluorescence staining for keratin expression confirmed the epithelial nature of the tumor cells. There was an increased expression of p16, β-catenin and proliferating cell nuclear antigen (PCNA) in the established cell line[NT014]. Smoke, administered to male strain A/J mice at a concentration of 140 mg/m³, 6 hours a day, 5 days/week for 4–5 months, increased plasma β-carotene level and lung tumor multiplicities and incidences but had no significant effect on lung β-carotene levels. β-carotene supplementation failed to modulate tumor development under all exposure conditions[NT026]. Smoke was administered to male strain A/J mice on a diet of Bowman–Birk protease inhibitor concentrate (BBIC) at a concentration of 1% in AIN-93G diet either during smoke exposure, after exposure or for 9 months. The mice were exposed to 89% cigarette sidestream and 11% mainstream smoke 6 hours a day, 5 days/week for 5 months and then allowed to recover for another 4 months in air. As a positive control, the mice were injected with 3-methylcholanthrene and fed a diet containing 1% BBIC. These animals were sacrificed 5 months later. In the animals treated with 3-methylcholanthrene, BBIC decreased lung tumor multiplicities, whereas in the smoke-exposed mice, BBIC did not modulate lung tumor development[NT028]. Aqueous extract of the STE, administered orally to female Sprague–Dawley rats at a dose of 25 mg/kg

for 90 days, produced an accumulation of indistinct filamentous material in the perisinusoidal spaces, disintegration of lipids, and a significant increase in heat stress/shock protein 90 expression[NT058]. Environmental tobacco smoke, administered by whole body exposure to male strain A/J mice at concentrations of 87 mg/m³ of total suspended particulate matter, 16 mg/m³ nicotine, and 246 ppm CO for 6 hours/day, 5 days/week 5 months, produced lung tumors. More than 80% of all tumors were adenomas, and the rest were adenocarcinomas[NT064]. Mainstream smoke, administered to male Balb/c mice for 4 months starting 10 or 30 days before the administration of ethyl carbamate, produced 7.6% decrease of lung adenoma multiplicity. The number of ethyl carbamate-induced lung tumors was not significantly affected by exposure to cigarette smoke when ethyl carbamate was injected intraperitoneally in single doses of 0.5 or 1 g/kg[NT073]. Smoke condensate, administered dermally to Balb/c mice, increased the density and changed the morphology of Langerhans' cells. The number of Langerhans' cells in epidermal sheets of treated mice was significantly higher than in the controls and remained elevated for 35 weeks. Langerhans' cells became less dendritic, or even rounded in shape, and smaller in size. The function of the morphologically altered Langerhans' cells was impaired. There was skin tumor development in all treated mice. After stopping the treatment, Langerhans' cells number in skin tumors and around lesions remained increased. Tumor regression occurred in 23% of tumors. The remaining tumors showed a 50% reduction in size[NT077]. Smoke, in pulmonary and liver microsomes of male NMRI mice, induced the enzymatic activities cata-lyzed by CYP1A1, CYP2B, CYP2C, CYP2D, CYP2E1, and CYP3A in liver microsomes. Immunoquantification of lung and liver CYP1A1, 2E1, and 3A demonstrated the following: CYP1A1 was induced in lung and liver; CYP3A subfamily was induced in liver and not detected in lung; and CYP2E1 was slightly induced in liver, whereas its pulmonary expression was more largely increased (6.8 fold) than CYP1A1 (twofold). This indicates that CYP2E1, which is known to be expressed in human lung, could actively participate in pulmonary carcinogenesis induced by cigarette smoke[NT080]. Six tobacco-specific *N*-nitrosamines and two major volatile *N*-nitrosamines of cigarette smoke, administered to female A/J mice, were active. *N*-nitrosodimethylamine was the most potent inducer of lung adenoma in the A/J mouse model, followed in order of decreasing potencies by 4-(methylnitrosamino)-1-(3-pyridyl)-1-butanone (NNK), 4-(methylnitrosamino)-1-(3-pyridyl)-1-butanol (iso-NNAL), *N*-nitrosopyrrolidine (NPYR), *N'*-nitrosonornicotine (NNN), and *N'*-nitrosoanabasine (NAB). NNK and 4-(methylnitrosamino)-4-(3-pyridyl)butyric acid (iso-NNAC) were inactive[NT087]. Iso-NNAC, administered to strain A mice, was inactive as a tumorigenic agent, and it did not induce DNA repair in primary rat hepatocytes[NT107]. Acetone/methanol extracts of sidestream and mainstream smoke condensates of a filtered commercial brand of blond cigarettes, administered on the shaved skin of female NMR1 mice twice a week for 3 months, produced no significant difference between the life span of mainstream smoke-treated and untreated mice. The life spans of sidestream smoke-treated mice were significantly shorter than those of mainstream smoke-treated mice. The numbers of tumors or lesions in mainstream smoke-treated mice were not increased dose-dependently. The initiation of lesions in sidestream smoke-treated mice was dose-dependent. The sidestream smoke-treated mice developed two to six times more skin tumors than the mainstream

smoke-treated mice. Comparing the treated groups with the negative controls, the overall carcinogenic effect observed was statistically significant. Comparing both treated groups with each other, the overall carcinogenic effect of sidestream smoke was much higher than that of mainstream smoke[NT113]. *N*-nitrosamines: 3-(methylnitrosamino)-propionic acid (NMPA), NNK, and iso-NNAC, evaluated in A/J mice, produced the following results in the lung (total dose in micromol mouse/lung tumors per mouse): NMPA (200/7.1 ± 2.9), NNK (2/15.7 ± 4.1), iso-NNAC (200/0.24 ± 0.43), and saline control (0.2 ± 0.4)[NT115]. Brown and black varieties of a pyrolyzed tobacco (masheri), was administered to Sprague–Dawley rats, Swiss mouse, and Syrian golden hamsters at a dose of 10% of diet. In Sprague–Dawley rats, only brown masheri was used, whereas in Swiss mice and Syrian golden hamsters, both varieties were used. Forestomach papillomas were induced in 37% of the rats, 42–47% of the mice, and 25–43% of the hamsters. No malignant changes were observed in any of the groups except two of the 23 male hamsters that showed forestomach carcinoma in the black masheri diet group[NT122]. NNN, NNK, NPYR, 5'-carboxy-*N'*-nitrosonornicotine (CNNN), *N*-nitrosoproline (NPRO), and 1-(3-pyridyl)-2-buten-1-one (PBO), administered to A/J mouse, produced the following results (dose in micromol per mouse/lung tumors per mouse): NNN (100/1.8 ± 1.4), NPYR (100/3.9 ± 1.5), CNNN (200/0.3 ± 0.5), CNNN (100/0.5 ± 0.6), NPRO (100/0.6 ± 0.7), NNK (20/7.2 ± 3.4), PBO (20/0.7 ± 1), and saline control (0.5 ± 0.7). NNK and NPYR were more tumorigenic than NNN. CNNN was nontumorigenic[NT123]. Smoke condensate, administered intragastrically to Swiss mice, did not produce any tumor. Bidi concentrate, at the same dose, induced liver hemangiomas, forestomach papilloma, and carcinomas of the esophagus and forestomach. Bidi concentrate had a higher benzo[a]pyrene level than cigarette smoke condensate[NT126]. NNK, iso-NNAL, and NNN, administrated dermally to female SENCAR mice at an initiator dose of 28 μmol/mouse in 10 subdoses administered every second day. Promotion commenced 10 days after the last initiator dose and consisted of twice weekly application of 2. μg of tetradecanoylphorbol acetate for 20 weeks. NNK induced a 79% incidence of skin tumors with an average of 1.6 tumors/mouse and a 59% incidence of lung adenomas. Iso-NNAL and NNN were not active. At a total initiator dose of 28 and 5.6 μmol/mouse, NNK induced a 59 and 24% incidence of skin tumors, respectively. In this dose response bioassay, NNK at a total initiator dose of 28 μmol induced a 63% incidence of lung adenomas. The numbers of lung adenomas induced at the lower doses employed were not significant. NNK, at a total initiation dose of 1.4 μmol, did not exhibit significant tumorigenic activity[NT129]. Fresh, whole cigarette smoke of Kentucky reference 2R1 cigarettes was administered intranasally to 2053 (C57BL/Cum × C3H/AnfCum)F1 female mice daily 5 days/week, for 110 weeks, produced a weak carcinogenic activity in mouse lung tissue, and an increased incidence of pigmented alveolar macrophage accumulation, otitis media, head and neck fibrosarcoma, and deposition of smoke particulates approx 125–200 mg total particulate matter/lung/day. The only lung cancers observed in 19 of 978 smoke-exposed mice were diagnosed as alveolar adenocarcinomas. A significant increase in the incidence of lung cancer was observed in one subset, but this difference was not found in the population as a whole or as a result of any other analyses[NT140]. Fresh mainstream smoke from one University of Kentucky reference cigarette (2R1), administered intranasally to male C57BL mice and F-344 rats daily under standardized condi-

tions, produced in mice, significantly elevated levels of blood COHb and pulmonary aryl hydrocarbon hydroxylase activity, and a fivefold to sevenfold increase in the number of bronchoalveolar lavage cells. The proportion of neutrophils increased to 18 ± 3% in smoke-exposed mice as compared to less than 1% in controls. Cessation of smoke treatments returned the proportion of neutrophils to those of controls within 5 weeks. Smoke exposure of rats for up to 32 weeks induced appreciable changes in the number and proportion of macrophages and neutrophils. Large brown macrophages were observed in smoke-exposed groups of both species. Bronchoalveolar lavage cells from smoke-treated mice but not rats released greater amounts of superoxides than controls under resting and phagocytically stimulated conditions. The activity of N-acetylglucosaminidase was increased in both species. The activity of 5'-nucleotidase was significantly reduced in macrophages from mice but not rats. The activity of leucine aminopeptidase remained unaltered in both species[NT141]. Tobacco alcoholic extract, administered intragastrically or in the diet of male Swiss mice, increased the incidence of lung and liver tumors. An additive effect of tobacco extract and hexachlorocyclohexane on liver tumor induction was found[NT154]. The weakly acidic fraction of cigarette smoke condensate subfractions II, administered dermally with 0.003% benzo[a]pyrene to noninbred Ha:ICR Swiss albino mice, produced significant cocarcinogenic activity (subfractions A-C and F-J); subfractions A, F, and H were the most active. Catechol was a major component of subfraction A and was also detected in subfractions B–D and F. Major components of the other subfractions included hydroquinone (B), coniferyl alcohol (C and H), hydroxyphenyl alcohols (D), alkyl-2-hydroxy-2-cyclopenten-1-ones (C, D, and F), hydroxyacetophenones (F), phenolic cyano compounds (F), and fatty acids (F). The results indicated the importance of catechol as a cocarcinogen in the weakly acidic fraction of cigarette smoke condensate[NT171]. Methanol (80%) insoluble fraction of aqueous extract of tobacco combined with the methanol soluble fraction was administered to mice treated with 7,12-dimethylbenz[a]anthracene. The subfraction (D) with a presumptive molecular weight greater than 13,000 produced a significantly higher tumor incidence and tumor yield, together with a significantly shorter latent period than the other subfractions. Subfraction D contained approx 12% of the total 80% methanol insoluble material. All of the other subfractions exhibited significant but less pronounced tumor copromoting activity[NT173]. Undifferentiated carcinomas of the salivary glands were found in two of 44 strain A mice injected intraperitoneally with an N-nitrosonornicotine. The presence of intranuclear rodlets in the salivary carcinomas provided the first demonstration of such structures in a nonneuronal tumor in mice. Two types of rodlets were exhibited: one was composed of fibrillar filaments arranged in bundles, and the other was much thicker and branching in form. Results indicated that these intranuclear rodlets were closely associated with nuclear chromatin or nucleoli[NT179]. NNK, NNN, and 4-(N-methyl-N-nitrosamino)-4-(3-pyridyl)butanal (NNA), administered to strain A mice, were active. NNK induced more lung adenomas per mouse than NNN, and NNA was less active than NNN. Two cases of undifferentiated carcinoma of the salivary glands occurred in the NNN experimental groups[NT181]. Smoke components, administered dermally to female ICR/Ha Swiss mice three times a week with 5 μg benzo[a]pyrene per application, enhanced the carcinogenicity of benzo[a]pyrene by catechol, pyrogallol, decane, undecane, pyrene, benzo[e]pyrene, and fluoranthene. The following compounds

inhibited benzo[a]pyrene carcinogenicity completely: esculin, quercetin, squalene, and oleic acid. Phenol, eugenol, resorcinol, hydroquinone, hexadecane, and limonene partially inhibited benzo[a]pyrene carcinogenicity. No direct correlation existed between tumor-promoting activity and cocarcinogenic activity. The cocarcinogens pyrogallol and catechol did not show tumor-promoting activity. Decane, tetradecane, anthralin, and phorbol myristate acetate showed both types of activities[NT183]. Acetone and alcohol extracts of the flue-cured tobacco, administered dermally to mice, produced weak activity. Chloroform/water extract produced tumor in 38% of the animals and was about fivefold more active than smoke condensate derived from an equal weight of tobacco[NT184]. NNN induced adenomas of the lung in mice. Bioassays of NNN in rats indicated carcinogenic activities on the esophagus and the nasal cavity[NT187]. Weakly acidic fraction of cigarette smoke particulate matter were tested on initiated mouse skin by long-term application. Two of these subfractions (40% of weakly acidic fraction) were inactive, and the 18 and 35% of weakly acidic fractions showed tumor-promoting activity. Catechol, hydroquinone, 3-hydroxypyridine, 6-methyl-3-hydroxypyridine, linolenic acid, and linoleic acid were inactive as tumor promoters in the experimental animal[NT188]. [5-(3)H]-(S)-NNN, in rat esophagus culture at a concentration of 1 μM, was predominantly metabolized to products of 2'-hydroxylation, 4-oxo-4-(3-pyridyl)butanoic acid (ketoacid), and 4-hydroxy-1-(3-pyridyl)-1-butanone. The major metabolite of (R)-NNN under these conditions was 4-hydroxy-4-(3-pyridyl)butanoic acid, a product of NNN 5'hydroxylation. The 2'-hydroxylation:5'-hydroxylation metabolite ratio ranged from 6.22 to 8.06 at various time intervals in the incubations with (S)-NNN. The corresponding ratios were 1.12-1.33 in the experiments with (R)-NNN. These differences were statistically significant ($p <$ 0.001). Because 2'-hydroxylation is thought to be the major metabolic activation pathway of NNN in the rat esophagus, the results demonstrated that (S)-NNN is metabolically activated more extensively than (R)-NNN and, therefore, may be more carcinogenic. [5-(3)H]-(R)-NNN, [5-(3)H]-(S)-NNN, or racemic [5-(3)H]NNN, administered intragastrically to rats at dose of 0.3 mg/kg, was metabolized to hydroxylacid and ketoacid. Products of 2'-hydroxylation predominated in the urine of the rats treated with (S)-NNN, whereas products of 5'-hydroxylation were more prevalent in the rats treated with (R)-NNN. 2'-Hydroxylation:5'-hydroxylation metabolite ratios ranged from 1.66 to 2.04 in the urine at various times after treatment with (S)-NNN, while the ratios were 0.398–0.450 for the rats treated with (R)-NNN ($p < 0.001$). The results indicated that the carcinogenicity of (S)-NNN, the predominant enantiomer in tobacco products, may be greater than that of (R)-NNN or racemic NNN[NT223].

Cardiovascular effect. Water extract of the dried leaf, administered intravenously to cats and rats at doses of 10–20 mg/kg, induced variable electrocardiogram patterns, including increases in the height of the QRS complexes, S-T segment elevation, occasional extrasystoles, and arrhythmias[NT588].

Cataractogenic effect. Cigarette smoke was administered to male Wistar rats for 90 days, with or without vitamin E supplement. The treatment significantly increased iron levels in the lenses of smoke-treated group. Smoke-treated rats and smoke-treated and vitamin-supplemented rats had significantly higher cadmium levels. Vitamin E treatment prevented iron accumulation in smoke-treated and vitamin-supplemented rats. Distinct histopathological changes observed in smoke-treated rats were not present in smoke-treated and vitamin-supplemented rats[NT236]. Cigarette and fire-wood smokes condensates were evaluated on isolated capsulated rat lenses incubated for varying periods, with and without antioxidants, in the presence and absence of light. The smoke condensates permeated the lens capsule and impart color and opacify to the lens in a light- and dose-dependent manner. Antioxidants offer partial inhibition against the damages. Smoke-induced damage possibly occurs through systemic absorption and transport of toxic components to several tissues, specially into the lens. The turnover is slow, leading to chronic accumulation causing oxidative damage to the constituent molecules and consequently to lenticular opacity[NT274].

Cell differentiation induction. Water extract of the dried leaf, administered to CBA/N strain mice at a concentration of 0.5%, was active on lymphocytes B[NT449]. A tobacco-specific carcinogen NNK, in cell culture, produced activation of the phosphatidylinositol 3'-kinase/Akt pathway (P13K/Akt). The pathway was evaluated in isogenic immortalized or tumorigenic human bronchial epithelial cells in vitro and in progressive murine lung lesions. Compared with immortalized cells, tumorigenic cells had greater activation of the P13K/Akt pathway, enhanced survival, and increased apoptosis in response to inhibition of the pathway. In vivo, increased activation of Akt and mammalian target of rapamycin were observed with increased phenotypic progression[NT005].

Cell metabolism induction. Methanol extract of STE, in collagen-producing cells, stimulated glycolysis by 80% in cartilage but was not affected in the other tissues. Medium alkaline phosphatase activity was unaffected. In the frontal bone and cartilage, [3H]hydroxyproline and [3H]proline contents were decreased. Neither was affected in the aorta.

Cell proliferation. Snuff extract in combination with DMBA, in primary embryonal mouse tongue culture, inhibited the proliferation of cells and decreased ornithine decarboxylase and hydrocarbon hydroxylase activities, compared to control[NT109]. NNN, in embryonic mouse tongue epithelial cells, increased [3H]dT uptake, and ornithine decarboxylase and aryl hydrocarbon hydroxylase activities. NNK produced further increases of [3H]dT uptake, cell count, and ornithine decarboxylase. The extract had an inhibitory effect on cell count, [3H]dT uptake, ornithine decarboxylase, and aryl hydrocarbon hydroxylase activities when administered alone or in combination with NNN or NNK[NT120]. Tobacco and tobacco smoke constituents, in ascites sarcoma BP8 cell culture, indicated that the most active constituents were unsaturated aldehydes and ketones, phenols, and indoles[NT189]. Smoke, administered to Sprague–Dawley rats at a dose of 10 cigarettes (smoke only), or the smoke of 10 cigarettes after iv infusion of endothelin A antagonist BQ-610 (smoke and BQ-610), produced significant cell proliferation in the airway epithelium and wall, in the peribronchiolar arterial endothelial compartment, and in the endothelial and wall compartments of the perialveolar ductular arteries. Pretreatment with BQ-610 reduced the peribronchiolar arterial endothelial and the perialveolar ductular arterial wall proliferation to control levels and reduced, but did not totally abrogate, the smoke-induced proliferation of the airway epithelial, airway wall, and perialveolar ductular arterial endothelial compartments. Results indicated that cigarette smoke-induced cell proliferation of the airways and pulmonary arterial vessels is at least partially mediated through stimulation of the endothelin-A receptors[NT255].

Cell signaling. Environmental tobacco smoke, administered to rats during gestation, the early neonatal period, or both, elicited induction of total adenylyl cyclase. In the brain, the specific coupling of β-adrenergic receptors to adenylyl cyclase was inhibited in the smoke-treated groups, despite a normal complement of β-receptor binding sites. In the heart, smoke evoked a decrease in M2-receptor expression. In both tissues, the effects of postnatal smoke, mimicking passive smoking, were equivalent to adenylyl cyclase level or greater than (M2-muscarinic cholinergic receptors) those seen with prenatal smoke mimicking active smoking. The effects of combined prenatal and postnatal exposure were equivalent to those seen with postnatal exposure alone. The smoke exposure evoked changes in cell signaling that recapitulate those caused by developmental nicotine treatment[NT208].

Cervical carcinoma. Smoke condensate, in human papillomavirus 18-immortalized ectocervical cells (HEC-18-1C), produced an invasive squamous cell carcinoma, from which was established a clonal line of cells (HEC-18-1CT). The moderate passage malignantly transformed HEC-18-1CT displayed severe dysplasia/carcinoma *in situ* in raft culture[NT620].

***C-fos* expression.** Mainstream smoke trapped in PBS solution, in quiescent Swiss 3T3 cells, produced dose-dependent expression of *c-fos* mRNA and protein. *C-fos* transcripts in cells exposed to 0.03 puffs (approx 1 cm^3) of smoke per medium, accumulated slowly but were still seen after 8 hours. The maximum expression rates were between 2 and 6 hours of exposure. An increase of *c-fos* message stability was observed in addition to slight transcriptional activation of the c-fos promoter[NT075].

Chemiluminescence. Cigarette smoke in determined quantity was streamed through physiologic saline solution, blood plasma, or ex vivo excised rat lung. The solutions and the supernatants from lung tissue homogenate produced a significant increase in chemiluminescence after *t*-butyl hydroperoxide induction[NT280].

Chromosome aberrations induction. Water extract of the dried leaf, in cell culture at a concentration of 15 mL, was active on

Chinese hamster ovary cells. The number of aberrant metaphases increased in cultures with 15 mL tobacco extract per milliliter of growth media[NT445]. Water extract of the dried leaf, administered to mice at a dose of 9.40 g/kg, 6 days a week for 10 months, was active on bone marrow. A combination of *Piper betle*, *Areca catechu*, and *Nicotiana tabacum* was used[NT524]. Seed, administered orally to adults with oral cancer and oral submucosal fibrosis and to healthy chewers, was active. An average of 6 quids of tobacco leaf, *Areca* nuts, and lime were chewed daily[NT521].

Chronic bronchitis. Cigarette smoke, administered to rats for 2 weeks, produced a significantly higher mean basal secretion of fucose in "bronchitic" rats than in the controls. In control and bronchitic animals, acute administrations of cigarette smoke, blown directly through the laryngeo-tracheal segment after equilibration, produced significant transient increases in the secretion of fucose, hexose, and protein but not albumin[NT299]. Cigarette smoke, administered to the specific pathogen-free rats at a dose of 25 cigarettes daily for 14 days and concurrently given N-acetylcysteine (NAC) as 1% of their drinking water, increased the thickness of the epithelium by 37–72% at three of the airway levels studied. The number of secretory cells was increased at all airway levels distal to the upper trachea 102–421%. Secretory cells containing neutral glycoproteins were reduced in number, but this was more than offset by a large increase in the number of secretory cells containing acidic glycoproteins at all airway levels[NT300].

Chronic obstructive pulmonary disease. Smoke-conditioned media, administered intranasally to Balb/c mice for 40 days, significantly increased bronchoalveolar lavage neutrophils, lymphocytes, chemokine, TNF-α, and mucin. There were changes in pulmonary reactivity to methacholine, inflammation, and cellular lung changes characteristic for human chronic obstructive pulmonary disease[NT025]. A polyphenol reagent isolated from cigarette smoke condensate primed purified human neutrophils. A mouse monoclonal antiidiotypic antibody directed against the polyphenols-reactive determinants on a rabbit polyclonal antitobacco glycoprotein antibody was generated and also primed neutrophils. After priming by the isolated polyphenol reagent or tobacco antiidiotypic antibody, there was a 2.5-fold to threefold increase in CD11b/18 expression and doubling of the number of formyl-methionyl-leucyl-phenylalanine receptors on the cells. The primed cells produced a twofold increase in production of superoxide and release of neutrophil elastase after stimulation with formyl-methionyl-leucyl-phenylalanine. The inflammatory process contributing to progression of chronic obstructive pulmonary disease in ex-smokers may be in part driven by tobacco antiidiotypic antibodies[NT041].

Chylomicron metabolism. Smoke, administered to rats injected intravenously with ^{14}C- and ^{3}H-labeled chylomicrons, produced no difference in the initial plasma clearance time of labeled chylomicrons between smoke-treated and control animals. Hepatic uptake of chylomicron cholesterol was slower in smoke-treated animals than in controls. More labeled chylomicrons remained in the heart of smoke-treated rats than controls[NT284].

Cimetidine kinetics. Low- or high-nicotine tar, administered orally and parenterally to rats for 10 minutes immediately after administration of cimetidine, produced lower plasma level after orally administered cimetidine in the absorption phase in the smoke inhaling groups than in the nonsmoking control group. It was particularly marked in the high-nicotine tar cigarette smoke-inhaling group. No significant difference was found in cimetidine plasma level between the cigarette smoke inhaling group and the nonsmoking control group when administered intraperitoneally or intravenously. The cigarette smoke inhalation produced suppression or a delay in cimetidine absorption from the gastrointestinal tract, and the degree of influence was dependent on the content of nicotine tar in the cigarette smoke[NT290].

Clastogenic activity. Water extract of the dried leaf, administered to mice at a dose of 9.4 g/kg, 6 days/week for 10 months, was active on bone marrow. A combination of aqueous extracts of *Piper betle*, *Areca catechu*, and *Nicotiana tabacum* was used[NT524]. Seed, administered orally to adults, produced an increase in micronuclei in healthy chewers and chewers with oral submucosal fibrosis. An average of 6 quids of tobacco leaf, *Areca* nuts, and lime were chewed daily[NT521]. Mainstream smoke, administered by whole-body exposure to male albino Swiss mice, produced a significant increase in the number of micronucleated bone marrow polychromatic erythrocytes. A high correlation was observed among the number of micronucleated polychromatic erythrocytes and the content of tar and nicotine[NT082]. Smoke, administered to pregnant BDF1 (C57B1 × DBA2) mice at a dose of 600 cm³ of smoke, four times of 15 minutes each with 1 minute intervals on day 16/17 of gestation, produced a two- to threefold increase in the number of micronucleated polychromatic erythrocytes in fetal liver and liver of newborn mice (1–5 hours after birth). Administration of smoke for 60 minutes/day repeatedly from day 11 of gestation produced slightly greater micronucleus response in fetuses. Smoke, administered transplacentally to newborn mice during the last trimester of pregnancy, produced greater clastogenic activity than in their 6-month-old mothers[NT118]. Smoke, administered to BDF1 mice at a dose of 600 cm³, two to six exposures of 30 minutes each, produced 3.5-fold increase of the number of micronucleated polychromatic erythrocytes in born marrow after 24 hours of exposure, and a two- to fivefold increase

in the peripheral blood of mice treated twice daily for 30 minutes, starting after 48 hours of exposure[NT124].

Central nervous system depressant activity. Ethanol (70%) extract of the fresh leaf, administered intraperitoneally to mice of both sexes at variable doses, produced strong activity. Initial excitation was followed by marked sedative effect[NT580].

Collagenase activity. Smoke was administered to Guinea pigs at a dose of 20 cigarettes per day for 8 weeks. At 6 and 8 weeks of exposure, lungs exhibited interstitial and peribronchiolar inflammation and moderate emphysematous changes. There was patchy expression of collagenase mRNA mainly in macrophages but also in alveolar epithelial and interstitial cells. Immunoreactive protein was detected in alveolar macrophages, in alveolar walls, and in interstitium. Collagenolytic activity increased beginning in the fourth week of exposure. Collagen concentration decreased from 50.7 ± 8.5 mg/g dry weight in control lungs to 40.2 ± 5 and 42.9 ± 6 at 6 and 8 weeks of exposure, respectively[NT260].

Comutagenic activity. Cigarette smoke condensate, in *Salmonella typhimurium* strains TA98 and TA98/1.8DNP6, specifically enhanced the mutagenicity of polyaromatic amines, such as 2-aminofluorene, 2-acetylaminofluorene, 4-acetylaminofluorene, and 2-aminoanthracene. Both black and blond tobacco proved to interact synergistically with 2-aminoanthracene mutagenicity. Administration of 2-aminoanthracene/smoke condensate mixtures, previously shown to be comutagenic in vitro, failed to demonstrate a synergistic effect in sister chromatid exchange induction in bone marrow cells of mice[NT103].

Connective tissue breakdown. Whole cigarette smoke, administered to C57-BL/6 mice, produced a dose-response increase in lavage neutrophils, desmosine, and hydroxyproline, but not lavage macrophages (MACs). The effect was evident after 6 hours of exposure to two cigarettes. Pretreatment with an antibody against polymorphonuclear leukocytes (PMNs) reduced lavage PMNs to undetectable levels after smoke exposure. It did not affect MAC numbers and prevented increases in lavage desmosine and hydroxyproline. Intraperitoneal injection of a commercial human α1-antitrypsin (α1AT) 24 hours before smoke exposure increased serum α1AT levels threefold and completely abolished smoke-induced connective tissue breakdown and the increase in lavage PMNs, without affecting MAC numbers[NT045].

CuZn-superoxide dismutase activity. Cigarette smoke was administered to the osteogenic disorder Shionogi (ODS) rats at doses of 4 mg/day, S4 or 40 mg/day, and S40 of ascorbic acid and exposed to smoke daily for 25 days. The treatment produced a significant decrease of CuZn-superoxide dismutase (SOD)[NT196].

Cyclin D1/2 expression. Smoke, administered to male strain A/J mice fed a diet with chemopreventive agents, produced a decrease in cyclin D1/2 expression. Expression of cyclin may be a useful marker in the identification of chemopreventive agents from tobacco smoke[NT030].

Cyclo-oxygenase activity. Aqueous cigarette tar extracts, in rat pulmonary alveolar macrophages, increased cyclo-oxygenase activity threefold above the initial activity within 2 hours of incubation and gradually decreased below the initial activity after 8 hours of incubation. Accumulated levels of prostaglandin-2 increased dramatically after 12 hours of incubation[NT233].

Cytochrome b5 induction. STE, in murine system at doses of 50 or 100 mg/kg body weight/day, elevated microsomal cytochrome b5, cytochrome P450, and malondialdehyde levels[NT059].

Cytochrome C oxidase inhibition. Smoke extract, in the mouse brain mitochondria culture in the presence or absence of vitamin C for 60 minutes, inhibited mitochondrial Adenosine triphosphatase (ATPase) and cytochrome C oxidase activities in a dose-dependent manner. The effect of extract on mitochondria swelling response to calcium stimulation was dependent on calcium concentrations. The extract treatment induced mitochondrial inner membrane damage and vacuolization of the matrix, whereas the outer mitochondrial membrane was preserved. Nicotine produced no significant damage[NT007].

Cytochrome P450 induction. STE, in murine system at doses of 50 or 100 mg/kg body weight/day, elevated microsomal cytochrome b5, cytochrome P450 (CYP), and malondialdehyde levels. These results indicated the inhibitory potential of STE on garlic-induced hepatic glutathion-S-transferase (GST)/GSH system besides significant augmentation on garlic-, mace- or black mustard-induced microsomal cytochromes[NT059]. Methyl chloride extract of the leaf, administered intragastrically to rats at a dose of 3 mg/animal daily for 21 months in DMSO solvent, was active. The rats were divided into two groups, one was fed a vitamin A diet, and the other a vitamin A-deficient diet. Treatment with the extract increased pulmonary CYP over controls in vitamin-deficient animals and among treated animals more so in the vitamin-deficient group[NT519]. Crude cigarette smoke condensate, in human liver microsomes, inhibited P450 1A2 cytochrome. The tobacco-specific nitrosamines were activated by a number of P450 enzymes. P450 1A2, 2A6, and 2E1 activated nitrosamines to genotoxic products[NT079]. Aged and diluted sidestream cigarette smoke, administered to timed pregnant rats and their pups four times a days from gestational day five to postnatal day 21, produced no alterations in mRNA in the fetal lung beginning at gestational day 17. Continued exposure significantly induced CYP1A1 but not other P450 genes as early as one day after birth. Results indicated that smoke-induced pulmonary

CYP1A1 in the first day of life fetal cytochrome P450 genes were not induced by maternal exposure to smoke. In the fetal lung, CYP1A1 and 1B1 can be induced by β-naphthoflavone[NT274]. Mainstream cigarette smoke, administered to F344 rats at a dose of 100 mg total particulate matter/m^3 for 2 or 8 weeks, induced CYP1A1 in respiratory and olfactory mucosae, liver, kidney, and lung. CYP1A2 levels increased slightly in the liver and olfactory mucosa. CYP2B1/2, which increased in the liver, decreased in the upper and lower respiratory tissues. Intense immunoreactivity was found in epithelia throughout the nasal cavity of smoke-exposed rats. Ethoxyresorufin O-demethylase activity (associated with CYP1A1/2) decreased approximately two-fold in olfactory mucosa but increased in nonnasal tissues. Methoxy- and pentoxy-resorufin O-dealkylase activities (associated with CYP1A2 and CYP2B1/2, respectively) decreased in olfactory and respiratory mucosae and lung (CYP2B1/2) but increased in liver[NT246]. Masheri, a pyrolyzed tobacco product, administered orally to Swiss mice, Sprague–Dawley rats, and Syrian golden hamsters at a dose of 10% diet for 20 months, produced a significant induction of cytochrome P450 in proximal and distal parts of the three species[NT100].

Cytotoxic effect. Gas phase of mainstream cigarette smoke, in monolayer culture of mouse lung epithelial cells, produced an increase in cytotoxicity in a dose-dependent manner. Cell viability of cultures exposed to gas phase with only the nonorganic components was equivalent to controls. Removal of volatile organic constituents resulted in almost elimination of cytotoxicity of the smoke[NT021]. Smoke condensate and tobacco extract, at high concentrations in Lewis lung adenocarcinoma cells and mice spleen lymphocytes, were cytotoxic. Smaller doses increased thymidine incorporation in both cell types. Lymphocytes were more susceptible to the toxic effect of tobacco products than lung cells. When smoke condensate and tobacco extract were mixed with Lewis lung adenocarcinoma cells and then inoculated into mice, they did not modify the size of the local Lewis lung adenocarcinoma-induced tumors or the number or appearance time of lung metastasis, although there was an increase in spleen weight[NT116]. Mainstream and sidestream smoke from the same cigarette, in monolayer cell culture of mouse fibroblast-like L-929 cells, produced a decrease of cytotoxicity with increasing smoke age (up to 8.7 seconds), smoke dilution, and the quantity of activated charcoal in filters. Acetate filters had little effect on cell mortality, and the age-of-smoke effect was not evident for mainstream smoke generated with a low puff volume and rapid dilution. The cytotoxicity of sidestream smoke also decreased rapidly with increasing smoke age and dilution[NT146]. Smoke condensate from the mainstream smoke of TOB-HT, IR4F, and 1R5F cigarettes, in human bronchial/tracheal epithelial cells, coronary artery endothelial cells, coronary artery smooth muscle cells, foreskin keratinocytes, and WB-344 rat liver epithelial cell line exposed for 1 hour, produced no inhibition of gap junction intercellular communication by TOB-HT in any of the human cell types tested at concentrations where 1R4F and IR5F did inhibit ($p < 0.05$). TOB-HT did not elevate lactate dehydrogenase release, when tested at concentrations where IR4F and IR5F did. Smoke condensate from TOB-HT cigarettes is less damaging to the structure or function of the cellular plasma membranes of a variety of human cell lines than from 1R4F and 1R5F tobacco burning reference cigarettes[NT226].

Dermal tumor. Smoke condensates were administered externally to female SENCAR mice at doses of 10, 20, or 40 mg Eclipse or 1R4F cigarette smoke condensates three times a week for 29 weeks. The treatment was initiated with a single topical application of 7,12-dimethylbenzanthracene. The treatment did not alter body weight, survival, or other indicators of subchronic toxicity. In 7,12-dimethylbenzanthracene-initiated mice, there were significant increases in both the number of tumor-bearing animals and dermal tumors at all 1R4F doses and the high-dose Eclipse[NT003].

Desensitization of nicotinic receptor. S-(-)-Nicotine (10 and 100 nM) diminished [^{3}H]overflow from ^{3}H-dopamine-preloaded rat striatal slices after subsequent superfusion with 10 µM S-(-)-nicotine (46 and 74%, respectively) or 10 µM S-(-)-nornicotine (59 and 81%, respectively). S-(-)-nornicotine (1 and 10 µM) diminished the response to subsequent superfusion with 10 µM S-(-)-nornicotine (85 and 97%, respectively) or 10 µM S-(-)-nicotine (82 and 88%, respectively). Thus, similar to S-(-)-nicotine, S-(-)-nornicotine-desensitized nicotinic receptors, but with approx 12-fold lower potency. Cross-desensitization suggested involvement of common nicotinic receptor subtypes[NT204].

Diltiazem kinetics. Cigarette smoke, administered to rats for 10 minutes using a Hamburg II smoking machine, immediately after oral administration of diltiazem (10 mg/kg), produced plasma diltiazem levels in the rats exposed to cigarette smoke reached the maximum (4.3 µg/kg) after 4 hours. In the nonsmoking nonrestrained rats, plasma diltiazem levels increased rapidly and reached the maximum (7.1 µg/kg) 2 hours after administration and decreased gradually thereafter. In the nonsmoking restrained rats, plasma diltiazem levels increased rapidly but showed almost constant levels between 1 hour and 8 hour after administration. The maximum level (5.4 µg/kg) was shown after 2 hours. Results indicated that absorption of orally administered diltiazem is inhibited and delayed by cigarette smoke[NT254].

Diuretic activity. Decoction of the dried leaf, administered nasogastrically to rats at a dose of 1 g/kg, produced strong activity[NT605].

DNA adduct formation. Mainstream Eclipse or 1R4F cigarettes smoke condensate was administered dermally to SENCAR mice at doses of 30, 60, or 120 mg/animal three times a week for 30 weeks. The treatment produced distinct time and dose-dependent diagonal radioactive zones in the DNA from lung, heart and skin tissues of 1R4F-treated mice. The relative adduct labeling values of lung, heart, and skin DNA from reference smoke condensate-treated animals were significantly greater than those of the solvent controls were. No diagonal radioactive zones were observed at any dose from the DNA of animals treated with smoke condensate from Eclipse[NT055]. Smoke condensate from cigarette and a reference tobacco-burning cigarette (1R4F) were administered dermally to CD-1 mice three times a week for 4 weeks at mass up to 180.0 mg "tar" per week per animal. Distinct diagonal radioactive zones in the DNA from both skin and lung tissues of animals dosed with reference cigarette smoke was produced. No corresponding diagonal radioactive zones were observed from the DNA of animals dosed with the test cigarette smoke or acetone (solvent control). The relative adduct labeling values of skin and lung DNA from reference-treated mice were significantly greater than those of the test cigarette-treated mice. The relative adduct labeling values of the test cigarette-treated animals were no greater than those of solvent controls[NT096]. Smoke condensate, administered topically to female ICR mice at four doses equivalent to three cigarettes daily, elicited aromatic adducts in most tissues, but not in white blood cells[NT111]. Cigarette smoke administered by inhalation, cigarette smoke condensate administered intraperitoneally, or neutral fraction in genetically responsive C57BL/6 (B6) and nonresponsive DBA/2 (D2) mice for 3–16 days, produced no detectable levels of benzo[a]pyrene-7,8-diol-9,10-epoxide

(BPDE)-DNA in lungs or liver. Aryl hydrocarbon hydroxylase (AHH) activity was induced in the lungs of B6 mice. Benzo[a]pyrene, administered intraperitoneally to mice at doses of 20–80 mg/kg, produced dose-dependent amount of BPDE-DNA-adducts in lung and liver. Administration of 4 mg/kg benzo[a]pyrene produced no effect. In B6 mice aryl hydrocarbon hydroxylase was induced in lungs and livers, but not in D2 mice, although the levels of BPDE-DNA-adducts were higher than in B6 mice[NT119]. Sidestream cigarette smoke, administered by a whole-body exposure to female Sprague–Dawley rats for 6 hours/day for 4 weeks, produced one major and several minor smoke-related adducts in lung, trachea, heart, and bladder[NT218]. Mainstream cigarette smoke, administered by whole-body exposure to female BD6 rats, 1 hour/day, 5 days/week for 8 months, produced no significant increase of DNA-protein cross-links in liver, lung, or heart. Cigarette smoke induced formation of DNA adducts in the lung and heart but not in the esophagus or liver. The combined ingestion of ethanol resulted in a significant formation of smoke-related DNA adducts in the esophagus and dramatic increase in the heart[NT245].

DNA damages. Environmental smoke was administered by whole-body exposure to adult female Balb/c mice in a regimen consisting of sequences of a 30 minutes exposure followed by a 90 minutes nonexposure. This regimen was performed once for the single exposure and repeated three times for the triple exposure. The exposure increased 8-hydroxy-2'-deoxyguanoside levels in the heart, lung, and liver. In some instances, the increased level returned to normal by the end of the nonexposure period, whereas other tissues showed a further increase following nonexposure[NT056]. NNK, administered to pregnant Swiss mice in a single or multiple doses, significantly increased lev-

els of 8-oxo-2'-deoxyguanosine in maternal lungs by 23 and 32%, respectively. In maternal liver, a 38% increase was observed after multiple dose treatment. In the fetuses, a 45% increase in 8-oxo-2'-deoxyguanosine levels was observed in liver after multiple doses[NT061]. Aqueous extract of smoke condensate, in rat lung culture in the absence of microsomes, produced radioactively labeled bulky reaction products accumulating in a time- and dose-dependent manner. Pretreatment of extract with radical scavengers/reducing agents (ascorbic acid, GSH), diminished adduct formation in a concentration-dependent manner. Adduct fractions derived from in vitro and in vivo experiments showed similar chromatographic behavior[NT091]. Smoke condensate, administered dermally to female ICR mice at a dose being equivalent of 4.5 cigarettes for 6 days, produced DNA damages in lung, heart, skin, and kidneys higher than in the liver. Spleen DNA was virtually adduct free. Preference for heart and lung was observed for mice treated for 1 and 3 days[NT128]. Cigarette tar, administered dermally to ICR mice at doses being equivalent to 1.5, 3, 6, and 9 cigarettes for 4, 3, 5, and 7 days, respectively, produced 12 distinct ^{32}P-labeled DNA adduct spots, and diagonal radioactive zone. One derivative in particular (adduct 1) increased rapidly during the early treatment phase and persisted to 8 days after treatment. The prominent adduct 1 was observed in the same location on the fingerprints of DNA samples from human smokers. Co-chromatography experiments suggested identity of human and mouse DNA adduct 1. Several other human and mouse adducts (adducts 3, 5, 6, and 9) appeared identical, and the diagonal radioactive zone was also present on DNA adduct maps from smokers[NT138]. Mainstream whole-smoke DMSO and phosphate buffer solutions induced DNA single-strand breakage in mice testicular cells. DMSO solution of cigarette smoke produced stronger cytotoxicity and genotoxicity than the phosphate buffer solution[NT211]. Cigarette smoke, administered in combination with asbestos to rats for 1, 2, and 14 days, increased in 2'-dioxyuridine-5'-triphosphate (dUTP)-biotin nick end labeling-positive, necrotic epithelial cells[NT219].

DNA deletion. Filtered and unfiltered smoke and smoke condensate were administered by whole-body exposure for 4 hours to pregnant pink eye-unstable C57BL/6J mutant mice or 15 mg/kg of smoke condensate during 10th day of gestation. A significant increase in the number of DNA deletions in the embryo, as evidenced by the spotted offspring in both smoke-exposed groups, was observed[NT053].

DNA synthesis stimulation. Smoke of the dried leaf, administered to rats at variable doses, was active. The effect of a combination of cigarette and hashish smoke on stress response was measured in rats held in a wire cage inside of a larger cage with a cat. Brains were measured for protein and catecholamine levels[NT590]. Whole Kentucky reference 2A1 cigarette smoke, administered to hybrid strain BC3F1/Cum (C57BL/Cum X C3H/AnfCum) mice, increased DNA replicative activity more than twofold within 1 week of beginning smoke exposure and remained elevated as long as smoke exposure was continued. Treatment of lung tissues in vitro with either the lung carcinogen 4-nitroquinoline-1-oxide or methylmethane sulfonate stimulated unscheduled DNA synthesis. Until the 10th to 12th week of smoke exposure, at which time the accumulated deposition of total particulate material in the lung was approx 40 mg, the level of unscheduled DNA synthesis (UDS) stimulated by the alkylating chemicals declined to approx 50% of that seen in lung tissue from sham-exposed control mice. If the mice were removed from smoke exposure, DNA replicative activity returned to normal levels within 1 week, but the UDS response to DNA damage remained depressed up to 5 months after ending smoke exposure[NT168].

DNA synthesis inhibition. Leaves, on agar plate at a concentration of 50%, produced weak activity on monkey kidney cells[NT574]. Smoke of the dried leaf, administered to rats at variable doses, produced weak activity[NT590].

Dominant-lethal mutations. Whole tobacco smoke was administered to male Balb/c, DF1 and H mice at two doses: low 1-hour treatment/day and high 2-hour treatment/day, 5 days/week for 8 weeks. Dominant-lethal mutations in both experimental groups of Balb/c, BDF1, and H mice were significantly induced ($p < 0.001$), but some strain differences existed. In Balb/c and BDF1 mice, the smoke-induced dominant-lethal mutations were found mainly in spermatocytes, spermatogonia, and gonial stem cells. In H mice, only spermatids and spermatocytes were affected. Exposure produced a twofold to threefold increase in the number of micronucleated polychromatic erythrocytes in the bone marrow of Balb/c and BDF1 mice in both dose groups. In H mice, this effect was observed only on days 19 and 38 of sampling. No cumulative or dose-dependent effects were detected[NT086].

Dopamine protection. Cigarette smoke, in 1-methyl-4-phenyl-1,2,3,6-tetrahydropyridine (MPTP) mouse model, partially protected against corpus striatal dopamine depletion by MPTP. This protection was associated with monoamine oxidase (MAO) inhibition in brain and liver and CYP induction. β-naphthoflavone pretreatment also partially protected against MPTP-induced depletion of striatal dopamine. The results indicated that both MAO inhibition and CYP induction may play a role in any biochemical protection afforded by cigarette smoke exposure against the development of Parkinson's disease[NT621].

Nicotine, 4-phenylpyridine, and hydrazine, administered to mice, prevented the decrease in dopamine metabolite levels induced by MPTP, but there was no significant effect on dopamine levels. The compounds did not inhibit monoamine oxidase (MAO) activity in cerebral tissue in vivo. In vitro, an extract produced significant inhibition of MAO A and B activities in the brain[NT102].

Dopaminergic activity. Smoke was administered intranasally to mice for 20 minutes twice daily for 3 days before methamphetamine treatment. The treatment significantly attenuated the neurotoxicity as judged by a lesser depletion of dopamine, dihydrophenylacetic acid, and homovanillic acid. The lesser effect of methamphetamine on the content of serotonin level was unaltered by prior inhalation of smoke[NT039]. Tobacco glycoside, administered to mice, increased behavior via dopamine 2 neuronal activity but not dopamine 1 activity in a dose-dependent manner. The results indicated that smoking can affect the human brain function via not only the nicotinic cholinergic neuron but also the dopamine 2 neuron[NT017].

Duodenal ulcer. Tobacco cigarette smoke, administered to mepirizole-treated rats, inhibited hyperemia at the ulcer margin after exposure[NT270].

E-cadherin expression. Smoke extract, on pig airway epithelial cells and mouse trachea, produced a decrease of E-cadherin expression on membrane and an increase of cytoplasmic expression at 12 and 24 hours after exposure. The expression at 24 hours was higher than at 12 hours[NT032].

Electron transport inhibition. Acetonitrile extracts of cigarette tar inhibited stage three and four respiration of intact mitochondria. Exposure of respiring submitochondrial particles to the acetonitrile extracts of cigarette tar results in a dose-dependent inhibition of oxygen consumption and reduced nicotinamide adenine dinucleotide oxidation. Intact mitochondria were less sensitive to extracts of tar than submitochondrial particles. The nicotinamide adenine dinucleotide (NADH)-ubiquinone (Q) reductase complex was more sensitive to inhibition by tar extract than the succinate-Q reductase and cytochrome complexes. Nicotine or catechol did not inhibit respiration of intact mitochondria. Treatment of submitochondrial particles with cigarette tar resulted in the formation of hydroxyl radicals[NT287].

Embryotoxic effect. Water extract of the dried leaf, administered by gastric intubation to pregnant rats, was active. Preimplantation and implantation periods were most sensitive[NT578].

Emphysematous influence. Smoke was administered to mice at a dose of one cigarette daily for up to 6 months. Some animals received 20 mg of human A1AT (Prolastin) every 48 hours. The treatments produced 63% protection against increased airspace size and abolished smoke-mediated increase in plasma TNF-α[NT018]. Smoke, administered by whole-body exposure to B6C3F1 mice and Fischer-344 rats at a concentration of 250 mg total particulate matter/m^3 for 6 hours/day, 5 days/week for 7 or 13 months, produced an enlargement of parenchymal air spaces in both mice and rats. The alveolar air space was increased significantly only in mice. Tissue loss was decreased at both time points in mice, but not in rats. Morphometric differences in the mice at 13 months were greater than at 7 months. Inflammatory lesions within the lungs of mice contained significantly more neutrophils than those lesions in rats[NT046]. Smoke, administered to macrophage elastase-deficient (MME-/-) mice, produced no increase in the numbers of macrophages in their lungs and did not develop emphysema[NT060]. Cigarette smoke, administered to male weanling rats at a dose of 20 nonfiltered commercial cigarettes/day, 5 days/week for 6 weeks, significantly decreased vitamin A levels in serum, lung, and liver. Histological examination revealed the presence of interstitial pneumonitis along with severe emphysema. There was a significant inverse relationship between vitamin A concentration in the lung and the severity of emphysema ($p <$ 0.03). Detachment or hyperplasia (and metaplasia) of the tracheal epithelium and liver vacuole formation also were evident in the smoke-treated rats[NT194]. Cigarette smoke was administered to rats immunized with rabbit antineutrophil antibody or antimonocyte/macrophage antibody and exposed to cigarette smoke 7 days/week for 2 months. Specific suppression of neutrophil accumulation and neutrophil-related elastinolytic burden in the lungs of the antineutrophil antibody-treated smoke-exposed rats was observed, in contrast to specific suppression of macrophage accumulation and macrophage-related elastinolytic burden in the lungs of the antimonocyte/macrophage antibody-treated smoke-exposed rats. Cigarette smoke exposure-induced lung elastin breakdown and emphysema in the lungs were not prevented in the lungs of antineutrophil antibody-treated smoke-exposed rats but was clearly prevented in lungs of the antimonocyte/macrophage antibody-treated smoke-exposed rats. Results indicate that macrophages rather than neutrophils were the critical pathogenic factor in cigarette smoke-induced emphysema[NT238]. Tobacco smoke was administered to weanling Wistar rats on vitamin E-depleted or normal diet for 4 weeks. The smoke induced emphysematous changes with significant increases in the mean linear intercept and the destructive index. This was supported by an increase in elastase-like activity and a decrease in elastase inhibitory capacity in bronchoalveolar lavage fluid in the normal diet group. In addition to vitamin E depletion, elastase-like activity, elastase inhibitory capacity in bronchoalveolar lavage fluid, and destructive index were comparable to that of tobacco-exposed animals on a normal diet. Mean linear intercept was markedly decreased with thickened epithelium and shrunk alveolar space[NT268].

Endogenous formation of tobacco-specific nitrosamines. (S)-Nicotine and $NaNO_2$ were administered intragastrically to rats at doses of 60 µmol/kg and 180 µmol/kg, respectively, and (S)-nicotine administered at a dose of 12 nmol/kg twice daily for 4 days. The treatments produced no metabolites of NNK;, and its glucuronide in the urine of treated rats. This indicated that endogenous conversion of nicotine to NNK did not occur. The urine contained NNN, N'-nitrosoanabasine (NAB), and N'-nitrosoanatabine (NAT). (S)-Nicotine used in this experiment demonstrated that it contained trace amounts of nornicotine, anabasine, and anatabine. (S)-Nicotine and synthetic (R,S)-nicotine with $NaNO_2$ supplement, administered to rats, produced NNN-, NAB-, and NAT-detectable levels in the urine of the rats treated with the (S)-nicotine and $NaNO_2$. NNN, but not NAB or NAT, was present in the urine of the rats treated with synthetic (R,S)-nicotine and $NaNO_2$. NNN probably formed via nitrosation of metabolically formed nornicotine. These results demonstrated that endogenous formation of tobacco-specific nitrosamines occurred in rats treated with tobacco alkaloids and $NaNO_2$[NT256].

Endothelial dysfunction. Cigarette smoke-treated Krebs buffer was evaluated on rat aortic rings. Agonist-stimulated endothelium-dependent vasorelaxation was measured. Relaxations to receptor-dependent agonists, acetylcholine, and adenosine 5'-diphosphate (ADP), as well as to a receptor-independent agonist, A23187 (Ca^{2+} ionophore) were significantly impaired by cigarette smoke. Cigarette smoke did not impair relaxations to sodium nitroprusside, indicating preserved guanylate cyclase activity. Cigarette smoke did not affect endothelial nitric oxide synthase (NOS) catalytic activity in homogenates from endothelial cells or aortas previously exposed to cigarette smoke-treated Krebs buffer. Treatment with superoxide dismutase or ifetroban and in a lesser degree by indomethacin prevented cigarette smoke-induced endothelial dysfunction[NT205].

Enzymatic activity. STE, administered to lactating mice and suckling neonates at doses of 50 or 100 mg/kg body weight/day, inhibited phytic acid-induced GST/GSH system efficiency and significantly augmented phytic acid- or butylated hydro-xyanisole-induced microsomal phase I enzymes[NT057]. STE, in murine system at doses of 50 or 100 mg/kg body weight/day, elevated microsomal cytochrome b5, CYP, and malondialdehyde levels. These results indicated the inhibitory potential of STE on garlic-induced hepatic GST/GSH system besides significant augmentation on garlic-, mace- or black mustard-induced microsomal cytochromes[NT059].

Epstein–Barr virus early antigen induction. Methanol extract of the dried leaf, in cell culture at a concentration of 1 μg/mL, was inactive. The assay was designed for tumor-promoting activity[NT414]. Two diastereoisomers of 2,7,11-cembratriene-4,6-diol (α- and β-CBT) from the neutral fractions of cigarette smoke condensate, in Raji cells, produced potent inhibitory effects on the induction of Epstein–Barr virus (EBV)-EA by 12-O-tetradecanoylphorbol-13-acetate (TPA). The doses of α- and β-CBT required for 50% inhibition of EBV-EA induction by TPA were 7.7 and 6.7 mg/mL, respectively. Application of α- and β-CBT to mouse skin before treatment with TPA, inhibited TPA-induced ornithine decarboxylase activity in a dose-dependent manner. Application of 16.5 μM/mouse of α- and β-CBT resulted

in a 50% and 40% reduction, respectively, of the maximum ornithine decarboxylase activity induced as a result of treatment with TPA. In initiation-promotion experiments, α-CBT markedly inhibited the promoting effect of TPA on skin tumor formation in mice that were initiated with 7,12-dimethylbenz[a]anthracene. The β-CBT was less effective. Application of 3.3 μM of α-CBT 40 minutes before treatment with TPA (1 μg) resulted in a 53% reduction in the number of papillomas per mouse[NT147].

Estrogenic effect. Tobacco smoke, administered to rats, induced no changes in the rat uterus weight or in oestrus cycle. It decreased estradiol (E2) concentration in the uterus tissue and increased and later decreased the proliferation index and percentage of the cells in the S-phase. The results indicated a phasic character of changes in the reproductive system under the effect of tobacco smoke and corroborated the concept of the role of smoking in the shifting the type of hormonal carcinogenesis from promotional to genotoxic[NT227]. Mainstream cigarette smoke, administered to female rats aged 2.5–3 and 6 months, 2 hours/day for 3 weeks or 3 months, did not induce any changes in uterine weight or estrous cycle. It decreased estradiol (E2) concentration in uterine tissue (especially in adult rats or in young rats after 3 months of experiment). No signs of aneuploidy were found in the uterus through proliferation index. The percentage of cells in S-phase were increased by 3 weeks and decreased by 3 months of experiment[NT240].

Fish poison. Water extract of the fresh leaf was active, LD$_{50}$ 0.23%[NT601].

Follicular fluid mutagenicity. In 24 patients, 12 smoking and 12 nonsmoking, who were treated in an in vitro fertilization program, the mutagenicity of follicular fluid was not influenced by the number of cigarettes smoked. However, urine samples of smoking patients showed a dose-dependent elevation of mutagenicity[NT319].

Foot-and-mouth disease. Tobacco transgenized with foot-and mouth disease virus (FMDV) serotype O using a recombinant tobacco mosaic viruses (TMV)F11 and TMVF14 was administered by parental injection to guinea pigs. The treatment produced a protection against FMDV challenge in case of using TMVF11, TMVF14, or the mixture TMVF11/TMVF14, but not wtTMV. The TMVF11/TMVF14 mixture protected all animals when challenged in 150 guinea pig 50% infection dosage. Oral administration of the mixture (3 mg total) protected 3/8 guinea pigs against the same FMDV challenge. Most of the suckling mice parentally injected with antiserum from guinea pigs immunized with the TMVF11/TMVF14 mixture, but not with wtTMV, were also protected against FMDV challenge with 10 suckling mouse LD_{50}[NT009].

Gastric mucosal exfoliant activity. Leaf, administered orally to adults at a dose of 200 mg/person, was active. Results were significant at $p < 0.05$[NT458].

Gastric mucosal hyperemia inhibition. Tobacco cigarette smoke, administered to rats at doses of 3 and 18 mL/minutes, significantly attenuated hyperemia and aggravated hypertonic saline-induced lesion in a dose-dependent manner. Administration of 18 mL/min of tobacco cigarette smoke and the dose of iv nicotine blocked injury-induced hyperemia. The treatment also aggravated saline-induced gastric damage and gastric mucosal damage induced by acidified aspirin or acidified ethanol[NT269].

Gastric mucus synthesis inhibition. Cigarette smoke, at concentrations of 2 or 4%, was administered to intact animals and animals with ulcers. The treatment significantly reduced the thickness of the mucous-secreting layer and gastric mucosal ornithine decarboxylase activity in animals with or without ulcers. The extract significantly reduced mucous synthesis and ornithine decarboxylase activity but not its mRNA expression in MKN-28 cells[NT217]. Cigarette smoke and its extract, in human MKN-28 cells, markedly decreased mucus synthesis in vivo and in vitro and suppressed ornithine decarboxylase activity[NT225].

Gastric secretory stimulation. Smoke of the dried leaf was administered to smoking adults with duodenal ulcers at variable doses. The treatment reduced the anti-secretory effect of cimetidine from 86 to 38% and inhibited pepsin secretion by 14% during smoking compared with 80% by non-smokers taking cimetidine. In a study with healthy adults, smoking had no effect on cimetidine-induced inhibition of pentagastrin-stimulated gastric acid secretion. The results were significant at $p < 0.05$[NT589].

Gastric ulcerations. Cigarette smoke was administered to rats at doses of 2 or 4% of for three 1-hour periods during a 24-hour starvation before ulcer induction. The treatment potentiated ulcer formation, which was accompanied by a reduction of gastric blood flow at the ulcer base and ulcer margin. Smoke exposure alone did not produce any macroscopic injury in the stomach but significantly decreased the basal gastric blood flow in a concentration-dependent manner, which was coupled with an increase in mucosal xanthine oxidase activity. The increment of constitutive NOS activity but not prostaglandin-E2 level was markedly attenuated by cigarette smoke exposure[NT247]. Tobacco cigarette smoke and subcutaneous nicotine, administered to rats, significantly attenuated the ulcer margin hyperemia in a dose-related manner. Repeated exposure to tobacco cigarette smoke increased ulcer size in the acute and the healing stages. Subcutaneous nicotine also increased the size of ulcers in the acute stage[NT272].

Gene expression. Aqueous extract of the smoke (smoke-bubbled phosphate-buffered saline), in Swiss 3T3 cell culture for 24 hours, produced differential gene expression, mainly antioxidant response genes, genes coding for transcription factor, cell cycle-related genes, and genes-mediators of an inflammatory/immune-regulatory response[NT029]. Cigarette smoke was administered to the ODS rats at doses of 4 mg/day, S4 or 40 mg/day, S40 of ascorbic acid, and exposed to smoke daily for 25 days. The treatment produced a significant decrease of SOD, MnSOD, catalase and protein disulfide isomerase (PDI) by high-dose ascorbic acid administration, and a nonsignificant decrease of plasma glutathione peroxidase. Cigarette smoke exposure slightly increased gene expression of PDI and catalase, but not significantly. The differently expressed 27 genes in the liver were found by differential display methods. From 27 genes, altered expression of plasma proteinase inhibitor, α-1-inhibitor III and CYP1A2 were confirmed by competitive RT-PCR[NT196]. Sidestream smoke was administered to male Wistar rats with a single intratracheal instillation of 2 mg of chrysotile or refractory ceramic fiber. The rats were exposed to smoke 5 days/week for 4 weeks. Administration of smoke alone increased IL-1(α) mRNA levels in alveolar macrophages. The smoke stimulated gene expression of inducible NOS in alveolar macrophages and IL-6 and basic fibroblast growth factor in lungs treated with chrysotile; IL-1(α) in alveolar macrophages and basic fibroblast growth factor in lungs did the same in lungs with refractory ceramic fiber[NT239].

Genotoxicity. Cigarette smoke, administered to male ICR mice, produced DNA single-strand breaks measured 15, 30, 60, 120, and 240 minutes after the exposure. Fifteen minutes after the animals were exposed for 1 minute to a sixfold dilution of smoke, the effect appeared in the lungs, stomach, and liver. The damage in the lungs and liver returned to almost control levels by 60 minutes and the stomach by 120 min-

utes. Kidney, brain, and bone marrow DNA were not damaged. Twelve- or 24-fold smoke dilution did not produce DNA damage. Single oral pretreatment (100 mg/kg) of either ascorbic acid or α-tocopherol acetate 1 hour before inhalation, prevented single-strand breaks in the stomach and liver, while α-tocopherol acetate but not ascorbic acid significantly reduced single-strand breaks in the lung. Five consecutive days of either ascorbic acid or α-tocopherol acetate (100 mg/kg/day) pretreatment completely prevented single-strand breaks in the lung, stomach, and liver[NT044]. Smoke condensate, in two hepatoma cell lines, induced a higher frequency of micronuclei in Hepa1c1c7 cells relative to TAOc1BP(r)c1 cells, which express 10-fold less aromatic hydrocarbon receptor (AhR). Smoke condensate, administered intraperitoneally to Ahr+/+ and Ahr–/– mice at doses of 0.5–10 µg/kg/day for 3 days, produced an increase in the incidence of micronucleated reticulocytes in Ahr+/+ mice, and no increase in the null allele animals. The frequency of micronucleated erythrocytes was slightly but significantly higher in Ahr+/+ relative to Ahr–/– mice[NT051]. Mainstream smoke from TOB-HT or 1R4F cigarettes, administered intranasally to male B6C3/F1 mice at concentrations of 0.16, 0.32, and 0.64 mg total particulate matter/L of air 1 hour/day 5 days/week for 4 weeks, produced an exposure-dependent increase of DNA adducts in lung and heart of animals exposed to 1R4F smoke at all concentrations. The concentration of DNA adducts in lung and heart of TOB-HT cigarette-treated mice was not significantly increased[NT066]. Aqueous suspension of the acetone extract of the paste-like tobacco preparation, administered orally to mice at single or multiple doses, induced significantly high frequencies of chromosome aberrations, micronuclei, and sister chromatid exchange. Single treatment with different doses revealed a distinct dose-dependent increase of the effect. There was a significant positive correlation between time-course of chronic treatment and frequencies of micronucleated cells. Incidences of chromosome aberrations, micronuclei, and sister chromatid exchange in bone marrow cells after repeated treatment for different periods did not differ significantly from each other and from the respective single treatment data for the same dose[NT092]. Aqueous extract of Swedish moist oral snuff, in human V79 lymphocytes, induced sister chromatid exchange and chromosome aberrations, with and without metabolic activation. No induction of point mutations was detected. The methylene chloride extract produced genotoxicity, but no induction of gene mutations in V79 cells was observed. The extract did not induce of micronuclei in mice or of sex-linked recessive lethal mutations in *Drosophila melanogaster*[NT097]. Smoke, in *Salmonella typhimurium* TA97a, TA100, and TA102, produced a threefold to ninefold increase in the frequency of his+ revertants. Activation by a postmitochondrial fraction from liver of rats pretreated with Aroclor-1254 or methylcholanthrene was required. Fractions from phenobarbital-pretreated or untreated rats had no effect. Vitamins A and E, but not C, inhibited the smoke-induced mutagenesis. Treatment of mice with smoke for 60 minutes/day increased the frequency of micronuclei in polychromatic erythrocytes in bone marrow and in fetal liver, and the number of micronucleated normochromatic erythrocytes in peripheral blood by four- to fivefold. Simultaneous treatment of mice with smoke and Na_2SeO_3 reduced the clastogenic effect of tobacco smoke. Ascorbic acid had no effect on clastogenicity but reduced toxicity as measured by body weight loss[NT105]. NNK, administered intravenously to pregnant C57Bl mice, diffused through the placenta and reached the fetal tissues. During the last days of gestation, nasal, pulmonary, and hepatic tissues developed the enzymatic capacity to activate NNK to alkylating species, which bind covalently to cellular macromolecules. Within 4 hours of the injection, a considerable proportion of NNK metabolites present in the fetal tissues were excreted in the amniotic fluid via the fetal urinary tract. Incubation of tissue slices with NNK indicated that the nose, the lung, and the liver of 13-day-old fetuses could reduce NNK to 4-(methylnitrosamino)-1-(3-pyridyl)butan-1-ol (NNA1), but could not activate NNK by α-carbon hydroxylation. Activating enzymes were competent in 18-day-old fetuses, and the activities increased during the first 6 days of life[NT158]. NNK and NNN, in *Salmonella* TA100, TA7004, 7005, and 7006 at concentrations of 250–2000 mg/plate, produced missense backmutations. NNN was active on TA100 and TA7004 but inactive in the presence of rat or hamster S9. NNK was mutagenic only in TA7004 strain with rat or hamster S9, but not in TA100. NNK and NNN, in dark mutant M-169 of *Vibrio fischeri* at concentrations up to 1 mg/mL, were active (Mutatox test). Nicotine, cotinine, *trans*-3-hydroxycotinine, cotinine-*N*-oxide, and nicotine-*N*-oxide were not mutagenic to *Salmonella* TA100 and TA7004 in the presence or absence of rat or hamster S9. The Mutatox test produced direct mutagenicity for COT, 3HC, and NNO, but not CNO. The latter was mutagenic in the Mutatox test with rat or hamster S9, but only rat S9 was effective for COT, NNO, and 3HC. Inhibitory potentiations of NNN by NIC and COT were observed on strain TA7004 and by NIC on strain TA100. There were no interactions on NNK in the presence of S9 for strain TA7004 or TA100. In contrast, a complex inhibition and enhancement behavior occurred in the Mutatox test for each interaction, but no effects were observed for CNO on NNK without S9, and few for NIC on NNK with hamster S9[NT206].

Glutathione formation induction. Methyl chloride extract of the leaf, administered intragastrically to rats at a dose of 3 mg/animal daily for 21 months in DMSO solvent, was active. The rats were divided into two groups: one was fed a vitamin A diet, and the other a vitamin A-deficient diet. Treatment with extract increased glutathione levels in both liver and lung in the vitamin-fed rats. In the vitamin-deficient group, hepatic and pulmonary glutathione levels were decreased by treatment with extract[NT519].

GSH peroxidase activity. Cigarette smoke was administered to the ODS rats at doses of 4 mg/day, S4 or 40 mg/day, S40 of ascorbic acid, and exposed to smoke daily for 25 days. The treatment produced a significant decrease of CuZn-SOD, MnSOD, catalase, and PDI by high-dose ascorbic acid administration, and nonsignificant decrease of plasma GSH peroxidase[NT196].

GST activity. Cigarette smoke, administered intranasally to young male C57BL mice fed 0, 5, and 100 ppm of vitamin E, 20 minutes/day for 8 weeks, produced no effect GST[NT153].

GST inhibition. Methyl chloride extract of the leaf, administered intragastrically to rats at a dose of 3 mg/animal daily for 21 months in DMSO solvent, was active. The rats were divided into two groups: one was fed a vitamin A diet, and the other a vitamin A-deficient diet. In the vitamin-deficient group, the treatment decreased GST levels in liver and lung vs control and vitamin-fed groups[NT519].

Glycation products formation. Reactive glycation products from an aqueous extract of tobacco and tobacco smoke reacted with proteins to form advanced glycation end products. The end products circulated in high concentrations in the plasma of patients with diabetes or renal insufficiency and have been linked to the accelerated vasculopathy seen in patients with these diseases. Glycotoxins (glycation products) exhibited a specific fluorescence when cross-linked to proteins and were mutagenic. Glycotoxins were transferred to the serum proteins of human smokers. Advanced glycation end products (AGE)-apolipoprotein (apo) B and serum AGE

levels in cigarette smokers were significantly higher than those in nonsmokers[NT248].

Hematopoiesis inhibition. Smoke, in bone-marrow culture in a long-term treatment, produced an inhibition of hematopoiesis. Nicotine significantly delayed the onset of hematopoietic loci and reduced their size, the number of long-term culture-initiating cells, nonadherent mature cells, and their progenitors but failed to influence the proliferation of committed hematopoietic progenitors when added into methylcellulose cultures. Exposure to nicotine decreased CD44 surface expression on primary bone marrow-derived fibroblast-like stromal cells and MS-5 stromal cell line but not on hematopoietic cells. Mainstream smoke altered the trafficking of hematopoietic stem/progenitor cells (HSPC) in vivo. Smoke exposure produced an inhibition of HSPC homing into bone marrow. Nicotine and cotinine treatment resulted in reduction of CD44 surface expression on lung micro-vascular endothelial cell line (LEI-SVO) and bone marrow-derived (STR-12) endothelial cell line. Nicotine increased E-selectin expression on LEISVO cells but not on STR-12 cells[NT035].

Heme oxygenase expression. Mainstream smoke trapped in phosphate-buffered saline solutions, in Swiss albino 3T3 fibroblasts, produced dose-dependent and transiently elevated expression of heme oxygenase. Heme oxygenase protein and its mRNA were detectable between 1 and 24 hours after exposure to 0.03 puffs (approx 1 cm^3/mL of medium). A nearly 50-fold increase in the amount of heme oxygenase mRNA was determined after 8 hours of exposure, compared to control levels. A decrease of more than 60% in glutathione levels was observed after the exposure. No elevated amounts of heme oxygenase mRNA appeared in smoke treated-cells when cysteine was exogenously added[NT083].

Hepatic enzymes activity. Tobacco smoke, administered by Hamburg II machine to mice at a dose of eight cigarettes per day for 2, 4, 8, or 31 days, significantly increased HbCO after 4 or 8 days of exposure and decreased after 31 days. The enzymate activities were significantly higher during the period of exposure[NT069].

Hepatic lipid peroxidation. Aqueous extract of STE activated macrophages with the resultant production of reactive oxygen species, including nitric oxide. Administration to rats at doses of 125–500 mg/kg induced dose-dependent increase in mitochondrial and microsomal lipid peroxidation, enhanced DNA single-strand breaks, and significantly increased the urinary excretion of the lipid metabolites malondialdehyde, formaldehyde, acetaldehyde, and acetone. Extract, administered orally to female Sprague–Dawley rats at a dose of 25 mg/kg daily for 105 days, increased lipid peroxidation 1.4- to 3.3-fold in hepatic mitochondria and microsome. Maximum increase in lipid peroxidation and DNA single-strand breaks occurred between 75 and 90 days of treatment. Maximum increase of urinary excretion of the four lipid metabolites malondialdehyde, formaldehyde, acetaldehyde, and acetone was observed between 60 and 75 days of treatment[NT242]. Aqueous STD, administered to rats at doses of 125, 250, and 500 mg/kg, produced dose-dependent increase of 1.8, 2.3, and 4.4-fold in mitochondrial and 1.5, 2.1, and 3.6-fold in microsomal lipid peroxidation at doses tested, respectively, relative to control values. At the same three doses of the extract, 1.3, 1.4, and 2.7-fold increases in hepatic DNA single-strand breaks occurred relative to control values. Administration also resulted in significant increases in excretion of urinary metabolites. Urinary excretion of the four lipid metabolites, malondialdehyde, formaldehyde, acetaldehyde, and acetone, were increased at every dose and time point with maximum increase between 12 and 24 hours after treatment[NT275]. Cigarette smoke, administered intranasally to young male C57BL mice fed 5 and 100 ppm of vitamin E, 20 minutes/day for 8 weeks, increased hepatic lipid peroxidation[NT153].

Histological changes. Mainstream smoke from a 1R4F and 2R4F research cigarette was administered intranasally to rats at doses of 0.06, 0.20, or 0.80 mg wet total particulate matter per liter of air for 1 hour/day, 5 days/week for 13 weeks. The treatment produced no significant differences between both tobacco types. After 13 weeks of the recovery period, there were no statistically significant differences in histopathological findings observed between the 1R4F and the 2R4F cigarettes. The complete toxicological assessment in this comparative inhalation study of 1R4F and 2R4F cigarettes suggests no overall biologically significant differences between the rats exposed to the two cigarettes[NT192]. Flue-cured tobacco was administered to rats at doses of 0.06, 0.20, or 0.80 mg wet total particulate matter per liter of air for 1 hour/day, 5 days/week, for 13 weeks. The only significant difference was increased epithelial hyperplasia of the anterior nasal cavity in males in the high-exposure group for the heat-exchanger cigarette. At the end of the exposure period, subsets of rats from each group were maintained without smoke exposures for an additional 13 week (recovery period). At the end of the recovery period, there were no statistically significant differences in histopathological findings between heat-exchanger-cured tobacco cigarette when compared to direct-fired cured tobacco cigarette[NT195].

Hypercholesterolemic activity. Leaf, administered by inhalation to adults of both sexes at variable concentrations, was active. Serum cholesterol was higher in persons smoking cigarettes in all age groups. The number of cigarettes smoked per day had a direct correlation with the serum total cholesterol, which increased as the number of cigarettes smoked per day increased[NT582].

Hyperplasia induction. Smoke condensate with nonpolar arotinoid, Ro 15-0778, in rodent respiratory epithelia organ culture antagonized the carcinogen-induced hyperplasia and metaplasia. In neonatal rat tracheas and fetal mouse lungs grown in vitro, 3,4-benzpyrene and cigarette smoke condensate induced an increased proliferation of epithelial cells associated with a loss of secretory activity and ciliary function. In explants pretreated with cigarette smoke condensate, Ro 15-0778 reversed the high proliferation rate and restored secretory differentiation and ciliary function[NT132]. Cigarette smoke condensate, in fetal mouse lung and neonatal rat tracheas organ cultures, induced a striking increase of epithelial mitosis within 12–14 days of treatment. The increase was associated with a loss of secretory activity and of ciliary function. Administration of etretinate with smoke condensate inhibited the increase in cell division and prevented the loss of secretory activity or ciliary function. In explants pretreated with cigarette smoke condensate, etretinate reduced the smoke condensate-induced increase in mitotic activity to normal levels and restored secretory differentiation and ciliary function[NT165].

Hypersecretion of mucous. Cigarette smoke, in rat larynx and trachea preparation exposed for 2 weeks, significantly increased the secretion of fucose-containing glycoconjugates above normal level[NT295].

Hypertensive activity. Water extract of the dried leaf, administered intravenously to cats and rats at doses of 1–4 mg/kg, produced an initial hypertension followed by hypotension[NT588].

Hypoxic pulmonary effect. Cigarette smoke, in isolated rat lungs perfused with blood, produced no change in pulmonary vascular resistance. The hypoxic pulmonary vasoconstriction was significantly enhanced by smoking. Indomethacin, an inhibitor of prostaglandins biosynthesis, administered in the perfusing blood (20 µg/mL) increased hypoxic pulmonary vasoconstriction in the nonsmoking lungs but not in lungs after smoking. Diethylcarbamazine citrate (DEC)

(1 mg/mL), an inhibitor of leukotrienes biosynthesis, decreased hypoxic pulmonary vasoconstriction before and after smoking. After perfusion with both indomethacin and DEC, hypoxic pulmonary vasoconstriction also decreased. Results indicated that leukotrienes act as mediators, whereas prostaglandins as modulators in hypoxic pulmonary vasoconstriction and prostaglandins and leukotrienes may play an important role in the increase of hypoxic pulmonary vasoconstriction by cigarette smoking[NT286]. Cigarette smoke extract, administered intravenously to Wistar rats during hypoxic ventilation, produced significant decrease in microvascular internal diameter of pulmonary arterioles and venules. After pretreatment of animal with smoke extract, much more remarkable pulmonary vasoconstriction was induced by hypoxia than before injection of the extract. During hypoxia, mean pulmonary arterial pressure increased by 13.53% before administration of smoke extract and by 30.57% after administration, respectively. Results indicated that smoke extract can strengthen pulmonary vasoconstriction and hypertension induced by acute alveolar hypoxia[NT288].

Immunogenicity. Tobacco was transferred by cholera toxin B (CTB) subunit of *Vibrion cholerae* encoding gene. An aliquot of total protein from the transgenic leaf tissue, administered intradermally to Balb/c (H2K-[d]) mice at a concentration of 5 µg/mL recombinant CTB, produced CTB-specific serum IgG in animals. Macrophages isolated from mice immunized with native or plant-expressed CTB showed enhanced secretion of IL-10. The secretion of lipopolysaccharide-induced IL-12 and TNF-α was inhibited. Results indicated that plant-expressed protein behaved like native CTB regarding effects on T-cell proliferation and cytokine levels[NT008]. Tobacco transgenized with recombinant FaeG protein (major subunit and adhesion of K88ad fimbriae), administered to mice, produced immunogenicity comparable to that generated with traditional approaches[NT012]. Tobacco, transgenized with an anti-hepatitis B virus surface antigen mouse IgG-1 monoclonal antibody, was active[NT015]. Extract of the leaf expressing Norwalk virus-like particles, administered intragastrically to CD1 mice, produced serum and secretory specific IgA[NT070]. Transgenic tobacco expressing genes encoding *Escherichia coli* heat-labile enterotoxin or *Escherichia coli* heat-labile enterotoxin fusion protein, administered intragastrically to mice, resulted in production of serum and gut mucosal anti-*Escherichia coli* heat-labile enterotoxin immunoglobulins that neutralized the enterotoxin in cell protection assay[NT074]. Transgenic tobacco leaf expressing recombinant hepatitis B surface antigen produced response qualitatively similar to those obtained by immunizing mice with commercial vaccine. T-cells were obtained from mice primed with the tobacco-derived recombinant hepatitis B surface antigenic peptide that represents part of the a determinant of hepatitis B surface antigen[NT076]. Tobacco smoke administered to mice for 3 days, 18 or 28 weeks before sheep red blood cell (SRBC) inoculation, produced "shorter-lived" splenomegaly. Mice exposed to smoke for 3 days or 18 weeks produced a reduction in both the magnitude and the duration of the primary immune response as evidenced by the pattern of expansion of splenic white pulp and "RNA-rich" white pulp volumes. Mice exposed to smoke for 28 weeks produced white pulp and "RNA-rich" white pulp volumes similar to those of control mice[NT170]. Extract of tobacco leaf and tobacco smoke components, administered to mice and rabbits, produced reaginic antibody in mice and precipitating antibody in rabbits. The results indicated that tobacco smoke extracts stimulated immune responses to tobacco leaf antigens in rabbits

and mice. The immunogen is apparently not a product of incineration because air passed through unlit cigarettes clearly extracted the antigenic component[NT174].

Immunostimulatory activity. Water extract of the dried leaf, administered to mice at a dose of 0.5%, was active on splenocytes and produced polyclonal AB response[NT449]. Mouse-tobacco hybrid calli and complete plants generated by somatic cell fusion of mouse spleen cells and tobacco mesophyll protoplasts produced mouse Ig-γ-3-heavy and λ-light chains[NT078]. Aqueous extract of the STD, in mouse lymphoid cells, produced a significant increase in the proliferation of spleen cells. The polyclonal IgM antibody responses were elevated in smoke-stimulated spleen cell cultures. Similar immunostimulatory results were found in the mesenteric lymph node cells. The extract stimulated the spleen cells of the immune defective CBA/N mice. The extract was mitogenic to B- and T-cells in the lipopolysaccharide-resistant C3H/HeJ mice spleen cells. The proliferation of T cells was not accompanied by secretion of IL-2 or expression of IL-2 receptors on T-cells. There was an increase of IL-1 activity in spleen cells. Activation of B- or T-lymphocytes did not result in the elevation of intracellular calcium levels[NT088].

Immunosuppressive activity. Water-soluble condensate of tobacco smoke, administered to C57Bl/6 mice at sublethal doses, inhibited the ability to respond to immunization with sheep erythrocytes by the formation of plaque-forming cells. Spleen cells from water-soluble condensate-treated mice were unable to mount a primary response to SRBC in vitro. There was a decrease in T-lymphocytes in the spleens of treated mice. T-cells from water-soluble condensate-treated mice were unable to cooperate with normal B-cells and macrophages in the response to SRBC. A less marked suppression of B-cell function was noted in condensate-treated mice. Although B-cells from such animals were able to co-operate with normal T-cells and macrophages to give a detectable primary response to SRBC, the response was depressed. Macrophages from water-soluble condensate-treated animals enhanced the response of normal T- and B-cells to SRBC[NT172].

Inflammation induction. Water extract of the leaf, administered intragastrically to mice at a dose of 4.9 g/kg 6 days per week for 5 months, was active. The extract consisted of 15 g *Areca catechu* nut, 10 g tobacco leaf, and either 3 or 10 g lime to which was added water extract of *Piper betle* leaf. Addition of the latter enhanced the effect, whereas the larger dose of lime antagonized the effect[NT612]. Ether extract of the dried leaf, administered externally to mice at a dose of 10 mL, was inactive[NT414].

Insecticidal activity. Alkaloid fraction and methanol extract of the leaf were active on *Culex pipens* larvae. Fifty or more percent lethality after 24–48 hours was obtained[NT613]. Acetone extract of the dried leaf, at variable doses, produced 80.6% mortality vs snout moths larva of rice[NT441]. Water extract of the dried leaf was active on *Phyllocnistis citrella*[NT616]. Methanol extract of the dried leaf, at a dose of 50 mg/mL, was inactive on *Rhinocephalus appendiculatus*. Inhibition of oviposition was used as a measure of ascaricidal activity[NT593]. Ethanol (95%) extract of the dried leaf, at a concentration of 50 μg/mL, was inactive on *Rhodnius neglectus*[NT456]. Methanol extract of the dried root, at a concentration of 50 μg/mL, was active on *Rhipicephalus appendiculatus*. The extract of dried stem was inactive. Inhibition of oviposition was used as a measure of ascaricidal activity[NT593].

Intercellular communication inhibition. Cigarette smoke condensate, administered by the microinjection-dye transfer technique to smooth muscle cells of human and rat, was able to inhibit intercellular communication in human and rat cells in a dose-dependent manner up to 60%[NT291].

Interferon-α/β production. Mainstream and sidestream smoke from Kentucky 2R1 reference cigarette, in murine L-929 cells were administered at the highest doses possible to generate a minimum toxic effect. The dose was then serially diluted to lower doses. The treatment produced viability of exposed cells equivalent to control cell cultures. Addition of polyriboinosinic–polyribocytidylic acid to the cells reduced the IFN production in viable smoke-exposed cells. Aging of smoke by delaying time of exposure of the cells to the smoke or filtration of smoke through activated charcoal has substantially decreased the alteration of IFN production by smoke exposure[NT142]. 4-aminobiphenyl, aniline-HCl, hydrazine sulfate, and 2-methylquinoline, administered intraperitoneally to mice, induced IFN production at 2, 24, or 48 hours after treatment. Mice treated with 4-aminobiphenyl showed some depression of IFN production 2 hours after treatment. Maximum inhibition of IFN induction was observed 24 hours after treatment and a return to control levels 48 hours after treatment. Mice treated with hydrazine sulfate showed maximum inhibition of IFN induction 24 hours after treatment, but no effects at any other treatment time. Treatment of mice with aniline-HCl resulted in marginal depression of IFN induction 24 hours after treatment. 2-methylquinoline had no effect[NT160]. 4-aminobiphenyl and aniline-HCl from sidestream cigarette smoke, in mouse embryo fibroblast cell cultures, produced severely reduced levels of α/β IFN after challenge with polyriboinosinic–polyribocytidylic acid when compared to control cultures. Treatment of additional cell cultures with 2-methylquinoline and intermediate-level component of sidestream tobacco smoke or hydrazine-sulfate also resulted in inhibition of IFN induction with polyriboinosinic acid–polyribocytidylic acid[NT164].

IL-12 activity stimulation. STD stimulated p40 and p35 promoter activity of the IL-12 (p70), and enhanced IFN-γ-induced p40 and p35 promoter activity. It had no effect on lipopolysaccharide-induced p35 and p40 promoter activity and diminished IFN-γ/lipopolysaccharide-induced p35 promoter activity. The results indicated that tobacco extract stimulation of bioactive IL-12 production is correlated with its effect on both p35 and p40 subunits. Stimulation of IL-12 production can increase the chances of oral inflammatory disease[NT016]. STD, in cell culture, decreased production of IL-12 p40 and p70 from lipopolysaccharide-stimulated peritoneal macrophages, lipopolysaccharide/IFN γ-stimulated peritoneal and splenic macrophages, and increased production of IL-12 p40 and p70 from IFN γ/CD40-stimulated splenic macrophages or IFN-γ-stimulated peritoneal macrophages. None of the effects resulted from nicotine, rutin, or chlorogenic acid. Nicotine, at a concentration of 100 µg/mL, significantly elevated production of IL-12 p40 and p70 from splenic macrophages stimulate by IFN-γ/lipopolisaccharide[NT031].

IL-I formation stimulation. Water extract of the dried leaf, administered to mice at a concentration of 0.05%, was active on splenocytes[NT449].

IL-II receptor gene stimulation. Water extract of the dried leaf, administered to mice at a concentration of 1%, was inactive on T-lymphocytes[NT449].

Intraepithelial mucosubstance effect. Diluted mainstream cigarette smoke was administered to F344 rats for 9 days for a 2-week period. After the last exposure, the treatment produced 270% more intraepithelial mucosubstances in the dorsal septum, 58% less intraepithelial mucosubstances in the midseptum, and amounts of intraepithelial mucosubstances in the ventral septum similar to controls. Smoke-exposed rats humanely killed 14 days after exposure still had increased amounts of intraepithelial mucosubstances in the dorsal septal region. There was no effect in regions of squamous metaplasia or amounts of intraepithelial mucosubstances in the midseptal and ventral septal regions that were different from air-exposed controls. Smoke exposure resulted in a significant increase in the unit length-labeling index at 1 day but not 14 days after exposure in the ventral and midseptal regions only[NT271].

Intraocular pressure reduction. Water extract of the dried leaf, administered intravenously to rabbits at a dose of 250 µg/animal, was active[NT512].

Irradiation-induced pneumonitis suppression. Diluted mainstream tobacco smoke was administered intranasally to rats at a concentration of approx 0.4 mg/L for 1 hour/day, 1–5 days/week for 10 weeks, 3 weeks before irradiation. The treatment produced less inflammation in the alveolar tissue in the irradiated smoke-exposed group than in the irradiated not exposed to smoke group. Mast cells were increased 100-fold in the lung interstitium and 30-fold in the peribronchial area in the irradiated not exposed to smoke group, whereas no increase was found in the irradiated smoke-exposed group or in the controls. The alveolar septa of the irradiated not-exposed group were thickened, with occurrence of inflammatory cells and mast cells, whereas the irradiated smoke-exposed group displayed no difference as compared to controls[NT282].

L-Ascorbic acid influence. Sidestream cigarette smoke, administered to male Wistar rats for 2 hours daily for 25 days, produced an increase of the excreted amount of L-ascorbic acid in the urine. At the end of the experimental period, the L-ascorbic acid content of the plasma and tissues, liver cytochrome P450 content, and the activities of drug-metabolizing enzymes in the test group were higher than the control[NT243].

Leukocyte dynamics. The effect of chronic smoking on the microcirculation immediately after exposure to smoke for 2, 4, and 6 weeks and after withholding smoke for 2 weeks from those previously exposed for 4 weeks was investigated. The mean rolling leucocytes at 2, 4, and 6 weeks were 11.10 ± 1.8, 23.7 ± 2.3, 40.2 ± 3.9 ($p < 0.001$). The rolling leukocytes, after smoking for 4 weeks and then having smoke withheld for 2 weeks, was 9.6 ± 1.4. The mean adherent leucocytes were 5 ± 0.7, 7.5 ± 1.1, 12.6 ± 1.8 ($p < 0.001$). The adherent leucocytes, after smoking for 4 weeks and then having smoke withheld for 2 weeks, was 3.5 ± 0.5. The results confirmed those of many previous studies of the adverse effects of cigarette smoking and that those deleterious effects are time-dependent. The reversibility of the deleterious effect of cigarette smoking after cessation of cigarette smoking before face-lift or flap reconstruction is at least 2 weeks. This information is also important for clinical management of patients who smoke and are scheduled for face-lift and flap reconstruction. Two weeks without cigarettes is a necessary period for successful elective plastic surgery[NT200].

Lipemic activity. Cigarette smoke extract, in macrophages with LDL culture at a dose of 100 μg/mL, stimulated cholesteryl oleate synthesis approximately equal to 12.5-fold. Enhancement in cholesteryl ester synthesis was dependent on the concentration of smoke-modified LDL and exhibited saturation kinetics. There was extensive fragmentation of apo B. This LDL modification depended on the incubation time and concentration of the smoke extract. Superoxide dismutase inhibited LDL modification by 52%, suggesting that superoxide anion is involved. The results indicated that smoke extract alters LDL into a form recognized and incorporated by macrophages[NT125]. En-

vironmental tobacco smoke, administered to rats, produced an increase in the rate of LDL accumulation. LDL accumulation was primarily dependent on LDL interaction with environmental tobacco smoke–plasma rather than the interaction of environmental tobacco smoke–plasma with the artery wall[NT261].

Lung aryl hydrocarbon hydroxylase activity. Cigarette smoke, administered intranasally to young male C57BL mice fed 5 and 100 ppm of vitamin E, 20 minutes/day for 8 weeks, produced no effect on hepatic aryl hydrocarbon hydroxylase. All of the mice on the vitamin E-free diet showed reduced lung aryl hydrocarbon hydroxylase activity. Lung aryl hydrocarbon hydroxylase activity was increased in all of the smoke-exposed mice[NT153].

Lymphocyte viability and proliferation. Acetaldehyde, benzene, butyraldehyde, isoprene, styrene, and toluene in mouse lymphocytes cell culture for 3 hours produced no effect on either viability or proliferation. Formaldehyde, catechol, acrylonitrile, propionaldehyde, and hydroquinone significantly inhibited T-lymphocyte and B-lymphocyte proliferation, inhibitory concentration $(IC)_{50}$ 1.19×10^{-5} M to 8.20×10^{-4} M. Acrolein and crotonaldehyde inhibited T-cell and B-cell proliferation and acted on viability with IC_{50} 2.06×10^{5} M to 4.26×10^{-5} M. Mixtures of acrolein, formaldehyde, and propionaldehyde or crotonaldehyde interactive effects at 0.5 and $1 \times IC_{50}$ were observed[NT022].

Malignant cell transformation. Smoke of cured leaf, administered to leaf-cutter ants at an undiluted concentration, was active on primary spermatocytes[NT404].

MAO inhibition. 2-Naphthylamine from smoke, in cell culture, inhibited mouse brain MAO A and B by mixed competitive- and noncompetitive-type inhibition[NT038].

Mastocytoma induction. Cigarette smoke condensate suspensions ("tars") from different cigarettes, administered to female CD-1 mice, produced cutaneous mastocytomas accompanied by diffuse dermal mast cell infiltration[NT145]. Cigarette smoke condensate suspensions ("tar"), administered to CAF1/J and ARS-HA (ICR) female mice on long-term application, produced a significant incidence of cutaneous mastocytomas. The skin mastocytomas were constantly accompanied by diffuse dermal mast cell infiltration, which was also seen in the tumor-free skin of the "tar"-treated mice[NT169].

Metabolizing enzymes induction. Masheri, a pyrolyzed tobacco product, administered orally to Swiss mice, Sprague–Dawley rats, and Syrian golden hamsters at a dose of 10% diet for 20 months, produced a significant induction of CYP and benzo(a) pyrene hydroxylase in proximal and distal parts of the three species. GSH and GST were depleted on masheri treatment in all three species only in proximal and distal parts of the intestine[NT100].

Metaplasia induction. Smoke condensate with nonpolar arotinoid, Ro 15-0778, in rodent respiratory epithelia organ culture, antagonized the carcinogen-induced hyperplasia and metaplasia. In neonatal rat tracheas and fetal mouse lungs grown in vitro, 3,4-benzpyrene and cigarette smoke condensate induced an increased proliferation of epithelial cells associated with a loss of secretory activity and ciliary function. In explants pretreated with cigarette smoke condensate, Ro 15-0778 reversed the high proliferation rate and restored secretory differentiation and ciliary function[NT132]. Cigarette smoke condensate, in fetal mouse lung and neonatal rat tracheas organ cultures, induced a striking increase of epithelial mitosis within 12–14 days of treatment. The increase was associated with a loss of secretory activity and of ciliary function. Administration of etretinate with smoke condensate inhibited the increase in cell division and prevented the loss of secretory

activity or ciliary function. In explants pretreated with cigarette smoke condensate, etretinate reduced the smoke condensate-induced increase in mitotic activity to normal levels and restored secretory differentiation and ciliary function[NT165].

Metaplasia induction. Water extract of the leaf, administered intragastrically to mice at a dose of 4.9 g/kg, was active. The extract consisted of 15.0 g *Areca catechu* nut, 10 g tobacco leaf, and either 3 or 10 g lime to which was added water extract of *Piper betle* leaf[NT612]. Cigarette smoke, administered to rats at a dose of 250 mg total particulate matter/m^3 6 hours/day for 5 days, increased the number of small mucous cells in the respiratory epithelium of the nasal septum in the early stages of squamous differentiation, but they were gradually replaced by squamous metaplastic cells. At 5 days after the withdrawal of cigarette smoke exposure, the morphology of the midseptal epithelium returned to that of a pseudostratified mucociliary epithelium and the epithelia lining the maxilloturbinates to that of a transitional epithelium[NT265].

Mitochondrial ATPase inhibition. Smoke extract, in the mouse brain mitochondria culture in the presence or absence of vitamin C for 60 minutes, inhibited mitochondrial ATPase and cytochrome C oxidase activities in a dose-dependent manner. The effect of extract on mitochondria swelling response to calcium stimulation was dependent on calcium concentrations. The extract treatment induced mitochondrial inner membrane damage and vacuolization of the matrix, whereas the outer mitochondrial membrane was preserved. Nicotine produced no significant damage[NT007].

Mitogenic activity. Water extract of the dried leaf, administered to mice at a concentration of 0.05%, was active on lymphocytes from mesenteric lymph node and lymphocytes B and T. Intracellular Ca^{2+} level was unchanged. The extract was active on splenocytes. There was an effect in cells from strains irresponsible to lipopolysaccharide[NT449].

Mitotic effect. STE, administered to the buccal mucosa of 15 female HMT rats, 6 months of age, weekly for 1 year, produced hyperorthokeratosis, acanthosis, numerous binucleate spinous cells, and subepithelial connective tissue hyalinization. Verrucous carcinoma and squamous cell carcinoma were not seen. Karyotyping revealed that lymphocytes of tobacco-treated, as well as control rats, had normal chromosome number and morphology. However, approx 25% of buccal epithelial cells of the tobacco-treated rats were tetraploid and 5% octaploid, compared with only 11% tetraploid and no octaploid in the controls. Results indicated that the mitotic process could be disturbed by tobacco treatment[NT297].

Molluscicidal activity. Water extract of the dried leaf, at a concentration of 168 ppm, produced equivocal effect on *Lymnaea luteola*[NT551].

Morphologic and pathological changes. Cigarette smoke inhalation and hydrocortisone acetate (HCA), administered to C57BL/6 male mice, induced in the lungs a marked reduction of pulmonary macrophage population that is normally elevated by smoke inhalation, an accumulation of surfactant and flocculent material in alveoli, a decrease in alveolar space surrounded by normal septal tissue, and an increase in hypertrophied alveolar parenchyma. Concomitant with altered lung morphology, lung volume and gas diffusing capacity were significantly compromised. Smoke inhalation or HCA administration alone had no ill effects[NT150]. Tobacco application (snuff water extract or smoking tar condensate) and herpes simplex virus (HSV)-1 inoculation, administered to mice for 2 months, produced epithelial dysplasia and other histomorphologic changes (hyperkeratosis, increased granular cell layer thickness, acanthosis, and increased inflammatory cell infiltration) in a significant number of animals. Tobacco or HSV-1 when administered alone did not induce dysplasia in the epithelium of labial mucosa. The result indicated that HSV-1 and tobacco could possibly act synergistically in the development of precancerous oral lesions and oral cancer[NT152]. Fresh smoke, administered to Balb/c mice at a daily equivalent of 30 high-tar filtered cigarettes for up to 95 weeks, produced an induction or production of significant numbers of malignant tumors of several types. Significant histopathological changes that consisted mainly of interstitial pneumonia and focal low-grade emphysema were observed[NT167]. Alveolar and bronchiolar spaces in the lungs of cigarette smokers contained numerous macrophages with pigmented cytoplasmic granules resulting from increased numbers of lysosomes and phagolysosomes and "smokers' inclusions" in the interstitial and alveolar macrophages of cigarette users. The inclusions have been referred to as "needle-shaped" and "fiber-like." Thin sectioning techniques impart varying lengths to the inclusions, suggesting that they have a disc, or platelet, configuration. Surgically resected lung tissue contained varying numbers of hexagonal plate-like particles that had features consistent with those of the aluminum silicate kaolinite, and energy-dispersive X-ray spectrometry confirmed the presence of these two elements. The origin of aluminum silicate inclusions in pulmonary macrophages has yet to be determined, although preliminary evidence strongly suggests that they were derived from inhaled tobacco smoke[NT190]. A mixture of mainstream and sidestream cigarette smoke, administered by whole-body exposure to Sprague–Dawley rats for 28 days, produced dramatic alterations of DNA adducts in bronchoalveolar lavaged cells, tracheal epithelium, lung, and heart. Oxidative damage to pulmonary DNA, hemoglobin adducts of 4-aminobiphenyl and benzo(a)pyrene-7,8-diol-9,10-

epoxide, micronucleated and polynucleated alveolar macrophages, and micronucleated polychromatic erythrocytes in bone marrow were also observed[NT209]. Mainstream smoke from an Eclipse and 1R4F reference cigarettes, administered to Sprague–Dawley rats of each gender at concentrations of 0, 0.16, 0.32, or 0.64 mg wet total particulate matter/liter air for 1 hour/day, 5 days/week for 13 weeks, produced a decrease of respiratory rate at all concentrations of 1R4F smoke and at the high concentration of Eclipse smoke. Tidal volume was depressed and minute volume was lower for all smoke-exposed rats. Carboxyhemoglobin and serum nicotine were directly related to the exposure concentrations of carbon monoxide and nicotine in an exposure-dependent manner. Body weights were slightly lower in smoke-exposed rats. The only treatment-related effect found in organ weights was an increase in heart weight in females in the Eclipse high-concentration exposure group. Nasal epithelial hyperplasia and ventral laryngeal squamous metaplasia were noted after exposure to either the 1R4F or Eclipse smoke. The degree of change was less in Eclipse smoke-exposed rats. Lung macrophages were increased to a similar extent in the Eclipse and 1R4F smoke-exposed groups. Brown/gold pigmented macrophages were detected in the lungs of rats exposed to 1R4F smoke, but not those exposed to Eclipse smoke[NT214].

mRNA expression. Cigarette smoke was administered to intact animals and animals with ulcers at concentrations of 2 or 4%. The treatment significantly reduced the thickness of the mucous secreting layer and gastric mucosal ornithine decarboxylase activity in animals with or without ulcers. The extract significantly reduced mucus synthesis and ornithine decarboxylase activity but not its mRNA expression in MKN-28 cells[NT217].

Murine CD4 T-cell costimulatory counterreceptors. STD, in splenic mononuclear cells at 1:10² to 1:10³ dilutions or 1–100 μg/mL nicotine for 48 and 72 hours of stimulation with anti-CD3, produced an increase of percentage and intensity of CTLA-4 expression and a decrease of CD28 expression during an exposure to a 1:10² dilution. Exposure to nicotine decreased the percentage of CD4+ T-cells expressing both CD28 and CTLA-4 and decreased the intensity of CD28 expression. Responding T-cells exposed to nicotine produced significantly less Th1 cytokines, IL-2 and IFN-γ, but significantly more Th2 cytokines, IL-4, and IL-10. Cytokine specific mRNA expression was only slightly affected by the exposure to nicotine[NT068].

Murine embryopathy. NNK, administered intraperitoneally to pregnant CD-1 mice during organogenesis at a dose of 100 mg/kg, produced open eye and one case of a cleft palate in 3 of 374 fetuses, which were not observed in 160 controls. With phenobarbital plus NNK, two fetuses had a cleft palate, two had exencephaly and one had a kinky tail, although phenobarbital controls showed no anomalies. NNK-initiated fetal postpartum lethality was enhanced by phenobarbital pretreatment. There were no fetal skeletal anomalies or alterations in resorptions or fetal body weight in any group. In embryo culture, gestational day 9.5 embryos exposed to and 10 μM of NNK had decreased yolk sac diameter, crown-rump length and somite development, and 100 μM of NNK decreased anterior neuropore closure and crown-rump length ($p <$ 0.05). Embryos exposed to 100 μM of NNK were assessed for K-*ras* codon 12 mutations and none was detected[NT050].

Mutagenic activity. Smoke of cured leaf, in broth culture was active on *Salmonella typhimurium*[NT402]. Environmental cigarette smoke, administered by whole-body to p53 mutant (UL53-3 × A/J)F₁ mice of both genders for up to 9.5 months, produced similar oxidative DNA damage in lung and heart of both mutants and wild-type littermate controls, proliferation of the bronchial epithelium, and levels of p53 oncoprotein as assessed after exposure for 28 days. Smoke-exposed mutant mice underwent a lower induction of apoptosis in bronchial epithelium, a greater formation of DNA adducts in lung and heart, and a more intense cytogenic damage. At the end of experiment, DNA adducts were not repaired in either wild-type or mutant mice after discontinuing exposure to smoke for 1 week. A weak but significant increase of lung tumor incidence and multiplicity was induced in p53 mutant mice after exposure to smoke for either 5 months. No tumorigenic effect was observed in their wild-type controls, carrying a 99.9% A/J background and 5% FVB genome[NT020]. Leaf, administered intragastrically to rats at a dose of 150 mg/animal twice daily 5 days-week for 15 weeks, was active on natural-killer (NK) cells. Activity of peripheral NK cells was assayed by lysis of YAC-1 lymphoma cells[NT525]. Smoke condensate, in combination with a 2 Gy dose of γ-rays, in C3H 10T1/2 cell system, induced a toxicity and transforming response that was largely additive in nature. Similar additive modes of interaction were observed when smoke condensate was combined with He4 ions at a dose that was equivalent in cell death to that used for γ-rays[NT089]. Smoke, at a concentration of 240 cm³ for 1 or 5 minutes, was active on Salmonella typhimurium TA98 in an S9 mix-type-dependent manner[NT124]. Black and brown masheri, a pyrolyzed tobacco product, were active on Salmonella typhimurium TA98 with metabolic activation and on V79 Chinese hamster cells producing 8-azaguanine resistant mutations. Both tobacco varieties induced statistically significant increase in micronuclei formations compared to the solvent controls and structural chromosomal aberrations in bone marrow cells of mice[NT130]. Smoke, at concentrations of 120–480 cm³ in a 16-1 glass chamber, for 1–10 minutes of

exposure and activated by S9 mix, induced a threefold to ninefold increase of spontaneous His+ reversion mutation rate in Salmonella typhimurium TA98, but not TA97a, TA100 and TA102. Smoke, administrated to BDF1 mice at a dose of 600 cm³, two exposures of 30 minutes each, produced a twofold dose-dependent elevation of the number of micronucleated polychromated erythrocytes in bone marrow. No cumulative effect was detected when mice were treated with tobacco smoke for 2 to 28 consecutive days. The effect observed 24 hours after tobacco-smoke exposure was abolished 48 hours later. Tobacco smoke (180 or 360 cm³), passed through the culture medium (with or without S9 mix) of human peripheral lymphocytes, did not increase the spontaneous rate of UDS[NT133]. Masheri extract was highly mutagenic in the presence of an exogenous metabolic system in the Ames test and in the micronucleus test, in a dose-dependent manner. It also induced 8-azaguanine-resistant mutants in Chinese hamster V79 cells. Dermal administration produced weak carcinogenic effect in Swiss nude mice. The saliva of masheri users produced high levels of NNN (14–43 ppb) and NPYR (2.2–8.3 ppb). The condensates collected after pipe smoking of a natural tobacco and a cavendish type tobacco produced an increase of the number of revertants induced with cavendish type tobacco on Salmonella typhimurium TA100 and TA98 in the presence of S9 activation in both strains compared to the natural tobacco. The increase in the number of revertants (approximately three times) was found when the tobacco was smoked after paper wrapping "savers"[NT148]. Alcoholic extract of the chewing tobacco, in Salmonella typhimurium TA98 culture, was active after activation with S9 mix. Extract induced 8-azaguanine-resistant mutation in V 79 Chinese hamster cells[NT154]. Urine concentrates from smokers, chewers, and nonsmokers, in

Salmonella typhimurium TA1538 with metabolic activation by S9, produced an effect by cigarette and bidi smokers' urine, whereas nonsmokers' urine was devoid of mutagenic effects. Urine of tobacco chewers produced variation in its mutagenic potential. Bidi smokers' urine showed maximum activity[NT155]. Bidi (Indian cigarette) smoke condensate, produced frameshift mutations in *Salmonella typhimurium* TA98 and TA1538, and induced 8-azaguanine-resistant mutations in V79 Chinese hamster cells in the presence of S9 mixture. Administration to Swiss mice induced elevated frequencies of micronucleated erythrocytes in the bone marrow[NT156]. A crude alcoholic extract of tobacco containing *N*-nitrosonornicotine and NNK, in histidine-deficient *Salmonella typhimurium* TA98 in the presence of 9000 × g supernatant fraction, was active[NT159].

NK-cell activity. Cigarette smoke, administered to mice preimmunized with a sublethal infection of influenza virus daily for 36 weeks, mounted a secondary immune response of normal height on subsequent challenge with the homologous virus strain. The response was less specific than that elicited in control mice, with high titers of cross-reacting antibody by hemagglutination inhibition to the following strain in the same antigenic series. Return of antibody to the previous level in the antigenic series was not observed[NT178]. Snuff, administered orally to male adult rats for 15 weeks, significantly decreased NK-cell activity in peripheral blood against murine NK-cell-sensitive target cells (YAC-1 lymphoma)[NT289].

Nervous system development. Water-soluble substances of cigarette smoke and combined effect of smoke and high temperature was investigated in pregnant rats at the 8th–11th day of gestation. The treatment produced changes of all indices correlated with embryonic nervous system development and morphological differentiation,

with an apparent dose-effect relationship ($p < 0.01$)[NT212].

Neuronal acetylcholine receptor blockade. Cembranoids ([4R]-2,7,11-cembratriene-4-6-diol and its diastereoisomer 4S), in SH-EP1-hα4β2 cell line heterologously expressing human α4β2-nicotine acetylcholine receptors (nAChRs), the SH-SY5Y neuroblastoma line naturally expressing human ganglionic α3β4-nAChRs, and the TE671/RD cell line naturally expressing embryonic muscle α1β1γδ-nAChRs, blocked carbamylcholine-induced (86)Rb(+) flux with IC_{50} in the low micromolar range. Tobacco ([4R]-2,7,11-cembratriene-4-6-diol and its diastereoisomer 4S) cembranoids blocked binding of the noncompetitive inhibitor [³H]tenocyclidine to nAChRs from *Torpedo californica* electric organ. IC_{50} values were in the submicromolar to low-micromolar range, with (4R)-2,7,11-cembratriene-4-6-diol displaying an order of magnitude higher potency than its diastereoisomer, 4S[NT210]. Presynaptic nAChRs mediated a calcium influx that enhanced the release of both glutamate and γ-aminobutyric acid (GABA). Fura-2 detection of calcium in single mossy fiber presynaptic terminals indicated that nAChRs directly mediated a calcium influx. In hippocampal neurons in primary culture, both spontaneous vesicular release and evoked release of glutamate and GABA were enhanced by nicotine. The nicotinic current displayed rapid desensitization kinetics, and the response to nicotine was inhibited by α-bungarotoxin and methylcaconitine, suggesting that nAChRs containing the α-7 subunit mediated the effect. Modulation of synaptic activity by presynaptic calcium influx may represent a physiological role of acetylcholine in the brain, as well as a mechanism of action of nicotine[NT237].

Neuroprotective effect. 2,3,6-trimethyl-1,4-naphthoquinone, administered to C57 BL/6 mice, protected against MPTP Parkinson's disease-mediated depletion of neo-striatal dopamine levels and lowered the brain MAO activity[NT037]. Smoke, administered to N-methyl-4-phenyl-1,2,3,6-tetrahydropyridine-treated C57 black mice, produced no protective effect[NT134]. Mainstream of cigarette smoke from 15 Kentucky 2R1F research cigarettes (28.6 mg tar, 1.74 mg nicotine/cigarette), administered to kainic acid-treated rats for 10 minutes daily, 6 days/week, for 4 weeks, indicated pre-exposure to smoke significantly reduced the seizures, mortality, and severe loss of cells in regions CA1 and CA3 of the hippocampus after kainic acid administration and attenuated the kainic acid-induced increased *Fos*-related antigen immunoreactivity in the hippocampus. In contrast, pretreatment with central nicotinic antagonist, mecamylamine (2 or 10 mg/kg, intraperitoneally) blocked the neuroprotective effects mediated by smoke in a dose-dependent manner. Results indicated that smoke exposure provided neuroprotection against the kainic acid insulted via nicotinic receptor activation[NT229]. 1,2,3,4-tetrahydro-β-carboline (TH β C), an endogenous or environmental neurotoxic factor putatively involved in the development of Parkinson's disease, reacted in vitro with some components of cigarette smoke. Significant differences in the recovery of some of TH β C-derivatives were obtained for Burley and Bright tobacco. Several of the reported compounds showed reversible and competitive MAO-A inhibitory properties. The detection of some of these compounds in rat brain after chronic administration of TH β C and a solution of cigarette smoke proved that the reported interactions also occur in vivo[NT241]. 1,2,3,4-tetrahydroisoquinoline (TIQ) and some components of tobacco smoke were investigated for their ability to inhibit rat brain MAO. 1-Cyano-TIQ (1CTIQ), N-(1'-cyanoethyl)-TIQ (CETIQ), N-(1'-cyanopropyl)-TIQ (CPTIQ), and N-(1'-cyanobutyl)-TIQ (CBTIQ) acted as competitive inhibitors for both MAO-A and MAO-B. K_i values ranged from 16.4 to 37.6 μM. N-(Cyanomethyl)-TIQ (CMTIQ) was not to be an inhibitor (K_i > 100.0 μM)[NT257]. 1,2,3,4-TIQ, a presumed proneutrotoxin linked with Parkinson's disease, interacted with some components of cigarette smoke. The in vitro formation of these compounds under physiological conditions occurred rapidly and with a high yield. Significant differences in the recovery of the different compounds were obtained for Burley tobacco compared to Bright tobacco. After chronic administration of TIQ and a solution of cigarette smoke to rats, the presence of some of these compounds was also detected in the brain[NT262].

Nicorandil kinetics. Cigarette smoke, administered to rats at a dose of 10 mg/kg for 8 minutes, produced the maximum nicorandil plasma levels in the rats inhaling standard cigarette and nicotine-less cigarette smoke 4.7 and 4.9 μg/mL, respectively, after 1–2 hours, compared to the controls. Nicorandil plasma level reached the maximum (7.6 μg/mL) after an hour and then decreased gradually[NT293].

NOS activity. Cigarette smoke or smoke extract, administered to ulcerated rats once daily for 3 days, produced concomitant and dose-dependent reduction of angiogenesis and constitutive NOS activity. The same treatments also delayed ulcer healing[NT232]. Sidestream smoke was administered to male Wistar rats with a single intratracheal instillation of 2 mg of chrysotile or refractory ceramic fiber. The rats were exposed to smoke 5 days/week for 4 weeks. Administration of smoke alone increased IL-1[α] mRNA levels in alveolar macrophages. The smoke stimulated the gene expression of inducible NOS in alveolar macrophages and IL-6 and basic fibroblast growth factor in lungs treated with chrysotile[NT239].

Non-Hodgkin's lymphoma. The 1450 cases of non-Hodgkin's lymphoma (NHL) and 1779 healthy controls from 11 Italian areas with different demographic and productive characteristics were included in a study, corresponding to approx 7 million residents. Odds ratios (ORs) adjusted for age, gender, residence area, educational level, and type of interview were estimated by unconditional logistic regression model. A statistically significant association (OR = 1.4, 95% confidence interval [CI] 1.1–1.7) was found for blond tobacco exposure and NHL risk. A dose-response relationship was limited to men younger than 52 years. Subjects starting smoking at an early age showed a higher risk in men younger than 65 years, whereas no clear trend was evident for the other age and gender subgroups. The analysis by Working Formulation categories showed the highest risks for follicular lymphoma in blond (OR = 2.1, 95% CI 1.4–3.2) and mixed (OR = 1.8, 95% CI 1.1–3) tobacco smokers and for large cell within the other Working Formulation group (OR = 1.6, 95% CI 1.1–2.4) only for blond tobacco[NT301].

NF-κB inhibition. Aqueous extract of mainstream smoke (smoke-bubbled phosphate-buffered saline), in Swiss 3T3 cells, decreased DNA binding of NF-κB during the first 2 hours of exposure and increased more than twofold over controls after 4–6 hours of exposure. There was lack of phosphorylation and degradation of IκB-α and a significant increase in thioredoxin reductase mRNA after 2–6 hours of exposure. Results indicated that the activity of NF-κB in smoke-treated cells was subject mainly to a redox-controlled mechanism dependent on the availability of reduced thioredoxin rather than being controlled by its normal regulator, IκB-α[NT040].

Oral tumorigenic effect. Snuff, administered to mice in the diet at concentrations of 25% gradually decreasing to 5% in a 14-month study, did not increase the tumor incidence. Administration to rats at a concentration of 5% for 18 months produced no result. Administration to hamsters at a dose of 20% for 2 years, produced forestomach tumors. Snuff, administered orally to hamster, produced a high incidence of squamous cell carcinomas. No carcinogenic activity was observed when snuff was inserted into the cheek pouch of the hamster or spread over the oral mucosa. This negative result was obtained in numerous experiments whether snuff was applied once only and left in place for several months or inserted repeatedly for up to 2 years. In the rat, a few tumors were observed when snuff was inserted into the artificial lip canal[NT052]. Tobacco smoke tar condensate or water-extract of snuff was administered dermally to mice in upper lips inoculated with latent HSV, for 2–3 months. Tar condensate induced reactivation of latent HSV in the ganglia of 10–20% of the animals, but snuff extract did not. The infectious virus was also detected in the lips after chronic application of tar condensate in 10% of the animals. Three months' exposure to tobacco produced epithelial dysplasia and other changes in a significant number of latent HSV-infected mice. Tobacco alone did not induce dysplasia in the labial epithelium of uninfected mice[NT137]. Nicotine, administered by surgically created canals in the mandibular lips of male Sprague–Dawley rats twice daily for 6 weeks, decreased the thromboxane B2 levels in nicotine treated tissues. Within the nicotine group, thromboxane B2 concentrations were lower at the nicotine site compared to the posterior site (18.3 ± 5.4 pg/mg). There was also a trend toward reduced 6-keto-PGF1α in the nicotine-treated tissues compared to saline-exposed sites. These alterations in cyclo-oxygenase metabolites were not accompanied by changes in epithelial proliferation or histologic parameters. 12(S)-hydroxyeicosatetraenoic acid and leukotriene B4 were not affected by nicotine[NT259].

Ornithine decarboxylase activity. Cigarette smoke was administered to intact animals and animals with ulcers at concentrations of 2 or 4%. The treatment significantly reduced the thickness of the mucous secreting layer and gastric mucosal ornithine decarboxylase activity in animals with or without ulcers. The extract significantly reduced mucus synthesis and ornithine decarboxylase activity but not its mRNA expression in MKN-28 cells[NT217]. Cigarette smoke and its extract, in human MKN-28 cells, markedly decreased mucus synthesis in vivo and in vitro and suppressed ornithine decarboxylase activity[NT225].

Ovarian toxicity. Cigarette smoke, administered to pregnant C57BL/6 and DBA/2 inbred strain mice during days 1–18 of pregnancy, did not affect the number of primordial follicles in the ovaries of the mothers. Counts were significantly decreased (31%) in the ovaries of DBA/2 offspring, and not significantly (20%) decreased in the ovaries of C57BL/6 offspring[NT151].

Oxidative stress. Smoke, administered to mice for 10 weeks, produced an increase in the levels of lipid peroxidation in the heart, catalase activity, and a decrease in glutathione level. Superoxide dismutase and heat-stable lactate dehydrogenase in serum activities were not affected[NT010]. Smoke, administered to mice, produced a significant decrease in total antioxidant capacity in bronchoalveolar lavage fluid and significant changes in oxidized glutathione, ascorbic acid, protein thiols, and 8 epi-PGF(2α). Treatment with smoke induced a 50% decrease in the inhibitory activity of human recombinant SLPI[NT036]. Peroxynitride formed by smoke in aqueous solutions, in Swiss 3T3 cells, sustained c-*fos* expression was obtained for smoke-bubbled PBS, peroxynitrite itself, and a compound known to stoichiometrically release superoxide and nitric oxide (NO) (3-morpholino-sydnonimine [SIN-1]). c-*fos* expression in cells

exposed to aqueous smoke fractions was inhibited by either the superoxide-scavenging enzyme superoxide dismutase, in combination with catalase, or the NO-scavenger oxyhemoglobin (HbO$_2$). Activation of guanylate cyclase in rat lung cells was observed only when bubbling was performed with filtered smoke and with whole smoke in the presence of SOD/catalase[NT065]. STD, in macrophage J774A.1 cell culture, produced an increase of lactate dehydrogenase in concentration- and time-dependent manner. The addition of 250 µg/mL dose produced 2.9-fold increase in the release of lactate dehydrogenase[NT072]. Tobacco smoke condensate, in rat pulmonary microvascular endothelial cell culture at a concentration of 20 µg/mL, significantly upregulated xanthine dehydrogenase/oxidase activity after 24 hours of exposure. Longer exposure (1 week) to a lower concentration of smoke (2 µg/mL) also produced an increase in xanthine dehydrogenase/oxidase activity. Unlike hypoxia, smoke treatment did not alter the phosphorylation of xanthine dehydrogenase/oxidase, but increased XO mRNA expression and the xanthine dehydrogenase/oxidase gene promoter activity. Actinomycin D blocked the activation of xanthine dehydrogenase/oxidase by smoke concentrate[NT198]. Gas-phase cigarette smoke, in rat lung tissue, produced infiltration of the terminal bronchioles by lymphocytes in the peribronchiolar region and a mild to moderate degree of emphysema in the alveolar spaces. The terminal bronchioles also produced marked lipid peroxidation, dilatation, and peribronchiolar fibrosis. The expression of inducible NOS, NF-κB, mitogen-activated protein kinases (MEK1, ERK2), phosphotyrosine protein, and c-*fos* was increased in the terminal bronchioles but protein kinase C (PKC), MEKK-1, c-*jun*, p38 and c-*myc* was not changed[NT207]. Smoke, administered to rats once only or daily for 1, 2, 7, or 28 days, did not change NOS-1 gene expression and protein levels. Levels of NOS-2 expression was twofold higher in smokers at day 1 and decreased to control values during 1 month with daily smoke exposure, whereas protein levels did not change. NOS-2 was diffusely expressed in the lung parenchyma, airways, and vessels. NOS-3 expression was increased approx 35% after 2 days of smoke exposure and remained increased to 28 days, whereas protein levels were increased by approx 60% at day 7 and remained elevated. NOS-3 was strongly expressed in vascular endothelium. Protein distribution was identical to mRNA tissue distribution, and these distributions were not changed by smoke[NT235].

p53 Mutations. Four head and neck squamous cell carcinomas from three patients using snuff and one patient not using snuff showed p53 mutations in tumors resected from two of three patients using snuff. No p53 mutations were observed in the tumor from the patient not using snuff. No K-*ras* (codons 12 and 13) or H-*ras* (codon 12) mutations were found in any of the tumors[NT071]. Smoke condensate, in sarcoma derived from Rat-1 cells transformed by smoke condensate-treated human fetal lung DNA, produced overexpression of p53 and contributed to the initiation of human lung carcinogenesis[NT085].

Pancreatic effect. Cigarette smoke, administered to anesthetized rats alone or in combination with iv ethanol infusion, reduced pancreatic blood flow temporarily and increased leukocyte–endothelium interaction (roller $p < 0.001$, sticker $p < 0.01$ vs baseline). Cigarette smoke potentiated the impairment of pancreatic capillary perfusion caused by ethanol, and both the number of rolling leukocytes and myeloperoxidase activity levels were increased compared with ethanol or nicotine administration alone[NT215]. Tobacco-specific nitrosamines, administered to rats, induced pancreatic acinar cell and ductal cell neoplasms. One of the tumors had a mixed ductal-squamous-islet cell components[NT296].

Parathion esterase activity. Cigarette smoke, administered intranasally to young male C57BL mice fed 0, 5, and 100 ppm of vitamin E, 20 minutes/day for 8 weeks, produced no effect parathion esterase or parathion desulfurase activities[NT153].

Periodontal disease. A total of 1085 people who smoke were examined for periodontal status. There was a significant dose-effect relationship between the exposure to tobacco smoke and the extent of periodontal disease assessed as attachment loss and tooth loss. There was a gene–environmental interaction. Subjects bearing at least one copy of the variant allele 2 at positions IL-1A-889 and IL-1B+3954 had an enhanced smoking-associated periodontitis as compared with their IL-1 genotype-negative counterparts[NT302]. Snuff, at a dose of 500 mg (1% nicotine), induced a rapid increase gingival blood flow that was higher than the increase in blood pressure, indicating an active vasodilatation, partly blocked by infraorbital nerve block anesthesia and more so by the superficial mucosal anesthesia. Piroxicam and dexchlorpheniramine had no effect[NT303]. In 240 patients, smoking had a 2.7 times greater probability to have established periodontal disease in smokers and 2.3 times in former smokers compared to nonsmokers, independent of age, sex, and plaque index. Among cases, probing depth, gingival recession, and clinical attachment level were greater in smokers than in former smokers or nonsmokers. The plaque index did not show differences. Bleeding on probing was less evident in smokers than in nonsmokers. There was a dose-dependent relationship between cigarette consumption and the probability of having advanced periodontal disease[NT304].

Plasma lipid profile. Tobacco was administered to 184 patients with head and neck cancer, 153 patients with oral precancerous conditions, and 52 controls. The treatment produced a significant decrease in plasma total cholesterol and HDL cholesterol in patients with cancer and oral precancerous conditions, compared to controls. The plasma very low-density lipoproteins (VLDL) and triglycerides levels were significantly lower in patients with cancer compared to the patients with oral precancerous conditions and controls. The results indicated that the tobacco habituates showed lower plasma lipid levels than the nonhabituates[NT002].

Polymorphonuclear cells. High-tar (16 mg tar/cigarette) filtered cigarettes, administered to Balb/c and C57 Black mice for up to 32 weeks, produced in Balb/c mice less phagocytic and degradative capacities of polymorphonuclear cells than those of C57 Black mice. Heat inactivation of complement within the serum reduced the differences between smoke-exposed animals and age-matched controls in both strains of mice. The treatment effects were seen at all times tested from 3 days to 32 weeks of tobacco smoke exposure. The results indicated that fc-receptor site activity of PMN cells was not significantly affected by smoke exposure but that complement interactions within the phagocytic process are significantly suppressed[NT161].

Prenatal influence. In 589 10-year-old children who have been observed from their gestation to tobacco smoke, half were females and 52% were African-American. During pregnancy, 52.6% of the mothers were smokers, 59.7% were smokers when their children were 10 years old. Six percent of the children (37/589) reported ever smoking cigarettes. Maternal smoking was significantly associated with an increased risk of the child's tobacco experimentation. Offspring exposed to more than half a pack per day during gestation had a 5.5-fold increased risk for early experimentation. Prenatal tobacco exposure had a direct and significant effect on the child's smoking and predicted child anxiety/depression and externalizing behaviors. Maternal current smoking had no significant effect[NT305]. Cell-free amniotic acid from groups of smokers and nonsmokers showed a presence of NNAL in 11/21 (52.4%) of smokers and in

2/30 (6.7%) of nonsmokers. There was not convincing evidence of NNAL-Gluc in the amniotic acid[NT307]. A total of 40 very-low-birth-weight infants (750–1500 g) of smoking during pregnancy (50%) and alcohol-consuming (42%) mothers were hospitalized and ventilated for respiratory distress syndrome. At birth, infants of mothers who smoked and consumed alcohol during pregnancy had significantly higher blood docosahexaenoic acid (DHA) than infants of nonsmoking and nondrinking mothers[NT308]. Mothers of 91 cases and 321 population controls matched for age, sex, and residence and smoking during pregnancy produced higher an odds ratio of 1.7 (95% CI 0.8, 3.8) of brain tumor in their children, although this was not statistically significant. Among nonsmoking mothers, the risk for light and heavy exposure to passive smoking was 1.7 (0.8, 3.6) and 2.2 (1.1, 4.5), respectively, and a statistically significant dose–response relationship was found[NT309]. Maternal use of masheri tobacco in pregnancy was associated with low birth-weight of the offspring, lower birth-weights in girls than in boys, and decreased male:female ratio in live newborns[NT310]. Mainstream and sidestream smoke, administered by inhalation to hamsters, retarded transport of preimplantation embryos through the hamster oviduct. Oviductal muscle contraction rate decreased significantly during a single exposure of animals to either mainstream or sidestream smoke, and contraction rate failed to return to initial control values during a 25-minute recovery period. Both preimplantation embryo transport and muscle contraction were more sensitive to sidestream than mainstream smoke[NT311].

Progesterone production inhibition. Nicotine, cotinine, and anabasine, together, or an aqueous extract of cigarette smoke, in MA-10 Leydig cells, produced a dose-dependent inhibition of progesterone and 20-α-dihydroprogesterone synthesis. The number of cells in the treated dishes was less than the controls. Growth of MA-10 cells was inhibited[NT306]. Cotinine, anabasine, a combination of nicotine, cotinine and anabasine, or an aqueous extract of cigarette smoke in human granulose cells produced an inhibition of progesterone synthesis. The alkaloids and some extract decreased the DNA content of the culture dish. Both cotinine and anabasine slightly stimulated the synthesis of normalized estradiol. Nicotine, combination of the three alkaloids, and cigarette smoke extract had no significant influence on estradiol production[NT318].

Prostaglandins formation. Aqueous cigarette tar extracts, in rat pulmonary alveolar macrophages, increased cyclo-oxygenase activity threefold above the initial activity within 2 hours of incubation and gradually decreased below the initial activity after 8 hours of incubation. Accumulated levels of prostaglandin-2 increased dramatically after 12 hours of incubation. Release of arachidonic acid from the cells was dramatically increased in cells incubated with smoke extracts in parallel to prostaglandins accumulation[NT233].

Prostate tumorigenic effect. Tobacco smoke was administered to rats with implanted bilaterally with Dunning R3327 tumor fragments at 10 weeks of age and smoke exposed for an hour each day, 5 days a week, for 9 or 20 weeks. The treatment produced only minor changes in the growth rates of both the control and the irradiated tumors. At the cellular level, smoking produced a small, but significant, increase in the fraction of tumor cells relative to controls. The main difference observed was in the mast cell numbers. Smoking produced a fourfold increase in mast-cell density. The combination of smoking and irradiation resulted in a 10-fold intermediate increase[NT228].

Protein synthesis stimulation. Smoke of the leaf, administered to rats at variable doses, was active. The effect of a combination of hashish and cigarette smoke on brain proteins and catecholamines was measured. This was compared with the effects of animals under stress[NT590].

Pulmonary arterial effects. Cigarette smoke, administered to 2- and 3-month-old rats at a dose of one cigarette 10 times a day, increased significantly the volume fractions of the fibroblasts, the collagenous bundles, and the elastic laminae of the pulmonary arteries. The volume fractions of smooth muscle cells and the remainder were decreased significantly in both groups compared to controls. An increase in the stiffness of the pulmonary arteries was found in both the 2- and 3-month smoke-exposed rats[NT281].

Pulmonary effect. Smoke, administered to mice at a dose of two cigarettes daily, 5 days/week for 2–4 months, decreased the number of dendritic cells in the lung tissue and reduced the percentage of B7.1-expressing dendritic cells. Inoculation with 2×10^8 pfu of a replication-deficient adenovirus three times 2 weeks apart during the last month of tobacco exposure, prevented the expansion and maximal activation of CD4 T-cells and reduced the number of both activated CD4 and CD8 T-cells. Smoke exposure shifted the activated CD4:CD8 T-cells ratio from 3 to 1.5, and decreased serum adenovirus-specific pan IgG, IgG1, and IgG2a levels[NT013]. NNK, in pulmonary cells, produced promutagenic adduct O-6-methylguanine. Administration of doses from 0.1 to 50 mg/kg increased the number of adducts (3- to 30-fold) in Clara cells those detected in type II cells and whole lung. Very low rates of repair of this adduct were detected in Clara cells, whereas efficient adduct removal occurred in type II cells. There was a strong correlation between the concentration of O-6-methylguanine in Clara cells and tumor incidence in the Fischer rat with NNK doses from 0.03 to 50 mg/kg. No differences in adduct concentration between type II and Clara cells from A/J mice were observed under conditions resulting in pulmonary tumor formation. Activation of the K-*ras* gene was detected in lung tumors from A/J mice. An early proliferative lesions observed in both mice and rats involved the alveolar areas. Ultrastructural examination of these lesions and adenomas revealed morphologic features characteristic of the type II cell[NT098]. Masheri (pyrolyzed tobacco), administered orally to Swiss mice, Sprague–Dawley rats, and Syrian golden hamsters at a dose of 10% of the diet for 20 months, produced significant increase in activities of phase I activating enzymes and a remarkable decrease in the phase II detoxification system in most extrahepatic tissues of the treated animals of the three species[NT099]. Cigarette smoke and hydrocortisone acetate (HCA), administered to C57BL/6J male mice, induced marked abnormalities in lungs, high congestion with surfactant and flocculent material in alveoli, prominent alveolar collapse, and septal hypertrophy. Results indicated that the genesis of abnormal conditions that resemble pulmonary alveolar proteinosis is potentiated by cumulative effects of different treatments (i.e., smoke, HCA, and stress), most significant being the interaction between cigarette smoke and the steroid[NT162]. Whole cigarette smoke from reference cigarettes administration produced the prompt (maximal activity was 6 hours), but fairly weak (similar to twofold), induction of murine pulmonary microsomal monooxygenase activity not unequivocally linked to the Ah locus. This activity can be detected by using as substrates either benzo(a)pyrene or ethoxyresorufin and can be inhibited by treatment with cycloheximide or actinomycin D. Whole-smoke condensate and fractions induced pulmonary monooxygenase activity, inhibited benzo(a)pyrene metabolism in vitro, were metabolized to forms mutagenic to *Salmonella typhimurium* TA153 and TA98, transformed C3H 10T1/2 cells in vitro, and

enhanced the carcinogenicity of benzo(a)-pyrene in murine pulmonary tissue. A potentially important observation was that whereas hepatic tissue is capable of activating whole cigarette smoke condensate to mutagenic forms in vitro, murine pulmonary tissue does not seem capable of such activation. Although these pulmonary-derived tissue homogenates had significant aryl hydrocarbon hydroxylase activity and can metabolize Aflatoxin B1, 2-aminofluorene, and 7, 8-dihydro-7,8-dihydroxybenzo(a)pyrene to mutagenic forms, these homogenates failed to activate both cigarette smoke condensate and the promutagen 6-aminochrysene[NT180]. Smoke, administered to Sprague–Dawley rats at a dose of seven cigarettes/day for 5 days/week during a total period of 12 months, produced early abnormalities in pulmonary function, with the forced expiratory volume in one second/forced vital capacity (FEV1/FVC) ratio, showing an acceleration of ageing effect, particularly between 4 and 8 months of exposure[NT253].

Pulmonary macrophage mobilization.
Smoke, administered to smoke-exposed and subsequently halothane anesthetized normal and to C57BL/6 mice, produced airway cilia shorter in stature and fewer in number. There was also disorientation of ciliary basal bodies. Airway macrophages were larger in size and contained more lysosomes and inclusions than phagocytes in airways of all other animals. Smoke inhalation alone produced a significant increase in the number of lung parenchymal macrophages when compared to the number of cells in sham-treated and control animals. The total macrophage population was significantly greater in lungs of smoke-exposed mice 48 hours after anesthesia than in lungs of smoke-exposed mice not subjected to halothane anesthesia and to those of sham-treated and control animals. Airway macrophage numbers were significantly elevated in smoke-exposed mice 48 hours

after halothane when compared to those of all other groups, but the number of parenchymal macrophages decreased in lungs[NT144].

Pulmonary surfactant activity. Smoke from Kentucky cigarette, administered intranasally to female Sprague–Dawley rats twice daily for 60 weeks, produced no difference in total phospholipids content of the bronchoalveolar lavage fluids and the lung tissues among the groups. Desaturated phosphatidylcholine levels in the bronchoalveolar lavage fluids were significantly decreased. The lung tissue desaturated phosphatidylcholine content in smoke-treated rats was not significantly different compared to controls. Phospholipids profile analysis did not reveal any significant differences among other major constituents of surfactant from control and smoke-treated rats[NT266].

Red blood cell labeling inhibition. Tobacco decreased the labeling of blood elements with technetium-99m and plasma proteins. This effect possibly resulted from either a direct or an indirect effect (reactive oxygen species [ROS]) of tobacco by oxidation of the stannous ion, possible damages caused in plasma membrane and/or possible chelating action on the stannous and/or pertechnetate ions[NT244].

Renal damages. Cigarette smoke condensate was administered to the oral mucosa of subtotally nephrectomized Sprague–Dawley rats, and to sham-operated Sprague–Dawley rats daily for 12 weeks. The treatment increased the indices of structural renal damage in the nephrectomized group. The cigarette smoke condensate increased the indices of glomerulosclerosis and tubulointerstitial damage in nephrectomized, but not sham-operated rats. This increase was completely prevented by renal denervation. Urinary albumin excretion went in parallel with the indices of glomerulosclerosis and tubulointerstitial damage and urinary endothelin-1 excretion was significantly increased in the nephrectomized animals[NT203].

Respiratory system toxicity. Smoke of cured leaf, administered by inhalation to adults at an undiluted concentration, was active on asthma[NT380].

RNA synthesis inhibition. Smoke of the leaf, administered to rats at variable doses, was active. The effect of a combination of cigarette and hashish smoke on stress response were measured in rats held in a wire cage inside of a larger cage with a cat. Brains were dissected and measured for protein and catecholamine levels[NT590].

Serotonin uptake. Cigarette smoke, administered to mice, increased serotonin concentration as a function of the frequency of exposure. Serotonin uptake by the skin was maximally increased after two 8-minute exposures. MAO activity for serotonin, but not for tyramine, was decreased by cigarette smoke exposure of more than 8 minutes[NT182].

Sister chromatid exchange inhibition. Water extract of the dried leaf, in cell culture at a concentration of 20 μL/mL, was active on Chinese hamster ovary cells. There was an elevation in frequency in cultures treated with 20 μL/mL of growth media[NT445]. Seed, administered orally to adults, was active in chewers with oral cancer or oral submucosal fibrosis and healthy chewers, compared to control. An average of 6 quids of tobacco leaf, *Areca* nut and lime were used daily[NT521]. Whole Kentucky reference 3A1 and American Blend cigarettes smoke were administered intranasally to B6C3F1 mice at a dose of 10% v/v 1, 4, 9, and 18 exposures/day (one exposure equal to one cigarette smoke) 5 days/week for 2 weeks. The treatment increased bone marrow sister chromatid exchange for both cigarette types in a dose-dependent manner. There was no effect on bone marrow cell replication kinetics[NT149]. Whole cigarette smoke, administered intranasally to B6C3F1/ Cum mice daily for 1 to 46 weeks, produced a twofold increase in sister chromatid exchange over sham-exposed control mice. In animals exposed either chronically or for 1 week to either type of smoke, the increase in sister chromatid exchange persisted for at least 1 week after cessation of smoke exposure[NT157]. Smoke, administered to young adult male mice, elevated pulmonary macrophage population. Pulmonary macrophages (free, attached, and septal or interstitial) divided only rarely. During the marked progressive increase in the labeled macrophage population in the lungs, the number of silver grains over the nuclei of labeled macrophages did not become significantly diluted. Results indicated that the markedly elevated macrophage population resulted from the immigration of cells from bone marrow rather than in situ division of resident macrophages[NT176]. Cigarette smoke, administered to adult male mice for 42 to 82 days, induced increased DNA activity in pulmonary tissue. No such induction was noted in the liver or spleen. An increase in DNA activity reflected a marked increase in the number of labeled pulmonary macrophages. At times, more than 50% of the total pool of labeled cells were identifiable as macrophages[NT177].

Skin tumorigenic effect. Aqueous extract of bidi tobacco, administered dermally according skin tumorigenesis protocol to hairless S/RV Cri-ba mice, did not exhibit carcinogenesis and effectively promoted skin papilloma formation in 7,12-dimethyl-benz[a]-anthracene-initiated mice. An increase in papilloma yield above the control was noted only after 30 weeks of promotion. At week 40 weeks of promotion with 5 mg and 50 mg extract, it was significantly higher than that in the control mice. Mild epidermal hyperplasia, increase in mitotic activity and dermal thickness induced by a single application of extract persisted on multiple treatment and correlated well with its tumor-promoting activity[NT084]. Brown and black varieties of pyrolyzed tobacco (mash-

eri) extracts were administered dermally to Swiss mice and Swiss bare mice. In Swiss mice, there was no tumorigenic effect but a marginal synergistic effect of 7,12-dimethyl-benz[a]anthracene (DMBA). The effect of black masheri extract was observed when DMBA was used as an initiator. In Swiss bare mice, black masheri extract induced tumors in 20–35% of the animals the two doses tested. In an initiation/promotion protocol with DMBA as an initiator, induction of tumors in 50–52% of the Swiss bare mice and a slight synergistic effect of black masheri extract were observed with a low dose of DMBA, suggesting a synergistic effect[NT121].

Small airway remodeling. Airway remodeling is usually attributed to the effects of cigarette smoke-induced inflammation in the airway wall, but little is known about its pathogenesis. Cigarette smoke, in rat tracheal explants at 24 hours after smoke exposure, produced a dose-dependent increase in gene expression of procollagen and a significant increase in tissue hydroxyproline, a measure of collagen content. Greater increases in procollagen gene expression were found with repeated smoke exposures. Results indicated that cigarette smoke can directly induce airway remodeling, specifically airway wall fibrosis, probably through active oxygen species-dependent transactivation of the epidermal growth factor receptor and subsequent NF-κB activation. Smoke-evoked inflammatory cells were not required for this process[NT193]. Cigarette smoke, in rat bronchioles previously exposed to smoke in vivo, induced a small but consistent degree of contraction of the airways in vitro, which could be reduced by an endothelin receptor antagonist in the animals which had no previous smoke exposure in vivo, and reduced by the oxidant scavengers SOD or catalase in the animals with previous smoke exposure. Results indicated that cigarette smoke induced acute small airways constriction through both endothelin release and direct oxidant effects[NT230]. Mainstream cigarette smoke, administered to rats at a dose of 250 mg total particulate matter/m^3 air for 6 hours/day, 5 days/week, for 2 weeks, increased the type II epithelial BrdU labeling index (LI). The axial airway and terminal bronchiolar LIs were enhanced only in the pump-labeled group. In the pump-labeled rats, the type II LI elevation was greater than the LI elevation in conducting airways, suggesting that the parenchyma may have been injured more than the conducting airways. The exposure did not increase the total number of mucosubstances-containing cells or the total number of axial airway epithelial cells, but there was a phenotype change in the mucosubstance cells. Neutral mucosubstance cells (periodic acid-Schiff-positive) were significantly decreased, while acid mucosubstance cells (Alcian blue-positive) were slightly increased by smoke exposure. Either cell replication and differentiation or differentiation alone may have changed the phenotype in the smoke cell population[NT231].

Spermatozoal effect. Filtered and non-filtered cigarette smoke, streamed at a rate of 100 mL/second into chamber with washed human spermatozoa, produced a dramatic drop in sperm motility, which caused sperm immobilization in about 15 minutes. This effect showed dose-response relationship with the amounts streamed or with the time of exposition and was almost the same for filtered or unfiltered smoke[NT312]. Semen of 119 tobacco chewers and 218 smokers selected from an idiopathically hypofertile population, produced some decrease in the ejaculating volume, density and total count compared to non-smokers, but statistically insignificant. No difference was found in motility and morphology[NT313]. Sperm of 103 smokers produced a significant decrease of density and motility compared with nonsmokers. Seventy-five percent of smokers vs 26% of nonsmokers had a sperm density under 40×10^6 sperm/mL. Morpho-

logic abnormalities, particularly bicephali, did not differ significantly[NT314]. Cigarette smoke, at doses of 10 cigarettes per day (57 cases), 11–20 (115 cases) or more than 20 (25 cases), produced significantly poorer sperm density, lower viability, motility and morphology in smokers. These parameters were worse in the heavy smoking groups[NT315]. The ejaculate content of seminal vesicles, prostate gland, and epididymis of 29 smokers and 25 chewers produced a significant decrease in vesicular and prostatic parameters in smokers compared to nonusers of tobacco, whereas these parameters were unchanged in chewers. The activity of α-1,4-glucosidase was significantly lowered in both types of tobacco users[NT316]. Serum levels of estradiol, prolactin, and total testosterone in 50 heavy smokers (median 23.5 cigarettes/day), produced higher levels of estradiol and prolactin, but not testosterone[NT317].

Sudden infant death syndrome. Water-soluble smoke extract, in cell culture supernatants of mouse fibroblasts (L-929 cell line), produced an increase in TNF-α from respiratory syncytial virus-infected cells. It decreased TNF-α from cells incubated with toxic shock syndrome toxin. Incubation with cigarette smoke extract decreased the NO production from respiratory syncytial virus-infected cells and increased the NO production from cells incubated with toxic shock syndrome toxin. Monocytes from a minority of individuals demonstrated extreme TNF-α responses and/or very high or very low NO. The proportion of samples in which extreme responses with a very high TNF-α and very low NO were detected was increased in the presence of the three agents to 20% compared with 0% observed with toxic shock syndrome toxin. One to 4% was observed with cigarette smoke extract or respiratory syncytial virus[NT047].

Symphatomimetic activity. Water extract of the dried leaf, administered intravenously to cats at doses of 0.05 and 10–20 mg/kg, enhanced the contractile response of the cat nictitating membrane evoked by preganglionic cervical sympathetic nerve stimulation. At higher doses it produced contractions and nictitating membrane contraction without nerve stimulation[NT588].

Systemic inflammatory cytokine production. Sidestream smoke was administered to mice at 60 and 120 minutes per day, 5 days/week for a 16 weeks. The treatment produced a significant increase in the pro-inflammatory cytokines, IL-6, TNF-α, and IL-1 β in 120-minutes smoke exposed mice. A decrease of the stroke volume, cardiac and hepatic antioxidant vitamin E levels, and heart pathology and increased peripheral arterial resistance were observed in 120-minute smoke-exposed mice. Hepatic lipid peroxides were increased on 60-minute smoke exposure[NT024].

Tachycardiac activity. Water extract of the dried leaf, administered intravenously to cats and rats at doses of 10–20 mg/kg, was active. Results were significant at $p < 0.05$ level[NT588].

T-cells influence. SSTE and nicotine were incubated in splenic mononuclear cells at concentrations of $1:10^2$ or $1:10^3$ dilutions of STD, or 10 or 100 µg/mL nicotine, during 4 days of stimulation with anti-CD3. The treatment sustained expression of IL-2, IFN-γ, IL-10, and IL-4 cytokine mRNA at 100 µg/mL nicotine. STD did not exhibit residual expression of cytokine mRNA. Restimulated STD exhibited maximum IL-2, IL-4, IFN- γ, and IL-10 mRNA at 48 hours[NT049]. STE, in splenic mononuclear cell culture at $1:10^2$ to $1:10^4$ dilutions, increased IL-2 production and decreased IL-10 at $1:10^2$ dilution. IFN-γ production was decreased at all concentrations. STE did not alter IL-4 production[NT062].

P-benzoquinone, a thiol-reactive benzene derivative from cigarette tar, was incubated in human peripheral blood mononuclear cells at a concentration of 10 µM. The treatment inhibited mitogen-induced IL-2 production by $76 \pm 7\%$ without affecting lymphocyte/macrophage agglutination or blast transformation. The effect of p-benzoquinone appeared to be specific for IL-2 production, since de novo induction of the IL-2 receptor α-chain (CD25) and intercellular adhesion molecule-1 (CD54) and upregulation of LFA-1 α/β (CD11a and CD18) were unaffected[NT063]. Smoke, administered by inhalation to mice, inhibited the antigen-specific T-cell proliferative response of lung-associated lymph nodes. Cell-mixing experiments demonstrated that the defect in smoke exposed mice resulted from an abnormality in T-lymphocyte function. The activity of antigen-presenting cells was similar in smoke-exposed and sham-smoke-exposed control animals[NT112]. Diluted, mainstream cigarette smoke was administered to rats for up to 30 months or nicotine at a concentration of 1 mg/kg body weight/24 hours via mini-osmotic pumps for 4 weeks. The treatment decreased antigen-mediated T-cells proliferation and constitutive activation of protein tyrosine kinase and phospholipase C-γ1 activities. Spleen cells from smoke-exposed and nicotine-treated animals have depleted inositol-1, 4,5-trisphosphate-sensitive Ca^{2+} stores and a decreased ability to raise intracellular Ca^{2+} levels in response to T-cell antigen receptor ligation. The results indicated that chronic smoking affects T-cell anergy by impairing the antigen receptor-mediated signal transduction pathways and depleting the inositol-1,4, 5-trisphosphate-sensitive Ca(2+) stores. Moreover, nicotine may account for or contribute to the immunosuppressive properties of cigarette smoke[NT222].

Teratogenic effect. Stem, administered orally to pigs, produced 80% congenital deformities if eaten between days 10 and 30 of pregnancy[NT439]. STE was administered to 65 pregnant CD-1 mice at the following doses: equivalent to 8 mg/kg nicotine (group ST), ethanol 1.8 g/kg (EtOH), a combination of ST and EtOH in the same dosages, or D-glucose (controls and ST alone) three times daily on 6–15 days of gestation. The mean maternal plasma drug levels were: nicotine, 321 ng/mL and ethanol, 0.105 g%. No significant differences were observed in maternal weight gain, litter size, or in the incidence of resorptions, deaths, and/or malformations. Fetal weights were reduced in the three treatment groups, with the greatest reduction (13% decrease) recorded in the ST group, and a 7% decrease in the ST/EtOH group. Placentas of the ST group weighed significantly less than controls. Ossification of the fetal skeleton, observed in 10 sites, was affected to the greatest extent in the ST group, followed by the EtOH and ST/EtOH groups. Craniofacial measurements were significantly affected in all three treatment groups, compared to controls[NT093]. Aqueous extract of STE was administered intragastrically to CD-1 mice at doses: ST/D-1 and ST/D-2, equivalent of 12 and 20 mg/nicotine kg body wt, respectively, three times daily for 5 weeks: 2 weeks before conception, during conception, and during gestational days 0–17. The weight gain was not significantly affected. The mean maternal plasma nicotine level for the low-dosage group was 363 ng/mL and 481 ng/mL for the high-dosage group. Maternal lethality for the low and high doses were at 9.6% and 28.2%, respectively. No significant differences were found between control and ST/D-1 maternal and/or fetal values. In ST/D-2 group, fetal weights were reduced by 5.4%; decreased ossification in femur measurements and in 9 of 10 characteristics measured; the frequency of resorptions was twofold higher than in controls; and the frequency of deaths and malformations was not affected. The low dose produced a negligible effect on the CD-1 mouse fetus. The high dose demonstrated growth retardation, increased embryotoxicity, and a significant

decrease in ossification[NT101]. Aqueous extract of the STE, administered intragastrically to CD-1 mice at doses of: 1× extract equivalent to 4 mg/mL nicotine/kg body weight; 3 × 12 mg nicotine, and 5 × 20 mg nicotine, three times daily for gestation days 1–17, produced no significant effect on the weight gain in comparison to treated control. Difference was significant in comparison to untreated controls. Placental weighs were unaffected by the extract. The lowest extract dosage produced a negligible effect on the CD-1 mouse and the fetus. The highest dose demonstrated embryotoxicity, growth retardation, few malformations, and maternal toxicity. The intermediate dose showed a range of effects between the highest and lowest doses to both the fetus and the mother[NT114]. NNK was administered intraperitoneally to A/J, C3B6F1, and Swiss outbred Cr:NIH(S) mice at a dose of 100 mg/kg on days 14, 16, and 18 of gestation to A/J and C3H/He mice and on days 15, 17, and 19 of gestation to the Swiss mice. There was significant incidences of tumors in the lungs of A/J progeny and in the livers of male C3B6F1 and Swiss progeny. A lung tumor incidence in male offspring of treated A/J mice vs control was not statistical significant but was significantly greater in progeny A/J mice of both sexes compared to controls. The incidence of liver tumors in the male C3B6F1 mice exposed transplacentally to NNK was 40%, compared with 17% in controls. No effect of postnatal sodium barbital or PCB was observed on transplacental NNK tumorigenicity in C3B6F1 mice. The combined incidence of liver carcinoma in male mice in all NNK-treated groups was significantly greater than in controls. In male Swiss mice exposed transplacentally to NNK, the incidence of liver tumors was 5%, compared to 0% in controls, and postnatal treatment with PCB on day 56 produced a significant increase in the incidence of NNK-induced liver tumors.

The combined incidence of liver tumors in the male offspring of the Swiss mice treated with NNK, with or without PCB, was 10%, compared to 0% in controls[NT117]. Aqueous extract of STE was administered intragastrically to pregnant Sprague–Dawley rats three times daily on gestational days 6–18 at doses equivalent to 1.33 mg nicotine/kg body weight (STD-1) or 6 mg nicotine/kg body weight (STD-2). The treatments reduced the weight gain of mothers, but fetal weights were reduced in the STD-2 group only. Placental weights, litter size, resorptions, deaths, and malformations were not significantly affected. Skeletal examinations revealed several dose-related differences between the smoke extract-treated and control groups. In the STD-1 group, reductions in ossification were seen in the nasal and femur width measurements only. In the STD-2 group, reductions in ossification were seen in femur length and width, in the number of ossification centers in the forelimb, and in the maxillary, mandibular, and nasal bone measurements[NT278]. STE was administered continuously via Alzet osmotic mini-pumps to CD-1 mice at doses of 3.2 mg/mL (dosage I) and 6.4 mg/mL (dosage II) for gestational days 7–14 and 6–13. The treatment produced plasma nicotine levels in the range of 29.4 ± 4.8 ng/mL to 44.3 ± 16 ng/mL for dosage I and in the range of 34.6 ± 10.9 ng/mL to 75.5 ± 19.9 ng/mL for the dosage II. Dosage I produced a tendency toward weight reduction, an increase in the incidence of hemorrhages and supernumerary ribs, and significant delay in ossification of the supraoccipital bone, the sacrococcygeal vertebrae, and the bones of the forefoot and hindfoot. Dosage II produced a significant (8.6%) weight reduction from normal and an increase in fetal deaths. There were no significant differences between placental weights. Weights of mothers were significantly reduced only at the higher doses[NT127].

Testosterone effect. Cigarette smoke diluted with 90% air, administered to 12 male adult rats for 2 hours/day for 60 days, produced significant decrease of the mean plasma testosterone level. The mean plasma luteinizing hormone and follicle-stimulating hormone levels of the two groups did not change significantly after exposure. Histological examination of the testes showed fewer Leydig cells and degeneration of the remaining cells. The results indicated that the decrease in plasma testosterone levels induced by exposure to smoke was not associated with changes in plasma gonadotrophin levels. The decrease in testosterone levels may be related to the toxic effects of smoke on Leydig cells[NT258].

Tourette's syndrome. Administration of nicotine (either 2 mg nicotine gum or 7 mg transdermal nicotine patch) potentiated the therapeutic properties of neuroleptics in treating patients with Tourette's syndrome, and a single patch may be effective for a variable number of days. These findings suggest that transdermal nicotine could serve as an effective adjunct to neuroleptic therapy[NT251].

Toxicity. Fresh tobacco smoke, administered to high leukemic AKR strain of mice at low levels for 1 day, produced significantly different mortality profiles associated with the sex of the animals and the age at which smoke exposure commenced. Females were more susceptible and died sooner than males, where a significant proportion of animals survived longer than age-matched controls. This prolongation of life appeared to result from a failure of the leukemic state to be mobilized in the smoke-exposed males. Exposure of both females and males to the smoke did not induce significant detectable immunological reactivity against the leukemic cells for the parameters tested. This possibly resulted from a significant enhancement of suppressor activity in the serum of the chronically exposed animals that also occurs in age-matched control animals[NT139]. Smoke of cured leaf, administered by inhalation to adults, was active[NT362]. Leaves, on agar plate at a concentration of 50%, produced changes in cell morphology of the monkey kidney cells[NT574]. Leaf, administered orally to adults, was active. Ultrastructure abnormalities included discontinuous and fragmented basement membrane, reduction in hemidesmosomes, and widened intercellular spaces of the esophageal mucosa[NT453]. Leaf, administered by inhalation to male adults at a dose of 15 g/day, was active vs various male sex gland functions in tobacco smokers. An 8-month-old infant ate two cigarette butts. On presentation 2.5 hours later, she was very lethargic and had depressed respiration, subsequently became somnolent with difficulty breathing. Urine toxicity screen was positive only for nicotine. She recovered with supportive treatment[NT511]. Fresh leaf, administered externally to adults, was active vs green tobacco sickness in tobacco workers[NT483]. The exposure of 47 patients to wet leaves resulted in nicotine toxicity, specifically nausea, vomiting, weakness, and dizziness. Mean time from exposure to onset of symptoms was 10 hours[NT452]. Smoke extract, in the mouse brain mitochondria culture in the presence or absence of vitamin C for 60 minutes, inhibited mitochondrial ATPase and cytochrome C oxidase activities in a dose-dependent manner. The effect of extract on mitochondria swelling response to calcium stimulation was dependent on calcium concentrations. The extract treatment induced mitochondrial inner membrane damage and vacuolization of the matrix, whereas the outer mitochondrial membrane was preserved. Nicotine produced no significant damage[NT007]. Nicotine, preincubated with normal human oral keratinocytes, altered the ligand-binding kinetics of their nicotinic acetylcholine receptors. It produced transcriptional and translational changes and changed the mRNA and protein levels of the cell cycle and cell differentiation markers Ki-67, PCNA, p21, cyclin D1, p53, filaggrin, loricrin, and cytokeratins 1 and 10. Environmental cigarette smoke or drinking water containing equivalent concentrations of nicotine that are pathophysiologically relevant, administered to rats and mice for 3 weeks, produced changes of the nicotinic acetylcholine receptors and the cell cycle and cell differentiation genes similar to those found in vitro[NT033].

Transglutaminase activity. Water-soluble extract of gas-phase cigarette smoke was incubated with mouse bone marrow-derived macrophage culture containing both tissue-type transglutaminase and factor XIII-associated transglutaminase for 15 minutes at 37°C. A dose-dependent decrease in tissue-type (thrombin-independent) transglutaminase activity was produced, as compared to control cells. Factor XIII (zymogen) was not inactivated after incubation of macrophages with smoke extracts. Smoke exposure had no effect on cell viability or adherence. The results indicated that bone marrow-derived macrophages contain factor XIII and tissue-type transglutaminase. Gas-phase cigarette smoke can inactivate tissue transglutaminase within viable murine bone marrow-derived macrophages but cannot inactive zymogenic factor XIII[NT131].

TNF-α production. Water-soluble cigarette smoke extract and/or respiratory syncytial virus (RSV), in cell culture, stimulated TNF-α release from monocytes by both RSV infection and smoke extract and an additive effect was observed. There was a decrease in NO release, significant only with smoke extract or a combination of smoke extract and RSV infection. Nicotine decreased both TNF-α and NO responses. The proportion of extreme responses with very high TNF-α and very low NO in the presence of both RSV and smoke extract increased to 20% compared with 5% observed with smoke extract or RSV alone[NT048]. Aqueous extract of the STE, in macrophage J774-A1 cell line and mouse splenocyte cultures at low concentrations, enhanced the production of both TNF-α and IL-1β and mitogen-induced murine splenocyte proliferation[NT054]. Tobacco smoke, in alveolar macrophages of C57BL/6 mice in vivo, produced a significant decrease in the production of TNF-α by alveolar macrophages with the stimulation of lipopolysaccharide. In vitro exposure of alveolar macrophages to tobacco smoke water-soluble extracts decreased the production of TNF-α up to 93% of control with stimulation of lipopolysaccharide without any decrease in cellular viability[NT095]. Smoke was administered to rats at a concentration of 10 mg/m³ of cigarette smoke for 8 hours daily and the recovered alveolar macrophages were incubated with chrysotile or ceramic fibers for 24 hours. TNF of alveolar macrophages that were not stimulated produced no difference between treated and control rats. In alveolar macrophages stimulated by chrysotile or ceramic fibers, production of TNF in smoke-exposed rats was higher than that of controls[NT279].

Tyrosinase inhibition. Methanol (80%) extract of the dried aerial parts, at a concentration of 100 μg/mL, produced weak activity[NT415].

UDP–glucuronyltransferase activity. Cigarette smoke, administered intranasally to young male C57BL mice fed 5 and 100 ppm of vitamin E, 20 min/day for 8 weeks, produced no effect on UDP–glucuronyltransferase[NT153].

Ulcer healing inhibition. Cigarette smoke or smoke extract, administered to ulcerated rats once daily for 3 days, produced concomitant and dose-dependent reduction of angiogenesis and constitutive NOS activity. The same treatments also delayed ulcer healing. Results indicated that cigarette smoke and its extract repressed the processes of new blood vessel formation and NOS activity during tissue repair in the gastric mucosa[NT232].

Urinary metabolites. Different biomarkers of NNK exposure and metabolism, including the urinary metabolite NNAL and the presumed detoxification product [4-(methylnitrosamino)-1-(3-pyridyl)but-1-yl]-β-O-D-glucosiduronic acid (NNAL-Gluc) were examined along with questionnaire data on lifestyle habits and diet in a metabolic epidemiological study of 34 black and 27 white healthy smokers. The results demonstrated that urinary NNAL-Gluc–NNAL ratios, a likely indicator of NNAL glucuronidation and detoxification, were significantly greater in whites than in blacks ($p < 0.02$). In addition, two phenotypes were apparent by probit analysis representing poor (ratio < 6) and extensive (ratio ≥ 6) glucuronidation groups. The proportion of blacks falling into the former, potentially high-risk group was significantly greater than that of whites ($p < 0.05$). The absolute levels of urinary NNAL, NNAL-Gluc, and cotinine were also greater in blacks than in whites when adjusted for the number of cigarettes smoked. None of the observed racial differences could be explained by dissimilarities in exposure or other sociodemographic or dietary factors. Also, it is unlikely that the dissimilarities are due to racial differences in preference for mentholated cigarettes, because chronic administration of menthol to NNK-treated rats did not result in either increases in urinary total NNAL or decreases in NNAL-Gluc–NNAL ratios. Altogether, these results suggest that racial differences in NNAL glucuronidation, a putative detoxification pathway for NNK, may explain in part the observed differences in cancer risk[NT250].

Vasoconstriction activity. Cigarette smoke, in isolated rat lungs perfused with blood, produced no change in pulmonary vascular resistance. The hypoxic pulmonary vasoconstriction was significantly enhanced by smoking. Indomethacin, an inhibitor of prostaglandins biosynthesis, administered in the perfusing blood, increased hypoxic pulmonary vasoconstriction in the nonsmoking lungs but not in lungs after smoking. Diethylcarbamazine citrate (1 mg/mL), an inhibitor of leukotrienes biosynthesis, decreased hypoxic pulmonary vasoconstriction before and after smoking. After perfusion with both indomethacin and diethylcarbamazine citrate, hypoxic pulmonary vasoconstriction also decreased. Results indicated that leukotrienes act as mediators whereas prostaglandins as modulators in hypoxic pulmonary vasoconstriction, and prostaglandins and leukotrienes may play an important role in the increase of hypoxic pulmonary vasoconstriction by cigarette smoking[NT286]. Cigarette smoke extract, administered intravenously to Wistar rats during hypoxic ventilation, produced significant decrease in microvascular internal diameter of pulmonary arterioles and venules. After pretreatment of animal with smoke extract, much more remarkable pulmonary vasoconstriction was induced by hypoxia than before injection of the extract. During hypoxia, mean pulmonary arterial pressure increased by 13.53% before administration of smoke extract and by 30.57% after administration, respectively. Results indicated that smoke extract can strengthen pulmonary vasoconstriction and hypertension induced by acute alveolar hypoxia[NT288].

Viral stimulant. Smoke of the leaf, administered by inhalation to mice at variable doses twice daily for 5 days followed by 2 nontreatment days, dosed for two to six cycles, was inactive on encephalomyocarditis virus, Herpes virus type 1, and influenza virus APR-8[NT587].

Vitamins A and C concentrations influence. Methyl chloride extract of the leaf, administered intragastrically to rats at a dose of 3 mg/animal daily for 21 months in DMSO solvent, was active. Rats were divided or two groups: one was fed a vitamin A diet, and one a vitamin A-deficient diet. Vitamin C levels in both liver and plasma elevated significantly in extract-treated animals, while vitamin A level decreased[NT519]. NNN and NNK, administered to Swiss and Balb/c male mice, produced a significant decrease in liver vitamin A levels by both nitrosamines. NNK treatment also produced a decrease in the levels of vitamin A in plasma[NT104].

Weight loss. Smoke of the leaf, administered by inhalation to mice at variable doses twice daily for 5 days followed by 2 nontreatment days, dosed for two to six cycles, was active[NT587]. Tobacco smoke, administered to 3-week-old Wistar rats on a vitamin E-depleted or normal diet, for 4 weeks, significantly suppressed body weight increases, particularly in the vitamin E-depleted group[NT268].

REFERENCES

NT001 Hatsukami, D. K., C. Lemmonds, Y. Zhang, et al. Evaluation of carcinogen exposure in people who used "reduced exposure" tobacco products. **J Natl Cancer Inst** 2004; 96(11): 844–852.

NT002 Patel, P.S., M. H. Shah, F. P. Jha, et al. Alterations in plasma lipid profile patterns in head and neck cancer and oral precancerous conditions. **Indian J Cancer** 2004; 41(1): 25–31.

NT003 Meckley, D. R., J. R. Hayes, K. R. Van Kampen, P. H. Ayres, A. T. Mosberg, and J. E. Swauger. Comparative study of smoke condensates from 1R4F cigarettes that burn tobacco versus ECLIPSE cigarettes that primarily heat tobacco in the SENCAR mouse dermal tumor promotion assay. **Food Chem Toxicol** 2004; 42(5): 851–863.

NT004 Nguyen Van Binh, P., D. Zhou, F. Baudouin, et al. *In vitro* and *in vivo* immunotoxic and immunomodulatory effects of nonsupplemented and selenium-supplemented cigarette smoke condensate. **Biomed Pharmacother** 2004; 58(2): 90–94.

NT005   West, K. A., I. R. Linnoila, S. A. Belinsky, C. C. Harris, and P. A. Dennis. Tobacco carcinogen-induced cellular transformation increases activation of the phosphatidylinositol 3'-kinase/Akt pathway in vitro and in vivo. **Cancer Res** 2004; 64(2): 446–451.

NT006   Witschi, H., I. Espiritu, D. Uyeminami, M. Suffia, and K. E. Pinkerton. Lung tumor response in strain a mice exposed to tobacco smoke: some dose–effect relationships. **Inhal Toxicol** 2004; 16(1): 27–32.

NT007   Yang, Y. M., and G. T. Liu. Injury of mouse brain mitochondria induced by cigarette smoke extract and effect of vitamin C on it in vitro. **Biomed Environ Sci** 2003; 16(3): 256–266.

NT008   Jani, D., N. K. Singh, S. Bhattacharya, et al. Studies on the immunogenic potential of plant-expressed cholera toxin B subunit. **Plant Cell Rep** 2004; 22(7): 471–477.

NT009   Wu, L., L. Jiang, Z. Zhou, et al. Expression of foot-and-mouth disease virus epitopes in tobacco by a tobacco mosaic virus-based vector. **Vaccine** 2003; 21(27–30): 4390–4398.

NT010   Sandhir, R., S. Subramanian, and A. Koul. Long-term smoking and ethanol exposure accentuates oxidative stress in hearts of mice. **Cardiovasc Toxicol** 2003; 3(2):135–140.

NT011   Jalas, J. R., X. Ding, and S. E. Murphy. Comparative metabolism of the tobacco-specific nitrosamines 4-(methylnitrosamino)-1-(3-pyridyl)-1-butanone and 4-(methylnitrosamino)-1-(3-pyridyl)-1-butanol by rat cytochrome P450 2A3 and human cytochrome P450 2A13. **Drug Metab Dispos** 2003; 31(10): 1199–1202.

NT012   Huang, Y., W. Liang, A. Pan, Z. Zhou, C. Huang, J. Chen, and D. Zhang. Production of FaeG, the major subunit of K88 fimbriae, in transgenic tobacco plants and its immunogenicity in mice. **Infect Immun** 2003; 71(9): 5436–5439.

NT013   Robbins, C. S., D. E. Dawe, S. I. Goncharova, et al. Cigarette smoke decreases pulmonary dendritic cells and impacts antiviral immune responsiveness. **Am J Respir Cell Mol Biol** 2004; 30(2): 202–211.

NT014   Zhou, H., G. M. Calaf, and T. K. Hei. Malignant transformation of human bronchial epithelial cells with the tobacco-specific nitrosamine, 4-(methylnitrosamino)-1-(3-pyridyl)-1-butanone. **Int J Cancer** 2003; 106(6): 821–826.

NT015   Ramirez, N., M. Rodriguez, M. Ayala, et al. Expression and characterization of an anti-(hepatitis B surface antigen) glycosylated mouse antibody in transgenic tobacco (Nicotiana tabacum) plants and its use in the immunopurification of its target antigen. **Biotechnol Appl Biochem** 2003; 38(Pt 3): 223–230.

NT016   Petro, T. M. Modulation of IL-12 p35 and p40 promoter activity by smokeless tobacco extract is associated with an effect upon activation of NF-kappaB but not IRF transcription factors. **Int Immunopharmacol** 2003; 3(5): 735–745.

NT017   Masuda, Y., S. Ohnuma, M. Kawagoe, and T. Sugiyama. A glycoside of Nicotina tabacum affects mouse dopaminergic behavior. **Methods Find Exp Clin Pharmacol** 2003; 25(1): 41–43.

NT018   Churg, A., R. D. Wang, C. Xie, and J. L. Wright. Alpha-1-Antitrypsin ameliorates cigarette smoke-induced emphysema in the mouse. **Am J Respir Crit Care Med** 2003;168(2): 199–207.

NT019   Koul, A., A. Singh, and R. Sandhir. Effect of alpha-tocopherol on the cardiac antioxidant defense system and atherogenic lipids in cigarette smoke-inhaling mice. **Inhal Toxicol** 2003; 15(5): 513–522.

NT020   De Flora, S., R. M. Balansky, F. D'Agostini, A. Izzotti, A. Camoirano, C. Bennicelli, Z. Zhang, Y. Wang, R. A. Lubet, and M. You. Molecular alterations and lung tumors in p53 mutant mice exposed to cigarette smoke. **Cancer Res** 2003; 63(4): 793–800.

NT021   Pouli, A. E., D. G. Hatzinikolaou, C. Piperi, A. Stavridou, M. C. Psallidopoulos, and J. C. Stavrides. The cytotoxic effect of volatile organic compounds of the gas phase of cigarette smoke on lung epithelial cells. **Free Radic Biol Med** 2003; 34(3): 345–355.

NT022   Poirier, M., M. Fournier, P. Brousseau, and A. Morin. Effects of volatile aromatics, aldehydes, and phenols in tobacco smoke on viability and proliferation of mouse lymphocytes. **J Toxicol Environ Health A** 2002; 65(19): 1437–1451.

NT023 Coggins, C.R. A minireview of chronic animal inhalation studies with mainstream cigarette smoke. **Inhal Toxicol** 2002; 14(10): 991–1002.

NT024 Zhang, J., Y. Liu, J. Shi, D. F. Larson, and R. R. Watson. Side-stream cigarette smoke induces dose–response in systemic inflammatory cytokine production and oxidative stress. **Exp Biol Med (Maywood)** 2002; 227(9): 823–829.

NT025 Miller, L. M., W. M. Foster, D. M. Dambach, et al. A murine model of cigarette smoke-induced pulmonary inflammation using intranasally administered smoke-conditioned medium. **Exp Lung Res** 2002; 28(6): 435–455.

NT026 Obermueller-Jevic, U.C., I. Espiritu, A. M. Corbacho, C. E. Cross, and H. Witschi. Lung tumor development in mice exposed to tobacco smoke and fed beta-carotene diets. **Toxicol Sci** 2002; 69(1): 23–29.

NT027 Matsunaga, K., T. W. Klein, H. Friedman, and Y. Yamamoto. Epigallocatechin gallate, a potential immunomodulatory agent of tea components, diminishes cigarette smoke condensate-induced suppression of anti-*Legionella pneumophila* activity and cytokine responses of alveolar macrophages. **Clin Diagn Lab Immunol** 2002; 9(4): 864–871.

NT028 Witschi, H., and I. Espiritu. Development of tobacco smoke-induced lung tumors in mice fed Bowman-Birk protease inhibitor concentrate (BBIC). **Cancer Lett** 2002; 183(2): 141–146.

NT029 Bosio, A., C. Knorr, U. Janssen, S. Gebel, H. J. Haussmann, and T. Muller. Kinetics of gene expression profiling in Swiss 3T3 cells exposed to aqueous extracts of cigarette smoke. **Carcinogenesis** 2002; 23(5): 741–748.

NT030 Witschi. H., I. Espiritu, M. Suffia, and K. E. Pinkerton. Expression of cyclin D1/2 in the lungs of strain A/J mice fed chemopreventive agents. **Carcinogenesis** 2002; 23(2): 289–294.

NT031 Petro, T. M., L. L. Anderson, J. S. Gowler, X. J. Liu, and S. D. Schwartz-

bach. Smokeless tobacco extract decreases IL-12 production from LPS-stimulated but increases IL-12 from IFN-gamma-stimulated macrophages. **Int Immunopharmacol** 2002; 2(2–3): 345–355.

NT032 Wang, X., T. Hao, and R. Wu. Effect of cigarette smoke extract on E-cadherin expression of airway epithelial cells. **Zhonghua Jie He He Hu Xi Za Zhi** 1999; 22(7): 414–416.

NT033 Arredondo, J., V. T. Nguyen, A. I. Chernyavsky, D. L. Jolkovsky, K. E. Pinkerton, and S. A. Grando. A receptor-mediated mechanism of nicotine toxicity in oral keratinocytes. **Lab Invest** 2001; 81(12): 1653–1668.

NT034 Cavarra, E., B. Bartalesi, M. Lucattelli, et al. Effects of cigarette smoke in mice with different levels of alpha(1)-proteinase inhibitor and sensitivity to oxidants. **Am J Respir Crit Care Med** 2001; 164(5): 886–890.

NT035 Khaldoyanidi, S., L. Sikora, I. Orlovskaya, V. Matrosova, V. Kozlov, and P. Sriramarao. Correlation between nicotine-induced inhibition of hematopoiesis and decreased CD44 expression on bone marrow stromal cells. **Blood** 2001; 98(2): 303–312.

NT036 Cavarra, E., M. Lucattelli, F. Gambelli, et al. Human SLPI inactivation after cigarette smoke exposure in a new in vivo model of pulmonary oxidative stress. **Am J Physiol Lung Cell Mol Physiol** 2001; 281(2): L412–L417.

NT037 Castagnoli, K. P., S. J. Steyn, J. P. Petzer, C. J. Van der Schyf, and N. Castagnoli Jr. Neuroprotection in the MPTP Parkinsonian C57BL/6 mouse model by a compound isolated from tobacco. **Chem Res Toxicol** 2001; 14(5): 523–527.

NT038 Hauptmann, N., and J. C. Shih. 2-Naphthylamine, a compound found in cigarette smoke, decreases both monoamine oxidase A and B catalytic activity. **Life Sci** 2001; 68(11): 1231–1241.

NT039 Bondy, S. C., S. F. Ali, and M. T. Kleinman. Exposure of mice to tobacco smoke attenuates the toxic effect of methamphetamine on dopamine systems. **Toxicol Lett** 2000; 118(1–2): 43–46.

NT040 Gebel, S., and T. Muller. The activity of NF-kappaB in Swiss 3T3 cells exposed to aqueous extracts of cigarette smoke is dependent on thioredoxin. **Toxicol Sci** 2001; 59(1): 75–81.

NT041 Koethe, S. M., J. R. Kuhnmuench, and C. G. Becker. Neutrophil priming by cigarette smoke condensate and a to-bacco anti-idiotypic antibody. **Am J Pathol** 2000; 157(5): 1735–1743.

NT042 Chen, S., J. Gong, F. Liu, and U. Mohammed. Naturally occurring polyphenolic antioxidants modulate IgE-mediated mast cell activation. **Immunology** 2000; 100(4): 471–480.

NT043 Seredenin, S. B., V. N. Zhukov, M. G. Miramedova, et al. A chamber for evaluating the free choice by laboratory rats and mice of a space containing tobacco smoke. **Eksp Klin Farmakol** 2000; 63(1): 66–70.

NT044 Tsuda, S., N. Matsusaka, S. Ueno, N. Susa, and Y. F. Sasaki. The influence of antioxidants on cigarette smoke-induced DNA single-strand breaks in mouse organs: a preliminary study with the alkaline single cell gel electrophoresis assay. **Toxicol Sci** 2000; 54(1): 104–109.

NT045 Dhami, R., B. Gilks, C. Xie, K. Zay, J. L. Wright, and A. Churg. Acute cigarette smoke-induced connective tissue breakdown is mediated by neutrophils and prevented by alpha1-antitrypsin. **Am J Respir Cell Mol Biol** 2000; 22(2): 244–252.

NT046 March, T.H., E. B. Barr, G. L. Finch, et al. Cigarette smoke exposure produces more evidence of emphysema in B6C3F1 mice than in F344 rats. **Toxicol Sci** 1999; 51(2): 289–299.

NT047 Raza, M. W., S. D. Essery, R. A. Elton, D. M. Weir, A. Busuttil, and C. Blackwell. Exposure to cigarette smoke, a major risk factor for sudden infant death syndrome: effects of cigarette smoke on inflammatory responses to viral infection and bacterial toxins. **FEMS Immunol Med Microbiol** 1999; 25(1–2): 145–154.

NT048 Raza, M. W., S. D. Essery, D. M. Weir, M. M. Ogilvie, R. A. Elton, and C. C. Blackwell. Infection with respiratory syncytial virus and water-soluble components of cigarette smoke alter production of tumour necrosis factor alpha and nitric oxide by human blood monocytes. **FEMS Immunol Med Microbiol** 1999; 24(4): 387–394.

NT049 Petro, T. M., S. D. Schwartzbach, and S. Zhang. Smokeless tobacco and nicotine bring about excessive cytokine responses of murine memory T-cells. **Int J Immunopharmacol** 1999; 21(2): 103–114.

NT050 Winn, L. M., P. M. Kim, and P. G. Wells. Investigation of the tobacco-specific carcinogen 4-(methylnitrosamino)-1-(3-pyridyl)-1–butanone for in vivo and in vitro murine embryopathy and embryonic ras mutations. **J Pharmacol Exp Ther** 1998; 287(3): 1128–1135.

NT051 Dertinger, S. D., A. E. Silverstone, and T. A. Gasiewicz. Influence of aromatic hydrocarbon receptor–mediated events on the genotoxicity of cigarette smoke condensate. **Carcinogenesis** 1998; 19(11): 2037–2042.

NT052 Grasso, P. and A. H. Mann. Smokeless tobacco and oral cancer: an assessment of evidence derived from laboratory animals. **Food Chem Toxicol** 1998; 36(11): 1015–1029.

NT053 Jalili, T., G. G. Murthy, and R. H. Schiestl. Cigarette smoke induces DNA deletions in the mouse embryo. **Cancer Res** 1998; 58(12): 2633–2638.

NT054 Seyedroudbari, S. A., and M. M. Khan. In vitro effects of smokeless tobacco extract on tumor necrosis factor-alpha (TNF-alpha) and interleukin-1beta (IL-1beta) production, and on lymphocyte proliferation. **Toxicon** 1998; 36(4): 631–637.

NT055 Brown, B., J. Kolesar, K. Lindberg, D. Meckley, A. Mosberg, and D. Doolittle. Comparative studies of DNA adduct formation in mice following dermal application of smoke condensates from cigarettes that burn or primarily heat tobacco. **Mutat Res** 1998; 414 (1–3): 21–30.

NT056 Howard, D. J., L. A. Briggs, and C. A. Pritsos. Oxidative DNA damage in mouse heart, liver, and lung tissue due to acute side-stream tobacco smoke exposure. **Arch Biochem Biophys** 1998; 352(2): 293–297.

NT057 Singh, A., and S. P. Singh. Postnatal effect of smokeless tobacco on phytic acid or the butylated hydroxyanisole–

modulated hepatic detoxication system and antioxidant defense mechanism in suckling neonates and lactating mice. **Cancer Lett** 1998; 122(1–2): 151–156.

NT058 Bagchi, M., D. Bagchi, E. Adickes, and S. J. Stohs. Chronic effects of smokeless tobacco extract on rat liver histopathology, and production of HSP-90. **J Environ Pathol Toxicol Oncol** 1995; 14(2): 61–68.

NT059 Singh, A., and S. P. Singh. Modulatory potential of smokeless tobacco on the garlic, mace or black mustard-altered hepatic detoxication system enzymes, sulfhydryl content and lipid peroxidation in murine system. **Cancer Lett** 1997; 118(1): 109–114.

NT060 Hautamaki, R. D., D. K. Kobayashi, R. M. Senior, and S. D. Shapiro. Requirement for macrophage elastase for cigarette smoke-induced emphysema in mice. **Science** 1997; 277(5334): 2002–2004.

NT061 Sipowicz, M. A., S. Amin, D. Desai, K. S. Kasprzak, and L. M. Anderson. Oxidative DNA damage in tissues of pregnant female mice and fetuses caused by the tobacco-specific nitrosamine, 4-(methylnitrosamino)-1-(3-pyridyl)-1-butanone (NNK). **Cancer Lett** 1997; 117(1): 87–91.

NT062 Petro, T. M., and S. Zhang. The effect of smokeless tobacco extract on murine T cell cytokine production. **Immunopharmacology** 1997; 36(1): 17–26.

NT063 Geiselhart, L. A., T. Christian, F. Minnear, and B. M. Freed. The cigarette tar component p-benzoquinone blocks T-lymphocyte activation by inhibiting interleukin-2 production, but not CD25, ICAM-1, or LFA-1 expression. **Toxicol Appl Pharmacol** 1997; 143(1): 30–36.

NT064 Witschi, H., I. Espiritu, J. L. Peake, K. Wu, R. R. Maronpot, and K. E. Pinkerton. The carcinogenicity of environmental tobacco smoke. **Carcinogenesis** 1997; 18(3): 575–586.

NT065 Muller, T., H. J. Haussmann, and G. Schepers. Evidence for peroxynitrite as an oxidative stress-inducing compound of aqueous cigarette smoke fractions. **Carcinogenesis** 1997; 18(2): 295–301.

NT066 Brown, B.G., C. K. Lee, B. R. Bombick, P. H. Ayres, A. T. Mosberg, and D. J. Doolittle. Comparative study of DNA adduct formation in mice following inhalation of smoke from cigarettes that burn or primarily heat tobacco. **Environ Mol Mutagen** 1997; 29(3): 303–311.

NT067 Attolini, L., M. Gantenbein, and B. Bruguerolle. Effects of tobacco smoke exposure on the kinetics of bupivacaine in mice. **Life Sci** 1997; 60(10): 725–734.

NT068 Zhang, S. and T. M. Petro. The effect of nicotine on murine CD4 T cell responses. **Int J Immunopharmacol** 1996; 18(8–9): 467–78.

NT069 Attolini, L., M. Gantenbein, P. H. Villard, B. Lacarelle, J. Catalin, and B. Bruguerolle. Effects of different exposure times to tobacco smoke intoxication on carboxyhemoglobin and hepatic enzymate activities in mice. **J Pharmacol Toxicol Methods** 1996; 35(4): 211–215.

NT070 Mason, H. S., J. M. Ball, J. J. Shi, X. Jiang, M. K. Estes, and C. J. Arntzen. Expression of Norwalk virus capsid protein in transgenic tobacco and potato and its oral immunogenicity in mice. **Proc Natl Acad Sci USA** 1996; 93(11): 5335–5340.

NT071 Lazarus, P., A. M. Idris, J. Kim, A. Calcagnotto, and D. Hoffmann. p53 mutations in head and neck squamous cell carcinomas from Sudanese snuff (toombak) users. **Cancer Detect Prev** 1996; 20(4): 270–278.

NT072 Bagchi, D., E. A. Hassoun, M. Bagchi, and S. J. Stohs. Protective effects of free radical scavengers and antioxidants against smokeless tobacco extract (STE)-induced oxidative stress in macrophage J774A.1. Cell cultures. **Arch Environ Contam Toxicol** 1995; 29(3): 424–428.

NT073 Balansky, R. M. Effects of cigarette smoke and disulfiram on tumorigenicity and clastogenicity of ethyl carbamate in mice. **Cancer Lett** 1995; 94(1): 91–95.

NT074 Haq, T. A., H. S. Mason, J. D. Clements, and C. J. Arntzen. Oral immunization with a recombinant bacterial antigen produced in transgenic plants. **Science** 1995; 268(5211): 714–716.

NT075   Muller, T. Expression of c-fos in quiescent Swiss 3T3 cells exposed to aqueous cigarette smoke fractions. **Cancer Res** 1995; 55(9): 1927–1932.

NT076   Thanavala, Y., Y. F. Yang, P. Lyons, H. S. Mason, and C. Arntzen. Immunogenicity of transgenic plant-derived hepatitis B surface antigen. **Proc Natl Acad Sci USA** 1995; 92(8): 3358–3361.

NT077   Zeid, N. A., and H. K. Muller. Tobacco smoke condensate cutaneous carcinogenesis: changes in Langerhans' cells and tumour regression. **Int J Exp Pathol** 1995; 76(1): 75–83.

NT078   Makonkawkeyoon, S., P. Smitamana, C. Hirunpetcharat, and N. Maneekarn. Production of mouse immunoglobulin G by a hybrid plant derived from tobacco-mouse cell fusions. **Experientia** 1995; 51(1): 19–25.

NT079   Guengerich F. P., T. Shimada, C. H. Yun, et al. Interactions of ingested food, beverage, and tobacco components involving human cytochrome P4501A2, 2A6, 2E1, and 3A4 enzymes. **Environ Health Perspect** 1994; 102(Suppl 9): 49–53.

NT080   Villard, P. H., E. Seree, B. Lacarelle, et al. Effect of cigarette smoke on hepatic and pulmonary cytochromes P450 in mouse: evidence for CYP2E1 induction in lung. **Biochem Biophys Res Commun** 1994; 202(3): 1731–1737.

NT081   Erenmemisoglu, A., C. Suer, and S. Temocin. Has nicotine a local anaesthetic action? **J Basic Clin Physiol Pharmacol** 1994; 5(2): 125–131.

NT082   Nersessian, A. K., and R. M. Arutyunyan. The comparative clastogenic activity of mainstream tobacco smoke from cigarettes widely consumed in Armenia. **Mutat Res** 1994; 321(1–2): 89–92.

NT083   Muller, T., and S. Gebel. Heme oxygenase expression in Swiss 3T3 cells following exposure to aqueous cigarette smoke fractions. **Carcinogenesis** 1994; 15(1): 67–72.

NT084   Bagwe, A. N., A. G. Ramchandani, and R. A. Bhisey. Skin-tumor-promoting activity of processed bidi tobacco

in hairless S/RV Cri-ba mice. **J Cancer Res Clin Oncol** 1994; 120(8): 485–489.

NT085   Li, Z.Q., H. J. Wei, X. M. Luo, et al. Specific overexpression of P53 in sarcoma derived from Rat-1 cells transformed by cigarette smoking condensate-treated human fetal lung DNA. **J Environ Pathol Toxicol Oncol** 1994; 13(3): 187–190.

NT086   Stoichev, I. I., D. K. Todorov, and L. T. Christova. Dominant-lethal mutations and micronucleus induction in male BALB/c, BDF1 and H mice by tobacco smoke. **Mutat Res** 1993; 319(4): 285–292.

NT087   Hoffmann, D., M. V. Djordjevic, A. Rivenson, E. Zang, D. Desai, and S. Amin. A study of tobacco carcinogenesis. LI. Relative potencies of tobacco-specific N-nitrosamines as inducers of lung tumours in A/J mice. **Cancer Lett** 1993; 71(1–3): 25–30.

NT088   Goud, S. N., L. Zhang, and A. M. Kaplan. Immunostimulatory potential of smokeless tobacco extract in *in vitro* cultures of murine lymphoid tissues. **Immunopharmacology** 1993; 25(2): 95–105.

NT089   Piao, C. Q., and T. K. Hei. The biological effectiveness of radon daughter alpha particles. I. Radon, cigarette smoke and oncogenic transformation. **Carcinogenesis** 1993; 14(3): 497–501.

NT090   Chung, F. L., and Y. Xu. Increased 8-oxodeoxyguanosine levels in lung DNA of A/J mice and F344 rats treated with the tobacco-specific nitrosamine 4-(methylnitrosamine)-1-(3-pyridyl)-1-butanone. **Carcinogenesis** 1992; 13(7): 1269–1272.

NT091   Randerath, E., T. F. Danna, and K. Randerath. DNA damage induced by cigarette smoke condensate *in vitro* as assayed by ^{32}P-postlabeling. Comparison with cigarette smoke-associated DNA adduct profiles *in vivo*. **Mutat Res** 1992; 268(1): 139–153.

NT092   Dash, B. C., and R. K. Das. Genotoxicity of 'gudakhu', a tobacco preparation. I. In mice *in vivo*. **Mutat Res** 1992; 280(1): 45–53.

NT093   Paulson, R. B., J. Shanfeld, J. Dean, D. Mullet, M. Fernandez, and J. O.

Paulson. Alcohol and smokeless tobacco effects on the CD-1 mouse fetus. **J Craniofac Genet Dev Biol** 1992; 12(2): 107–117.

NT094   Lenz, L.G., W. K. Ramp, R. J. Galvin, and W. M. Pierce Jr. Inhibition of cell metabolism by a smokeless tobacco extract: tissue and species specificity. **Proc Soc Exp Biol Med** 1992; 199(2): 211–217.

NT095   Higashimoto, Y., Y. Shimada, Y. Fukuchi, et al. Inhibition of mouse alveolar macrophage production of tumor necrosis factor alpha by acute *in vivo* and *in vitro* exposure to tobacco smoke. **Respiration** 1992; 59(2): 77–80.

NT096   Lee, C. K., B. G. Brown, E. A. Reed, et al. DNA adduct formation in mice following dermal application of smoke condensates from cigarettes that burn or heat tobacco. **Environ Mol Mutagen** 1992; 20(4): 313–319.

NT097   Jansson, T., L. Romert, J. Magnusson, and D. Jenssen. Genotoxicity testing of extracts of a Swedish moist oral snuff. **Mutat Res** 1991; 261(2): 101–115.

NT098   Belinsky, S. A., T. R. Devereux, C. M. White, J. F. Foley, R. R. Maronpot, and M. W. Anderson. Role of Clara cells and type II cells in the development of pulmonary tumors in rats and mice following exposure to a tobacco-specific nitrosamine. **Exp Lung Res** 1991; 17(2): 263–278.

NT099   Nair, U. J., N. Ammigan, J. J. Kayal, and S. V. Bhide. Species differences in hepatic pulmonary and upper gastrointestinal tract biotransformation enzymes on long-term feeding of masheri—a pyrolyzed tobacco product. **Dig Dis Sci** 1991; 36(3): 293–298.

NT100   Nair, U. J., N. Ammigan, J. R. Kulkarni, and S. V. Bhide. Species difference in intestinal drug metabolising enzymes in mouse, rat and hamster and their inducibility by masheri, a pyrolysed tobacco product. **Indian J Exp Biol** 1991; 29(3): 256–258.

NT101   Paulson, R.B., J. Shanfeld, L. Prause, S. Iranpour, and J. O. Paulson. Pre- and post-conceptional tobacco effects on the CD-1 mouse fetus. **J Craniofac Genet Dev Biol** 1991; 11(1): 48–58.

NT102   Carr, L. A., and J. K. Basham. Effects of tobacco smoke constituents on

MPTP-induced toxicity and monoamine oxidase activity in the mouse brain. **Life Sci** 1991; 48(12): 1173–1177.

NT103   Crebelli, R., L. Conti, S. Fuselli, P. Leopardi, A. Zijno, and A. Carere. Further studies on the comutagenic activity of cigarette smoke condensate. **Mutat Res** 1991; 259(1): 29–36.

NT104   Padma, P. R., A. J. Amonkar, and S. V. Bhide. Effect of long-term treatment of two tobacco-specific N-nitrosamines on the vitamin A status of mice. **Nutr Cancer** 1991; 15(3–4): 217–220.

NT105   Balansky, R. M., P. M. Blagoeva, and Z. I. Mircheva. Modulation of genotoxic activity of tobacco smoke. **IARC Sci Publ** 1991; (105): 535–537.

NT106   Hoffmann, D., A. A. Melikian, and K. D. Brunnemann. Studies in tobacco carcinogenesis. **IARC Sci Publ** 1991; (105): 482–484.

NT107   Brunnemann, K. D., M. V. Djordjevic, R. Feng, and D. Hoffmann. Analysis and pyrolysis of some N-nitrosamino acids in tobacco and tobacco smoke. **IARC Sci Publ** 1991; (105): 477–481.

NT108   Beregi, E., O. Regius, K. Rajczy, M. Boross, and L. Penzes. Effect of cigarette smoke and 2-mercaptoethanol administration on age-related alterations and immunological parameters. **Gerontology** 1991; 37(6): 326–334.

NT109   Gijare, P. S., K. V. Rao, and S. V. Bhide. Inhibitory effects of snuff extract on ornithine decarboxylase and aryl hydrocarbon hydroxylase activities in relation to cell proliferation of mouse tongue epithelial cells. **Indian J Exp Biol** 1990; 28(11): 1012–1026.

NT110   Uejima, Y., Y. Fukuchi, T. Nagase, et al. Influences of inhaled tobacco smoke on the senescence accelerated mouse (SAM). **Eur Respir J** 1990; 3(9): 1029–1036.

NT111   Reddy, M. V., and K. Randerath. A comparison of DNA adduct formation in white blood cells and internal organs of mice exposed to benzo[a]pyrene, dibenzo[c,g]carbazole, safrole and cigarette smoke condensate. **Mutat Res** 1990; 241(1): 37–48.

NT112   Chang, J. C., S. G. Distler, and A. M. Kaplan. Tobacco smoke suppresses T cells but not antigen-presenting cells in the lung-associated lymph nodes. **Toxicol Appl Pharmacol** 1990; 102(3): 514–523.

NT113 Mohtashamipur, E., A. Mohtashamipur, P. G. Germann, H. Ernst, K. Norpoth, and U. Mohr. Comparative carcinogenicity of cigarette mainstream and sidestream smoke condensates on the mouse skin. **J Cancer Res Clin Oncol** 1990; 116(6): 604–608.

NT114 Paulson, R., J. Shanfeld, L. Sachs, T. Price, and J. Paulson. Effect of smokeless tobacco on the development of the CD-1 mouse fetus. **Teratology** 1989; 40(5): 483–494.

NT115 Rivenson, A., M. V. Djordjevic, S. Amin, and R. Hoffmann. A study of tobacco carcinogenesis XLIV. Bioassay in A/J mice of some N-nitrosamines. **Cancer Lett** 1989; 47(1–2): 111–114.

NT116 Martinez, R. D., L. Eisenbach, and M. Feldman. Cytotoxic and proliferative effect of tobacco products on Lewis lung adenocarcinoma cells and spleen lymphocytes. **Allergol Immunopathol (Madr)** 1989; 17(5): 257–261.

NT117 Anderson, L. M., S. S. Hecht, D. E. Dixon, et al. Evaluation of the transplacental tumorigenicity of the tobacco-specific carcinogen 4-(methylnitrosamino)-1-(3-pyridyl)-1-butanone in mice. **Cancer Res** 1989; 49(14): 3770–3775.

NT118 Balansky, R. M., and P. M. Blagoeva. Tobacco smoke-induced clastogenicity in mouse fetuses and in newborn mice. **Mutat Res** 1989; 223(1): 1–6.

NT119 Bjelogrlic, N., M. Iscan, H. Raunio, O. Pelkonen, and K. Vahakangas. Benzo[a]pyrene-DNA-adducts and monooxygenase activities in mice treated with benzo[a]pyrene, cigarette smoke or cigarette smoke condensate. **Chem Biol Interact** 1989; 70(1–2): 51–61.

NT120 Gijare, P. S., K. V. Rao, and S. V. Bhide. Effects of tobacco-specific nitrosamines and snuff extract on cell proliferation and activities of ornithine decarboxylase and aryl hydrocarbon hydroxylase in mouse tongue primary epithelial cell cultures. **J Cancer Res Clin Oncol** 1989; 115(6): 558–563.

NT121 Kulkarni, J., V. S. Lalitha, and S. Bhide. Weak carcinogenic effect of masheri, a pyrolysed tobacco product, in mouse skin tumor models. **J Cancer Res Clin Oncol** 1989; 115(2): 166–169.

NT122 Kulkarni, J. R., V. S. Lalitha, and S. V. Bhide. Carcinogenicity studies of masheri, a pyrolysed product of tobacco. **Carcinogenesis** 1988; 9(11): 2137–2138.

NT123 Hecht, S. S., A. Abbaspour, and D. Hoffman. A study of tobacco carcinogenesis. XLII. Bioassay in A/J mice of some structural analogues of tobacco-specific nitrosamines. **Cancer Lett** 1988; 42(1–2): 141–145.

NT124 Balansky, R. M., P. M. Blagoeva, and Z. I. Mircheva. The mutagenic and clastogenic activity of tobacco smoke. **Mutat Res** 1988; 208(3–4): 237–241.

NT125 Yokode, M., T. Kita, H. Arai, C. Kawai, S. Narumiya, and M. Fujiwara. Cholesteryl ester accumulation in macrophages incubated with low density lipoprotein pretreated with cigarette smoke extract. **Proc Natl Acad Sci USA** 1988; 85(7): 2344–2348.

NT126 Pakhale, S. S., S. Sarkar, K. Jayant, and S. V. Bhide. Carcinogenicity of Indian bidi and cigarette smoke condensate in Swiss albino mice. **J Cancer Res Clin Oncol** 1988; 114(6): 647–649.

NT127 Paulson, R., J. Shanfeld, L. Sachs, M. Ismail, and J. Paulson. Effect of smokeless tobacco on the development of the CD-1 mouse fetus. **Teratog Carcinog Mutagen** 1988; 8(2): 81–93.

NT128 Randerath, E., D. Mittal, and K. Randerath. Tissue distribution of covalent DNA damage in mice treated dermally with cigarette 'tar': preference for lung and heart DNA. **Carcinogenesis** 1988; 9(1): 75–80.

NT129 LaVoie, E. J., G. Prokopczyk, J. Rigotty, A. Czech, A. Rivenson, and J. D. Adams. Tumorigenic activity of the tobacco-specific nitrosamines 4-(methylnitrosamino)-1-(3-pyridyl)-1-butanone (NNK), 4-(methylnitrosamino)-4-(3-pyridyl)-1-butanol (iso-NNAL) and N'-nitrosonornicotine (NNN) on topical application to Sencar mice. **Cancer Lett** 1987; 37(3): 277–283.

NT130 Kulkarni, J. R., S. Sarkar, and S. V. Bhide. Mutagenicity of extracts of brown and black masheri, pyrolysed products of tobacco using short-term tests. **Mutagenesis** 1987; 2(4): 263–266.

NT131 Roth, W. J., H. B. Fleit, S. I. Chung, and A. Janoff. Characterization of two distinct transglutaminases of murine bone marrow-derived macrophages: effects of exposure of viable cells to cigarette smoke on enzyme activity. **J Leukoc Biol** 1987; 42(1): 9–20.

NT132 Lasnitzki, I., and W. Bollag. Prevention and reversal by a non-polar arotinoid (Ro 15-0778) of 3,4-benzpyrene- and cigarette smoke condensate-induced hyperplasia and metaplasia of rodent respiratory epithelia grown *in vitro*. **Eur J Cancer Clin Oncol** 1987; 23(6): 861–865.

NT133 Balansky, R. M., P. M. Blagoeva, and Z. I. Mircheva. Investigation of the mutagenic activity of tobacco smoke. **Mutat Res** 1987; 188(1): 13–19.

NT134 Perry, T. L., S. Hansen, and K. Jones. Exposure to cigarette smoke does not decrease the neurotoxicity of N-methyl-4-phenyl-1,2,3,6-tetrahydropyridine in mice. **Neurosci Lett** 1987; 74(2): 217–220.

NT135 Watson, E. S., A. B. Jones, M. K. Ashfaq, and J. T. Barrett. Spectrophotometric evaluation of carboxyhemoglobin in blood of mice after exposure to marijuana or tobacco smoke in a modified Walton horizontal smoke exposure machine. **J Anal Toxicol** 1987;11(1): 19–23.

NT136 Bhide, S. V., J. Kulkarni, U. J. Nair, B. Spiegelhalder, and R. Preussmann. Mutagenicity and carcinogenicity of masheri, a pyrolysed tobacco product, and its content of tobacco-specific nitrosamines. **IARC Sci Publ** 1987; (84): 460–462.

NT137 Park, N. H., E. G. Herbosa, and J. P. Sapp. Effect of tar condensate from smoking tobacco and water-extract of snuff on the oral mucosa of mice with latent herpes simplex virus. **Arch Oral Biol** 1987; 32(1): 47–53.

NT138 Randerath, E., T. A. Avitts, M. V. Reddy, R. H. Miller, R. B. Everson, and K. Randerath. Comparative ^{32}P-analysis of cigarette smoke-induced DNA damage in human tissues and mouse skin. **Cancer Res** 1986; 46(11): 5869–5877.

NT139 Nguyen D. T., and D. Keast. Effects of chronic daily exposure to tobacco smoke on the high leukemic AKR strain of mice. **Cancer Res** 1986; 46(7): 3334–3340.

NT140 Henry, C. J., and R. E. Kouri. Chronic inhalation studies in mice. II. Effects of long-term exposure to 2R1 cigarette smoke on (C57BL/Cum x C3H/AnfCum)F$_1$ mice. **J Natl Cancer Inst** 1986; 77(1): 203–212.

NT141 Gairola, C. G. Free lung cell response of mice and rats to mainstream cigarette smoke exposure. **Toxicol Appl Pharmacol** 1986; 84(3): 567–575.

NT142 Sonnenfeld, G., and R. W. Hudgens. Effect of sidestream and mainstream smoke exposure on *in vitro* interferon-alpha/beta production by L-929 cells. **Cancer Res** 1986; 46(6): 2779–2783.

NT143 Lehrer, S. B., R. P. Stankus, and J. E. Salvaggio. Tobacco smoke sensitivity: a result of allergy? **Ann Allergy** 1986; 56(5): 369–381.

NT144 Hegab, E. S., and D. H. Matulionis. Pulmonary macrophage mobilization in cigarette smoke-exposed mice after halothane anesthesia. **Anesth Analg** 1986; 65(1): 37–45.

NT145 Tanaka, T. and A. Rivenson. Mastocytoma induced by cigarette smoke particulates: "cigarette tar". **Arch Dermatol Res** 1986; 279(2): 130–135.

NT146 Sonnenfeld, G., R. B. Griffith, and R. W. Hudgens. The effect of smoke generation and manipulation variables on the cytotoxicity of mainstream and sidestream cigarette smoke to monolayer cultures of L-929 cells. **Arch Toxicol** 1985; 58(2): 120–122.

NT147 Saito, Y., H. Takizawa, S. Konishi, D. Yoshida, and S. Mizusaki. Identification of cembratriene-4,6-diol as antitumor-promoting agent from cigarette smoke condensate. **Carcinogenesis** 1985; 6(8): 1189–1194.

NT148 Cerna, M. and K. J. Angelis. Mutagenicity in the *Salmonella*/microsome assay of tobacco condensates formed during pipe smoking. **Mutat Res** 1985; 143(3): 161–164.

NT149 Putman, D. L., R. M. David, J. M. Melhorn, D. R. Dansie, C. J. Stone, and C. J. Henry. Dose-responsive increase in sister-chromatid exchanges in bone-marrow cells of mice exposed nose-only to whole cigarette smoke. **Mutat Res** 1985; 156(3): 181–186.

NT150 Matulionis, D. H., E. Kimmel, and L. Diamond. Morphologic and physiologic response of lungs to steroid and cigarette smoke: an animal model. **Environ Res** 1985; 36(2): 298–313.

NT151 Vahakangas, K., H. Rajaniemi, and O. Pelkonen. Ovarian toxicity of cigarette smoke exposure during pregnancy in mice. **Toxicol Lett** 1985; 25(1): 75–80.

NT152 Park, N. H., E. G. Herbosa, K. Niukian, and G. Shklar. Combined effect of herpes simplex virus and tobacco on the histopathologic changes in lips of mice. **Oral Surg Oral Med Oral Pathol** 1985; 59(2): 154–158.

NT153 Graziano, M. J., C. Gairola, and H. W. Dorough. Effects of cigarette smoke and dietary vitamin E levels on selected lung and hepatic biotransformation enzymes in mice. **Drug Nutr Interact** 1985; 3(4): 213–222.

NT154 Shah, A. S., A. V. Sarode, and S. V. Bhide. Experimental studies on mutagenic and carcinogenic effects of tobacco chewing. **J Cancer Res Clin Oncol** 1985; 109(3): 203–207.

NT155 Menon, M. M., and S. V. Bhide. Mutagenicity of urine of bidi and cigarette smokers and tobacco chewers. **Carcinogenesis** 1984; 5(11): 1523–1524.

NT156 Shirname, L. P., M. M. Menon, S. S. Pakhale, and S. V. Bhide. Mutagenicity of smoke condensate of bidi—an indigenous cigarette of India. **Carcinogenesis** 1984; 5(9): 1179–1181.

NT157 Benedict, W. F., A. Banerjee, K. K. Kangalingam, D. R. Dansie, R. E. Kouri, and C. J. Henry. Increased sister-chromatid exchange in bone-marrow cells of mice exposed to whole cigarette smoke. **Mutat Res** 1984; 136(1): 73–80.

NT158 Tjalve, H., A. Castonguay, and S. S. Hecht. Fate of the tobacco-specific carcinogen 4-(methylnitrosamino)-1-(3-pyridyl)-1-butanone in pregnant and newborn C57BL mice. **IARC Sci Publ** 1984; (57): 787–796.

NT159 Bhide, S. V., A. S. Shah, J. Nair, and D. Nagarajrao. Epidemiological and experimental studies on tobacco-related oral cancer in India. **IARC Sci Publ** 1984; (57): 851–857.

NT160 Sonnenfeld, G., and R. W. Hudgens. Effect of carcinogenic components of cigarette smoke on in vivo production of murine interferon. **Cancer Res** 1983; 43(10): 4720–4722.

NT161 Keast, D., and K. Taylor. The effects of chronic tobacco smoke exposure from high-tar cigarettes on the phagocytic and killing capacity of polymorphonuclear cells of mice. **Environ Res** 1983; 31(1): 66–75.

NT162 Matulionis, D. H. Pulmonary tissue and cigarette smoke. 2. Parenchymal response. **Environ Res** 1983; 31(1): 176–188.

NT163 Francus, T., G. W. Siskind, and C. G. Becker. Role of antigen structure in the regulation of IgE isotype expression. **Proc Natl Acad Sci USA** 1983; 80(11): 3430–3434.

NT164 Sonnenfeld, G. Effect of sidestream tobacco smoke components on alpha/beta interferon production. **Oncology** 1983; 40(1): 52–56.

NT165 Lasnitzki, I., and W. Bollag. Prevention and reversal by a retinoid of 3,4-benzpyrene- and cigarette smoke condensate-induced hyperplasia and metaplasia of rodent respiratory epithelia in organ culture. **Cancer Treat Rep** 1982; 66(6): 1375–1380.

NT166 Hoffmann, D., J. D. Adams, K. D. Brunnemann, A. Rivenson, and S. S. Hecht. Tobacco specific N-nitrosamines: occurrence and bioassays. **IARC Sci Publ** 1982; (41): 309–318.

NT167 Keast, D., D. J. Ayre, and J. M. Papadimitriou. A survey of pathological changes associated with long-term high tar tobacco smoke exposure in a murine model. **J Pathol** 1981; 135(4): 249–257.

NT168 Rasmussen, R. E., C. H. Boyd, D. R. Dansie, R. E. Kouri, and C. J. Henry. DNA replication and unscheduled DNA synthesis in lungs of mice exposed to cigarette smoke. **Cancer Res** 1981; 41(7): 2583–2588.

NT169   Ohmori, T., H. Mori, and A. Rivenson. A study of tobacco carcinogenesis XX: mastocytoma induction in mice by cigarette smoke particulates ("cigarette tar"). **Am J Pathol** 1981; 102(3): 381–387.

NT170   Ayre, D. J., D. Keast, and J. M. Papadimitriou. Effects of tobacco smoke exposure on splenic architecture and weight, during the primary immune response of BALB/c mice. **J Pathol** 1981; 133(1): 53–59.

NT171   Hecht, S. S., S. Carmella, H. Mori, and D. Hoffmann. A study of tobacco carcinogenesis. XX. Role of catechol as a major cocarcinogen in the weakly acidic fraction of smoke condensate. **J Natl Cancer Inst** 1981; 66(1): 163–169.

NT172   Jacob, C. V., G. T. Stelzer, and J. H. Wallace. The influence of cigarette tobacco smoke products on the immune response. The cellular basis of immunosuppression by a water-soluble condensate of tobacco smoke. **Immunology** 1980; 40(4): 621–627.

NT173   Bock, F. G., and D. F. Clausen. Further fractionation and co-promoting activity of the large molecular weight components of aqueous tobacco extracts. **Carcinogenesis** 1980; 1(4): 317–321.

NT174   Lehrer, S. B., M. R. Wilson, and J. E. Salvaggio. Immunogenicity of tobacco smoke components in rabbits and mice. **Int Arch Allergy Appl Immunol** 1980; 62(1): 16–22.

NT175   Herscowitz, H. B., and R. B. Cooper. Effect of cigarette smoke exposure on maturation of the antibody response in spleens of newborn mice. **Pediatr Res** 1979; 13(9): 987–991.

NT176   Matulionis, D. H. Reaction of macrophages to cigarette smoke. II. Immigration of macrophages to the lungs. **Arch Environ Health** 1979; 34(5): 298–301.

NT177   Matulionis, D. H. Reaction of macrophages to cigarette smoke. I. Recruitment of pulmonary macrophages. **Arch Environ Health** 1979; 34(5): 293–298.

NT178   Mackenzie, J. S., and R. L. Flower. The effect of long-term exposure to cigarette smoke on the height and specificity of the secondary immune response to influenza virus in a murine model system. **J Hyg (Lond)** 1979; 83(1): 135–141.

NT179   Hirota, N. Intranuclear rodlets in undifferentiated carcinomas of salivary glands in strain A mice in a study involving a tobacco specific nitrosamine, N-nitrosonornicotine. **Cancer Lett** 1979; 6(6): 365–369.

NT180   Kouri, R. E., T. H. Rude, R. D. Curren, K. R. Brandt, R. G. Sosnowski, L. M. Schechtman, W. F. Benedict, and C. J. Henry. Biological activity of tobacco smoke and tobacco smoke-related chemicals. **Environ Health Perspect** 1979; 29: 63–69.

NT181   Hecht, S. S., C. B. Chen, N. Hirota, R. M. Ornaf, T. C. Tso, and D. Hoffmann. Tobacco-specific nitrosamines: formation from nicotine in vitro and during tobacco curing and carcinogenicity in strain A mice. **J Natl Cancer Inst** 1978; 60(4): 819–824.

NT182   Essman, W. B. Serotonin and monoamine oxidase in mouse skin: effects of cigarette smoke exposure. **J Med** 1977; 8(2): 95–101.

NT183   Van Duuren, B. L., and B. M. Goldschmidt. Cocarcinogenic and tumor-promoting agents in tobacco carcinogenesis. **J Natl Cancer Inst** 1976; 56(6): 1237–1242.

NT184   Chortyk, O. T., and F. G. Bock. Tumor-promoting activity of certain extracts of tobacco. **J Natl Cancer Inst** 1976; 56(5): 1041–1045.

NT185   Keller, K. F., and R. J. Doyle. A mechanism for tobacco smoke-induced allergy. **J Allergy Clin Immunol** 1976; 57(3): 278–282.

NT186   Justus, D. E., and D. A. Adams. Evaluation of tobacco hypersensitivity responses in the mouse. A potential animal model for critical study of tobacco allergy. **Int Arch Allergy Appl Immunol** 1976; 51(6): 687–695.

NT187   Hoffmann, D., S. S. Hecht, R. M. Ornaf, E. L. Wynder, and T. C. Tso. Chemical studies on tobacco smoke. XLII. Nitrosonornicotine: presence in tobacco, formation and carcinogenicity. **IARC Sci Publ** 1976; (14): 307–320.

NT188   Hecht, S. S., R. L. Thorne, R. R. Maronpot, and D. Hoffmann. A study of tobacco carcinogenesis. XIII. Tumor-promoting subfractions of the weakly acidic fraction. **J Natl Cancer Inst** 1975; 55(6): 1329–1336.

NT189 Pilotti, A., K. Ancker, E. Arrhenius, and C. Enzell. Effects of tobacco and tobacco smoke constituents on cell multiplication in vitro. **Toxicology** 1975; 5(1): 49–62.

NT190 Brody, A. R., and J. E. Craighead. Cytoplasmic inclusions in pulmonary macrophages of cigarette smokers. **Lab Invest** 1975; 32(2): 125–132.

NT191 Onoue, S., Y. Ohmori, K. Endo, S. Yamada, R. Kimura, and T. Yajima. Vasoactive intestinal peptide and pituitary adenylate cyclase-activating polypeptide attenuate the cigarette smoke extract-induced apoptotic death of rat alveolar L2 cells. **Eur J Biochem** 2004; 271(9): 1757–1767.

NT192 Higuchi, M. A., J. Sagartz, W. K. Shreve, and P. H. Ayres. Comparative subchronic inhalation study of smoke from the 1R4F and 2R4F reference cigarettes. **Inhal Toxicol** 2004; 16(1): 1–20.

NT193 Wang, R. D., H. Tai, C. Xie, X. Wang, J. L. Wright, and A. Churg. Cigarette smoke produces airway wall remodeling in rat tracheal explants. **Am J Respir Crit Care Med** 2003; 168(10): 1232–1236.

NT194 Li, T., A. Molteni, P. Latkovich, W. Castellani, and R. C. Baybutt. Vitamin A depletion induced by cigarette smoke is associated with the development of emphysema in rats. **J Nutr** 2003; 133(8): 2629–2634.

NT195 Kinsler, S., D. H. Pence, W. K. Shreve, A. T. Mosberg, P. H. Ayres, and J. W. Sagartz. Rat subchronic inhalation study of smoke from cigarettes containing flue-cured tobacco cured either by direct-fired or heat-exchanger curing processes. **Inhal Toxicol** 2003;15(8): 819–854.

NT196 Ueta, E., Y. Tadokoro, T. Yamamoto, et al. The effect of cigarette smoke exposure and ascorbic acid intake on gene expression of antioxidant enzymes and other related enzymes in the livers and lungs of Shionogi rats with osteogenic disorders. **Toxicol Sci** 2003; 73(2): 339–347.

NT197 Wang, H. Y., V. Y. Shin, S. Y. Leung, S. T. Yuen, and C. H. Cho. Involvement of bcl-2 and caspase-3 in apoptosis induced by cigarette smoke extract in the gastric epithelial cell. **Toxicol Pathol** 2003; 31(2): 220–226.

NT198 Kayyali, U. S., R. Budhiraja, C. M. Pennella, S. Cooray, J. J. Lanzillo, R. Chalkley, and P. M. Hassoun. Upregulation of xanthine oxidase by tobacco smoke condensate in pulmonary endothelial cells. **Toxicol Appl Pharmacol** 2003; 188(1): 59–68.

NT199 Delibas, N., R. Ozcankaya, I. Altuntas, and R. Sutcu. Effect of cigarette smoke on lipid peroxidation, antioxidant enzymes and NMDA receptor subunits 2A and 2B concentration in rat hippocampus. **Cell Biochem Funct** 2003; 21(1): 69–73.

NT200 Chen, S. H., Y. H. Lee, F. C. Wei, J. Y. Huang, and H. C. Chen. *In vivo* evaluation of leucocyte dynamics in cremaster muscle in rats after exposure to cigarette smoke. **Scand J Plast Reconstr Surg Hand Surg** 2002; 36(6): 321–325.

NT201 Smith, K. R., D. L. Uyeminami, U. P. Kodavanti, J. D. Crapo, L. Y. Chang, and K. E. Pinkerton. Inhibition of tobacco smoke-induced lung inflammation by a catalytic antioxidant. **Free Radic Biol Med** 2002; 33(8): 1106–1114.

NT202 Mullick, A. E., J. M. McDonald, G. Melkonian, P. Talbot, K. E. Pinkerton, and J. C. Rutledge. Reactive carbonyls from tobacco smoke increase arterial endothelial layer injury. **Am J Physiol Heart Circ Physiol** 2002; 283(2): H591–H597.

NT203 Odoni, G., H. Ogata, C. Viedt, K. Amann, E. Ritz, and S. R. Orth. Cigarette smoke condensate aggravates renal injury in the renal ablation model. **Kidney Int** 2002; 61(6): 2090–2098.

NT204 Dwoskin, L. P., L. H. Teng, and P. A. Crooks. Nornicotine, a nicotine metabolite and tobacco alkaloid: desensitization of nicotinic receptor-stimulated dopamine release from rat striatum. **Eur J Pharmacol** 2001; 428(1): 69–79.

NT205 Raij, L., E. G. DeMaster, and E. A. Jaimes. Cigarette smoke-induced endothelium dysfunction: role of superoxide anion. **J Hypertens** 2001; 19(5): 891–897.

NT206 Yim, S. H., and S. S. Hee. Bacterial mutagenicity of some tobacco aromatic nitrogen bases and their mixtures. **Mutat Res** 2001; 492(1–2): 13–27.

NT207 Chang, W. C., Y. C. Lee, C. L. Liu, et al. Increased expression of iNOS and c-fos via regulation of protein tyrosine phosphorylation and MEK1/ERK2 proteins in terminal bronchiole lesions in the lungs of rats exposed to cigarette smoke. **Arch Toxicol** 2001; 75(1): 28–35.

NT208 Slotkin, T. A., K. E. Pinkerton, M. C. Garofolo, J. T. Auman, E. C. McCook, and F. J. Seidler. Perinatal exposure to environmental tobacco smoke induces adenylyl cyclase and alters receptor-mediated cell signaling in brain and heart of neonatal rats. **Brain Res** 2001; 898(1): 73–81.

NT209 Izzotti, A., R. M. Balansky, F. Dagostini, et al. Modulation of biomarkers by chemopreventive agents in smoke-exposed rats. **Cancer Res** 2001; 61(6): 2472–2479.

NT210 Ferchmin, P. A., R. J. Lukas, R. M. Hann, et al. Tobacco cembranoids block behavioral sensitization to nicotine and inhibit neuronal acetylcholine receptor function. **J Neurosci Res** 2001; 64(1): 18–25.

NT211 Zhang, Z., Z. Heng, A. Li, and R. Zhao. Study on the effects of DNA damage induced by cigarette smoke in male mice testicular cells using comet assay. **Wei Sheng Yan Jiu** 2001; 30(1): 28–30.

NT212 Feng, H., Y. Li, Z. Xu, and J. Wu. Effects of high temperature and cigarette smoke on the development of nervous system in early rat embryos. **Wei Sheng Yan Jiu** 2001; 30(1): 25–27.

NT213 D'Agostini, F., R. M. Balansky, A. Izzotti, R. A. Lubet, G. J. Kelloff, and S. De Flora. Modulation of apoptosis by cigarette smoke and cancer chemopreventive agents in the respiratory tract of rats. **Carcinogenesis** 2001; 22(3): 375–380.

NT214 Ayres, P. H., J. R. Hayes, M. A. Higuchi, A. T. Mosberg, and J. W. Sagartz. Subchronic inhalation by rats of mainstream smoke from a cigarette that primarily heats tobacco compared to a cigarette that burns tobacco. **Inhal Toxicol** 2001; 13(2): 149–186.

NT215 Hartwig, W., J. Werner, E. Ryschich, et al. Cigarette smoke enhances ethanol–induced pancreatic injury. **Pancreas** 2000; 21(3): 272–278.

NT216 Trauth, J. A., F. J. Seidler, and T. A. Slotkin. Persistent and delayed behavioral changes after nicotine treatment in adolescent rats. **Brain Res** 2000; 880(1–2): 167–172.

NT217 Ma, L., W. P. Wang, J. Y. Chow, S. K. Lam, and C. H. Cho. The role of polyamines in gastric mucus synthesis inhibited by cigarette smoke or its extract. **Gut** 2000; 47(2): 170–177.

NT218 Arif, J. M., C. G. Gairola, G. J. Kelloff, R. A. Lubet, and R. C. Gupta. Inhibition of cigarette smoke-related DNA adducts in rat tissues by indole-3-carbinol. **Mutat Res** 2000; 452(1): 11–18.

NT219 Jung, M., W. P. Davis, D. J. Taatjes, A. Churg, and B. T. Mossman. Asbestos and cigarette smoke cause increased DNA strand breaks and necrosis in bronchiolar epithelial cells in vivo. **Free Radic Biol Med** 2000; 28(8): 1295–1299.

NT220 Baskaran, S., S. Lakshmi, and P. R. Prasad. Effect of cigarette smoke on lipid peroxidation and antioxidant enzymes in albino rat. **Indian J Exp Biol** 1999; 37(12): 1196–1200.

NT221 Wang, H., L. Ma, Y. Li, and C. H. Cho. Exposure to cigarette smoke increases apoptosis in the rat gastric mucosa through a reactive oxygen species–mediated and p53–independent pathway. **Free Radic Biol Med** 2000; 28(7): 1125–1131.

NT222 Kalra, R., S. P. Singh, S. M. Savage, G. L. Finch, and M. L. Sopori. Effects of cigarette smoke on immune response: chronic exposure to cigarette smoke impairs antigen–mediated signaling in T cells and depletes IP3–sensitive Ca(2+) stores. **J Pharmacol Exp Ther** 2000; 293(1): 166–171.

NT223   McIntee, E. J., and S. S. Hecht. Metabolism of N'–nitrosonornicotine enantiomers by cultured rat esophagus and *in vivo* in rats. **Chem Res Toxicol** 2000; 13(3): 192–199.

NT224   Lee, C. Z., F. H. Royce, M. S. Denison, and K. E. Pinkerton. Effect of *in utero* and postnatal exposure to environmental tobacco smoke on the developmental expression of pulmonary cytochrome P450 monooxygenases. **J Biochem Mol Toxicol** 2000; 14(3): 121–130.

NT225   Ma, L., E. S. Liu, J. Y. Chow, J. Y. Wang, and C. H. Cho. Interactions of EGF and ornithine decarboxylase activity in the regulation of gastric mucus synthesis in cigarette smoke exposed rats. **Chin J Physiol** 1999; 42(3): 137–143.

NT226   McKarns, S. C., D. W. Bombick, M. J. Morton, and D. J. Doolittle. Gap junction intercellular communication and cytotoxicity in normal human cells after exposure to smoke condensates from cigarettes that burn or primarily heat tobacco. **Toxicol In Vitro** 2000; 14(1): 41–51.

NT227   Bershtein, L. M., E. V. Tsyrlina, V. B. Gamaiunova, et al. Effect of tobacco smoke on the level of estrogens and DNA in the rat uterus. **Ross Fiziol Zh Im I M Sechenova** 1999; 85(11): 1440–1444.

NT228   Johansson, S., M. Landstrom, L. Bjermer, and R. Henriksson. Effects of tobacco smoke on tumor growth and radiation response of dunning R3327 prostate adenocarcinoma in rats. **Prostate** 2000; 42(4): 253–259.

NT229   Kim, H. C., W. K. Jhoo, K. H. Ko, et al. Prolonged exposure to cigarette smoke blocks the neurotoxicity induced by kainic acid in rats. **Life Sci** 2000; 66(4): 317–326.

NT230   Wright, J. L., J. P. Sun, and A. Churg. Cigarette smoke exposure causes constriction of rat lung. **Eur Respir J** 1999; 14(5): 1095–1099.

NT231   March, T. H., L. M. Kolar, E. B. Barr, G. L. Finch, M. G. Menache, and K. J. Nikula. Enhanced pulmonary epithelial replication and axial airway mucosubstance changes in F344 rats exposed short-term to mainstream

cigarette smoke. **Toxicol Appl Pharmacol** 1999; 161(2): 171–179.

NT232   Ma, L., J. Y. Chow, E. S. Liu, and C. H. Cho. Cigarette smoke and its extract delays ulcer healing and reduces nitric oxide synthase activity and angiogenesis in rat stomach. **Clin Exp Pharmacol Physiol** 1999; 26(10): 828–829.

NT233   Hwang, D., P. Chanmugam, M. Boudreau, K. H. Sohn, K. Stone, and W. A. Pryor. Activation and inactivation of cyclo-oxygenase in rat alveolar macrophages by aqueous cigarette tar extracts. **Free Radic Biol Med** 1999; 27(5–6): 673–682.

NT234   Ozlu, T., M. Cay, A. Akbulut, H. Yekeler, M. Naziroglu, and M. Aksakal. The facilitating effect of cigarette smoke on the colonization of instilled bacteria into the tracheal lumen in rats and the improving influence of supplementary vitamin E on this process. **Respirology** 1999; 4(3): 245–248.

NT235   Wright, J. L., J. Dai, K. Zay, K. Price, C. B. Gilks, and A. Churg. Effects of cigarette smoke on nitric oxide synthase expression in the rat lung. **Lab Invest** 1999; 79(8): 975–983.

NT236   Avunduk, A. M., S. Yardimci, M. C. Avunduk, and L. Kurnaz. Cadmium and iron accumulation in rat lens after cigarette smoke exposure and the effect of vitamin E (alpha-tocopherol) treatment. **Curr Eye Res** 1999; 18(6): 403–407.

NT237   Radcliffe, K. A., J. L. Fisher, R. Gray, and J. A. Dani. Nicotinic modulation of glutamate and GABA synaptic transmission of hippocampal neurons. **Ann NY Acad Sci** 1999; 868: 591–610.

NT238   Ofulue, A. F., and M. Ko. Effects of depletion of neutrophils or macrophages on development of cigarette smoke-induced emphysema. **Am J Physiol** 1999; 277(1 Pt 1): L97–L105.

NT239   Morimoto, Y., T. Tsuda, H. Hori, et al. Combined effect of cigarette smoke and mineral fibers on the gene expression of cytokine mRNA. **Environ Health Perspect** 1999; 107(6): 495–500.

NT240   Berstein, L. M., E. V. Tsyrlina, V. B. Gamajunova, et al. Study of tobacco smoke influence on content of estrogens and DNA flow cytometry data in uterine tissue of rats of different age. **Horm Metab Res** 1999; 31(1): 27–30.

NT241   Soto-Otero, R., E. Mendez-Alvarez, R. Riguera-Vega, E. Quinoa-Cabana, I. Sanchez-Sellero, and M. Lopez-Rivadulla Lamas. Studies on the interaction between 1,2,3,4-tetrahydro-beta-carboline and cigarette smoke: a potential mechanism of neuroprotection for Parkinson's disease. **Brain Res** 1998; 802(1–2): 155–162.

NT242   Bagchi, M., D. Bagchi, E. A. Hassoun, and S. J. Stohs. Subchronic effects of smokeless tobacco extract (STE) on hepatic lipid peroxidation, DNA damage and excretion of urinary metabolites in rats. **Toxicology** 1998; 127(1–3): 29–38.

NT243   Kurata, T., E. Suzuki, M. Hayashi, and M. Kaminao. Physiological role of L-ascorbic acid in rats exposed to cigarette smoke. **Biosci Biotechnol Biochem** 1998; 62(5): 842–845.

NT244   Vidal, M. V., B. Gutfilen, L.M. da Fonseca, and M. Bernardo-Filho. Influence of tobacco on the labelling of red blood cells and plasma proteins with technetium-99m. **J Exp Clin Cancer Res** 1998; 17(1): 41–46.

NT245   Izzotti, A., R. M. Balansky, P. M. Blagoeva, et al. DNA alterations in rat organs after chronic exposure to cigarette smoke and/or ethanol ingestion. **FASEB J** 1998; 12(9): 753–758.

NT246   Wardlaw, S. A., K. J. Nikula, D. A. Kracko, G. L. Finch, J. R. Thornton-Manning, and A. R. Dahl. Effect of cigarette smoke on CYP1A1, CYP1A2 and CYP2B1/2 of nasal mucosae in F344 rats. **Carcinogenesis** 1998; 19(4): 655–662.

NT247   Ma, L., J. Y. Chow, and C. H. Cho. Mechanistic study of adverse actions of cigarette smoke exposure on acetic acid-induced gastric ulceration in rats. **Life Sci** 1998; 62(3): 257–266.

NT248   Cerami, C., H. Founds, I. Nicholl, et al. Tobacco smoke is a source of toxic reactive glycation products. **Proc Natl Acad Sci USA** 1997; 94(25): 13915–13920.

NT249   Gilks, C. B., K. Price, J. L. Wright, and A. Churg. Antioxidant gene expression in rat lung after exposure to cigarette smoke. **Am J Pathol** 1998; 152(1): 269–278.

NT250   Richie, J. P. Jr, S. G. Carmella, J. E. Muscat, D. G. Scott, S. A. Akerkar, and S. S. Hecht. Differences in the urinary metabolites of the tobacco-specific lung carcinogen 4-(methylnitrosamino)-1-(3-pyridyl)-1-butanone in black and white smokers. **Cancer Epidemiol Biomarkers Prev** 1997; 6(10): 783–790.

NT251   Sanberg, P. R., A. A. Silver, R. D. Shytle, et al. Nicotine for the treatment of Tourette's syndrome. **Pharmacol Ther** 1997; 74(1): 21–25.

NT252   Kamisaki, Y., K. Wada, K. Nakamoto, Y. Kishimoto, K. Ashida, and T. Itoh. Substances in the aqueous fraction of cigarette smoke inhibit lipid peroxidation in synaptosomes of rat cerebral cortex. **Biochem Mol Biol Int** 1997; 42(1): 1–10.

NT253   Wright, J. L., J. P. Sun, and S. Vedal. A longitudinal analysis of pulmonary function in rats during a 12 month cigarette smoke exposure. **Eur Respir J** 1997; 10(5): 1115–1159.

NT254   Matsuka, N., K. Furuno, K. Eto, R. Oishi, and Y. Gomita. Effects of cigarette smoke inhalation on plasma diltiazem levels in rats. **Methods Find Exp Clin Pharmacol** 1997; 19(3): 173–179.

NT255   Dadmanesh, F., and J. L. Wright. Endothelin-A receptor antagonist BQ-610 blocks cigarette smoke-induced mitogenesis in rat airways and vessels. **Am J Physiol** 1997; 272(4 Pt 1): L614–L618.

NT256   Carmella, S. G., A. Borukhova, D. Desai, and S. S. Hecht. Evidence for endogenous formation of tobacco–specific nitrosamines in rats treated with tobacco alkaloids and sodium nitrite. **Carcinogenesis** 1997; 18(3): 587–592.

NT257   Mendez-Alvarez, E., R. Soto-Otero, I. Sanchez-Sellero, and M. Lopez-Rivadulla Lamas. Inhibition of brain monoamine oxidase by adducts of 1,2,3,4-tetrahydroisoquinoline with components of cigarette smoke. **Life Sci** 1997; 60(19): 1719–1727.

NT258   Yardimci, S., A. Atan, T. Delibasi, K. Sunguroglu, and M. C. Guven. Long-term effects of cigarette-smoke exposure on plasma testosterone, luteinizing hormone and follicle-stimulating hormone levels in male rats. **Br J Urol** 1997; 79(1): 66–69.

NT259　Ringdahl, B. E., G. K. Johnson, R. B. Ali, and C. C. Organ. Effect of nicotine on arachidonic acid metabolites and epithelial parameters in rat oral mucosa. **J Oral Pathol Med** 1997; 26(1): 40–45.

NT260　Selman, M., M. Montano, C. Ramos, et al. Tobacco smoke-induced lung emphysema in guinea pigs is associated with increased interstitial collagenase. **Am J Physiol** 1996; 271(5 Pt 1): L734–L743.

NT261　Roberts, K. A., A. A. Rezai, K. E. Pinkerton, and J. C. Rutledge. Effect of environmental tobacco smoke on LDL accumulation in the artery wall. **Circulation** 1996; 94(9): 2248–2253.

NT262　Soto-Otero, R., R. Riguera-Vega, E. Mendez-Alvarez, I. Sanchez-Sellero, and M. Lopez-Rivadulla Lamas. Interaction of 1,2,3,4-tetrahydroisoquinoline with some components of cigarette smoke: potential implications for Parkinson's Disease. **Biochem Biophys Res Commun** 1996; 222(2): 607–611.

NT263　Anand, C. V., U. Anand, and R. Agarwal. Anti-oxidant enzymes, gamma-glutamyl transpeptidase and lipid peroxidation in kidney of rats exposed to cigarette smoke. **Indian J Exp Biol** 1996; 34(5): 486–488.

NT264　Li, X. Y., I. Rahman, K. Donaldson, and W. MacNee. Mechanisms of cigarette smoke induced increased airspace permeability. **Thorax** 1996; 51(5): 465–471.

NT265　Tesfaigzi, J., J. Th'ng, J. A. Hotchkiss, J. R. Harkema, and P. S. Wright. A small proline–rich protein, SPRR1, is upregulated early during tobacco smoke-induced squamous metaplasia in rat nasal epithelia. **Am J Respir Cell Mol Biol** 1996; 14(5):478–486.

NT266　Subramaniam, S., P. Bummer, and C. G. Gairola. Biochemical and biophysical characterization of pulmonary surfactant in rats exposed chronically to cigarette smoke. **Fundam Appl Toxicol** 1995; 27(1): 63–69.

NT267　Yasuda, K., M. Takashima, and I. Sawaragi. Influence of a cigarette smoke extract on the hormonal regulation of platelet-activating factor acetylhydrolase in rats. **Biol Reprod** 1995; 53(2): 244–252.

NT268　Uejima, Y., Y. Fukuchi, T., Nagase, T. Matsuse, M. Yamaoka, and H. Orimo. Influences of tobacco smoke, and vitamin E depletion on the distal lung of weanling rats. **Exp Lung Res** 1995; 21(4): 631–642.

NT269　Iwata, F., X. Y. Zhang, and F. W. Leung. Aggravation of gastric mucosal lesions in rat stomach by tobacco cigarette smoke. **Dig Dis Sci** 1995; 40(5): 1118–1124.

NT270　Iwata, F., O. U. Scremin, and F. W. Leung. Tobacco cigarette smoke attenuates duodenal ulcer margin hyperemia in the rat. Comparison of IAP clearance and hydrogen gas clearance techniques for measurements of gastrointestinal blood flow. **Dig Dis Sci** 1995; 40(5): 1112–1117.

NT271　Hotchkiss, J. A., W. A. Evans, B. T. Chen, G. L. Finch, and J. R. Harkema. Regional differences in the effects of mainstream cigarette smoke on stored mucosubstances and DNA synthesis in F344 rat nasal respiratory epithelium. **Toxicol Appl Pharmacol** 1995; 131(2): 316–324.

NT272　Iwata, F., and F. W. Leung. Tobacco cigarette smoke aggravates gastric ulcer in rats by attenuation of ulcer margin hyperemia. **Am J Physiol** 1995; 268(1 Pt 1): G153–G160.

NT273　Leichter, J. Decreased birth weight and attainment of postnatal catch-up growth in offspring of rats exposed to cigarette smoke during gestation. **Growth Dev Aging** 1995; 59(1–2): 63–66.

NT274　Shalini, V. K., M. Luthra, L. Srinivas, et al. Oxidative damage to the eye lens caused by cigarette smoke and fuel smoke condensates. **Indian J Biochem Biophys** 1994; 31(4): 261–266.

NT275　Bagchi, M., D. Bagchi, E. A. Hassoun, and S. J. Stohs. Smokeless tobacco induced increases in hepatic lipid peroxidation, DNA damage and excretion of urinary lipid metabolites. **Int J Exp Pathol** 1994; 75(3): 197–202.

NT276   Skowronski, R. J., and D. Feldman. Inhibition of aldosterone synthesis in rat adrenal cells by nicotine and related constituents of tobacco smoke. **Endocrinology** 1994; 134(5): 2171–2177.

NT277   Paulson, R. B., J. Shanfeld, C. J. Vorhees, J. Cole, A. Sweazy, and J. O. Paulson. Behavioral effects of smokeless tobacco on the neonate and young Sprague Dawley rat. **Teratology** 1994; 49(4): 293–305.

NT278   Paulson, R. B., J. Shanfeld, D. Mullet, J. Cole, and J. O. Paulson. Prenatal smokeless tobacco effects on the rat fetus. **J Craniofac Genet Dev Biol** 1994; 14(1): 16–25.

NT279   Morimoto, Y., M. Kido, I. Tanaka, A. Fujino, T. Higashi, and Y. Yokosaki. Synergistic effects of mineral fibres and cigarette smoke on the production of tumour necrosis factor by alveolar macrophages of rats. **Br J Ind Med** 1993; 50(10): 955–960.

NT280   Torok, B. Chemoluminescence induced by t-butyl hydroperoxide increases under the effect of cigarette smoke (preliminary report). **Orv Hetil** 1993; 134(37): 2045–2047.

NT281   Liu, S. Q., and Y. C. Fung. Changes in the structure and mechanical properties of pulmonary arteries of rats exposed to cigarette smoke. **Am Rev Respir Dis** 1993; 148(3): 768–777.

NT282   Bjermer, L., Y. Cai, K. Nilsson, S. Hellstrom, and R. Henriksson. Tobacco smoke exposure suppresses radiation-induced inflammation in the lung: a study of bronchoalveolar lavage and ultrastructural morphology in the rat. **Eur Respir J** 1993; 6(8): 1173–1180.

NT283   Skold, C. M., K. Andersson, J. Hed, and A. Eklund. Short-term *in vivo* exposure to cigarette-smoke increases the fluorescence in rat alveolar macrophages. **Eur Respir J** 1993; 6(8): 1169–1172.

NT284   Pan, X. M., I. Staprans, T. E. Read, and J. H. Rapp. Cigarette smoke alters chylomicron metabolism in rats. **J Vasc Surg** 1993; 18(2): 161–167.

NT285   Lai, Y. L., and L. Diamond. Cigarette smoke exposure does not prevent cadmium-induced alterations in rat lungs.

J Toxicol Environ Health 1992; 35(1): 63–76.

NT286   Yang, G. T., and D. X. Wang. Influence of cigarette smoking on the hypoxic pulmonary vasoconstriction in isolated rat lungs—the role of prostaglandins and leukotrienes. **J Tongji Med Univ** 1992; 12(1): 6–10.

NT287   Pryor, W. A., N. C. Arbour, B. Upham, and D. F. Church. The inhibitory effect of extracts of cigarette tar on electron transport of mitochondria and submitochondrial particles. **Free Rad Biol Med** 1992; 12(5): 365–372.

NT288   Pi, Y. Q. Effect of cigarette smoke extract on hypoxic pulmonary vasoconstriction. **Zhonghua Jie He He Hu Xi Za Zhi** 1991; 14(6): 356–358, 377–378.

NT289   Johansson, S. L., J. M. Hirsch, and D. R. Johnson. Effect of repeated oral administration of tobacco snuff on natural killer-cell activity in the rat. **Arch Oral Biol** 1991; 36(6): 473–476.

NT290   Eto, K., Y. Gomita, K. Furuno, K. Yao, M. Moriyama, and Y. Araki. Influences of cigarette smoke inhalation on pharmacokinetics of cimetidine in rats. **Drug Metab Drug Interact** 1991; 9(2): 103–114.

NT291   Zwijsen, R. M., L. H. de Haan, J. S. Oosting, H. L. Pekelharing, and J. H. Koeman. Inhibition of intercellular communication in smooth muscle cells of humans and rats by low density lipoprotein, cigarette smoke condensate and TPA. **Atherosclerosis** 1990; 85(1): 71–80.

NT292   Lee, L. Y. Inhibitory effect of gas phase cigarette smoke on breathing: role of hydroxyl radical. **Respir Physiol** 1990; 82(2): 227–238.

NT293   Gomita, Y., K. Eto, K. Furuno, and Y. Araki. Effects of standard cigarette and nicotine-less cigarette smoke inhalings on nicorandil plasma levels in rats. **Pharmacology** 1990; 40(6): 312–317.

NT294   Osawa, Y., B. Tochigi, M. Tochigi, et al. Aromatase inhibitors in cigarette smoke, tobacco leaves and other plants. **J Enzyme Inhib** 1990; 4(2): 187–200.

NT295   Rogers, D. F., N. C. Turner, C. Marriott, and P. K. Jeffery. Oral N-acetylcysteine or S-carboxymethyl-cysteine inhibits cigarette smoke-in-duced hypersecretion of mucus in rat larynx and trachea in situ. **Eur Respir J** 1989; 2(10): 955–960.

NT296 Pour, P. M., and A. Rivenson. Induc-tion of a mixed ductal-squamous-islet cell carcinoma in a rat treated with a tobacco-specific carcinogen. **Am J Pathol** 1989; 134(3): 627–631.

NT297 Chen, S. Y. Effects of smokeless to-bacco on the buccal mucosa of HMT rats. **J Oral Pathol Med** 1989; 18(2): 108–112.

NT298 Mousa, S. A., V. J. Aloyo, and G. R. Van Loon. Tolerance to tobacco smoke- and nicotine-induced analgesia in rats. **Pharmacol Biochem Behav** 1988; 31(2): 265–268.

NT299 Rogers, D. F., N. C. Turner, C. Marriott, and P. K. Jeffery. Cigarette smoke-induced 'chronic bronchitis': a study *in situ* of laryngo–tracheal hyper-secretion in the rat. **Clin Sci (Lond)** 1987; 72(5): 629–637.

NT300 Rogers, D. F., and P. K. Jeffery. Inhibi-tion by oral N-acetylcysteine of ciga-rette smoke-induced "bronchitis" in the rat. **Exp Lung Res** 1986; 10(3): 267–283.

NT301 Stagnaro, E., R. Tumino, S. Parodi, et al. Non-Hodgkin's lymphoma and type of tobacco smoke. **Cancer Epidemiol Biomarkers Prev** 2004; 13(3): 431–437.

NT302 Meisel, P., C. Schwahn, D. Gesch, O. Bernhardt, U. John, and T. Kocher. Dose-dependent relation of smoking and the interleukin-1 gene polymor-phism in periodontal tissue. **J Perio-dontol** 2004; 75(2): 236–242.

NT303 Mavropoulos, A., H. Aartd, and P. Brodin. The involvement of nervous and some inflammatory response mechanisms in the acute snuff-induced gingival hyperaemia in humans. **J Clin Periodontol** 2002; 29(9): 855–864.

NT304 Calsina, G., J. M. Ramon, and J. J. Echeverria. Effects of smoking on peri-odontal tissues. **J Periodontol** 2002; 29(8): 771–776.

NT305 Cornelius, M. D., S. L. Leech, L. Goldsmidt, and N. L. Day. Prenatal tobacco exposure: is a risk factor for early tobacco experimentation? **Nico-tine Tob Res** 2000; 2(1): 45–52.

NT306 Gocze, P. M., and D. A. Freeman. Cytotoxic effects of cigarette smoke alkaloids inhibit the progesterone pro-duction and cell growth of cultured MA-10 Leydig tumor cells. **Eur J Obstet Gynecol Reprod Biol** 2000, 93(1): 77–83.

NT307 Milunsky, A., S. G. Carmella, M. Ye, and S. S. Hecht. A tobacco-specific carcinogen in the fetus. **Prenat Diagn** 2000; 20(4): 307–310.

NT308 Smuts, C. M., H. Y. Tichelaar, M. A. Dhansay, M. Faber, J. Smith, and G. F. Kirsten. Smoking and alcohol use dur-ing pregnancy affects preterm infants' docosahexaenoic acid (DHA) status. **Acta Paediatr** 1999; 88(7): 757–762.

NT309 Filippini, G., M. Farinotti, G. Lovicu, P. Maisonneuve, and P. Boyle. Moth-ers' active and passive smoking during pregnancy and risk of brain tumours in children. **Int J Cancer** 1994; 57(6): 769–774.

NT310 Krischnamurty, S., and S. Joshi. Gen-der differences and low birth weight with maternal smokeless tobacco use in pregnancy. **J Trop Pediatr** 1993; 39(4): 253–254.

NT311 DiCarlantonio, G., and P. Talbot. In-halation of mainstream and sidestream cigarette smoke retards embryo trans-port and slow muscle contraction in oviducts of hamsters (*Mesocricetus auratus*). **Biol Reprod** 1999; 61(3): 651–656.

NT312 Makler, A., J. Reiss. J.Stoller, Z. Blumenfeld, and J. M. Brandes. Use of sealed minichamber for direct observa-tion and evaluation of the *in vitro* ef-fect of cigarette smoke on sperm motility. **Fertil Steril** 1993; 59(3): 645–651.

NT313 Dikshit, R. K., J. G. Buch, and S. M. Mansuri. Effect of tobacco consump-tion on semen quality of a population of hypofertile males. **Fertil Steril** 1987; 48(2): 334–336.

NT314 Kulikauskas, V., D. Blaustein, and R. J. Ablin. Cigarette smoking and its possible effects on sperm. **Fertil Steril** 1985; 44(4): 526–528.

NT315 Merino, G., S. C. Lira, and J. C. Mertinez-Chequer. Effects of cigarette smoking on semen characteristics of a population in Mexico. **Arch Androl** 1998; 41(1): 11–15.

NT316   Pakrashi, A. and S. Chatterjee. Effect of tobacco consumption on the function of male accessory sex glands. **Int J Androl** 1995; 18(5): 232–236.

NT317   Attia, A. M., M. R. el-Dakhly, F. A. Halawa, N. F. Ragab, and M. M. Mossa. Cigarette smoking and male reproduction. **Arch Androl** 1989; 23(1): 45–49.

NT318   Gocze, P. M., I. Szabo, and D. A. Freeman. Influence of nicotine, cotinine, anabasine and cigarette smoke extract on human granulose cell progesterone and estradiol synthesis. **Gynecol Endocrinol** 1999; 13(4): 266–272.

NT319   Bos, R. P., C. H. van Heijst, H. M. Hollanders, J. L. Theuws, R. F. Thijssen, and T. K. Eskes. Is there influence of smoking on the mutagenicity of follicular fluid? **Fertil Steril** 199; 52(5): 774–777.

NT320   Dymicki, M. and R. L. Stedman. Composition studies on tobacco. I. Beta-sitosteryl D-glucoside from flue-cured tobacco leaves. **Tobacco** 1958; 147(3): 21.

NT321   Kisaki, T., S. Mizusaki, and E. Tamaki. Phytochemical studies on tobacco alkaloids. 11. A new alkaloid in *Nicotiana tabacum* roots. **Phytochemistry** 1968; 7: 323–327.

NT322   Osman, S., and J. Barson. The volatile bases of cigar smoke. **Phytochemistry** 1964; 3(5): 587–590.

NT323   Poindexter Jr, E. H., and R. D. Carpenter. The isolation of harmane and norharmane from tobacco and cigarette smoke. **Phytochemistry** 1962; 1(3): 215–221.

NT324   Noguchi, M., H. Sakum, and E. Tamaki. The isolation and identification of nicotianine: a new amino acid from tobacco leaves. **Phytochemistry** 1968; 7(10): 1861–1866.

NT325   Reid, W. W. Accumulation of squalens-2,3-oxide during inhibition of phytosterol biosynthesis in *Nicotiana tabacum*. **Phytochemistry** 1968; 7(3): 451–452.

NT326   Chamberlain, W. J., and R. L. Stedman. Composition studies of tobacco. XXVIII. 2,3,6-trimethyl-1,4-aphthoquinone in cigarette smoke. **Phytochemistry** 1968; 7: 1201–1203.

NT327   Irvine, W. J., and M. J. Saxby. The constituents of certain tobacco types. I. **Phytochemistry** 1968; 7: 277–281.

NT328   Wahlberg, I., I. Forsblom, C. Vogt, et al. Tobacco chemistry. Five new cembranoids from tobacco. **J Org Chem** 1985; 50(23): 4527–4538.

NT329   Vainio, H., and E. Heseitine. Tobacco and cancer. **Cancer Res** 1986; 46(1): 444–447.

NT330   Koseki, K., F. Saito, N. Kawashima, and M. Noma. New cembranoic diterpene with IAA inhibitory activity from *Nicotina tabacum*. **Agr Biol Chem** 1986; 50(7): 1917–1918.

NT331   Tazaki, H., H. Kodama, T. Fujimori, and A. Ohnishi. Hydroxysolanascone glucosides from flue–cured tobacco leaves. **Agr Biol Chem** 1986; 50(9): 2231–2235.

NT332   Wahlberg, I., R. Arndt, T. Nishida, and C. R. Enzell. Tobacco chemistry. Syntheses and stereostructures of six tobacco seco-cembranoids. **Acta Chem Scand Ser B** 1986; 40: 123–134.

NT333   Wahlberg, I., A. M. Eklund, C. Vogt, C. R. Enzell, and J. E. Berg. Tobacco chemistry. Two new 7,8-epoxycembranods from tobacco. **Acta Chem Scand Ser B** 1986; 40(10): 855–860.

NT334   Uegaki, R., T. Fujimori, N. Ueda, and A. Ohnishi. Cembrane-derived diterpenoid having a carbotricyclic skeleton. **Phytochemistry** 1987; 26(11): 3029–3031.

NT335   Wahlberg, I., C. Vogt, A. M. Eklund, and C. R. Enzell. Tobacco chemistry. Two new 20–norcembranoids from tobacco. **Acta Chem Scand Ser B** 1987; 41(10): 749–753.

NT336   Koseki, Y., Y. Tanabe, S. Kubo, and M. Noma. New diterpene from *Nicotiana tabacum* and its use as a tobacco flavorant. Patent-Japan Kokai Tokkyo Koho-62 148,439 1987; 3 pp.

NT337   Arndt, R, I. Wahilberg, C. R. Enzell, and J. E. Berg. Tobacco chemistry. Structure determination and biomimetic syntheses of two new tobacco cembranoids. **Acta Chem Scand Ser B** 1988; 42(5): 294–302.

NT338   Wahilberg, I., A. M. Eklund, K. Nordfors, C. Vogt, C. R. Enzell, and J. E. Berg. Tobacco chemistry. Five new labdanic compounds from tobacco. **Acta Crystallogr Ser B** 1988; 42(10): 708–716.

NT339   Isogai, A., N. Fukuchi, M. Hayashi, H. Kamada, H. Harada, and A. Suzuki. Structure of a new opine, mikimopine, in hairy root induced by *Agrobacterium rhizogenes.* **Agr Biol Chem** 1988; 52(12): 3235–3237.

NT340   Tazaki, H., H. Kodama, A. Ohnishi, and T. Fujimori. Structures of new solanascone glucosides from flue–cured tobacco leaves. **Agr Biol Chem** 1989; 53(11): 3037–3038.

NT341   Arndt, R., J. E. Berg, and I. Wahlberg. Tobacco chemistry. Structure determination and biomimetic studies of five new tobacco cembranoids. **Acta Chem Scand** 1990; 44(8): 814–825.

NT342   Olsson, E., A. M. Eklund, and I. Wahlberg. Tobacco chemistry. Five new cembratrientriols from tobacco. **Acta Chem Scand** 1991; 45(1): 92–98.

NT343   Tazaki, H., H. Kodama, A. Ohnishi, and T. Fujimori. Structure of sesquiterpenoid glucoside from flue–cured tobacco leaves. **Agr Biol Chem** 1991; 55(7): 1889–1890.

NT344   Vogt, C., J. E. Berg, and I. Wahlberg. Tobacco chemistry. Four new epoxycembranoids from tobacco. **Acta Chem Scand** 1992; 46(8): 789–795.

NT345   Eklund, A. M., J. E. Berg, and I. Wahlberg. Tobacco chemistry. 4,6,8-Trihydroxy-11-capnosene-2,10-dione, a new cembrane-derived bicyclic diterpenoid from tobacco. **Acta Chem Scand** 1992; 46(4): 367–371.

NT346   Forsblom, I., J. E. Berg, and I. Wahlberg. Tobacco chemistry. Two new cembratrienetriols from tobacco. **Acta Chem Scand** 1993; 47(1): 80–88.

NT347   Olsson, E., J. E. Berg, and I. Wahlberg. Eight new cembranoids from tobacco-structural elucidation and conformational studies. **Tetrahedron** 1993; 49(22): 4975–4992.

NT348   Eklund, A. M. and I. Wahlberg. Tobacco chemistry. Seven new cembrane-derived compounds from tobacco. **Acta Chem Scand** 1994; 48(10): 850–856.

NT349   Pettersson, T., A. M. Eklund, and I. Wahlberg. New lactones from tobacco. **J Agr Food Chem** 1993; 41(11): 2097–2103.

NT350   Balint, R., G. Cooper, M. Staebell, and P.Filner. N-Caffeoyl-4-amino-N-butyric acid, a new flower-specific metabolite in cultured tobacco cells and tobacco plants. **J Biol Chem** 1987; 262(23): 11026–11031.

NT351   Shvets, S. A., P. K. Kintya, and O. N. Gutsu. Steroid glycosides of *Nicotiana tabacum* seeds. I. The structures of nicotianosides A, B, and E. **Chem Nat Comp** 1994; 30(6): 684–688.

NT352   Shvets, S. A., P. K. Kintya, O. N. Gutsu, and V. I. Grishkovets. Steroid glycosides of the seeds of *Nicotiana tabacum.* II. The structures of nicotianosides C and F. **Chem Nat Comp** 1995; 31(3): 332–335.

NT353   Shinozaki, Y., T. Tobita, M. Mizutani, and T. Matsuzaki. Isolation and identification of two new diterpene glycosides from *Nicotiana tabacum.* **Biosci Biotech Biochem** 1996; 60(5): 903–905.

NT354   Ohshima, N., H. Nishitani, S. Nishikawa, K. Okumura, and H. Taguchi. 1-O-nicotinoyl-beta-D-glucopyranose in cultured tobacco cells. **Phytochemistry** 1997; 44(8): 1483–1484.

NT355   Zook, M., K. Johnson, T. Hohn, and R. Hammerschmidt. Structural characterization of 15-hydroxytrychodiene, a sesquiterpenoid produced by tansformed tobacco cell suspension cultures expressing a trichodiene synthase gene from *Fusarium sporotrichoides.* **Phytochemistry** 1996; 43(6): 1235–1237.

NT356   Eklund, A.M., I. Forsblom, J. E. Berg, C. Damberg, and I. Wahlberg. Tobacco chemistry. Four new cyclized cembranoids from tobacco. **Acta Chem Scand Ser A** 1998; 52(10): 1254–1262.

NT357   Carter, C., R. A. Graham, and R. W. Thornburg. Nectarin is a novel, soluble germin-like protein pexpressed in the nectar of *Nicotiana* sp. **Plant Mol Biol** 1999; 41(2): 207–216.

NT358   Zargari, A. Medicinal plants. Vol 3, 5th Ed, Tehran Unversity Publications, No 1810/3, Tehran, Iran 1992; 889 pp.

NT359   Gaines, T. P., and J. D. Miles. Protein composition and classification of tobacco. **J Agr Food Chem** 1975; 23(4): 690.

NT360   Mahmoud, A. E. S., and Y. A. Mohamed. An extractive-spectrophotometric method for the determination of nicotine. **Planta Med** 1975; 27: 140.

NT361   Springer, J. P., J. Clardy, R. H. Cox, H. G. Culter, and R. J. Cole. The struc-

ture of a new type of plant growth inhibitor extracted from immature tobacco leaves. **Tetrahedron Lett** 1975;
1975: 2737.

NT362   Rylander, R. Review of studies on environmental tobacco smoke. **Scand J
Resp Dis Suppl** 1974; 91: 10.

NT363   Bazhanova, N. V., and A. G.
Gevorkyan. Daily change of the con-
tents of photosynthesizing pigments in
hydroponic plant leaves. **Sobshch Inst
Agrokhim Probl Gidroponiki Akad
Nauk Arm SSR** 1974; 14: 89.

NT364   Hussey, J. S. Some useful plants of early
New England. **Econ Bot** 1974; 28: 311.

NT365   Mokhnachew, I. G., and S. W.
Kamenshchikova. Chlorogenic acid in
tobacco. **Tabak (Moscow)** 1974;
1974(4): 35.

NT366   Chirek, Z. Physiological and biochemical effects of morphactin IT
3233 on callus and tumor tissues of
Nicotiana tabacum cultured *in vitro*. III.
Transamination process catalyzed by
aminotransferase 1-alanine:2-oxogluta-
rate. **Acta Soc Bot Pol** 1974; 43: 169.

NT367   Aasen, A. J., C. H. G. Vogt, and C. R.
Enzell. Tobacco chemistry. Structure
and synthesis of drim-8-en-7-one, a
new tobacco constituent. **Acta Chem
Scand Ser B** 1975; 29: 51.

NT368   Grunwald, C. Phytosterols in tobacco
leaves at various stages of physiological maturity. **Phytochemistry** 1975;
14: 79–82.

NT369   Demole, A., and C. Demole. A chemical study of burley tobacco flavour
(*Nicotiana tabacum*). V. Identification
and synthesis of the novel terpenoid
alkaloids 1,3,6,6-tetramethyl-5,6,7,8-
tetrahydro-8-one and 3-6-6-trimethyl-
5-6-dihydro-7H-2-pyrindin-7-one.
Helv Chim Acta 1975; 58: 523.

NT370   Powell, B. L., J. W. Pickering, S. H.
Wender, and E. C. Smith. Isoperoxi-
dases from tobacco tissue cultures.
Phytochemistry 1975; 14: 1715–1717.

NT371   Schneider, H. A. W., and W. W.
Beisenherz. Determination of the sites
of synthesis of chlorophyll synthesiz-
ing enzymes in cell cultures of *Nicotiana tabacum*. **Biochem Biophys Res
Commun** 1974; 60: 468.

NT372   Demole, E., and P. Enggist. A chemical study of burley tobacco flavour

(*Nicotiana tabacum*). VI. Identification
and synthesis of four irregular terpenoids related to solanone, including a
'prenylsolanone'. **Helv Chim Acta**
1975; 58: 1602.

NT373   Aasen, A. J., J. R. Hlubucek, and C. R.
Enzell. Tobacco chemistry. The structures of four stereoisomeric 8,12-XI-
epoxylabd-14-en-13-XI-ols isolated
from Greek *Nicotiana tabacum*. **Acta
Chem Scand Ser B** 175; 29: 589.

NT374   Fujimori, T., R. Kasuga, H. Kaneko,
and M. Noguchi. A new acetylenic
diol, 3-hydroxy-7,8-dihydro-betaionol,
from burley *Nicotiana tabacum*. **Phytochemistry** 1975; 14: 2095.

NT375   Aasen, A. J., J. R. Hlubucek and C. R.
Enzell. Tobacco chemistry. (7S)-10-
oxo-4-XI-methyl-7-isopropyl-5E-
undecen-4-olide, a new thunbergan-
type nor-isoprenoid isolated from Greek
Nicotiana tabacum. **Acta Chem Scand
Ser B** 175; 29: 677.

NT376   Blomberg, L., and G. Widmark. Separation of fresh tobacco smoke on a
packed polar gas chromatographic column prior to on-line analysis by gas
chromatography-mass spectrometry
using a non-polar capillary column. **J
Chromatogr** 1975; 106: 59.

NT377   Leete, E. Biosynthesis of azetidine-2-
carboxylic acid from methionine in
Nicotiana tabacum. **Phytochemistry**
1975; 14: 1983–1984.

NT378   Hoffmann, D., S. S. Hecht, R. M.
Ornaf, and E. L. Wynder. N'-nitro-
sonornicotine in tobacco. **Science**
1974; 186: 265.

NT379   Lichtenthaler, H. K., and V. Straub.
The formation of lipoquinones in tissue
cultures. **Planta Med Suppl** 1975; 198.

NT380   Woolf, C. R. Clinical findings, sputum
examinations and pulmonary function
tests related to the smoking habit of
500 women. **Chest** 1974; 66: 652.

NT381   Gayard, P., J. Orehek, C. Grimaud,
and J. Charpin. Bronchoconstriction
due to the inhalation of tobacco
smoke: comparison of effects in the
normal and the asthmatic subject. **Bull
Physio Pathol Respir** 1974; 10: 451.

NT382   Tomita, Y., and A. Uomori. Biosynthesis of isoprenoids. III. Mechanism of
alkylation during biosynthesis of stigmasterol in tissue cultures of higher

plants. **J Chem Soc Perkin Trans I** 1973; 2656.

NT383   Mader, M. Change of the peroxidase-isoenzyme-pattern in callus cultures independent of the differentiation. **Planta Med Suppl** 1975; 153.

NT384   Al-Khateeb, F. A. L. Effect of light quality on protein synthesis and peroxidase-indoleacetic oxidase activity in cultured tobacco pith tissues. **Diss Abstr Int B** 1974; 35: 2035.

NT385   Kanamaru, K., K. Kato, and M. Noguchi. Isolation and identification of gamma-L-glutamyl-L-glutamic acid from tobacco cells in suspension culture. **Agr Biol Chem** 1974; 38: 2285.

NT386   Kaul, K., and P. S. Sabbarwal. Kinetin induced changes in delta-aminolevulinic acid dehydratase of tobacco callus. **Plant Physiol** 174; 54: 644.

NT387   Maeder, P., and M. Bopp. Regulation and significance of peroxidase pattern variations during shoot differentiation in callus cultures of *Nicotiana tabacum*. **Planta** 1975; 123: 257.

NT388   Laurent'eva, L. M., and M. P. Pyatniskii. Quantitative determination of citric acid in tobacco. Patent-USSR-454,458 1974.

NT389   Leu, S. L. K., S. H. Wender, and E. C. Smith. Effect of darkness on isoperoxidases in tobacco tissue cultures. **Phytochemistry** 1975; 14: 2551–2554.

NT390   Chirek, Z. Physiological and biochemical effects of morphactin IT3233 on callus and tumor tissues of *Nicotiana tabacum* cultured *in vitro*. IV. Beta-indolylacetic acid oxidase activity. Oat *Coleoptile*. **Acta Soc Bot Pol** 1974; 43: 177.

NT391   Izman, G. V., N. A. Sherstyannykh, and L. G. Astaghova. Analysis of the tobacco haploids, produced by culturing anthers *in vitro*, in regards to their content of alkaloids and volatile acids. **Genetika (Moscow)** 1975; 11(3): 50.

NT392   Kemp, J. D. Protein metabolism in cultured plant tissues. V. Identification of the nonprecursor pool as L-leucine. **Physiol Plant** 1975; 35: 53.

NT393   Fujimori, T., R. K. Asuga, and M. Nouchi. Isolation of R-(-)-3-hydroxy-beta-ionone from burley tobacco. **Agr Biol Chem** 1974; 38: 891.

NT394   Thorpe, T. A., and D. D. Meier. Starch metabolism in shoot-forming tobacco callus. **J Exp Bot** 1974; 25: 288.

NT395   Konstantinova, T. N., L. V. Golfstein, O. I. Molodyuk, T. V. Bavrina, and N. P. Aksenova. Study of histones of calluses with vegetative and generative morphogenesis in trapezoid tobacco. **Dokl Akad Nauk SSR** 1974; 216: 226.

NT396   Ackermann, L. Evidence of a glycoprotein, until now unknown, in tissue culture of *Nicotiana tabacum*. **C R Seances Soc Biol Ses Fil** 1974; 168: 344.

NT397   Feng, K. A., and J. W. Unger. Presence of adenosine triphosphate in tobacco (*Nicotiana tabacum*) tissue grown in nutrient medium containing various concentrations of kinetin. **Experientia** 1975; 31: 31.

NT398   Chuman, T., H. Kaneko, T. Fukuzumi, and M. Noguchi. Isolation of two terpenoid acids, 4-isopropyl-7-methyl-5E, 7-octadienoic acid and 3-isopropyl-6-methyl - 4E, 6 - methyl - 4E, 6 -heptadienoic acid from Turkish tobacco. **Agr Biol Chem** 1974; 38: 2295.

NT399   Fujimori, T., R. Kasuga, H. Kaneko, and M. Noguchi. Isolation of 3-(4,8,12-trimethyltridecyl)-furan (phytofuran) from burley tobacco. **Agr Biol Chem** 1974; 38: 2293.

NT400   Wojnarowicz, C. Tobacco seed oil. **Tluszcze Jadalne** 1974; 18: 7.

NT401   Legrand, M., B. Fritig, and L. Hirth. Metabolism of phenylpropanoids in the leaf veins of healthy hypersensitive tobacco or tobacco infected by tobacco mosaic virus. **C R Acad Sci Ser D** 1974; 279: 1043.

NT402   Kier, L. D., E. Yamasaki, and and B. N. Ames. Detection of mutagenic activity in cigarette smoke condensates. **Proc Natl Acad Sci USA** 1974; 71: 4159.

NT403   Van Cantfort, J., and J. Gielen. Organ specificity of aryl hydrocarbon hydroxylase induction by cigarette smoke in rats and mice. **Biochem Pharmacol** 1975; 24: 1253.

NT404   Benedict, W. F., N. Rucker, J. Faust, and R. E. Kouri. Malignant transformation of mouse cells by cigarette smoke condensate. **Cancer Res** 1975; 35: 857.

NT405 Perkins, D. L., and L. S. Ciereszko. Effect of macrocyclic diterpene from tobacco on *Tetrahymena pyriformis*. **Proc Okla Acad Sci** 1974; 54: 34–35.

NT406 Demole, E., and C. Demole. A chemical study of burley tobacco flavour (*Nicotiana tabacum*). VII. Identification and synthesis of twelve irregular terpenoids related to solanone, including 7,8-dioxabicyclo[3,2,1]-octane and 4,9-dioxabicyclo[3.3.1]nonane derivatives. **Helv Chim Acta** 1975; 58: 1867.

NT407 Bharadwaj, B. V., S. Takayama, T. Yamada, and A. Tanimura. N'-nitrosonornicotine in Japanese tobacco products. **Gann** 1975; 66: 585.

NT408 Randolph, H. R. Gas chromatographic determination of nicotine in an isopropyl alcohol extract of smoke particulate matter. **Tobacco** 1974; 176: 44.

NT409 Yung, K. H., and D. H. Northcote. Enzymes in the walls of mesophyll cells of tobacco leaves. **Biochem J** 1975; 151: 141.

NT410 Semenova, N. I., V. V. Chenikov. E. N. Shopovalov, and A. D. Zelenskaya. Effect of isoquercitrin on the taste indexes of tobacco. **Ezv Vyssh Uchebn Zaved Pishch Tekhnol** 1974; 1974(5): 167–168.

NT411 Lichtenthaler, H. K., V. Straub, and K. H. Grumbach. Unequal formation of prenyl-lipids in a plant tissue culture and in leaves of *Nicotiana tabacum*. **Plant Sci Lett** 1975; 4: 61.

NT412 Moree-Testa, P., M. Donzel, M. H. Bergerol, and M. M. Luzinier. Determination of pyridinic and pyrazinic compounds in tobacco and cigarette smoke. **Ann Tab Sect** 1974; 1(12): 27.

NT413 Richter, M. Composition of essential oils in tobacco. III. Analysis of phenolic fraction. **Ber Inst Tabakforsch (Dresden)** 1974; 21: 52.

NT414 Ilham, M., M. Yaday, and A. W. Norhanom. Tumour-promoting activity of plants used in Malaysian traditional medicine. **Nat Prod Sci** 1995; 1(1): 31–42.

NT415 Shin, N. H., K. S. Lee, S. H. Kang, K. R. Ming, S. H. Lee, and Y. S. Kim. Inhibitory effect of herbal extracts on DOPA oxidase activity of tyrosinase. **Nat Prod Sci** 1997; 3(2): 111–121.

NT416 Park, K. H., J. D. Park, K. H. Hyun, M. Nakayama, and T. Yokota. Brassinosteroids and monoglycerides with brassinosteroid–like activity in immature seeds of *Oryza sativa* and *Perilla frutescens* and in cultured cells of *Nicotiana tabacum*. **Biosci Biotech Biochem** 1994; 58(12): 2241–2243.

NT417 Aragozzini, F., R. Gualandris, E. Maconi, and R. Craveri. Coenzyme Q-10 in plant cell cultures. **Ann Microbiol Enzimol** 1984; 34(1): 75–81.

NT418 Reuveny, Z. Regulation of ATP sulfurylase in cultured tobacco cells. **Diss Abstr Int B** 1976; 36: 4450.

NT419 Rennenberg, H. Glutathione in conditioned media of tobacco suspension cultures. **Phytochemistry** 1976; 15: 1433–1434.

NT420 Chuman, T., and M. Noguchi. The structure of a new terpenoid acid 6(S)-isopropyl-3 epsilon methyl-3-epsilon-hydroxy-9-oxo-4E-decenid acid, isolated from Turkish tobacco. **Agr Biol Chem** 1976; 40: 1793–1796.

NT421 Nishio, M., C. S. Zushi, and T. Ischii. Mass fragmentation determination of indole-3-acetic acid in callus tissues of *Panax ginseng* and *Nicotiana tabacum*. **Chem Pharm Bull** 1976; 24: 2038.

NT422 Janski, A. M. Purification and characterization of a sugar unspecific nuclease from tobacco suspension cultures. **Diss Abstr Int B** 1976; 36: 6128.

NT423 Kamenshchikova, S. V., and I. G. Moknachev. Hydrogen cyanide in tobacco smoke. **Tabak (Moscow)** 1975; 1975(2): 49.

NT424 Colledge, A., and W. W. Reid. The phytochemistry of the genus *Nicotiana*. Part V. The biosynthesis of is–abienol and phytosterols in *Nicotiana tabacum* PB. **Ann Tab Sect 2** 1974; 1974(11): 177.

NT425 Harrell, T. G., K. L. Rush, and A. J. Sensabaugh Jr. Colorimetric method for the determination of ammonia in tobacco smoke. **Tob Sci** 1975; 19: 154.

NT426 Ieda, T., T. Matsumoto, and M. Noguchi. Culture conditions of higher plant cells in suspension culture. Part 7. Formation of ubiquinone by tobacco plant cells in suspension culture. **Phytochemistry** 1976; 15: 568–569.

NT427   Noguchi, M., T. Matsumoto, K. Okunishi, and T. Ikeda. Production of ubiquinone 10 from callus. Patent-Japan Kokai-76 32,788 1976.

NT428   Fujimori, T., R. Kasuga, H. Matsuhira, H. Kaneko, and M. Noguchi. Neutral aroma constituents in burley tobacco. **Agr Biol Chem** 1976; 40: 303.

NT429   Aasen, A. J., A. Pilotti, C. R. Enzell, J. E. Berg, and A. M. Pilotti. Tobacco chemistry 31. (1S,4S,8R,11S,12R)-8,12-epoxy-2E,6E-thunbergadiene-4,11-diol, a new constituent of Greek tobacco. **Acta Chem Scand Ser B** 1976; 30: 999.

NT430   Demole, E. and P. Enggist. A chemical study of Virginia tobacco flavour (*Nicotiana tabacum*). I. Isolation and synthesis of two bicyclodamascenones. **Helv Chim Acta** 1976; 59: 1938.

NT431   Chuman, T., H. Kaneko, and T. Fukuzumi. Acidic aroma constituents of Turkish tobacco: terpenoid acids related to tobacco thunberganoids. **Agr Biol Chem** 1976; 40: 587.

NT432   Lance, B., R. C. Durley, D. M. Rreid, T. A. Thorpe, and R. P. Pharis. Metabolism of (^{3}H)gibberellin A-20 in light and dark-grown tobacco callus cultures. **Plant Physiol** 1976; 58: 387.

NT433   Nishinari, N., and T. Yamaki. Relation between cell division and endogenous auxin in synchronously-cultured tobacco cells. **Bot Mag (Tokyo)** 1976; 89: 73.

NT434   Novotny. M., M. L. Lee, and K. D. Bartle. A possible chemical basis for the higher mutagenicity of marijuana smoke as compared to tobacco smoke. **Experientia** 1976; 32: 280.

NT435   Yasumatsu, N., M. Eda, Y. Tsujino, and M. Noguchi. Isolation of oxygenated derivatives of solanesol from burley tobacco. **Agr Biol Chem** 1976: 40: 1757.

NT436   Hutchinson, C. R., M. T. S. Hsia, and R. A. Carver. Biosynthetic studies with $^{13}CO_2$ secondary plant metabolites. *Nicotiana* alkaloids. 1. Initial experiments. **J Am Chem Soc** 1976; 98: 6006.

NT437   Leete, E., and S. A. Slattery. Incorporation of (2-^{14}C) nicotinic acid into the tobacco alkaloids. Biosynthesis of anatabine and alpha, beta-dipyridyl. **J Am Chem Soc** 1976; 98: 6326.

NT438   Viesca-Trevino, C. Estudios sobre etnobotanica y antropologia medica. Inst Mexicano Para Est Pl Medic, Mexico 1976: 104.

NT439   Noma, M., and M. Noguchi. Occurrence of nicotianamine in higher plants. **Phytochemistry** 1976; 15: 1701–1702.

NT440   Nagaraj, G., and M. K. Chakraborty. Alkaloids and volatile acids of natu tobacco (*Nicotiana tabacum*) **Indian J Chem** 1979; 17B (6): 648–649.

NT441   Zao, S. H., and X. Zhang. On the antifeedant and toxicities of natural organic insecticides against snout moth's larva of rice. **Chin J Agr Sci** 1982; 1982(2): 55–60.

NT442   Shimazaki, M., and A. Ohta. Asymmetric synthesis of (-)-(E)-5-hydroxy-5-isopropyl-3-hepten-2-one, a cembrane-derived compound from Greek tobacco. **Synthesis** 1992; 1992(10): 957–958.

NT443   Hodges, L. C., G. W. Robinson, and K. Green. Extract of tobacco callus with antiglaucoma activity. **Phytother Res** 1991; 5(1): 15–18.

NT444   Nielsen, M. T., and R. F. Severson. Inheritance of diterpene constituent in tobacco trichome exudates. **Crop Sci** 1992; 32(5): 1148–1150.

NT445   Miedzybrodzka, M. B. W., and M. M. Yeoman. Effect of culture origin and conditions of duvatrienedol accumulation in shoot cultures of tobacco. **J Exp Bot** 1992; 43(256): 1419–1427.

NT446   Trivgedi, A. H., B. J. Dave, and S. G. Adhvaryu. Genotoxic effects of tobacco extract on Chinese hamster ovary cells. **Cancer Lett** 1993; 70(1/2): 107–112.

NT447   Guedes, M. E. M., J. Kuc, R. Hammerschmidt, and R. Bostock. Accumulation of six sesquiterpenoid phytoalexins in tobacco leaves infiltrated with *Pseudomonas lachrymans*. **Phytochemistry** 1982; 21(12): 2987–2988.

NT448   Hayashi, K., Y. Shimizu, and H. Takahara. Extraction of nerve growth factor biosynthesis promoters from tobacco. Patent-Japan Kokai Tokkyo Koho-04 210,643 1992; 5 pp.

NT449   Goud, S. N., L. Zhang, and A. M. Kaplan. Immunostimulatory potential of smokeless tobacco extract in *in vitro* cultures of murine lymphoid tissues. **Immunopharmacology** 1993; 25(2): 95–105.

NT450 Demian, B. A. Trace analysis of vanillin in tobacco. **J Liq Chromatogr** 1993; 16(161): 3563–3574.

NT451 Ollson, E., A. Holth, E. Kumlin, L. Bohlin, and I. Wahlberg. Structure-related inhibiting activity of some tobacco cembranoids on the prostaglandin synthesis *in vitro*. **Planta Med** 1993; 59(4): 293–295.

NT452 Anon. Green tobacco sickness in tobacco harvesters-Kentucky 1992. **Morbid Mortal Wkly Rep** 1993; 42(13): 237–240.

NT453 Shankaran, K., S. V. Kandarkar, Q. Q. Contractor, R. H. Kalro, and H. G. Desai. Ultrastructural changes in esophageal mucosa of chronic tobacco chewers. **Indian J Med Res** 1993; 98(1): 15–19.

NT454 Vogeli, U., R. Vogeli-Lange, and J. Chappell. Inhibition of phytoalexin biosynthesis in elicitoritreated tobacco cell-suspension cultures by calcium/calmodulin antagonists. **Plant Physiol** 1992; 100: 1369–1376.

NT455 Holdsworth, D., and L. Balun. Medicinal plants of the East and West Sepik provinces, Papua New Guinea. **Int J Pharmacog** 30(3): 218–222.

NT456 Schmeda-Hirschmann, G., and A. Rojas de Arias. A screening method for natural products on triatomine drugs. **Phytother Res** 1992; 6(2): 68–73.

NT457 Wibberley, M. S., J. R. Lenton, and S. J. Neill. Sesquiterpenoid phytoalexins produced by hairy roots of *Nicotiana tabacum*. **Phytochemistry** 1994; 37(2): 349–351.

NT458 Parkih, S. S., K. B. Chopra, R. H. Kalro, and H. G. Desai. The effect of chewing toacco on portal hypertensive gastric mucosa. **J Clin Gastroenterol** 1994; 18(4): 348–350.

NT459 Tabata, M., E. Sezik, G. Honda, et al. Traditional medicine in Turkey. III. Folk medicine in East Anatolia, Van and Biltis provinces. **Int J Pharmacog** 1994; 32(1): 3–12.

NT460 Misuzaki, S., D. Yoshida, and Y. Saito. Antineoplastic agent. Patent-PCT Int Apl-86 02,835 1986; 26 pp.

NT461 Selvaraj, G., R. K. Jain, D. J. Olson, R. Hirji, S. Jana, and L. R. Hogge. Glycinebetaine in oilseed rape and flax leaves: detection by liquid chromatography/continuous flow secondary ion-mass spectrometry. **Phytochemistry** 1995; 38(5): 1143–1146.

NT462 Tazaki, H., H. Kodama, M. Fujimori, and A. Onishi. Extraction of 15-hydroxysolanascone-beta-glucoside, and flavoring agent of tobacco. Patent-Japan Kokai Tokkyo Koho-61 227,587 1986; 4 pp.

NT463 Bhattarai, N. K. Medical ethnobotany in the Karnali zone, Nepal. **Econ Bot** 1992; 46(3): 257–261.

NT464 Giron, L. M., V. Freire, A. Alonzo, and A. Caceres. Ethnobotancal survey of the medicinal flora used by the Caribs of Guatemala. **J Ethnopharmacol** 1991; 34(2i3): 173–187.

NT465 Barrett, B. Medicinal plants of Nicaragua's atlantic coast. **Econ Bot** 1994; 48(1): 8–20.

NT466 Loewenthal, R., and J. Peer. Traditional methods used in the treatment of ophthalmic diseases among the Turkana tribe in north west Kenya. **J Ethnopharmacol** 1991; 33(3): 27–229.

NT467 Singh, V. K., Z. A. Ali, and M. K. Siddioui. Ethnomedicines in the Bahraich district of Uttar Pradesh, India. **Fitoterapia** 1996; 67(1): 65–76.

NT468 Coee, F. G., and G. J. Anderson. Ethnobotany of the Garifuna of eastern Nicaragua. **Econ Bot** 1996; 50(1): 71–107.

NT469 Flores, J. S., and R. V. Ricalde. The secretions and exudates of plants used in Mayan traditional medicine. **J Herbs Spices Med Plants** 1996; 4(1): 53–59.

NT470 Comerford, S. C. Medicinal plants of two Mayan healers from San Andres, Peten, Guatemala. **Econ Bot** 1996; 50(3): 327–336.

NT471 Smith, I. K. Evidence for o-acetylserine in *Nicotiana tabacum*. **Phytochemistry** 1977; 16: 1293–1294.

NT472 Ishiguro, S., and S. Sugawara. Comparison of volatile N-containing compounds in the smoke of Lamina and Midrib of flue-cured tobacco leaves. **Agr Biol Chem** 1977; 41: 377.

NT473 Chuman, T., M. Noguchi, A. Okhubo, and S. Toda. The structure of a novel acid '3 XI-hydroxy-4 XI, 9-dimethyl-6E, 9E-dodecadienedioic acid' isolated from Turkish tobacco. **Tetrahedron Lett** 1977; 1977: 3045–3048.

NT474   Zelcer, A. and E. Galun. Culture of newly isolated tobacco protoplasts: precursor incorporation into protein, RNA and DNA. **Plant Sci Lett** 1976; 7: 331.

NT475   Deki, M. Determination of solanesol in tobacco extracts by thin layer chromatography and high pressure liquid chromatography. **Kanzei Chuo Bunsekishoho** 1977; 17: 9.

NT476   Behr, D., I. Wahlberg, T. Nishida, and C. R. Enzell. Tobacco chemistry. 34. (3E,6E)-2,6-dimethyl-10-oxo-3, 6-undecadien-2-ol and (2E)-3-methyl-4-oxo-2-nonen-8-ol. Two new constituents of Greek *Nicotiana tabacum*. **Acta Chem Scand Ser B** 1977; 31: 573.

NT477   Anderson, R. C., D. M. Gunn, J. Murray-Rust, P. Murry-Rust, and J. S. Roberts. Vetispirane sesquiterpene glucosides from flue-cured Virginia tobacco: structure, absolute stereochemistry, and synthesis. X-ray structure of the P-bromobenzenesulphonate of one of the derived aglycones. **Chem Commun** 1977; 1977: 27.

NT478   Behr, D., I. Wahlberg, and C. R. Enzell. Tobacco chemistry. Structure elucidation and synthesis of 3,3-dimethyl-7-hydroxy-2-octanone, a new seco nor-carotenoid constituent of Greek tobacco. **Acta Chem Scand Ser B** 1977; 31: 793.

NT479   Behr, D., I. Wahlberg, T. Nishida, and C. R. Enzell. Tobacco chemistry. Structure elucidation and synthesis of 5(13),7E-megastigmadien-6,9-diol, a new constituent of Greek tobacco. **Acta Chem Scand Ser B** 1977; 31: 609.

NT480   Itoh, T., T. Tamura, and T. Matsumoto. Triterpene alcohols in the seeds of *Solanaceae*. **Phytochemistry** 1977; 16: 1723–1726.

NT481   Desmarchelier, C., A. Gurni, G. Ciccia, and A. M. Giuletti. Ritual and medicinal plants of the Ese'ejas of the Amazonian rainforest (Madre de Dios, Peru). **J Ethnopharmacol** 1996; 52(1): 45–51.

NT482   Akinpelu, D. A. and E. M. Obuotor. Antibacterial activity of *Nicotiana tabacum* leaves. **Fitoterapia** 2000; 1(2): 199–200.

NT483   Ballard, T., J. Ehlers, E. Freund, M. Auslander, V. Brandt, and W. Halperin. Green tobacco sickness: occupational nicotine poisoning in tobacco workers. **Arch Environ Health** 1995; 50(5): 384–389.

NT484   Ulbelen, A., G. Iskender, G. Topcu, and S. Atmaca. Flavonoids of the cured tobacco leaves from black sea area. **J Fac Pharm Istancul Univ** 1981; 17: 71–76.

NT485   Pakrashi, A., and S. Chatterjee. Effect of tobacco consumption on the function of male accessory sex glands. **Int J Androl** 1995; 18(5): 232–236.

NT486   Anon. Cigarette smoking and spontaneous abortion. **Br Med J** 1978; 1: 259.

NT487   Demole, E., and P. Enggist. A chemical study of Virginia tobacco flavour (*Nicotinia tabacum*). II. Isolation and synthesis of cis-2-isopropenyl-8-methyl-1,2,3,4-tetrahydro-1-naphthalemol and 3-isopropenyl-5-methyl-1,2-dihydronaphthalene. **Helv Chim Acta** 1978; 61: 1335.

NT488   Fujimori, T., R. Kasuga, H. Kaneko, and M. Noguchi. Isolation of solavetivone from *Nicotiana tabacum*. **Phytochemistry** 1977; 16: 392.

NT489   Kawashima, N., N. Inoue, and M. Noma. Saccharopine from tobacco leaves. **Phytochemistry** 1978; 17: 991A.

NT490   Itoh, T., T. Ishii, T. Tamura, and T. Matsumoto. Four new and other 4-alpha-methylserols in the seeds of Solanaceae. **Phytochemistry** 1978; 17: 971–977.

NT491   Jeong, T. M., M. S. Yang, and H. H. Nah. Sterols compositions in three *Solanaceae* seed oils. **Hanguk Nonghwa Hakhoe Chi** 1978; 21(1): 51–57.

NT492   Chilton, W. S., J. Temple, M. Marzke, and M. D. Chilton. Succinamopine: A new crown gall opine. **J Bacteriol** 1984; 157(2): 357–362.

NT493   Puangnak, W. and S. Vorabhleuk. Studies on organic acids in Thai flue-cured tobaccos and their relationship to quality. **Thai J Agr Sci** 1984; 17(2): 103–118.

NT494 Sinnwell, V., V. Heemann, A. M. Bylov, W. Hass, C. Kahrec, and F. Seehofer. A new cembranoid from tobacco, IV. **Z Naturforsch Ser C** 1985; 39(11/12): 1023–1026.

NT495 Plowman, T. The ethnobotany of coca (*Erythroxylum spp., Erythroxylaceae*). Advances in Economic botany ethnobotany in the Neotropics G. T. Prance, and J. A. Kallunki (eds.) New York Botanical Garden, Bronx, NY 1984; 1: 62–111.

NT496 Anon. 3-Hydroxysolamascone-beta-sophoroside. Patent-Japan Kokai Tokkyo Koho-59 141,595: 4 pp (1984).

NT497 Gupta, M. and T. Chatterjee. Effects of citrinin on cigarette smoke inhaled and nicotine treated mice. **Indian Drugs** 1981; 18: 309–316.

NT498 Anderson, R. C., A. G. Kelly, and J. S. Roberts. Two new acidic constituents of flu-cured Virginia tobacco. **J Agr Food** 1983; 31(2): 458–459.

NT499 Tiburcio, A. F., R. Ingersoll, and A. W. Galston. Modified alkaloid pattern in developing tobacco callus. **Plant Sci** 1985; 38(3): 207–212.

NT500 Takagi, Y., T. Fujimori, H. Kaneko, and K. Kato. Isolation of new tobacco constituents, 8,9–dihydroxymegastigmatrienone, from Japanese domestic suifu tobacco. **Agr Biol Chem** 1981; 45(3): 787–788.

NT501 Wahlberg, I., E. B. Walsh, I. Forsblom, et al. Tobacco chemistry 64. A new sucrose ester from Greek tobacco. **Acta Chem Scand Ser B** 1986; 40(9): 724–730.

NT502 Nyiredy, S. Z., G. A. Gross, and O. Sticher. Minor alkaloids from *Nicotiana tabacum*. **J Nat Prod** 1986; 49(6): 1156–1157.

NT503 Behr, D., I. Wahlberg, T. Nishida, and C. R. Enzell. Tobacco chemistry. 47. (3S,6R,7E,9R)- and (3S,6R,7E,9S)-4,7-megastigmadiene-3,9-diol. Two new nor-carotenoids of Greek tobacco. **Acta Chem Scand Ser B** 1978; 32(6): 391–394.

NT504 Eda, S., K. Miyabe, Y. Akiyama, A. Ohnishi, and K. Kato. A pectic polysaccharide from cell walls of tobacco (*Nicotiana tabacum*) mesophyll. **Carbohydr Res** 1986; 158(12): 205–216.

NT505 Takagi, Y., T. Fujimori, H. Kaneko, and K. Kato. C-15 and C-17 aldehydes from Japanese domestic tobacco, *Nicotiana tabacum* cv. Suifu. **Acta Biol Chem** 1981; 45(3): 769–770.

NT506 Burton, H. R., R. A. Andersen, P. D. Fleming, and L. R. Walton. Changes in chemical composition of burley tobacco during senescence and curing. 2. **J Agr Food Chem** 1988; 36(3): 579–584.

NT507 Begley, M. J., L. Crombie, D. Mc Namara, D. F. Firth, S. Smith, and P. C. Bevan. Cembrenediols in the cutting of tobacco. X-ray crystal structures of beta-cembrenediol and alpha-cembreneketol. **Phytochemistry** 1988; 27(6): 1695–1703.

NT508 Saitoh, F., M. Noma, and N. Kawashima. The alkaloid contents of sixty *Nicotiana* species. **Phytochemistry** 1985; 24(3): 477–480.

NT509 Kolossa, E., B. Deus-Neumann, and M. H. Zenk. Radioimmunoassays for the quantitative determination of cembratrienediol. **Planta Med** 1987; 53(5): 449–456.

NT510 Whitehead, I. M., D. R. Trelfall, and D. F. Ewing. 5-Epi-aristolochene is a common precursor of the sesquiterpenoid phytoalexins capsidiol and debneyol. **Phytochemistry** 1989; 28(3): 775–779.

NT511 Borys, D. J., S. C. Setzer, L. J. Ling. CNS depression in an infant after the ingestion of tobacco: A case report. **Vet Hum Toxicol** 1988; 30(1): 20–22.

NT512 Deutsch, H. M., K. Green, and L. H. Zalkow. Water soluble high molecular weight components from plants with potent intraocular pressure lowering activity. **Curr Eye Res** 1987; 6(7): 949–950.

NT513 Goncalo, M., J. Couto, and S. Goncalo. Allergic contact dermatitis from *Nicotiana tabacum*. **Contact Dermatitis** 1990; 22(3): 188–189.

NT514 Walhberg, I., A. M. Eklund, and C. R. Enzell. Tobacco chemistry. Six new cembrane-derived compounds from tobacco. **Acta Chem Scand** 1990; 44(5): 504–512.

NT515 Frega, N., F. Bocci, L. S. Conte, and F. Testa. Chemical composition of tobacco seeds (*Nicotiana tabacum* L.). **J Am Oil Chem Soc** 1991; 68(1): 29–33.

NT516 Caceres, A., B. R. Lopez, M. A. Giron, and H. Logemann. Plants used in Guatemala for the treatment of dermatophytic infections. I. Screening for antomycotic activity of 44 plant extracts. **J Ethnopharmacol** 1991; 31(3): 263–276.

NT517 Nagaraju, N., and K. N. Rao. A survey of plant crude drugs of Rayalaseema, Andhra Pradesh, India. **J Ethnopharmacol** 1990; 29(2): 137–158.

NT518 Sun, J. S., Z. Q. Zhu, S. Q. Li, and Y. Zhu. Studies on 6-benzuladenine localization in callus cells of tobacco. **Zhiwa Xuebao** 1986; 25(5): 480–482.

NT519 Song, Y. N., M. Shibuya, Y. Ebizuka and U. Sankawa. Indentification of plant factors inducing virulence gene expression in Agrobacterium tumefaciens. **Chem Pharm Bull** 1991; 39(9): 2347–2350.

NT520 Songstad, D. D., W. G. W. Kurz, and C. L. Nessler. Tyramine accumulation in Nicotiana tabacum transformed with a chimeric tryptophan decarboxylase gene. **Phytochemistry** 1991; 30(10): 3245–3246.

NT521 Adhvaryu, S. G., B. J. Dave, and A. H. Trivedi. Cytogenetic surveillance of tobacco-areca nut (mava) chewers, including patients with oral cancers and premalignant conditions. **Mutat Res** 1991; 261(1): 41–49.

NT522 Matsuzaki, T. and A. Koiwai. Antioxidative beta-diketones in stigma lipids of tobacco. **Agr Biol Chem** 1988; 52(9): 2341–2342.

NT523 Cusack, M. and W. S. Pierpoint. Similarities between sweet protein thaumatin and A pathogenesis-related protein from tobacco. **Phytochemistry** 1988; 27(12): 3817–3821.

NT524 Sen, S., G. Talukder, and A. Sharma. Betel cytotoxicity: further evidence from mouse bone marrow cells. **Int J Pharmacog** 1991; 29(2): 130–140.

NT525 Johansson, S. L., J. M. Hirsch, and D. R. Johnson. Effect of repeated oral administration of tobacco snuff on natural killer-cell activity in the rat. **Arch Oral Biol** 1991; 36(6): 473–476.

NT526 Bowman, D. T., W. W. Weeks, and C. A. Wilkinson. Stability of alkaloid production in flue–cured tobacco. **Comp Sci** 1991; 31(5): 1121–1124.

NT527 Grasso, S. and R. J. Shepherd. Isolation and partial characterization of virus inhibitors from plant species taxonomically related to Phytolacca. **Phytopathology** 1978; 68: 199.

NT528 Fujimori, T., R. Kasuga, H. Kaneko, Set al. Isolation and structure determination of solanascone, a new tetracyclic sesquiterpene ketone from Nicotiana tabacum. **Tennen Yuki Kagobutsu Toronkai Koen Yoshishu** 1978; 417.

NT529 Demole, E., P. Enggist, M. Winter, et al. Megastigma-5,8-dien-4-one, an aroma constituent of the yellow passion fruit and Virginia tobacco. **Helv Chim Acta** 1979; 62: 67.

NT530 Chuman, T., and M. Noguchi. Isolation of new terpenoid acids (-)-3-methyl-6-isopropyl-9-oxo-2E,4E-decadienoic acid and 3-isopropyl-6-oxo-2Z-heptenoic acid from Turkish tobacco. **Agr Biol Chem** 1975; 39: 1169.

NT531 Matsushita, H., Y. Tsujino, D. Yoshida, A. Saito, K. Kato, and M. Noguchi. New minor alkaloids in flue-cured tobacco leaf (Nicotiana tabacum cv BY-260-9). **Agr Biol Chem** 1979; 43: 193–194.

NT532 Behr, D., I. Wahlberg, T. Nishid, and C. R. Enzell. Tobacco chemistry. 45. (2E,6S)-2,6-dimethyl-2,7-octadiene-1,6-diol, a new monoterpenoid from Greek tobacco. **Acta Chem Scand Ser B** 1978; 32: 228–234.

NT533 Chuman, T., and M. Noguchi. Isolation of a new terpenoid acid 2-methyl-5-isopropyl-1-cyclopentene-1-carboxylic acid from Turkish tobacco. **Agr Biol Chem** 1975; 39: 567–568.

NT534 Takagi, Y., T. Fujimori, H. Kaneko, T. Fukuzumi, and M. Noguchi. Isolation of a new tobacco constituent, (3S,5R, 6S,9Zeta)-3-hydroxy-5,6-epoxy-beta-ionol, from Japanese domestic suifu tobacco. **Agr Biol Chem** 1978; 42: 1785–1787.

NT535 Demole, E., and P. Enggist. Indentification of twenty-one novel constituents of oriental tobacco flavour (Nicotiana tabacum L.) including (E)-3-methyl-non-2-en-4-one,15-olide, 8-alpha,13:9-alpha,13-diepoxy-15,16-dinorlabdane,(z)-octadec-9-en-18-olide, and (E)-2-ethylidene-6,10,14-trimethyl, trans-2-ethylidene. **Helv Chim Acta** 1978; 61: 2318–2327.

NT536 Behr, D., I, Wahlberg, A. J. Aasen, et al. Tobacco chemistry. 44. (1S,2E,4R, 6E,8R,11S,12R): and (1s,2E,4S,6E, 8R,11S,12R)-8,11-eposy-2,6-thunbergadiene-4,12-diol. Two new diterpenoids of Greek tobacco. **Acta Chem Scand Ser B** 1978; 32: 221–227.

NT537 Takagi, Y., T. Chuman, T. Fujimori, H. Kaneko, T. Fukuzumi, and M. Noguchi. Isolation of new nor–isoprenoids related to tobacco thunberganoids from Japanese domestic suifu tobacco. **Agr Biol Chem** 1978; 42: 327–331.

NT538 Coxon, D. T., A. M. C. Davies, G. R. Fenwick, R. Self, J. L. Firmin, D. Lipkin and N. F. Janes. Agropine, a new amino acid derivative from crown gall tumors. **Tetrahedron Lett** 1980; 21: 495–498.

NT539 Takagi, Y., T. Fujimori, H. Kaneko, and K. Kato. Phytuberol from Japanese domesto tobacco, *Nicotiana tabacum* cv. Suifu. **Agr Biol Chem** 1979; 43: 2395–2396.

NT540 Chortyk, O. T., R. F. Severson, and R. F. Arrendale. Isolation and quantitation of terpenoid and lipid constituents of tobacco. **Lloydia** 1978; 41(6): 647–648.

NT541 Takagi, Y., T. Fujimori, H. Kaneko, and K. Kato. Cembrene, from Japanese domestic tobacco *Nicotiana tabacum*. **Agr Biol Chem** 1980; 44: 467–468.

NT542 Kung, S. D., J. A. Saunder, T. C. Tso, D. A. Vaughan, M. Womack, R. C. Staples, and G. R. Beecher. Tobacco as a potential food source and smoke material nutritional evaluation of tobacco leaf protein. **J Food Sci** 1980; 45: 320–327.

NT543 De Salles, L. The water soluble fraction of cigarette smoke condensate identification of the principal components. **Ann Tab Sect** 1976; 1(14): 119–124.

NT544 Court, W. A., and J. G. Hendel. Determination of nonvolatile organic and fatty acids in flue–cured tobacco by gas liquid chromatography. **J Chromatogr Sci** 1978; 16: 314–317.

NT545 Kawashima, N., and Y. Tanabe. Comparison of the primary structure of the large and small subunits of fraction 1 protein from *Solanaceae* plants and other families. **Biochem Syst Ecol** 1975; 2: 193–199.

NT546 Behr, D., I. Wahlberg, T. Nishida, C. R. Enzell, J. Berg, and A. Pilotti. Tobacco chemistry. New cembranic diterpenoids from Greek tobacco. **Acta Chem Scand Ser B** 1980; 34: 195–202.

NT547 Uegaki, R., T. Fujimori, H. Kaneko, K. Kato, and M. Noguchi. Isolaton of dehydrololiolide and 3-oxo-actinidol from *Nicotiana tabacum*. **Agr Biol Chem** 1979; 43(5): 1149–1150.

NT548 Kodama, H., T. Fujimori, and K. Kato. Non-volatile constituents in tobacco. Part 1. Isolation of a new terpene clucoside,3-hydroxy-5,6-epoxy-beta-ionyl-beta-D-glucopyranoside from flue–cured tobacco. **Agr Biol Chem** 1981; 45: 941–944.

NT549 Wahlberg, I., D. Behr, A. M. Eklund, T. Nishida, and C. R. Enzell. Tobacco chemistry. Seven new nor-cembranoids isolated from Greek tobacco. **Acta Chem Scand Ser B** 1980; 34(34): 675–683.

NT550 Miyano, M., N. Yasumatsu, H. Matsushita, and K. Nishida. 1-(6-hydroxyoctanoyl)nornicotine and 1-(7-hydroxyoctanoyl)nornicotine, two new alkaloids from Japanese deomestic tobacco. **Agr Biol Chem** 1981; 45: 1029–1032.

NT551 Rao, V. P., D. Chowdary, and R. Narayanan. Effect of aqueous tobacco extract on the bioenergetis parameters of the snail host, *Lymnaea luteola*. **Proc Tent Int Congress Trop Med & Malaria** 1980; 355–.

NT552 Wahlberg, I., D. Behr, A. M. Eklund, T. Nishida, C. R. Enzell, and J. E. Berg. Tobacco chemistry. 54. (1S,2E,4S,6E, 8S,11R,12S)-8-11-epoxy-cembradiene-1,12-diol, a new constituent of Greek tobacco. **Acta Chem Scand Ser B** 1982; 36: 37–41.

NT553 Wahlberg, I., I. Wallin, C. Narbonne, N. Toshiaki, C. R. Enzell, and J. E. Berg. Tobacco chemistry. Three new cemebranoids from Greek tobacco. The stereochemistry of (1S,2E,4S, 6R,7E,11E)-2,7,11-cembratriene-4,6-diol. **Acta Chem Scand Ser B** 1982; 36: 147–153.

NT554 Katz, T., T. P. Pitner, R. D. Kinser, R. N. Gerfuson, and W. N. Einolf. Isolation and indentification of two new seco-cembranoids from cigarette smoke. **Tetrahedron Lett** 1981; 22: 4771–4774.

NT555 Siddiqui, I. R., N. Rosa, and G. L. Benzing. An amadori compound from tobacco. **Carbohydr Res** 1981; 98: 57–63.

NT556 Jujimori, T., Y. Takagi, and K. Kato. Isolation of 8,9-dehydrotheaspirone from Nicotiana tabacum. **Agr Biol Chem** 1981; 45: 2925–2926.

NT557 Uegaki, R., T. Fujimori, H. Kaneko, and K. Kato. Isolation of geranyl-geraniadiene from Nicotiana tabacum cv. burley. **Agr Biol Chem** 1980; 44: 2215.

NT558 Kodama, H., T. Fujimori, and K. Kato. Non-volatile constituents on tobacco. Isolation of a new perpene glucoside, loliolide-beta—D-glucopyranoside from flue-cured tobacco. **Agr Biol Chem** 1982; 46: 1409–1411.

NT559 Bolt, A. J. N., S. W. Purkis, and J. S. Sadd. A damascene derivative from Nicotiana tabacum. **Phytochemistry** 1983; 22(2): 613–614.

NT560 Park, O. S. Isolation of solanesol from Korean native tobacco. **Korean J Pharmacol** 1981; 12: 211–214.

NT561 Wahlberg, I., A. M. Eklund, T. Nishida, C. R. Enzell, and J. E. Berg. Tobacco chemistry. 58. 7,8-Epoxy-4-basmen-6-one, a tobacco diterpenoid having a novel skeleton. **Tetrahedron Lett** 1983; 24(8): 843–846.

NT562 Leete, E. Biosynthesis and metabolism of the tobacco alkaloids. Alkaloids: Chemical and Biological Perspectives. John Wiley and Sons, NY, 1983: 85–152.

NT563 Matsuzaki, T., A. Koiwai, and N. Kawashima. Isolation of tetra-, penta-, and hepta-acyl glycerides from stigmas of Nicotiana tabacum. **Agr Biol Chem** 1983; 47(1): 77–82.

NT564 Grady, K. L., and J. A. Bassham. 1-Aminocyclopropane-1-carboxylic acid concentrations in shoot-forming and non-shoot forming tobacco callus cultures. **Plant Physiol** 1982; 70: 919–921.

NT565 Nishikawaji, S., T. Fujimori, S. Matsushima, and K. Kato. Sesquiterpenoids

from flue-cured tobacco leaves. **Phytochemistry** 1983; 22(8): 1819–1820.

NT566 Matsushima S., T. Ohsumi, and S. Sugawara. Composition of trace alkaloids in tobacco lean lamina. **Agr Biol Chem** 1983; 47(3): 507–510.

NT567 Heemann, V., A. M. Bylov, U. Brummer, W. Hass, and F. Seehofer. 3,7,11,15-Cembratetraen-6-ol, a new cembranoid from tobacco, III. **Z Naturforsch Ser C** 1983; 38(7/8): 517–518.

NT568 Kodama, H., T. Fujimori, and K. Kato. Structure determination of new sesquiterpene glycosides from flue–cured tobacco by two dimensional NMR. Proc 26th Symposium on the Chemistry of Natural Products, Kyoto, Japan 1983; 26: 1–8.

NT569 Wahlberg, I., K. Nordfors, C. Vogt, T. Nishida, and C. R. Enzell. Tobacco chemistry. Five new hydroperoxy-cembratrinediols from tobacco. **Acta Chem Scand Ser B** 1983; 37(7): 653–656.

NT570 Bylov, A. M., U. Brummer, W. Hass, F. Seehofer, V. Heemann, and V. Sinnwell. New cembranoids from tobacco, II. **Z Naturforsch Ser C** 1983; 38(7/8): 515–516.

NT571 Gore, N. R., and J. L. Wray. Leucine: tRNA ligase from cultured cells of Nicotiana tabacum var. xanthi. Evidence for de novo synthesis and for loss of functional enzyme molecules. **Plant Physiol** 1978; 61(1): 20–24.

NT572 Kodama, H., T. Fujimori, and K. Kato. Glucosides of ionone-related compounds in several Nicotiana species. **Phytochemistry** 1984; 23(3): 583–585.

NT573 Kodama, H., T. Fujimori, and K. Kato. A nor-sesquiterpene glycoside, rishitin-beta-sophoroside, from tobacco. **Phytochemistry** 1984; 23(3): 690–692.

NT574 Hirsch, J. M., B. Svennerholm, and A. Vahlne. Inhibition of herpes simplex virus replication by tobacco extracts. **Cancer Res** 1984; 44(5): 1991–1997.

NT575 Wahlberg, I., R. Arndt, I. Wallin, C. Vogt, T. Nishida, and C. R. Enzell. Tobacco chemistry. Six new cembra-trienetriols from tobacco. **Acta Chem Scand Ser B** 1984; 38(1): 21–30.

NT576 Misawa, M. Production of natural substances by plant cell cultures described in Japanese Patents. Plant Tissue Culture its Bio–Technol Appl Int Congr 1st 1976; 17–26.

NT577 Yamada, Y., Y. Hara, M. Senda, M. Nishihara, and M. Kito. Phospholipids of membranes of cultured cells and the products of protoplast fusion. **Phytochemistry** 1979; 18: 423–426.

NT578 Sheveleva, G. A., and A. P. Kiryushchenkov. Effect of nicotine on fetal development and offspring (of treated rats). **Akush Ginekol** 1981; 6: 31–34.

NT579 Thelestam, M., M. Curvall, and C. R. Enzell. Effect of tobacco smoke compounds on the plasma membrane of cultured human lung fibroblasts. **Toxicology** 1980; 15: 203–217.

NT580 Adesina, S. K. Studies on some plants used as anticonvulsants in Amerindian and African traditional medicine. **Fitoterapia** 1982; 53: 147–162.

NT581 Mousdale, D. M. A. Reversed-phase ion-pair high-performance liquid chromatography of the plant hormones indolyl-3-acetic, and abscisic acid. **J Chromatogr** 1981; 209: 489–493.

NT582 Agarwal, J. L., A. K. Sisodia, C. D. Pande. An effect of cigarette smoking on serum total cholesterol level. **Ann Natl Acad Med Sci (India)** 1982; 18(1): 15–20.

NT583 Chang, C. C., C. M. Chen, B. R. Adams, and B. M. Trost. Leucinopine. A characteristic compound of some crown gall tumors. **Proc Nat Acad Sci USA** 1983; 80: 3573–3576.

NT584 Nemity, W. Agents to wean smokers from nicotine. Patent-Ger Offen-1,911,112: 1970; 8 pp.

NT585 Luna, L. E. The concept of plants as teachers among four Mestizo shamans of Iquitos, northeastern Peru. **J Ethnopharmacol** 1984; 11(2): 135–156.

NT586 Kargbo, T. K. Traditional practices affecting the health of women and children in Africa. Unpublished manuscript, 1984.

NT587 Bredon, M., A. M. Quero, and A. German. Tobacco smoke influence on mice resistance to different viral diseases. **Ann Pharm Fr** 1982; 40(2): 153–165.

NT588 Ojewole, J. A. O., A. D. Adekile, and O. O. Odebiyi. Pharmacological studies on a Nigerian herbal preparation: 1. Cardiovascular actions of cow's urine concoction (cuc) and it individual components. **Int J Crude Drug Res** 1982; 20: 71–85.

NT589 Boyd, E. J. S., J. A. Wilson, and K. G. Wormsley. Smoking impairs therapeutic gastric inhibition. **Lancet** 1983; 8316: 95–97.

NT590 Khan, N. A. and S. S. Hasan. Effect of *Cannabis* hemp (hashish) on normal and rats subjected to psychological stress. **Proc Indian Acad Sci Anim** 1984; 93(2): 121–129.

NT591 Adesina, S. K. Studies on a Nigerian herbal anticonvulsant recipe. **Int J Crude Drug Res** 1982; 20: 93–100.

NT592 Hedberg, I., O. Hedberg, P. J. Madati, K. E. Mshigeni, E. N. Mshiu, and G. Samuelsson. Inventory of plants used in traditional medicine in Tanzania. II. Plants of the families *Dilleniaceae–Opilliaceae*. **J Ethnopharmacol** 1983; 9(1): 105–127.

NT593 Van Puyvelde, L., D. Geysen, F. X. Ayobangira, E. Hakizamungu, A. Nshimiyimana, and A. Kalisa. Screening of medicinal plants of Rwanda for ascaricidal activity. **J Ethnopharmacol** 1985; 13(2): 209–215.

NT594 Singh, Y. N. Traditional medicine in Fiji: Some herbal folk cures by Fiji Indians. **J Ethnopharmacol** 1986; 15(1): 57–88.

NT595 Barrieri, R. L., P. M. Mc Shane, and K. J. Ryan. Constituents of cigarette smoke inhibit human granulose cell aromatase. **Farmatsiya (Sofia)** 1986; 46(2): 232–236.

NT596 Matsuzaki, T., and A. Koiwai. Germination inhibition in stigma extracts of tobacco and indentification of MeABA, ABA and ABA-Beta-D-glucopyranoside. **Agr Biol Chem** 1986; 50(9): 2193–2199.

NT597 Wahlberg, I., A. M. Eklund, C. R. Enzell, and J. E. Berg. Tobacco chemistry. (5R,6S,7E,9S)-7-megastigmene-5,6-9-triol, a new constituent of Greek tobacco. **Acta Chem Scand Ser B** 1987; 41(6): 455–458.

NT598 Weniger, B., M. Rouzier, R. Daguilh, D. Henrys, J. H. Henrys, and R. Anton.

Popular medicine of the central plateau of Haiti. Ethnopharmacological inventory. **J Ethnopharmacol** 1986; 17(1): 13–30.

NT599 Hoffman, D., J. D. Adams, D. Lisk, I. Fisenne, and K. D. Brunnemann. Toxic and carcinogenic agents in dry and moist snuff. **J Nat Cancer Inst** 1987; 79(6): 1281–1286.

NT600 Arenas, P. Medicine and magic among the Maka Indians of the Paraguayan Chaco. **J Ethnopharmacol** 1987; 21(3): 279–295.

NT601 Kulakkattolickal, A. Piscicidal plants of Nepal: Preliminary toxicity screening using grass carp (*Ctenopharyngodon idella*) fingerlings. **J Ethnopharmacol** 1987; 21(1): 1–9.

NT602 Whitehead, I. M., D. F. Ewing, and D. R. Threlfall. Sesquiterpenoids related to the phytoalexin debneyol from elicited cell suspension cultures of *Nicotiana tabacum*. **Phytochemistry** 1988; 27(5): 1365–1370.

NT603 Becker, C. G., D. P. Hajjar, and J. M. Hefton. Tobacco constituents are mitogenic for arterial smooth-muscle cells. **Am J Pathol** 1985; 120(1): 1–5.

NT604 Leifertova, I., and M. Lisa. The antifungal properties of higher plants affecting some species of the genus *Aspergillus*. **Folia Pharm (Prague)** 1979; 2: 29–54.

NT605 Caceres, A., L. M. Giron, and A. M. Martinez. Diuretic activity of plants used for the treatment of urinary ailments in Guatemala. **J Ethnopharmacol** 1987; 19(3): 233–245.

NT606 Ramirez, V. R., L. J. Mostacero, A. E. Garcia, et al. Vegetales empleados en Medicina Tradicional Norperuana. Banco Agrario Del Peru & NACL Univ Trujillo, Peru, June 1988: 54 pp.

NT607 Caceres, A., L. M. Giron, S. R. Alvarado, and M. F. Torres. Screening of antimicrobial activity of plants popularly used in Guatemala for the treatment of dermatomucosal diseases. **J Ethnopharmacol** 1987; 20(3): 223–237.

NT608 Tanaka, H., R. Uegaki, T. Fujimori, and K. Kato. Antibacterial activity of sesquiterpenoids from tobacco leaves elicited by *Pseudomonas solanacearum* and tobacco mosaic virus. **Nippon Shokubutsu Byori Gakkaiho** 1983; 49(4): 501–507.

NT609 Hirschmann, G. S., and A. Rojas De Arias. A survey of medicinal plants of Minas Gerais, Brazil. **J Ethnopharmacol** 1990; 29(2): 159–172.

NT610 Grunweller, S., E. Schroder, and J. Kesselmeier. Biological activities of furostanol saponins from *Nicotiana tabacum*. **Phytochemistry** 1990; 29(8): 2485–2490.

NT611 Holdsworth, D., and H. Sakulas. Medicinal plants of the Morobe province part II. The Aseki valley. **Int J Crude Drug Res** 1986; 24(1): 31–40.

NT612 Sen, S., G. Talukder, and A. Sharma. Potentiation of betel-induced alterations of mouse glandular stomach mucosa by tobacco in studies simulating betel addiction. **Int J Crude Drug Res** 1987; 25(4): 209–215.

NT613 Yamaguchi, K., T. Suzuki, A. Katayama, M. Sasa, and S. Iida. Insectidcidal action of Japanese plants. II. A general method of detecting effective fractions and its application to 24 species of insecticidal plants. **Botyu Kagaku** 1950; 15: 62–70.

NT614 Roig, Y., and J. T. Mesa. Plantas Medicinales, Aromaticas o Venenosas de Cuba. Ministerio de Agricultura, Republica de Cuba, Havana. Book 1945; 872 pp.

NT615 Humphreys, F. R. The occurrence and industrial productin of rutin in southeastern Australia. **Econ Bot** 1964; 18: 195–253.

NT616 Bhasin, H. D. Annual report of the entomologist to Government, Punjab, Lyallpur, for the year 1924–25. Report Operations Dept Agr Punjab 1926; 1(II): 69–121.

NT617 Prance, G. T. An ethnobotanical comparison of four tribes of Amazonian Indians. **Acta Amazonica** 1972; 2(2): 7–27.

NT618 Moller, M. S. G. Custom, pregnancy and child bearing in Tanganyika. **J Trop Pediatrics Afr Child Health** 1961; 7(3): 66–78.

NT619 Schultes, R. E., and R. F. Raffauf. The Healing Forest: medicinal and toxic plants of the northwest Amazonia. Dioscorides Press, Portland, OR. 1995; 432–436.

NT620 Nakao, Y., X. Yang, M. Yokoyama, M. M. Pater, and A. Pater. Malignant transformation of human ectocervical cells immortalized by HPV 18: *in vitro* model of carcinogenesis by cigarette smoke. **Carcinogenesis** 1996; 17(3): 577–83.

NT621 Shahi, G. S., N. P. Das, and S. M. Moochhala. 1-Methyl-4-phenyl-1,2,3, 6-tetrahydropyridine-induced neurotoxicity: partial protection against striato-nigral dopamine depletion in C57BL/6J mice by cigarette smoke exposure and by beta-naphthoflavone-pretreatment. **Neurosci Lett** 1991; 127(2): 247–250.

NT622 Aasen, A. J., T. Chuman, and C. R. Enzell. (6S)-6-isopropyl-3-methyl-9-oxo-2E, 4E-decadenoic acid from Turkish *Nicotiana tabacum*, assignment of absolute configuration. **Agr Biol Chem** 1975; 39; 2085.

NT623 Wahlberg, I., A. M. Ecklund, T. Nishida, and C. R. Enzell. Tobacco chemistry. Two new nor-drimanes from Greek tobacco. **Acta Chem Scand Ser B** 1981; 35: 307–310.

NT624 Nagai, N., Y. Kojima, M. Shimosaka, and M. Okazaki. Effects of kinetin on L-phenylalanine ammonia–lyase activity in tobacco cell culture. **Agr Biol Chem** 1988; 52(10): 2617–2619.

NT625 Kodama, H., T. Fujimori, and K. Kato. Three new sesquiterpenoid glycosides from tobacco. **Agr Biol Chem** 1985; 49(9): 2537–2541.

NT626 Ferguson, F. N., F. F. Whidby., E. B. Sanders, et al. Isolation and characterization of 2,3-dimethyl-6-(4,8,12-trimethyltridecyl)-1,4-naphthoquinone from tobacco, and smoke. **Tetrahedron Lett** 1978; 1978: 2645–2648.

NT627 Maisch, R., B. Knoop, and R. Beiderbeck. Absorbent culture of tobacco cell suspensions with different absorbents. **Z Naturforsch Ser C** 1986; 41(11/12): 1040–1044.

10 | Olea europaea

L.

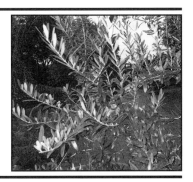

Common Names

Aceituna	Spain	Olijf	Netherlands
Alyvos	Lithuania	Oliondo	Spain
Aseituna	Netherlands Antilles	Olipuus	Estonia
Azeitona	Portugal	Oliv	Sweden
Culoare masline	Romania	Oliva europska	Slovakia
Dege e ullirit	Albania	Oliva	Czech Republic
Elia	Greece	Oliva	Ethiopia
Euroopa olipuu	Estonia	Oliva	Hungary
Eylbert	Israel	Oliva	Italy
Jaitun	India	Oliva	Portugal
Jitabdoogh	Armenia	Oliva	Romania
Jiteni	Armenia	Oliva	Russia
Julipe	India	Oliva	Spain
Maslin	Romania	Oliva	Ukraine
Maslina	Bulgaria	Olivas	Latvia
Maslina	Croatia	Olive	England
Maslina	Serbia	Olive	France
Maslina	Ukraine	Olive	Germany
Masline	Israel	Olive	Guyana
Masliniu	Romania	Olive	The Isle of Man (Manx)
Maslinov	Croatia	Olive	United States
Maslinov	Serbia	Oliveira	Portugal
Mohlware	South Africa	Oliven	Denmark
Ngjyre ulliri	Albania	Oliven	Norway
Oastre	Spain	Olivenbaum	Germany
Olajbogyo	Hungary	Olivera	Spain
Olajfa	Hungary	Olivgront	Sweden
Olbaum	Germany	Olivo	Spain
Oleifi	Netherlands Antilles	Olivove drevo	Czech Republic
Olewydden	England	Olivovnik europsky	Slovakia
Oliba	Spain	Olivovnik	Czech Republic
Olifa	Iceland	Olivy	Czech Republic
Oliif	Spain	Oliwka	Poland
Oliivi	Finland	Oljka	Slovenia

From: *Medicinal Plants of the World, vol. 3: Chemical Constituents, Traditional and Modern Medicinal Uses*
By: I. A. Ross © Humana Press Inc., Totowa, NJ

Oljypuu	Finland	Ullir	Albania
Olyf	Cornwall	Zaitun	Indonesia
Olyva	Ukraine	Zayit	Israel
Oulivie	France	Zaytun	Arabic countries
Oulivie	France	Zebbug	Malta
Qolli	Boliwia	Zeituni	Mozambique
Qolli	Peru	Zeituni	Tanzania
Rabell	Spain	Zeituni	Zaire
Saidun	India	Zetis	Georgia
Saidun	Sri Lanka	Zetiskhili	Georgia
Uliva	Switzerland	Zeyatin	Turkmenistan
Ullastre	Spain	Zeytin	Turkey
Ulli	Albania	Zeytoon	Armenia

BOTANICAL DESCRIPTION

Olea europaea is a large evergreen shrub of the OLEACEAE family. In its native state, it is a multistemmed evergreen tree, 6–9 m high, with equal or slightly less spread. The trunk is massive, especially in older plantings; gray, gnarled, bumpy, and contorted. Most trees have round, spreading crowns, but tall, cylindrical trees are grown in some parts of Italy, and trees may be trellised in intensive plantings. Leaves are 7.5 cm long, narrow, opposite, lanceolate or linear, with entire margins and acute tips, silver-green, underside lighter. Small creamy white flowers are borne in inflorescences of 15 flowers in axillary clusters of 1-year wood; blooms in spring. Trees produced flowers in 2–3 years, but seedlings have a long juvenile period. Most flowers undergo pistil abortion, leaving only one to two fruits per axil at harvest. Olives are self-fruitful but bear heavier crops when cross-pollinated. Wind is the pollinator. Fruits are drupes: edible olives, 4 cm across; green in late summer, maturing to black; drops when ripe. Trees have a tendency toward heavy alternate bearing, unless fruit are thinned in the "on" year. Olives require 6–8 months for maturation, but table olives are picked earlier when firm and oil olives are left on trees until oil content reaches 20–30%.

ORIGIN AND DISTRIBUTION

The name *Olea europaea* applies to both the wild and domestic olive. The wild olive or oleaster has a disjunctive distribution in the Mediterranean region and the Near East down to South Africa and has been cultivated by man since ancient times. The olive was spread throughout Mediterranean Europe and North Africa very early, owing to its ease of propagation by seed, cuttings, or "ovules" (callus growths on trunks that produce rooted shoots). Trees are extremely long-lived (up to 1000 years) and tolerant of drought, salinity, and almost total neglect and have been reliable producers of food and oil for thousands of years. Oil was used for cooking as well as burning in lamps; several references are made to olive oil lamps in the Bible and other ancient writings. Evidence of olive stones from archaeological sites in the Near East and Cyprus suggests that olives have been consumed since approx 9000 BC, although it is only from 3500 BC that there is clear evidence of domestication. Olives are most commonly linked to Greece, and this country has a long tradition of olive cultivation and use. By 1300 BC, Greek palaces had rooms devoted to storing jars full of olive oil.

Although the primary area of olive cultivation still lies in the Mediterranean region, olives are also cultivated in other parts of the world, such as California and South Africa.

TRADITIONAL MEDICINAL USES

Arabic countries. In Unani medicine, dried plant is taken by fumigation as an abortifacient[OE179].

Argentina. Decoctions of the dried fruit and of the dried leaf are taken orally for diarrhea and to treat respiratory and urinary tract infections[OE131].

Brazil. Hot water extract of the fresh leaf is taken orally to treat hypertension and to induce diuresis[OE183].

Canary Islands. An infusion prepared from the fresh or dried leaf is taken orally as a hypoglycemic agent. Leaves are taken orally as a hypotensive and administered *per rectum* for hemorrhoids[OE145]. Hot water extract of dried leaves of *Olea europaea* and *Foeniculum vulgare* is taken orally as a hypotensive agent[OE184].

East Africa. Infusion of the trunk bark, pounded and soaked overnight, is taken orally for tapeworm infestation[OE121].

Greece. Hot water extract of the leaf is taken orally for high blood pressure[OE102].

Iran. Decoctions of the dried bark, applied externally or decoction of the dried leaf taken orally, are used for hypertension. Fresh fruit fixed oil is used as food and laxative. Seed oil is taken orally as a cholagogue; to remove gallstones; in nephritis associated with lead intoxication, spasms associated with systemic intoxication, dry coughing, and intestinal occlusion and obstructions; and as a vermicide. Taken with lemon juice, it is used to prevent vomiting associated with rancid olive oil remaining in the intestine. The oil is applied externally as an emollient before taking a sunbath, prophylaxis for irritations caused by sunburn, and for snake and insect bites. To prevent hair loss, oil is applied every night on the scalp then shampooed the next morning[OE110].

Italy. Extract of the fruit's essential oil is taken orally as a cholagogue and laxative

and to treat renal lithiasis. It is used externally to treat sores, burns, and rheumatism; to promote circulation; and as a hemostat. Water extract of the fruit's essential oil is used externally to treat sunburns. Decoction of the fruit essential oil is taken orally as a diuretic and hypotensive[OE140]. Fruit-fixed oil is taken orally by adults for intestinal obstructions. Tincture of the leaf is taken orally as a febrifuge[OE111]. Infusion of the dried leaf is taken orally as a hypotensive[OE191] and is used for its anti-hypertensive properties[OE193]. Infusion of the fresh leaf is taken orally as an anti-inflammatory[OE053]. Infusion of the leaf is taken orally as a hypotensive and applied externally as a vulnerary, emollient for ingrown nails, and restorer of epthelium[OE128].

Japan. Hot water extract of the dried bark is taken orally as an antipyretic, for rheumatism, as a tonic, and for scrofula[OE158].

Jordan. Seed oil is taken orally as a laxative and applied externally as an emollient and pectoral[OE142].

Kenya. Stem, fresh, and dried twigs of *Olea europaea* ssp. *africana* are used as a chewing stick[OE168,OE127].

Madeira. Infusion of leaves of *Olea europaea* var. *maderensis* is taken orally as an antihypertensive[OE139].

Mexico. Decoction of dried leaves is taken orally for diabetes[OE147].

Morocco. Leaves are taken orally for stomach and intestinal diseases and used as a mouth cleanser. Essential oil made from the leaves is taken orally for constipation, liver pain, and tonic and applied externally for hair care[OE144].

Oman. Decoction of the bark is taken orally for constipation. Barks and leaves are applied externally for skin rash. Fruit resin mixed with the gall bladder of sheep or goat is applied ophthalmically for cataract. The fruit is applied externally for fractured limb. Cataplasm prepared from leaves is applied externally for ulcers[OE126].

Peru. Hot water extract of the dried bark is taken orally for urinary retention, herpes simplex, and constipation and to expel biliary calculi[OE189].

Reunion Island. Hot water extract of the dried *Olea europaea* ssp. *africana* plant is taken orally for diabetes, diarrhea, rheumatism, fever, and gastroenteritis in infants[OE098].

South Africa. Hot water extract of the dried bark of *Olea europaea* ssp. *africana* is taken orally as antirheumatic and antifebrile agents[OE159, OE072] and as a tonic[OE072].

Spain. Infusion of the leaf is taken orally for hypertension. Extract of the leaf is taken orally for gastrointestinal colic. Leaves are eaten for diabetes. Fruits are eaten for pain and wasp sting[OE138].

Trinidad. Hot water extract of the lead is taken orally to increase milk supply of nursing mother. On first day, the mother drinks tea of *Stachytarpheta jamaicensis* leaves, on the second day, she drinks tea made from olive leaves and milk, and on the third day she will be able to nurse the baby[OE198].

Tunisia. Extract of the dried leaf is taken orally for diabetes and as a hypotensive[OE181].

Turkey. The fruit is used externally as a skin cleanser[OE141].

Ukraine. Hot water extract of dried plant is taken orally for bronchial asthma[OE174].

United States. Infusion of the fruit-fixed oil is taken orally to treat hypertension and agitation. Extract of the fruit-fixed oil is taken orally as a mild laxative and vermicide and taken externally as a counterirritant[OE167].

Yugoslavia. Hot water extract of the dried leaf is taken orally for diabetes[OE175].

CHEMICAL CONSTITUENTS

(ppm unless otherwise indicated)
(E)-2-Decenal: Pl[OE222]
(E)-2-Eptenal: Pl[OE222]
(E)-2-Hexenal: Pl[OE222]
(E)-2-Nonenal: Pl[OE222]
(E)-2-Octenal: Pl[OE222]
(E,E)-2,4-Decadienal: Pl[OE222]
3,4-Dihydroxyphenylethyl 4-formyl-3-formylmethyl-4-hexenoate: Lf[OE221]
Acetaldehyde: Call Tiss[OE038]

Acetic acid: Call Tiss[OE038]
Acetone: Call Tiss[OE038]
Aconitic acid: Fr[OE029]
Aesculetin: St 209.2[OE091]
Aesculin: St 2.9[OE091]
Africanal, (+): Heartwood[OE090]
Alkanes, N: Sd Oil[OE058]
Allergen: Pollen[OE078]
Amyrin, α: Fixed oil[OE084]
Amyrin, β: Lf[OE030], Fr[OE065], Fixed oil[OE042]
Apigenin: Lf[OE011,OE225]
Apigenin-4'-O-rhamnosyl-glucoside: Lf 15[OE053]
Apigenin-7-di-O-β-D-xyloside: Lf[OE032]
Apigenin-7-O-glucoside: Dried Lf[OE225]
Arachidic acid: Sd oil 0.3%[OE034]
Avenasterol, 5-dehydro: Fr fixed oil[OE201]
Avenasterol, 7-dehydro: Fr fixed oil[OE201]
Behenic acid: Sd oil 0.3–0.4%[OE034]
Benzoic acid, 4-hydroxy: Fr[OE048]
Brassicasterol: Fr fixed oil[OE041]
Butan-1-al, 3-methyl: Call Tiss[OE038]
Butanol, 3-methyl: Call Tiss[OE038]
Butyl acetate: Call Tiss[OE038]
Butyrospermol: Fr[OE065], Fr fixed oil[OE042], Fixed oil[OE084]
Caffeic acid: Fr[OE048], Sd oil[OE050], Fr fixed oil[OE039]
Campest-7-en-ol: Fr fixed oil[OE041]
Campesterol: Fr fixed oil[OE031], Fixed oil[OE084]
Carotene, α, hydroxy: Fr fixed oil[OE077]
Carotene, α: Fr fixed oil[OE077]
Carotene, β: Fr fixed oil[OE077]
Carotene, γ: Fr fixed oil[OE077]
Carotene: Lf[OE017]
Chlorogenic acid: Lf[OE044]
Chlorophyll A: Fr fixed oil[OE077]
Chlorophyll B: Lf[OE157], Fr fixed oil[OE077]
Cholesterol, 24-methylene: Fixed oil[OE084]
Cholesterol: Fr fixed oil[OE041]
Choline: Fr[OE004], Lf[OE012]
Chrysanthemin: Fr[OE066]
Chrysoeriol: Lf 16.6[OE053]
Chrysoeriol-7-O-β-d-glucoside: Lf[OE091]
Chrysoeriol-7-O-glucoside: Lf[OE228]
Cinchonidine: Lf[OE006]
Cinchonine, dihydro: Lf 25[OE005]
Cinchonine: Lf 20–170[OE005]
Cinnamic acid ethyl ester: Fr fixed oil[OE086]
Cinnamic acid: Fr fixed oil[OE039]
Citric acid, iso: Fr, Lf[OE029]
Citric acid: Fr, Lf[OE029]

Citrostadienol, 28-iso: Fixed oil[OE084]

Citrostadienol: Fr[OE064], Fixed oil[OE084]

Cornoside: Kernel 250[OE043], Fr[OE034]

Cosmosiin: Lf[OE091]

Coumaric acid, para: Fr fixed oil[OE039]

Cryptoxanthene: Fr fixed oil[OE077]

Cyanidin: Fr[OE008]

Cyanidin-3-O-β-D-rutinoside: Fr[OE066]

Cyanidin-3-O-β-D-glucosyl-rutinoside: Fr[OE066]

Cycloartanol, 23-trans-dehydro, 31-nor, 24-methyl: Fixed oil[OE084]

Cycloartanol, 24-methylene: Fr[OE065], Fr fixed oil[OE075], Fixed oil[OE084]

Cycloartenol, 24-methylene: Fr fixed oil[OE042]

Cycloartenol, 31-nor: Fr[OE064]

Cycloartenol: Fr[OE065], Fr fixed oil[OE042], Fixed oil[OE084]

Cyclobranol: Fr fixed oil[OE075], Fr[OE065], Fixed oil[OE084]

Cycloeucalenol: Fr[OE064], Fixed oil[OE084]

Cycloolivil, (+): Bk 8.7–15[OE158]

Cyclosadol: Fr fixed oil[OE075], Fixed oil[OE084]

Cynaroside: Lf[OE091]

Dammaradienol: Fixed oil[OE084]

Delphinidin-3-rhamnoglucside-7-xyloside: Fr[OE094]

Eicosenoic acid: Sd oil 0.2–0.3%[OE034]

Elenoic acid glucoside: Fr[OE083]

Elenoic acid, deacetoxy: Fr Pu[OE151]

Elenoic acid: Fr[OE055]

Elenolide: Fr, Lf, St Bk 22[OE016], Fr Ju 58[OE067]

Eleutheroside: Lf+Twigs[OE172]

Ergosta-7-trans-22-dien-3-β-ol: Fixed oil[OE084]

Erythrodiol: Lf[OE073], Fr fixed oil 7.2%[OE041], Fr[OE063], Fruitpeel[OE047]

Essential oil: Lf[OE017]

Estrone: Kernel 34[OE088]

Ethan-1-ol, 2-phenyl, 3'-4'-dihydroxy: Lf 73.5[OE020]

Ethanol, 2-(3-4-dihydroxy-phenyl): Fr[OE056]

Ethanol, β-(3-4-dihydroxy-phenyl): Fr fixed oil[OE003]

Ethanol, para-hydroxy-phenyl: Sd oil[OE024]

Ethyl acetate: Call Tiss[OE038]

Ethyl propionate: Call Tiss[OE038]

Euphol: Fr[OE093]

Ferulic acid: Fr fixed oil[OE039]

Flavone, 4'-hydroxy: Fr[OE008]

Fraxiresinol-1-β-D-glucoside, (+): Bk 31[OE021]

Fraxiresinol-1-O-β-d-glucoside, (+): Bk 31[OE021]

Fructose: Sd[OE059]

Fucosterol, 28-iso: Fixed oil[OE084]

Fucosterol, iso: Fr fixed oil[OE031]

Fucosterol: Fr fixed oil[OE041], Fixed oil[OE084]

Fumaric acid: Fr, Lf[OE029]

Gallic acid: Fr fixed oil[OE039]

Germanicol: Fixed oil[OE084]

Glucose: Sd[OE059]

Glutaric acid, 3-[1-(formyl)-trans-1-propenyl]: Fr 4.6[OE025]

Glutaric acid, 3-[1-(hydroxy-methyl)-trans-1-propenyl]: Fr 6.9[OE025]

Gramisterol: Fr[OE064], Fixed oil[OE084]

Hemicellulose B: Fr Pu[OE081]

Heptane, 3-4-dimethyl: Call Tiss[OE038]

Hesperidin: Dried Lf[OE225]

Hex-3-en-al: Call Tiss[OE038]

Hexacosan-1-ol: Fr fixed oil[OE068]

Hexadecanoic acid, 10-16-dihydroxy: Lf 2.08[OE007]

Hexan-1-al: Call Tiss[OE038]

Hexan-1-ol: Call Tiss[OE038]

Hexanal: Flavor[OE222]

Hexane, N: Call Tiss[OE038]

Hex-cis-2-en-1-ol: Call Tiss[OE038]

Hex-cis-3-en-1-ol acetate: Call Tiss[OE038]

Hex-cis-3-en-1-ol: Call Tiss[OE038]

Hex-trans-2-en-1-al: Call Tiss[OE038]

Hex-trans-2-en-1-ol: Call Tiss[OE038]

Hex-trans-3-en-1-ol: Call Tiss[OE038]

Hexyl acetate: Call Tiss[OE038]

Hydroxytyrosol: Fr[OE224]

Inositol, myo: Sd[OE059]

Kaempferol: St 1.2[OE091], Lf[OE225]

Lanost-9(11)-en-3-β-ol, 31-nor, 24-methyl: Fixed oil[OE084]

Lanost-en-3-β-ol, 24-methylene: Fr[OE093]

Ligstral: Lf[OE151]

Ligstroside, 10-hydroxy: Lf[OE151]

Ligstroside: Fr[OE055], Kernel 0.15%[OE043], Lf 32.3[OE022]

Linoleic acid: Sd oil 7.5-12.2%[OE034]

Linolenic acid: Sd oil 0.7-0.8[OE034]

Loganin, 7-epi: Lf[OE151]

Loganin, keto: Lf[OE151]

Lophenol, 24(25)-dehydro, 24-ethyl: Fixed oil[OE084]

Lophenol, 24(25)-dehydro, 24-methyl: Fixed oil[OE084]

Lophenol, 24-ethyl: Fixed oil[OE084]

Lophenol, 24-methyl: Fixed oil[OE084]

Lophenol, trans-23-dehydro, 24-ethyl: Fixed oil[OE084]

Lophenol, *trans*-23-dehydro, 24-methyl: Fixed oil[OE084]

Lophenol: Fr[OE064]

Lutein: Fr fixed oil[OE077]

Lutein-5-6-epoxide: Fr fixed oil[OE077]

Luteolin: Lf[OE014], Fr[OE079]

Luteolin-4'-β-D-glucoside: Lf 10[OE053]

Luteolin-4'-O-β-D-glucoside: Lf[OE091]

Luteolin-7-O-glucoside: Lf[OE225]

Malic acid: Fr, Lf[OE029]

Mannitol: Branch[OE054], Lf[OE017], Lf & St 1.5%[OE089], Sd[OE059]

Maslinic acid, 2-α-3-β-diacetoxy: Fr[OE037]

Maslinic acid, δ: Lf[OE018]

Maslinic acid: Fruitpeel[OE047], Lf[OE030]

Neoxanthene: Fr fixed oil[OE077]

Nonal-1-al: Call Tiss[OE038]

Nonanal: Pl[OE222]

Nonanoic acid methyl ester: Call Tiss[OE038]

Nuezhenide oleoside: Sd[OE033], Endosperm[OE151]

Nuezhenide: Sd[OE033], Endosperm[OE151]

Obtusifoliol: Fr[OE064], Fixed oil[OE084]

Octadecanoic acid, 9-10-18-trihydroxy: Lf 1.28%[OE007]

Octan-1-al: Call Tiss[OE038]

Octan-2-ol: Call Tiss[OE038]

Octane, N: Call Tiss[OE038]

Ole e-10: Pl[OE207]

Ole e-7: Pl[OE027]

Olea europaea compound 5: Sd oil[OE024]

Olea europaea compound 5-A: Sd oil[OE024]

Olea europaea compound 6: Sd oil[OE024]

Olea europaea compound 7: Sd oil[OE024]

Olea europaea compound 7-A: Sd oil[OE024]

Olea europaea derivative 2-A: Fr[OE026]

Olea europaea derivative 2-B: Fr[OE026]

Olea europaea derivative 3: Fr[OE026]

Olea europaea phenolic glucoside 7: Lf[OE028]

Olea europaea secoiridoid 2: Lf 15[OE020]

Olea europaea secoiridoid 3: Lf 17.25[OE020]

Olea galactoglucomann: Pu[OE186]

Olea secoirioid 5: Fr Ju 1875[OE023]

Olea substance A: Lf[OE046]

Olea xyloglucan: Pu[OE097]

Oleacein: Lf[OE052]

Oleanolic acid, 3-acetoxy: Fr[OE037]

Oleanolic acid: Lf[OE157], Fr peel[OE047]

Oleic acid: Sd oil 70.2–75.1%[OE034]

Oleocyanin: Fr[OE015]

Oleoeurop: Fr 6.6%[OE001]

Oleoside methyl ester: Lf[OE151]

Oleoside: Lf[OE151]

Oleoside-11-methyl ester: Lf 15[OE028]

Oleoside-7-methyl ester: Lf 15[OE070]

Oleuropein, dimethyl: Fr[OE083], Bk 15[OE070], Lf[OE151], Kernel[OE043]

Oleuropein: Lf[OE002], Pl[OE010], Branch[OE049], Fr[OE055], Sh[OE085], Sd oil 0.566%[OE057], Kernel 1.03%[OE043], Buds[OE087], Rt, St[OE009], Bk 0.15%[OE070]

Oleuroside: Lf 293.5[OE022]

Olivil, (–): Bk 15[OE158]

Olivin: Lf[OE014]

Olivin-4'-di-glucoside: Lf[OE014]

Palmitic acid: Sd oil 12.3–15.4%[OE034]

Palmitoleic acid: Sd oil 1–2.2%[OE034]

Parkeol, 24-dihydro, 24-methylene: Fr fixed oil[OE075], Fr[OE093], Fixed oil[OE084]

Parkeol: Fixed oil[OE084]

Pentan-2-one: Call Tiss[OE038]

Peroxidase: Lf[OE017]

Phaeophorbide A: Fr fixed oil[OE077]

Phaeophorbide B: Fr fixed oil[OE077]

Phaeophytin A: Fr fixed oil[OE077]

Phaeophytin B: Fr fixed oil[OE077]

Phenol, 4-4-vinyl: Fr fixed oil[OE086]

Phenylacetic acid, para-hydroxy: Fr Ju[OE074]

Phenylethanol, 3-4-dihydroxy: Fr[OE051]

Phenylethanol, 4-hydroxy, glucoside: Fr[OE034]

Phenyl-glycol, 3-4-dihydroxy: Fr[OE051]

Phytoene: Fr fixed oil[OE077]

Phytofluene: Fr fixed oil[OE077]

Phytol: Fr[OE062]

Pinoresinol, 1-acetoxy, (+): Bk[OE092]

Pinoresinol, 1-acetoxy, 4'-β-D-glucoside (+): Bk 5.3[OE061]

Pinoresinol, 1-acetoxy, 4'-β-D-glucoside-4''-O-methyl ether, (+): Bk 55[OE021]

Pinoresinol, 1-acetoxy, 4'-O-β-D-glucoside (+): Bk 50.9[OE021]

Pinoresinol, 1-acetoxy, 4''-methyl ether-4'-O-β-D-glucoside (+): Bk 55[OE021]

Pinoresinol, 1-acetoxy-4''-O-methyl ether (+): Bk 46.4[OE158]

Pinoresinol, 1-hydroxy, (+): Bk 138.4[OE158]

Pinoresinol, 1-hydroxy, 1-β-D-glucoside (+): Bk[OE092]

Pinoresinol, 1-hydroxy, 1-O-β-D-glucoside, (+): Bk 50.1[OE021]

Pinoresinol, 1-hydroxy, 4'-β-D-glucoside (+): Bk 11.2[OE021]

Pinoresinol, 1-hydroxy, 4'-methyl ether (+): Bk[OE092]

Pinoresinol, 1-hydroxy-4''-O-methyl ether (+): Bk 23.2[OE158]

Pinoresinol-4'-β-D-glucoside, (+): Bk[OE096]

Quercetin: St1.7[OE091], Lf, Fr[OE079,OE225]
Quercetin-3-O-rhamnoside: Lf[OE228]
Quercitrin: Lf[OE040]
Raffinose: Sd[OE059]
Rhoifolin, iso: Lf[OE069]
Rutin: Lf[OE225,OE044], Husk[OE151]
Salidroside: Sd[OE033]
Saponins: Pl[OE098]
Scopoletin, iso: Bk 32.9[OE095]
Scopoletin: Bk 32.9[OE095]
Scopolin: Bk 180.3[OE072]
Sedoheptulose: Sd[OE019]
Sitosterol, β: Fr fixed oil[OE042], Lf[OE030], Fixed oil[OE084]
Squalene: Lf[OE013], Fr fixed oil[OE036]
Stearic acid: Sd oil 1.5%[OE034]
Sterols: Pl[OE098]
Stigmast-7-enol: Fr fixed oil[OE041]
Stigmasta-5-24(25)-dien-3-β-ol: Fixed oil[OE084]
Stigmasterol: Fr fixed oil[OE031], Fixed oil[OE084]
Succinic acid: Fr, Lf[OE029]
Sucrose: Sd[OE059]
Syringic acid: Fruit fixed oil[OE039]
Tannin: Lf[OE017]
Taraxasterol, pseudo: Fr[OE093]
Taraxerol: Fixed oil[OE084], Fr[OE093]
Tetracosan-1-ol: Fr fixed oil[OE068]
Tirucalla-7-24-dien-3-β-ol: Fr[OE093], Fixed oil[OE084]
Tirucallol: Fr fixed oil[OE075], Fixed oil[OE084]
Tocopherol, α: Fr[OE076]
Tocopherol, β: Fr[OE076]
Tocopherol, δ: Fr[OE076]
Tocopherol, γ: Fr[OE076]
Triacylglycerol: Fr oil[OE212]
Tyrosine: Fr fixed oil[OE003]
Tyrosol, hydroxy: Fr fixed oil[OE035], Sd oil[OE050]
Tyrosol: Fr[OE034], Fixed oil 3.3[OE082], Sd oil[OE050]
Ursolic acid: Fl 0.5%[OE045], Fr Peel[OE047]
Uvaol: Fr[OE063], Fr fixed oil 2.1%[OE041], Lf[OE073], Fr peel[OE047]
Vanillic acid: Fr[OE048], Fr fixed oil[OE050]
Veratric acid: Fr Ju[OE074]
Verbascoside: Fr[OE071], Lf[OE151], Kernel[OE043]
Vitamin D: Fr[OE004], Lf[OE017]
Xyloglucan (*Olea europaea*): Fr peel[OE080]

PHARMACOLOGICAL ACTIVITIES AND CLINICAL TRIALS

Acetoaceyl-CoA ligase stimulation. Fruit fixed oil, administered intragastrically to rats at a dose of 2 mL/kg, was active[OE192].

Acetoaceyl-CoA thiolase stimulation. Fruit fixed oil, administered intragastrically to rats at a dose of 2 mL/kg, was active[OE192].

Acetylglucoseaminidase inhibition. Water extract of the fresh twig of *Olea europaea* ssp. *africana*, at a concentration of 500 µg/mL, was active on *Porphyromonas gingivalis*[OE127].

Allergenic activity. Fixed oil, administered externally to adults, was inactive. Most cases of atopy were reclassified as cases of irritation[OE114]. Dried pollen, administered by a patch test to adults of both sexes, was active. Skin reaction test, conducted on 1573 patients suspected of respiratory allergy, was positive in 1144 cases. Positive skin reactions to olive pollen among atopic patients of the population where olive trees are abundant was high (66%), and lower (29%) where trees are scarce ($p < 0.003$)[OE205]. Ole e-1 in polyactide coglycolide microparticles, administered intraperitoneally to Balb/c mice, induced specific and long-lasting antibodies that were predominantly of the immunoglobulin (Ig)G-2 isotype. Splenic cells from the immunized mice secreted in vitro interferon-γ, but not interleukin -4, indicating that Ole e-1 containing polyactide coglycolide microparticles elicit a specific T-helper 1-type immune response[OE208]. Depigmented and glutaraldehyde-polymerized pollen extracts, administered by injections to 45 adults at doses of 44 or 4.4 µg/mL, produced a dose-dependent effect[OE209]. Pollen extract, administered preseasonally to patients with rhinitis and/or asthma, monosensitized to olive, was active. Eighty-three percent of the patients reached the proposed maximal dose of 75 Bethesda units (45.0 µg Ole e-1) with a rate of 0.8% of systemic reactions. There was an improvement in the treated group both in nasal ($p < 0.05$) and bronchial ($p < 0.05$) symptoms, and the consumption of antihistamines and β 2-agonists decreased. A decrease in specific IgE and an increase in IgG-1 and IgG-4 were found[OE210]. Crude protein extracts of the pollen were used to carry out skin prick tests on 30 patients with allergies to evaluate the clinical importance of differences between olive cultivars. Ole e-1 was present in all cultivars, although significant quantitative differences were detected[OE211]. The association between sensitization to allergens of olive pollen and confirmed plant-derived food allergy and hypersensitivity of food allergy reaction was studied on 134 patients with *Olea* pollinosis. Adverse reactions were observed in 40 patients, 21 of whom were classified as aral allergy syndrome and 19 as anaphylaxis. All of the patients showed positive skin prick test (SPT) against one or more of *Olea* allergens. Sensitization to Ole e-7 was more frequent ($p < 0.02$) in anaphylactic patients. In this group, significant association with *Olea* pollen allergens were found between positive SPT to *Rosaceae* fruits and Ole e-3 ($p < 0.045$) and Ole e-7 ($p < 0.03$), *Cucurbitaceae* and Ole e-7 ($p < 0.03$) and *Actinidiaceae* with Ole e-3 ($p < 0.04$)[OE217]. *Olea* pollens were tested on 119 patients with seasonal rhinitis and/or asthma and a positive SPT, 10 atopic patients without pollinosis and a negative SPT. All of the patients had positive skin responses to at least one of the allergen tested. A combination of Ole e-1 and Ole e-2, together with a minor allergen Ole e-6 and Oe e-7, disclosed the same diagnostic value that was obtained with the use of crude olive pollen extract[OE218]. Natural and recombinant Ole e-1 allergens of the *Olea* pollen, administered intraperitoneally to Balb/c mice, induced high level of specific IgE and IgG-1 vs low IgG-2 antibody levels[OE220]. The pollen, in peripheral blood mononuclear cell culture of Ole e-1-sensitized patients, was active. The results indicated that it is possible to find T cells reactive to Ole e-1 peptides with and without significant levels of Ole e-1 IgE antibodies. The percentage of response was higher in patients with IgE antibodies 71.4 vs 25%[OE226]. The effect of pollen on children

monosensitized to *Olea*, with rhinitis and/or bronchial asthma, and SPT positive only to pollens was investigated. Six of seven children showed a perennial pattern of symptoms in comparison to 7 of 23 and 3 of 12, respectively, in subjects with *Parietaria* and *Gramineae* pollinosis. All of the patients with perennial nasal symptoms of the *Olea europaea* group exhibited a late nasal response after specific nasal provocation test[OE227]. The glycerinated allergenic extract, administered to 23 atopic rhinitis and/or asthmatic patients monosensitized to *Olea* and tested by skin prick test for *Olea europaea*, *Fraxinus excelsior*, and *Ligustrum vulgare*, produced a statistically significant correlation between results of SPT and of specific IgE assayed pollens[OE230]. An extract of the pollen was administered sublingually to group of nine patients with rhinitis and/or rhinoconjunctivitis. The subjects treated with extract presented a slightly lower incidence of nasal symptoms of sneezing and obstruction and developed less dyspnea ($p < 0.05$) than the control group. No differences were observed in the immunological determinations. Differences in SPT displayed a slight significance between the two groups at the end of trial[OE231]. The extract modified with glutaraldehyde was administered to patients with pollinosis, suffering from seasonal rhinoconjunctivitis or rhinoconjunctivitis and seasonal asthma, and treated with conjunctival provocation test with two types of antigen: *Lolium perenne* and *Olea*. These extract were tolerated quite well and produced no alterations in specific IgG-4 or IgE levels. There was a significant decrease in allergen-specific skin reactivity and increased response thresholds to the CPT ($p < 0.01$). A high correlation between skin and conjunctival provocation tests was observed at some stages[OE233]. A commercial extract, administered to 30 patients, produced a significant decrease in the specific skin reactivity (skin index geometrical mean from 2.73 to 0.88, $p < 0.001$), the specific IgE from 7.76 to 4.74 peripheral resistance unit/ mL, p < 0.001. The specific IgG in basic condition was detectable only in 9 of 30 patients. After immunotherapy they were found in almost all patients with a remarkable increase (from 5.48 to 266.89 arbitrary unit/mL, p < 0.001). No correlation was found among the changes in the considered parameters[OE235]. Fixed oil, administered externally on human adults, produced irritation[OE114].

Analgesic activity. Fruit essential oil, administered externally to adults, was active. Biological activity reported has been patented[OE194].

Anti-arrhythmic activity Ethanol (95%), glycerin, and glycerin/ethanol extracts of the leaf, administered intragastrically to rats at a dose of 25 mg/kg, were active vs aconitine-induced arrhythmia[OE085]. Ethanol (95%) and glycerin extracts of the seed oil, administered intragastrically to rats at a dose of 25 mg/kg, were active[OE085].

Anti-atherosclerotic activity. Extracts of leaves of three isolates (Greek olive leaves [GO], African wild olive leaves [AO], and Cape Town olive leaves [CT]), administered to Dahl salt-sensitive, insulin-resistant rats at a dose of 60 mg/kg for 6 weeks, were active[OE214].

Antibacterial activity. Decoction of the dried fruit, on agar plate, was inactive on *Pseudomonas aeruginosa*[OE131]. Water extract of the dried fruit, on agar plate, was active on *Salmonella typhi*, inhibitory concentration (IC)$_{50}$ 10.3 µg/mL[OE113]. Water extract of the dried fruit, on agar plate at a concentration of 62.5 mg/mL, was inactive on *Escherichia coli* and *Staphylococcus aureus*[OE129]. Water extract of the dried fruit, on agar plate at a concentration of 1 mg/mL, was inactive on *Salmonella typhi*[OE113]. Hot water extract of the dried fruit, on agar plate at a concentration of 62.5 mg/mL, was inactive on *Escherichia coli* and *Staphylococcus aureus*[OE129]. Ethanol (100%) extract of the fresh leaf, on agar plate, at a concentration of 2.5 mg/disc, was inactive on *Escherichia coli*, *Proteus mirabilis*, *Pseudomonas aeruginosa*, *Staphylococcus aureus*, and *Staphylococcus epidermidis*[OE153]. Water extracts of the dried stem bark and dried stem wood of *Olea europaea* ssp. *africana*, on agar plate, were active on *Streptococcus viridans*[OE195]. Aliphatic long-chain aldehydes from olive flavor did not exhibit significant antibacterial activity on standard and freshly isolated bacterial strains that may be causal agents of human intestinal and respiratory tract infections. The α- and β-unsaturated aldehydes have a broad antimicrobial spectrum and produced similar activity on Gram-positive and Gram-negative microorganisms[OE222]. Two olive secoiridoides (oleuropein and hydroxytyrosol) were tested for in vitro susceptibility to five ATCC standard bacteria strains (*Haemophilus influenzae* ATCC 9006, *Moraxella catarrhalis* ATCC 8176, *Salmonella typhi* ATCC 6539, *Vibrio paraemolyticus* ATCC 17802, and *Staphylococcus aureus* ATCC 25923) and 44 fresh clinical isolates (*Haemophilus influenzae*, eight strains; *Moraxella catarrhalis*, six strains; *Salmonella* sp., 15 strains; *Vibrio cholerae*, one strain; *Vibrio alginolyticus*, two strains; *Vibrio parahaemolyticus*, one strain; *Staphylococcus aureus*, five penicillin-susceptible strains and six penicillin-resistant strains). The minimum inhibitory concentrations (MICs) was evidence of the broad antimicrobial activity of hydroxytyrosol, MIC values between 0.24 and 7.85 µg/mL for ATCC strains and between 0.97 and 31.0 µg/mL for clinical isolates. Oleuropein inhibited the growth of several strains, MIC values between 62.5 and 500 µg/mL for ATCC strains and between 31.25 and 250.0 µg/mL for clinical isolates; oleuropein was ineffective against *Haemophilus influenzae* and *Moraxella catarrhalis*[OE224].

Anticlastogenic activity. Polyphenolic extract of the leaf, in bone marrow of mouse before and after X-ray irradiation, was determined by using the micronucleus test. With treatment before X-irradiation, the most effective compounds were: rutin > dimethylsulfoxide (DMSO) > olive leaves (OL) > propylthiouracil (PTU) > diosmin. These results indicated a linear correlation ($R^2 = 0.965$) between anticlastogenic activity and antioxidant capacity. The magnitude of protection with treatment after X-irradiation was lower, and the most effective compounds were, in order: *Olea* leaves > diosmin > rutin; DMSO and PTU lacked radioprotective activity. *Olea* leaf is the only substance that showed a significant anticlastogenic activity both before and after X-irradiation[OE215].

Anticonvulsant activity. Water extract of the dried leaf and stem, administered intraperitoneally to mice at a dose of 0.6 mL/animal, was inactive vs picrotoxins-induced convulsions[OE186].

Anticrustacean activity. Ethanol (10%) extract of the fresh leaf was active on *Artemia salina*, lethal dose$_{50}$ 164 μg/mL. The assay system was intended to predict for antitumor activity[OE153].

Antidysrrhythmic activity. Oleanolic acid and uvaol, isolated from the leaves of *Olea europaea* ssp. *africana*, administered at a dose of 40 mg/kg, were active on ischemia and reperfusion arrhytmias[OE206].

Antifungal activity. Hot water extract of the dried fruit, on agar plate at a concentration of 62.5 mg/mL, was inactive on *Aspergillus niger*[OE129]. Ethanol (50%) extract of the dried leaf, on agar plate at a concentration of 500 mg/mL, was active on *Botrytis cinerea*, and inactive on *Aspergillus fumigatus*, *Aspergillus niger*, *Fusarium oxysporum*, *Penicillum digitatum*, *Rhizopus nigricans*, and *Trichophyton mentagrophytes*. The dose was expressed as dry weight of plant[OE185].

Antihypercholesterolemic activity. Glycerin/ethanol extract of the fresh leaf, administered intragastrically to rats at a dose of 500 mg/kg for 15 days, was active vs diet- and triton-induced hypercholesterolemia[OE122].

Antihyperglycemic activity. Powder of the dried leaf, administered intragastrically to rats at a dose of 0.75 g/kg, was inactive vs streptozotocin-induced hyperglycemia[OE143]. Water extract of the dried leaf, administered intragastrically to male rats at a dose of 0.5 g/kg, reduced blood glucose levels of normal or alloxan-induced diabetic rats[OE118]. Decoction of the dried leaf, administered intragastrically to male rabbits, at a dose of 4 mg/kg, was inactive. A dose of 32 mg/kg was active on rats vs alloxan-induced hyperglycemia[OE147]. Infusion of the dried leaf, administered in drinking water of male rats at a dose of 5%, was inactive vs streptozocin-induced diabetes[OE155]. Water extract of the *Olea europaea* var. *oleaster* dried leaf, administered intragastrically to rats of both sexes at a dose of 15 mL/kg, was active on plasma[OE152].

Antihypertensive activity. Glycerin/ethanol extract of the leaf, administered intragastrically to rats at a dose of 250 mg/kg, was active vs desoxycorticosterone acetate-induced hypertension[OE085]. Ethanol/chloroform (25%) extract of the dried leaf, administered orally to adults, produced a slow decline in blood pressure in moderate hypertension after prolonged treatment[OE107]. Water extract of the dried leaf, administered orally to adults, was active[OE017]. Infusion of the dried leaf, administered intravenously to rats at a dose of 5%, produced no effect on normal blood pressure but decreased the hypertension caused by rennin and norepinephrine[OE104]. Seed oil, administered intragastrically to rats at a dose of 1 mL/day for 3 months, was active vs angiotensin II-induced hypertension and inactive vs rennin-induced hypertension[OE190]. Ethanol/chloroform (25%) extract of the dried fruit, administered orally to adults, produced a slow decline in blood pressure in moderate hypertension after prolonged treatment[OE107]. Glycerin/ethanol extract of the seed oil, administered intragastrically to rats at a dose of 125 mg/kg, was active vs desoxycorticos-terone acetate-induced hypertension[OE085]. The extracts of leaves of three isolates: GO, AO, and CT, administered to Dahl salt-sensitive, insulin-resistant rats at a dose of 60 mg/kg body weight for 6 weeks, were active[OE214]. The aqueous extract of the leaf, administered to patients with essential hypertension at a dose of 400 ng × 4/24 hours for 3 months, produced a significant decrease in blood pressure ($p < 0.001$)[OE229]. A specially prepared leaf extract (EFLA 943), administered orally to L-NAME (NG-nitro-L-arginine methyl ester) rendered hypertensive rats at variable doses, produced a dose-dependent effect against the rise in blood pressure induced by L-NAME, best effect being induced by a dose of 100 mg/kg of the extract. In rats previously rendered hypertensive by L-NAME for 6 weeks and then treated with that dose of the extract for a further 6 weeks without discontinuation of L-NAME, normalization of the blood pressure was observed[OE216].

Antihyperuricemic activity. Decoction of the dried leaf, administered orally to adults at a dose of 3 mL/person, was active. Infusion of the dried leaf, administered orally to adults at a dose of 5 mL/person, was active[OE108].

Anti-inflammatory activity. Seed oil, administered orally to adults at a dose of 20 mL/day, was active. Ten patients with rheumatoid arthritis were given the oil for 12 weeks while abstaining from nonsteroidal antiinflammatory drugs. Prostaglandin E_2 level decreased in three patients and 6-keto-prostaglandin F_1-α level increased in two patients[OE161]. Water extract of the dried leaf, administered intragastrically to rats, was active vs carrageenin-induced paw edema[OE112].

Antimycobacterial activity. Ethanol (95%) extract of the plant, in broth culture at a dilution of 1:80, was active on *Mycobacterium tuberculosis* H37RVTMC 102[OE169].

Antioxidant activity. Ethanol (defatted with petroleum ether) extract of the dried leaf, at a concentration of 0.1%, was active vs olive oil rancidity[OE105]. Methanol extract of the dried leaf, at variable concentrations, was active[OE123]. Maslinic acid obtained from olive pomace, administered to rats, was active on the susceptibility of plasma or hepatocyte membranes to lipid peroxidation induced by hydroxyl radical. Endogenous plasma lipoperoxide (LPO) levels and susceptibility to LPO were decreased in animals treated with maslinic acid after exposure to hydroxyl radicals by Fe^{2+}/H_2O_2. Coincubation with maslinic acid prevented hepatocyte membrane LPO[OE213]. The extracts of leaves of three isolates—GO, AO, CT—administered to Dahl salt-sensitive, insulin-resistant rats at a dose of 60 mg/kg for 6 weeks, were active[OE214].

Antipyretic activity. Ethanol (50%) extract of the plant, administered intraperitoneally to guinea pigs, was inactive[OE103].

Anti-thrombotic effect. Olive oil extract of the fruit, administered intragastrically to male rabbits at a dose of 150 g/kg, was active. Lipid profile was improved with decreased platelet hyperactivity and subendothelial thrombogenicity and less severe morphological lesion of the endothelium and vascular wall[OE154].

Anti-thyroid activity. Pickled green olives, administered orally to adults at a dose of 200 g/person, were inactive on iodine uptake by the thyroid[OE202].

Anti-ulcer activity. Water extract of the dried leaf, administered intragastrically to mice, was active against aspirin-induced gastric ulcers[OE112].

Antiviral activity. Water extract of the dried fruit, in cell culture at a concentration of 10%, was inactive on herpes virus-type 2, influenza, poliovirus, and vaccina[OE182]. Tincture of the dried fruit, administered orally to adults of both sexes at a dose of 60 mL/person, was active on herpes virus. PCT patent number W096/14064 reported treatment of six subjects with herpes virus infections. The activity was highly dose dependent. Biological activity has been patented[OE115].

Anti-yeast activity. Ethanol (50%) extract of the dried fruit, on agar plate at a concentration of 500 mg/mL, was inactive on *Candida albicans* and *Saccharomyces pastorianus*. The dose was expressed as dry weight of plant[OE185]. Ethanol extract of the fresh leaf, on agar plate at a concentration of 2.5 mg/disc, was inactive on *Candida albicans*[OE153].

Apoptosis induction. Allergens, in cell culture, induced apoptosis in peripheral blood mononuclear cells from atopic patients with positive reactivity to the allergens. Peripheral blood mononuclear cells from atopic patients proliferated more vigorously than cells from normal subjects after culture in vitro. The percentage of apoptosis increased when atopic subjects had been previously treated with immunotherapy[OE223].

Arachidonate 12-lipoxygenase inhibition. Essential oil of the unripe fruit was active on platelets, IC_{50} 7 µg/mL [OE056].

Arachidonate 5-lipoxygenase inhibition. Essential oil of the unripe fruit was active, IC_{50} 8.3 µg/mL[OE056].

Arachidonate metabolism inhibition. Seed oil, administered to mice at a dose of 10% of diet, reduced arachidonic acid in mice lung and spleen without affecting prostaglandins[OE187].

Arginine arylamidase inhibition. Water extract of the fresh twig of *Olea europaea* ssp. *africana*, at a concentration of 100 µg/mL, was active on *Porphyromonas gingivalis*[OE127].

Bile secretion increase. Fixed oil, administered to rats at a dose of 9% of diet, was inactive[OE135].

Bradycardiac activity. Water extract of the dried leaf, administered intravenously to dogs, was active[OE017].

Carcinogenesis inhibition. Fixed oil, applied externally to female mice at a dose of 150 µg/animal, was active vs ultraviolet (UV)-induced tumors[OE156]. Olive oil extract, administered in the ration of male rats at a

dose of 7.4 mL/kg, was active[OE148]. Seed oil, administered to C3H mice at a dose of 10% of diet for more than 50 weeks, was inactive[OE176].

Cercarial penetration inhibition. Seed oil, applied externally to mice at an undiluted concentration, was inactive on *Schistoma mansoni*[OE199].

Cholesterol level decrease. Fixed oil, administered to rats at a dose of 20% of diet, was inactive[OE120].

Cholesterol level increase. Fixed oil, administered to rats at a dose of 9% of diet, was active on liver[OE135].

Chronotropic effect negative. Ethanol (50%) extract of the fresh leaf, administered by gastric intubation to rats at a dose of 40 mL/kg, produced weak activity. Results were significant at $p < 0.05$ level[OE183]. Glycerin/ethanol extract of the fresh leaf, administered intragastrically to dogs at a dose of 20 mg/kg, produced an increase in length of sinusal cycle (16%), sinoatrial conduction time (27%), and sinus node recovery time (31%)[OE165].

Chronotropic effect positive. Glycerin/ethanol extract of the leaf and seed oil, administered intragastrically to desoxycorticosterone acetate-induced hypertensive rats at doses of 500 and 125 mg/kg, respectively, was active[OE085].

Complement alternative pathway inhibition. Ethyl acetate and methanol extracts of the fresh leaf, administered at concentration of 50 µg/mL, were inactive on red blod cells[OE053].

Complement classical pathway inhibition. Ethyl acetate and methanol extracts of the fresh leaf were active on red blood cells, IC_{50} greater than 7.7 µg/mL and greater than 5.8 µg/mL, respectively[OE053].

Cyclo-oxygenase inhibition. Essential oil of the unripe fruit, at a concentration of 100 µg/mL, produced weak activity on platelets[OE056].

Cytotoxic activity. Seed oil, in cell culture at a concentration of 300 µg/mL, was active on human colon cancer HT29 cell line[OE203]. Water extract of the dried fruit, in cell culture at a concentration of 10%, was inactive on HeLa cells[OE182]. Methanol extract of the dried leaf, in cell culture at a concentration of 100 μg/mL, was inactive on hamster-chinese-V79 cells[OE130]. Ethanol extract of the fresh leaf, in cell culture was inactive on CA-A549, human colon cancer cell line HT29, and CA-mammary MCF-7[OE153]. Methanol extract of the dried leaves and twigs, in cell culture, produced weak activity on CA-9KB, ED_{50} 31 μg/mL[OE204]. Methanol extract of the dried leaves and twigs, in cell culture, was inactive on leuk-P388, effective dose $(ED)_{50}$ greater than 100 μg/mL[OE204]. Decoction of the dried leaf, administered orally to adults, at a dose of 3 mL/person, produced weak activity. Infusion of the dried leaf, administered orally to adults, at a dose of 5 mL/person, produced weak activity[OE108]. Water extract of the *Olea europaea* var. *oleaster* dried leaf, administered intragastrically to rats of both sexes at a dose of 15 mL/kg, was active on plasma[OE152].

Dermatitis-producing effect. Fruit-fixed oil, applied externally to adults at an undiluted concentration, was active[OE164].

Diuretic activity. Decoction and infusion of the dried leaf, administered orally to adults at a dose of 5 mL/person for 20–25 days, increased daily urinary output by 100–145 mL, and did not affect blood/sodium, potassium, and chloride[OE108]. Ethanol (50%) extract of the fresh leaf, administered intragastrically to rats at a dose of 40 mL/kg, was active. Five parts of fresh plant material in 100 parts water/ethanol was used[OE160]. The extracts of leaves of three isolates—GO, AO, and CT—administered to Dahl salt-sensitive, insulin-resistant rats at a dose of 60 mg/kg for 6 weeks, were active[OE214].

DNA-binding effect. Methanol extract of dried leaves and twigs, at a concentration of 1 μg/mL, was inactive[OE204].

Dromotropic effect (negative). Glycerin/ethanol extract of the fresh leaf, adminis-

tered intragastrically to dogs at a dose of 30 μg/kg, increased intra-atrial (20%), nodal (41%), his-Purkinje (14%), intraventricular (12%), and conduction times[OE165].

Effective refractory period increase. Glycerin/ethanol extract of the fresh leaf, administered intragastrically to dogs at a dose of 30 mg/kg, increased duration of ventricular effective refractory period (21%)[OE165].

Estrogenic effect. Seed oil, administered orally to female mice at a dose of 10% of diet, was active[OE101]. Seed oil, administered subcutaneously to ovariectomized female mice, produced activity equivalent to 0.25 units of estrone[OE197].

Fibrinogen level decrease. Seed oil, administered orally to female adults at a dose of 6 mg/person, lowered fibrinogen and raised plasminogen activator inhibitor levels in women with high baseline fibrinogen levels[OE134].

Gallbladder effect. Seed oil, administered orally to 11 young normocholesterolemic males at a dose of 100 g/day, was active. The subjects received 3 weeks of a low-fat diet followed by 3 weeks of a diet enriched with 100 g/daily of olive oil. Mean total cholesterol, total apolipoprotein (apo) B, low-density lipoprotein (LDL) cholesterol, and triglycerides decreased significantly after the olive oil diet. High-density lipoprotein (HDL) cholesterol, apo A-1, cholesterol saturation of bile, and gallbladder volumes were unchanged[OE188].

Hematological effect. Decoction of the dried leaf, administered orally to adults at a dose of 3 mL/person, did not alter blood surface tension and viscosity. Infusion of the dried leaf, administered orally to adults at a dose of 5 mL/person, produced no change in the blood levels of sodium, potassium, and chloride[OE108].

3-Hydroxy-3-methylglutaryl coenzyme A reductase inhibition. Seed oil, administered intragastrically to rats at a dose of 2 mL/kg, was active[OE192].

3-Hydroxy-3-methylglutaryl coenzyme A synthase inhibition. Seed oil, administered intragastrically to rats at a dose of 2 mL/kg, was active[OE192].

Hydrogen peroxide release inhibition. Seed oil, administered to rats at a concentration of 8% of diet, was active on macrophages. Capsaicin or curcumin enhanced the effect[OE132].

Hypercholesterolemic activity. Fruit fixed oil, administered orally to adults at a dose of 60 g/day, was active. The result was equivalent to the effect of daily intake of 200–400 mg of squalene[OE036].

Hyperthermic effect. Hot water extract of the dried leaf, administered intraperitoneally to the guinea pig, was inactive[OE200]. Water extract, administered intravenously to the guinea pig, was active[OE017].

Hypocholesterolemic activity. Fixed oil, administered to rats at a dose of 17% of diet, decreased HDL cholesterol level[OE196]. Seed oil, administered orally to 11 young males who were normocholesterolemic at a dose of 100 g/day, was active. The subjects received 3 weeks of a low-fat diet followed by 3 weeks of a diet enriched with 100 g/daily of olive oil. Mean total cholesterol, total apo B, LDL cholesterol, and triglycerides decreased significantly after the olive oil diet. HDL cholesterol, apo A-1, cholesterol saturation of bile, and gallbladder volumes were unchanged[OE188].

Hypoglycemic activity. Ethanol extract, defatted with petroleum ether extract, of the dried leaf, administered by gastric intubation to rabbits, produced a 17–23% decrease in blood sugar levels reaching a maximum in 6 hours and returning to normal in 48 hours[OE106]. Decoction of the dried leaf, administered intragastrically to rats at a dose of 0.5 g /kg, was active. Leaves collected in July, August, and September had no effect[OE124]. Water extract of the *Olea europaea* var. *oleaster* dried leaf, administered intragastrically to rats of both sexes at a dose of 15 mL/kg, was active on

plasma[OE152]. The extracts of leaves of three isolates (GO, AO, and CT), administered to Dahl salt-sensitive, insulin-resistant rats at a dose of 60 mg/kg for 6 weeks, were active[OE214]. Aqueous leaf extract, administered repeatedly to male and female rats at doses of 37.5, 75, 150, 300, 600, and 1200 mg/kg daily for 60 days, induced an increase of weight, hypotension, hypoglycemia, and hypouricemia[OE232]. Seed oil, administered orally to 11 young males who were normocholesterolemic at a dose of 100 g/day, was active. The subjects received 3 weeks of a low-fat diet followed by 3 weeks of a diet enriched with 100 g/daily of olive oil. Mean total cholesterol, total apo B, LDL cholesterol, and triglycerides decreased significantly after the olive oil diet. HDL cholesterol, apo A-1, cholesterol saturation of bile, and gallbladder volumes were unchanged[OE188].

Hypotensive activity. Hot water and water extracts, administered intravenously to cats, were active[OE099,OE100]. Chloroform, methanol, and petroleum ether extracts of the dried fruit, administered intravenously to cats and rabbits, were inactive. The acetone and ethanol (95%) extracts produced weak activity. Water extract of the dried fruit, administered intravenously to rats, cats, dogs, and rabbits at a dose of 0.8 mL/kg, were active[OE012,OE178,OE177]. Ethanol (50%) extract of the fresh leaf, administered by gastric intubation to rats at a dose of 40 mL/kg, was active. Results were significant at $p < 0.05$ level[OE183]. Ethanol (95%), glycerin, and ethanol/glycerin extracts of the seed oil, administered intragastrically to rats at a dose of 100 mg/kg, were active. Maximum effect was seen 60–120 minutes after administration of extract[OE085]. Aqueous extract of the leaf, administered repeatedly to male and female rats at doses of 37.5, 75, 150, 300, 600, and 1200 mg/kg daily for 60 days, produced an increase of weight, hypotension, hypoglycemia, and hypouricemia[OE232].

Hypothermic activity. Ethanol extract of the plant, administered intraperitoneally to guinea pigs, was inactive[OE103].

Hypouricemic activity. An aqueous leaf extract, administered repeatedly to male and female rats at doses of 37.5, 75, 150, 300, 600, and 1200 mg/kg daily for 60 days, produced an increase of weight, hypotension, hypoglycemia, and hypouricemia[OE232].

Immunosuppressant activity. Seed oil, administered in ration of mice, was active[OE163].

Inotropic effect positive. Glycerin/ethanol extract of the leaf, administered to rabbits at a dose of 5 mg/mL, was active on heart[OE085]. Ethanol (95%), glycerin, and ethanol/glycerin extracts of the seed oil, administered to rabbits at a dose of 5 mg/mL, were active on heart[OE085].

Insulin level increase. Powder of the dried leaf, administered intragastrically to rats at a dose of 0.75 g/kg, was inactive[OE143].

Insulin-potentiating effect. Water extract of the *Olea europaea* var. *oleaster* dried leaf, administered intragastrically to rats of both sexes at a dose of 15 mL/kg, was active on plasma[OE152].

Insulin release stimulation. Fruit-fixed oil, in cell culture, was active on pancreatic islets[OE119]. Decoction of the dried leaf, in cell culture at a concentration of 0.4 µg/mL, was active on adrenal gland[OE124].

Intercellular adhesion molecule-1 inhibition. Fixed oil of embryos, administered orally to human adults, decreased the expression of intercellular adhesion molecule-1[OE117].

LDL oxidation inhibition. Seed oil, administered orally to male adults at a dose of 30.5% of diet, produced weak activity vs copper catalyzed oxidation[OE116].

LDL-receptor degradation inhibition. Seed oil, administered orally to adult males, produced weak activity[OE109].

Lipid peroxide formation stimulation. Seed oil, administered to rats fed a diet with given composition of fat at a dose of 15% of diet for 6 weeks, was inactive on rat liver microsomes. Malondialdehyde concentration was unchanged among animals given different oils. Vitamin E level decreased among those fed soybean oil[OE125]. Seed oil, administered to rats at a dose of 10% of diet, was inactive. High-cholesterol diet with olive oil did not stimulate lipid peroxidation[OE150].

Lymphocyte proliferation inhibition. Fixed oil, administered to rats at a dose of 20% of diet, was active on hypogastric nerve-vas deferens[OE120].

Molluscicidal activity. Methanol extract of the leaf, at a concentration of 2000 ppm for 2 hours of exposure, was active on *Biomphalaria glabrata*[OE173].

Monophasic action potential. Glycerin/ethanol extract of the fresh leaf, administered intragastrically to dogs at a dose of 30 mg/kg, increased duration of ventricular monophasic action potential (16%)[OE165].

Mutagenic activity. Ethanol (100%) extract of the fresh leaf, on agar plate, was active on *Salmonella typhimurium* T1530[OE153].

Natural-killer cell enhancement. Fixed oil of embryos, administered orally to adults, was inactive[OE117]. Nonsaponifiable fraction of fruit fixed oil and seed oil, administered to rats at a dose of 0.3% of diet, were active. The polyphenol stripped seed oil was inactive[OE170].

Oxygen radical inhibition. Seed oil, administered to rats at a concentration of 8% of diet, was active on macrophages. Capsaicin or curcumin enhanced the effect[OE132].

Phagocytosis stimulation. Ethanol (95%) extract and unsaponifiable fraction of the dried leaf, administered intraperitoneally to male mice at a dose of 0.5 mL/animal, were inactive[OE180].

Platelet aggregation inhibition. Methanol extract of the fruit, at a concentration of 500 µg/mL, produced weak activity on human platelets vs collagen-induced aggregation[OE146]. Seed oil, administered intragastrically to rats at a dose of 5 mL/kg for 2 months, was active. Aortas from the treated rats released higher amounts of antiaggregatory substances vs adenosine 5'-diphosphate-induced aggregation[OE190].

Prostaglandin induction. Seed oil, administered to rats at a concentration of 5% of diet, was active[OE162].

Protease inhibition. Water extract of the dried twig of *Olea europaea* ssp. *africana*, was inactive on *Bacteroides intermedius*, IC_{50} 100 µg/mL and *Treponema denticola*, IC_{50} greater than 250 µg/mL, and active on *Bacteroides gingivalis*, IC_{50} 75 µg/mL[OE168].

Serum HDL-lowering effect. Seed fixed oil, administered to male hamsters at a concentration of 19% of diet, was inactive[OE149].

Serum LDL-lowering effect Seed oil, administered orally to male adults at a dose of 30.5% of diet, produced weak activity[OE116].

Spasmogenic activity. Water extract of the dried leaf, administered to rats at a dose of 0.1 µg/mL was active on ileum and a dose of 0.3 µg/mL was active on ileum vs acetylcholine-induced contractions[OE137].

Spasmolytic activity. Ethanol (95%), ethanol/glycerin, and glycerin extracts of the leaf, administered to guinea pigs at a dose of 50 mg/kg, was active vs vasopressin-induced coronary spasms as determined from electrocardiogram[OE085]. Ethanol (30%) extract of the dried leaf, administered to rabbits at a concentration of 1 mg/mL, was active on aorta vs K^+-induced contractions[OE136]. Decoction of the dried leaf, administered to rats, was active on aorta, IC_{50} 1.12 mg/mL. The effect of the lyophilized extract on phenylephrine-induced contraction and endothelium was present. Decoction of the dried leaf, administered to rats, was active on the aorta vs phenylephrine-induced contraction, IC_{50} 1.16 mg/mL. Water extract of the dried leaf, administered to rats at a dose of 3 mg/mL, was active on trachea vs acetylcholine-induced contractions[OE137].

Superoxide production inhibition. Seed oil, administered to rats at a concentration

of 8% of diet, was active on macrophages. Capsaicin or curcumin enhanced the effect[OE132].

Thromboxane B-2 synthesis induction. Seed oil, administered orally to 10 patients with rheumatoid arthritis at a dose of 20 mL/day for 12 weeks, produced mixed clinical results. The patients abstained from nonsteroidal anti-inflammatory drugs during the trial period. Thromboxane B-2 level increased in four patients[OE161].

Thyroid activity. A freeze-dried aqueous extract of the leaf, administered to rats, was active. The results suggest a stimulatory action of the extract on the thyroid, unrelated to the pituitary[OE219].

Toxic effect. Water extract of the dried leaf, administered orally to adults, was inactive[OE017]. Infusion of the dried leaf, administered in drinking water to male rats at a dose of 5%, was inactive[OE155].

Tumor-promoting effect. Seed oil, administered in ration to rats at a dose of 3.4% of diet, was active. Rats were given 7,12-dimethylbenz[a]anthracene to induce tumorigenesis[OE166].

Tyrosinase inhibition. Ethanol (50%) extract of the fresh leaf, at a concentration of 0.5 mg/mL, was inactive[OE133].

Vasodilator effect. The decoction of leaves caused relaxation of isolated rat aorta preparations both in the presence (IC_{50} 1.12 ± 0.33 mg/mL) and in the absence (IC_{50} 1.67 ± 0.16 mg/mL) of endothelium[OE234]

Weight increase. Aqueous leaf extract, administered repeatedly to male and female rats at doses of 37.5, 75, 150, 300, 600, and 1200 mg/kg/24 hours for 60 days, produced an increase of weight, hypotension, hypoglycemia, and hypouricemia[OE232].

REFERENCES

OE001   Ragazzi, E., and G. Veronese. Presence of demethyloleoeuropeine in olives of various cultures. **Ann Chim (Rome)** 1973; 63: 21.

OE002   Panizzi, L., M. L. Scarpati, and G. Oriente. The constitution of oleuropein. A bitter glucoside of the olive with hypotensive action. **Ric Sci** 1958; 28: 994.

OE003 Ragazzi, E., and G. Veronese. Phenolic components of olive oils. **Riv Ital Sostanze Grasse** 1973; 50: 443.

OE004 Vlostov, L. I. Sterol, and choline levels in some edible fruits. **Rast Resur** 1972; 8: 557.

OE005 Schneider, G., and W. Kleiner. Cinchona alkaloids of the olive tree leaves. **Planta Med** 1972; 22: 109.

OE006 Schneider, G., and W. Kleinert. Cinchonine alkaloids in leaves of the olive tree. **Naturwissenschaften** 1971; 58: 524A.

OE007 Meakins, G. D., and R. Swindells. Structures of two acids from olive leaves. **J Chem Soc** 1959; 1959: 1044–1047.

OE008 Cantarelli, C. The polyphenols of olives and olive oils. **Riv Ital Sostanze Grasse** 1961; 38: 69–72.

OE009 Shasha, B., and J. Leibowitz. Oleoropepin from *Olea europaea*. **Bull Res Counc Israel** 1959; A8: 92.

OE010 Bourquelot, E., and J. Vintilesco. "Oleuropein", a new glucoside from *Olea europaea* L. **J Pharm Chim** 1938; 28: 303–314.

OE011 Kriventsov, V. I., L. G. Dolganenko, and L. I. Dranik. Flavonoids of *Olea europaea* leaves. **Khim Prir Soedin** 1974; 10(1): 97.

OE012 Samuelson, G. The blood pressure-lowering factor in leaves of *Olea europaea*. **Farm Rev** 1951; 50: 229–240.

OE013 Roncero, A. V., and L. Janer. Squalene in olive tree leaves. **Grasas Aceites (Seville)** 1962; 13: 242–243.

OE014 Bockova, H., J. Holubek, and Z. Cekan. Constituents of olive tree (*Olea europaea* L.). **Collect Czech Chem Commun** 1964; 29(6): 1484–1491.

OE015 Musajo, L. The olive anthocyanin, oleocyanin. **Gazz Chim Ital** 1940; 70: 293–300.

OE016 Beverman, H. C., L. A. Van Dick, J. Levisalles, A. Melera, and W. L. C. Veer. The structure of elenolide. **Bull Soc Chim Fr** 1961; 1961 (10): 1812–1820.

OE017 Cavanna, D., and M. Pirona. Hypotensor action of leaves of *Olea europaea*. **Boll Chim Farm** 1950; 89: 3–8.

OE018 Caputo, R., L. Mangoni, P. Monaco, and L. Previtera. New triterpenes from the leaves of *Olea europaea*. **Phytochemistry** 1974; 13: 2825–2827.

OE019 Kull, U. The occurrence of sedoheptulose in seeds and vegetative parts of several Angiosperms. **Phytochemistry** 1968; 7(5): 783–785.

OE020 Griboldi, P., G. Jommi, and L. Verotta. Secoiridoids from *Olea europaea*. **Phytochemistry** 1986; 25(4): 865–869.

OE021 Tsukamoto, H., S. Hisada, and S. Nishibe. Lignans from bark of the *Olea* plants. II. **Chem Pharm Bull** 1985; 33(3): 1232–1241.

OE022 Kuwajima, H., T. Uemura, K. Takaishi, K. Inoue, and H. Inouye. A secoiridoid glucoside from *Olea europaea*. **Phytochemistry** 1988; 27(6): 1757–1759.

OE023 Lo Scalzo, R., and M. L. Scarpati. A new secoiridoid from olive wastewaters. **J Nat Prod** 1993; 56(4): 621–623.

OE024 Montedoro, G., M. Servilli, M. Baldioli, R. Selvaggini, E. Miniati, and A. Macchioni. Simple and hydrolyzable compounds in virgin olive oil. 3. Spectroscopic characterizations of the secoiridoid derivatives. **J Agr Food Chem** 1993; 41(11): 2226–2234.

OE025 Gil, M., A. Haidour, and J. L. Ramos. Two glutaric acid derivatives from olives. **Phytochemistry** 1998; 49(5): 1311–1315.

OE026 Bianco, A. D., I. Muzzalupo, A. Piperno, G. Romeo, and N. Uccella. Bioactive derivatives oleuropein from olive fruits. **J Agr Food Chem** 1999; 47(9): 3531–3534.

OE027 Tefera, M. L., M. Villalba, E. Batanero, and R. Rodriguez. Identification, isolation, and characterization of ole E-7, a new allergen of olive tree pollen. **J Allergy Clin Immunol** 1999; 104(4): 797–802.

OE028 de Nino, A., F. Mazzotti, S. P. Morrone, E. Perri, A. Raffaelli, and G. Sindona. Characterization of cassanese olive cultivar through the identification of new trace components by ion spray tandem mass spectrometry. **J Mass Spectrom** 1999; 34(1): 10–16.

OE029 Donaire, J. P., A. J. Sanchez, J. Lopez-Gorge, and L. Recalde. Biochemical and physiological studies in the olive tree. Part II. Metabolic changes in fruit and leaf during ripening in the olive. **Phytochemistry** 1975; 14: 1167–1169.

OE030 Mussini, P., F. Orsini, and F. Pelizzoni. Triterpenes in leaves of *Olea europaea.* **Phytochemistry** 1975; 14: 1135A.

OE031 Ghimenti, G., and G. Taponeco. Terpenic dialcohols in olive oil and their modification during the course of refining. **Riv Soc Ital Sci Aliment** 1974; 3: 335.

OE032 Krivensov, V. I., L. G. Dolganenko, and L. I Dranik. Flavonoids of the leaves of *Olea europaea.* **Chem Nat Comp** 1974; 10(1): 101.

OE033 Maestro-Duran, R., R. Leon-Cabello, V. Ruiz-Gutierrez, P. Fiestas, and A. Vazquez-Roncero. Bitter phenolic glucosides from seeds of olive (*Olea europaea*). **Grasas Aceites (Seville)** 1994; 45(5): 332–335.

OE034 Limiroli, R., R. Consonni, A. Ranalli, G. Bianchi, and L. Zetta. 1H NMR study of phenolics in the vegetation water of tree cultivars of *Olea europaea*: similarities and differences. **J Agr Food Chem** 1996; 44(8): 2040–2048.

OE034 Thakur, B. S., and T. R. Chadha. Comparative studies of the fatty acids compositions of olive (*Olea europaea*) oil extracted from pulp and kernel. **Gartenbauwissenschaft** 1991; 56(1): 31–33.

OE035 Petroni, A., M. Blasevitch, N. Papini, M. Salami, A. Sala, and C. Galli. Inhibition of leukocyte leukotriene B4 production by an olive oil-derived phenol identified by mass-spectrometry. **Thrombosis Res** 1997; 87(3): 315–322.

OE036 Newmark, H. L. Squalene, olive oil, and cancer risk: a review and hypothesis. **Cancer Epidemiol Biomark Prevent** 1997; 6(12): 1101–1103.

OE037 Gil, M., A. Haidour, and J. L. Ramos. Identification of two triterpenoids in solid wastes from olive cake. **J Agr Food Chem** 1997; 45(11): 4490–4494.

OE038 Williams, M., M. T. Morales, R. Aparicio, and J. L. Harwood. Analysis of volatiles from callus cultures of olive *Olea europaea.* **Phytochemistry** 1998; 47(7): 1253–1259.

OE039 Visioli, F., and C. Galli. Olive oil phenols and their potential effects on human health. **J Agr Food Chem** 1998; 46(10): 4292–4296.

OE040 Males, Z., and D. Tuckar. Quantitative and qualitative analysis of the flavonoids of *Olea europaea* leaves. **Farm Gras** 1998; 54(1): 1–4.

OE041 Cucurachi, A., L. Camera, F. Angerosa, and M. Solinas. Erhythrodiol content of dark green olive oils. **Riv Ital Sostanze Grasse** 1975; 52: 266.

OE042 Paquot, C., and H. Kaller. Evolutions of the sterols and the triterpenoid alcohols during the ripening of the fruits of the olive tree. **C R Acad Sci Ser C** 1976; 282: 1041.

OE043 Bianco, A., R. Lo Scalzo, and M. L. Scarpati. Isolation of cornoside from *Olea europaea* and its transformation into halleridone. **Phytochemsitry** 1993; 32(2): 455–457.

OE044 Heimler D., A. Pieroni, M. Tattini, and A. Cimato. Determination of flavonoids, flavonoid glycosides and bioflavonoids in *Olea europaea* L. leaves. **Chromatographia** 1992; 33(7/8): 369–373.

OE045 Mamedova, M. E., and S. M. Aslanov. Contents of ursolic acid in flowers of *Olea europaea* L. (Azerbaijan). **Rast Resur** 1992; 28(3): 79–81.

OE046 Yahiaoui, R., A. Guechi, E. Lukasova, and L. Girre. Mutagenic and membranal effect of a phytotoxic molecule isolated from olive leaves parasitized by the fungus *Cycloconium oleaginum* Cast. **Mycopathologia** 1994; 126(2): 121–129.

OE047 Bianchi, G., N. Pozzi, and G. Vlahov. Pentacyclic triterpene acids in olives. **Phytochemistry** 1994; 37(1): 205–207.

OE048 Visioli, F., F. F. Vinceri, and C. Galli. "Waste waters" from olive oil production are rich in natural antioxidants. **Experientia** 1995; 51(1): 32–34.

OE049 Nakajima, S., T. Kitamura, N. Baba, J. Iwasa, and T. Ichikawa. Oleuropein, a secoiridoid glucoside from olive, as a feeding stimulant to the olive weevil (*Dyscerus perforatus*). **Biosci Biotech Biochem** 1995; 59(4): 769–770.

OE050 Akasbi, M., D. W. Shoeman, and A. S. Csallany. High-performance liquid chromatography of selected phenolic compounds in olive oils. **J Amer Oil Chem Soc** 1993; 70(4): 367–370.

OE051   Bianchi, G., and N. Pozzi. 3,4-Dihydroxyphenylglycol, a major C6-C2 phenolic in *Olea europaea* fruits. **Phytochemistry** 1994; 35(5): 1335–1337.

OE052   Hansen, K., A. Andersen, S. B. Christensen, S. R. Jensen, U. Nyman, and U. W. Smitt. Isolation of an angiotensin converting enzyme (ACE) inhibitor from *Olea europaea* and *Olea lancea*. **Phytomedicine** 1996; 2(4): 319–325.

OE053   Pieroni, A., D. Heimler, L. Pieters, B. Van Poel, and A. J. Vlietnick. *In vitro* anti-complementary activity of flavonoids from olive (*Olea europaea*) leaves. **Pharmazie** 1996; 51(10): 765–768.

OE054   Lopez-Gonzalez, J. D. Extraction and purification of polyhydroxylated compounds from olive branches. Patent-Span-414,205, 1976.

OE055   Ryan, D., K. Robards, P. Prenzler, D. Jardine, T. Herlt, and M. Antolovich. Liquid chromatography with electrospray ionization mass spectrometric detection of phenolic compounds from *Olea europaea*. **J Chromatogr A** 1999; 855(2): 529–537.

OE056   Kohyama, N., T. Nagata, S. I. Fujimoto, and K. Sekiya. Inhibition of arachidonate lipoxygenase activities by 2-(3-4-dihydroxyphenyl) ethanol, a phenolic compounds from olives. **Biosci Biotech Biochem** 1997; 61(2): 347–350.

OE057   Perri, E., A. Raffaelli, and G. Sindona. Quantitation of oleuropein in virgin olive oil by ionspray mass spectrometry-selected reaction monitoring. **J Agr Food Chem** 1999; 47(10): 4156–4160.

OE058   Rovellini, P., and N. Cortesi. Identification of three intermediates compounds in the biosynthesis of secoiridoids as oleoside-type in different anatomic parts of *Olea europaea* L. by HPLC-electrospray-mass spectrometry. **Riv Ital Sostanze Grasse** 1998; 75(12): 543–550.

OE059   Rivas, M. M. Sugars and polyols in olive seed. I. Identification by paper chromatography and gas-liquid-chromatography. **Grasas Aceites (Seville)** 1983; 34(1): 13–16.

OE060   Kubo, I., and A. Matsumoto. Secreted oleanolic acid on the cuticle *Olea europaea* (*Oleaceae*), a chemical barrier to fungal attack. **Experientia** 1984; 32(7): 2730–2735.

OE061   Chiba, M., K. Okabe, S. Hisada, K. Shima, T. Takemoto, and S. Nishibe. Elucidation of the structure of new lignan glucoside from *Olea europaea* by carbon-13 nuclear magnetic resonance spectroscopy. **Chem Pharm Bull** 1979; 27: 2868–2873.

OE062   Baganuzzi, V. Distribution of alcoholic components of the unsaponifiable matter in the olive drupe. Note V. Aliphatic alcohols. **Riv Ital Sostanze Grasse** 1980; 57(7): 341–345.

OE063   Camurati, F., A. Rizzolo, and E. Fedeli. Chemical components of anatomical parts of the fruit of *Olea europaea*. Part I. Lipid extracts. **Riv Ital Sostanze Grasse** 1980; 57(8): 369–377.

OE064   Paganuzzi, V. Distribution of the alcoholic components of the unsaponifiable matter in the olive drupe. Note IV. 4-Methylsterols. **Riv Ital Sostanze Grasse** 1980; 57(6): 291–294.

OE065   Paganuzzi, V. Distribution of the alcoholic components of the nonsaponifiable matter within the olive drupe. III. Triterpene alcohols. **Riv Ital Sostanze Grasse** 1980; 57(3): 145–149.

OE066   Maestro, D. R., and R. A. Vazquez. Anthocyanic pigments in rupe manzanillo olives. **Grasas Aceites (Seville)** 1976; 27(4): 237–243.

OE067   Veer, W. L. C. Preparing elenolide and elenolic acid from *Oleaceae*. Patent-Dutch-90,043 1959.

OE068   Dimitrios, B., S. Gregorios, K. Miltiadis, and M. Stavros. Tetracosanol and hexacosanol content of Greek olive oils. **Grasas Aceites (Seville)** 1983; 34(6): 402–404.

OE069   Harborne, J. B., and P. S. Green. A chemotaxonomic survey of flavonoids in leaves of the *Oleaceae*. **Bot J Linn Soc** 1980; 81: 155–167.

OE070   Tsukamoto, H., S. Hisada, and S. Nishibe. Isolation of secoiridoid glucosides from the bark of *Olea europaea*. **Shoyakugaku Zasshi** 1985; 39(1): 90–92.

OE071   Fleuriet, A., J. J. Macheix, C. Andary, and P. Villemur. Identification and determination of verbascoside by high-performance liquid chromatography in the fruit of six cultivars of *Olea europaea* L. **C R Acad Sci Ser III** 1984; 299(7): 253–256.

OE072 Tsukamoto, H., S. Hisada, and S. Nishibe. Coumarin and secoiridoid glucosides from bark of *Olea europaea* and *Olea capensis*. **Chem Pharm Bull** 1985; 33(1): 396–399.

OE073 Cortesi, N., C. Mosconi, and E. Fedeli. High-performance liquid chromatography in the analysis of *Olea europaea* leaf extracts. **Riv Ital Sostanze Grasse** 1984; 61(10): 549–557.

OE074 Balic, V., and O. Cera. Acidic phenolic fraction of the juice of olives determined by a gas chromatographic method. **Grasas Aceites (Seville)** 1984; 35(3): 178–180.

OE075 Paganuzzi, V. Modifications of triterpene alcohol composition caused by olive oil refining. **Riv Ital Sostanze Grasse** 1983; 60(8): 489–499.

OE076 Golubes, V. N., Z. D. Gusar, E. S. Mamedov. Tocopherols of *Olea europaea*. **Chem Nat Comp** 1987; 23(1): 119–120.

OE077 Golubes, V. N., Z. D. Gusar, E. S. Mamedov. Pigments of *Olea europaea*. **Chem Nat Comp** 1986; 22(2): 225–226.

OE078 Rubio, N., A. Brieva, and B. Alcazar. Purification of allergens by high-performance liquid chromatography. IV. Purification of the allergen of olive pollen (*Olea europaea*). **J Chromatogr** 1987; 403(1): 312–318.

OE079 Movsumov, I. S., A. M. Aliev, and Z. D. Tagieva. Pharmacochemical studies of olives grown in the Azerbaijan Soviet Socialist Republic. **Farmatsiya (Moscow)** 1987; 36(2): 32–34.

OE080 Gil-Serrano, A., and P. Tejero-Mateo. A xyloglucan from olive pulp. **Carohydr Res** 1988; 181(1): 278–281.

OE081 Serrano, G., M. Mateos, and M. Tejero. Olive polysaccharides. IX. Characterization of hemicellulose B from the pulp of Hojiblanca variety of olive. **An Quim Ser C** 1987; 83(1): 135–136.

OE082 Forcadell, M. L., M. Comas, X. Miquel, and M. C. De La Torre. Tyrosol and hydroxytrosol determination in virgin olive oils. **Rev Fr Corps Gras** 1987; 34(12): 547–549.

OE083 Amiot, M. J., A. Fleuriet, and J. J. Macheix. Accumulation of oleuropein derivatives during olive maturation. **Phytochemistry** 1989; 28(1): 67–69.

OE084 Itoh, T., K. Yoshida, T. Yatsu, T. Tamura, and T. Matsumoto. Triterpene alcohols and sterols of Spanish olive oil. **J Amer Oil Chem Soc** 1981; 58(4): 545–550.

OE085 Circosta, C., F. Occhiuto, A. Gregorio, S. Toigo, and A. Pasquale. Cardiovascular activity of the young shoots and leaves of *Olea europaea* L. and of oleuropein. **Plant Med Phytother** 1990; 24(4): 264–277.

OE086 Saez, J. J. S., M. D. H. Garraleta, and T. B. Otero. Identification of cinnamic acid ethyl ester and 4-vinylphenol in off-flavour olive oils. **Ann Chim Acta** 1991; 247(2): 295–297.

OE087 Ficarra, P., R. Ficarra, A. De Pasquale, M. T. Monforte, and M. L. Calabro. HPLC analysis of oleuropein and some flavonoids in leaf and bud of *Olea europaea*. **Farmaco** 1991; 46(6): 803–815.

OE088 Amin, E. S., and A. R. Bassiuny. Estrone in *Olea europaea* kernel. **Phytochemistry** 1979; 18: 344.

OE089 Martinez Nieto, L., D. Morales Villena, and J. M. Jimenez Castillo. Mannitol extraction from olive tree pruning residues. Study of some physicochemical properties of the aqueous extract. **Afinidad** 1978; 35: 487–489.

OE090 Viviers, P. M., D. Ferreira, and D. G. Roux. (+)-Africanal, a new lignan of aryltetrahydronaphthalene class. **Tetrahedron Lett** 1979; 1979: 3773–3776.

OE091 Tomas, F., and F. Ferrers. Flavonoids of *Olea europaea*. **An Quim Ser C** 1980; 76: 292–293.

OE091 Nishibe, S., H. Tsukamoto, I. Agata, S. Hisada, K. Shima, and T. Takemoto. Isolation of phenolic compounds from stems of *Olea europaea*. **Shokugaku Zasshi** 1981; 35: 251–254.

OE092 Tsukamoto, H., S. Hisada, and S. Nishibe. Studies on the lignans from Oleaceae plants. Proc 26th Symposium on the Chemistry of Natural Products, Kyoto, Japan 1983; 26: 181–188.

OE093 Paganuzzi, V. Use of silver nitrate TLC in the analysis of olive oil triterpene alcohols. I. Oils obtained from various anatomical parts of the olives. **Riv Ital Sostanze Grasse** 1981; 58(8): 285–393.

OE094 Tanchev, S., N. Joncheva, N. Genov, and M. Codounis. Identification of anthocyanins contained in olives. **Georgike Ereuna** 1980; 4(1): 4–13.

OE095 Tsukamoto, H., S. Hisada, S. Nishibe, D. G. Roux, and J. P. Rourke. Coumarins from *Olea africana* and *Olea capensis*. **Phytochemistry** 1984; 23(3): 699–700.

OE096 Nishibe, S., H. Tsukamoto, S. Hisada, T. Nikaido, T. Ohmoto, and U. Sankawa. Inhibition of cyclic AMP phosphodiesterase by lignans and coumarins of *Olea* and *Fraxinus* barks. **Shoyakugaku Zasshi** 1986; 40(1): 89–94.

OE097 Tejero Mateo, M. P., A. Gil Serrano, and J. Fernandez-Blanos. Polysaccharides in olives. VII. Study a galactoglucomannan isolated from olive pulp of the variety Gordal. **Ann Quim Ser C** 1986; 82(2): 158–161.

OE098 Vera, R., J. Smadja, and J. Y. Conan. Preliminary assay of some plants with alkaloids from Reunion Islands. **Plant Med Phytother** 1990; 24(1): 50–65.

OE099 Janku, I., H. Ravkova, O. Motl, and Z. Blavek. The blood pressure lowering principle of olive extracts. **Arch Int Pharmacodyn Ther** 1957; 112; 342–347.

OE100 Kosak, R., and P. Stern. Pharmacology of the hypotensive principle of olive leaves. **Planta Med** 1959; 7: 118.

OE101 Booth, A. N., E. M. Bickoff, and G. O. Kohler. Estrogen-like activity in vegetable oils and mill by-products. **Science** 1960; 131; 1807.

OE102 Lawrendiadis, G. Contribution to the knowledge of the medicinal plants of Greece. **Planta Med** 1961; 9: 164.

OE103 Delphaut, J., J. Balansard, and P. Roure. Pharmacodynamic investigations of some plant drugs alleged to have an antipyretic action. **C R Seances Soc Biol Ses Fil** 1941; 135; 1458–1460.

OE104 Kosak, R., and P. Stern. Examination of the hypotensive activity of *folium olivae*. **Acta Pharm Jugosl** 1956; 6: 121–132.

OE105 Vazquez Roncero, A., and F. Mazuelos Vela. Natural antioxidants in the leaves of olive trees. **Grasas Aceites (Seville)** 1958; 8: 247–249.

OE106 Manceau, P., G. Netien, and P. Jardon. Hypoglucemic action of extract of olive leaves. **C R Soc Biol** 1942; 136: 810–811.

OE107 Luibl, E. Leaves of the olive tree in hypertension. **Med Monatschr** 1958; 12: 181–182.

OE108 Capretti, G., and E. Bonaconza. Effect of infusion of decoctions of olive leaves (*Olea europaea*) on some physical constants of blood (viscosity and surface tension) and on some components of metabolism (uric acid, chlorides, sodium, potassium and cholesterol). **Giorn Clin Med** 1949; 30: 630–642.

OE109 Nicolatew, N., N. Lemort, L. Adorni, et al. Comparison between extra virgin olive and oleic acid rich sunflowers oil: effects on postprandial lipemia and LDL susceptibility to oxidation. **Ann Nutr Metab** 1998; 42(5): 251–260.

OE110 Zargari, A. Medicinal plants, vol 3, 5th ed., Tehran University Publications, no 1810/3, Tehran, Iran, 1992; 3: 889.

OE111 Gastaldo, P. Official compendium of the Italian flora. XVI. **Fitoterapia** 1974; 45: 199–217.

OE112 Fehri, B., J. M. Aiache, S. Mrad, S. Korbi, and J. L. Lamaison. *Olea europaea* L.: stimulant, anti-ulcer and anti-inflammatory effects. **Boll Chim Farm** 1996; 135(1): 42–49.

OE113 Perez, C., and C. Anesini. *In vitro* antibacterial activity of Argentine folk medicinal plants against *Salmonella typhi*. **J Ethnopharmacol** 1994; 44(1): 41–46.

OE114 Kranke, B., P. Komericki, and W. Aberer. Olive oil-contact sensitizer or irritant? **Contact Dermatitis** 1997; 36(1): 5–10.

OE115 Frederickson, W. R. Antiviral compositions comprising secoiridoids obtained from *Oleaceae*. Patent-PCT Int Appl -96 14,064 1996; 20 pp.

OE116 Carmena, R., J. F. Ascaso, G. Camejo, et al. Effect of olive and sunflower oils on low density lipoprotein level, composition, size, oxidation and interaction with arterial proteoglycans. **Atherosclerosis** 1996; 125(2): 243–255.

OE117 Yaqoob, P., J. A. Knapper, D. H. Webb, C. M. Williams, E. A. Newsholme, and P. C. Calder. Effect of olive oil on immune function in middle-aged men. **Amer J Clin Nutr** 1998; 67(1): 129–135.

OE118   Trovato, A., A. M. Forestieri, L. Iak, R. Barbera, M. T. Monforte, and E. M. Galati. Hypoglycemic activity of different extracts of *Olea europaea* L. in the rats. **Plant Med Phytother** 1993; 26(4): 300–308.

OE119   Pininato, M. C., R. Curi, U. F. Machado, and A. R. Carpinelli. Soybean-and olive oils-enriched diets increase insulin secretion to glucose stimulus in isolated pancreatic rat islets. **Physiol Behav** 1998; 65(2): 289–294.

OE120   Jeffery, N. M., P. Yaqoob, E. A. Newsholme, and P. C. Calder. The effects of olive oil upon rat serum lipid levels and lymphocyte functions appear to be due to oleic acid. **Ann Nutr Metab** 1996; 40(2): 71–80.

OE121   Kokwaro, J. O. Medicinal plants of East Africa. East Afr Literature Bureau, Nairobi 1976.

OE122   De Pasquale, R., M. T. Monforte, A. Trozzi, A. Raccuia, S. Tommansini, and S. Ragusa. Effects of leaves and shoots of *Olea europaea* L. and oleuropein on experimental hypercholesterolemia in rat. **Plant Med Phytother** 1991; 25(2/3): 134–140.

OE123   Le Tutour, B. and D. Guedon. Antioxidative activities of *Olea europaea* leaves and related phenolic compounds. **Phytochemistry** 1992; 31(4): 1173–1178.

OE124   Gonzalez, M., A. Zarzuelo, M. J. Gamez, M. P. Utrilla, J. Jimenez, and I. Osuna. Hypoglycemic activity of olive leaf. **Planta Med** 1992; 58(6): 513–515.

OE125   Nardii, M., C. Scaccini, M. D'Aquino, P. Benedetti, M. A. Di Felice, and G. Tomassi. Lipid peroxidation in liver microsomes of rats fed soybean, olive and coconut oil. **J Nutr Biochem** 1993; 4(1): 39–44.

OE126   Ghazanfar, S. A., and M. A. Al-Sabahi. Medicinal plants of northern and central Oman (Arabia). **Econ Bot** 1993; 47(1): 89–98.

OE127   Homer, K. A., F. Manji, and D. Beighton. Inhibition of peptidase and glycosidase activities of *Porphyromonas gingivalis*, *Bacteroides intermedius* and *Treponema denticola* by plant extracts. **J Clin Periodontol** 1992; 19(5): 305–310.

OE128   De Feo, V., and F. Senatore. Medicinal plants and phytotherapy in the Amalfitan Coast, Salerno province, Campania, southern Italy. **J Ethnopharmacol** 1993; 39(1): 39–51.

OE129   Anesini, C., and C. Perez. Screening of plants used in Argentine folk medicine for antimicrobial activity. **J Ethnopharmacol** 1993; 39(2): 119–128.

OE130   Hirobe, C., D. Palevitch, K. Takeya, and H. Itokawa. Screening test for antitumor activity of crude drugs. (IV). Studies on cytotoxic activity of Israeli medicinal plants. **Nat Med** 1994; 48(2): 168–170.

OE131   Perez, C., and C. Anesini. Inhibition of *Pseudomonas aeruginosa* by Argentinean medicinal plants. **Fitoterapia** 1994; 65(2): 169–172.

OE132   Joe, B., and B. R. Lokesh. Role of capsaicin, curcumin and dietary N-3 fatty acids in lowering the generation of reactive oxygen species in rat peritoneal macrophages. **Biochim Biophys Acta** 1994; 1124(2): 255–263.

OE133   Matsuda, H., S. Nakamura, and M. Kubo. Studies on cuticle drugs from natural sources. II. Inhibitory effect of *Prunus* plants on melanin biosynthesis. **Biol Pharm Bull** 1994; 17(10): 1417–1420.

OE134   Oosthuizen, W., H. H. Vorster, J. C. Jerling, et al. Both fish oil and olive oil lowered plasma fibrinogen in women with high baseline fibrinogen levels. **Thrombosis Homeostasis** 1994; 72(4): 557–562.

OE135   Smit, M. J., H. Wolters, A. M. Temmerman, F. Kuipers, A. C. Beynen, and R. J. Vonk. Effects of dietary corn and olive oil versus coconut fat on biliary cholesterol secretion in rats. **Int J Vitam Nutr Res** 1994; 64(1): 75–80.

OE136   Rauwald, H. W., O. Brehm, and K. P. Odenthal. Screening of nine vasoactive medicinal plants for their possible calcium antagonistic activity. Strategy of selection and isolation for the active principles of *Olea europaea* and *Pseucedanum ostrithium*. **Phytother Res** 1994; 8(3): 135–140.

OE137 Fehri, B., S. Mrad, J. M. Alache, and J. L. Lamaison. Effects of *Olea europaea* L. extract on the rat isolated ileum and trachea. **Phytother Res** 1995; 9(6): 435–439.

OE138 Martinez-Lirola, M. J., M. R. Gonzalez-Tejero, and J. Molero-Mesa. Ethnobotanical resources in the province of Almeria, Spain, Campos de Nijar. **Econ Bot** 1996; 50(1): 40–56.

OE139 Rivera, D., and C. Obon. The ethnopharmacology of Madeira and Porto Santo Islands, a review. **J Ethnopharmacol** 1995; 46(2): 73–93.

OE140 De Feo, V., R. Aquino, A. Menghini, E. Ramundo, and F. Senatoare. Traditional phytotherapy in the Peninsula Sorrentina, Campania, southern Italy. **J Ethnopharmacol** 1992; 36(2): 113–125.

OE141 Fujita, T., E. Sezik, M. Tabata, et al. Traditional medicine in Turkey. VII. Folk medicine in middle and west Black Sea regions. **Econ Bot** 1995; 49(4): 406–422.

OE142 Al-Khalil, S. A survey of plants used in Jordanian traditional medicine. **Int J Pharmacol** 1995; 33(4): 317–323.

OE143 Eskander, E. F., and H. W. Jun. Hypoglycaemic and hyperinsulinemic effects of some Egyptian herbs used for the treatment of diabetes mellitus (type II) in rats. **Egypt J Pharm Sci** 1995; 36(1–6): 331–342.

OE144 Bellakhdar, J., R. Claisse, J. Fleurentin, and C. Yonos. Repertory of standard herbal drugs in the Moroccan pharmacopoeia. **J Ethnopharmacol** 1991; 35(2): 123–143.

OE145 Darias, V., S. Abdala, D. Martin, and F. Ramos. Hypoglycaemic plants from Canary Islands. **Phytother Res Suppl** 1996; 10: S3–S5.

OE146 Okazaki, K., S. Nakayama, K. Kawazoe, and Y. Takaishi. Antiaggregant effects on human platelets of culinary herbs. **Phytother Res** 1998; 12(8): 603–605.

OE147 Alarcorn-Aguilara, F. J., R. Roman-Ramos, S. Perez-Gutierrez, A. Aguilar-Contreras, C. C. Contreras-Weber, and J. L. Flores-Saenz. Study of the anti-hyperglycemic effect of plants used as antidiabetics. **J Ethnopharmacol** 1998; 61(2): 101–110.

OE148 Bartioli, R., F. Fernandez-Banarez, E. Navarro, et al. Effect of olive oil on early and late events of colon carcinogenesis in rats: modulation of arachidonic acid metabolism and local prostaglandin E2 synthesis. **Gut** 2000; 46(2): 191–199.

OE149 Van Tol, A., A. E. H. Terpsta, P. Van Der Berg, and A. C. Beynen. Dietary corn oil versus olive oil enhances HDL protein turnover and lowers HDL cholesterol levels in hamsters. **Atherosclerosis** 1999; 147(1): 87–94.

OE150 Bulur, H., G. Ozdemirler, B. Oz, G. Toker, M. Ozturk, and M. Uysal. High cholesterol diet supplemented with sunflower seed oil but not olive oil stimulates lipid peroxidation in plasma, liver, and aorta of rats. **J Nurt Biochem** 1999; 6(10): 547–550.

OE151 Rovellini, P., and N. Cortesi. Identification of three intermediates compounds in the biosynthesis of secoiridoids as oleoside-type in different anatomic parts of *Olea europaea*. **Riv Ital Sostanze Grasse** 1998; 75(12): 543–550.

OE152 Bennani-Kabchi, N., H. Fdhil, Y. Cherrah, et al. Effects of *Olea europaea* var. *oleaster* leaves in hypercholesterolemic insulin-resistant sand rats. **Therapie** 1999; 54(6): 717–723.

OE153 Alkofahi, A., R. Batshoun, W. Owais, and N. Najib. Biological activity of some Jordanian medicinal plant extracts. **Fitoterapia** 1997; 68(2): 163–168.

OE154 De la Cruz, J. P., A. Villabobos, J. A. Carmona, M. Martin-Romero, J. M. Smith-Agreda, and F. Sanchez de la Cuesta. Antithrombotic potential of olive oil administration in rabbits with elevated cholesterol. **Thrombosis Res** 2000; 100(4): 305–315.

OE155 Onderoglu, S., S. Sozer, K. M. Erbil, R. Ortac, and F. Lermioglu. The evaluation of long-term effects of cinnamon bark and olive leaf on toxicity induced by streptozotocin administration to rats. **J Pharm Pharmacol** 1999; 51(11): 1305–1312.

OE156 Budiyanto, A., N. U. Ahmed, Z. Wu, et al. Protective effect of topically applied olive oil against photocarcinogenesis following UVB exposure of mice. **Carcinogenesis** 2000; 21(11): 2085–2090.

OE157 Susnik-Rybarski, I., F. Mihelic, and S. Durakovic. Antioxidation properties of substances isolated from olive leaves. **Hrana Ishrana** 1983; 24(1/2): 11–15.

OE158 Tsukamoto, H., S. Hisada, and S. Nishibe. Lignans from bark of the *Olea* plants. I. **Chem Pharm Bull** 1984; 32(7): 2730–2735.

OE159 Tsukamoto, H., S. Hisada, S. Nishibe, and D. Roux. Phenolic glucosides from *Olea europaea subsp. africana.* **Phytochemistry** 1984; 23(12): 155–167.

OE160 De la Ribeiro, R., F. Barros, M. Margarida, et al. Acute diuretic effects in conscious rats produced by some medicinal plants used in the state of Sao Paulo, Brasil. **J Ethnopharmacol** 1988; 24(1): 19–29.

OE161 Jantti, J., E. Seppala, H. Vapaatalo, and H. Isomaki. Evening primrose oil and olive oil in treatment of rheumatoid arthritis. **Clin Rheumatol** 1989; 8(2): 238–244.

OE162 Blankenship, J. W., R. Jenks, A. M. MacMurray, L. B. Sandberg, and R. J. Boucek. Uniqueness of dietary olive oil in stimulating aortic prostacyclin production in post-weanling rats. **Prostaglandins Leukotrienes Essent Fatty Acids** 1989; 36(1): 31–34.

OE163 Watson, J., D. Godfrey, W. H. Stimson, J. J. F. Belch, and R. D. Sturrock. The therapeutic affects of dietary fatty acid supplementation in the autoimmune disease of the MRL-MP-1PR mouse. **Int J Immunopharmacol** 1988; 10(4): 467–471.

OE164 Padoan, S. M., A. Pettersson, and A. Svensson. Olive oil as a cause of contact allergy in patients with venous eczema, and occupationally. **Contact Dermatitis** 1990; 23(2): 73–76.

OE165 Occhiuto, F., C. Circosta, A. Gregorio, and G. Busa. *Olea europaea* L. and oleuropein: effects on excito-conduction and on monophasic action potential in anesthetized dogs. **Phytother Res** 190; 4(4): 140–143.

OE166 Lasekan, J. B., M. K. Clayton, A. Gendron-Fitzpatrick, and D. M. Ney. Dietary olive and safflower oils in promotion of DMBA-induced mammary tumorigenesis in rats. **Nutr Cancer** 1990; 13(3): 153–163.

OE167 Giordano, J., and P. J. Levine. Botanical preparations used in Italian folk medicine: possible pharmacological and chemical basis of effect. **Social Pharmacol** 1989; 3(1/2): 83–110.

OE168 Homer, K. A., F. Manji, and D. Beighton. Inhibition of protease activities of periodontopathic bacteria by extracts of plants used in Kenya as chewing sticks (mswaki). **Arch Oral Biol** 1990; 35(6): 421–424.

OE169 Grange, J. M., and R. W. Davey. Detection of antituberculous activity in plant extracts. **J Appl Bacteriol** 1990; 68(6): 587–591.

OE170 Huang, Y. S., P. Redden, X. Lin, R. Smith, S. MacKinnon, and D. F. Horrobin. Effect of dietary olive oil non-glyceride fraction of plasma cholesterol level and live phospholipid fatty acid composition. **Nutr Res** 1991; 11(5): 439–448.

OE171 Tarzuelo, A., J. Duarte, J. Jimenez, M. Gonzalez, and M. P. Utrilla. Vasodilator effect of olive leaf. **Planta Med** 1991; 57(5): 417–419.

OE172 Plouvier, V. Occurrence and distribution of syringoside, calycanthoside and similar coumarinic glycosides in several botanical groups. **C R Acad Sci Ser II** 1985; 301(4): 117–120.

OE173 Kubo, I., and A. Matsumoto. Moluscicides from olive *Olea europaea* and their efficient isolation by countercurrent chromatographies. **J Agr Food Chem** 1984; 32(3): 687–688.

OE174 Vardanian, S. A. Phytotherapy of bronchial asthma in medieval Armenian medicine. **Ter Arkh** 1978; 50: 133–136.

OE175 Tucakov, J. Ethnophytotherapy of diabetes. **SRP Arh Celok Lek** 1978; 106: 159–173.

OE176 Tinsley, I. J., G. Wilson, and R. R. Lowry. Tissue fatty acid changes and tumor incidence in C3H mice ingesting cotton seed oil. **Lipids** 1982; 17: 115–117.

OE177 Lasserre, B., R. Kaiser, P. Huu Chanh, N. Ifansyah, J. Gleye, and C. Moulis. Effects on rats of aqueous extracts of plants used in folk medicine as antihypertensive agents. **Naturwissenschaften** 1983; 70(2): 95–96.

OE178 Funayama, S., and H. Hikino. Hypotensive principles from plants. **Heterocycles** 1981; 15: 1239–1256.

OE179 Razzack, H. M. A. The concept of birth control in Unani medical literature. Unpublished manuscript of the author 1980; 64 pp.

OE180 Delaveau, P., P. Lallouette, and A. M. Tessier. Stimulation of the phagocytic activity of reticuloedothelial system by plant drugs. **Planta Med** 1980; 40: 49–54.

OE181 Boukef, K., H. R. Souissi, and G. Balansard. Contribution to the study on plants used in traditional medicine in Tunisia. **Plant Med Phytother** 1982; 16(4): 260–279.

OE182 May, G., and G. Willuhn. Antiviral activity of aqueous extracts from medicinal plants in tissue cultures. **Arzneim-Forsch** 1978; 28(1): 1–7.

OE183 De la Ribeiro, R., M. M. R. Fiuza de Melo, F. de Barros, C. Gomes, and G. Trolin. Acute antihypertensive effect in conscious rats produced by some medicinal plants used in the state of Sao Paolo. **J Ethnopharmacol** 1986; 15(3): 261–269.

OE184 Darias, V., L. Bravo, E. Barquin, D. M. Herrera, and C. Fraile. Contribution to the ethnopharmacological study of the Canary Islands. **J Ethnopharmacol** 1986; 15(2): 169–193.

OE185 Guerin, J, C., and H. P. Reveillere. Antifungal activity of plant extracts used in therapy. II. Study of 40 plant extracts against 9 fungi species. **Ann Pharm Fr** 1985; 43(1): 77–81.

OE186 Abdul-Ghani, A. S., S. G. El-Lati, A. I. Sacaan, M. S. Suleiman, and R. M. Amin. Anticonvulsant effects of some Arab medicinal plants. **Int J Crude Drug Res** 1987; 25(1): 39–43.

OE186 Tejero-Mateo, M. P., A. Gil-Serrao, and J. Fernandez-Bolanos. Polysaccharides in olives. VI. Study of a galactoglucomannan isolated from olive pulp of the variety Gordal. **Ann Quim Ser C** 1986; 82(2): 155–157.

OE187 Lokesh, B., H. L. Hsieh, and J. E. Kinsella. Olive oil enriched diets decreases arachidonic acid without affecting prostaglandin synthesis in mouse lung and spleen. **Nutr Res** 1988; 8(5): 499–507.

OE188 Baggio, G., A. Pagnan, M. Muraca, et al. Olive-oil-enriched diet: effect on serum lipoprotein levels and biliary cholesterol saturation. **Amer J Clin Nutr** 1988; 47(6): 960–964.

OE189 Ramirez, V. R., L. J. Mostacero, A. E. Garcia, et al. Vegetales empleades en medicina tradicional Norperuana. Banco Agrario del Peru & NACL Univ Trujillo, Trujillo, Peru 1988; 54 pp.

OE190 Scholkens, B. A., D. Gehring, V. Schlotte, and U. Weithmann. Evening primrose oil, a dietary prostaglandin precursor, diminishes vascular reactivity to rennin and angiotensin II in rats. **Prostaglandins Leukotrienes Med** 1982; 8(3): 273–285.

OE191 Antonone, R., F. De Simone, P. Morrica, and E. Ramundo. Traditional phytotherapy in the Roccamonfina volcanic group, Campania, southern Italy. **J Ethnopharmacol** 1988; 22(3): 295–306.

OE192 Salam, W. H., L. M. Cagen, and M. Heimberg. Regulation of hepatic cholesterol biosynthesis by fatty acids: effect of feeding olive oil on cytoplasmic acetoacetyl-coenzyme A thiolase, beta-hydroxy-beta-methylglutaryl-coA synthase, and acetoacetyl-coenzyme A ligase. **Biochem Biohys Res Commun** 1988; 153(1): 422–427.

OE193 Lokar, L. C., and L. Poldini. Herbal remedies in the traditional medicine of the Venezi Giulia region (northeast Italy). **J Ethnopharmacol** 1988; 22(3): 231–239.

OE194 Arora, V. Topical composition for relieving aches and pains. Patent-US-5,223,257 1993; 2 pp.

OE195 Gebre-Mariam, T., Y. Bekele, A. Hymete, and A. S. Nikoiayev. Comparative antimicrobial activity and phytochemical screening of some Ethiopian chewing sticks. **Indian Drugs** 1993; 30(5): 225–229.

OE196 De Bruin, T. W. A., C. B. Brouwer, M. L. S. Trip, H. Jansen, and D. W. Erkelens. Different postprandial metabolism of olive oil and soyean oil: a possible mechanism of the high-density lipoprotein conserving effect of olive oil. **Amer J Clin Nutr** 1993; 58(4): 477–483.

OE197 Vague, J., J. C. Garrigues, J. Berthet, and G. Favier. The oestrogenic effect of several plant oils. **Ann Endocrinol** 1959; 18: 745–751.

OE198 Simpson, G. E. Folk medicine in Trinidad. **J Amer Folklore** 1962; 75: 326–340.

OE199 Hunter III, G. W., H. A. Kemp, H. E. Smalley, O. P. Wilkins, and C. F. Dixon. Studies on schistosomiasis. XII. Some ointments protecting mice against the *Cercariae* of *Schistoma mansoni*. **Amer J Trop Med Hyg** 1956; 5: 713–736.

OE200 Delphaut, J., J. Balansard, and P. Roure. Pharmacodynamic investigations of some plant drugs alleged to have any antipyretic action. **C R Soc Biol** 1941; 135: 1458–1460.

OE201 Tiscornia, E., and G. C. Bertini. Composition of the stearolic fractions of *Olea europaea, Carthamus tinctorius,* and *Helianthus annuus*. **Riv Ital Sostanze Grasse** 1974; 51(2): 50–61.

OE202 Greer, M. A., and E. B. Astwood. The antithyroid effect of certain foods in man as determined with radioactive iodine. **Endocrinology** 1948: 43: 105–119.

OE203 Salerno, J. W., and D. E. Smith. The use of sesame oil and other vegetable oils in the inhibition of human colon cancer growth *in vitro*. **Anticancer Res** 1991; 11(1): 209–215.

OE204 Pezzuto, J. M., C. T. Che, D. D. McPherson, et al. DNA as an affinity probe useful in the detection and isolation of biologically active natural products. **J Nat Prod** 1991; 54(6): 152–153.

OE205 Geller-Bernstein, C., G. Arad, N. Keynan, C. Lahoz, B. Cardaga, and Y. Waisel. Hypersensitivity to pollen of *Olea europaea* in Israel. **Allergy** 1996; 51(5): 356–359.

OE206 Somova, L. I., F. O. Shode, and M. Mipando. Cardiotonic and antidysrhythmic effects of oleanolic and ursolic acids, methyl maslinate and uvanol. **Phytomedicine** 2004; 11(2-3): 121–129.

OE207 Barral, P., E. Batanero, O. Palomares, J. Quiralte, M. Villalba, and R. Rodriguez. A major allergen from pollen defines a novel family of plant proteins and shows intra-and interspecies cross-reactivity. **J Immunol** 2004; 172(6): 3644–3651.

OE208 Batanero, E., P. Barral, M. Villalba, and R. Rodriguez. Encapsulation of Ole e-1 in biodegradable microparticles induces Th1 response in mice: a potential vaccine for allergy. **J Control Release** 2003; 92(3): 395–398.

OE209 Guerra, F., J. C. Daza, and E. Almeda. Immunotherapy with a depigmented, polymerized vaccine of *Olea europaea* pollen allergens. Significantly reduces specific bronchial and skin test reactivity in sensitized patients after one year of treatment. **I Investig Allergol Clin Immunol** 2003; 13(2): 108–117.

OE210 Gonzalez, P., F. Florido, B. Saenz de San Pedro, F. de la Torre, P. Rico, and S. Martin. Immunotherapy with an extract of *Olea europaea* quantified in mass unit. Evaluation of the safety and efficacy after one year of treatment. **J Investig Allergol Clin Immunol** 2002; 12(4): 263–271.

OE211 Castro, A. J., J. de Dios Alche, J. Cuevas, P. J. Romero, V. Alche, and M. L. Rodriguez-Garcia. Pollen from different olive tree cultivars containing varying amounts of the major allergen Ole e-1. **Int Arch Allergy Immunol** 2003; 131(3): 164–173.

OE212 Perona, J. S., J. Canizares, E. Montero, J. M. Sanchez-Dominguez, and V. Ruiz-Gutierrez. Plasma lipid modifications in elderly people after administration of two virgin olive oils of the same variety (*Olea europaea* var. *hojiblanca*) with different triacylglycerol composition. **Br J Nutr** 2003; 89(6): 819–826.

OE213 Montilla, M. P., A. Agil, M. C. Navarro, et al. Antioxidant activity of maslnic acid, a triterpene derivative obtained from *Olea europaea*. **Planta Med** 2003; 69(5): 472–474.

OE214 Somova, L. I., F. O. Shode, P. Ramnanan, and A. Nadar. Antihypertensive, antiatherosclerotic and antioxidant activity of triterpenoids isolated from *Olea europaea, subspecies africana* leaves. **J Ethnopharmacol** 2003; 84(2–3): 299–305.

OE215 Benavente-Garcia, O., J. Castillo, J. Lorente, and M. Alcaraz. Radioprotective effects *in vivo* of phenolics extracted from *Olea europaea* L. leaves against X-ray-induced chromosomal damage: comparative study versus flavonoids and sulfur-containing compounds. **J Med Food** 2002; 5(3): 125–135.

OE216	Khayyal, M. T., M. A. el-Ghazaly, D. M. Abdallah, N. N. Nassar, S. N. Okpanyi, and M. H. Kreuter. Blood pressure lowering effect of an olive leaf extract (*Olea europaea*) in L-NAME induced hypertension in rats. **Arzneimittelforschung** 2002; 52(11): 797–802.

OE217	Florido-Lopez, J. F., J Quiralte-Enriquez, J. M. Arias de Saavendra, B. Saenz de San Pedro, and E. Martin Casanez. An allergen from *Olea europaea* pollen (Ole e 7) is associated with plant-derived food anaphylaxis. **Allergy** 2002; 71: 53–59.

OE218	Quiralte, J., F. Florido, J. M. Arias de Saavedra, et al. Olive allergen-specific IgE responses in patients with *Olea europaea* pollinosis. **Allergy Suppl** 2002; 71: 47–52.

OE219	Al-Quarawi, A. A., M. A. Al-Damegh, and S. A. El-Mougy. Effect of freeze-dried extract of *Olea europaea* on the pituitary-thyroid axis in rats. **Phytother Res** 2002; 16(3): 286–287.

OE220	Batanero, E., P. Barral, M. Villalba, and R. Rodriguez. Sensitization of mice with olive pollen allergen Ole e 1 induces a Th2 response. **Int Arch Allergy Immunol** 2002; 127(4): 269–275.

OE221	Paia-Martins, F., and M. H. Gordon. Isolation and characterization of the antioxidant component 3,4-dihydroxyphenylethyl 4-formyl-3-formylmethyl-4-hexenoate from olive (*Olea europaea*) leaves. **J Agric Food Chem** 2001; 49(9): 4214–4219.

OE222	Bisignano, G., M. G. Lagana, D. Trombetta, et al. *In vitro* antibacterial activity of some aliphatic aldehydes from *Olea europaea* L. **FEMS Microbiol Lett** 2001; 198(1): 9–13.

OE223	Guerra, F., J. Carracedo, J. A. Madueno, P. Sanchez-Guijo, and R. Ramirez. Allergens induce apoptosis in lymphocytes from atopic patients. **Hum Immunol** 1999; 60(9): 840–847.

OE224	Bisignano, G., A. Tomaino, R. LoCascio, G. Crisafi, N. Uccella, and A. Saija. On the *in vitro* antimicrobial activity of oleuropein and hydroxytyrosol. **J Pharm Pharmacol** 1999; 51(8): 971–974.

OE225	de Laurentis, N., L. Stefanizzi, M. A. Mililloand, and G. Tantillo. Flavonoids from leaves of *Olea europaea* L. cultivars. **Ann Pharm Fr** 1998; 56(6): 268–273.

OE226	Cardaba, B., V. Del Pozo, A. Jurado, et al. Olive pollen allergy: searching for immunodominant T-cell epitopes on the Ole e 1 molecule. **Clin Exp Allergy** 1998; 28(4): 413–422.

OE227	Liccardi, G., M. Russ, A. Piccolo, et al. The perennial pattern of clinical symptoms in children monosensitized to *Olea europaea* pollen allergens in comparison with subjects with *Parietaria* and *Gramineae* pollinosis. **Allergy Asthma Proc** 1997; 18(2): 99–105.

OE228	Pieroni, A., D. Heimler, L. Pieters, B. van Poel, and A. J. Vlietinck. *In vitro* anti-complementary activity of favonoids from olive (*Olea europaea* L.) leaves. **Pharmazie** 1996; 51(1): 765–768.

OE229	Cherif, S., N. Rahal, M. Haouala, et al. A clinical trial of a titrated *Olea* extract in the treatment of essential arterial hypertension. **J Pharm Belg** 1996; 51(2): 69–71.

OE230	Lccardi, G., M. Russo, M. Saggese, M. D'Amato, and G. D'Amato. Evaluation of serum specific IgE and skin responsiveness to allergenic extracts of *Oleaceae* pollens (*Olea europaea*, *Fraxinus excelsior* and *Ligustrum vulgare*) in patients with respiratory allergy. **Allergol Immunopathol (Madr)** 1995; 23(1): 41–46.

OE231	Casanovas, M., F. Guerra, C. Moreno, R. Miguel, F. Maranon, and J. C. Daza. Double-blind, placebo-controlled clinical trial of preseasonal treatment with allergenic extracts of *Olea europaea* pollen administered sublingually. **J Investig Allergol Clin Immunol** 1994; 4(6): 305–314.

OE232	Fehri, B., J. M. Aiache, A. Memmi, et al. Hypotension, hypoglycemia and hypouricemia recorded after repeated administration of aqueous leaf extract of *Olea europaea* L. **J Pharm Belg** 1994; 49(2): 101–108.

OE233   Guerra, F., C. Moreno, J. C. Daza, R.
        Miguel, M. Garcia, and P. Sanchez-
        Guijo. Linear monitoring of pa-
        tients sensitive to *Olea* and grass
        pollens treated with immunotherapy
        based on glutaraldehyde-modified
        (allergoid) extracts. **J Investig Al-
        lergol Clin Immunol** 1993; 3(4):
        182–190.

OE234   Zarzuelo, A., J. Duarte, J. Jimenez, M.
        Gonzalez, and M. P. Utrila. Vasodila-
        tor effect of the olive leaf. **Planta Med**
        1991; 57(5): 417–419.
OE235   Macchia, L., M. F. Caiaffa, G.
        DiFelice, et al. Changes in skin reactiv-
        ity, specific IgE and IgG levels after one
        year of immunotherapy in olive polli-
        nosis. **Allergy** 1991; 46(6): 410–418.

11 | Oryza sativa
L.

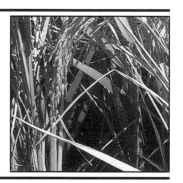

Common Names

Aisskssiinainikimm	United States	Ilayisi	Africa
Aleysi	Suriname	Karga	India
Aloruz	Arabic countries	Klao	Thailand
Araisa	Samoa	Loso	Congo
Arisi	India	Luama	Vietnam
Aros	Netherlands Antilles	Mchele	Mozambique
Aroz	France	Mchele	Tanzania
Arros	Spain	Mchele	Zaire
Arroz colorado	Argentina	Mpunga	Africa
Arroz macho	Argentina	Mupunga	Botswana
Arroz preto	Brazil	Mupunga	Zambia
Arroz rojo	Bolivia	Mupunga	Zimbabwe
Arroz rojo	Colombia	Nasi	Indonesia
Arroz rojo	Costa Rica	No	China
Arroz rojo	Cuba	Orez	Romania
Arroz rojo	Ecuador	Oriz	Albania
Arroz rojo	Honduras	Oriz	Bulgaria
Arroz rojo	Mexico	Oriz	Macedonia
Arroz rojo	Nicaragua	Orizen	Bulgaria
Arroz rojo	Panama	Orizov	Bulgaria
Arroz rojo	Paraguay	Padi ketek	Indonesia
Arroz rojo	Peru	Paparean	Indonesia
Arroz rojo	Puerto Rico	Pirinac	Yugoslavia
Arroz rojo	Venezuela	Pirinac	Croatia
Arroz vermelho	Brazil	Pirinac	Serbia
Arroz	Portugal	Pirinac	Turkey
Arroz	Spain	Pirinc	Turkey
Aruz	Ecuador	Pugas	Hawaii
Bariis	Somalia	Pugas	Pacific Islands
Beras	Malaysia	Raihi	New Zealand
Birhni	India	Reesa	India
Bugas	Philippines	Reis	England
Com cay lua	Vietnam	Reis	Germany
Erus	Malaysia	Reise	The Isle of Man (Manx)

From: *Medicinal Plants of the World, vol. 3: Chemical Constituents, Traditional and Modern Medicinal Uses*
By: I. A. Ross © Humana Press Inc., Totowa, NJ

Reisi	South Africa	Riso	Italy
Rice	Guyana	Riz	France
Rice	India	Riz	Rwanda
Rice	United Kingdom	Rizs	Hungary
Rice	United States	Ruzi	Greece
Riisi	Finland	Rys	Netherlands
Rijst	Netherlands	Rys	South Africa
Ris	Denmark	Ryz	Poland
Ris	Faeroe Islands	Ryze	Czech Republic
Ris	France	Salebyeo	Korea
Ris	Norway	Sragne	Cambodia
Ris	Russia	Tao	China
Ris	Sweden	Umupunga	Africa
Ris	Switzerland	Vary	Madagascar
Ris	Ukraine	Wild rice	Australia
Risgryn	Sweden		

BOTANICAL DESCRIPTION

Oryza sativa is a perennial, cultivated as an annual of the POACEAE (GRAMINEAE) family. The root system of the plant is fibrous, with roots rising from the lower nodes of the culm. The plant tiller usually bears four or five culms, to 0.6–2.4 m high. Each culm has 10–20 internodes and is surrounded by sheaths of leaves. Leaf blades are narrow, flat, 30–50 cm long and 7–25 mm wide, slightly pubescent with spiny hairs on the margin. The inflorescence is a panicle, 7.5–37.5 cm long, varying from close and compact in some, to loose and spreading in others; exerting or partially exerting. Panicle branches arise in whorls, each branch bears 75–150 spikelets, each with single floret. Large numbers of spikelets are usually associated with smaller size and a densely packed arrangement. The flower consists of two lodicules, six stamens, and two plumose stigmas on two styles, surrounded by the floral bracks and two small outer glumes. Lemma and palea surrounding the kernel, variously colored: golden yellow, red, purple, brown and black, becoming straw or light yellow when the grain ripens. Grain varying in size from 5 to 14 mm long and 2–3.7 mm broad. The length/breadth ratio defining size and shape of the grain. Kernel is usually white, sometimes red, purple, or brown.

ORIGIN AND DISTRIBUTION

Rice is one of the oldest food crops. Currently, it does not seem possible to determine the place of domestication, but it probably occurred in India or China. Its cultivation in India, Indochina, China, Indonesia, and East Africa is prehistoric. It is now distributed throughout the tropics and warm parts of temperate regions of the world. The temperate zone varieties were named *japonica*, and the tropical zone varieties *indica*.

TRADITIONAL MEDICINAL USES

China. Hot water extract of the dried straw is taken orally for hepatitis[OS117].

India. Hot water extract of the grain is taken orally for jaundice[OS136]. Powdered grain is taken orally for typhoid fever. The grain is kept for a month with "birbahuti" (cochineal insects) before given[OS064].

Indonesia. The charred stem is immersed in water, and the liquid is taken orally by pregnant women as an abortifacient[OS003]. The stem ash is eaten twice daily as an abortifacient[OS125].

Iran. The grain is taken orally for intestinal inflammation and administered rectally for diarrhea. The grain flour is used externally to reduce topical inflammation, to remove rash and erythema, and to treat genital irritation in children resulting from contact with urine, and it is mixed with talc powder to prevent dryness of the skin[OS024].

Japan. The fresh grain is taken orally as a general nutrient[OS054].

Malaysia. Infusion of the root is taken orally to facilitate parturition[OS062].

Mexico. The grain is taken orally to treat diarrhea[OS070].

Nepal. Water obtained from rice wash "chaulani" is taken orally to relieve vaginitis[OS065]. To relieve leukorrhea, approx 10 g of the flowers of fire-flame bush *Woodfordia fruticosa* (L.) Kurz. is boiled in 600–700 mL of rice wash and the decoction is cooled and taken orally twice daily for at least 2 weeks[OS063].

Nicaragua. The grain is taken orally for diarrhea and externally for skin rashes[OS069].

Peru. Hot water extract of the dried fruit is used externally for acne and orally for gastric irritation, diarrhea, and bloody dysentery[OS139].

Philippines. Decoction of the dried seed hull in used in steam baths for postpartum care. Also, added to the bath are *Paspalum scrobiculatum*, monkey bones, deer antler, incense, *Commophora myrrha*, salt, and rice[OS130].

Taiwan. Hot water extract of the dried root is taken orally for liver diseases[OS138].

Thailand. Hot water extract of the fresh seedling is taken orally as a tonic[OS145].

CHEMICAL CONSTITUENTS

(ppm unless otherwise indicated)

15,16-Epoxy-3-oxa-kauran-2-one: Lf[OS159]
15,16-Epoxy-3 α-palmitoyloxy-kauran-2-one: Lf[OS159]
15,16-Epoxy-3 β-dyfroxy-kauran-2-one: Lf[OS159]
15,16-Epoxy-3 β-myristoyloxy-kauran-2-one: Lf[OS159]
15,16-Epoxy-3 β-palmitoyloxy-kauran-2-one: Lf[OS159]
15,16-Epoxy-kauran-2,3-dione: Lf[OS159]
3-Dehydro-6-deoxoteasterone: Pl[OS158]
3-Dehydroteasterone: Pl[OS158]
6-Deoxoteasterone: Pl[OS158]
Abscisic acid: Sd[OS007]
Aconitic acid: Aer[OS043]
Aconitic acid, *trans*: Aer[OS112]
Alanine, D: Lf[OS099]
Alanyl-glycine, D: Lf[OS099]
Aluminum: Lf[OS027]
Arabino-hexono-1-4-lactone, D, 3-deoxy: Pl[OS015]
Arabino-1-4-lactone, D: Pl[OS015]
Arabinol, iso: Aer[OS006,OS005]
Arundoin: Aer[OS006,OS005]
Asparagine: Rt[OS026]
Asparatic acid: Pl[OS117]
Auxin: Sh[OS081]
Benzoic acid, 4-hydroxy: St[OS044]
Brassicasterol, 22-dihydro: Bran 69.6[OS080]
Caffeic acid: St[OS044]
Campesterol: Aer[OS127,OS006]
Campesterol ferulate: Bran 69.6[OS080], Sd oil[OS055]
Castasterone: Sh 13.60 ppt[OS088], Aer 13.6[OS089], Sd[OS033]
Castasterone, 6-deoxy: Sd[OS033]
Chrysanthemin: Seedling Rt[OS030]
Coumaric acid, para: St[OS044]
Cyanidin: Sd[OS157]
Cyanidin 3-O-β-D-glucoside: Pl[OS045]
Cyanidin diglycoside: Lf[OS144]
Cyanidin monoglycoside: Sd[OS144]
Cyanidin-5-glycoside: Lf[OS002]
Cycloartanol ferulate: Sd oil[OS042]
Cycloartanol, 24-methylene, ferulate: Sd oil[OS042], Bran 278.7[OS080]
Cycloartenol ferulate: Sd oil[OS042], Bran 139.3[OS080]
Cycloartenol ferulic acid ester: Bran[OS047]
Cycloeucalenol: Sd oil[OS076]
Cylindrin: Aer[OS006,OS005]
Daucosterol: Sd Hu[OS079]
Diazepam: Sd[OS035]
Diazepam, N-demethyl: Sd[OS035]
DNA topoisomerase 1: Seedling[OS109]
Dolichosterone: Sh 8.40 ppt[OS088]
Erythrono-1-4-lactone, D: Pl[OS015]
Erythrono-1-4-lactone, D, 2-C-hydroxy-methyl: Pl[OS015]

Erythrono-1-4-lactone, D, 2-C- methyl: Pl[OS015]
Ferulic acid: St[OS044], Bran[OS084]
Glucan, α: Pl[OS098]
Glutamic acid: Straw[OS117]
Glutathione: Rt[OS052]
Glycine: Straw[OS117]
Kaur-15-ene, ent: Sh[OS058]
Kaur-16-ene, ent: Sh[OS058]
Leucine: Straw[OS117]
Leucine, iso: Straw[OS117]
Linoleic acid, 12-13-epoxy: Lf[OS037]
Lutexin: Lf[OS009]
Lutonaretin: Lf[OS009]
Lysine: Straw[OS117]
Lyxono-1-1-lactone, D: Pl[OS015]
Lyxono-1-4-lactone, D-2-deoxy: Pl[OS015]
Malvidin: Sd[OS157]
Melatonin: Sd 1498[OS156]
Methionine: Straw[OS117]
Momilactone A: Lf[OS017]
Momilactone B: Pl[OS116]
Momilactone C: Husk[OS077]
Nicotianamine: Seedling[OS121]
Olein, mono: Sd[OS033]
Oryza antifungal protein: Sd[OS021]
Oryza protein φ: Bran 0.07%[OS065]
Oryza sativa lectin: Fr[OS010]
Oryza sativa phytoglycolipid: Sd Ct[OS094]
Oryza sativa polysaccharides RBS: Fr[OS012]
Oryza sativa substance RBF-PM: Sd[OS118]
Oryza sativa substance RBF-X: Sd[OS118]
Oryzabran A: Sd Ct[OS137]
Oryzabran B: Sd Ct[OS137]
Oryzabran C: Sd Ct[OS137]
Oryzabran D: Sd Ct[OS137]
Oryzacystatin A: Sd[OS066]
Oryzacystatin I: Sd[OS056]
Oryzacystatin II: Sd[OS056]
Oryzalexin A: Lf 1.0[OS120]
Oryzalexin B: Lf[OS123]
Oryzalexin C: Lf[OS123]
Oryzalexin D: Lf[OS017]
Oryzalexin F: Lf 2.3[OS019]
Oryzalexin S: Lf[OS017]
Oryzalide A: Lf 1.2[OS016]
Oryzanol: Sd oil[OS048]
Oryzanol, γ: Sd oil[OS032,OS042]
Oryzaran A: Rt[OS096]
Oryzaran B: Rt[OS096]
Oryzaran C: Rt[OS096]
Oryzaran D: Rt[OS096]
Oryzatensin: Sd[OS022]

Oryzenin: Sd[OS071]
Paeonidin-3-O- β-D-glucoside: Seedling Rt[OS030]
Palmitin, mono: Sd[OS033]
Pantoyllactone primeveroside: Seedling[OS023]
Phytic acid: Sd[OS038], Bran[OS051]
Phytin: Sd Hu[OS095], Fr[OS111], Epicarp 4.42%[OS113], Sd[OS090]
Phytocassane A: Call Tiss[OS029]
Phytocassane B: Call Tiss[OS029]
Phytocassane C: Call Tiss[OS029]
Phytocassane D: Call Tiss[OS029]
Phytocassane E: Call Tiss[OS029]
Prolamine: Sd[OS040]
Protein: Sd[OS114]
Protein (*Oryza sativa*): Straw 47[OS011]
Protocatechuic acid: St[OS044]
Pyridoxine, 5-O-(β-D-glucopyranosyl): Fr[OS078]
Pyrrolidine, 1 (2 acetyl): Sd[OS110]
Pyrroline, 1 (2 acetyl): Fr 1.52[OS103]
Quinic acid: Lf[OS025]
Resorcinol, 5-(heptadec-12-enyl): Seedling[OS031]
Resorcinol, 5-heptadecyl: Seedling[OS031]
Resorcinol, 5-pentadecyl: Seedling[OS031]
Resorcinol, 5-tridecyl: Seedling[OS031]
Rhamnono-1-4-lactone, L: Pl[OS015]
Rice antifungal protein 1: Seedling[OS018]
Sakuranetin: Lf[OS034,OS017]
Salicyclic acid: Sh 61[OS053], Seedling 37.19[OS060]
Satiomem: Sd[OS020]
Serine: Straw[OS117]
Shikimic acid: Lf[OS025]
Sitosterol, β: Aer[OS127,OS006]
Sitosterol, β cellopentaoside: Sd[OS115]
Sitosterol, β cellotetraoside: Sd[OS115]
Sitosterol, β ferulate: Sd oil[OS042], Bran 96.9[OS080]
Squalene: Sd[OS146], Sh[OS058]
Stigmasterol: Aer[OS127]
Stigmasterol ferulate: Sd oil[OS042]
Teasterone: Sd[OS033]
Thiamine: Sd[OS057]
Threonine: Straw[OS117]
Tocopherol, α: Fixed oil[OS042]
Tocopherol, β: Fixed oil[OS042]
Tocopherol, δ: Fixed oil[OS042]
Tocopherol, γ: Fixed oil[OS042]
Tocotrienol, α: Fixed oil[OS042]
Tocotrienol, β: Fixed oil[OS042]
Tocotrienol, δ: Fixed oil[OS042]
Tocotrienol, γ: Fixed oil[OS042]

Tricin: Straw[OS117]
Tricin-5-O- β-D-Glucoside: Pl[OS008]
Tyrosine: Straw [OS117]
Valine: Straw[OS117]
Vanillic acid: St[OS044]
Violanthin: Lf, St[OS097]
Vitexin: Lf [OS009]
Vitexin, Iso: Lf [OS009]
Wax (*Oryza sativa*): Fixed oil[OS028]

PHARMACOLOGICAL ACTIVITIES AND CLINICAL TRIALS

5-α Reductase inhibition. Water extract of the grain, applied externally on adults at a concentration of 10%, was active. The biological activity has been patented[OS072].

Anaphylactic activity. Methanol extract of grains, administered intraperitoneally to rats at a dose of 1 g/kg, dose-dependently inhibited systemic anaphylaxis induced by compound 48/80. When the extract was pretreated at concentrations ranging from 0.001 to 1 mg/g body weight, the serum histamine levels were reduced in a dose-dependent manner. It also inhibited local anaphylaxis activated by anti-dinitrophenyl immunoglobulin E (IgE). The extract dose-dependently inhibited the histamine released from rat peritoneal mast cells activated by compound 48/80 or antidinitrophenyl IgE. The level of cyclic adenosine monophosphate in the rat peritoneal mast cells, when the extract was added, significantly increased compared with the basal cells[OS082]. Methanol extract of the dried seed, in cell culture at variable concentrations, inhibited compound of IgE-induced release from rat peritoneal mast cells. The methanol extract, administered intragastrically to rats at a dose of 1 g/kg, inhibited the rate of passive cutaneous anaphylaxis reaction. Intraperitoneal administration inhibited systemic anaphylaxis induced by compound 48/80[OS083].

Anti-acne activity. Water extract of the grain, applied externally on adults at a concentration of 10%, was active. The biological activity has been patented[OS072].

Antibacterial activity. Ethanol (95%) and water extracts of the dried grain, on agar plate at a concentration of 50 μL/plate, were active on *Staphylococcus aureus*[OS067].

Antidiarrheal activity. A mixture consisted of rice powder and various electrolytes dissolved in 1 L of water was successful in treating 82% of 38 adult patients and 80% children with diarrhea due to *Vibrio cholerae*. The mixture was also successful in treating 89% of patients with diarrhea resulting from *Escherichia coli*[OS131]. Rice flour, used as a rehydration therapy instead of glucose, was active[OS049]. Water extract of the grain, administered intragastrically to rats, was active. The extract was tested as an oral rehydration solution for the treatment of bacterial diarrhea. The solution inhibited secretions by inhibiting chloride channel secretion in the small intestine[OS075]. Rice powder, administered orally to 96 children with diarrhea in a study to evaluate the efficacy of cereal-based oral rehydration therapy compared with World Health Organization oral rehydration therapy recovery, produced 3.5 vs 40% in controls[OS068]. Rice water, with NaCl, KCl, and CaCl$_2$ added was used for rehydration in mild to acute diarrhea. The efficacy was as great as World Health Organization oral rehydration solutions[OS059].

Antidysenteric activity. Cooked rice, fed to pigs infected with *Serpulina hyodysenteriae*, produced drier colonic contents and feces and lighter large intestines, and the contents of their large intestines had increased pH values and decreased total volatile fatty acid concentrations than on other diets. None of the pigs fed the cooked-rice diet developed colonic changes or disease, whereas most pigs on the other diets developed mucohemorrhagic colitis and dysentery[OS148].

Antifungal activity. Acetone extract of the fresh leaf, on agar plate at a concentration of 200 ppm, was active on *Pyricularia oryzae* cultivars Fukuyuki and Fukunishiki using the acidic part and inactive on cultivars Sasanishiki using the acid and neutral parts and on Fukunishiki and Fukuyuki using the neutral part[OS037].

Antihistamine activity. Methanol extract of grains, in cell culture at a concentration of 10 mg/mL, was active on mast cells vs inhibition of histamine release induced by compound 48/80. The extract, administered intragastrically to rats at a dose of 1 g/kg, was active vs inhibition of histamine release induced by compound 48/80[OS082].

Antihypercholesterolemic activity. Fixed oil in the ration of adults, at a dose of 35 g/day, was active. Twelve patients with high serum cholesterol or triglycerides used rice bran oil instead of their usual cooking oil (palm oil) and in similar quantities. Serum cholesterol and triglycerides were reduced after 15 days of use. No reduction was seen in the control group using the normal cooking oil[OS100]. Fixed oil, taken orally by adults, was active. Fifteen patients with elevated low-density lipoprotein (LDL) cholesterol were treated with rice bran oil, which comprised two-thirds of the fat of a diet with 30% fat. The patients showed lower levels of LDL cholesterol, and plasma cholesterol levels were similar to those obtained from patients consuming canola, corn, and olive oils[OS138]. Rice bran, taken orally by adults at a dose of 100 g/day, produced a reduction in LDL, high-density lipoprotein , and very low-density lipoprotein cholesterol. The treatment was administered to 11 patients with moderately to high blood cholesterol levels for two 3-week periods. Before the treatment phase, a control diet without bran was provided for 2 weeks[OS039]. Seed oil, in the ration of rats at a concentration of 10% of the diet, was active. Rats fed bran oil with cholesterol supplementation had lower serum cholesterol than those fed similar levels of peanut oil. High-density lipoprotein level was higher in the rice bran oil group[OS102].

Antihyperglycemic activity. Dried grains, taken orally by adults of both sexes, was active. The hypoglycemic response of three traditional sorghum (both whole and dehulled) recipes namely missiroti, upma, and dhokla were studied on six patients with noninsulin-dependent diabetes. Consumption of whole sorghum recipes resulted in significantly lower plasma glucose levels, lower percent peak rise, and lower area-under-the-curve in patients with diabetes when compared with the consumption of dehulled sorghum and wheat recipes. The least glycemic response was observed with whole sorghum semolina (75.6 mg), followed by whole sorghum missiroti (77.8 mg) and whole sorghum dhokla (84.5 mg). No significant difference ($p < 0.05$) was seen in the mean peak rise of plasma glucose levels of the subjects fed with wheat and dehulled recipes[OS073]. The cooked grain, taken orally by adults, was inactive vs glucose-induced hyperglycemia[OS140]. The grain, taken orally by eight healthy individuals with normal glucose tolerance at a dose of 25 g/person, was active[OS041]. Water extract of the dried grain, administered intragastrically to mice at a dose of 1 g/kg, was inactive. The dose was given 1 hour after streptozotocin and twice daily for 3 subsequent days. Blood glucose was 255.3 vs 236.3 mg/dL for controls vs streptozotocin-induced hyperglycemia[OS108].

Antihyperlipemic activity. Fixed oil in the ration of adults, at a dose of 35 g/day, was active. Twelve patients with high serum cholesterol or triglycerides used rice brain oil instead of their usual cooking oil (palm oil) and in similar quantities. Serum cholesterol and triglycerides were reduced after 15 days of use. No reduction was seen in the control group using the normal cooking oil[OS100].

Anti-inflammatory activity. Methanol extract of the bran, used externally on the mouse ear, was active vs 12-O-tetradecanoylphorbol-13-acetate-induced ear inflammation[OS080]. Rice germ oil, used externally on rabbits three times a day for 2 days, prevented subsequent sodium dodecyl sulfate-induced blistering, erythema, and edema. The biological activity has been patented[OS107].

Antimutagenic activity. Water extract of the dried seed coat did not affect the mutagenicities of coffee, black tea, whisky, or several mutagenic compounds[OS129].

Antioxidant activity. Bran, at a concentration of 65 mg/mL, was active. Superoxide radicals were generated using the hypoxanthine-xanthine oxidase system[OS046]. Chloroform/methanol and methanol (50%) extracts of the dried seed hulls were active[OS093].

Antisecretory effect. Water extract of the dried grain was active on the small intestinal crypt cells vs cyclic adenosine monophosphate-induced secretion stimulation[OS061].

Antispasmodic activity. Ethanol (50%) extract of grain was active on the guinea pig ileum vs acetylcholine- and histamine-induced spasms[OS001].

Anti-thyroid activity. Boiled rice taken orally by adults at a dose of 350 g/person was inactive on iodine uptake by the thyroid[OS147].

Anti-tumor activity. Bran, administered intraperitoneally to mice at a dose of 100 mg/kg, was active on Sarcoma 180 (solid). The biological activity has been patented[OS119]. Fermented grains, in the ration of rats, were active. Miso, a paste made from the seeds of *Oryza sativa* and *G lycine max* (soybean), was fed *ad libitum*. The incidence of cancers in the miso treated rats was 20% less than controls vs 7,12-dimethylbenz-[a]anthracene -induced carcinogenesis[OS104]. Water extract of dried seed hull, administered intraperitoneally to mice, was active on Sarcoma 180 (ASC). A glycoprotein fraction has been tested. The biological activity reported has been patented[OS133].

Anti-ulcer activity. A cerebroside fraction of rice bran, administered intraperitoneally to mice at a dose of 100 mg/kg, was inac-

tive vs water immersion stress-induced ulcers[OS122]. Freshly harvested grains (milled and unmilled) and fresh bran, in the ration of rats, was active vs pylorus ligation-induced ulcers[OS101].

Antiviral activity. Aqueous low-speed supernatant and juice of the fresh seed, at a concentration of 10%, were active on virus-top necrosis in plants[OS092].

Anti-yeast activity. Ethanol (80%) extract of the dried entire plant, on agar plate at a concentration of 1 mg/mL, was inactive on *Candida albicans*[OS126].

Apoptosis induction. Lipoprotein fraction of the bran, in cell culture at a concentration of 100 µg/mL, was active vs human endometrial adenocarcinoma cells[OS085].

Atopic dermatitis effect. Rice bran broth, administered to 17 patients with atopic dermatitis as bath therapy, was safe and clinically useful. The rice bran broth was dissolved in the bathtub as a medicinal bath. One of the patients discontinued therapy after developing redness and itching of the skin just after bathing. The other 16 patients continued the bath for 2–5 months and recorded skin conditions once a month. The efficacy of the therapy in alleviating skin symptoms was excellent in four patients, good in seven, slightly effective in four, and effective in one. Recurrence of initial symptoms was not detected in any patients during the rice bran broth bathing[OS149].

Bioavailability of starch. Cooked rice was administered to colectomized rats by gastric intubation and the recovery of starch in the ileal digesta measured after 10 hours of ingestion. Significant starch (11–15%) was recovered from animals fed peas, lima beans, or kidney beans; 0.2–0.4% of starch from rice. Oligosaccharide extraction, the size of the test meal, and the amount of starch did not affect starch biovailability[OS150].

cAMP accumulation. Methanol extract of the grain, in cell culture at a concentration of 1 mg/mL, was active on mast cells[OS082].

Carcinogenesis inhibition. Polysaccharide fraction of the dried seed hulls, administered to rats by gastric intubation, was active vs tumor induction with *N*-ethyl-*N*-nitro-*N*-nitrosoguanidine[OS132]. Rice bran, administered orally to male rats at a concentration of 4% of the diet, was active. A 1:1 combination of wheat bran and psyllium, at a total level of 8% dietary fiber, offers the highest protection against colon tumor development[OS141].

Cell proliferation inhibition. Lipoprotein fraction of bran, in cell culture at a concentration of 100 µg/mL, was active vs Sawano cells[OS085].

Cytotoxic activity. Dried seedling hulls, in cell culture, was active on Cells-HSOS-1, Cells-Jurkat, Cells-X63-AG8, and Leuk-P388[OS050]. Ethanol (50%) extract of the grain, in cell culture, was inactive on CA-9KB, effective dose$_{50}$ greater than 20 µg/mL[OS001]. Water extract of the dried grain, in cell culture at a concentration 500 µg/mL, was inactive on CA-mammary-microalveolar cells[OS105]. Water extract of the freeze-dried grains, in cell culture, was active on Leuk-P815. The toxic activity of the tumor was evaluated by culturing mastocytoma P815 with macrophage cells and measuring the incorporation of ^{3}H-thymidine[OS106].

Dermatitis-producing effect. A case of dermatitis in a female adult was reported after contact with the fresh leaf[OS128].

Diabetes inhibition of development. Methanol/ethanol/ketone extract of bran, in the ration of male rats at a dose of 0.5 g/kg, was active vs streptozotocin-induced diabetes[OS086].

Estrogenic effect. Polished rice, in the ration of immature female rats, was active[OS143]. Saponifiable fraction of the embryo, administered subcutaneously to female mice, was active[OS142]. Seed oil, administered orally to female mice at a dose of 10% of the diet, was active[OS004].

Feeding deterrent. The fresh sap and chromatographic fraction of the fresh sap were active on *Nilaparvata lugens OS127*.

Feeding stimulant. Flavonoid fraction of the dried entire plant was active on *Laodelphax striatellus*, *Sogatella furcifera*, and *Nilaparvata lugens*[OS013]. Methanol extract of the fresh leaf, at a concentration of 2%, was active on *Laodelphax striatellus*, *Nilaparvata lugens* and *Sogatella furcifera*. The results were significant at *p* less than 0.01 level[OS014].

Fungal stimulant. Dried entire plant, at a concentration of 100 ppm, was active on *Gerlachia oryzae*[OS015].

Glutamate–pyruvate–transminase inhibition. Ethanol (50%) extract of the dried root, in cell culture at a concentration of 1 mg/mL, was inactive on hepatocytes vs prostaglandin E-1- and CCl$_4$-induced hepatotoxicity[OS138].

Glycemic index. Rice, consumed by patients with noninsulin-dependent diabetes mellitus, correlated positively with in vitro starch digestibility of food slurry and negatively with amylase content of the food. Glutinous rice had the highest values and mung bean noodles the lowest[OS152]. Rice and combinations of rice and legumes, consumed by 36 patients with noninsulin-dependent diabetes mellitus, produced significantly lower blood glucose response 2 hours postprandially as compared with blood glucose responses to a 50 g glucose load for the same group. A higher glycemic index was obtained for rice with peas; all other combinations yielded lower glycemic indices. No significant difference was observed for triglyceride responses of the different foods[OS153].

Hair-growth stimulant. Water extract of the grain, applied externally on adults at a concentration of 10%, was active. The biological activity has been patented[OS072].

Hypocholesterolemic activity. Unsaponifiable fraction of seed oil, administered orally to rats at a dose of 0.4% of the diet, was active[OS134]. Seed oil, administered orally to adults and by gastric intubation to dogs, was active[OS124].

Hypoglycemic activity. Dried grain, taken orally by human adults at a dose of 162 g/person, was active, results were significant at p less than 0.001 level[OS091]. Water extract of the dried seed coat of cultivar Fukuyuki, administered intraperitoneally to mice at a dose of 100 mg/kg, was active[OS137].

Hypotensive activity. Ethanol (50%) extract of the grain, administered intravenously to dogs at a dose of 50 mg/kg, was active[OS001].

Interleukin induction. Water extract of freeze-dried grain was active. Interleukin-1 activity was measured by the interleukin-1 dependent growth of a T-helper cell line[OS106].

Lipid metabolism effects. Grains, in the ration of rats at a dose of 68 g/animal daily for 3 months, were active vs rats fed tapioca. Total serum cholesterol and triglycerides were higher than animals fed tapioca. Glucose-6-phosphate levels were lower, and triglyceride lipase and lipoprotein lipase were increased over levels found in the tapioca group[OS087]. Seed oil, in the ration of rats at a concentration of 10% of the diet, was active. Liver triglycerides were lower in rats fed rice brain oil than those fed peanut oil[OS102].

Lymphocyte stimulation. Bran fiber hemicellulose, administered to rats at a dose of 10% of the diet, produced weak activity on sperm cells[OS036].

Metabolism and gastric emptying. Polished rice, consumed by 13 healthy adults, produced no correlation between gastric emptying and blood glucose or plasma insulin after the meal. Three meals of equal energy content consisting of mashed potatoes, polished rice, or white beans were investigated. Blood glucose and plasma insulin were measured after overnight fast and after ingestion of the test meals. Gastric empty-

ing of mashed potatoes was faster than that of polished rice and of white beans. Blood glucose and plasma insulin responses to the meal with mash potatoes were greater than that of polished rice, which also produced a greater glucose response than that of white beans. The glucose and insulin responses to potatoes and rice were strongly related to gastric emptying rate, but other factors dominates the control of these responses to white beans[OS154].

Mutagenic activity. Seed oil was inactive on *Salmonella typhimurium* TA100 and TA98. Metabolic activation had no effect on the results[OS135].

Parkinson's disease. Unpolished rice, in combination with *Carica papaya*, seaweeds, and effective micro-organisms, produced potential neuroprotective effects. The treatment was investigated using the 6-hydroxydopamine-lesion rat model of Parkinson's disease. The nigrostriated dopaminergic neurons were unilaterally lesioned with 6-hydroxydopamine in rats that were treated. Seven days after lesion, the integrity (number of tyrosine hydroxylase-positive cells in the substantia nigra pars compacta) and functionality (dopamine and its metabolites 3,4-dihydroxyphenylacetic acid and homovanillic acid content in the striata) of nigrostriatal dopaminergic neurons were assessed[OS155].

Passive cutaneous anaphylaxis inhibition. Methanol extract of the grain, administered intragastrically to rats at a dose of 1 g/kg, was active vs anti-2,4-dinitrophenyl immunoglobulin administration followed by intravenous antigenic challenge[OS082].

Protein secretion stimulation. Decoction of the grain, administered intraperitoneally to mice at a dose of 100 mg/kg, increased protein content of saliva in streptozotocin-induced diabetic mice. The results were significant at $p < 0.01$ level[OS074].

Radical scavenging effect. Bran was active when scavenging of 1,1-diphenyl 1,2-

picrylhydrazine radicals was assayed, inhibitory concentration$_{50}$ was 0.875 mg/mL; scavenging of hydroxyl radicals, inhibitory concentration$_{50}$ 2.79 mg/mL and for superoxide, lethal concentration$_{50}$ 0.73 mg/mL[OS046].

Radioprotective effect. Rice seeds of cultivars Katakutara and Kusabue, kept in the seed hull and irradiated with γ-radiation, showed greater germination than those that had been dehulled and irradiated[OS093].

Salivary secretion. Decoction of the grain, administered intraperitoneally to mice at a dose of 100 mg/kg, was inactive vs pilocarpine-induced salivary flow in streptozotocin-diabetic mice[OS074].

Toxicity assessment. Ethanol (50%) extract of the grain, administered intraperitoneally to mice, produced LD$_{50}$ 750 mg/kg and maximum tolerated dose 500 mg/kg[OS001].

Ulcerogenic activity. Fixed oil of the dried seed husks, in the ration of rats, was active vs pylorus ligation-induced ulcers. The ulcers were reversible using cysteine[OS101].

Vitamin modification. Boiled white rice, administered to rats as the only diet for 23 days, produced significantly lower fecal concentrations of the main menaquinone-producing bacterial species (*Bacteroides fragilis* and *Bacteroides vulgatus*) than animals on either rice and bean diet or a stock diet. The rats on the boiled white rice diet developed symptoms of severe vitamin K deficiency within 23 days. Inclusion of autoclaved black-eye beans (*Vigna unguiculata*) in the diet prevented the bleeding syndrome[OS151].

White blood cell stimulant. The hemicellulose of bran fiber, administered to rats at a dose of 10% of the diet, produced weak activity on leukocytes[OS036].

White blood cell-macrophage stimulant. Water extract of the freeze-dried grain, at a concentration of 2 μg/mL, was active. Nitrite formation was used as an index of the macrophage-stimulating activity to screen effective foods[OS106].

REFERENCES

OS001 Dhar, M. L., M. M. Dhar, B. N. Dhawan, B. N. Mehrotra, and C. Ray. Screening of Indian plants for biological activity: Part I. **Indian J Exp Biol** 1968; 6: 232–247.

OS002 Hayashi, K. Anthocyanins. XIII. Several anthocyanins containing cyanidin as the aglycone. **Acta Phytochim** 1944; 14: 55.

OS003 Steenis-Kruseman, M. J. Van. Select Indonesian medicinal plants. **Organiz Sci Res Indonesia Bull** 1953; 18: 1.

OS004 Booth, A. N., E. M. Bickoff, and G. O. Kohler. Estrogen-like activity in vegetable oils and mill by-products. **Science** 1960; 131: 1807.

OS005 Ohmoto, T., M. Ikuse, and S. Natori. Triterpenoids of the *Gramineae*. **Phytochemistry** 1970; 9: 2137.

OS006 Ohmoto, T., T. Nikaido, K. Nakadai, and E. Tohyama. Triterpenoids and the related compounds from *Gardenia*. VII. **Yakugaku Zasshi** 1970; 90; 390.

OS007 Ortani, T. Nitrogen metabolism in crop plants. IX. Identification of (DL)-ascorbic acid in the immature seeds of several species of *Gramineae*. **Nippon Sakumotsu Gakkai Kiji** 1971; 40(1): 34–39.

OS008 Glennie, C. W., and J. B. Harborne. Flavone and flavonol 5-glucosides. **Phytochemistry** 1971; 10(6): 1325–1329.

OS009 Harborne, J. B., and E. Hall. Plant polyphenols—XII. The occurrence of tricin and of glycoflavones in grasses. **Phytochemistry** 1964; 3(3): 421-428.

OS010 Kortanakul, C., and J. Boonjawat. Rice bran lectin and its agglutination with nitrogen-fixing bacteria isolated from the rhizosphere of rice. Abstr 3rd Congress of the Federation of Asian and Oceanian Biochemists Bangkok Thailand, 1983: 74.

OS011 Pongpan, A., W. Avirutnant, and P. Chumsri. Some Thai plants as substrates for microbial protein production. **Mahidol Univ J Pharm Sci** 1983; 10(1): 15–18.

OS012 Ito, E., S. Takeo, H. Kado, et al. Studies on an antitumor polysaccharide RBS derived from rice bran. I. Preparation, physico-chemical properties and biological activities of RBS. **Yakugaku Zasshi** 1985; 105(2): 188–193.

OS013 Besson, E., G. Dellamonica, J. Chopin, et al. C-glycosylflavones from *Oryza sativa*. **Phytochemistry** 1985; 24(5): 1061–1064.

OS014 Kim, M., H. S. Koh, and H. Fukami. Isolation of c-glycosylflavones as probing stimulant of planthoppers in rice plant. **J Chem Ecol** 1985; 11(4): 441–452.

OS015 Koiso, Y., I. Ito, S. Y. Huang, et al. The effect of rice plant components on rice plant pathogen. I. Isolation of anastomosis promoting factors for conidia of G. *oryzae* from a rice plant (1.) **Yakugaku Zasshi** 1986; 106(5): 383–390.

OS016 Watanabe, M., Y. Sakai, T. Teraoka, et al. Novel C19-kaurane type of diterpenes (oryzalide A), a new antimicrobial compound isolated from healthy leaves of a bacterial leaf blight resistant cultivar of rice plant. **Agr Biol Chem** 1990; 54(4): 1103–1105.

OS017 Kodama, O., W. X. Li, S. Tamogami, and T. Akatsuka. Oryzalexin S, a novel stemarane-type diterpene rice phytolexin. **Biosci Biotech Biochem** 1992; 56(6): 1002–1003.

OS018 Liu, H., H. Y. Gu, X. Chen, S. J. Tang, N. S. Pan, and Z. L. Chen. Isolation and partial characterization of an antifungal protein from rice. **Curr Plant Sci Biotechnol Agr** 1993; 15: 11–17.

OS019 Kato, H., O. Kodama, and T. Akatsuka. Oryzalexin F, a diterpene phytoalexin from UV-irradiated rice leaves. **Phytochemistry** 1994; 36(2): 299–301.

OS020 Upreti, R. K., S. Ahmad, S. Shukla, and A. M. Kidwai. Experimental anorexigenic effect of a membrane proteoglycan isolated from plants. **J Ethnopharmacol** 1994; 42(1): 53–61.

OS021 Liu, H., H. Y. Hu, X. Chen, N. S. Pan, and Z. L. Chen. Isolation, purification, and characterization of an antifungal protein from rice. **Gaojishu Tongxun** 1994; 4(2): 22–26.

OS022 Takahashi, M., S. Moriguchi, M. Yoshikawa, and R. Sasaki. Isolation and characterization of oryzatensin: A novel bioactive peptide with ileum-contracting and immunomodulating

activities derived from rice albumin. **Biochem Mol Biol Int** 1994; 33(6): 1151–1158.

OS023 Scaglioni, L., A. Selva, L. Cattaruzza, and F. Menegus. Pantoyllactone primeveroside structure and its distribution with pantoyllactone glucoside in rice seedling organs. **Nat Prod Lett** 2000; 14(3): 159–166.

OS024 Zagari, A. Medicinal Plants. Vol 4, 5th Edition. Tehran University Publications, No 1810/4, Tehran, Iran Book 1992; 4: 969 pp.

OS025 Yoshida, S., K. Tazaki, and T. Minamikawa. Occurrence of shikimic and quinic acids in angiosperms. **Phytochemistry** 1975; 14: 195–197.

OS026 Kanamori, T., and H. Matsumoto. Role of glutamine in asparagine biosynthesis in rice plant roots. **Z Pflanzenphysiol** 1974; 74: 264.

OS027 Lancaster, L. A., and B. Rajadurai. An automated procedure for the determination of aluminum in soil and plant digests. **J Sci Food Agr** 1974; 25: 381.

OS028 Naser, A. M., M. A. El-Azmirly, and A. Z. Gomaa. Industrial application of the Egyptian rice germ oil in the field of surface coatings. I. Separation and modification of rice germ wax. **J Oil Colour Chen Ass** 1975; 58: 131.

OS029 Ogasawara, N., J. Koga, T. Yamauchi, and M. Shimura. Antifungal terpene compounds and process for producing the same. **Patent-Pct Int Appl-96 24,681** 1996: 68 pp.

OS030 Tsai, T. C., and S. H. Chen. The structure identification of two major anthocyanins in wu-no-tao (*Oryza sativa*). **Shipin Kexue** 1996; 23(3): 444–452.

OS031 Bouillant, M. L., C. Jacoud, I. Zanella, J. Favre-Bonvin, and R. Bally. Identification of 5-(12-heptadecenyl)-resorcinol in rice root exudates. **Phytochemistry** 1994; 35(3): 769–771.

OS032 Das, P. K., A. Chaudhuri, T. N. B. Kaimal, and U. T. Bhalerao. Isolation of gamma-oryzanol through calcium ion induced precipitation of anionic micellar aggregates. **J Agr Food Chem** 1998; 46(8): 3073–3080.

OS033 Park, K. H., J. D. Park, K. H. Hyun, M. Nakayama, and T. Yokota. Brassinosteroids and monoglycerides with brassinosteroid-like activity in immature seeds of *Oryza sativa* and *Perilla frutescens* and in cultured cells of *Nicotiana tabacum*. **Biosci Biotech Biochem** 1994; 58(12): 2241–2243.

OS034 Kodama, O., J. Miyakawa, T. Akatsuka, and S. Kiyosawa. Sakuranetin, a flavanone phytoalexin from ultraviolet-irradiated rice leaves. **Phytochemistry** 1992; 31(11): 3807–3809.

OS035 Unseld, E., D. R. Krishna, C. Fischer, and U. L. Klotz. Detection of desmethyldiazepam and diazepam in brain of different species and plants. **Biochem Pharmacol** 1989; 38(15): 2473–2478.

OS036 Takenaka, S., and Y. Itoyama. Rice bean hemicellulose increases the peripheral blood lymphocytes in rats. **Life Sci** 1993; 52(1): 9–12.

OS037 Kato, T., Y. Yamaguchi, T. Namai, and T. Hirukawa. Oxygenated fatty acids with anti-rice blast fungus activity in rice plants. **Biosci Biotech Biochem** 1993; 57(2): 283–287.

OS038 Gahlawat, P., and S. Sehgal. Phytic acid, saponins, and polyphenols in weaning food prepared from oven-heated green gram and cereals. **Cereal Chem** 1992; 69(4): 463–464.

OS039 Hegsted, M., M. M. Windhauser, M. S. Morris, and S. B. Lester. Stabilized rice bran and oat bran lower cholesterol in humans. **Nutr Res** 1993; 13(4): 387–398.

OS040 Ando, H., H. Iizuka, and T. Mitsunaga. Prolamin in rice grains. **Kinki Daigaku Nogakubu Kiyo** 1992; 25: 51–54.

OS041 Miller, J. B., E. Pang, and L. Bramall. Rice: A high or low glycemic index food? **Amer J Clin Nutr** 1992; 56(6): 1034–1036.

OS042 Rogers, E. J., S. M. Rice, R. J. Nicolosi, D. R. Carpenter, C. A. McClelland, and L. J. Romanczyk Jr. Identification and quantitation of gamma-oryzanol components and simultaneous assessment of tocols in rice bran oil. **J Amer Chem Soc** 1993; 70(3): 301–307.

OS043 Rustamani, M. A., K. Kanehisa, and H. Tsumuki. Aconitic acid content of some cereals and its effect on aphids. **Appl Entomol Zool** 1992; 27(1): 79–87.

OS044 Shahjahan, M., M. Mosihuzzaman, and A. Mian. Phenolic acids in rice plant (*Oryza sativa*). **J Bangladesh Chem Soc** 1992; 5(1): 59–63.

OS045 Nakashima, R., K. Hakamoto, Y. Katagiri, T. Mizutani, N. Ueda, and J. Yamamoto. Structure determination of a pigment from *Oryza sativa* Linn. (Kurogome). **Chem Express** 1993; 8(6): 393–396.

OS046 Osato, J. A., L. A. Santiago, G. M. Remo, M. S. Cuadra, and A. Mori. Antimicrobial and antioxidant activities of unripe papaya. **Life Sci** 1993; 53(17): 1383–1389.

OS047 Hiraga, Y., N. Nakata, H. Jin, et al. Effect of the rice bran-derived phytosterol cycloartenol ferulic acid ester on the central nervous system. **Arzneim-Forsch** 1993; 43(7): 715–721.

OS048 Mao, X. H., R. P. Xu, S. G. Wang, et al. Simultaneous extraction of oryzanol and yazhouning from crude rice bran oil. **Patent-Faming Zhuanli Shenqing Gongkai Shuomingshu**—1,067,448 1992: 14 pp.

OS049 Islam, M. A., D. Mahalanabis, and N. Majid. Use of rice-based oral rehydration solution in a large diarrhoea treatment centre in Bangladesh: in-house production, use and relative cost. **J Trop Med Hyg** 1994; 97(6): 341–346.

OS050 Okai, Y., T. Eksttikul, O. Svendsby, M. Izukz, K. Ito, and N. Minamiura. Antitumor activity in an extract of Thai rice seedlings. **J Ferment Bioeng** 1993; 76(5): 367–370.

OS051 Lehrfeld, J. HPLC separation and quantitation of phytic acid and some inositol phosphates in foods. **J Agr Food Chem** 1994; 42(12): 2726–2731.

OS052 Obata, H., K. Imai, N. Inoue, and M. Umebayashi. A highly sensitive quantitative determination of glutathione in plant roots by high performance gel filtration chromatography and fluorometic detection after pre-column derivatization with *N*-(7-dimethylamino-4-methyl coumarinyl)-maleimide. **Phytochem Anal** 1994; 5(5): 239–242.

OS053 Scott, I. M., and H. Yamamoto. Mass spectrometric quantification of salicylic acid in plant tissues. **Phytochemistry** 1994; 37(2): 336.

OS054 Hattori, A., H. Migitaka, M. Ligo, et al. Identification of melatonin in plants and its effects on plasma melatonin levels and binding to melatonin receptors in vertebrates. **Biochem Mol Biol Int** 1995; 35(3): 627–634.

OS055 Norton, R. A. Quantitation of steryl ferulate and p-coumarate esters from corn and rice. **Lipids** 1995; 30(3): 269–274.

OS056 Aoki, H., T. Akaike, K. Abe, et al. Antiviral effect of oryzacystatin, a proteinase inhibitor in rice, against Herpes Simplex Virus Type I *in vitro* and *in vivo*. **Antimicrob Agents Chemother** 1995; 39(4): 846–849.

OS057 Ohta, H., M. Maeda, Y. Nogata, K. Yoza, Y. Takeda, and Y. Osaiima. A simple determination of thiamin in rice (*Oryza sativa* L.) by high-performance liquid chromatography with post-column derivatization. **J Liq Chromatogr** 1993; 16(12): 2617–2629.

OS058 Moore, T. C., H. Yamane, N. Murofushi, and N. Takahashi. Concentrations of ENT-kaurene and squalene in vegetative rice shoots. **J Plant Growth Regul** 1988; 7(3): 145–151.

OS059 Lebenthal, E., U. Khin-Maung, D. D. K. Rolston, et al. Composition and preliminary evaluation of a hydrolyzed rice-based oral rehydration solution for the treatment of acute diarrhea in children. **J Amer Coll Nutr** 1995; 14(3): 299–303.

OS060 Silverman, P., M. Seskar, D. Kanter, P. Schweizer, J. P. Metraux, and I. Raskin. Salicylic acid in rice: Biosynthesis, conjugation and possible role. **Plant Physiol** 1995; 108(2): 633–639.

OS061 Macleod, R. J., H. P. J. Bennett, and J. R. Hamilton. Inhibition of intestinal secretion by rice. **Lancet** 1995; 346(8967): 90–92.

OS062 Ahmad, F. B., and D. K. Holdsworth. Traditional medicinal plants of Sabah, Malaysia. Part III. The Rungus people of Kudat. **Int J Pharmacog** 1995; 33(3): 262–264.

OS063 Bhattarai, N. K. Folk herbal remedies for gynaecological complaints in Central Nepal. **Int J Pharmacog** 1994; 32(1): 13–26.

OS064 Singh, V. K., and Z. A. Ali. Folk medicines in primary health care: Common plants used for the treatment of fevers in India. **Fitoterapia** 1994; 65(1): 68–74.

OS065 Toki, S. Preparation of antitumor protein PHI from rice bran. Patent-Japan Kokai Tokkyo Koho-63 179,899 1988; 10 pp.

OS066 Izquierdo-Pulido, M. L., T. A. Haard, J. Hung, and N. F. Haard. Oryzacystatin and other proteinase inhibitors in rice grain: Potential use as a fish processing aid. **J Agr Food Chem** 1994; 42(3): 616–622.

OS067 Perez, C., and C. Anesini. Antibacterial activity of alimentary plants against *Staphylococcus aureus* growth. **Amer J Chinese Med** 1994; 22(2): 169–174.

OS068 Mustafa, S. A., Z. E. A. Karrar, and J. I. A. Suliman. Cereal-based oral rehydration solutions in Sudanese children with diarrhoea: A comparative clinical trial of rice-based and sorghum-based oral rehydration solutions. **Ann Trop Paediat** 1995; 15(4): 313–319.

OS069 Coee, F. G., and G. J. Anderson. Ethnobotany of the Garifuna of Eastern Nicaragua. **Econ Bot** 1996; 50(1): 71–107.

OS070 Heinrich, M., H. Rimpler, and N. A. Barrera. Indigenous phytotherapy of gastrointestinal disorders in a lowland Mixe community (Oaxaca, Mexico): Ethnopharmacologic evaluation. **J Ethnopharmacol** 1992; 36(1): 63–80.

OS071 Liao, Z. K., J. Jiang, and X. P. Xu. The technical method for preparation of phytic acid and oryzenin. **Huaxi Yaoxue Zazhi** 1996; 11(1): 46–70.

OS072 Tokuyama, T. 5-Alpha-reductase inhibitor from rice for therapeutic use. Patent-Japan Kokai Tokkyo Koho-07 157,436 1993: 7 pp.

OS073 Lakshmi, K. B., and V. Vimala. Hypoglycemic effect of selected sorghum recipes. **Nutr Res** 1996; 16(10): 1651–1658.

OS074 Kimura, M., I. Kimura, and F. J. Chen. Combined potentiating effects of byakko-ka-ninjin-to, its constituents, rhizomes of anemarrhena, asphodeloides, timosaponin a-III, and calcium on pilocarpine-induced saliva secretion in streptozotocin-diabetic mice. **Biol Pharm Bull** 1996; 19(7): 926–931.

OS075 Goldberg, E. D., and J. R. Saltzman. Rice inhibits intestinal secretions. **Nutr Rev** 1996; 54(1): 36–37.

OS076 Itoh, T., K. Uchikawa, T. Tamura, and T. Matsumoto. Two new 4-alpha methylsterols in the seeds of *Brassica napus*. **Phytochemistry** 1977; 16: 1448 –1449.

OS077 Tsunakawa, M., A. Ohba, N. Sasaki, et al. Momilactone C, a minor constituent of growth inhibitors in rice husk. **Chem Lett** 1976; 1976: 1157.

OS078 Yasumoto, K., H. Tsuji, K. Iwami, and H. Mitsuda. Isolation from rice bran of a bound form of vitamin B-6 and its identification as 5'-O-(beta-D-glucopyranosyl) pyridoxine. **Agr Biol Chem** 1977; 41: 1061.

OS079 Ahn, E. M., M. H. Lee, Y. D. Rho, and N. I. Baek. Isolation of daucosterol from the rice hull of *Oryza sativa* L. **Han'guk Nonghwa Hakhoe Chi** 1998; 41(6): 486–488.

OS080 Yasukawa, K., T. Akihisa, Y. Kimura, T. Tamuara, and M. Takido. Inhibitory effect of cycloartenol ferulate, a component of rice bran, on tumor promotion in two-stage carcinogenesis in mouse skin. **Biol Pharm Bull** 1998; 21(10): 1072–1076.

OS081 Kim, Y. S., D. H. Kim, and J. Jung. Isolation of a novel auxin receptor from soluble fractions of rice (*Oryza sativa* L.) shoots. **FEBS Lett** 1998; 438(3): 241–244.

OS082 Kim, H. M., C. S. Kangk, E. H. Lee, and T. Y. Shin. The evaluation of the antianaphylactic effect of *Oryza sativa* L. subsp. *hsien ting* in rats. **Pharmacol Res** 1999; 40(1): 31–36.

OS083 Kim, H. M., D. K. Yi, and H. Y. Shin. The evaluation of the antianaphylactic effect of *Oryza sativa* L. in rats. **Amer J Chinese Med** 1999; 27(1): 63–71.

OS084 Taniguchi, H., A. Hosoda, T. Tsuno, Y. Maruta, and E. Nomura. Preparation of ferulic acid and its application for the synthesis of cancer chemopreventive agents. **Anticancer Res** 1999; 19(5A): 3757–3761.

OS085 Fan, H., T. Morioka, and E. Ito. Induction of apoptosis and growth inhibition of cultured human endometrial adeno-carcinoma cells (sawano) by an antitumor lipoprotein fraction of rice bran. **Gynecol Oncol** 2000; 76(2): 170–175.

OS086 Ohara, I., D. Agr, R. Tabuchi, K. Onai, and M. H. Econ. Effects of modified rice bran on serum lipids on taste preference in streptozotocin-induced diabetic rats. **Nutr Res** 2000; 20(1): 59–68.

OS087 Premakumari, K., and P. A. Kurup. Lipid metabolism in rats fed rice and tapioca. **Indian J Med Res** 1982; 76: 488–493.

OS088 Abe, H., K. Nakamura, T. Morishita, M. Uchiyama, S. Takatsuto, and N. Ikekawa. Endogenous brassinosteroids of the rice plant: Castasterone and dolichosterone. **Agr Biol Chem** 1984; 48(4): 1103–1104.

OS089 Ikekawa, N., S. Takatsuto, T. Kitsuwa, H. Saito, T. Morishita, and H. Abe. Analysis of natural brassinosteroids by gas chromatography and gas chromatography-mass spectrometry. **J Chromatogr** 1984; 290(1): 289–302.

OS090 Tashmenov, R. S., K. A. Sabirov, and S. M. Makhkamov. Improved process for extraction of phytin. **Khim Farm Zh** 1984; 18(10): 1229–1231.

OS091 Kamath, P. S., J. B. Dilawari, S. Raghavan, R. P. Batta, S. Mukewar, and R. J. Dash. Plasma insulin response to legumes and carbohydrate foods. **Indian J Med Res** 1982; 76: 583–590.

OS092 Roy, A. N., B. P. Sinha, and K. C. Gupta. The inhibitory effect of plant juices on the infectivity of top necrosis virus of pea. **Indian J Microbiol** 1979; 19: 198–201.

OS093 Osawa, T., T. Narasimhan, S. Kawakishi, M. Namiki, and T. Tashiro. Antioxidative defense systems in rice hull against damage caused by oxygen radicals. **Agr Biol Chem** 1985; 49(10): 3085–3087.

OS094 Ito, S., M. Kojima, and Y. Fujino. Occurrence of phytoglycolipid in rice bran. **Agr Biol Chem** 1985; 49(6): 1873–1875.

OS095 Anon. Isolation of phytin from rice bran. Patent-Japan Kokai Tokkyo Koho-60 58,993 1985: 2 pp.

OS096 Hikino, H., M. Murakami, Y. Oshima, and C. Konno. Isolation and hypoglycemic activity of oryzarans A, B, C and D: Glycans of *Oryza sativa* roots.1. **Planta Med** 1986; 52(6): 490–492.

OS097 Kaneta, M., and N. Sugiyama. Identification of flavone compounds in eighteen *Gramineae* species. **Agr Biol Chem** 1973; 37: 2663–2665.

OS098 Kato, Y., and K. Matsuda. An alpha-glucan from suspension-cultured rice cells. **Plant Cell Physiol** 1987; 28(3): 439–446.

OS099 Manabe, H. Distribution of d-alanyl-glycine and related compounds in *Oryza* species. **Phytochemistry** 1986; 25(9): 2233–2235.

OS100 Raghuram, T. C., U. B. Rao, and C. Rukmini. Studies on hypolipidemic effects of dietary rice bran oil in human subjects. **Nutr Rep Int** 1989; 39(5): 889–895.

OS101 Jayaraj, A. P., F. I. Tovey, C. G. Clark, K. R. Rees, J. S. White, and M. R. Lewin. The ulcerogenic and protective action of rice and rice fractions in experimental peptic ulceration. **Clin Sci** 1987; 72(4): 463–466.

OS102 Seetharamaiah, G. S., and N. Chandrasekhara. Studies on hypocholesterolemic activity of rice bran oil. **Atherosclerosis** 1989; 78(2/3): 219–223.

OS103 Harada, N., N. Okazaki, Y. Kizaki, and S. Kobayashi. Identification and distribution of an aroma component in rice. **Nippon Jozo Kyokaishi** 1990; 85(5): 350–352.

OS104 Baggott, J. E., T. Ha, W. H. Vaughn, M. M. Juliana, J. M. Hardin, and C. J. Grubbs. Effect of miso (Japanese soybean paste) and NaCl on DMBA-induced rat mammary tumors. **Nutr Cancer** 1990; 14(2): 103–109.

OS105 Sato, A. Studies on anti-tumor activity of crude drugs. I. The effects of aqueous extracts of some crude drugs in short term screening test. **Yakugaku Zasshi** 1989; 109(6): 407–423.

OS106 Miwa, M., Z. L. Kong, K. Shinohara, and M. Watanabe. Macrophage stimulating activity of foods. **Agr Biol Chem** 1990; 54(7): 1863–1866.

OS107 Klosa, J. Rice oil for protection of skin from aging, folding and detergents. Patent-Ger Offen-3,938,284 1990: 5 pp.

OS108 Kim, C. J., S. K. Cho, M. S. Shin, et al. Hypoglycemic activity of medicinal plants. **Arch Pharm Res** 1990; 13(4): 371–373.

OS109 Yoshida, T., T. Nakata, and E. Ichishima. DNA topoisomerase I from rice: Enzyme synthesis in germination and partial purification from cultured cells. **Phytochemistry** 1991; 30(12): 3885–3887.

OS110 Tanchotikul, U., and T. C. Y. Hsieh. An improved method for quantification of 2-acetyl-1-pyrroline, a "popcorn"-like aroma, in aromatic rice by high-resolution gas chromatography/mass spectrometry/selected ion monitoring. **J Agr Food Chem** 1991; 39(5): 944–947.

OS111 Shao, J. H, and J. G. Wu. Phytin extraction from rice bran and preparation of inositol. **Hua Hsueh Chih Ji** 1990; 31(11): 518–521.

OS112 Koh, H. S., M. Kim, T. Obata, H. Fukami, and S. Ishii. Antifeedant in barnyard grass against the brown planthopper-trans-aconitic acid. Rice Brown Planthopper (*Pap Semin*) 1976 Food Fert Technol Center Asian Pac Reg, Taipei, Taiwan.

OS113 Akbarov, R. R., K. S. Mukhaedova, and S. T. Akramov. Method for obtaining phytin from rice middlings. **Khim Prir Soedin** 1979; 15(4): 540–543.

OS114 Wu, P. L., Q. S. Gao, H. S. Chen, Y. L. Shan, A. Z. Niu, and W. Du. Rapid determination and screening technique of protein content of single grains in rice breeding. **Chung-Kuo Nunh Yeh K'O Hsueh (Peking)** 1979; 4: 51–55.

OS115 Fujino, Y., and M. Ohnishi. Novel sterylglycosides. Cellotetraosyl sitosterol and cellopentaosyl sitosterol in rice grain. **Proc Japan Acad Serv B** 1979; 55: 243–246.

OS116 Cartwright, D. W., P. Langcake, R. J. Pryce, D. P. Leworthy, and J. P. Ride. Isolation and characterization of two phytoalexins from rice as monilactones A and B. **Phytochemistry** 1981; 20: 535–537.

OS117 Tan, W. J., A. H. l. Hung, and T. H. Han. Chemical constituents of straw of *Oryza sativa*. **Chung Ts'ao Yao** 1980; 11: 440–441.

OS118 Kawai, K., K. Sugawara, and T. Moringag. Antitumor substance. Patent-Eur Appl-27,514 1981; 45 pp.

OS119 Ito, E. Antitumor agents from rice bran. Patent-Japan Kokai Tokkyo Koho-81 29,519 1981; 12 pp.

OS120 Akatsuka, T., O. Kodama, H. Kato, Y. Kono, and S. Takeuchi. 3-Hydroxy-7-oxo-sandaaraco-primaradiene (Oryzalexin A), a new phytolexin isolated from rice blast leaves. Agr Biol Chem 1983; 47(2): 445–447.

OS121 Fushiya, S., K. Takahaashi, S. Nakatsuyama, Y, Sato, S. Nozoe, and S. Takagi. Co-occurrence of nicotianamine and avenic acids in Avena sativa and Oryza sativa. Phytochemistry 1982; 21: 1907–1908.

OS122 Okuyama, E., and M. Yamazaki. The principles of Tetragonia tetragonoides having anti-ulcerogenic activity. Ll. Isolation and structure of cerebrosides. Chem Pharm Bull 1983; 31(7): 2209–2219.

OS123 Kono, Y., S. Takeuchi, O. Kodama, and T. Akatsuka. Absolute configuration of Oryzalexin A and structures of its related phytoalexins isolated from rice blast leaves infected with Pyricularia oryzae. Agr Biol Chem 1984; 48(1): 253–255.

OS124 Chindavanig, A. Effect of vegetable oils on plasma cholesterol in man and dog. Thesis-Master Department of Biochemistry, Mahidol University, Bangkok, Thailand, 1971; 58 pp.

OS125 Hirschhorn, H. H. Botanical remedies of the former Dutch East Indies (Indonesia). 1. Eumycetes, Pteridophyta, Gymnospermae, Angiospermae (monocotyledons only). J Ethnopharmacol 1983; 7(2): 123–156.

OS126 Al-Shamma, A., and L. A. Mitscher. Comprehensive survey of indigenous Iraqi plants for potential economic value. 1. Screening results of 327 species for alkaloids and antimicrobial agents. J Nat Prod 1979; 42(6): 633–642.

OS127 Shigematsu, Y., N. Murofushl, K. Ito, C. Kaneda, S. Kawabe, and N. Takahashi. Sterols and asparagines in the rice plant, endogenous factors related resistance against the brown planthopper. Agr Biol Chem 1982; 46(11): 2877–2879.

OS128 Nakamura, T. Contact dermatitis to Oryza. Contact Dermatitis 1983; 9(1): 80.

OS129 Suwa, Y., T. Kobayashi, N. Kiyotan, and H. Yoshizumi. Antimutagenic agent and method of inactivating the mutagenicity of foods and beverages by using this agent. Patent-Eur Pat Appl-124,891 1984; 36 pp.

OS130 Velazco, E. A. Herbal and traditional practices related to maternal and child health care. Rural Reconstruction Review 1980; 35–39.

OS131 Molla, A. M., M. Hossain, S. A. Sarker, A. Molla, and W. B. Greenough III. Rice-powder electrolyte solution as oral therapy in diarrhoea due to Vibrio cholerae and Escherichia coli. Lancet 1982; 1(8285): 1317–1319.

OS132 Minaguchi, S., E. Sudoh, M. Takeshita, et al. Effects of various immunopotentiators on ENNG-induced carcinogenesis in rats. Igaku No Ayumi 1985; 133(5): 321–322.

OS133 Yamazaki, N., T. Otomo, and K. Kawai. Antitumor glycoprotein extraction from rice bran. Patent-Japan Kokai Tokkyo Koho-61 143,323. 1986; 9 pp.

OS134 Sharma, R. D. and C. Rukmini. Hypocholesterolemic activity of unsaponifiable matter or rice bran oil. Indian J Med Res. 1987; 3: 278–281.

OS135 Polasa, K., and C. Rukmini. Mutagenicity tests of cashewnut shell liquid, rice-bran oil and other vegetable oils using the Salmonella typhimurium/microsome system. Food Chem Toxicol 1987; 25(10): 763–766.

OS136 Hemadri, K., and S. S. Rao. Jaundice: Tribal medicine. Ancient Sci Life 1984; 3(4): 209–212.

OS137 Hikino, H., M. Takahashi, Y. Oshima, and C. Konno. Isolation and hypoglycemic activity of Oryza brans A, B, C and D, glycans of Oryza sativa bran. Planta Med 1988; 54(1): 1–3.

OS138 Yanfg, L. L., K. Y. Yen, Y. Kiso, and H. Kikino. Antihepatotoxic actions of Formosan plant drugs. J Ethnopharmacol 1987; 19(1): 103–110.

OS139 Ramirez, V. R., L. J. Mostacero, A. E. Garcia, et al. Vegetales empleados en medicina tradicional norperuana. Banco Agrario Del Peru & NACL Univ Trujillo, Peru 1988; 54 pp.

OS140 Dilavari, J. B., V. K. A. Kumar, S. Khurana, R. Bhatnagar, and R. J. Dash. Effect of legumes on blood sugar in diabetes mellitus. **Indian J Med Res** 1987; 85(2): 184–187.

OS141 Alabaster, O., Z. C. Tang, A. Frost, and N. Shivapurkar. Potential synergism between wheat bran and psyllium: Enhanced inhibition of colon cancer. **Cancer Lett** 1993; 75(1): 53–58.

OS142 Ashikari, H. Estrone-like substance present in rice embryo. **Arb Med Fakultat Okayama** 1940; 6: 448.

OS143 Reiss, M., and S. Pereny. Estruation effect of feeding polished rice on rats. **Endocrinologie** 1928; 1: 411–418.

OS144 Krishnamoorthy, V. and T. R. Seshadri. Survey of anthocyanins from Indian sources: Part III. **J Sci Ind Res-B** 1962; 21: 591–593.

OS145 Wasuwat, S. A list of Thai medicinal plants. Research Report, ASRCT, No 1 on Res. Project 17. 1967; 22 pp.

OS146 Fitelson, J. The occurrence of squalene in natural fats. **J Ass Offic Agr Chem** 1943; 26: 506–511.

OS147 Greer, M. A., and E. B. Astwood. The antithyroid effect of certain foods in man as determined with radioactive iodine. **Endocrinology** 1948; 43: 105–119.

OS148 Siba, P. M., D. W. Pethick, and D. J. Hampson. Pigs experimentally infected with *Serpulina hyodysenteriae* can be protected from developing swine dysentery by feeding them a highly digestible diet. **Epidemiol Infect** 1966; 116(2): 207–216.

OS149 Jujiwaki, T., and K. Furusho. The effects of rice bran broth bathing in patients with atopic dermatitis. **Acta Paediatr Jpn** 1992; 3495): 505–510.

OS150 Hildebrandt, L. A., and J. A. Marlett. Starch bioavailability in the upper gastrointestinal tract of colectomized rats. **J Nutr** 1991; 121(7): 1141.

OS151 Mathers, J. C., F. Fernandez, M. J. Hill, P. T. McCarthy, M. J. Shearer, and A. Oxley. Dietary modification of potential vitamin K supply from enteric bacterial menaquinones in rats. **Br j Nutr** 1990; 63(3): 639–652.

OS152 Juliano, B. O., C. M. Perez, S. Komindr, and S. Banphotkasem. Properties of Thai cooked rice and noodles differing in glycemic index in non-insulin-dependent diabetics. **Plant Foods Hum Nutr** 1989; 39(4): 369–374.

OS153 Mani, U. V., S. Bhatt, N. C. Mehta, S. N. Pradhan, V. Shah, and I. Mani. Glycemic index of traditional Indian carbohydrate foods. **J Am Coll Nutr** 1990; 9(6): 573–577.

OS154 Torsdottir, I., M. Alpsten, D. Andersson, R. J. Brummer, and H. Anderson. Effect of different starchy foods in composite meals on gastric emptying rate and glucose metabolism. I. Comparisons between potatoes, rice and white beans. **Hum Nutr Clin Nutr** 1984; 38(5): 329–338.

OS155 Datla, K. P., R. D. Bennett, V. Zbarsky, et al. The antioxidant drink 'effective microorganism-X (EM-X)" pre-treatment attenuates the loss of nigrostriatal dopaminergic neurons in 6-hydroxydopamine-lesion rat model of Parkinson's disease. **J Pharm Pharmacol** 2004; 56(5): 649–654.

OS156 Badria, F. A. Melatonin, sertonin, and tryptamine in some Egyptian food and medicinal plants. **J Med Food** 2002; 5(3): 153–157.

OS157 Hyun, J. W., and H. S. Chung. Cyanidin and Malvidin from *Oryza sativa* cv. Heugjinjubyeo mediate cytotoxicity against human monocytic leukemia cells by arrest of G(2)/M phase and induction of apoptosis. **J Agric Food Chem** 2004; 52(8): 2213–2217.

OS158 Hong, Z., M. Ueguchi-Tanaka, K. Umemura, Set al. A rice brassinosteroids-deficient mutant, ebisu-dwarf (d2), is caused by a loss of function of a new member of cytochrome P450. **Plant Cell** 2003; 15(12): 2900–2910.

OS159 Kono, Y., A. Kojima, R. Nagai, et al. Antibacterial diterpenes and their fatty acid conjugates from rice leaves. **Phytochemistry** 2004; 65(9): 1291–1298.

12 | Plantago ovata

Forsk.

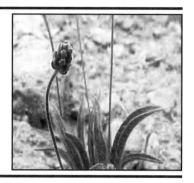

Common Names

Ashwagolam	India	Lisn al kalb	Arabic countries
Babka	Poland	Obeko	Japan
Barhanj	Arabic countries	Plantago	United States
Bidr qtn	Arabic countries	Plantain	United States
Blond psyllium	Arabic countries	Psillo indiano	Germany
Buzar qatona	Arabic countries	Qurayta	Arabic countries
Ch-chientzu	China	Rebla	Arabic countries
Common plantain	Arabic countries	Spangur	India
Hab zargah	Arabic countries	Spogel	Iran
Isphghol	India	Warak sabun masasah	Arabic countries

BOTANICAL DESCRIPTION

Plantago ovata is a stemless, soft, hairy annual herb of the PLANTAGINACEAE family that grows to a height of 30–45 cm. The leaves are 7.5–23 cm long, 0.5–1 cm broad, narrowly linear, linear lanceolate or filiform, opposite, finely acuminate entire or distantly toothed, attenuated at the base and usually three-nerved. The root system has a well-developed taproot with few fibrous secondary roots. A number of flowering shoots arise from the base of the plant. The flower spikes turn reddish brown at ripening, the lower leaves dry, and the upper leaves yellow. Plants flower approx 60 days after planting. Flowers are numerous, small, and white, in ovoid or cylindrical spikes 1.3–3.8 cm long, bracts 4 mm long and broad. The corolla gives attachment to four protruded stamina, ovary free with one or two cells, containing one or more ovules. The style capillar and terminated by a single subulate stigma. The fruit is a small pyxidium covered by the persistent corolla and enclosed in capsules that open at maturity. They are composed of a proper integument which covers a fleshy endosperm at the center of which is a cylindrical axile and a homotype embryo, ovoid-oblong or boat-shaped, smooth and yellowish brown, acute at one end 2–3 mm long, pale-green brown with a darker elongated spot on the convex side. On the concave side, the hilium is covered with the remains of a thin white membrane. It has no odor or taste, but the herbage is demulcent, bitter, and somewhat astringent. Seeds are hard, translucent, boat-shaped structure, up to 8 mm long and

From: *Medicinal Plants of the World, vol. 3: Chemical Constituents, Traditional and Modern Medicinal Uses*
By: I. A. Ross © Humana Press Inc., Totowa, NJ

1 mm broad. The surface is glossy and shining, with a pinkish brown color. There is an oval spot in the center of convex (dorsal) surface. On the concave (ventral) surface is a deep furrow is seen with a hilum that appears as a red spot in the center.

ORIGIN AND DISTRIBUTION

Plantago ovata originated from Europe to Southern Mediterranean to Eastern Asia (India, Iraq, Iran, Spain, and Canary Islands). It is produced commercially in several European countries, Pakistan, and India. Seed produced from *Plantago ovata* is known in trading circles as white or blonde psyllium, Indian Plantago, or Isabgol; the common name in India for *Plantago ovata*, comes from the Persian words "isap" and "ghol" which mean horse ear, which is descriptive of the shape of the seed. India dominates the world market in the production and export of psyllium. In India, *Plantago ovata* is cultivated mainly in North Gujarat as a "Rabi" or post-rainy season crop. An important environmental requirement of this crop is a dry open place. Psyllium research and field trials in the United States have been conducted mainly in Arizona and Washington. A major cultural problem limiting psyllium production in the upper midwest is the shattering characteristic of the mature crop. Some success has been achieved by crossbreeding high-yielding Indian varieties with varieties that are more shatter-tolerant.

TRADITIONAL MEDICINAL USES

India. Decoction of dried seeds is taken orally for diarrhea[PO030] and as a demulcent[PO052]. Seeds are taken externally as an emollient poultice, for constipations, and for gastric complaints[PO052].

Iran. Water extract of the dried seed is administered externally for its inflammatory and emollient effects. Mixed with coconut juice, it is used as a diuretic. Dried seeds are taken orally for diarrhea and indigestion associated with bile secretion abnormalities. Mucilage of the dried seed is used externally as an emollient. Seedcoat of the dried seed is taken orally as a bulk laxative. Acetic acid extract of the dried seed is used externally for rheumatoid arthritis and gout. Infusion of the dried seed is taken orally for urinary tract inflammations[PO005].

Spain. Leaf is taken orally by infusion for cold[PO045]

Thailand. Hot water extract of the dried seed husks is taken orally as a demulcent and for diarrhea[PO061].

CHEMICAL CONSTITUENTS

(ppm unless otherwise indicated)
Alanine, (DL): Sd[PO062]
Amyrin, α: Sd[PO073]
Amyrin, β: Sd[PO073]
Asparagine, l, (–): Sd[PO062]
Aucubin glucoside: Sd[PO073]
Campesterol: Sd[PO073]
Cystine, l: Sd[PO062]
Docosane, N: Sd Ct[PO004]
Dotriacontane, iso: Sd Ct[PO004]
Dotriacontane, N: Sd Ct[PO004]
Eicosane, N: Sd Ct[PO004]
Fixed oil (*Plantago ovata*): Endosperm 8.8%[PO070]
Fructose: Sd[PO073]
Glucose: Sd[PO073]
Glutamic acid: Sd[PO062]
Glycine: Sd[PO062]
Heneicosane, N: Sd Ct[PO004]
Hentriacontane, iso: Sd Ct[PO004]
Hentriacontane, N: Sd Ct[PO004]
Heptacosane, N: Sd Ct[PO004]
Heptadecane, iso: Sd Ct[PO004]
Heptadecane, N: Sd Ct[PO004]
Hexacosane, N: Sd Ct[PO004]
Hexadecane, ante-iso: Sd Ct[PO004]
Hexadecane, iso: Sd Ct[PO004]
Hexadecane, N: Sd Ct[PO004]
Indicaine: Sd[PO073]
Leucine, nor, (DL): Sd[PO062]
Linoleic acid: Sd oil 53.4%[PO070], Sd Ct[PO004]
Linolenic acid: Sd Ct[PO004]
Luteolin: Lf[PO102]
Lysine, l: Sd[PO062]
Myristic acid: Sd Ct[PO004]
Nonacosane, iso: Sd Ct[PO004]
Nonacosane, N: Sd Ct[PO004]

Nonadecane, N: Sd Ct[PO004]
Octadecane, ante-iso: Sd Ct[PO004]
Octadecane, iso: Sd Ct[PO004]
Octadecane, N: Sd Ct[PO004]
Octadec-cis-12-enoic acid, 9-oxo: Sd oil[PO049]
Oleic acid: Sd oil[PO070], Sd Ct[PO004]
Palmitic acid: Sd Ct[PO004]
Pentacosane, iso: Sd Ct[PO004]
Pentacosane, N: Sd Ct[PO004]
Plantago ovata mucilage: Sd husk[PO060]
Plantagonine: Sd[PO073]
Planteose: Sd[PO002]
Ricinoleic acid, iso: Sd oil[PO049]
Sitosterol, β: Sd[PO073]
Stearic acid: Sd Ct[PO004]
Stigmasterol: Sd[PO073]
Sucrose: Sd[PO073]
Tetracosane, N: Sd Ct[PO004]
Triacontane, N: Sd Ct[PO004]
Tricosane, N: Sd Ct[PO004]
Tritriacontane, iso: Sd Ct[PO004]
Tritriacontane, N: Sd Ct[PO004]
Tyrosine: Sd[PO062]
Valine, (DL): Sd[PO062]

PHARMACOLOGICAL ACTIVITIES AND CLINICAL TRIALS

Abortifacient effect. Dried seeds, administered intravaginally to pregnant women, were active[PO063]. The seedcoat, administered intrauterine to pregnant women at a dose of 350 g/person, was active[PO059].

Absorption effect. Dried seed husks, administered orally to adults at a dose of 3.5 g/person, decreased the bioavailability of carbamazepine[PO044].

Allergenic activity. Fiber of the dried seed, administered orally to female adults, was active. Total serum immunoglobulin (Ig) E was elevated in a 40-year-old woman with allergic cutaneous and respiratory symptoms associated with chronic psyllium ingestion[PO037]. Dried seedcoat, administered orally to adults, was active. A 60-year-old female suffered an anaphylactic reaction after ingestion of a psyllium-containing cereal[PO054]. Skin prick result from psyllium powder and specific IgE antibodies were positive in a 31-year-old atopic woman who

prepared a laxative containing Plantago ovata seeds twice daily (Plantaben) prescribed to her paralytic mother. Methacholine inhalation test revealed mild bronchial hyperresponsiveness (PC_{20} = 1.5 mg/mL), which elicited an isolated early asthmatic response[PO086]. Two years after initiating regular psyllium-containing laxative use, a 40-year-old woman suffered with pruritic macular, an urticarial rash involving the entire body including the palms, soles, and oropharynx sparing only the face. There was an associated sensation of chest and throat tightness and lip swelling. The signs and symptoms resolved on discontinuation of the psyllium and occurred immediately after the patient initiated a challenge test. The total serum IgE was elevated, and the modified radioallergosorbent test (RAST) for psyllium-specific IgE was positive (Plantago ovata antigen)[PO093].

Anaphylactic response. Dried seeds, administered orally to female adults, produced wheezing, throat and chest tightness, urticaria, itching, nasal congestion, and vomiting after ingestion of the psyllium[PO021]. A severe anaphylactic reaction was produced by the ingestion of psyllium, a major constituent of several bulk laxatives. The hypersensitivity was confirmed by skin testing and RAST[PO101].

Anti-artherosclerotic effect. Husks, administered to African green monkeys at a concentration of 10% of diet, were active. The monkeys were fed a high cholesterol diet[PO025].

Antibacterial activity. Water extract of the dried seed, on agar plate at concentration of 10 mg/mL, was inactive on Corynebacterium diphtheriae, Diplococcus pneumoniae, Staphylococcus aureus, and Streptococcus viridans and produced weak activity on Streptococcus pyogenes[PO057].

Antidiabetic activity. Dietary psyllium fiber, administered to patients with type 2 diabetes at three doses of 5 g each daily before meals, produced no significant changes in patient's weight. Fasting plasma glucose, total cholesterol, low-density lipoprotein (LDL) cholesterol, and triglyceride levels showed a reduction ($p < 0.05$), whereas high-density lipoprotein (HDL) cholesterol increased significantly ($p < 0.01$) after the treatment. The 125 subjects were given a 6-week period of diet counseling, followed by a 6-week of treatment period[PO079].

Antidiarrheal activity. Ethanol extract (50%) of the dried seed, administered to guinea pigs and rabbits at a dose of 300 mg/kg, was inactive on the ileum vs *Escherichia coli*-enterotoxin-induced diarrhea[PO030]. The fiber, administered intragastrically to 10 calves with diarrhea at a dose of 18.89 g/L, was equivocal, and breath hydrogen was decreased[PO034]. Seedcoat, administered orally to human adults at a dose of 30 g/day, was active[PO028].

Antigalactogogue effect. Dried kernel, administered to cows at a concentration of 50% of diet, was inactive[PO066].

Antihypercholesterolemic activity. Seeds, administered orally to 20 adults with mild hypercholesterolemia at a dose of 5.1 g/day for 40 days, reduced LDL cholesterol by 8% and total cholesterol by 6%[PO022]. Dried seed fiber, in the ration of Syrian hamster at a dose of 7.5% of diet, was active[PO038]. Dried seed fiber, administered orally to adults at a dose of 10.2 g/day, was active[PO040]. Dried seed fiber, administered orally to 50 healthy children 2 to 11 years of age at a dose of 6.4 g/day for 12 weeks, was active[PO042]. The hydrophobic colloid of the dried seed, administered in the ration of sea quails at a dose of 10% of diet, was active vs diet-inducing hypercholesterolemia[PO019]. The seed hull, administered in the ration of genetically diabetic mice at a dose of 2.5% of diet for 18 weeks, was active. Total cholesterol was lower, and HDL-cholesterol higher in psyllium-fed than in placebo-fed animals[PO051]. The seed hull, administered orally to 286 adults with hypercholesterolemia at a dose of 10.2 g/day, was active[PO014]. Husks, administered to male rats at a dose of 10% of diet, reduced total cholesterol and increased HDL-cholesterol levels in animals fed a high-cholesterol diet[PO009]. The husk, administered orally to 25 children of both sexes with hypercholesterolemia at a dose of 58 g/day for 6 weeks, was active on the blood. Significant reduction in total and LDL cholesterol levels was noted during the treatment period[PO010]. The seed, administered to male rats at a dose of 10% of diet, reduced total cholesterol and increased HDL cholesterol levels in animals fed a high-cholesterol diet[PO009]. The seed, administered orally to 28 adults of both sexes with mild hypercholesterolemia at a dose of 8.06 g/day for 3 months, was active. After the treatment, serum total cholesterol, LDL cholesterol, and artherogenic index significantly decreased, but the level of HDL cholesterol, triglyceride, and urea nitrogen was not affected[PO015]. Husk, administered orally to adults of both sexes at a dose of 3 g/day, was active on the blood. A meta-analysis was done to determine the effect of consumption of psyllium-enriched cereal products on blood total cholesterol, LDL and HDL cholesterol levels to estimate the magnitude of the effect among 404 adults with mild to moderate hypercholesterolemia who consumed a low-fat diet. Female subjects were divided into two groups to provide a rough estimate of the effect of menopausal status (premenopausal < 50 years, postmenopausal > 50 years) on blood lipids. The meta-analysis indicated that subjects who consumed a psyllium cereal had lower total cholesterol and LDL cholesterol concentrations (differences of 0.31 mmol/L [5%] on 0.35 mmol/L [9%], respectively) than subjects who ingested a control cereal. HDL cholesterol concentrations were unaffected. There was no effect of sex, age, or menopausal status on blood lipids. The results indicated that consuming a psyllium-enriched cereal as part of a low-fat diet improves the blood lipid profile on hypercholesterolemic adults over that which can be achieved with a low-fat diet alone[PO011]. Seed oil, administered by gastric intubation to cholesterol fed rabbits at a dose of 5 mL/animal, was active[PO071]. Seedcoat, administered orally to nine adults with hyperlipoproteinemia at a dose of 30 g/day for 11 days, decreased serum and LDL cholesterol. The treatment increased HDL cholesterol precursors and fecal elimination of cholesterol and bile acids[PO050].

Antihyperglycemic activity. The seed hull, administered to genetically diabetic mice at a dose of 2.5% of diet for 18 weeks, produced higher levels of insulin than in the control and placebo group[PO051]. Psyllium decreased the amount of dialyzable glucose when added at a concentration of 20% to in vitro mix of bran cereal and human saliva. Bran, administered orally to adults at a dose of 10% of diet, lowered the glycemic index of a bran cereal meal when taken just before or concurrently with meal in both diabetic and normal volunteers[PO056].

Antihyperlipemic activity. The seed hull, administered to genetically diabetic mice at a dose of 2.5% of diet for 18 weeks, was inactive[PO051]. Husks and seeds, administered in ration of male rats at a dose of 10%, were active on the liver and reduced the lipid levels in animals fed a high-cholesterol diet[PO009]. Seedcoat, administered orally to nine adults with hyperlipoproteinemia at a dose of 30 g/day for 11 days, decreased serum cholesterol, lowered LDL, and slightly increased HDL. Serum triglycerides were unchanged. Cholesterol precursors and fecal elimination of cholesterol and bile acids were increased[PO050].

Antihypertriglyceridemic effect. Fiber of the fresh seed husks, administered orally to adults of both sexes at a dose of 7 g/day, was active. Triglyceride level continued to drop 90 days after treatment was discontinued. Results were significant at $p < 0.01$ level[PO039].

Antihypocholesterolemic activity. $CHCl_3/$ MeOH (9:1) extract of the husks, administered orally to nine patients with primary hypercholesterolemia at a dose of 10.2 g/day, produced a decrease in total cholesterol and LDL levels[PO026]. Husks, administered in the ration of African green monkeys at a concentration of 10% of diet, were active. Plasma cholesterol concentrations were reduced by decreasing LDL synthesis[PO020]. Monkeys fed the high-cholesterol diet showed a 39% decrease in serum cholesterol[PO025]. Dried husks fiber, administered orally to adults of both sexes at doses of 13.7% of diet, was active[PO032].

Antileukemic activity. Aucubin, in combination with caffeic acid, chlorogenic acid, ferulic acid, *p*-coumaric acid, and vanillic acid, exhibited weak antileukemic activity (inhibitory concentration $[IC]_{50}$ 26–56 µg/mL, international system of units 2–11) on human leukemia and lymphoma cell lines. Water-insoluble compounds, such as triterpenoids (oleanolic acid and ursolic acid), monotepene (linalool), and flavonoid (luteolin) produced strong activity[PO077].

Anti-nematodal activity. Water extract of the dried seed, at various concentrations, was active on *Meloidogyne incognita*[PO064].

Anti-yeast activity. Ethanol (80%) extract of the dried entire plant, on agar plate at a concentration of 1 mg/mL, was inactive on *Candida albicans*[PO065].

Appetite suppressant. Dried seeds powder, administered orally to adults at a dose of 20 g/person 3 hours before feeding, produced a significant increase in sense of fullness and a decrease in fat consumption[PO043].

Bile acid synthesis stimulation. Fiber, administered in ration of male rats at a dose of 5% of the diet, produced a higher total bile acid pool size compared to rats fed cellulose. It also lowered the hydrophobicity of the bile acid pool[PO036].

Bile secretion increase. Dried seeds, administered orally to 20 male adults with mild hypercholesterolemia at a dose of 5.1 g/day for 40 days, were active[PO022]. Fiber, administered in the ration of male rats at a dose of 5% of diet, was active[PO036].

Carcinogenesis inhibition. Fiber, administered orally to male rats at a concentration of 4%, was active. Wheat bran and psyllium (1:1), at a total level of 18% dietary fiber, offered the highest protection against colon tumor development[PO069].

Cervical dilator. Isaptent, prepared from granulated *Plantago ovata* seed husk, administered as a cervical dilator to 804 women between 15 and 45 years of age, achieved satisfactory dilatation in 94% of the cases. The cervical dilatation bore no relationship to age, parity, and gestation period of the subjects. There was no apparent damage to the cervix, and the vaginal flora remained unchanged in the randomly selected subjects[PO059].

Cholesterol absorption inhibition. Fiber, administered in ration of male hamsters at a concentration of 7.5% of diet, was inactive[PO033]. Seeds, administered orally to 20 male adults with mild hypercholesterolemia at a dose of 5.1 g/day for 40 days, were active[PO022].

Cholesterol level decrease. The husks and seeds were administered orally to six normal adult males and five adult males with ileostomy and six normal adult males and four adult males with ileostomy, respectively, at a dose of 10 g/day for 3 weeks. The husk had no effect on cholesterol or triglyceride concentrations in either normal or ileostomy subjects. Total and HDL cholesterol concentrations were reduced on average by 6.4 and 9.3%, respectively, in normal group after seed supplementation. No effect on fecal bile acid excretion in the normal subjects was found after both regimens. Ileostomy bile acids were increased (on average 25%) after seed supplementation, whereas no effect on cholesterol concentrations was found. These results suggest that psyllium seed may be more effective than the husk in

reducing serum cholesterol, that this cholesterol-lowering effect is not mediated by increased fecal bile acid losses, and increased ileal losses of bile acids may be compensated for by enhanced reabsorption into the colon[PO007]. Fiber, administered to Syrian hamsters at a dose of 7.5% of diet, was active. Major effect was exerted at the level of LDL-cholesterol production. Minor effect resulted from an increase in receptor-mediated LDL clearance by the tissues[PO038]. Husk, administered orally to adults of both sexes with hyperlipidemia at a dose of 11.9 g/day, produced lowered total, LDL, and HDL cholesterol[PO047]. Short-term dietary fibers, *Plantago ovata*, and guar gum preparations decreased serum cholesterol, mainly LDL cholesterol, as compared to low-fiber or nonviscous high-fiber periods, through enhancing cholesterol elimination as fecal bile acids. These changes were associated with significant increases in serum levels of cholesterol precursors, whereas that of cholestanol was decreased[PO099].

Chronic constipation. Seeds, administered orally to 149 patients, ages 18–81 years with chronic constipation at a dose of 15–30 g/day for at least 6 weeks, produced improvement or symptom-free in 85% of the patients. Eight percent of patients with slow transit and 63% of patients with a disorder of defecation did not respond to dietary fiber[PO089]. A double-blind study comprising 20 patients with chronic constipation, of whom 10 had associated irritable bowel syndrome, was conducted. All of the patients receiving *Plantago* had good results against one in the placebo group. Frequency of stools increased from 2.5 ± 1 vs 8 ± 2.2 stool per week, $p < 0.001$ for paired data. Fecal weight increase and colonic transit time decrease was observed in the treated group[PO096].

Cocarcinogenic activity. Seeds, administered in ration of rats at a dose of 20%, produced an increased incidence of colon tumors induced with 1, 2-dimethyl hydantoin in male rats only. A mixture of pure compounds was used to obtain the reported effect[PO067]. Bran, administered to rats at a concentration of 4% of the diet, was active vs N-methynitroso-induced carcinogenesis in the breast. Greatest effect was obtained with coadministration of wheat bran[PO013].

Colonic tumor. Seeds, administered in a fiber supplemented diet at a concentration of 5% of the diet to rats with trinitrobenzenesulfonic acid-induced colitis, indicated that dietary fiber supplementation facilitated recovery from intestinal insult. This was evidenced both histologically by a preservation of intestinal cytoarchitecture and biochemically by a significant reduction in colonic meloperoxidase activity and by restoration of colonic glutathione levels. The intestinal content of fiber-fed colitic rats showed significantly higher production of short-chain fatty acids, mainly butyrate and propionate[PO075]. Seeds, administered to 20 patients resected for colorectal cancer at a dose of 20 g/day for 3 months, increased fecal concentrations of butyrate by $42 \pm 12\%$ from 13.2 ± 1.2 to 19.3 ± 3 mmol/L, acetate by $25 \pm 6\%$, propionate by $28 \pm 9\%$, and total short-chain fatty acids by $25 \pm 6\%$. Concentrations were increased during the 3-month fiber treatment but reversed to pretreatment levels within 1 to 2 months after cessation of fiber supplementation. The relative concentration of butyrate was not altered owing to a simultaneous increase in acetate and propionate. Fecal pH decreased initially but was normalized after 2 months of fiber supplements. Fiber therapy increased the 24-hour productions of butyrate by $47 \pm 10\%$ ($p < 0.0001$) and acetate by 50 $\pm 7\%$ ($p < 0.0001$) in 16.6% fecal homogenates with added *Plantago ovata* seeds (20 mg/mL), but short-chain fatty acid productions returned to pretreatment levels after discontinuation of additional fiber intakes[PO083].

Colorectal effects. Seed, administered orally to 20 patients of both sexes at a dose of 20 g/day for 3 months, was active on co-

lon. The treatment, in patients resected for colorectal cancer, increased the intake of fiber by 17.9 ± 0.8 g/day from basal levels of 19.22 ± 1.7 g/day. Fecal samples were obtained on eight occasions, twice before treatment and thrice during and thrice after treatment. One month of fiber therapy increased fecal concentration of butyrate by $42 \pm 12\%$ (from 13.2 ± 1.2 to 19.3 ± 3 mmol/L), acetate by $25 \pm 6\%$, propionate by $28 \pm 9\%$, and total short chain fatty acids by $25 \pm 6\%$. Concentrations were increased during the 3-month fiber treatment but reversed to pretreatment levels within 1–2 months. After cessation of fiber supplementation, the relative concentration (ratio) of butyrate was not altered owing to a simultaneous increase in acetate and propionate. Fecal pH decreased initially but was normalized after 2 months of fiber supplements. Fiber therapy increased the 24-hour productions of butyrate by $47 \pm 10\%$ and acetate by $50 \pm 7\%$ in 16.6% fecal homogenates with added *Plantago ovata* seed. Short-chain fatty acid productions returned to pretreatment levels after discontinuation of additional fiber intake. Oral intake of *Plantago ovata* seeds adapted the colonic flora to increase the production of butyrate and acetate from this fiber and increased fecal concentration of butyrate by 42% in patients resected for colonic cancer. The effects depended on continuity of the treatment[PO008]. Husk, administered orally to adults of both sexes at a dose of 7.4 g/day, was active in a double-blind, randomized crossover study with 14 healthy volunteers, to evaluate the effect of psyllium on postprandial serum glucose, triglycerides and insulin levels, gastric fullness, hunger feeling, and food intake. Gastric emptying was measured using a standard double-radiolabeled 450-kcal meal and feelings by visual analogical scales. No delay in the gastric emptying of the solid and liquid phases of the meal was observed. After the meal, hunger feelings and energy intake were significantly lower during the psyllium session than during the placebo session (13% and 17%, respectively, $p < 0.05$). Postprandial increase in serum glucose, triglycerides, and insulin levels was less with psyllium than with placebo ($p < 0.05$). Psyllium reduced hunger feelings and energy intake in normal volunteers at reasonable dose and without requiring mixing with the meal. It does not act by slowing the gastric emptying of hydrosoluble nutrients but by increase in the time allowed for intestinal absorption, as suggested by the flattening of the postprandial serum glucose, insulin, and triglyceride curves[PO016]. Seeds and husks, administered to rats at doses of 100 to 200 g/kg, produced elevated total acetate in the cecal content or feces, total fecal bile acid excretion was stimulated and β-glucuronidase (EC3.2.1.31) activity reduced. The seeds increased fecal fresh weight to 100%, fecal dry weight to 50%, and fecal water content to 50%. The husks, at the high concentration only, had such effect. Fecal bacterial mass as estimated from the 2,6-diaminoplimelic acid output was increased to the greatest extent by the seed-containing diet and by the high concentration of the husks. Length and weight of the small intestine were not greatly affected by the seeds, but both variables increased significantly in the large intestine. Mucosal digestive enzyme activities were inhibited to different degrees by both fibers in the jejunum and occasionally activated in the ileum[PO097].

Digestibility. The effect of *Plantago ovata* seed containing supplement (*Plantaginis ovatae* semen and testa) on appetite variables and nutrient and energy intake in 17 subjects was investigated. There were three study periods of 3 days each in which the subjects were given *Plantago* (20 g granules with 200 mL water), placebo (20 g granules with 200 mL water) or water 3 hours premeal and the same dose immediately premeal. There was a significant difference in fullness at 1

hour postmeal between *Plantago* and placebo and also *Plantago* and water. Total fat intake was significantly lower in grams per day and as a percentage of energy on the day of the meal after *Plantago* compared with water[PO091].

Esophageal obstruction. A case was reported of a 41-year-old woman with chest pain and regurgitation after swallowing a tablespoonful of *Plantago ovata* in granules. She kept the granules in her mouth for a few seconds before swallowing with 250 mL of water. Flexible endoscopy revealed a consistent mass blocking the inferior esophagus. A mild hiatus hernia was subsequently discovered. Most of the cases that were reported with this problem took the granules with insufficient liquid[PO074].

Ethinylestradiol pharmacokinetics. Seed, at a concentration of 65% of the diet and seed cuticle at a concentration of 2.2%, administered orally at the same time with ethinylestradiol to rabbits, decreased between 29% and 35% the extent of ethinylestradiol absorbed (represented by the pharmacokinetic parameters area under the curve and the maximum plasma concentration) without affecting the rate of the absorption process (represented by the time to reach maximum concentration and the absorption rate constant)[PO088].

Food consumption reduction. Seed hull, administered to mice at a concentration of 52.5% of diet, was inactive. No differences in psyllium-fed and placebo-fed groups and for normal and diabetic rats were detected[PO051].

Gallbladder effect. Seeds, administered orally to 20 adult males with mild hypercholesterolemia at a dose of 5.1 g/day for 40 days, reduced postprandial residual volume and increased volume of bile emptied[PO022].

Gallstone prevention. Psyllium was investigated in a double-blind clinical trial to compare the effect of rational diet plus ursodeoxycholic acid vs a rational diet supplemented with psyllium in obese subjects undergoing a weight-reduction diet. Patients with body mass index of 30 kg/m² or more and with normal gallbladder and biliary tree ultrasound were included. Weight-reduction diet was individually calculated for each patient, according to his energy expenditure. Patients were randomly assigned to group I (diet with 750 mg ursodeoxycholic acid and fiber placebo) or group II (diet with 15 g of psyllium and ursodeoxycholic acid placebo) for 2 months. Weight reduction was similar in both groups, gallstone disease was observed in one patient of group I (5.5%) and two patients of group II ($p > 0.05$). All of the patients with gallstone disease lost a minimum of 4 kg during the study period[PO081].

Gastric digestibility. Ispaghula, mucilage from *Plantago*, administered orally to seven healthy subjects at a dose of 18 g/day for two 15-day periods, indicated that whole gut transit time and gas excretion in breath and flatus were not different during periods of ispaghula and placebo ingestion. Fecal wet and dry weights increased significantly during ispaghula ingestion. Fecal short-chain fatty acid concentrations and the molar proportions of propionic and acetic acids also increased. Most of the ispaghula had reached the cecum 4 hours after ingestion in an intact highly polymerized form. During ispaghula ingestion, the increase in the fecal output of neutral sugars was accounted for by the fecal excretion of arabinose and xylose in an intact highly polymerized form[PO092]. Ispaghula, administered at doses of 5, 15, or 50 g/kg to rats on a basal diet of 45 g nonstarch polysaccharides/kg for 28 days, increased stool dry weight and apparent wet weight. Fecal water-holding capacity (amount of water held per gram dry fecal material at 0.2 mPa) was unchanged. Fecal short-chain fatty acids concentration did not change, but short-chain fatty acid output increased. The molar proportion of

short-chain fatty acid as propionic acid increased and fecal pH was reduced. Values from pooled fecal samples indicated that approx 50% of the ingested ispaghula was excreted by the 50-g ispaghula/kg diet group[PO095].

Gastric emptying time. Dried husk of the seed, administered orally to 12 healthy adults at a dose of 10 g/person, delayed gastric emptying from the third hour after a meal. It increased satiety and decreased hunger 6 hours after a meal[PO024].

Gastrointestinal enzymes effect. Seed and husk, incubated in vitro with gastrointestinal enzymes in buffer solutions at concentrations of 1–5% for 10–30 min at 37°C, had no effect on pepsin, trypsin, and α-amylase, only stimulating effect on chymotrypsin, lipase, and lactase[PO098].

Glucose tolerance test. Psyllium mucilage, administered to eight healthy volunteers at doses of 10, 20, and 30 g of mucilage in 75 g of glucose, produced a significant relationship between dose of psyllium mucilage and its attenuating effect of hyperglycemia. Serum glucose levels were measured at 0, 30, 60, 120, and 180 minutes. Maximum peak of glucose at 30 minutes and the area under a curve of glucose were significantly lower in the test with 20 and 30 g of mucilage than the test with 0 and 10 g[PO084].

Glycemic index. Psyllium, administered to 12 patients with noninsulin-dependent diabetes mellitus and 10 healthy volunteers, reduced the glycemic index of carbohydrate food. Each subject was evaluated after three meal tests with an intake of 90 g of white bread (50 g of carbohydrates). In one test, the subjects were also given 15 g of psyllium mucilage and in another 200 mg of acarbose. Only bread was ingested in the control group. Serum glucose and insulin concentrations were measured every 30 minutes from 0–180 minutes. In the noninsulin-dependent diabetes mellitus patients, area-under-the-curve (AUC)-glucose in the test with acarbose (1.9 ± 0.7 mmol/L) and with psyllium (4.3 ± 1.2 mmol/L) was significantly lower than in the control test (7.4 ± 1.5 mmol/L). The glycemic index of bread plus acarbose was 26 ± 13 and of bread plus psyllium 59 ± 10. AUC-insulin and insulin index behaved similarly. In healthy individuals, AUC-glucose and glycemic index did not significantly change with the treatments; however, insulinic index with acarbose was 17 ± 16 and with psyllium was 68 ± 15[PO080].

Hepatic encephalopathy. Psyllium, administered to eight patients with diabetes with chronic portal systemic encephalopathy, produced a significant increase in the number of bowel movements. In this crossover study, for one group, a meat protein diet was consumed and neomycin plus laxatives was given. The other group received vegetable protein supplemented with psyllium fiber to reach 35 g of fiber per day. At the end of the experimental period, fasting glucose levels were 204 ± 86 mg% in the meat protein diet group and 127 ± 8 mg% in the vegetable protein diet group. In all cases, fasting glucose levels decreased at the end of the vegetable diet period, regardless of the previous treatment. An improvement of greater than or equal to 25 mg% of fasting glucose levels was observed in seven of the eight patients after the vegetable protein diet and in no case after the meat protein diet (p < 0.0078). The parameters of encephalography were comparable at the end of both of meat protein diet and the vegetable protein diet[PO105].

3-Hydroxy-3-methylglutaryl coenzyme A reductase inhibition. Husks, administered to African green monkeys at a concentration of 10% of diet, were active. The monkeys were fed a high cholesterol diet[PO025].

Water extract of the plant, administered orally to rabbits at a dose of 0.5 g/kg, produced a significant decrease in anti-hemag-glutinating antibody titer in primary response. Intraperitoneal injection of 0.25 g/kg of the extract to mice prior to immunization with sheep red blood cells resulted in a significant decrease in hemagglutinating antibody titre. Oral and intraperitoneal administration of 0.25 and 0.5 g/kg resulted in an increase in white blood cells and spleen leukocyte counts. The spleen weight also increased with intraperitoneal injection (0.25 and 0.5 g/kg) and oral administration of 0.5 g/kg of *Plantago ovata*. Results suggest that *Plantago ovata* can suppress the humoral immune responses, especially in primary immune response[PO078].

Hypercholesterolemic activity. Fiber of the fresh seed husks, administered orally adults of both sexes at a dose of 7 g/day, was active. Results were significant at p < 0.05 level[PO039]. Psyllium, administered orally to 14 subjects with polygenic hypercholesterolemia at a dose of 3.4 g three times daily before meals, produced a reduction of 8% in total cholesterol and 11% in LDL cholesterol. The subjects with secondary dyslipidemias were excluded from this study. The subjects were given an isocaloric diet, with less than 10% of the calories provided as saturated fats, polyunsaturated:saturated relation greater than 1 and daily intake of less than 300 mg of cholesterol. The study was divided in two stages: The first, from week –6 to 0, evaluated exclusively the response to diet, and the second, from week 0 to 12, evaluated the response to psyllium. No significant changes in triglycerides and HDL cholesterol were observed[PO104].

Hypocholesterolemic activity. Fiber, administered orally to males with hyperlipidemia, produced a 5.7% decrease in LDL cholesterol level. Fiber, administered orally to healthy adults of both sexes at a dose of 15 g/person, was inactive[PO027]. Husks, administered in ration of adults at a dose of 114 g/day for 6 weeks, decreased the total cholesterol and LDL cholesterol levels[PO018]. Fiber, administered in ration of male hamsters at a dose 7.5% of diet, enhanced the loss of sterol by the liver[PO033]. Fiber, administered orally to human adults at a dose of 20 g/person, increased fecal fat loss and decreased fat digestibility coefficient in healthy volunteers[PO035]. Seed hull, administered to mice at a dose of 2.5% of diet, was inactive. Aside from a transient decrease at 4 and 10 weeks of an 18-week feeding period, total cholesterol was similar in psyllium-fed and placebo-fed animals. HDL level was similar in the two groups[PO051]. Fiber of the fresh seed husks, administered orally to adults of both sexes at a dose of 7 g/day, produced a drop in LDL and total cholesterol levels. The levels continued to decrease 90 days after treatment stopped[PO039]. Seed oil, administered orally to rabbits at a dose of 5 mL/animal, was active[PO001]. Administration by gastric intubation was inactive[PO071].

Hypoglycemic activity. Seed administered orally to 18 patients with noninsulin-dependent diabetes at a dose of 13.6 g/day in two equal doses lowered glucose level by 14 % after breakfast and 20% after dinner[PO055]. Seed hull, administered to mice at a dose of 2.5% of the diet for 18 weeks, produced a transient decrease in 10 weeks in psyllium-fed animals relative to placebo-fed animals[PO051].

Hypolipidemic activity. Seed hull, administered to mice at a dose of 2.5% of diet for 18 weeks, was inactive[PO051]. The husk, administered orally to male Hartley guinea pigs at doses of 7.5 or 10 g/100 g of *Plantago ovata* for 4 weeks, exerted a hypolipidemic effect by affecting bile acid absorption and altering hepatic cholesterol metabolism[PO076].

Insulin release inhibition. Seed administered orally to 18 patients with noninsulin-dependent diabetes at a dose of 13.6 g/day lowered insulin levels by 17%[PO055].

Internal bleeding hemorrhoids. Fiber, administered orally to 50 patients with bleeding internal hemorrhoids for 15 days, decreased the number of bleeding episodes. During the 15 days of treatment, the average number of bleeding episodes was 4.8 ± 3.8 vs 6.4 ± 3 for the control group. During the following 15 days, it decreased to 3.1 ± 2.7 vs 5.5 ± 3.2 ($p < 0.05$) in the control group, and in the last 10 days of treatment a further reduction to 1.1 ± 1.4 was found vs 5.5 ± 2.9 ($p < 0.01$). The number of congested hemorrhoid cushions diminished from 2.6 ± 1 to 1.6 ± 2.2 after fiber treatment ($p < 0.01$), and no differences were found in the control group. In the fiber group, hemorrhoids bled on contact in 5 out of 22 patients before treatment and in none after treatment, no differences were found in the control group[PO082].

Laxative effect. Seed hull, taken orally by adults at a dose of 7 g/person, increased weekly fecal mass without influencing transit time or frequency[PO023]. Seedcoat, administered orally to 80 patients at a dose of 6.4 g/person three times daily, was active in a blinded placebo controlled study of efficacy of extract in treatment of irritable bowel syndrome[PO048]. Water extract of the dried kernel, administered orally to 40-year-old adults of both sexes, was active[PO058]. Seed powder, administered orally to adults of both sexes, was active. Biological activity reported has been patented[PO006]. Dried seeds, administered orally to adults at a dose of 0.5 g/person, were active. Placing the seeds in water increased their volume, 90% alcohol produced a decrease in volume to normal seed size, and linseed oil had no effect on volume. The seed mucilage remained in gel form and is considered preferable to the solid form because it is more easily digested[PO072]. Dried seed powder, administered orally to 35 patients with chronic constipation at a dose of 50 mg/person, was active in a controlled, double-blind study[PO012]. Fiber, administered orally to adults, was active. Psyllium fiber and sennosides were prepared into a wafer to be used as a laxative. Biological activity reported has been patented[PO029]. Mixture of the *Plantago ovata* and *Cassia senna* fibers, taken orally by adults at a dose of 10 mL/person, were active for constipation[PO031]. Fiber, administered orally to adults of both sexes at a dose of 30 g, was inactive vs loperamide-induced constipation on healthy volunteers. No effect on colon transit was seen. There was an increase in stool weight[PO041].

Lipid metabolism effect. Fiber of the fresh seed husk, administered orally to adults of both sexes at a dose of 7 g/day, was active. LDL/HDL ratio dropped during treatment and for 90 days thereafter. Results were significant at $p < 0.05$ level[PO039].

Sterol metabolism. Psyllium husk, administered orally to six normal subjects and five subjects with ileostomy at a dose of 10 g/day for 3 weeks and psyllium seeds administered to six normal subjects and four subjects with ileostomy at a dose of 10 g/day, indicated that psyllium seed might be more effective than the husk in reducing serum cholesterol. The cholesterol-lowering effect is not mediated by increased fecal bile acid losses, and increased ileal losses of bile acids might be compensated for by enhanced reabsorption in the colon. The husk had no effect on cholesterol or triglyceride concentrations in either normal or ileostomy subjects. Total and HDL cholesterol concentrations were reduced on average by 6.4 and 9.3%, respectively, in the normal group after seed supplementation. No effect on fecal bile acid excretion in the normal subjects was found after both regimes. Ileostomy bile acids were increased (on average 25%) after seed supplementation, whereas no effect on cholesterol concentrations was found[PO090].

Taurocholic acid adsorption. Husk and seed, inoculated with human fecal culture and incubated with taurocholic acid, produced 53% incorporation if taurocholic acid for the husk and 59% for the seed[PO090].

Toxic effect. Dried kernel of the seed, administered to cows at a dose of 50% of diet, was inactive[PO066].

Ulcerative colitis. *Plantago ovata* seeds, administered orally to 105 patients with ulcerative colitis in remission at a dose of 10 g twice daily, produced a 40% (14 of 35 patients) failure rate after 12 months. The patients were randomized into groups that also received mesalamine (500 mg twice daily) and *Plantago ovata* seeds plus mesalamine at the same dose. The primary efficacy was maintenance of remission for 12 months. Of the 105 patients, 102 were included in the final analysis. After the 12-month treatment period, the failure rate was 35% (13 of 37) in the mesalamine group and 30% (9 of 30) in the *Plantago ovata* plus mesalamine group. Probability of continued remission was similar (Mantel-Cox test, $p = 0.67$; intent-to-treat analysis). A significant increase in fecal butyrate levels ($p = 0.018$) was observed after *Plantago ovata* seed administration[PO087].

Weight increase. Seed hull, administered in ration of mice at a concentration of 2.5% of diet for 18 weeks, was active. No differences in psyllium-fed and placebo-fed groups in both diabetic and normal animals were found[PO051].

Weight loss. Mucilage, administered orally to human adults at a dose of 3 g/person, was active. Twenty-eight obese women were divided into two groups and given mucilage twice daily in conjunction with an 800-calorie hypoglucidic diet, or diet only, in a crossover design. Weight loss was similar for both groups in the first period. In the second period, the group given mucilage lost more weight than the diet-only group, indicating that the weight-reducing effect of mucilage only becomes important as compliance with the diet decreases owing to time[PO053].

Wound healing. Husk mucopolysaccharides, administered as a sachet (Askina Cavity) or in a hydrocolloid mixture (Askina Hydro), produced a gradual and sustained absorbency over 7-day period, amounting to four to six times their weight in water. Adherence of wound bacteria to the mucopolysaccharides started after 2 hours and was more pronounced after 3 hours. Semi-quantitative measurements of bacterial adherence used centrifugation and subsequent optical density determinations of supernatant. These confirmed the strong adherence potential of psyllium particles. Lactic acid dehydrogenase staining of pretreated cultured human skin explants did not reveal toxicity of the mucopolysaccharides derived from psyllium husk. Langerhans' cell migration from the epidermis was negligible, and interleukin-1 β expression in the explants was not significant, supporting the low allergenic potential of psyllium. The characteristics of mucopolysaccharides granulate derived from husk in Askina Cavity (sachet) and Askina Hydro (hydrocolloid mixture) related to fluid absorption, bacterial adherence, biocompatibility, stimulation of macrophages, irritancy response, and allergenicity showed an optimal profile, supporting the good clinical performance[PO085].

REFERENCES

PO001 Siddiqui, H. H., K. K. Kapur, and C. K. Atal. Indian seeds oils. Effect of *Plantago ovata* embryo oil on serum cholesterol levels in rabbits. **Indian J Pharmacy** 1964; 26: 266.

PO002 Wattiez, N., and M. Hans. A holoside extracted from the seeds of *Plantago major* L. and *Plantago ovata* Forsk (*P. isphagulata* Roxb.). **Bull Acad Roy Med Belg** 1943; 8: 386–396.

PO003 Khorana, M. L., V. G. Prabbu, and M. R. R. Rao. Pharmacology of an alcoholic extract of *Plantago ovata*. **Indian J Pharmacy** 1958; 29: 3–6.

PO004 Gelpi, E., H. Schneider, V. M. Doctor, J. Tennison, and J. Oro. Gas chromatographic–mass spectrometric identifications of the hydrocarbons and fatty acids of *Plantago ovata* seeds. **Phytochemistry** 1969; 8(10): 2077–2081.

PO005 Zagari, A. Medicinal plants. Vol. 4, 5th ed, Tehran University Publications, No 1810/4, Tehran, Iran, 1992; 4: 969.

PO006 Sander, E. H. Psyllium-hydrocolloid gum compositions and fiber supplements. Paten-Can Pat Appl-2,100,295 1994; 17 p.

PO007 Gelissen, C., B. Brodie, and M. A. Eastwood. Effect of *Plantago ovata* (psyllium) husk and seeds on sterol metabolism: studies in normal and ileostomy subjects, **Amer J Clin Nutr** 1994; 59(2): 395–400.

PO008 Nordgaard, I., H. Hove, M. R. Clausen, and P. B. Mortensen. Colonic production of butyrate in patients with previous colonic cancer during long-term treatment with dietary fiber (*Plantago ovata* seeds). **Scand J Gastroenterol** 1996; 31(10): 1011–1020.

PO009 Kritschevsky, D., S. A. Tepper, and D. M. Klurfeld. Influence of psyllium preparations on plasma and liver lipids of cholesterol-fed plants. **Artery** 1995; 21(6): 303–311.

PO010 Davidson, M. H., L. D. Dugan, J. H. Burns, D. Sugimoto, K. Story, and K. Drennan. A psyllium-enriched cereal for treatment of hypercholesterolemia in children: a controlled, double blind, crossover study. **Amer J Clin Nutr** 1996; 63(1): 96–102.

PO011 Olson, B. H., S. M. Anderson, M. P. Becker, et al. Psyllium-enriched cereals lower blood total cholesterol and LDL cholesterol, but not HDL cholesterol, in hypercholesterolemic adults: results of a meta-analysis. **J Nutr** 1997; 127(10): 1973–1980.

PO012 Odes, H. S., and Z. Madar. A double-blind trial of a celandine, *Aloe vera* and psyllium laxative preparation in adult patients with constipation. **Digestion** 1991; 49(2): 65–71.

PO013 Cohen, L. A., Z. Zhao, E. A. Zhang, T. T. Wynn, B. Simi, and A. Rivenson. Wheat bran and psyllium diets: effects on N-methylnitrosourea-induced mammary tumorigenesis in F344 rats. **J Nat Cancer Inst** 1996; 88(13): 898–907.

PO014 Davidson, M. H., K. C. Maki, J. C. Kong, et al. Long-term effects of consuming food containing psyllium seed husk on serum lipids in subjects with hypercholesterolemia. **Amer J Clin Nutr** 1998; 67(3): 367–376.

PO015 Segawa, K., T. Kataoka, and Y. Fukuo. Cholesterol-lowering effects of psyllium seed associated with urea metabolism. **Biol Pharm Bull** 1998; 21(2): 184–187.

PO016 Riguad, D., F. Paycha, A. Muelemans, M. Merrouche, and M. Mignon. Effect of psyllium on gastric emptying, hunger feeling, and food intake in normal volunteers: a double-blind study. **European J Clin Nutr** 1998; 52(4): 239–245.

PO017 Arlian, L. G., D. L. Vyszenski-Noher, A. T. Lawrence, K. R. Schrotel, and H. L. Ritz. Antigenic and allergenic analysis of psyllium seed components. **J Allergy Clin Immunol** 1992; 89(4): 866–876.

PO018 Anderson J. W., S. Riddell-Mason, N. J. Gustafson, S. F. Smith, and M. Mackey. Cholesterol-lowering effects of psyllium-enriched cereal as an adjunct to a prudent diet in the treatment of mild to moderate hypercholesterolemia. **Amer J Clin Nutr** 1992; 56(1): 93–98.

PO019 Day, C. E. Activity of psyllium hydrophilic colloid for reducing serum cholesterol in sea quail fed diet supplemented with cholesterol. **Artery** 1991; 18(3): 163–167.

PO020 Mc Call, M. R., T. Mehta, C. W. Leathers, and D. M. Foster. Psyllium husk II. Effect on the metabolism of apoliprotein B in African green monkeys. **Amer J Clin Nutr** 1992; 56(2): 385–393.

PO021 James, J. M., S. K. Cooke, A. Barnett, and H. A. Sampson. Anaphylactic reactions to a psyllium-containing cereal. **J Allergy Clin Immunol** 1991; 88(3): 402–408.

PO022 Everson, G. T., B. P. Daggy, C. Mc Kinley, and J. A. Story. Effect of psyllium hydrophilic mucilloid on LDL-cholesterol and bile acid synthesis in hypercholesterolemic men. **J Lipid Res** 1992; 33(8): 1183–1192.

PO023 Tomlin, J., and N. W. Read. A comparative study of the effects on colon function caused by feeding ispaghula husk and polydextrose. **Aliment Pharmacol Ther** 1988; 2(6): 513–519.

PO024 Bergmann, J. F., O. Chassany, A. Petit, R. Triki, C. Caulin, and J. M. Segrestaa. Correlation between echographic gastric emptying and appetite: Influence of psyllium. **Gut** 1992; 33(8): 1042–1043.

PO025 Mc Call, M. R., T. Mehta, C. W. Leathers, and D. M. Foster. Psyllium husk I. Effect on plasma lipoprotein, cholesterol metabolism, and artherosclerosis in African green monkeys. **Amer J Clin Nutr** 1992; 56(2): 376–384.

PO026 Smith, M. A., and A. A. Aso. Comparison of psyllium hydrophilic mucilloid and bile salt binding resin therapy for hypercholesterolemia. Abstr Endocrine Society 144th Annual Meeting June 1992; 62.

PO027 Hopewell, R., R. Yeater, and I. Ullrich. Soluble fiber: Effect on carbohydrate and lipid metabolism. **Progress Food Nutr Sci** 1993; 17(2): 159–182.

PO028 Eherer, A. J., A. Santa, A. Carol, J. Porter, and J. S. Fordtran. Effect of psyllium, calcium polycarbophil, and wheat bran on secretory diarrhea induced by phenolphthalein. **Gastroenterology** 1993; 104(4): 1007–1012.

PO029 Colliopoulos, J. Psyllium-based laxative compositions. Patent-US-5,232, 699 1993; 6 p.

PO030 Gupta, S., J. N. S. Yadava, and J. S. Tandon. Antisecretory (antidiarrheal) activity of Indian medicinal plants against Escherichia coli enterotoxin-induced secretion in rabbit and Guinea pig ileal loop models. **Int J Pharmacog** 1993; 31(3): 198–204.

PO031 Passmore, A. P., K. Wilson-Davies, C. Stoker, and M. E. Scott. Chronic constipation in long stay elderly patients: a comparison of lactulose and a senna-fiber combination. **Brit Med J** 1993; 307(6907): 769–771.

PO032 Wolever, T., D. Jenkins, S. Mueller, et al. Method of administration influences the serum cholesterol lowering effect of psyllium. **Amer J Clin Nutr** 1994; 59(5): 1055–1059.

PO033 Turley, S.D., B. P. Daggy, and J. M. Dietschy. Psyllium augments the cholesterol-lowering action of cholestyramine in hamsters by enhancing sterol loss from the liver. **Gastroenterology** 1994; 107(2): 444–452.

PO034 Naylor, J. M. and T. Lieber. Effect of psyllium on plasma concentration of glucose, breath hydrogen concentration, and fecal composition in calves with diarrhea treated orally with electrolyte solutions. **Amer J Vet Res** 1995; 56(1): 56–59.

PO035 Ganji, V. and C. V. Kies. Psyllium husk fiber supplementation to soybean and coconut oil diets of humans: effect on rat digestibility and fecal fatty acid excretion. **Eur J Clin Nutr** 1994; 48(8): 595–597.

PO036 Matheson, H. B. and J. A. Story. Dietary psyllium hydrocolloid and pectin increase bile acid pool size and change bile acid composition in rats. **J Nutr** 1994; 124(8): 1161–1165.

PO037 Freeman, G. L. Psyllium hypersensitivity. **Ann Allergy** 1994; 73(6): 490–492.

PO038 Turley, S. D., and J. M. Dietschy. Mechanisms of LDL-cholesterol lowering action of psyllium hydrophilic mucilloid in the hamster. **Biochim Biophys Acta** 1995; 1255(2): 177–184.

PO039 Gupta, B. R., C. G. Agrawal, G. P. Singh, and A. Ghatak. Lipid-lowering efficacy of psyllium hydrophilic mucilloid in non insulin dependent diabetes mellitus with hyperlipidaemia. **Indian J Med Res** 1994; 100(5): 237–241.

PO040 Chan, E. K., and D J. Schroeder. Psyllium in hypercholesterolemia. **Ann Pharmacother** 1995; 29(6): 625–627.

PO041 Ewe, K., B. Uberschaer, and A. G. Press. Influence of senna, fiber, and fiber+senna on colonic transit in lopermaide-induced constipation. **Pharmacology** 1993; 47(1): 242–248.

PO042 Williams, C. L., M. Bollella, A. Spark, and D. Puder. Soluble fiber enhances the hypercholesterolemic effect of the step I diet in childhood. **J Amer Coll Nutr** 1995; 14(3): 251–257.

PO043 Turnbull, W. H., and H. G. Thomas. The effect of a *Plantago ovata* seed containing preparation of appetite variables, nutrient, and energy intake. **Int J Obesity** 1995; 19(5): 338–342.

PO044 Etman, M. A. Effect of a bulk forming laxative on the bioavailability of carbamazepine in man. **Drug Dev Ind Pharm** 1995; 21(16): 1901–190.

PO045 Martinez-Lirola, M. J., M. R. Gonzalez-Tejero, and J. Molero-Mesa. Ethnobotanical resources in the province of Almeria, Spain: Campos de Nijar. **Econ Bot** 1996; 50(1): 40–56.

PO046 Arjmandi, B. H., E. Sohn, S. Juma, S. R. Murthy, and B. P. Daggy. Native and partially hydrolyzed psyllium has comparable effects on cholesterol metabolism in rats. **J Nutr** 1997; 127(3): 463–469.

PO047 Jenkins, D., T. Wolever, E. Vidgen, et al. Effect of psyllium in hypercholesterolemia at two monounsaturated fatty acid intakes. **Amer J Clin Nutr** 1997; 65(5): 1524–1533.

PO048 Prior, A., and P. J. Whorwell. Double blind study of Ispaghula in irritable bowel syndrome. **Gut** 1987; 28: 1510–1513.

PO049 Jamal, S., I. Ahmad, R. Agarwal, M. Ahamad, and S. M. Osman. A novel oxo fatty acid in *Plantago ovata* seed oil. **Phytochemistry** 1987; 26(11): 3067–3069.

PO050 Miettinen, T. A., and S. Tarpila. Serum lipids and cholesterol metabolism during guar gum, *Plantago ovata* and high fiber treatments. **Clinica Chim Acta** 1989; 183: 253–262.

PO051 Watters, K., and P. Blaisdell. Reduction of glycemic and lipid levels in DB/DB diabetic mice by psyllium plant fiber. **Diabetes** 1989; 38(12): 1528–1533.

PO052 Shah, G. L. and G. V. Gopal. Ethnomedical notes from the tribal inhabitants of the north Gujarat (India). **J Econ Taxon Botany** 1985; 6(1): 193–201.

PO053 Enzi, G., E. M. Inelmen, and G. Crepaldi. Effect of a hydrophilic mucilage in the treatment of obese patients. **Pharmacotherapeutica** 1980; 2(7): 421–428.

PO054 Lantner, R. R., B. R. Espiritu, P. Zumerchik, and M. C. Tobin. Anaphylaxis following ingestion of a psyllium-containing cereal. **JAMA** 1990; 264(19): 2534–2536.

PO055 Pastors, J. G., P. W. Blaisdell, T. K. Balm, C. M. Asplin, and S. L. Pohl. Psyllium fiber reduces rise in postprandial glucose and insulin concentrations in patients with non-insulin–dependent diabetes. **Amer J Clin Nutr** 1991; 53(6): 1431–1435.

PO056   Wolever, T. M. S., V. Vuksan, H. Eshuis, et al. Effect of method of administration of psyllium on glycemic response and carbohydrate digestibility. **J Amer Coll Nutr** 1991; 10(4): 364–371.

PO057   Naovi, S. A. H., M. S. Y. Khan, and S. B. Vohora. Anti-bacterial, anti-fungal and anthelmintic investigations on Indian medicinal plants. **Fitoterapia** 1991; 62(3): 221–228.

PO058   Ricci, P. D., and R. Angeli. *Plantago ovata* and defecation disorders in the aged. Effects of the administration of powdered *Plantago ovata* on defecation disorders in the aged. **Clin Ter** 1978; 86: 434–439.

PO059   Khanna, N. M., J. P. S. Sarin, R. C. Nandi, et al. Isaptent—a new cervical dilator. **Contraception** 1980; 21: 29–40.

PO060   Sandhu, J. S., G. J. Hudson, and J. F. Kennedy. The gel nature and structure of the carbohydrate of Ispaghula husk. **Carbohydr Res** 1981; 93: 247–259.

PO061   Jewvachdamrongkul, Y., T. Dechatiwongtse, D. Pecharaply, J. Bansiddhi, and P. Kanchanapee. Identification of some Thai medicinal plants. **Mahidol Univ J Pharm Sci** 1982; 9(3): 65–73.

PO062   Patel, R. B., C. G. Rana, M. R. Patel, H. K. Dhyani, and H. V. Chauhan. Chromatographic screening of proteins of seeds of *Plantago ovata* Forsk. **Indian Drugs Pharm Ind** 1981; 16: 3–5.

PO063   Roy, P. Mid trimester abortion by slow dilatation with Isapgol tents (Dilexc). **Patna J Med** 1982; 56(5): 95–97.

PO064   Vijayalakshimi, K., S. D. Mishra, and S. K. Prasad. Nematocidal properties of some indigenous plant materials against second stage juveniles of *Meloidogyne incognita* (koffoid and white) chitwood. **Indian J Entomol** 1979; 41(4): 326–331.

PO065   Al–Shamma, A., and L. A. Mitscher. Comprehensive survey of indigenous Iraqi plants for potential economic value. I. Screening results of 327 species for alkaloids and antimicrobial agents. **J Nat Prod** 1979; 42: 633–642.

PO066   Shukla, P. C., M. C. Desai, L. P. Purohit, and H. B. Desai. Use of Isabgul (*Plantago ovata* Forsk.) gola in

the concentrate mixture of milk cows. **Gujarat Agr Univ Res** 1983; 9(1): 33–36.

PO067   Toth, B. Effect of Metamucil on tumor formation by 1,2-dimethylhydrazine dihydrochloride in mice. **Food Chem Toxicol** 1984; 22(7): 573–578.

PO068   Dooley, D. P., M. Rhodes, and D. Drehner. Psyllium worm. **Amer J Gastroenterol** 1993; 88(1): 153–154.

PO069   Alabaster, O., Z. C. Tang, A. Frost, and N. Shivapurkar. Potential synergism between wheat bran and psyllium: enhanced inhibition of colon cancer. **Cancer Lett** 1993; 75(1): 53–58.

PO070   Atal, C. K., K. K. Kapoor, and H. H. Siddiqui. Studies on Indian seed oils. Part I. Preliminary screening of linoleic acid rich oils. **Indian J Pharmacy** 1964; 26; 163–164.

PO071   Siddiqui, H. H., K. K. Kapoor, and C. K. Atal. Studies on Indian seed oils. Part II. Effect of *Plantago ovata* embryo oil on raised serum cholesterol levels in rabbits. **Indian J Pharmacy** 1964; 26: 1663–1664.

PO072   Wasicky, B. Investigations of the seeds of *Plantago ovata*, *P. psyllium*, and *P. major* variety cruenta as laxatives. **Planta Med** 1961; 9: 232–244.

PO073   Balbaa, S. I., M. S. Karawaya, and M. S. Afifi. Pharmacognostical study of the seeds of certain *Plantago* species growing in Egypt. **UAR J Pharm Sci** 1971; 12(1): 35–52.

PO074   Salguero Molpeceres O., M. C. Seijas Ruiz-Coello, J. Hernandez-Nunez, D. Caballos Villar, L. Diaz Picazo, and L. Ayerbe Garcia-Monzon. Esophageal obstruction caused by dietary fiber from *Plantago ovata*, a complication preventable by adequate information. **Gastroenterologia y Hepatologia** 2003; 26(4): 248–250.

PO075   Rodriguez-Cabezaz, M. E., J. Galvez, M. D. Lorente, et al. Dietary fiber down-regulates colonic tumor necrosis factor alpha and nitric oxide production in trinitrobenzenesulfonic acid–induced colitis rats. **J Nutr** 2002; 132(11): 3263–3271.

PO076   Romero, A. L., K. L. West, T. Zern, and M. L. Fernandez. The seeds from *Plantago ovata* lower plasma lipids by altering hepatic ad bile acid metabolism in guinea pigs. **J Nutr** 2002; 132(6): 1194–1198.

PO077 Chiang, L. C., W. Chiang, M. Y. Chiang, L. T. Ng, and C. C. Lin. Antileukemic activity of selected natural products in Taiwan. **Amer J Chin Med** 2003; 31(1): 37–46.

PO078 Rezaeipoor, R., S. Saednia, and M. Kamalinejad. The effect of *Plantago ovata* on humoral immune responses in experimental animals. **J Ethnopharmacol** 2000; 72(1–2): 283–286.

PO079 Rodriguez-Moran, M., F. Guerrero-Romero, and G. Lazcano-Burciaga. Lipid- and glucose-lowering efficacy of *Plantago psyllium* in type II diabetes. **J Diabet Complic** 1998; 12(5): 273–278.

PO080 Frati-Munari, A. C., W. Benitez Pinto, C. Raul Ariza Andraca, and M. Casarrubias. Lowering glycemic index of food by acarbose and *Plantago psyllium* mucilage. **Arch Med Res** 1998; 29(2): 137–141.

PO081 Moran, S., M. Uribe, M. E. Prado, et al. Effects of fiber administration in the prevention of gallstones in obese patients on a reducing diet. A clinical trial. **Revista de Gastroenterologia de Mexico** 1997; 62(4): 266–272.

PO082 Perez-Miranda, M., A. Gomez-Cedenilla, T. Leon-Colombo, J. Pajares, and J. Mate-Jimenez. Effect of fiber supplements on internal bleeding hemorrhoids. **Hepato-Gastroener** 1996; 43(12): 1504–1507.

PO083 Nordgaard, I., H. Howe, M. R. Clausen, and P. B. Mortensen. Colonic production of butyrate in patients with previous colonic cancer during long-term treatment with dietary fiber. **Scand J Gastroenter** 1996; 31(10): 1011–1020.

PO084 Frati-Munai, A. C., M. A. Flores-Garduno, R. Ariza-Andraca, S. Islas-Andrade, and A. Chavez-Negrete. Effect of different doses of *Plantago psyllium* mucilage on the glucose tolerance test. **Archivos de Investigacion Medica** 1989; 20(2): 147–152.

PO085 Westerhof, W., P. K. Das, E. Middlelkoop, J. Verschoor, L. Storey, and C. Regnier. Mucopolysaccharides from psyllium involved in wound healing. **Drugs Under Exp Clin Res** 2001; 27(5–6): 165–175.

PO086 Aleman, A. M., S. Quirce, C. Bombin, and J. Sastre. Asthma related to inhalation of *Plantago ovata*. **Med Clin** 2001; 116(1): 20–22.

PO087 Fernandez-Banares, F., J. Hinojosa, J. L. Sanchez-Lombrana, et al. Randomized clinical trial of *Plantago ovata* seeds (dietary fiber) as compared with mesalamine in maintaining remission in ulcerative colitis. Spanish Group for the Study of Crohn's Disease and Ulcerative Colitis (GETECCU). **Amer J Gastroenterol** 1999; 94(2): 427–433.

PO088 Fernanzed, N., M. J. Diez, M. T. Teran, J. J. Garcia, A. P. Calle, and M. Sierra. Influence of two commercial fibers in the pharmacokinetics of ethinylestradiol in rabbits. **J Pharmacol Exp Therap** 1998; 286; 870–874.

PO089 Voderholzer, W.A., W. Schatke, B. E. Muhldorfer, A. G. Klauser, B. Birkner, and S. A. Muller-Lissner. Clinical response to dietary fiber treatment of chronic constipation. **Amer J Gastroenterol** 1997; 92(1): 95–98.

PO090 Gelissen, I. C., and M. A. Eastwood. Taurocholic acid adsorption during non-starch polysaccharide fermentation: an *in vitro* study. **Brit J Nutr** 1995; 74(2): 221–228.

PO091 Turnbull, W. H., and H. G. Thomas. The effect of a *Plantago ovata* seed containing preparation on appetite variables, nutrient and energy intake. **Int J Obesity Rel Metab Disord** 1995; 19(5): 338–342.

PO092 Marteau, P., B. Flourie, C. Cherbut, et al. Digestibility and bulking effect of ispaghula husk in healthy humans. **Gut** 1994; 35(12): 1747–1752.

PO093 Freeman, G. L. Psyllium hypersensitivity. **Ann Allergy** 1994; 73(6): 490–492.

PO094 Gelissen, I. C., B. Brodie, and M. A. Eastwood. Effect of *Plantago ovata* (psyllium) husk and seeds on sterol metabolism: studies in normal and ileostomy subjects. **Amer J Clin Nutr** 1994; 59(2): 395–400.

PO095 Edwards, C. A., J. Bowen, W. G. Brydon, and M. A. Eastwood. The effect of ispaghula on rat caecal fermentation and stool output. **Brit J Nutr** 1992; 68(2): 473–482.

PO096   Tomas-Ridicci, M., R. Anon, M. Minguez, A. Zaragoza, J. Ballester, and A. Benages. The efficacy of *Plantago ovata* as a regulator of intestinal transit. A double-blind study compared to placebo. **Revista Espanola de Enfermedades Digestivas** 1992; 82(1): 17–22.

PO097   Leng-Peschlow, E. *Plantago ovata* seeds as dietary fiber supplement: physiological and metabolic effects in rats. **Br J Nutr** 1991; 66(2): 331–349.

PO098   Leng-Peschlow, E. Interference of dietary fibers with gastrointestinal enzymes *in vitro*. **Digestion** 1989; 44(4): 200–210.

PO099   Miettinen, T. A. and S. Tarpila. Serum lipids and cholesterol metabolism during guar gum, *Plantago ovata* and high fiber treatments. **Clin Chim Acta** 1989; 183; 253–262.

PO100   Faber, P., and A. Strenge–Hesse. Relevance of rhein excretion into breast milk. **Pharmacology** 1988; 1(Suppl 36): 212–220.

PO101   Suhonen, R., I. Kantola, and F. Bjorksten. Anaphylactic shock due to ingestion of psyllium laxative. **Allergy** 1983; 38(5): 363–365.

PO102   Harborne, J. B., and C. A. Williams. Comparative biochemistry of flavonoids. XIII. 6-Hydroxyluteolin and scutellarein as phyletic markers in higher plants. **Phytochemistry** 1971; 10: 367–378.

PO103   Machado, L., O. Zetterstrom, and E. Fagerberg. Occupational allergy in nurses to a bulk laxative. **Allergy** 1979; 34(1): 51–55.

PO104   Lerman Garber, I., M. Lagunas, J. C. Sierra Perez, et al. The effect of psyllium *plantago* in slightly to moderately hypercholesterolemic patients. **Archives del Instituto de Cardiologia de Mexico** 1990; 606): 535–539.

PO105   Uribe, M., M. Dibildox, S. Malpica, et al. Beneficial effect of vegetable protein diet supplemented with psyllium *plantago* in patients with hepatic encephalopathy and diabetes mellitus. **Gastroenterology** 1985; 88(4): 901–907.

13 | Saccharum officinarum

L.

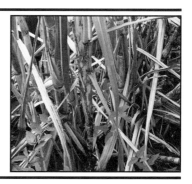

Common Names

'O:yz	Laos	Harilik suhkruroog	Estonia
Aankha	India	Havupunkit	Finland
Ak	Pakistan	Hong gan zhe	China
Ampeu	Cambodia	Iikh	India
Azucar, cane de	Canary Islands	Ikhhu	Pakistan
Azucar, cane de	Guatemala	Kaneh	Israel
Bagasse	China	Kansha	Japan
Cana comun	Spain	Khand	Pakistan
Cana de assucar	Portugal	Ko	Hawaii
Cana de azucar	Canary Islands	Kushiar	Pakistan
Cana de azucar	Guatemala	Mia	Vietnam
Cana de azucar	Mexico	Moba	Tanzania
Cana de azucar	Spain	Naishekar	Iran
Cana dulce	Canary Islands	Noble cane	United States
Cana dulce	Spain	Oi daeng	Thailand
Canaduz	Spain	Oi	Thailand
Canamiel	Spain	Qasab al sukkar	Arabic countries
Cane, sugar	India	Qasab es sukkar	Arabic countries
Canna da zucchero	Italy	Saccar	Nepal
Canna mele	Italy	Sahacar	Nepal
Canne de sucre	France	Sahachar	Nepal
Cay mia	Vietnam	Sakhara	India
Cha'ncat	Mexico	Sakharnyi trostnik	Russia
Cukornad	Hungary	kul'turnyi	
Cukrova trtina	Czech Republic	Sakharnyi trostnik	Russia
Dulce, cana	Canary Islands	lekarstvennyi	
Gan zhe	China	Satou kibi	Japan
Ganiesi	Nicaragua	Shecerna trska	Croatia
Ganna	Nepal	Shecerna trska	Serbia
Ganna	Pakistan	Sladkornitrs	Slovenia
Gannaa	India	Sockerror	Sweden
Gannaa	Pakistan	Sokeriruoko	Finland
Gendari	Pakistan	Sugar cane	Barbados
Guo zhe	China	Sugar cane	Guyana

From: *Medicinal Plants of the World, vol. 3: Chemical Constituents, Traditional and Modern Medicinal Uses*
By: I. A. Ross © Humana Press Inc., Totowa, NJ

Sugar cane	India	Tebu	Indonesia
Sugar cane	Indonesia	Tebu	Malaysia
Sugar cane	Iran	Tiwu	Sudan
Sugar cane	Jamaica	To pi'avare	Rarotonga
Sugar cane	Tanzania	Ton oi	Thailand
Sugar cane	Trinidad	Tubo	Philippines
Sugarcane	Hawaii	Tue	Papua-New Guinea
Sugarcane, blue ribbon	United States	Ukha	India
Suikerriet	Netherlands	Ukhu	Nepal
Sukkerroer	Denmark	Usa	India
Sukkerror	Norway	Uuka	India
Teboe	Indonesia	Zuckerrohr	Germany
Tebu telur	Malaysia		

BOTANICAL DESCRIPTION

Saccharum officinarum is a tropical perennial grass of the GRAMINEAE family. It is 3–4 m tall, approx 5 cm in diameter, with unbranched stems, which have many nodes and short conspicuous internodes filled with solid, juicy pulp. Each stem produces its own root system. Two types of roots develop: the first type, from the primordia of the cutting after planting, are thin and branched, and the second type, from the primordia of the tillers, which are thick, fleshy, and less branched. With age, all roots become brown, shrivel, and die. Leaves are up to 1.5 m long, falling from the lower stems when they wither. Each leaf consists of linear-lanceolate blade, up to 10 cm wide in the base, narrowing into sheath clasping the stem, sharp serrate on the margin and siliceous. The midrib is prominent and broad, white and concave on the upper surface, and green below. Flowers are clustered in large, dense, feathery, ovoid, terminal panicles up to 1 m or more, with many fragile, jointed branches. Spikelets are paired; one is pedicellate and the other sessile, with silver silky hairs spreading from the base, twice as long as the body of spikelet. Both spikelets are two-flowered: the lower empty, and the upper bisexual. Glumes are equal, mostly chartaceous, lemma of upper floret is awnless. The seeds are ovate, yellowish-brown, approx 1 mm long, dry one-seeded fruits.

ORIGIN AND DISTRIBUTION

Native to Old World tropics, probably New Guinea. It is cultivated for the sugar-rich stems or canes in the most parts of Southeast Asia, Africa, India, South America, China, islands of the Pacific and Caribbean, and other tropical regions.

TRADITIONAL MEDICINAL USES

Brazil. Hot water extract of the fresh leaf is taken orally to treat hypertension or induce diuresis[SO113].

Canary Islands. Hot water extract of the fresh fruit juice is taken orally for cystitis and hot water extract of the fresh stem is used ophthalmically for conjunctivitis[SO121].

Guatemala. Hot water extract of the dried leaf is taken orally for renal inflammation and as a diuretic[SO118]. Hot water extract of the dried stalk is used externally for skin diseases and irritations, mouth lesions, stomatitis, dermatitis, and inflammations[SO119].

Hawaii. Water extract of the shoot is taken orally for asthma[SO129].

India. Decoction of the juice, 2–3 g *Diospyros melanoxylon* gum and water are boiled and taken orally three times daily for 3 days for typhoid. No food is taken during treatment. Juice is mixed with *Ficus religiosa* roots and made into pills the size of small peas. Pills are taken mornings and evenings for 3 days for malaria[SO117]. Ten grams of 3-year-old fresh stem and 0.5 g of sulfur are mixed thoroughly, made into pills the size of a peanut, and taken orally. Three pills daily are taken by women for approx 40 days to produce permanent sterility[SO122].

Indonesia. Extract of the plant is used as an abortifacient[SO079]. A 4–5 cm long piece of black cane stalk is pounded with half of a young pineapple, ragi (rice, garlic, *Alpinia galangal*, cinnamon, ginger, and *Capsicum annuum*) and diluted with water. The extract is taken twice daily as an abortifacient[SO110].

Mexico. Ethanol (95%) extract of the stem is used as a mouthwash for toothaches. The extract is rubbed on affected area of nettle stings[SO111].

Nepal. Hot water extract of the stem is taken orally by men as an aphrodisiac[SO078].

Pakistan. Juice of the stem is taken orally in large quantities as an anaphrodisiac[SO079].

Papua-New Guinea. Fresh stem is chewed for diarrhea and vomiting sickness[SO100].

Rarotonga. Juice of the fresh stem is taken orally to treat bronchitis[SO125].

Saudi Arabia. Boiled molasses is used to sterilize wounds[SO124].

Taiwan. Decoction of the dried root is taken orally to treat diabetes mellitus[SO126].

Tanzania. Decoction of the dried stems of sugar cane and *Pachystela msolo* is taken orally as a galactogogue[SO114].

CHEMICAL CONSTITUENTS

(*ppm unless otherwise indicated*)

2-[4-(3-Hydroxy-1-propenyl)-2,6-dimethoxyphenoxy]-3-hydroxy-3-(4-hydroxy-3,5-dimethoxyphenyl)propyl-β-D-glucopyranoside: Pl[SO004]

3-[5-(Threo) 2,3-dihydro-2-(4-hydroxy-3-methoxyphenyl)-3-hydroxymethyl-7-methoxybenzofuranyl]-propanoic acid: Pl[SO004]

3-Hydroxy-1-(4-hydroxy-3,5-dimethoxyphenyl)-2-[4-(3-hydroxy-1-(E)-propenyl)-2,6-dimethoxyphenoxy]propyl-β-D-glucopyranoside: Pl[SO044]

3-Hydroxy-1-(4-hydroxy-3-methoxyphenyl)-2-[4-(3-hydroxy-1-(E)-propenyl)-2-methoxyphenoxy]propyl-β-D-glucopyranoside: Pl[SO044]

3-Hydroxy-1-(4-hydroxy-3-methoxyphenyl)-2-[4-(3-hydroxy-1-(E)-propenyl)-2,6-dimethoxyphenoxy]propyl-β-D-glucopyranoside: Pl[SO044]

3-Hydroxy-4,5-dimethoxyphenyl-β-D-glucopyranoside: Pl[SO044]

4-(β-D-glucopyranosyloxy)-3,5-dimethoxyphenyl-propanone: Pl[SO004]

4-[(Erythro) 2,3-dihydro-3(hydroxymethyl)-5-(3-hydropropyl)-7-methoxy-2-benzofuranyl]-2,6-dimethoxyphenyl-β-D-glucopyranoside: Pl[SO004]

4-[Ethane-2-[3-(4-hydroxy-3-methoxyphenyl)-2-propen]oxy]-2,6-dimethoxyphenyl-β-D-glucopyranoside: Pl[SO044]

4-[Ethane-2-[3-(4-hydroxy-3-methoxyphenyl)-2-propen]oxy]-2-methoxyphenyl-β-D-glucopyranoside: Pl[SO044]

9-O-β-D-xylopyranoside of icariol A2: Pl[SO004]

Abscisic acid: St[SO091]

α-Galactosidase: Immature Stalk[SO019]

α-Mannosidase: Immature Stalk[SO019]

Apigenin, 5-7-dimethyl: 4'-O-β-D-glucoside: Lf[SO102]

Apigenin, 5-O-methyl: Fl[SO104]

Apigenin: St[SO128]

Arabinose: St[SO101]

Arundoin: Lf wax[SO096]

Benzoic acid: St[SO086]

β-D-fructfuranosyl-α-D-(6-syringyl)-glucopyranoside: Pl[SO044]

β-D-fructfuranosyl-α-D-(6-vanilloyl)-glucopyranoside: Pl[SO044]

β-Galactosidase: Immature Stalk[SO019]

β-Glucosidase: Immature Stalk[SO019]

β-N-acetylglucosaminidase: Immature Stalk[SO019]

β-xylosidase: Immature Stalk[SO018]

Calcium: Pl Ju[SO087]

Campesterol: Bract[SO093], St[SO085]

Coumarin: St[SO086]

Cylindrin: Lf wax[SO096]

Dehydrodiconiferyl alcohol-9'-β-D-glucopyranoside: Pl[SO044]

Dotriacontanoic acid: Wax[SO043]

Feruloyl-α-L-arabinofuranosyl(phenylpropanoid-1-3)-O-β-D-xylopyranosyl(1-4)-D-xylopyranose, O-β-D-xylopyranosyl(1-4)-O-(5-O-*trans*): St[SO095]

Flavone, 5-7-dimethoxy-3'-O-β-D-glucoside: St[SO088]

Flavone,3'-4'-5-7-tetrahydroxy-3-6-dimethoxy: Fl[SO104]

Flavone,7-hyroxy-5-methoxy: 3'-O-β-D-galactoside: St[SO088]

Fructose: St[SO101]

Galactose: St[SO101]

Gibberellin A-1: St[SO091]

Gibberellin A-19: St[SO091]

Gibberellin A-20: St[SO091]

Gibberellin A-29: St[SO091]

Gibberellin A-3: St[SO091]

Glucose: St[SO101]

Invertase: Immature Stalk[SO019]

Lupeol, O-methyl: Lf wax[SO096]

Luteolin: St[SO128]

Melibiose: Immature Stalk[SO019]

Mg inorganic: Pl Ju[SO087]

Octacosanoid acid: Wax[SO043]

Octacosanol: Wax[SO016]

O-Nitrophenyl-β-D-xylopyrosinase: Immature Stalk[SO018]

Orientin, 3'-7-dimethyl ether: St[SO108]

Orientin, iso, 3'-7-dimethoxy: Pl[SO092]

Orientin, iso, 3'-7-dimethyl ether: St[SO108]

Orientin, iso: St[SO128]

Orientin: St[SO128]

Peonidin-3-O-β-D-galactoside: St[SO089]

Phenyl-O-D-glucoside, 3-4-6-trimethohy: St[SO082]

Phenyl-O-D-glucoside, 3-4-dimethoxy: St[SO082]

Phosphorus inorganic: Pl Ju[SO087]

Phytosterol: Bract 0.36-0.43%[SO093]

P-Nitrophenyl-β-D-xylopyrosinase: Immature Stalk[SO018]

Potassium inorganic: Fr Ju (unripe)[SO103], Pl Ju[SO087]

Protein (*Saccharum officinarum*): Bagasse (press mud) 40.0%[SO081]

Raffinose: Immature Stalk[SO019]

Saccharan A: St[SO099], Stalk[SO094]

Saccharan B: St[SO099], Stalk[SO094]

Saccharan C: St[SO099], Stalk[SO094]

Saccharan D: St[SO099], Stalk[SO094]

Saccharan E: St[SO099], Stalk[SO094]

Saccharan F: St[SO099], Stalk[SO094]

Saccharum officinarum glucan B-O: Bagasse[SO115]

Schaftoside, iso: St[SO128]

Schaftoside: St[SO128]

Sitosterol, β: St[SO085], Bract[SO093]

Stachyose: Immature Stalk[SO019]

Stigmasterol: St[SO085], Bract[SO093]

Sucrose: St[SO086]

Sugar, invert: St[SO084]

Sulfur inorganic: Pl Ju[SO087]

Swertiajaponin: St[SO128]

Swertisin: St[SO108]

Taraxerol methyl ether: Lf wax[SO096]

Tetracontanoic acid: Wax[SO043]

Traicontanoic acid: Wax[SO043]

Tricin: St[SO128]

Tricin-7-glucoside sulfate: St[SO128]

Tricin-7-glucoside: St[SO108]

Tricin-7-O-(2"-O-rhamnosyl)-galacturonide: St[SO108]

Tricin-7-O-β-D-glucopyranoside: Pl[SO092]

Tricin-7-rhamnosyl-galacturonide: St[SO128]

Vanilloyl-1-O-β-D-glucoside: Rt[SO083]

Vicenin: Pl[SO092]

Xylopyranose, D, O-(5-O-feruloyl-α-L-arabinofuranosyl)-(1-3)-O-β-D-Xylopyranosyl-(1-4): St[SO107]

Xylose: St[SO101]

PHARMACOLOGICAL ACTIVITIES AND CLINICAL TRIALS

Abortifacient effect. Ethanol (50%) extract of the dried leaf, administered intragastrically to rats at a dose of 200 mg/kg, was active[SO112].

Acetylcholine release. Policosanol produced some interactions in the modulation of the acetylcholine (ACh) release at the mouse neuromuscular junction. Policosanol enhanced to a small extent either the spontaneous or the evoked ACh release. An increase in the rate of the conformational change induced at the nicotinic receptor-channel complex by ACh was also observed[SO053].

Allergenic effect. Twenty-two children with asthma aged from 7 to 14 years old, and 12 "normal" control children aged from 8 to 13 years were submitted to nonspecific bronchoprovocation test with metacholine before and during the sugar cane burning. The metacholine concentrations used were 0.025, 0.25, 1, 2.5, 10, and 25 mg/mL. The results were expressed as concentration of metacholine that induces a fall of 20% or more in the forced expiratory volume in the first second (FEV1; PC$_{20}$). The PC$_{20}$ average for children with asthma was significantly lower than the control group, before (asthmatic children [A] = 3.68, control children [C] = 25.62 mg/mL) and during the burning (A = 4.11, C = 25.25 mg/mL) ($p < 0.05$). There were no significant differences when PC$_{20}$ values before and during burning were compared in each group. The same was observed regarding FEV1, forced vital capacity (FVC), and forced expiratory flux (FEF) between 25 and 75% of FVC (25–75%)[SO028]. Specific immunoglobulin (Ig) E antibodies to sugar cane pollen were investigated in 74 Okinawan children who suffered from allergic disorders. Two (2.7%) with asthma of the 74 patients had specific IgE antibodies to sugar cane pollen, house dust, and *Dermatophagoides farinae*. They had no histories of their symptoms being aggravated when sugar cane flowers bloom[SO059]. The interaction of a complement activating glucan from sugar cane (Bo) with Igs was studied. Bo precipitated a small fraction of IgG from human serum. In combination with this fraction, it activated complement by the classical pathway, not in its absence. The results indicated that normal human serum contains natural antibodies against Bo, which form complement-activating immune complexes with Bo by binding it to their F(ab) region. The antibodies did not cross-react with dextran, a glucan from barley, and surface constituents of *Escherichia coli*[SO067]. The immunostimulating polysaccharide (Bo) from sugar cane activated complement in whole human and guinea pig serum in vitro by the classical pathway. Complement consumption was also demonstrated in guinea pigs on iintravenous injection. Complement in sera from two severely patients with hypogammaglobulinemia was not activated by polysaccharide but was made reactive by the addition of purified human IgG[SO68]. Three glucan contaminants of crude cane sugar and invert sugar solutions, applied intradermally into human skin, produced localized wheals and erythema reactions. The glucans were active on intradermal injection into both dextran-sensitive and dextran-resistant rats and, like dextrans, were active on subcutaneous injection into dextran-sensitive animals[SO072].

Analgesic effect. FAM, a mixture of fatty acids from wax oil, in the hot-plate model and in the acetic acid-induced writhing test in mice, produced analgesic properties[SO005]. Ethanol (95%) extracts of the fresh leaf, administered intragastrically to mice at a dose of 1 g/kg, were active vs benzoyl peroxide-induced writhing. Extract of the fresh shoot was inactive. Both extracts were inactive vs tail flick response to hot water[SO120].

Antibacterial activity. Tincture of dried stalk (extract of 10 g plant material in 100 mL ethanol), on agar plate at a concentration of 30 µL/disc, was inactive on *Pseudomonas aeruginosa*, *Staphylococcus aureus*, and produced weak activity on *Escherichia coli*[SO119].

Antihepatotoxic activity. Water extract of the dried stem (bagasse), administered intraperitoneally to mice at a dose of 25 mg/kg, was active vs CCl$_4$-induced hepatotoxicity[SO105].

Antihypercholesterolemic effect. Policosanol, administered orally to normocholesterolemic New Zealand rabbits at doses of 5–200 mg/kg for 4 weeks, significantly reduced total cholesterol and low-density lipoprotein cholesterol (LDL-C) serum levels in a dose-dependent manner. Serum triglyceride (TG) levels of the treated and control animals were significantly different, but the reduction observed was not dose-dependent. High-density lipoprotein cholesterol (HDL-C) levels remained unchanged. The results indicated that the reduction in total cholesterol values induced by policosanol was mainly mediated through a decrease in LDL-C levels[SO16]. Policosanol was administered to patients who were obese (body mass index [BMI] $\geq$ 30) with type II hypercholesterolemia at a dose of 5 mg once daily with the evening meal for 3 years. The treatment significantly lowered serum LDL-C ($p < 0.01$ vs placebo), the primary efficacy variable (24.3%), and total cholesterol (15.8%) after 1 year of treatment. There was an increase in HDL-C (21.9%). The effects were persistent during the trial. At the completion of the study, policosanol had lowered LDL-C by 31.8% and total cholesterol by 20.1%, whereas it markedly raised HDL-C (24.6%). Thirty patients (18 placebos and 12 policosanol) discontinued the study: 15 (11 placebos and 4 policosanol) because of adverse events and 12 (9 placebos and 3 policosanol) because of serious adverse events (SAE), most vascular. Policosanol was safe and well tolerated, not impairing significantly any safety indicator. Average body weight was slightly reduced during the study, indicating a general acceptable compliance with dietary recommendations, but policosanol did not show any drug effect on body weight[SO020]. Policosanol, administered to 239 patients with type 2 diabetes at a dose of 5 mg/day or placebo for 2 years, significantly reduced LDL-C (21.1%), total cholesterol (17.5%), and TGs (16%) after 1 year. There was an increase in HDL-C levels (10.7%). The effects of the treatment persisted during the study. At the completion of the study, policosanol lowered LDL-C (29.5%), total cholesterol (21.9%), and TGs (16.9%) and elevated HDL-C (12.4%). No significant changes on lipid profile variables of the placebo group occurred during the study. The frequency of serious adverse events, most vascular, in policosanol patients (6/119, 5%) was lower than in respective placebo (26/120, 43.3%). No drug-related impairment of safety indicators, particularly on glycemic control, was observed. A reduction of systolic and diastolic blood pressures was observed in patients receiving policosanol compared with placebo[SO021]. D-003 (a mixture of high-molecular-weight aliphatic primary acids purified from sugar cane wax) was administered to rabbits fed a casein diet at doses of 5, 50, and 100 mg/kg/day for 4 weeks. The 50 and 100 mg doses significantly decreased total cholesterol and LDL-C. TGs were not affected. At the completion of the study, HDL-C levels significantly increased at all the doses assayed. D-003 inhibited *de novo* synthesis of cholesterol, since the incorporation of ^3H_2O into sterols in the liver and proximal small bowel was significantly depressed. D-003 significantly raised the rate of removal of [^{125}I]-LDL from serum and significantly elevated [^{125}I]-LDL binding activity to liver homogenates[SO025]. Policosanol was administered to older patients (60–80 years) with type II hypercholesterolemia at a dose of 10 mg tablets once daily with the evening meal for 8 weeks. The treatment was less effective than atorvastatin (10 mg/day) in reducing serum LDL-C and total cholesterol levels. Policosanol, but not atorvastatin, significantly increased serum HDL-C levels, whereas both drugs similarly reduced atherogenic ratios and serum TGs. Policosanol was better tolerated than atorvastatin as revealed by patient withdrawal analysis and overall frequency of adverse events[SO037]. Policosanol was administered to 56 postmenopausal women at a dose of 5 mg/day for 8 weeks and doubled to 10 mg/day during the next 8 weeks. The treatment significantly decreased LDL-C, total cholesterol, the ratios of LDL-C to HDL-C, and total cholesterol to HDL-C when compared with baseline and placebo. HDL-C levels were significantly elevated by 7.4% at the completion of the study. The drug was safe and well tolerated. No drug-related adverse effects were observed. Five patients taking placebo (17.9%) and 13 patients taking policosanol (46.4%) reported improvements in habitual symptoms and health perception during the study[SO046].

Antihyperglycemic activity. Ethanol (95%) extract of the dried leaf, administered intragastrically to rabbits at a dose of 1 g/kg, produced weak activity vs alloxan-induced hyperglycemia. The effect did not increase proportionally with the dose[SO080]. Ethanol (20%) extract of the fresh stem, administered intragastrically to rats at a dose of 60 mg/animal, was active vs glucose administration[SO082].

Anti-implantation effect. Ethanol (50%) extract of the dried leaf, administered intragastrically to hamsters at a dose of 100 mg/kg, was active[SO112].

Anti-inflammatory effect. FAM, administrated orally to rats, produced anti-inflammatory activity in the cotton pellet granuloma assay and in the carrageenin-induced pleurisy test. The effect was also produced in the peritoneal capillary permeability test in mice[SO005].

Anti-thrombotic activity. D-003, administered orally to rats at a single dose of 200 mg/kg, but not at 25 mg/kg, significantly increased plasma levels of 6 keto PGF1-α levels, a stable metabolite of prostacyclin PGI(2) from collagen-stimulated blood (4 μg/mL) compared with control group. Levels of 6 keto PGF1-α levels determined after 10 days of oral treatment with both doses of D-003 were significantly larger than the controls. Single and repeated oral doses of D-003 significantly reduced the thromboxane TxB(2) plasma levels obtained from whole blood stimulated by collagen and the weight of venous thrombus experimentally induced in rats. TxB(2)/6 keto PGF1-α ratio significantly decreased in animals treated with D-003. D-003 at single doses (400 mg/kg but not 200 mg/kg) significantly protected from death induced by endovenous infusion of collagen plus epinephrine in mice[SO040]. D-003, administered orally to guinea pigs and rats at single or repeated doses of 25–200 mg/kg for 3 days, inhibited platelet aggregation induced by collagen (2.2 μg/mL) and adenosine 5'-triphosphate (ADP) (2 μmol/L) in rats, and collagen (0.25 μg/mL) induced aggregation in guinea pigs in a dose-dependent manner. Single doses of D-003 (5–500 mg/kg), administered orally 2 hours before induction of arterial thrombosis, significantly inhibited the reduction of rectal temperature. D-003 administered at a single dose (50–200 mg/kg) 2 hours before the experiment significantly increased the bleeding time in a dose-dependent manner. The time-course effects of D-003 on platelet aggregation, arterial thrombus formation, and bleeding time showed no effect 0.5 hour after dosing, and maximal effects exhibited 1–2 hours after treatment. There was no significant effect 4 hours after treatment[SO050].

Anti-yeast activity. Tincture of the dried stalk (extract of 10 g plant material in 100 mL ethanol), on agar plate at a concentration of 30 μL/disc, was inactive on *Candida albicans*[SO119].

Arterial blood pressure. Policosanol, administered orally to spontaneously hypertensive rats (SHR) at doses of 25, 50, and 200 mg/kg, did not significantly change arterial pressure. Pretreatment with 200 mg/kg of policosanol significantly increased propranolol-induced hypotensive effects. The effect of nifedipine remained unchanged. The results indicated that policosanol did not antagonize the hypotensive effect of β-blockers, but it can increase the hypotensive effect of β-blockers without modifying cardiac frequency[SO012].

Arterial thrombosis. Policosanol, in the venous thrombosis models at a concentration of 25 mg/kg, significantly decreased the thrombus weight, the protective effect persisting until 4 hours after its oral administration and reduced rectal temperature variation induced by arterial thrombosis. At the same dose, policosanol increased 6-keto-PGF1-α serum levels in rats[SO015].

Atherosclerotic lesions protection. Policosanol (with acacia gum as vehicle) was administered orally to male New Zealand rabbits on a cholesterol-rich diet at doses of 25 or 200 mg/kg for 60 days. The control animals developed marked hypercholesterolemia, macroscopic lesions, and arterial intimal thickening. Intima thickness was significantly less (32.5 ± 7 and 25.4 ± 4 μM) in hypercholesterolemic rabbits treated with policosanol than in controls (57.6 ± 9 μM). In most policosanol-treated animals, atherosclerotic lesions were not present. In others, thickness of fatty streaks had less foam cell layers than in controls[SO051]. Policosanol, administered orally to 50 male Wistar rats at doses of 0.5, 2.5, 5, and 25 mg/kg daily for 8 days, produced a significant reduction of the atherosclerotic lesions in animals treated with lipofundin[SO058].

Bone resorption inhibition. D-003 was administered to ovariectomized or sham operated Sprague–Dawley female rats at doses of 50 and 200 mg/kg/day for 3 months. The treatment prevented a decrease in trabecular number and thickness and increases in trabecular separation, osteoclast number, and surface compared with ovariectomized controls. D-003 prevented the bone loss and decreased bone resorption induced by ovariectomy. It failed to increase osteoblast surface compared with control ovariectomized rats[SO024]. A polysaccharide fraction of *Saccharum officinarum* was administered to normal rats and rats fed a high-sugar diet. Feeding the high-sugar diet induced an elevation of serum glucose and significant accumulation of lipid peroxides in the serum and liver. The accumulation of lipid peroxides was inhibited by combined feeding with the polysaccharide fraction. Pathological examination showed that endothelial cell swelling in the ascending aorta in one third of rats receiving the high-sugar diet control but no pathological change was observed in all of the rats concurrently treated with the polysaccharide fraction[SO017]. Sugar cane wax was administered to rats fed a restricted, semipurified diet containing a 50%-reduced level of carbohydrate and oil diet but normal levels of protein, minerals, and vita-

mins. The rats fed this diet did not exhibit osteoporosis as the rats without sugar cane wax in the diet. The sugar cane wax, containing a long-chain carbohydrate with an hydroxy radical, prevented the development of osteoporosis via a nonestrogenic mechanism[SO033].

Carcinogenicity. Policosanol (Ateromixol), administered orally to Swiss mice of both sexes at doses of 50–500 mg/kg for 18 months, produced no differences in daily clinical observations, weight gain, food consumption, and mortality (survival analysis) between groups. Histopathological study indicated that the frequency of neoplastic (benign and malignant) lesions was similar in the control and policosanol-treated groups. No drug-related increase in the occurrence of malignant or benign neoplasm and no acceleration in tumor growth in any specific group were observed[SO057]. Water extract of the stem, administered subcutaneously to female rats at a dose of 35 mg/animal for 77 weeks, was inactive[SO090].

Cardiovascular disease prevention. Policosanols, administered at 5 to 20 mg/day, decreased the risk of atheroma formation by reducing platelet aggregation, endothelial damage, and foam cell formation in animals. It lowered total cholesterol and LDL-C levels by 13 to 23% and 19 to 31%, respectively, while increasing HDL-C from 8 to 29%. Policosanols improved lipid profiles by reducing hepatic cholesterol biosynthesis while enhancing LDL clearance. When compared with statins, policosanols exhibited comparable cholesterol-lowering effects at much smaller doses[SO029].

Carotid artery thickening effect. Policosanol was administered to rabbits with collars around the left carotid at doses of 5 and 25 mg/kg for 7 and 15 days or 20 mg/kg lovastatin for 15 days. There was a significant reduction in neointima in the treated animals compared with controls. The reduction in lovastatin-treated animals was significantly lower than in policosanol-treated groups. The reduction in smooth muscle cell proliferation observed in policosanol-treated rabbits was significantly larger than in lovastatin-treated animals[SO049]. Policosanol, administered orally to rabbits at doses of 5 and 25 mg/kg, prevented intimal thickening. Collars were placed around the left carotid for 15 days. To evaluate intimal thickening, the cross-sectional area of intima and media were measured. Neointima was significantly reduced in policosanol-treated animals compared with controls. The smooth muscle cell proliferation was studied by the immunohistochemical detection of proliferating cell nuclear antigen, and a significant reduction was observed in policosanol-treated rabbits[SO054].

Cerebral ischemia. Policosanol, administered to Mongolian gerbils at a dose of 200 mg/kg immediately after unilateral carotid ligation and at 12- or 24-hour intervals for 48 hours, significantly inhibited mortality and clinical symptoms when compared with controls. Lower dose (100 mg/kg) was not effective. Control animals showed swelling (tissue vacuolization) and necrosis of neurons in all areas of the brain studied (frontal cortex, hippocampus, striatum, and olfactory tubercle), showing a similar injury profile. In the group treated with 200 mg/kg policosanol, swelling and necrosis were significantly reduced when compared with the control group. In another experimental model, policosanol at a dose of 200 mg/kg (n = 19) significantly reduced the edema compared with the control group, with a cerebral water content identical to that of the sham-operated animals. The policosanol-treated group (n = 10) showed significantly higher cyclic adenosine monophosphate (cAMP) levels (2.68 pmol/g of tissue) than the positive control (1.91 pmol/g of tissue) and similar to those of nonligated gerbils (2.97 pmol/g of tissue)[SO052]. Policosanol, administered orally to Mongo-

lian gerbils at doses of 25, 50, and 200 mg/kg, significantly reduced serum thromboxane B2 levels. The highest dose significantly increased 6-keto-PGF1-α. The results indicated that policosanol, at 200 mg/kg, significantly protected against cerebral ischemia induced by unilateral ligation of common carotid artery in Mongolian gerbils. Administration of ineffective doses of policosanol (25 mg/kg) and aspirin (30 mg/kg) significantly protected animals indicating a synergism between them[SO061].

Cholesterol synthesis inhibition. D-003, in cultured fibroblasts at doses of 0.05-50 μg/mL for 12 hours, inhibited cholesterol biosynthesis from ^{14}C-labeled acetate (33–68%) in a dose-dependent manner[SO046]. Policosanol, in human lung fibroblasts for 48 hours before the experiment, produced a dose-dependent inhibition of ^{14}C-acetate incorporation into total cholesterol. Labeled mevalonate incorporation was not inhibited. LDL processing was markedly enhanced. LDL binding, internalization, and degradation were significantly increased after policosanol treatment. Cholesterol generation was not inhibited at the lowest dose of policosanol assayed, but LDL processing was significantly increased[SO060]. Polysaccharide fraction of the dried stem, administered intraperitoneally to rats at a dose of 40 mg/kg, was inactive vs high-sugar diet[SO116].

Chronotropic effect negative. Ethanol (50%) extract of the fresh leaf, administered intragastrically to rats at a dose of 40 mg/kg, was active[SO113].

Coagulative effect. D-003, a mixture of aliphatic primary acid from sugar cane wax, administered orally to beagle dogs at doses of 200 or 400 mg/kg for 9 months, significantly reduced total cholesterol, inhibited platelet aggregation, and increased bleeding time compared with levels in controls. Data analyses of body weight gain, food consumption, clinical observations, the remaining blood biochemistry, and hematology indicators, including coagulation parameters (prothrombin time and kaolin-activated thromboplastin time), organ weight ratios, and histopathological findings, showed no trends with D-003 doses or significant differences between treated animals and controls[SO001].

Cytotoxic activity. Fresh plant juice, in cell culture was inactive, ED_{50} 6.25%[SO109]. Dried retina, in cell culture at undiluted concentration was active on macrophages[SO106]. D-003 at doses of 5 or 25 mg/kg for 18 hours, significantly decreased the percentage of turgent cells and hepatocytes with necrosis and increased the percentage of normal hepatocytes with respect to positive controls in a dose-dependent manner. Necrotic areas and inflammatory infiltrates were observed in the liver of 90% positive (paracetamol-treated) controls. D-003 dramatically reduced both necrotic areas and inflammatory infiltrate and was present in 10% animals treated in the two experimental series. There were no histological alterations in liver sections of negative controls[SO003]. D-003 was administered to male Sprague–Dawley rats with acute hepatotoxicity induced by intraperitoneal injection of carbon tetrachloride (1 mL/kg). Treatment with D-003 at 25 or 100 mg/kg for 18 hours significantly decreased the percentage of ballooned cells and hepatocytes with lipidic inclusions. It increased the percentage of normal hepatocytes compared with that in positive controls in a dose-dependent manner. The percent inhibitions of the occurrence of ballooned cells and hepatocytes with lipids were marked (75 and 50%, respectively) with the high dose (100 mg/kg). The percentage of turgent hepatocytes was significantly reduced compared with positive controls, but this effect was not dose-dependent. No histological alterations in the liver sections of negative controls were found. Necrotic areas and inflammatory in-

filtrate were observed in the liver of 87.5% of positive controls. D-003 dramatically reduced both necrotic areas and inflammatory infiltrate and was present in only 12.5% animals treated with 25 mg/kg of D-003 and in none (0%) of the animals treated with 100 mg/kg[SO007].

Dental caries development influence. Two groups of sugar cane cutters and sisal plant workers, with similar socioeconomic backgrounds, had similar levels of fluoride in drinking water, consuming similar amounts of refined sugar per day but had a significant difference in the number of pieces of sugar cane chewed per day. Sugar cane cutters had significantly higher mean decayed missing teeth (DMT)/decayed missing surface (DMS) scores than sisal plant workers. Analysis of variance revealed a weakly significant effect of sugar cane chewing on the caries scores ($p = 0.02$ from DMT and $p = 0.05$ for DMS). The results of the study indicated that sugar cane chewing in large quantities for a long period has a caries-promoting effect in populations with a low-caries prevalence[SO063].

Diabetogenic effect. Chromatographic fraction of the fresh stem, administered intragastrically to rats at a dose of 1 g/kg, was active. The fraction inhibited the elevation of serum TG, lipid peroxides, and insulin of rats fed on a high-sugar diet for 61 days[SO127].

Diuretic activity. Decoction of the dried leaf, administered nasogastrically to rats at a dose of 1 g/kg, was inactive[SO118]. Ethanol (50%) extract of the fresh leaf, administered intragastrically to rats at a dose of 40 mL/kg, was active. Five parts fresh plant material in 100 parts water/ethanol was used[SO098].

Esophageal motility. Forty healthy volunteers (20 aged 20–30 years, 10 aged 50–60 years, and 10 aged 70–80 years) were submitted to esophageal manometry during 10 swallows of water, 10 swallows of sugar cane syrup, and 10 "dry" swallows. Basal pressure of the upper esophageal sphincter and the lower esophageal sphincter, amplitude, duration and velocity of contraction, and the duration of the lower esophageal sphincter relaxation were measured. Water and sugar cane syrup did not differ regarding quantitative contraction parameters, but sugar cane syrup led to a higher incidence of synchronous contractions. The three age groups had similar amplitude and velocity of con-tractile waves. The oldest group had markedly more frequent synchronous contractions and failures of contraction after both water and sugar cane syrup swallows. This was associated with a high incidence of scintigraphic transit abnormalities in this group[SO055].

Fecal steroid and lipid excretion. Fiber supplements from sugar cane residue (bagasse), administered to volunteers for 12 weeks, increased stool weights and stool fat excretion. Bagasse increased the daily loss of acid steroids and decreased transit time without alteration in fecal flora. The increased excretion of bile acids and fatty acids failed to lower the plasma cholesterol and TGs after 12 weeks[SO076].

Foam-cell formation. Policosanol was administered to 18 Wistar rats with carrageenan-induced granulomas at doses of 2.5 or 25 mg/kg for 20 days. The treatment produced a significant reduction of the foam-cell formation in granulomas (extravascular medium)[SO056].

Gastrointestinal effect. Sugar-cane fiber (bagasse) was administered to normal ambulant volunteers at a dose of 10.5 g of bagasse containing 5.1 g of crude fiber to a normal diet containing 3.7 g of crude dietary fiber daily for 9 months. The treatment raised the mean fecal weight from 88.3 ± 6.4 g to 139.7 ± 10.2 g/day ($p < 0.005$). There was a significant rise in fecal solids and fecal water, although the percentage of water in the stools remained unchanged. Bagasse supplements accelerated gastrointestinal transit when measured by the carmine marker technique. Daily supplements of bagasse increased the total daily excretion of fecal bacteria, but there were no changes in bacteria excreted per gram of feces. The composition of the bacterial flora showed no change. There was increased excretion of fecal acid sterols on the bagasse supplement, but this failed to occur with bran. No changes attributable to fiber supplements occurred in the plasma TGs or cholesterol[SO073].

Glutamate–oxaloacetate–transaminase inhibition. Polysaccharide fraction of the dried stem, administered intraperitoneally to rats at a dose of 40 mg/kg, was active vs high-sugar diet[SO116].

Glutamate–oxaloacetate–transaminase stimulation. Polysaccharide fraction of the dried stem, administered intragastrically to rats at a dose of 1 g/kg, was active vs high-sugar diet[SO116].

Glutamate–pyruvate–transaminase inhibition. Polysaccharide fraction of the dried stem, administered intraperitoneally to rats at a dose of 40 mg/kg, was inactive[SO116].

Glutamate–pyruvate–transaminase stimulation. Polysaccharide fraction of the dried stem, administered intragastrically to rats at a dose of 1 g/kg, was active vs high-sugar diet[SO116].

Growth-promoting effect. Sugar cane extract, administered orally to 1-week-old chicken at a dose of 500 mg/kg/day for 3 or 6 days, produced significantly higher body weight and gain in body weight/day and a lower food conversion ratio within the growing period of 6 weeks than physiological saline-administered control chickens[SO038]. A black phenolic-carbohydrate complex (nonsugar, nondialyzable components of cane molasses fractions), administered to male weanling rats at a dose of 0.03% of diet, significantly increased the growth rate above that of rats fed the basal diet alone. The alkaline cleaved, nondialyzable-free hemicellulose stimulated growth when incorporated into rat diets at the 0.03% levels. Acid hydrolysis of the complex yielded an insoluble product identified as lignin and represented 18–20% of the entire complex[SO074].

Hemoglobin effect. Molasses, administered to 40 male weaning rats, 21 days of age, at a dose of 12.5% molasses in casein diet with 10.14% protein, produced a small but not significant increase in hemoglobin levels compared to the control groups[SO048].

Hepatotoxicity. D-003 was administered to male Sprague–Dawley rats with liver damage induced by paracetamol orally at a dose of 600 mg/kg, or intraperitoneally at a dose of 200 mg/kg[SO003].

3-Hydroxy-3-methylglutaryl coenzyme A reductase activity. Policosanol, in Vero fibroblast cell culture at concentrations of 0.5–50 µg/mL, decreased in a dose-dependent manner, cholesterol biosynthesis from [^{14}C]-acetate and ^{3}H-water, but not from [^{14}C]-mevalonate. There was no evidence for a competitive or noncompetitive inhibition of 3-hydroxy-3-methylglutaryl coenzyme A (HMG-CoA) reductase activity. Treatment of intact cells with policosanol in the presence of lipid-depleted medium produced a suppressive effect on enzyme activity, indicating a modulatory effect of policosanol on reductase activity[SO009]. Policosanol downregulated cellular expression of HMG-CoA reductase and, thus, has the potential to suppress isoprenylation reactions much like statins do. Policosanol did not directly inhibit HMG-CoA reductase, and even in high concentrations, it failed to downregulate this enzyme by more than 50%, thus likely accounting for the safety of policosanol[SO041].

Hypocholesterolemic activity. A mixture of high molecular-weight primary aliphatic alcohols from sugar cane (Lesstanol, provided by Johnson & Barana), administered intragastrically to normocholesterolemic rabbits at a dose of 100 mg/kg at 48 hour intervals for 4 weeks, produced no effect on food intake and body weight. Plasma LDL increased and plasma TG levels decreased in all groups. The results did not confirm a hypocholesterolemic effect of policosanol[SO022].

Hypoglycemic activity. Ethanol (95%) extract of the dried leaf, administered intragastrically to rabbits at a dose of 1 g/kg, produced weak activity[SO080]. Juice of the dried stalk, administered intraperitoneally to mice at a dose of 200 mg/kg, was active[SO094]. Polysaccharide fraction of the dried stem, administered intraperitoneally to rats at a dose of 40 mg/kg, was inactive vs high-sugar diet[SO116].

Hypolipemic activity. Polysaccharide fraction of the dried stem, administered intragastrically to rats at a dose of 1 g/kg, was active vs high-sugar diet. Intraperitoneal administration at a dose of 40 mg/kg was active[SO116].

Hypotensive activity. Ethanol (50%) extract of the fresh leaf, administered intragastrically to rats at a dose of 40 mL/kg, was active[SO113].

Immunostimulating effect. Sugar cane extract, administrated orally to 3-week-old chickens at a dose of 500 mg/kg/day for 3 days before or after irradiation, enhanced both primary and secondary immune responses in chickens immunized with sheep red blood cells and *Brucella abortus*. Cell-mediated immunity was measured by delayed-type hypersensitivity to human γ-globulin[SO002]. Sugar cane extract, administered orally to 2- or 10-month-old chickens at a dose of 500 mg/kg/day for 3 days before immunized with sheep red blood cells, *Brucella abortus*, and *Salmonella enteritidis* organisms, produced significantly increased and prolonged antibody responses to these antigens, compared with control chickens. Chickens treated with extract revealed enhanced delayed type hypersensitivity responses to human γ globulin[SO036]. Sugar cane extract, in chicken polymorphonuclear cell culture of the peripheral blood at doses of 250–1 mg/mL for 24 hours, significantly increased the phagocytosis[SO038]. Water extract of the dried stem, administered intragastrically to mice at a dose of 200 mg/kg, prolonged the survival time of animals irradiated by deep X-ray. Intraperitoneal administration to mice, at a dose of 25 mg/kg, increased spleen weight and antagonized the immunosuppressive actions of prednisolone and cyclophosphamide. Intraperitoneal administration to mice at a dose of 25 mg/kg, prolonged the survival time of animals irradiated by deep X-ray and was inactive on graft vs host reaction model[SO105].

Immunosuppression prevention. Sugar cane extract was administered orally to 3-week-old inbred chickens at a dose of 500 mg/kg/day for 3 days before or after injection of cyclophosphamide; on the last day, the chickens were immunized intravenously with sheep red blood cells (SRBC) and *Brucella abortus*. The treatment produced a significant increase in body weight, gain in body weight per day, relative weight of the bursa of Fabricius, and antibody responses to SRBC and *Brucella abortus* than untreated control chickens. There were significantly higher values in body weight, gain in body weight per day, and relative bursal weight, and antibody responses to both antigens, when compared to chickens treated with cyclophosphamide alone. In histological examination, chickens that were given the extract showed a typical bursa with well-constituted follicles, and chickens treated with extract and cyclophosphamide showed a well-reconstituted bursa with almost normal structure[SO023].

Insulin antagonist. Ethanol (20%) extract of the fresh stem, administered intragastrically to rats at a dose of 60 mg/animal, was active vs glucose administration. Insulin elevation was inhibited[SO082H13208].

Lipid metabolism. Polysaccharide fraction of the dried stem, administered intragastrically to rats at a dose of 1 g/kg daily for 14 weeks, was active vs high-sugar diet. The effect was measured in the liver. Intraperitoneal administration at doses of 20 and 40 mg/kg for 14 weeks was active. The higher dose produced an increase of liver phospholipids[SO116]. Sugar cane carbohydrate was administered to rats at doses: a. starch (54%) + cane sugar (0%); b. starch (44%) + cane sugar (10%); c. starch (10%) + cane sugar (44%); and d. only cane sugar (54%) for 8 weeks. The beneficial effect of the unsaturated fat in lowering the serum cholesterol level was nullified by an excess of cane sugar in the diet. In the liver, there was an increase of 40–50% of cholesterol, as the cane sugar level in the diet was raised, irrespective of the type of dietary fat[SO075]. D-003 was administered orally to normocholesterolemic rabbits at doses of 5 mg/kg/day alone or with fluvastatin at 5 mg/kg/day each for 30 days. D-003 produced a decrease of LDL-C by 81.5% ($p < 0.01$) and the combined therapy reduced LDL-C values by 75.9%. D-003 and combined therapy significantly lowered serum total cholesterol by 48.4% ($p < 0.01$) and 45.3%, respectively, compared to controls. The responses of LDL-C and total cholesterol to combined therapy were statistically similar but less pronounced than those reached by D-003 alone. D-003 and combined therapy increased HDL-C 21.5% and 19%, respectively; the changes were significant vs the control. Combined therapy, but not D-003 alone, lowered TGs (13.0%, $p < 0.05$ vs control). The effects of combined therapy on HDL-C were similar to those of D-003 alone. All groups showed similar food consumption and body weight gain, health status being unaffected by the treatments[SO027]. Octa-6, a policosanol mixture from sugar cane wax, was administered orally to 50 male golden Syrian hamsters at a dose of 25 mg/kg body weight for 4 weeks. The treatment produced no difference between Octa-6 and Ricewax (a policosanol mixture from rice wax, 50 mg/kg BW) treatments in any of the lipid parameters measured, and both had similar levels of TG, total cholesterol, and HDL-C as the control. Octa-6, but not Ricewax increased non-HDL-C as compared with the control[SO032].

Lipoprotein oxidation inhibition. Policosanol was administered orally to rats at doses of 250–500 mg/kg/day for up to 4 weeks. There was no change in cholesterol, TGs, and phospholipid content of lipoprotein very low-density lipoprotein + LDL fractions. Policosanol significantly prolonged the lag time and reduced the propagation rate of diene generation and thiobarbituric acid-reactive substances content. Policosanol increased lysine reactivity in Cu^{2+}-treated lipoprotein fractions[SO011]. Policosanol, administered orally to rats at doses of 100 and 250 mg/kg for up to 4 weeks, produced a partial prevention of rat in vitro microsomal lipid peroxidation. The formation of thiobarbituric acid-reactive substances in microsomes isolated from treated rats was significantly decreased by about 50%, when peroxidation was initiated by Fe^{3+}/ADP/nicontinamide adenine dinucleotide phosphate (NADPH), Fe^{2+}/ascorbate, and CCl4/NADPH-generating system. Oral administration of policosanol in rats provided a partial inhibition of lipid peroxidation[SO013]. D-003, administered orally to rats at doses of 0.5, 5, 50, and 100 mg/kg for 4 weeks, produced at doses 5, 50, and 100 mg/kg significant inhibition of copper-mediated conjugated-diene generation in a concentration-dependent manner. D-003 increased lag phase by 53.1, 115.3, and 119.3%, respectively, and decreased the rate of conjugate-diene generation by 16.6, 21.5, and 19.6%, respectively. D-003 inhibited azo-compound-initiated and macrophage-mediated lipid peroxidation as judged by the

significant decrease in thiobarbituric acid reactive substance generation. In all the systems, the maximum effect was attained at 50 mg/kg. There was a parallel attenuation in the reduction of lysine amino groups and a significant reduction of carbonyl content after oxidation of lipoprotein samples[SO043]. Policosanol, administered to patients with type II hypercholesterolemia at doses of 20 mg/day or 40 mg/day, did not produce significant additional cholesterol-lowering efficacy at higher dose over the 20 mg/day dose[SO045].

Metabolic effect. A case of 22 infants with acute diarrhea was studied. Eleven infants aged 4–10 months were given nasogastric infusion, and 11 infants aged 5–17 months received intravenous fluid. The absorption of nasogastric infusion fluid was remarkable as was observed by the amount of stool loss, weight gain, reduction of serum specific gravity, and urea nitrogen. Biochemical study showed high incidence of hypernatremia. Nasogastric infusion fluid containing a table salt and cane sugar provided effective volume. Electrolyte imbalance and metabolic acidosis were gradually corrected at a similar rate to bicarbonate-containing solution. Balance study indicated that nasogastric infusion retained less nitrogen and sodium during the course of treatment as compared to intravenous infusion. All of the infants recovered from diarrheal disease once dehydration was corrected without complications[SO071].

Migraine. Sixty patients with migraine completed elimination diets after a 5-day period of withdrawal from their normal diet. Fifty-two (87%) of the patients had been using oral contraceptive steroids, tobacco, and/or ergotamine for an average of 3 years, 22 years, and 7.4 years, respectively. The foods causing reactions were wheat (78%), orange (65%), eggs (45%), tea and coffee (40% each), chocolate and milk (37% each), beef (35%), and corn, cane sugar, and yeast (33% each). When averages of 10 common foods were avoided, there was a dramatic fall in the number of headaches per month, 85% of patients becoming headache-free. The 25% of patients with hypertension became normotensive[SO070].

Myocardial necrosis inhibition. D-003 was administered orally to rats with isoproterenol-induced myocardial necrosis at single (25–400 mg/kg) or repeated doses of 5–200 mg/kg. Single doses dose-dependently decreased necrosis area, percent of infarct area, and the presence of polymorphonuclear cells (PMNs) in myocardial tissue, but only the reductions induced by 200 and 400 mg/kg were significant. D-003 administered repeatedly for 10 days decreased all myocardial necrosis indicators in a dose-dependent manner, with results effective from 25 mg/kg to the highest dose tested, indicating that the repeated dose scheme was more effective to prevent the damage[SO031].

Ophthalmic surgical swabs. Four locally available plant materials have been studied and adapted for use as suitable surgical swabs for various ophthalmic surgical procedures. Corn, millet and sugar cane stems, and the banana leaf frond provided cheap, easily available, and suitable materials for use as alternative surgical swabs to the much used and tested German Spontex swabs[SO064].

Platelet aggregation. Policosanol, in patients with type II hypercholesterolemia and positive pleiotropic properties (inhibition of platelet aggregation and lipid peroxidation), reduced thromboxane A(2) and malondialdehyde (MDA) serum levels. In rats, the percentage of inhibition of adenosine diphosphate-induced aggregation (preincubation with nitroprusside) was higher in platelet-rich plasma of policosanol-treated animals than in control animals. Pretreatment with single doses of policosanol significantly increased the nitroprusside-induced hypotensive effect[SO006]. D-003, administered orally to Sprague–Dawley rats of both sexes at doses of 250, 500, and 1000 mg/kg/day for 6 months, significantly inhibited platelet aggregation. Bleeding time was increased after 3 months of treatment with D-003. The increase was maintained for 6 months and was reversible after washout. Coagulation factors, such as prothrombin time and kaolin-activated thromboplastin-time, which were determined in eight male animals from each group, were unaffected. Data analyses of body weight gain, food consumption, clinical observations, blood biochemistry, hematology, organ weight ratios, and histopathological findings did not show trends related to D-003 dose or significant differences between control and treated groups. The highest studied dose of D-003 (1 mg/kg/day) represented a nontoxic dose level in the chronic toxicity study in rats[SO008]. Policosanol, administered orally to rats at doses of 5–20 mg/kg, inhibited the decrease in circulating platelet counts and collagen-induced malondialdehyde concentration in plasma. Policosanol (25 mg/kg) inhibited the clotted whole-blood thromboxane B2 formation. Administration of 50–200 mg/kg, in a single dose, inhibited ADP-induced platelet aggregation in platelet-rich plasma, whereas a lower dose (25 mg/kg) did not change responses to ADP significantly, but rats treated with this dose for 4 weeks showed a significant inhibition of platelet aggregation in PRP when a submaximal ADP concentration was administered[SO062].

Postprandial glycemic response reduction. Sugar cane bioflavonoid was administered to 10 healthy, nonsmoking, normal-weight young adults with normal glucose tolerance at doses of 15, 50, or 100 mg of bioflavonoid. The treatment produced no significant differences among the mean glycemic index (GI) values of the three extract test meals. The bioflavonoid extract effectively reduced the GI value of a high-GI starchy meal by up to 37% without any apparent side effects[SO026].

Serum and liver cholesterol influence. Partially purified Okinawan sugar cane wax and fatty alcohol, administered to Wistar rats at a dose of 0.5% of diet, significantly lowered the concentrations of serum and liver cholesterol in the rats. There were no significant differences observed in phospholipid and TG levels either in serum or liver among the experimental groups. No significant differences in the amount of feces excreted by the three experimental diet groups and no significant differences in the excretion of cholesterol were found[SO066]. Okinawan sugar cane rind, administered to Wistar rats, produced no significant differences in the food intakes and the liver weight between the rats fed sugar cane rind and other groups. The addition of 1% cholesterol to the diet produced a significant increase in body weight gain but the supplementation of sugar cane rind (2%) showed an effect on weight control of rats. The serum cholesterol and TG levels of the rats given sugar cane rind were lowered significantly. The lipid levels in the liver were almost the same when compared with the control groups. The amount of feces excreted by the rats fed with sugar cane rind was approx 37% more than that of the control group, and the fecal excretion of neutral sterols was significantly higher[SO069].

Spinal cord ischemia. D-003, administered to New Zealand rabbits at doses of 25 and 200 mg/kg for 10 days, significantly increased the mean scores reached 4 hours after reperfusion, although no dose relation was observed. Twenty-four hours after reperfusion, no deaths occurred in both sham and D-003 treated groups; meanwhile, in positive controls, the mortality rate was 38.5%. In addition, 100% of sham, 69% and 77% of rabbits treated with D-003 at 25 and 200 mg/kg, respectively, did not show histopathological changes. One hundred percent of positive control animals showed severe damage. Animals treated with both doses of

D-003 showed prostacyclin PGI(2) levels significantly larger than those of positive and negative controls and a dose-related effect[SO030].

Toxicity. D-003, a mixture of higher aliphatic primary acids purified from sugar cane wax, administered to Wistar rats at a dose of 2000 mg/kg, was investigated according to the Acute Toxic Class (ATC) method (an alternative for the classical LD$_{50}$ test). The results obtained in this study defined D-003 oral acute toxicity as unclassified. D-003, administered orally to rats of both sexes at doses of 50, 200, and 1250 mg/kg for 90 days, produced no evidence of treatment-related toxicity. Data analysis of body weight gain, food consumption, clinical observations, blood biochemical, hematology, organ weight ratios, and histopathological findings did not produce significant differences between control and treated groups. The results indicated that D-003 orally administered to rats was safe and that no drug-related toxicity was detected even at the highest doses investigated in both acute (200 mg/kg) and subchronic (1205 mg/kg) studies[SO010]. D-003 was administered intragastrically to CEN/NMRI mice (6–8 animals per sex per group) at doses of 5, 50, or 500 mg/kg for 90 days. The treatment did not increase the frequency of micronucleated polychromatic erythrocytes evaluated only in female mice or the ratio of polychromatic to normochromatic erythrocytes, compared with the controls. D-003 did not change the sperm count or the frequency of all types of abnormal head shapes, compared with the controls. D-003, administered to mice of both sexes at a dose of 2 g/kg for 6 days, produced no cytotoxic and genotoxic effects. D-003, administered intragastrically to five male Sprague–Dawley rats at a dose of 1.25 g/kg for 90 days, produced no single-strand breaks or alkali-labile site induction on DNA in liver cells using Comet assay[SO034]. D-003 (suspended in

1% acacia gum solution), administered intragastrically to rats at doses of 5, 100, and 1000 g/kg/day on days 6 through 15 of gestation, produced no evidence of maternal or developmental toxicity. Maternal clinical signs of toxicity were not observed, and the analysis of initial body weight and the body weight gain during the treatment period were comparable among the groups treated with D-003 and control. D-003 produced no adverse effects on reproductive performance or on embryonic or fetal development, including visceral and skeletal examination[SO039]. D-003, in the neutral red (NR) assay and in the Ames test at doses up to 1 mg/mL for up to 72 hours, produced no cytotoxic evidences. D-003 (5–5000 μg/plate) did not increase the frequency of reverse mutations in the Ames test in both alternatives with or without S9 mix metabolic activation and a preincubation step[SO042]. Policosanol, administered intragastrically to 24 beagle dogs (12 males and 12 females) at doses of 30 and 180 mg/kg daily for 52 weeks, produced no mortality in any group. Policosanol was well tolerated, and no toxic symptoms were observed. All groups showed similar weight gain and food consumption. Lipid profile determinations showed that policosanol decreased total cholesterol by approx 20% from 8 to 52 weeks. TGs and HDL-C were not changed significantly. No blood biochemistry or histopathological disturbances were observed[SO014]. Policosanol, administered orally to Sprague–Dawley rats at doses of 50, 500, 2500, or 5000 mg/kg for 6 months, produced no significant differences in blood biochemistry, hematology, organ weight ratios, and histopathological findings compared with controls, nor any tendency with the dose. Body weight gain and food consumption in the groups receiving 2500 or 5000 mg/kg tended to be lower than in the control group, but difference was not significant. No drug-related toxicity symptoms were de-tected. Eight of treated rats (six males and two females) died during the study, five of them (four males and one female) from among those receiving the highest dose (5000 mg/kg). All deaths were related to gavage manipulation of higher doses[SO035].

Voluntary ethanol intake effect. SKV, an Ayurvedic formula produced by the fermentation of cane sugar with raisins and 12 herbal ingredients, decreased the voluntary ethanol ingestion in the rats and increased food intake. Electrocardiogram and electroencephalogram studies in alcoholic rats showed cardiac depression; augmentation of frequency and amplitude of the α, Δ, and φ waves; and weakness in the β waves. The changes were reversed during SKV-induced voluntary alcohol restriction. The involvement in the electrocardiogram and electroencephalogram wave patterns was associated with improvement in blood glucose and plasma protein levels and reduction in γ-glutamyl transpeptidase activities[SO065].

Weight loss. Polysaccharide fraction of the dried stem, administered intragastrically to rats at a dose of 1 g/kg daily for 14 weeks, was inactive vs high-sugar diet. Intraperitoneal administration at doses of 20 and 40 mg/kg for 14 weeks was active[SO116].

REFERENCES

SO001 Gamez, R., R. Mas, M. Noa, et al. Effects of chronic administration of D-003, a mixture of sugar cane wax high molecular acids, in beagle dogs. **Drugs Exp Clin Res** 2004; 30(2): 75–88.

SO002 Amer, S., K.J. Na, M. El-Abasy, M. Motobu, Y. Koyama, K. Koge, and Y. Hirota. Immunostimulating effects of sugar cane extract on X-ray radiation induced immunosuppression in the chicken. **Int Immunopharmacol** 2004; 4(1): 71–77.

SO003 Mendoza, S., M. Noa, R. Mas, and N. Mendoza. Effect of D-003, a mixture of high molecular weight primary acids from sugar cane wax, on paracetamol-induced liver damage in rats. **Int J Tissue React** 2003; 25(3): 91–98.

SO004   Takara, K., D. Matsui, K. Wada, T. Ichiba, I. Chinen, and Y. Nakasone. New phenolic compounds from Kokuto, non-centrifuged cane sugar. **Biosci Biotechnol Biochem** 2003; 67(2): 376–379.

SO005   Ledon, N., A. Casaco, V. Rodriguez, et al. Anti-inflammatory and analgesic effects of a mixture of fatty acids isolated and purified from sugar cane wax oil. **Planta Med** 2003; 69(4): 367–369.

SO006   Arruzazabala, M.L., D. Carbajal D, R. Mas R, S. Valdes, and V. Molina V. Pharmacological interaction between Policosanol and nitroprusside in rats. **J Med Food** 2001; 4(2): 67–70.

SO007   Noa, M., S. Mendoza, R. Mas, and N. Mendoza. Effect of D-003, a mixture of high molecular weight primary acids from sugar cane wax, on CL4C-induced liver acute injury in rats. **Drugs Exp Clin Res** 2002; 28(5): 177–183.

SO008   Gamez, R., R. Mas, M. Noa, et al. Six-month toxicity study of oral administration of D-003 in Sprague Dawley rats. **Drugs R D** 2002; 3(6): 375–386.

SO009   Menendez, R., A.M. Amor, I. Rodeiro, et al. Policosanol modulates HMG-CoA reductase activity in cultured fibroblasts. **Arch Med Res** 200; 32(1): 8–12.

SO010   Gamez, R., R. Mas, M. Noa, et al. Acute and oral subchronic toxicity of D-003 in rats. **Toxicol Lett** 2000; 118(1-2): 31–41.

SO011   Menendez, R., V. Fraga, A.M. Amor, R.M. Gonzalez, and R. Mas. Oral administration of policosanol inhibits *in vitro* copper ion-induced rat lipoprotein peroxidation. **Physiol Behav** 1999; 67(1): 1–7.

SO012   Molina Cuevas, V., M.L. Arruzazabala, D. Carbajal Quintana, R. Mas Ferreiro, and S. Valdes Garcia. Effect of policosanol on arterial blood pressure in rats. Study of the pharmacological interaction with nifedipine and propranolol. **Arch Med Res** 1998; 29(1): 21–24.

SO013   Fraga, V., R. Menendez, A.M. Amor, R.M. Gonzalez, S. Jimenez, and R. Mas. Effect of policosanol on *in vitro* and *in vivo* rat liver microsomal lipid peroxidation. **Arch Med Res** 1997; 28(3): 355–360.

SO014   Mesa, A. R., R. Mas, M. Noa, et al. Toxicity of policosanol in beagle dogs: one-year study. **Toxicol Lett** 1994; 73(2): 81–90.

SO015   Carbajal, D., M. L. Arruzazabala, R. Mas, V. Molina, and S.Valdes. Effect of policosanol on experimental thrombosis models. **Prostaglandins Leukot Essent Fatty Acids** 1994; 50(5): 249–251.

SO016   Arruzazabala, M. L., D. Carbajal, R. Mas, V. Molina, S. Valdes, and A. Laguna. Cholesterol-lowering effects of policosanol in rabbits. **Biol Res** 1994; 27(3-4): 205–208.

SO017   Hikino, H., M. Takahashi, C. Konno, A. Ishimori, T. Kawamura, and T. Namiki. Effect of glycans of *Saccharum officinarum* on carbohydrate and lipid metabolism of rats. **J Ethnopharmacol** 1985; 14(2–3): 261–268.

SO018   Chinen, I., K. Oouchi, H. Tamaki, and N. Fukuda. Purification and properties of thermostable beta-xylosidase from immature stalks of *Saccharum officinarum* L. (sugar cane). **J Biochem (Tokyo)** 1982; 92(6): 1873–1881.

SO019   Chinen, I., T. Nakamura, and N. Fukuda. Purification and properties of alpha-galactosidase from immature stalks of *Saccharum officinarum* (sugar cane). **J Biochem (Tokyo)** 1981; 90(5): 1453–1461.

SO020   Mas, R., G. Castano, J. Fernandez, et al. Long-term effects of policosanol on obese patients with Type II hypercholesterolemia. Asia Pacific **J Clin Nutr** 2004; 13(Suppl): S102.

SO021   Mas, R., G. Castano, J. Fernandez, et al. Long-term effects of policosanol on older patients with Type 2 diabetes. **Asia Pacific J Clin Nutr** 2004; 13(Suppl): S101.

SO022   Murphy, K. J., D. A. Saint, and P. R. Howe. Lack of effect of sugar cane and sunflower seed policosanols on plasma cholesterol in rabbits. **Asia Pacific J Clin Nutr** 2004; 13(Suppl): S69.

SO023   El-Abasy, M., M. Motobu, K. Nakamura, K. Koge, T. Onodera, O. Vainio, P. Toivanen, and Y. Hirota. Preventive and therapeutic effects of sugar cane extract on cyclophosphamide-induced immunosuppression in chickens. **Int Immunopharmacol** 2004; 4(8): 983–990.

SO024 Noa, M., R. Mas, S. Mendoza, R. Gamez, and N. Mendoza. Effects of D-003, a mixture of high molecular weight aliphatic acids from sugar cane wax, on bones from ovariectomized rats. **Drugs Exp Clin Res** 2004; 30(1): 35–41.

SO025 Menendez, R., R. Mas, J. Perez, R.M. Gonzalez, and S. Jimenez. Oral administration of D-003, a mixture of very long chain fatty acids prevents casein-induced endogenous hypercholesterolemia in rabbits. **Can J Physiol Pharmacol** 2004; 82(1): 22–29.

SO026 Holt, S., V.D. Jong, E. Faramus, T. Lang, and J. Brand Miller. A bioflavonoid in sugar cane can reduce the postprandial glycaemic response to a high-GI starchy food. **Asia Pacific J Clin Nutr** 2003; 12(Suppl): S66.

SO027 Mendoza, S., R. Gamez, R. Mas, and E. Goicochea. Effects of D-003, a mixture of long-chain aliphatic primary acids, fluvastatin and the combined therapy of D-003 plus fluvastatin on the lipid profile of normocholesterolemic rabbits. **Int J Tissue React** 2003; 25(3): 81–89.

SO028 Barba, T. F., C.A. Barba, D. Sole, and C.K. Naspitz. Non-specific broncho-provocation with metacholine in children before and during sugar cane burning in Catanduva-SP. **J Pediatr (Rio J)** 1998; 74(3): 228–232.

SO029 Varady, K. A., Y. Wang, and P. J. Jones. Role of policosanols in the prevention and treatment of cardiovascular disease. **Nutr Rev** 2003; 61(11): 376–383.

SO030 Carbajal, D., M. L. Arruzazabala, M. Noa, et al. Protective effect of D-003 on experimental spinal cord ischemia in rabbits. **Prostaglandins Leuko Essent Fatty Acids** 2004; 70(1): 1–6.

SO031 Carbajal, D., M. Noa, V. Molina, et al. Effect of D-003 on isoproterenol-induced myocardial necrosis in rats. **J Med Food** 2003; 6(1): 13–18.

SO032 Wang, Y.W., P.J. Jones, I. Pischel, and C. Fairow. Effects of policosanols and phytosterols on lipid levels and cholesterol biosynthesis in hamsters. **Lipids** 2003; 38(2): 165–170.

SO033 Tamaki, H., S. L. Man, Y. Ohta, N. Katsuyama, and I. Chinen. Inhibition of osteoporosis in rats fed with sugar cane wax. **Biosci Biotechnol Biochem** 2003; 67(2): 423–425.

SO034 Gamez, R., J. E. Gonzalez, I. Rodeiro, et al. *In vivo* genotoxic evaluation of D-003, a mixture of very long chain aliphatic acids. **J Med Food** 2001; 4(2): 85–91.

SO035 Gamez, R., C. L. Aleman, R. Mas, et al. A 6-month study on the toxicity of high doses of Policosanol orally administered to Sprague-Dawley rats. **J Med Food** 2001; 4(2): 57–65.

SO036 El-Abasy, M., M. Motobu, T. Sameshima, K. Koge, T. Onodera, and Y. Hirota. Adjuvant effects of sugar cane extracts (SCE) in chickens. **J Vet Med Sci** 2003; 65(1): 117–119.

SO037 Castano, G., R. Mas, L. Fernandez, et al. Comparison of the efficacy and tolerability of policosanol with atorvastatin in elderly patients with type II hypercholesterolaemia. **Drugs Aging** 2003; 20(2): 153–163.

SO038 El-Abasy, M., M. Motobu, K. Shimura, et al. Immunostimulating and growth-promoting effects of sugar cane extract (SCE) in chickens. **J Vet Med Sci** 2002; 64(11): 1061–1063.

SO039 Rodriguez, M. D., R. Gamez, J. E. Gonzalez, H. Garcia, C. P. Acosta, and E. Goicochea. Lack of developmental toxicity of D-003: a mixture of long-chain fatty acids in rats. **Food Chem Toxicol** 2003; 41(1): 89–93.

SO040 Molina, V., M. L. Arruzazabala M. L, D. Carbajal, and R. Mas. D-003, a potential antithrombotic compound isolated from sugar cane wax with effects on arachidonic acid metabolites. **Prostaglandins Leuko Essent Fatty Acids** 2002; 67(1): 19–24.

SO041 McCarty, M.F. Policosanol safely down-regulates HMG-CoA reductase—potential as a component of the Esselstyn regimen. **Med Hypotheses** 2002; 59(3): 268–279.

SO042 Gamez, R., I. Rodeiro, I. Fernandez, and P.C. Acosta. Preliminary evaluation of the cytotoxic and genotoxic potential of D-003: mixture of very long chain fatty acids. **Teratog Carcinog Mutagen** 2002; 22(3): 175–181.

SO043 Menendez, R., R. Mas, A. M. Amor, et al. Inhibition of rat lipoprotein lipid peroxidation by the oral administration of D-003, a mixture of very long-chain saturated fatty acids. **Can J Physiol Pharmacol** 2002; 80(1): 13–21.

SO044 Takara, K., D. Matsui, K. Wada, T. Ichiba, and Y. Nakasone. New antioxidative phenolic glycosides isolated from Kokuto non-centrifuged cane sugar. **Biosci Biotechnol Biochem** 2002; 66(1): 29–35.

SO045 Castano, G., R. Mas, L. Fernandez, J. Illnait, R. Gamez, and E. Alvarez. Effects of policosanol 20 versus 40 mg/day in the treatment of patients with type II hypercholesterolemia: a 6-month double-blind study. **Int J Clin Pharmacol Res** 2001; 21(1): 43–57.

SO046 Mirkin, A., R. Mas, M. Martinto, et al. Efficacy and tolerability of policosanol in hypercholesterolemic postmenopausal women. **Int J Clin Pharmacol Res** 2001; 21(1): 31–41.

SO047 Menendez, R., R. Mas, A. M. Amor, I. Rodeiros, R. M. Gonzalez, and J. L. Alfonso. Inhibition of cholesterol biosynthesis in cultured fibroblasts by D-003, a mixture of very long chain saturated fatty acids. **Pharmacol Res** 2001; 44(4): 299–304.

SO048 Costa, M. J., L. H. Moraes, F. M. Bion, M. A. Rivera, L. S. Moura, and M. L. Conceicao. Efficacy evaluation of the molasses supplementation in normal and depleted rats diet. **Arch Latinoam Nutr** 2000; 50(4): 341–345.

SO049 Noa, M., R. Mas, and R. Mesa. A comparative study of policosanol vs lovastatin on intimal thickening in rabbit cuffed carotid artery. **Pharmacol Res** 2001; 43(1): 31–37.

SO050 Molina, V., M. L. Arruzazabala, D. Carbajal, R. Mas, and S. Valdes. Antiplatelet and antithrombotic effect of D-003. **Pharmacol Res** 2000; 42(2): 137–143.

SO051 Arruzazabala, M. L., M. Noa, R. Menendez, R. Mas, D. Carbajal, S. Valdes, and V. Molina. Protective effect of policosanol on atherosclerotic lesions in rabbits with exogenous hypercholesterolemia. **Braz J Med Biol Res** 2000; 33(7): 835–840.

SO052 Molina, V., M. L. Arruzazabala, D. Carbajal, et al. Effect of policosanol on

cerebral ischemia in Mongolian gerbils. **Braz J Med Biol Res** 1999; 32(10): 1269–1276.

SO053 Re, L., S. Barocci, C. Capitani, et al. Effects of some natural extracts on the acetylcholine release at the mouse neuromuscular junction. **Pharmacol Res** 1999; 39(3): 239–245.

SO054 Noa, M., R. Mas, and R. Mesa. Effect of policosanol on intimal thickening in rabbit cuffed carotid artery. **Int J Cardiol** 1998; 67(2): 125–132.

SO055 Ferriolli, E., R. O. Dantas, R. B. Oliveira, and F. J. Braga. The influence of ageing on oesophageal motility after ingestion of liquids with different viscosities. **Eur J Gastroenterol Hepatol** 1996; 8(8): 793–798.

SO056 Noa, M., M. C. de la Rosa, and R. Mas. Effect of policosanol on foam-cell formation in carrageenan-induced granulomas in rats. **J Pharm Pharmacol** 1996; 48(3): 306–309.

SO057 Aleman, C. L., M. N. Puig, E. C. Elias, et al. Carcinogenicity of policosanol in mice: an 18-month study. **Food Chem Toxicol** 1995; 33(7): 573–578.

SO058 Noa, M., R. Mas, M. C. de la Rosa, and J. Magraner. Effect of policosanol on lipofundin-induced atherosclerotic lesions in rats. **J Pharm Pharmacol** 1995; 47(4): 289–291.

SO059 Agata, H., N. Kondo, A. Yomo, et al. Sensitization to sugar cane pollen in Okinawan allergic children. **Asian Pacific J Allergy Immunol** 1994; 12(2): 151–154.

SO060 Menendez, R., S. I. Fernandez, A. Del Rio, et al. Policosanol inhibits cholesterol biosynthesis and enhances low density lipoprotein processing in cultured human fibroblasts. **Biol Res** 1994; 27(3–4): 199–203.

SO061 Arruzazabala, M. L., V. Molina, D. Carbajal, S. Valdes, and R. Mas. Effect of policosanol on cerebral ischemia in Mongolian gerbils: role of prostacyclin and thromboxane A2. **Prostaglandins Leuko Essent Fatty Acids** 1993; 49(3): 695–697.

SO062 Arruzazabala, M. L., D. Carbajal, R. Mas, M. Garcia, and V. Fraga. Effects of Policosanol on platelet aggregation in rats. **Thromb Res** 1993; 69(3): 321–327.

SO063 Frencken, J. E., P. Rugarabamu, and J. Mulder. The effect of sugar cane chewing on the development of dental caries. **J Dent Res** 1989; 68(6): 1102–1104.

SO064 Oji, E. O. Locally available plant materials for use as ophthalmic surgical swabs. **Ann R Coll Surg Engl** 1986; 68(6): 307–309.

SO065 Shanmugasundaram, E. R., and K. R. Shanmugasundaram. An Indian herbal formula (SKV) for controlling voluntary ethanol intake in rats with chronic alcoholism. **J Ethnopharmacol** 1986; 17(2): 171–182.

SO066 Sho, H., I. Chinen, and N. Fukuda. Effects of Okinawan sugar cane wax and fatty alcohol on serum and liver lipids in the rat. **J Nutr Sci Vitaminol (Tokyo)** 1984; 30(6): 553–559.

SO067 Li, X. Y., R. Nolte, and W. Vogt. Natural antibodies against a polysaccharide (Bo) from sugar cane mediate its complement-activating effect. **Immunobiology** 1983; 164(2): 110–117.

SO068 Li, X., and W. Vogt. Activation of the classical complement pathway by a polysaccharide from sugar cane. **Immunopharmacology** 1982; 5(1): 31–38.

SO069 Sho, H., I. Chinen, K. Uchihara, and N. Fukuda. Effects of Okinawan sugar cane rind on serum and liver cholesterol and triglyceride levels in the rat. **J Nutr Sci Vitaminol (Tokyo)** 1981; 27(5): 463–470.

SO070 Grant, E.C. Food allergies and migraine. **Lancet** 1979; 1(8123): 966–969.

SO071 Varavithya, W., P. Posayanond, K. Tontisirin, L. Chernjitra, and C. Kashemsant. Oral hydration in infantile diarrhoea. **Southeast Asian J Trop Med Public Health** 1978; 9(3): 414–419.

SO072 West, G. B. Glucans and dextrans in rats and man. **Int Arch Allergy Appl Immunol** 1978; 56(4): 380–382.

SO073 Baird, I. M., R. L. Walters, P. S. Davies, M. J. Hill, B. S. Drasar, and D. A. Southgate. The effects of two dietary fiber supplements on gastrointestinal transit, stool weight and frequency, and bacterial flora, and fecal bile acids in normal subjects. **Metabolism** 1977; 26(2): 117–128.

SO074 Fahey, G. C., J. E. Williams, and G.A. McLaren. Influence of molasses lignin-hemicellulose fractions in rat nutrition. **J Nutr** 1976; 106(10): 1447–1451.

SO075 Dumaswala, U. J., R. U. Dumaswala, and A. Venkataraman. The relative effect of dietary fats and carbohydrates on lipid metabolism in the albino rat. 1: **Ital J Biochem** 1976; 25(4): 289–303.

SO076 Walters, R. L., I. M. Baird, P. S. Davies, et al. Effects of two types of dietary fibre on faecal steroid and lipid excretion. **Br Med J** 1975; 2(5970): 536–538.

SO077 Suwal, P. N. Medicinal plants of Nepal. Ministry of Forests, Department of Medicinal Plants, Thapathali, Kathmandu, Nepal 1970.

SO078 Couvee. Compilation of herbs, plants, crops supposed to be effective in various complaints and illness. **J Sci Res** 1952; 1S: 1.

SO079 Ahmad, Y.S. A note on the plants of medicinal value found in Pakistan. Government of Pakistan Press, Karachi, 1957.

SO080 Lin, Y. C., J. T. Huang and H. C. Hsiu. Studies on the hypoglycemic activity of the medicinal herbs. **Formosan Med Assoc** 1964; 63(8): 400–404.

SO081 Pongpan, A., W. Avirutnant, and P. Chumsri. Some Thai plants as substrates for microbial protein production. **Mahidol Univ J Pharm Sci** 1983; 10(1): 15–18.

SO082 Kimura, Y., H. Okua, N. Shoji, T. Taemto, and S. Arichi. Effects of non-sugar fraction in black sugar on lipid and carbohydrate metabolism. Part II. New compounds inhibiting elevation of plasma insulin. **Planta Med** 1984; 1984(5): 469–473.

SO083 Yadava, V. S., and K. Misra. Vanilloyl-1-O-beta-D-glucoside acetate from the roots of *Saccharum officinarum*. **Indian J Chem Ser B** 1989; 28(1): 875–877.

SO084 Morita, I., S. Morishita, T. Tatsumi, and S. Kako. Invert sugar having high inversion. Patent-Japan Kokai-74 134,852 1974.

SO085 Doepke, W., and U. Hess. Obtaining phytosterol mixtures from oil fraction sof sugar cane waxes. **Patent-Ger (East)** 1974; 104,513.

SO086 Ferber, L., and F. G. Carpenter. Plant pigments as colorants in cane sugar. **US Agr Res Serv South Reg ARS** 1975; 51: 23.

SO087 Da Gloria, N. A., and A. A. Rodella. Inorganic quantitative analysis of sugar cane juice, vinasse, and molasses. I. Calcium, magnesium, potassium, sulfur and phosphorus determination in single extract. **An Esc Super Agr Luiz Dr Queiroz Univ Sao Paulo** 1972; 29: 5.

SO088 Dubey, R. C., and K. Misra. Flavonoids of sugar cane. **J Indian Chem Soc** 1974; 51: 653.

SO089 Misra, K. and R. C. Dubey. Anthocyanin of sugarcane. Curr Sci 1974; 43: 544A.

SO090 Kapadia, G. J., E. B. Chung, B. Ghosh, et al. Carcinogenicity of some folk medicinal herbs in rats. **J Nat Cancer Inst** 1978; 60: 683–686.

SO091 Kuhnie, J. A., P. H. Moore, W. F. Haddon, and M. M. Fitch. Identification of gibberellins from sugar cane plants. J **Plant Growth Regul** 1983; 2(1): 59–71.

SO092 Patron, N. H., P. Smith, and T. J. Mabry. Identification of flavonoid compounds in HPLC separation of sugar cane colorants. **Int Sugar J** 1985; 87(1043): 213–215.

SO093 Goswami, P. C., H. D. Singh, and J. N. Baruah. Isolation of phytosterols from sugarcane press mud and microbial conversion of the phytosterols to 17-ketosteroids. **Curr Sci** 1984; 53917): 917–919.

SO094 Taahashi, M., C. Konno, and H. Hikino. Isolation and hypoglycemic activity of saccharin A, B, C, D, E, and F, glycans of Saccharum officinarum stalks. **Planta Med** 1985; 1985(3): 258–260.

SO095 Kato, A., J. I. Azuma, and T. Koshijima. Isolation and identification of a new feruloylated tetrasaccharide from bagasse lignin-carbohydrate complex containing phenolic acid. **Agr Biol Chem** 1987; 51(6): 1691–1693.

SO096 Smith, R. M., and M. Martin-Smith. Triterpen methyl ethers in leaf waxes of Saccharum and related genera. **Phytochemistry** 1978; 17(8): 1307–1312.

SO097 Seetharam, K. A., and J.S. Pasricha. Condiments and contact dermatitis of the finger-tips. **Indian J Dermatol Venerol Leprol** 1987; 53(6): 325–328.

SO098 De A Ribeiro, R., F. Barros, M. Margarida, et al. Acute diuretic effects in conscious rats produced by some medicinal plants used in the state of Sao Paulo, Brasil. **J Ethnopharmacol** 1988; 24(1): 19–29.

SO099 Takagi, S. Isolation of polysaccharides as pharmaceuticals from sugarcane and its molasses. Patent-Japan Kokai Tokkyo Koho-61 83,130 1986; 13 pp.

SO100 Holdsworth, D., and T. Rali. A survey of medicinal plants of the southern Highlands, Papua New Guinea. **Int J Crude Drug Res** 1989; 27(1): 1–8.

SO101 Vicente, C., J. L. Mateos, M. M. Pedrosa, and M.E. Legaz. High-performance liquid chromatographic determination of sugars and polyols in extracts of lichens and sugarcane juice. **J Chromatogr** 1991; 553(1/2): 271–283.

SO102 Misra, C. S., and K. Misra. Dimethyl apigenin 4'-O-beta-D-glucopyranoside from Saccharum officinarum leaves. **Curr Sci** 1978; 47: 152.

SO103 Irvine, J. E. Variation of non-sucrose solids in sugarcane. I. Potassium. **Sugar J** 1978; 41(5): 28–30.

SO104 Misra, K., and C. S. Misra. Flavonoids of Saccharum officinarum flowers. **Indian J Chem Ser B** 1979; 18: 88.

SO105 Jin, Y. N., H. Z. Liang, C. Y. Cao, Z. W. Wang, R. S. Shu, and X. Y. Li. Immunological activity of bagasse polysaccharides. Chung-Kuo Yao Li Hsueh Pao 1981; 2: 269–275.

SO106 Bhattacharjee, J. W., R. P. Saxena, and S.H. Zaidi. Experimental studies on the toxicity of bagasse. **Environ Res** 1980; 23: 68–76.

SO107 Kato, A., J. Azuma, and T. Koshijima. A new feruloylated trisaccharide from bagasse. **Chem Lett** 1983; 1983(1): 137–140.

SO108 Mabry, T. J., Y. L. Liu, J. Pearce, et al. New flavonoids from sugarcane (Saccharum). **J Nat Prod** 1984; 47(1): 127–130.

SO109 Achamaas, G., and R. Thawornset. Phytochemical and anticancer screening of Schefflera leucantha and Saccharum officinarum. Undergraduate Special Project Report 1980; 69 pp.

SO110 Hirschhorn, H. H. Botanical remedies of the former Dutch East Indies (Indonesia). I. Eumycetes, Pteridpohyta, Gymnospermae, Angiospermae (Monocotyledons only). J Ethnopharmacol 1983; 7(2): 123–156.

SO111 Martinez, M. A. Medicinal plants used in a Totonac community of the Sierra Norte del Puebla: Tuzamapan de Galeana, Puebla, Mexico. J Ethnopharmacol 1984; 11(2): 203–221.

SO112 Aswal, B. S., D. S. Bahakuni, A. K. Goel, K. Kar, B. N. Mehrotra, and K.C. Mukherjee. Screening of Indian plants for biological activity: part X. Indian J Exp Biol 1984; 22(6): 312–332.

SO113 De A Ribeiro, R., M. M. R. Fiuza de Melo, F. de Baroz, C. Gomes, and G. Troln. Acute antihypertensive effect in conscious rats produced by some medicinal plants used in the state of Sao Paulo. J Ethnopharmacol 1986; 15(3): 261–269.

SO114 Hedberg, I., O. Hedberg, P. J. Madati, K. E. Mshigeni, E. N. Mshiu, and G. Samuelsson. Inventory of plants used in traditional medicine in Tanzania. Part III. Plants of the families Papillionaceae-Vitaceae. J Ethnopharmacol 1983; 9(2/3): 237–260.

SO115 Li, X., B. Damerau, and W. Vogt. Influence of a bagasse glucan (B-O) on leukocyte aggregation and accumulation. Chung-Kuo Yao Li Hsueh Pao 1985; 6(2): 137–140.

SO116 Hikino, H., M. Takahashi, C. Konno, A. Ishimori, T. Kawamura, and T. Namiki. Effect of glycans of Saccharum officinarum on carbohydrate and lipid metabolism of rats. J Ethnopharmacol 1985; 14(2/3): 261–268.

SO117 Anis, M., and M. Iqbal. Antipyretic utility of some Indian plants in traditional medicine. Fitoterapia 1986; 57(1): 52–55.

SO118 Caceres, A., L. M. Giron, and A. M. Martinez. Diuretic activity of plants used for the treatment of urinary ailments in Guatemala. J Ethnopharmacol 1987; 19(3): 233–245.

SO119 Caceres, A., L. M. Giron, S. R. Alvarado, and M.F. Torres. Screening of antimicrobial activity of plants popularly used in Guatemala for the treatment of dermatomucosal diseases. J Ethnopharmacol 1987; 20(3): 223–237.

SO120 Costa, M., L. C. di Stasi, M. Kirizawa, S. L. J. Mendacolli, C. Gomez, and G. Trolin. Screening in mice of some medicinal plants used for analgesic purposes in the state of Sao Paulo. J Ethnopharmacol 1989; 27(1/2): 25–33.

SO121 Darias, V., L. Bravo, R. Rabanal, C. Sanchez Mateo, R. M. Gonzalez Luis, and A. M. Hernandez Perez. New contribution to the ethnopharmacological study of the Canary Islands. J Ethnopharmacol 1989; 25(1): 77–92.

SO122 Vedavathy, S., K. N. Rao, M. Rajaiah, and N. Nagaraju. Folklore information from Ryalaseema region, Andhra Pradesh for family planning and birth control. Int J Pharmacog 1991; 29(2): 113–116.

SO123 Aleman, C. L., R. Mas, C. Hernandez, I. Rodeiro, E. Cerejido, M. Noa, A. Capote, R. Menedez, A. Amor, V. Fraga, V. Sotolongo, and S. Jimenez. A 12-month study of policosanol oral toxicity in Sprague Dawley rats. Toxicol Lett 1994; 70(1): 77–87.

SO124 Seabrook, W. B. adventures in Arabia among the Bedouins, Druses, Whirling Dervishes & Yezidee devil worshipers. Blue Ribbon Book, New York 1927; 99–105

SO125 Holdsworth, D. K. Traditional medicinal plants of Rarotonga, Cook Islands. Part II. Int J Pharmacog 1991; 29(1): 71–79.

SO126 Lin, C. C. Crude drugs used for the treatment of diabetes mellitus in Taiwan. Amer J Chin Med 1992; 20(3/4): 269–279.

SO127 Kimura, Y., H. Okuda, and S. Arichi. Effects of non-sugar fraction in black sugar on lipid and carbohydrate metabolism: part I. Planta Med 1984; 1984(4): 465–468

SO128 McGhie, T. Analysis of sugarcane flavonoids by capillary zone electrophoresis. J Chromatogr 1993; 534(1): 107–112.

SO129 Hope, B. E., D. G. Massey, and G. Massey-Fournier. Hawaiian Materia Medica for asthma. Hawaiian Med J 1993; 52(6): 160–166.

14 | Serenoa repens

(Bantam) Small

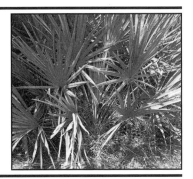

Common Names

American dwarf palm tree	United States	Palmetta Della Florida	Italy
		Palmetto de la sierra	Spain
Cabbage palm	United States	Palmetto fan palm	United States
Chou palmiste	France	Palmetto, dark	United States
Corifa del Malabar	Italy	Palmier nain	France
Grote waaier palm	Netherlands	Palmier pitic	Romania
Ju zhong lu	China	Palmito	Portugal
Kaapiopalmu	Finland	Palmito	Spain
Karlikova palma	Ukraine	Sabal du Mexique	France
Karlikovaya palma	Russia	Sabal du Texas	France
Kis legyezopalma	Hungary	Sabal	United States
Niska palma	Bulgaria	Sagepalme	Germany
Palma enana Americana	Spain	Sagepalmefruchte	Germany
		Sagpalmetto	Sweden
Palma nana	Italy	Saw palmetto	United Kingdom
Palma sabal	Spain	Saw palmetto	United States
Palmeen	The Isle of Man (Manx)	Serenoa palmu	Finland
Palmet	Netherlands	Solfjaderspalm	Sweden

BOTANICAL DESCRIPTION

The saw palmetto is a creeping, horizontal periennial of the PALMAE family. Saw palmetto usually grows as a small shrub to a height of 0.6–2.1 m. Occasionally, it grows as a small tree with erect or oblique stems, 6–7.5 m tall. In its procumbent form, saw palmetto branches form a tangled mass, with the root crown projecting above to support the foliage. The stem systems run parallel to the soil surface, eventually branching beneath the substrate to form rhi-zomes. The bright-green, fan-shaped ever-green leaves are approx 1 m wide, with 15 to 30 divisions that are roundish in outline and are borne on slender stalks edged with spines. The white, small flowers are borne on stalked panicles that grow from the leaf axils. The flower spike is thickly hairy and considerably shorter than the leaves. The petioles are armed with sharp spines, giving saw palmetto its common name. The fruit is a fleshy, elipsoid drupe, 1.2–2.5 cm long, one-seeded, which is green or yellow before

From: *Medicinal Plants of the World, vol. 3: Chemical Constituents, Traditional and Modern Medicinal Uses*
By: I. A. Ross © Humana Press Inc., Totowa, NJ

ripening but becomes reddish brown or blackish brown as it matures.

ORIGIN AND DISTRIBUTION

This palm is native to the southeastern United States, from Florida to North Carolina. It grows in coastal dune areas and inland pine woodlands, often forming dense, impenetrable thickets in the understory of pines, such as slash pine (*Pinus elliottii*) and longleaf pine (*Pinus palustris*).

TRADITIONAL MEDICINAL USES

Germany. The fruit is taken orally as a source of estrogen[SR077].

North America. Hot water extract of the fruit is taken orally as a sedative[SR127].

United States. Hot water extract of the fruit is taken orally for prostate inflammation[SR123] and for benign prostatic hyperplasia[SR098,SR109]. Fluid extract of the fruit is taken orally for dysmenorrhea[SR126]. Hot water extract of the fruit is used to treat colds and for irritated throat. A teaspoon of berries in a cup of boiling water is cooled and taken 1 or 2 cups a day[SR128].

CHEMICAL CONSTITUENTS

(ppm unless otherwise indicated)
1-Monolaurin: Dried Fr[SR034]
1-Monomyristin: Dried Fr[SR034]
Anthranilic acid: Fr[SR078]
Arachic acid: Fr[SR100]
Campesterol: Fr[SR124]
Capric acid: Fr Pu, Sd[SR113], Sd oil[SR080]
Caprinic acid: Fr[SR120]
Caproic acid ethyl ester: Fr[SR112]
Caproic acid: Sd oil[SR080], Fr 1.5%[SR117]
Caprylic acid ethyl ester: Fr[SR112]
Caprylic acid: Fr[SR100], Sd oil[SR100]
Carotene: Sd oil[SR080]
Coumaric acid, para: Fr Ju (unriped)[SR104]
Cycloartenol, 24-methylene: Fr[SR105]
Cycloartenol: Fr[SR105]
Daucosterol: Fr 47[SR077]
Decanoid acid: Fr[SR120]
Dotriaconta-2-*cis*-6-*cis*-10-*cis*-14-*cis*-18-*trans*-22-*trans*-26-*trans*-octaen-1-ol,3-7-11-15-19-23-27-31-octamethyl: Fr 270[SR120]

Eicosenoic acid: Fr[SR100]
Farnesol: Fr[SR105]
Geraniol, geranyl: Fr 16[SR120]
Geranyl-geraniol: Fr[SR105]
Glycerol: Sd oil[SR080]
Hexacosan-1-ol: Fr 170[SR117]
Hexatriaconta-2-*cis*-6-*cis*-10-*cis*-14-*cis*-18-*cis*-22-*trans*-26-*trans*-30-*trans*-34-*trans*-nonaen-1-ol,3-7-11-15-19-23-31-35-nonamethyl: Fr 19[SR120]
Lauric acid: Fr[SR130], Fr Pu, Sd[SR113]
Laurin, 1-mono: Fr[SR034]
Linoleic acid: Fr[SR101], Sd[SR113]
Linolenic acid: Fr Pu, Sd[SR113]
Lupen-3-one: Fr[SR124]
Lupeol: Fr[SR120]
Mannitol: Sd oil[SR080]
Myristic acid ethyl ester: Fr[SR112]
Myristic acid: Fr[SR100], Sd[SR113]
Myristin, 1-mono: Fr[SR034]
Octacosan-1-ol: Fr 0.46%[SR117]
Oleic acid: Fr[SR106], Sd[SR113]
Palmitic acid: Fr 9.5%[SR117], Sd[SR113]
Palmitoleic acid: Fr[SR100]
Phytol: Fr[SR120]
Populnin: Fr[SR121]
Quercitrin, iso: Fr[SR121]
Rhoifolin: Fr[SR121]
Rutin: Fr[SR121]
Serenoa polyprenol 2: Fr 5[SR120]
Serenoa polyprenol 3: Fr 35[SR120]
Serenoa polysaccharide: Fr[SR074]
Serenoa triacylglycerols: Fr Pu, Sd[SR113]
Sitosterol, β, 6-O-caprinoyl-β-D-glucoside: Fr[SR121]
Sitosterol, β, 6-O-lauryl-β-D-glucoside: Fr[SR121]
Sitosterol, β, 6-O-myristyl-β-D-glucoside: Fr[SR121]
Sitosterol, β, diglucoside: Fr[SR121]
Sitosterol, β, laurate: Fr[SR121]
Sitosterol, β, myristate: Fr[SR121]
Sitosterol, β, palmitate: Fr[SR121]
Sitosterol, β: Fr[SR124]
Stearic acid: Fr 1.8%[SR117]
Sterols (3): Mesocarp, Epicarp[SR079]
Stigmasterol acetate: Fr[SR105]
Stigmasterol: Fr[SR124]
Tetracosan-1-ol: Fr 40[SR117]
Triacontan-1-ol: Fr[SR123]
Tridecanoid acid: Fr[SR101]
Undecanoid acid: Fr[SR130]
Valerianic acid ethyl ester: Fr[SR112]

PHARMACOLOGICAL ACTIVITIES AND CLINICAL TRIALS

Adaptation to resistance training. AN-DRO-6 mixture, containing 300 mg androstenedione, 150 mg dehydroepiandrosterone, 750 mg *Tribulus terrestris*, 625 mg chrysin, 300 mg indole-3-carbinol, and 540 mg saw palmetto, administered daily to 10 young men 3 days/week for 8 weeks, did not increase serum testosterone (T) concentrations, reduced the estrogenic effect of androstenedione, and did not augment the adaptations to resistance training[SR062].

α-Adrenoreceptor blocking. Lipid fraction of the dried fruit was active. The biological activity has been patented[SR100]. Extract of the dried fruit, administered to male adults at a concentration of 125 μg/mL, inhibited ^{3}H-prozosin binding to cloned human prostatic adrenoreceptors[SR063].

Androgenic effect. Extract, administered to patients with benign prostatic hyperplasia (BPH) at a dose of 320 mg/day for 3 months, produced a statistically significant reduction of dihydrotestosterone (DHT) (2363 ± 553 pg/g tissue, $p < 0.001$) and epidermal growth factor (6.98 ± 2.48 ng/g tissue, $p < 0.01$) and increased T values (1023 ± 101 pg/g tissue, $p < 0.001$) mainly in the periurethral region of the BPH tissue. The biochemical effects were similar to those obtained with finasteride. This enlargement is responsible for urinary obstruction with respect to the subcapsular region[SR030]. Permixon, in the prostatic cell lines LNCaP and PC3, respectively, responsive and unresponsive to androgen stimulation, induced a double proliferative/differentiative effect in LNCaP cell line not observed in PC3 cells. In PC3 cells cotransfected with wild-type androgen receptors and catalase reporter genes under the control of an androgen-responsive element, the extract inhibited androgen-induced catalase transcription[SR036]. Permixon, the liposterolic

extract, in 11 different tissue specimens, reduced the mean uptake of DHT and T by 40.9% and 41.9%, respectively, in all tissue specimens[SR044]. Lipidic extract, in human foreskin fibroblasts, was incubated with [^{3}H] T or [^{3}H] DHT at different dilutions (5.7–28.6 U/mL. One unit was defined as the amount of extract required to inhibit 50% of the specific binding (inhibitory concentration [IC]$_{50}$) of [^{3}H]1881 to rat prostate cytosol. A dilution of 28.6 U/mL significantly altered the formation of DHT and strongly inhibited 3-ketosteroid reductase-mediated conversion of DHT to 5-α-androstane-3 α, 17-β-diol. Dilution of 7.1 U/mL extract resulted in 50% inhibition of the binding of 2×10^{-9} M [^{3}H]DHT to its receptor. Sucrose gradient centrifugation of the radioactive cell lysate of fibroblasts demonstrated that 28.6 U/mL extract abolished 70% of the 3.6 S receptor-complex radioactive peak. The results indicated that the extract inhibited 5-α-reductase, 3-ketosteroid reductase and receptor binding of androgens[SR046]. Permixon, administered to rats with [^{3}H]methyltrienolone as a ligand at a concentration of 5 nM, inhibited competitively the binding to the cytosolic receptor of the rat prostate[SR047]. Saw palmetto herbal blend, administered to men with symptomatic BPH for 6 months, reduced the prostatic tissue DHT levels by 32% from 6.49 to 4.40 ng/g in the saw palmetto group ($p < 0.005$), with no significant change in the placebo group[SR058]. A 24-year-old woman with androgenetic alopecia who became sensitized to topical minoxidil after using an extemporaneous preparation of minoxidil 4% with retinoic acid in a propylene glycol base, subsequently became sensitized to saw palmetto, a topical herbal extract commonly promoted for hair-loss treatment[SR012]. The liposterolic extract of *Serenoa repens* (LSESr) and β-sitosterol, administered to healthy males between the ages of 23 and

64 years, with mild-to-moderate androgenetic alopecia, produced a highly positive response to treatment. The blinded investigative staff assessment report indicated that 60% of the study subjects dosed with the active study formulation were rated as improved at the final visit[SR018]. Extract of the dried fruit, administered intragastrically to male rats at a dose of 300 mg/day, inhibited the decrease in prostate weight induced by castration[SR117]. Lipid fraction in cell culture was active on fibroblasts of human skin and the prostate gland[SR108]. Hexane extract of the dried fruit, administered intragastrically to rats at a dose of 1.8 g/day, was inactive vs T- and DHT-stimulated prostate growth in castrated rats[SR084].

Androgenic receptor-binding activity. Ethanol (95%) extract of the dried fruit, at a concentration of 100 µg/mL, was inactive vs displacement of DHT from rat prostate androgen receptors. Administration to rats produced weak activity vs ^{3}H-methyltrienolone binding to cytosolic androgen receptors in the ventral prostate of castrated rats, IC_{50} 1 mg/mL[SR089]. Ethanol (95%) extract of the dried fruit, in cell culture, was inactive on human skin[SR110]. Steroid fraction of the extract, administered to rats, was active on prostate gland, IC_{50} 0.33 mg/mL[SR103]. Ethanol (95%) extract of the dried fruit, administered to male rats, was inactive vs binding of labeled DHT to the rat prostatic androgen receptor[SR084]. Hexane extract of the dried fruit, administered to adults, reduced DHT binding to receptor in cultured genital skin fibroblasts, IC_{50} 7.1 U/mL[SR082]. Premixon, a liposterolic extract of the plant, inhibited competitively the binding of DHT to the cytosolic receptor of the rat prostate[SR047].

Anti-androgenic effect. Sterol fraction of the dried fruit, in cell culture, was active on CA-PC3 and reduced androgen-induced reporter gene expression in transcriptional assay; IC_{50} 50 µg/mL[SR036]. Administration to adults inhibited uptake of DHT in foreskin, uterus, and vaginal skin[SR044] and was active on fibroblasts, IC_{50} 7.1 U/mL[SR046]. Ethanol (95%) extract of the dried fruit, administered intragastrically to rats at a concentration of 300 mg/mL, reduced the weight of the ventral prostate or seminal vesicle in castrated rats after administration of exogenous T[SR089].

Anticrustacean activity. Ethanol (95%) extract of the dried fruit produced weak activity on *Artemia salina*, lethal concentration $(LC)_{50}$ 31.5 µg/mL[SR034].

Anti-edematous activity. Ethanol (95%) extract of the dried fruit, administered externally to mice at a concentration of 500 µg, reduced croton oil ear edema by 42%[SR089]. Hexane extract of the dried fruit (PA-109), administered intragastrically to rats at a dose of 5 g/kg, was active vs dextran-induced pedal enema[SR088].

Anti-estrogenic activity. *Serenoa repens* extract, administered to 35 patients with benign prostatic hypertrophy at a dose of 160 mg twice daily for 3 months, produced negative result of nuclear fraction of estrogen receptors for high-affinity low-capacity binding and the low-affinity high-capacity binding classes in 17 cases and cytosolic fraction of estrogen receptors in 6 of 18 cases. Both estrogen receptors were detected in all 15 samples examined, but in the treated group, nuclear fraction of estrogen receptors were significantly ($p < 0.01$) lower than in the untreated group. The cytosolic fraction of estrogen receptors remained almost unchanged. Similar results were obtained for progesterone receptors: the nuclear fraction of the treated group prostatic samples was significantly ($p < 0.01$) lower than that of the untreated group[SR043]. The fruit, taken orally by 35 adults with BPH at a dose of 160 mg/person, three times a day for 3 months, suppressed expression of nuclear estrogen receptors and androgen receptors[SR043]. Hexane extract of the dried fruit, administered intragastrically to 35 adults at a dose of 320 mg/day for 3 months, inhibited nuclear estrogen receptors in prostatic tissue samples[SR114].

Anti-inflammatory activity. Ethanol (95%) extract of the fruit, administered by gastric intubation to guinea pigs at a dose of 5 g/kg, was active vs carrageenan-induced pedal edema[SR121]. Hexane extract, administered by gastric intubation to guinea pigs at a dose of 1 mL/kg, was active vs ultraviolet (UV)-induced erythema. The treatment was effective for up to 5 hours of exposure. A dose of 5 mL/kg was protective against UV erythema after 7 hours of exposure. A dose of 3 mL/kg, administered to mice, was active vs centrifugation-induced tail edema. The extract was administered for 5 days before induction. A dose of 10 mL/kg, administered to rats, was active vs histamine-induced cutaneous capillary permeability increase. The effect peaked in 3 hours. There was no significant activity after 24 hours, and the activity was highly dose-dependent. The dose was also active vs serotonin-, bradykinin-, 48/80-, and dextrose-induced papules, and immunoglobulin (Ig) E-dependent passive cutaneous anaphylaxis. The extract was given 30 minutes before induction. A dose of 5 mL/kg, administered to rats by gastric intubation, was active vs dextran-induced generalized edema, histamine-induced papules in adrenalectomized rats, and IgE-dependent passive cutaneous anaphylaxis in adrenalectomized rats[SR125]. The extract, SG 291 (Talso, Talso uno) from the fruits, produced dual inhibition of the cyclo-oxygenase (IC$_{50}$ 28.1 µg/mL) and 5-lipoxygenase pathway (IC$_{50}$ 18 µg/mL). Fraction A (acid lipophilic compounds) inhibited the biosynthesis of cyclo-oxygenase (CO) and 5-lipoxygenase (5-LO) metabolites in the same intensity as the native extract, SG 291. The fractions B and C (fatty alcohols and sterols), and β-sitosterol produced no inhibitory effect on both enzymes of the arachidonic acid pathways. Results indicated that CO- and 5-LO-inhibiting principle of the extract SG 291 must be localized in the acidic lipophilic fraction. The CO and 5-LO inhibitory effects is an explanation for the in vivo observed antiphlogistic and antiedematous activity of the lipophilic extract SG 291[SR042]. Hexane extract of the dried fruit, administered intragastrically to guinea pigs at a dose of 1 mL/kg, was active vs UV-induced erythema for up to 5 hours of exposure. A dose of 5 mL/kg was effective after 7 hours after exposure. A dose of 5 mL/kg was active vs dextran-induced generalized edema, histamine-induced papules, and IgE-dependent passive cutaneous anaphylaxis in adrenalectomized rats. A dose of 10 mg/kg was active vs histamine-induced cutaneous capillary permeability increase, dextran- and 48/80-induced papules, and IgE-dependent passive cutaneous anaphylaxis and inactive vs bradykinin- and serotonin-induced papules. Administration to mice at a dose of 3 mL/kg was active vs centrifugation-induced tail edema. The extract was given for 5 days before induction[SR125]. Ethanol extract of the dried fruit, administered intragastrically to rats at a dose of 5 g/kg[SR121], and water extract, administered intravenously at a dose of 0.3 mg/kg[SR074], were active vs carrageenan-induced pedal edema.

Antioxidant activity. Ether extract of the dried fruit, administered externally to adults as an ingredient in cosmetic, was active. The biological activity has been patented[SR122].

Antiphlogistic activity. Water extract of the fruit and an acidic polysaccharide produced strong antiphlogistic activity. The polysaccharide had an average molecular weight (MW) of 100,000 and contained as main sugar components galactose (38.4%), arabinose (18.7%), and uronic acid (14%)[SR074].

Apoptosis induction. Permixon, in the stroma and epithelium of normal prostate and of BPH tissues from patients treated with or without Permixon, produced cell numbers and proliferative indices higher in BPH than in normal prostates. Apoptosis values were similar. In normal prostates, there was no significant difference between apoptotic and proliferative indices. In the BPH-treated group, Permixon significantly inhibited proliferation and induced cell death in both epithelium and stroma[SR024]. Permixon, in cultures of fibroblast and epithelial cells from the prostate, epididymis, testes, kidney, skin, and breast at a concentration of 10 µg/mL, produced no changes in the morphology of prostate cells, including accumulation of lipid in the cytoplasm and damage to the nuclear and mitochondrial membranes. Permixon increased the apoptotic index for prostate epithelial cells by 35 and 12% in the prostate stromal/fibroblast. A lesser apoptotic effect was found in skin fibroblast (3%). None of the other primary cultures showed any increase in apoptosis compared with the controls[SR025].

Aromatase inhibition. Ether extract of the dried fruit, administered to adults at concentrations of 91 and 132 µg/mL, produced weak activity on microsomes[SR089].

Calcium ion release inhibition. Hexane extract of the dried fruit, in cell culture at a concentration of 10 µg/mL, was active vs prolactin-induced calcium ion increase in Chinese hamster ovary cells[SR021].

Category III prostatitis/chronic pelvic pain syndrome. Extract, administered to men 24 to 58 years old (mean age 43.2), diagnosed with category III prostatitis (CP)/chronic pelvic pain syndrome (CPPS), at a dose of 325 mg daily for 1 year, produced no appreciable long-term improvement. There was a decrease of mean total National Institutes of Health Chronic Prostatitis Symptom Index score from from 24.7 to 24.6 in the saw palmetto arm ($p = 0.41$). There were three cases of headache in the saw palmetto group. At the end of the trial, 13 of 32

(41%) of the patients opted to continue therapy[SR050].

Cell-growth effect. Saw palmetto berry extract, in prostatic 267B-1, BRFF-41T, and LNCaP cell lines for 3 days, inhibited proliferation, IC_{50} 20–30 nL/mL of medium for 267B-1 and BRFF-41T and approx 10-fold more for the LNCaP cell line. The effect on the cell lines was not irreversible. Concentration of 200 nL extract equivalent/mL inhibited normal prostate cells by 20–25%. Growth of other nonprostatic cancer cell lines, i.e., Jurkat and HT-29 was affected by approx 50 and 40%, respectively. Administration of the extract and DHT to LNCaP cells decreased significantly the IC_{50} concentration compared to LNCaP cells grown in the presence of serum and extract. The reduced cellular growth after treatment of the cell lines with the extract may relate to decreased expression of Cox-2 and may result from changes observed in the expression of Bcl-2. Expression of Cox-1 under similar conditions was not affected because of its constitutive expression[SR053].

Cell proliferation effect. Permixon, in biopsies of human prostate, did not affect basal prostate cell proliferation, with the exception of two prostate specimens in which a significant inhibition of basal proliferation was observed with the highest concentration (30 µg/mL) and inhibited basic fibroblast growth factor (b-FGF)-induced proliferation of human prostate cell cultures. This effect was significant for the highest concentration of Permixon. In some prostate samples, a similar inhibition was also noted with lower concentrations. Unsaturated fatty acids ranging from 1 to 30 ng/mL did not affect the basal prostate cell proliferation; a slight increase in cell proliferation was noted in one prostate specimen. Doses of 1, 10, or 30 µg/mL markedly inhibited the b-FGF-induced cell proliferation to the basal value. Lupenone, hexacosanol, and the unsaponified fraction of Permixon markedly inhibited the b-FGF-induced cell proliferation, whereas a minimal effect on basal cell proliferation was noted. b-FGF induced a 2.5-fold increase in human prostate cell proliferation; the glandular epithelium was mainly affected, minimal labeling being recorded in the other regions of the prostate. Similar results were observed with epidermal growth factor (EGF), although the increase in cell proliferation was not recorded in some cases. Lovastatin antagonized both the basal proliferation and the growth factor-stimulated proliferation of human prostate epithelium. Geraniol and farnesol increased cell proliferation only in some prostate specimens, this effect being antagonized by lovastatin[SR032].

Coagulative effect. Permixon, administered to 108 patients at a dose of 320 mg/day for at least 8 weeks before the procedure of transurethral resection of prostate, produced significantly lower bleeding than in the control (124 vs 287 mL, respectively), and the need of transfusion decreased remarkably. The duration of postoperative catheterization (3 vs 5 days, respectively) and the evaluated hematological parameters (red cells 4.5 vs 4 million, hemoglobin 13.4 vs 11.9 g, hematocrit 40 vs 35%) were significantly lower than in the control group[SR001].

Cyclo-oxygenase inhibition. Ethanol (95%) extract of the dried fruit, administered to sheep, was active on microsomes, IC_{50} 28.1 µg/mL[SR089].

Cytochrome P450 2D6 and 3A4 activities. Saw palmetto extract, administered to healthy volunteers (six men and six women) for 14 days at generally recommended doses, did not alter the disposition of coadministered dextromethorphan and alprazolam primarily dependent on the CYP2D6 or CYP3A4 pathways for elimination[SR004].

Cytotoxic activity. Extract from saw palmetto, in LNCaP cell culture, produced cell death. Myristoleic acid had been identified as one of the cytotoxic components in the extract. The cell death exhibited apoptotic and necrotic nuclear morphology. Cell death was also partially associated with caspase activation[SR022]. The extract, in human urological cancer cell lines, PC-3, LNCaP, and SKRC-1, at concentrations of 1–10 µg/mL, effectively suppressed the invasion activity of PC-3 cells into Matrigel, whereas that of LNCaP and SKRC-1 cells was unaffected by the extract. The extract did not affect the viability, adhesion ability, or motility of the cell lines. Urokinase plasminogen activator (uPA) was more strongly expressed on the membrane fraction of PC-3 cells than that of LNCaP or SKRC-1 cells. The purified uPA activity was inhibited by the extract from *Serenoa repens* in a dose-dependent manner, indicating that the suppression of PC-3 cell invasion by the extract is based on an inhibition of the uPA activity, which is necessary for tumor cell invasion[SR023]. The compounds (1-monolaurin and 1-monomyristin) fractionated from ethanol extract (95%) of the powdered, dried berries, produced moderate biological activities in the brine shrimp lethality test and against renal (A-498) and pancreatic (PACA-2) human tumor cells. Borderline cytotoxicity was exhibited against human prostatic (PC-3) cells[SR034]. Hexane extract of the dried fruit, in cell culture at a concentration of 100 µg/mL, was inactive on Chinese hamster ovary cells[SR021].

Diuretic activity. Fruit, administered in the ration of mice, combined with tomato fruit, promoted urination. The biological activity has been patented[SR097].

DNA content in prostate epithelial cells. Saw palmetto herbal blend, administered to 20 men with symptomatic BPH, mean age 65 years and International Prostate Symptom Score (IPSS) 18 for 6 months, produced no significant change from baseline in the nuclear morphometric descriptors (e.g., size, shape, DNA content, and textural features). After 6 months, 25 of the 60 nuclear morphometric descriptors were significantly different compared with baseline. The multivariate model had an area under the receiver operating characteristic curve of 94% and an accuracy of 85%. Results indicated that treatment appeared to alter the DNA chromatin structure and organization in prostate epithelial cells[SR052].

Drug–dietary supplement interaction. A survey was conducted on dietary supplement use in 458 veteran outpatients currently taking prescription medications. Self-reported dietary supplement use was cross-referenced with each patient's prescription medication list, and potential interactions were identified from several tertiary sources and medical literature searches. A total of 197 patients (43%) were currently taking at least one dietary supplement with prescription medication(s). The most common products included vitamins and minerals, garlic, Ginkgo biloba, saw palmetto, and ginseng. Among these, 89 (45%) had a potential for drug-dietary supplement interactions of any significance. Most of these interactions ($n = 84$ [94%]) were not serious based on limited available evidence, giving an incidence of 6% (5/89) of potentially severe interactions among patients taking interacting drugs and dietary supplements and 3% (5/197) among patients taking coincident dietary supplements and medications[SR048].

Early urodynamic effect. Permixon was administered to 75 patients with lower urinary tract symptoms resulting from mild-to-moderate BPH (mean IPSS 8.2), aged 52–78 years, at a dose of 160 mg twice daily for 9 weeks. Maximum urinary flow rate increased 6% ($p < 0.001$), and there was a reduction in detrusor pressure at maximum flow (12.8%, $p < 0.001$), opening detrusor pressure (12.6%, $p < 0.001$), and residual urine volume (12.6%, $p < 0.05$). The IPSS

and quality-of-life score both decreased significantly from baseline in the active treatment group (26.8% and 18.2%, respectively, $p < 0.001$). There were also improvements in prostate volume (2.7%) and maximum detrusor pressure (5.2%) in the Permixon group. Three patients receiving Permixon experienced gastrointestinal disturbances but these did not lead to withdrawal or require additional therapy. In patients with mild/moderate BPH, Permixon treatment reduced intravesical obstruction and produced a rapid improvement in urodynamic parameters and symptoms. The drug was well tolerated[SR010].

Estradiol/T-induced prostate enlargement. The LSESr was administered to rats: shams treated with LSESr (sham rats), castrated animals treated with estradiol, castrated animals treated with T, castrated animals treated with estradiol/T, and castrated treated with LSESr for 3 months. A significant increase of the weight of prostates in the estradiol/T-treated castrated rats was observed in comparison with sham-operated rats. The increase reached a maximum in 30 days and remained at a plateau or slightly declined thereafter. The increase of prostate total weight induced by the hormone treatment was inhibited by the administration of LSESr. The weight was significantly lower at days 60 and 90 for the dorsal and lateral regions of the prostate. The weight of the ventral region of the prostate was significantly lower after 30 and 60 days treatment with LSESr[SR037].

Estrogenic effect. Hexane extract of the fruit, at a concentration of 5 nM, inhibited the binding of mibolerone and methyltrienolone to androgen receptors[SR087].

Fertility effect. Tetrahydrofuran extract of the fruit, administered orally to hamster at a concentration of 9 mg/mL, reduced sperm penetration[SR115]. Zona-free hamster oocytes, pretreated with 0.6 mg/mL of St. John's wort at a concentration of 0.06 mg/mL, resulted in zero penetration after incubation with *Serenoa repens* extract for 1 hour. Sperm exposed to 0.6 mg/mL of St. John's wort resulted in DNA denaturation and mutation of the BRCA1 exon 11 gene[SR028].

Follicle-stimulating hormone release inhibition. Extract of the dried fruit, administered orally to male adults at a dose of 160 mg/person twice daily for 30 days, was inactive[SR045].

Gene expression inhibition. Hexane extract of the fruit, taken orally by male adults at a dose of 320 mg/day, significantly reduced nuclear estrogen and androgen receptors in the prostate[SR087].

Growth inhibition. Fruit, administered to immature rats at a dose of 50% of the diet for 75 days, produced uniform retardation in skeletal and organ development. Growth of suckling rats whose dam received the berries was depressed. Adult rats were not affected by the diet[SR081].

Hair stimulant effect. Hexane extract of the dried fruit, administered externally to adults, was active. Biological activity has been patented. This patent claims usefulness for alopecia[SR096].

Hepatotoxic activity. Ether extract of the dried fruit, administered orally to male adults at a dose of 320 mg/day, was active on the liver[SR094].

Hormonal effects. A commercial product, PC-SPES, composed of *Chrysantemum morifolium*, *Ganoderma lucidum*, *Glycyrrhiza glabra*, *Isatis indigotica*, *Panax pseudoginseng*, *Rabdosia rubescens*, *Scutellaria baicalensis*, and *Serenoa repens* was tested in hormone-insensitive cell lines LNCAP-BCL-2, PC-3, and DU-145 at variable concentrations. LNCAP, the only hormone-sensitive cell line, was affected by the lowest dose of PC-SPES tested[SR119].

Hydroxysteroid(17-β) dehydrogenase inhibition. Hexane extract of the dried fruit, administered to adult males, was active on fibroblasts isolated from BPH tissue, IC$_{50}$ 200 μg/mL. The extract was active on prostate epithelial cells isolated from BPH tissue, IC$_{50}$ 40 μg/mL, fibroblasts isolated from adenocarcinoma, IC$_{50}$ 70 μg/mL, and prostate epithelial cells isolated from adenocarcinoma tissue, IC$_{50}$ 90 μg/mL[SR038].

Hydroxysteroid(3-α) dehydrogenase inhibition. Sterol fraction of the dried fruit, administered to adults at a concentration of 5.7 U/mL, was active on fibroblasts[SR046].

Immunostimulant activity. Polysaccharide fraction of the fruit, administered intraperitoneally to mice at a dose of 10 mg/animal, was active vs clearance of colloidal carbon[SR066]. The treatment increased serum androstenedione concentrations after 2, 5, and 8 weeks ($p < 0.05$), while serum concentrations of free and total T were unchanged. Serum estradiol was elevated at weeks 2, 5, and 8 in ANDRO-6 ($p < 0.05$). Serum estrone was elevated at weeks 5 and 8 ($p < 0.05$). Muscle strength was also increased ($p < 0.05$). The acute effect of one-third of the daily dose of ANDRO-6 was studied in 10 men (23 ± 4 years). Serum androstenedione concentrations were elevated ($p < 0.05$) from 150 to 360 minutes after ingestion, and serum free or total T concentrations were unchanged[SR062]. Water-soluble, acidic branched-chain heteroglycanes isolated from the water or alkaline-water extracts produced significant immunostimulating activities[SR066,SR067].

Insulin-like growth factor 1 signaling suppression. Saw palmetto extract, in the P69 prostate epithelial cell line at a concentration of 150 μg/mL for 24 hours, decreased insulin-like growth factor-I (IGF-1)-induced proliferation of P69 cells and induced cleavage of the enzyme poly(adenosine 5'-diphosphate [ADP]-ribose)polymerase, an index of apoptosis. Treatment of serum-starved P69 cells with 150 μg/mL for 6 hours, reduced IGF-1-induced phosphorylation of Akt and Akt activity. The extract reduced IGF-1-induced phosphorylation of the adapter protein insulin receptor substrate-1 and decreased downstream effects of Akt activation, including increased cyclin D1 levels and phosphorylation of glycogen synthase kinase-3 and p70(s6k). There was no effect on IGF-1-induced phosphorylation of MAPK, IGF-1 receptor, or Shc. Treatment of starved cells with the extract alone induced phosphorylation the proapoptotic kinase/c-Jun N-terminal kinase[SR049].

Intraoperative hemorrhage. A case was reported of severe intraoperative hemorrhage in a patient who was taking saw palmetto. His bleeding time, which was prolonged, normalized a few days after he discontinued saw palmetto treatment[SR057].

Leukotriene B4 production inhibition. The lipidic extract (LESSr), in calcium ionophore A23187-stimulated human polymorphonuclear neutrophils at a concentration of 5 µg/mL, significantly inhibited the production of the 5-lipoxygenase metabolites 5-HETE, 20-COOH LTB4, LTB4, and 20-OH LTB4. This effect of LESSr was also observed in the presence of exogenous arachidonic acid (20 µg/mL) and when formyl-methionyl-leucyl-phenylalanine was used as the antagonist, indicating that inhibition of LTB4 production by the extract was unrelated to phospholipase A2 blockade and independent of the stimulating agent[SR033].

Lipoxygenase (platelet) inhibition. Hexane extract of the dried fruit, administered to rats at a concentration of 700 mg/mL, had no effect on arachidonic acid transformation[SR125].

Lipoxygenase 5 inhibition. Extract of the dried fruit, in cell culture, was active on platelets, IC_{50} 18 µg/mL[SR129].

Low urinary tract symptoms. Permixon, administered to 685 patients with BPH with IPSS greater than or equal to 10 and 124 patients with severe low urinary tract symptoms (LUTS) (IPSS >19) at a dose of 320 mg/day or tamsulosin 0.4 mg/day for 12 months, decreased total IPSS by 7.8 with Permixon and 5.8 with tamsulosin (p = 0.051). The irritative symptoms improved significantly more (p = 0.049) with Permixon (–2.9 vs –1.9 than tamsulosin). The superiority of Permixon in reducing irritative symptoms appeared as soon as month 3 and was maintained up to month 12 (p = 0.03)[NT002]. Fifty men with previously untreated LUTS and a IPSS greater than or equal to 10 were treated with a commercially available extract at a dose of 160 mg twice daily for 6 months. The mean IPSS improved from 19.5 ± 5.5 to 12.5 ± 7.0 (p < 0.001) among the 46 men who completed the study. An improvement in symptom score of 50% or greater after treatment for 2, 4, and 6 months was noted in 21% (10 of 48), 30% (14 of 47), and 46% (21 of 46) of the patients, respectively. There was no significant change in peak urinary flow rate, postvoid residual urine volume, detrusor pressure at peak flow, and mean serum prostate-specific antigen (PSA) level[SR031]. Saw palmetto extract, administered to 85 men 45 years of age or older, with IPSS greater than or equal to 8, for 6 months, produced a decrease of the mean symptom score from 16.7 to 12.3 in the saw palmetto group, compared with 15.8 to 13.6 in the placebo group (p = 0.038). The quality-of-life score improved to a greater degree in the saw palmetto group, but this difference was not statistically significant. No change occurred in the sexual function questionnaire results in either group. The peak flow rate increased by 1 mL/s and 1.4 mL/s in the saw palmetto and placebo groups, respectively (p = 0.73)[SR054].

Lymphohistiocytic adenoma activity. The lipidosterolic extract of saw palmetto, in cells infiltrating the adenoma (lymphocyte T, lymphocyte B, and macrophages with a high proportion of lymphocyte T), modified the inflammatory process. Many of the inflammatory markers, such as lymphoquines (interleukin [IL]-1, IL-2, IL-4, IL-6, and IL-13) and some growth factors (EGF, transforming growth factor [TGF]-α, interferon [IFN]-γ, TGF-β) were elevated in the adenoma tissue[SR016].

Mast cell accumulation. Permixon, administered to adult Wistar rats at a dose of 100 mg/kg body weight every second day for 90 days, produced significant changes with acinar epithelium becoming flat or low cuboidal in the central region of ventral prostate. In the same region, mean mast cell number per optical field in the control, low-dose and high-dose groups were, respectively, 4.7 ± 0.7, 3.4 ± 1 and 2.4 ± 0.6, showing a dose-dependent, statistically significant decrease. Administration of Permixon significantly reduced mast cell accumulation and provoked epithelium atrophy within the central area of the rat ventral prostate[SR017].

Mutagenic activity. Tetrahydrofuran extract of the fruit, at a concentration of 9 mg/mL, was inactive on *Gambusia affinis* sperm[SR115].

Phagocytosis rate increase. Polysaccharide fraction of the fruit, administered to adults at a concentration of 10 µg/mL, was active on polymorphonuclear leukocytes[SR067].

Pharmacokinetics. Hexane extract of the fruit, administered rectally to 12 healthy male adults at a dose of 640 mg, produced bioavailability similar to that observed for the oral formulations. Extract, administered orally to healthy males at a dose of 320 mg (1×320 mg capsule, new formulation; or 2×160 mg, reference preparation) for 1 month, produced a rapid absorption with a peak time (T_{max}) of 1.5–1.58 hour and peak plasma level (C_{max}) of 2.54–2.67 µg/mL. The area under the curve value ranged from 7.99 to 8.42 µg/hour/mL. The plasma concentration-time profile of both preparation was nearly identical. Both preparations can be considered as bioequivalent[SR099]. Hexane extract, administered orally to healthy males at a dose of 320 mg, produced plasma level concentration-time profile almost identical with reference preparation dose (160 mg). The ratio of area under the curve (AUC) (extent of absorption) was 1.026 (90% confidence interval 0.992–1.062). The ratio of C_{max} (rate of absorption) was 0.982 (90% confidence interval 0.930–1.038). The difference of T_{max} was 0 hours (90% confidence interval from 0 to 0.25 hour)[SR086].

Phospholipase A2 inhibition. The extract on the pancreas, inhibited the hydrolysis of diplamitoyl-phosphatidylcholine by *Naja naja* pancreas phosphatase A2, IC_{50} 54 µg/mL. The extract inhibited the hydrolysis of diplamitoyl-phosphatidylcholine on the pig pancreas, IC_{50} 35 µg/mL. Hexane extract, in cell culture, was inactive on cultured prostatic cells[SR083].

Potassium channel blocking activity. Hexane extract, in Chinese hamster ovary cells overexpressing the prolactin receptor at a concentration of 30 µg/mL, was active[SR021].

Prolactin receptor signal transduction. The lipidosterolic extract, in Chinese hamster ovary cells, reduced the basal activity of a K^+ channel and of protein kinase (PK) C. Pretreatment of the cells with the extract for 6–36 hours abolished the effects of prolactin on Ca^{2+}, K^+ conductance and PKC. The results indicated that the extract can block prolactin-induced prostate growth by inhibiting several steps of prolactin receptor signal transduction[SR021].

Prostaglandin inhibition. Ethanol (95%) extract of the dried fruit, at variable concentrations, was active[SR121].

Prostate cancer effect. Saw palmetto, vitamin E, and selenium supplements were used by 26.5% of the questioned men diagnosed with prostate cancer[SR051]. PC-SPES, an herbal mixture of chrysanthemum, isatis, licorice, *Ganoderma lucidum*, *Panax pseudoginseng*, *Rabdosia rubescens*, saw palmetto, and *Scutellaria* was administered to two patients with hormone-refractory prostate cancer with metastatic disease. treatment with total androgen blockade progressing to an androgen-independent status, decreased the PSA value for both patients from an initial value of 100 and 386 ng/mL to 24 and 114 ng/mL after 1 year and 4 months, respectively, remaining stable. No gynecomastia or hot flashes were observed in these patients and the treatment was well tolerated. PC-SPES has shown a strong estrogenic in vitro and in vivo activity as an alternative tool in the management of prostate cancer patients. The results indicated that PC-SPES might have some potential activity against hormone-independent prostate cancers[SR061]. An extract of saw palmetto, administered to 20 mature male dogs with benign prostatic hyperplasia, at doses of 1500 mg/day or 300 mg/day for 91 days, did not affect prostatic weight, prostatic volume, or prostatic histologic scores, libido, semen characteristics, radiographs of the caudal portion of the abdomen, prostatic ultrasonographs, or serum T concentrations. Results of complete blood cell counts, serum biochemical analyses or urinalysis, and body weights did not change during treatment[SR026].

Prostate hypertophy. Permixon, administered to 30 patients at a dose of 320 mg/day for 30 days, produced significant differences in the number of voidings, strangury, maximum and mean flow, and residual urine compared to placebo group[SR071]. The extract, administered to 40 patients with moderate BPH at a dose of 160 mg twice daily for 3 months, produced significant improvements in the number of daytime voidings, nocturia, incomplete voidings, dysuria, and urine retention. Transrectal and superpubic ultrasound indicated the residual urine content dropped from 110 mL at the beginning of the study to 45 mL at the end. There was no significant change in the size of the prostate in either group[SR072].

Prostate-specific gene expression and proliferation. PC-SPEC ethanol extract, a multi-herbal mixture, in androgen-dependent LNCaP cell culture at concentrations of 1 or 5 µL/mL for 72 hours, produced a 72–80% reduction in cell growth and a similar decrease in cell viability by the higher concentration. These results contrasted with cells incubated with same concentration of individual herbal extract, which supressed growth in the order: *Dendranthema morifolium* Tzvel (85.2% reduction) greater than *Panax pseudoginseng* (80.9%) greater than *Glycyrrhiza uralensis* Fisch (73%) greater than *Rabdosia rubescens* Hara (70.8%) greater than *Scutellaria baicalensis* Georgi (66.5%) greater than *Ganoderma lucidum* Karst (63.5%) greater than *Isatis indgotica* Fort (50.0%) greater than *Serenoa repens* (14.5%). *Serenoa repens* lowered intracellular and secreted PSA level[SR020].

Prostatic adenoma. Permixon (PA 109), admininistered for 1 month to 110 patients with a prostatic adenoma, produced a greater effect in nocturia, urinary output, postmicturitional residue and subjective criterias: dysuria, patients' opinions than placebo, especially in the objective criteria. In a supplementary study of 47 patients, with a mean follow-up of 14.5 months and over 2.5 years in some cases, permixon produced good effect for micturitional disorders associated with nonsurgical adenomas of the prostate[SR076]. The extract, administered to 22 patients at a dose of 320 mg/day for 60 days, produced significant differences for volume voided, maximum and mean urine flow, dysuria, and nocturia compared with placebo group. There were no side effects[SR070].

Prostatic hyperplasia. Permixon was administered to 4280 patients during 14 clinical trials. The trials were of different sizes (22–1100 patients) and duration (21–720 days). Permixon produced a significant improvement in peak flow rate and reduction in nocturia above placebo, and a five-point reduction in the IPSS[SR003]. Permixon, administered orally to patients with BPH at a dose of 160 mg twice daily for 3 months, produced a decrease in the number of lymphocytes B as compared to control (Permixon-treated 58.2 ± 53.7 and control 91.4 ± 44.1). Tumor necrosis factor-α and IL-1β were dramatically lower in the Permixon-treated group. Other parameters did not show significant changes. IPSS in the Permixon-treated group was significantly reduced ($p < 0.006$) from 20 ± 5.9 to 14.9 ± 3.8[SR005]. Serenoa repens extract, at a dose of 320 mg for 12 weeks, was administered to 100 men aged under 80 years with BPH symptoms and a maximum urinary flow rate of 5–15 mL/s for a voiding volume of 150 mL. The extract produced no significant difference in the IPSS, peak urinary flow rate or for the Rosen International Index of Erectile Function questionnaire[SR007]. Hexane extract of the fruit, taken orally by male adults at a dose of 320 mg/day, was active in a 3-year prospective multicenter study that evaluated the use of the extract in treating 435 patients. Symptomatic improvement included a 50% reduction in residual urine and a 6.1 mL/second increase in peak urine flow. The deterioration rate was significantly lower in the treated patients[SR111]. The extract, administered to male rats, inhibited estradiol/T-induced prostate enlargement[SR087]. Permixon, administered to 155 men with BPH at a dose of 160 mg twice daily for 2 years, produced a significant improvement of IPSS and quality of life from baseline at each evaluation time point. At the end of the study and at each evaluation, maximum urinary flow also improved significantly. Prostate size decreased. Sexual function remained stable during the first year of treatment and significantly improved ($p = 0.001$) during the second year. PSA was not affected, and no changes in plasma hormone levels were observed. Nine patients reported 10 adverse events, none related to treatment. Improvements in efficacy parameters began at 6 months and were maintained up to 24 months[SR008]. Libeprosta, the lipidosterolic extract of Serenoa repens, administered to 100 male outpatients with LUTS suggestive of BPH, at doses of two 80 mg tablets twice daily or two 80-mg tablets three times daily, significantly reduced the IPSS mean total score from baseline values ($p < 0.001$) by the both regimens. Significant improvements from baseline also occurred in quality-of-life scores, maximum and mean urinary flow rates, and residual urine volume ($p < 0.05$). The decrease in residual urine with both regimens was highly significant ($p < 0.001$). No significant differences in efficacy were noted between the two dose groups. No treatment-related complications or clinical adverse events occurred[SR009]. Saw palmetto, in combination with tamsulosin (TAM), and TAM alone were evaluated in patients with IPSS greater than or equal to 13 and a maximum urinary flow rate 7–15 mL/second. A dose of 160 mg of saw palmetto/TAM (SR/TAM) or 0.4 mg of TAM were administered twice daily for 52 weeks. There was no statistically significant difference between the two groups for the major end points and the secondary end points. For the major end points total IPSS between the baseline value and the final evaluation were TAM –5.2, TAM/SR –6 ($p = 0.286$). For the secondary end points, changes in the voiding scores ($p = 0.239$), filling scores ($p = 0.475$) of IPSS, maximum urinary flow rate ($p = 0.564$), percentage of respondents according to the IPSS ($p = 0.361$), improvement in quality of life ($p = 0.091$)[SR013]. Permixon, administered to men with symptomatic BPH at doses of 320 mg per day ($N = 350$) or TAM 0.4 mg per day ($N = 354$) for 1 year, produced a decrease of IPSS by 4.4 and no differences in either irritative or obstructive symptom improvements. The increase in maximum urinary flow rate was similar in both treatment groups (1.8 mL/second Permixon, 1.9 mL/second TAM). Serum prostate-specific and antigen remained stable, whereas prostate volume decreased slightly in the Permixon-treated patients. The two compounds were well tolerated; however, ejaculation disorders occurred more frequently in the TAM group[SR014]. Preparations of saw palmetto, administered to 3139 men in 21 randomized trials lasting 4–48 weeks, improved urinary symptom scores, symptoms, and flow measures compared with the placebo. Compared with finasteride, *Serenoa repens* produced similar improvements in urinary symptom scores and peak urine flow. Adverse effects resulting from *Serenoa repens* were mild and infrequent. Withdrawal rates in the men assigned to placebo, *Serenoa repens* or finasteride were 7%, 9%, and 11%, respectively[SR015]. Permixon, administered to 26 patients with prostatic hyperplasia (total PSA < 4 ng/mL) before meal with a small quantity of water at a total daily dose of 320 mg twice daily for 5 years, significantly reduced the disease symptoms and improved quality of life. Five years of treatment decreased mean IPSS by 8.8 ± 0.18 (75.5%), quality of life by 1.31 ± 0.08 (53.3%), and size of the prostate by 10.81 ± 0.55 cm³ (29.8%). Neither the symptoms nor quality of life became worse for these five years. The size of the prostate reduced in 16 patients, was unchanged in 9 patients, and increased in 1 patient. Maximal urinary flow rate increased by 35%. Residual urine increased during the treatment in one patient. Permixon intolerance was not observed[SR019].

Prostatic hypoplasia. The extract of saw palmetto, crushed whole berry derived from saw palmetto fruit, or a combination of the saw palmetto extract and cernitin, administered to castrated rats receiving T, decreased the size of the prostate to roughly the same size as in the noncastrated rats, a size that was significantly smaller than castrated rats treated with T in the same manner ($p < 0.01$). Both nutraceuticals generally decreased body weight[SR006].

Protein kinase C inhibition. Hexane extract, at a concentration of 30 µg/mL on Chinese hamster ovary cells overexpressing the prolactin receptor, was active[SR021].

Protein synthesis stimulation. Sterol fraction of the extract, in cell culture at a concentration of 25 µg/mL, produced weak activity on CA-LNCAP. A concentration of 50 µg/mL was active on CA-PC3[SR036].

PSA production inhibition. Ethanol (70%) extract of PC-SPES (a Chinese herb combination of chrysanthemum, dyers woad, licorice, reishi, san-qi ginseng, rabdosia, saw palmetto, and baikal skullcap), in cultured prostate cancer cell line at variable doses for 24 hours, produced a significant effect in supressing cell growth in all the cell lines[SR119].

Radioactivity distribution. The N-hexane lipido/sterolic extract (LSESr) supplemented with [¹⁴C]-labeled oleic or lauric acids or β-sitosterol was administered orally to rats. The highest level of radioactivity uptake was LSESr supplemented with [¹⁴C]-labeled oleic acid. Ratios of radioactivity in tissues compared to plasma showed an uptake of radioactivity greater in prostate as compared with other genital organs, i.e., the seminal vesicles or to other organs such as liver[SR035].

Rectal bioavailability and pharmacokinetics. *Serenoa repens* extract, administered rectally to 12 healthy male volunteers at a dose of 640 mg/person, produced the mean maximum concentration in plasma of nearly 2.60 µg/mL approx 3 hours after administration, with mean value for the area under the curve AUC 10 µg/hour/mL. The bioavailability and pharmacokinetic profile were similar to those observed after oral administration. T_{max} occurred approx 1 hour later, and plasma concentration 8 hours after drug administration was still quantified. The drug tolerability was good, and no adverse effect was observed[SR068]. *Serenoa repens* capsules, administered orally at a dose of 160 mg four times daily or rectally 640 mg daily for 30 days to 60 patients with BPH, produced no significant differences in diminution of scores assigned to dysuria, pollakiuria, prostate dimension, and micturition residue between the two groups[SR069].

Reductase, 5-α inhibition. Permixon was evaluated in cultures of fibroblast and epithelial cells from the prostate, epididymis, testes, kidney, skin, and breast at a concentration of 10 µg/mL. The extract inhibited 5-αR type I and II isoenzymes activity in prostate cells, but other cells showed no inhibition of 5-αR activity[SR025]. Saw palmetto extract, in pig prostatic tissue, inhibited 5-α-reductase enzyme, which catalyzes the conversion of T into DHT in prostatic microsomes of growing pigs. Peaks for the 5-α-reductase activity were found at pH 5.5 and 8, which indicates the presence of both type 1 and type 2 isozymes. Kinetic parameters of porcine 5-α-reductase in the presence of *Serenoa repens* extracts revealed uncompetitive, noncompetitive, and mixed types of inhibitions[SR029]. Ethanol (95%) extract of the fruit, administered to adults at a concentration of 500 µg/mL, was active on prostate glands when assayed in epithelium and stroma of BPH tissue[SR106]. Fixed oil of the fruit, administered orally to male adults at a dose of 320 mg/day, was active[SR116]. Hexane extract of the fruit, at concentrations of 50 and 100 mg/L, was active. A concentration of 20 mg/L was inactive[SR101]. Ether extract of the dried fruit, at concentrations of 59 and 71 µg/mL, produced weak activity[SR089]. Hexane extract of the dried fruit, was active on reductase type 1 and 2, IC_{50} 4.0 and 7 µg/mL, respectively[SR039]. Permixon, administered to adults at a dose of 10 µg/mL, was active on prostate gland[SR075]. CO_2 extract of the dried fruit was active, minimum inhibitory concentration 1:500[SR102]. Hexane extract of the fruit (Permixon), in cell culture was active vs cocultures of prostatic epithelial cells and fibroblasts[SR118]. Hexane extract of the fruit, administered to male adults, was active[SR082]. Administration of the extract to male rats was active, IC_{50} 5.6 µg/mL. Oral administra-

tion to male adults at a dose of 320 mg/day was inactive on serum[SR084]. Hexane extract of the fruit, administered orally to male adult at a dose of 160 mg/day, was inactive on serum[SR041]. Lipid fraction of the extract, in cell culture was active on human prostate cancer cell line DU-145; administered orally to adults at a dose of 320 mg/person/day for 3 months, was inactive[SR108].

Respiration inhibition (cellular)-state 4. Extract of the fruit, in cell culture, was active on platelets. IC_{50} 28.1 µg/mL[SR129].

Serum PSA. PC-SPES, a Chinese herb combination of chrysanthemum, dyers woad, licorice, reishi, san-qi ginseng, rabdosia, saw palmetto, and baikal skullcap, produced positive results. The respondents experienced a decline in serum PSA, most to the undetectable range. Of these patients, 88% maintained a low PSA concentration, whereas 12% had a rise from nadir. In a second study, 93% of the respondents with positive results and only 7% reporting a rise in PSA after the initial lowering with PC-SPES was found. There were some side effects[SR060].

Serum sex hormones effect. DION (300 mg androstenedione, 150 mg dehydroepiandrosterone, 540 mg saw palmetto, 300 mg indole-3-carbinol, 625 mg chrysin, 750 mg *Tribulus terrestris*), administered daily to healthy 30- to 59-year-old men for 28 days, produced no change in serum concentrations of total T and PSA. DION increased the concentrations of serum androstenedione (342%), free T (38%), DHT (71%), and estradiol (103%). Serum high-density lipoprotein (HDL) cholesterol concentrations were reduced by 5 mg/dL in DION (p < 0.05). Increases in serum free T (r^2 = 0.01), androstenedione (r^2 = 0.01), DHT (r^2 = 0.03), or estradiol (r^2 = 0.07) concentrations in DION were not related to age. The ingestion of androstenedione combined with herbal products increased serum-free T concentrations in older men, but herbal products did not prevent the conversion of ingested androstenedione to estradiol and DHT[SR055]. Nutritional supplement (AND-HB) containing 300 mg androstenediol, 480 mg saw palmetto, 450 mg indole-3-carbinol, 300 mg chrysin, 1500 mg γ-linolenic acid and 1350 mg *Tribulus terrestris*, administrated per day to the men stratified into age groups: 30 year olds, 40 year olds, and 50 year olds for 28 days, produced no difference in basal serum total T, estradiol, and PSA concentrations between age groups. Basal serum-free T concentrations were higher ($p < 0.05$) in the 30- (70.5 ± 3.6 pmol/L) than in the 50-year-olds (50.8 ± 4.5 pmol/L). Basal serum androstenedione and DHT concentrations were significantly higher in the 30-year-olds than in the 40- or 50-year-olds. Basal serum hormone concentrations did not differ between the treatment groups. Serum concentrations of total T and PSA were unchanged by supplementation. Ingestion of AND-HB resulted in increased ($p < 0.05$) serum androstenedione (174%), free T (37%), DHT (57%) and estradiol (86%) throughout the treatment period. There was no relationship between the increases in serum-free T, androstenedione, DHT, or estradiol and age ($r^2 = 0.08$, 0.03, 0.05, and 0.02, respectively). Serum HDL cholesterol concentrations were reduced ($p < 0.05$) by 0.14 mM/L in AND-HB[SR056]. Permixon, administered to healthy male volunteers aged 20–30 years at a dose of 80 mg twice a day for 1 week, produced no effect on the serum DHT level. No significant difference was found between finasteride and Permixon with respect to serum T, except on days 3 and 6, respectively ($p \leq 0.05$). The corresponding serum T levels remained within the normal ranges[SR041].

Smooth muscle relaxant activity. Hexane extract of the dried fruit, administered to guinea pigs at a concentration of 0.15 mg/mL, was active on bladder and ileum vs KCl-induced contractions[SR085]. Administration to

rats, at a concentration of 0.33 mg/mL, was active vs contractions of ductus differens induced by electrical stimulation[SR085].

Spasmolytic activity. Lipidic extract of the fruit relaxed vanadate-induced contractions on rat uterus incubated in a calcium-free solution, effective concentration ($EC)_{50}$ = 11.41 ± 1.38 µg/mL. The effect was not modified by 3 µM concentration of indomethacin, EC_{50} = 8.77 ± 1.28 vs 11.41 ± 1.38 µg/mL, and 5 µg/mL concentration of actinomycin D, EC_{50} = 8.23 ± 2.19 vs 11.41 ± 1.38 µg/mL. The inhibitor of intracellular calcium mobilization TMB-8 (0.1 mM), Na^+/Ca^{2+} exchanger inhibitor amiloride (0.1 mM), calcium chelator BAPTA-AM (50 mM), PKA inhibitor TPCK (10 µM), and protein synthesis inhibitor cycloheximide (10 µg/mL), significantly shifted to the right the dose-response curve of the extract (EC_{50} = 17.83 ± 1.87 µg/mL, 18.61 ± 2.50 µg/mL, 35.28 ± 9.13 µg/mL, 33.99 ± 3.07 µg/mL, and 27.31 ± 4.93 µg/mL, respectively, vs 11.41 ± 1.38 µg/mL)[SR064]. Total lipidic (L) and saponifiable (S) extracts of the fruit, at concentrations of 0.1–1 mg/mL, relaxed the tonic norepinephrine-induced contraction on the rat aorta, EC_{50} 0.53 ± 0.05 mg/mL (L) and 0.5 ± 0.04 mg/mL (S), and by KCl on rat uterus. The extracts, at concentrations of 0.3–1 mg/mL, antagonized the dose–response curve of contractions induced by acetylcholine on urinary bladder. DL-Propranolol (1 µM) but not the inactive (R)-(+)-propranolol (1 µM), potentiated the extracts relaxant effect by lowering the EC_{50} 0.35 ± 0.2 vs 0.20 ± 0.01 mg/mL (L) and 0.43 ± 0.02 vs 0.19 ± 0.02 mg/mL, $p < 0.01$, (S). Cycloheximide, at a concentration of 10 µg/mL, antagonized the effect of saw palmetto extracts. Actinomycin D (5 µg/mL) significantly ($p \leq 0.01$) antagonized the effect of the total lipidic extract without modifying the effect of the saponifiable extract. The relaxant effect of both extracts was not modified by the tyrosine kinase inhibitor genistein (10 µM) or the ornithine decarboxylase inhibitor α-difluoromethyl-ornithine (10 mM)[SR065]. Ethanol (95%) extract of the fruit, administered to guinea pigs at a concentration of 0.15 mg/mL, was active on the bladder and ileum vs KCl-induced contractions. Administration to rats at a concentration of 0.3 mg/mL, was active on vas deferens vs norepinephrine-induced contractions[SR109].

Sperm motility inhibition. Saw palmetto (Permixon, *Sabal serrulatum*), incubated with washed sperm at a concentration of 0.6 mg/mL for 24 and 48 hours, inhibited sperm motility[SR027].

Testosterone effects. A liposterolic extract of *Serenoa repens* was administered to 20 men aged 50 to 75 years with BPH at a dose of 160 mg twice daily for 30 days. The extract produced no changes in plasma levels of T, FSH, and luteinizing hormone. The results indicated that *Serenoa* extract, which is useful in the treatment of BPH, does not act via systemic changes of hormone levels[SR045].

Testosterone metabolism. The lipido-sterol extract (LSESr, Permixon) was studied in primary cultures of epithelial cells and fibroblasts separated from benign prostate hypertrophy and prostate cancer tissues. The extract inhibited the formation of the T metabolites androstenedione δ 4 and 5 α-DHT [SR038]. The lipophilic extracts of fruits inhibited T 5µ-reductase (EC 1.3.99.5) (5µR). For fatty acid-like 5µR inhibition a strongly polar end-group and a molecular skeleton allowing nonpolar interactions with the enzyme were required. The result indicated that 5µR activity in prostatic tissue may be influenced by the lipid environment[SR073]. Three different saw palmetto extract preparations, administered to 12 healthy young men at a dose of 320 mg daily for 8 days, did not result in α1-adrenoceptor subtype occupancy in the radioreceptor assay. Although the extracts produced minor

reductions of supine blood pressure, they did not affect blood pressure during orthostatic stress testing and did not alter heart rate under either conditions. Plasma catecholamines remained largely unaltered[SR059]. The extracts of saw palmetto inhibited radioligand binding to human α1-adrenoceptors and antagonist-induced [^{3}H]inositol phosphate formation. Saturation binding experiments in the presence of a single saw palmetto extract concentration indicated a noncompetitive antagonism. The relationship between active concentrations in vitro and recommended therapeutic doses for the saw palmetto extracts was slightly lower than that for several chemically defined α 1-adrenoceptor antagonists[SR063]. N-hexane lipid/sterol extract inhibition of a type 1 5-α-R expressed in a baculovirus-directed-insect cell system was noncompetitive. When expressed in terms of recommended therapeutic doses, was threefold greater for the n-hexane lipid/sterol extract than for finasteride[SR040].

Thromboxane A2 synthesis inhibition. Ethanol (95%) extract of the dried fruit, administered to rats, was active on leukocytes vs A23187 stimulation, IC_{50} 15.2 µg/mL[SR089].

Toxic effect. Ethanol (95%) extract of the dried fruit, administered to adult males at a dose of 320 mg/day, was inactive[SR091, SR095]. Ether extract of the fruit, administered orally to male adults at a dose of 320 mg/day, was inactive[SR090,SR093,SR031]. Ether extract of the fruit, administered orally with *Urtica dioica* to male adults at a dose of 320 mg/day for 24 weeks, was inactive[SR092]. Hexane extract of the fruit, administered orally to male adults at a dose of 320 mg/day, was inactive[SR076,SR107].

Type 1 and 2 5-α-reductase activity. The lipidosterol extract of seeds was investigated in the baculovirus-directed insect cell expression system Sf9 expressing the corresponding type 1 and type 2 human genes.

The extract produced an inhibition of 5-αR1 and 5-αR2 activities in the presence of free fatty (oleic, lauric, linoleic, and myristic) acids only. Esterified fatty acids, alcohols, and sterols assayed were inactive. A specificity of the fatty acids in 5-αR1 or 5-αR2 inhibition has been found. Palmitic and stearic acids were inactive on the two isoforms. Lauric acid was active on 5-αR1 ($IC_{50} = 17 \pm 3$ μg/mL) and 5-αR2 ($IC_{50} = 19 \pm 9$ μg/mL). The inhibitory activity of myristic acid was evaluated on 5-αR2 only and found active on this isoform ($IC_{50} = 4 \pm 2$ μg/mL)[SR011]. LSESr markedly inhibited both isozymes (K_i [type 1] = 8.4 nM and 7.2 μg/mL, respectively; K_i [type 2] = 7.4 nM and 4.9 μg/mL, respectively). Results indicated that LSESr displayed non-competitive inhibition of the type 1 isozyme and uncompetitive inhibition of the type 2 isozyme[SR039].

Vasoconstriction activity. Fruit, administered to immature rats at a dose of 50% of the diet for 75 days after weaning, resulted in peripheral vasoconstriction leading to gangrene in the extremities within 40 days, and the loss of whole limbs in some cases[SR081].

Weight loss. Fruit, administered to rats at a dose of 50% of the diet for 75 days, was inactive[SR081].

REFERENCES

SR001 Pecoraro, S., A. Annecchiarico, M. C. Gambardella, and G. Sepe. Efficacy of pretreatment with Serenoa repens on bleeding associated with transurethral resection of prostate. **Minerva Urol Nefrol** 2004; 56(1): 73–78.

SR002 Debruyne, F., P. Boyle, F. Calais Da Silva, et al. Evaluation of the clinical benefit of permixon and tamsulosin in severe BPH patients-PERMAL study subset analysis. **Eur Urol** 2004; 45(6): 773–779.

SR003 Boyle, P., C. Robertson, F. Lowe, and C. Roehrborn. Updated meta-analysis of clinical trials of Serenoa repens extract in the treatment of symptomatic

benign prostatic hyperplasia. **BJU Int** 2004; 93(6): 751–756.

SR004 Markowitz, J. S., J. L. Donovan, C. L. Devane, et al. Multiple doses of saw palmetto (Serenoa repens) did not alter cytochrome P450 2D6 and 3A4 activity in normal volunteers. **Clin Pharmacol Ther** 2003; 74(6): 536–542.

SR005 Vela Navarrete, R., J. V. Garcia Cardoso, A. Barat, F. Manzarbeitia, and A. Lopez Farre. BPH and inflammation: pharmacological effects of Permixon on histological and molecular inflammatory markers. Results of a double blind pilot clinical assay. **Eur Urol** 2003; 44(5): 549–555.

SR006 Talpur, N., B. Echard, D. Bagchi, M. Bagchi, and H. G. Preuss. Comparison of Saw Palmetto (extract and whole berry) and Cernitin on prostate growth in rats. **Mol Cell Biochem** 2003; 250(1–2): 21–26.

SR007 Willetts, K. E., M. S. Clements, S. Champion, S. Ehsman, and J. A. Eden. Serenoa repens extract for benign prostate hyperplasia: a randomized controlled trial. **BJU Int** 2003; 92(3): 267–270.

SR008 Pytel, Y. A., A. Vinarov, N. Lopatkin, A. Sivkov, L. Gorilovsky, and J. P. Raynaud. Long-term clinical and biologic effects of the lipidosterolic extract of Serenoa repens in patients with symptomatic benign prostatic hyperplasia. **Adv Ther** 2002; 19(6): 297–306.

SR009 Giannakopoulos, X., D. Baltogiannis, D. Giannakis, et al. The lipidosterolic extract of Serenoa repens in the treatment of benign prostatic hyperplasia: a comparison of two dosage regimens. **Adv Ther** 2002; 19(6): 285–296.

SR010 Al-Shukri, S. H., P. Deschaseaux, I. V. Kuzmin, and R. R. Amdiy. Early urodynamic effects of the lipido-sterolic extract of Serenoa repens (Permixon®) in patients with lower urinary tract symptoms due to benign prostatic hyperplasia. **Prostate Cancer Prostatic Dis** 2000; 3(3): 195–199.

SR011 Raynaud, J. P., H. Cousse, and P. M. Martin. Inhibition of type 1 and type 2 5alpha-reductase activity by free fatty acids, active ingredients of Permixon. **J Steroid Biochem Mol Biol** 2002; 82(2–3): 233–239.

SR012 Sinclair, R. D., R. S. Mallari, and B. Tate. Sensitization to saw palmetto and minoxidil in separate topical extemporaneous treatments for androgenetic alopecia. **Austr J Dermatol** 2002; 43(4): 311–312.

SR013 Glemain, P., C. Coulange, T. Billebaud, B. Gattegno, R. Muszynski, G. Loeb, and the OCOS Groupe de l'essai. Tamsulosin with or without *Serenoa repens* in benign prostatic hyperplasia: the OCOS trial. **Prog Urol** 2002; 12(3): 395–403.

SR014 Debruyne, F., G. Koch, P. Boyle, et al., and the Groupe d'etude PERMAL. Comparison of a phytotherapeutic agent (Permixon) with an alpha-blocker (Tamsulosin) in the treatment of benign prostatic hyperplasia: a 1-year randomized international study. **Prog Urol** 2002; 12(3): 384–392.

SR015 Wilt, T., A. Ishani, and R. Mac Donald. *Serenoa repens* for benign prostatic hyperplasia. **Cochrane Database Syst Rev** 2002; (3): CD001423.

SR016 Vela Navarrete, R., J. Garcia Cardoso, A. Lopez Farre, et al. Benign prostatic hyperplasia: biological significance of lymphohistiocytic infiltration of the adenoma. **Acta Urol Esp** 2002; 26(3): 163–173.

SR017 Mitropoulos, D., A. Kyroudi A, A. Zervas, et al. *In vivo* effect of the lipido-sterolic extract of *Serenoa repens* (Permixon) on mast cell accumulation and glandular epithelium trophism in the rat prostate. **World J Urol** 2002; 19(6): 457–461.

SR018 Prager, N., K. Bickett, N. French, and G. Marcovici. A randomized, double-blind, placebo-controlled trial to determine the effectiveness of botanically derived inhibitors of 5-alpha-reductase in the treatment of androgenetic alopecia. **J Altern Complement Med** 2002; 8(2): 143–152.

SR019 Aliaev, I. G., A. Z. Vinarov, K. L. Lokshin, and L. G. Spivak. Five-year experience in treating patients with prostatic hyperplasia patients with permixone (*Serenoa repens* "Pierre Fabre Medicament). **Urologia** 2002; (1): 23–25.

SR020 Hsieh, T. C., and J. M. Wu. Mechanism of action of herbal supplement PC-SPES: elucidation of effects of individual herbs of PC-SPES on proliferation and prostate specific gene expression in androgen-dependent LNCaP cells. **Int J Oncol** 2002; 20(3): 583–588.

SR021 Vacher, P., N. Prevarskaya, R. Skryma, M. C. Audy, A. M. Vacher, M. F. Odessa, and B. Dufy. The lipidosterolic extract from *Serenoa repens* interferes with prolactin receptor signal transduction. **J Biomed Sci** 1995; 2(4): 357–365.

SR022 Iguchi K., N. Okumura, S. Usui, H. Sajiki, K. Hirota, and K. Hirano. Myristoleic acid, a cytotoxic component in the extract from *Serenoa repens*, induces apoptosis and necrosis in human prostatic LNCaP cells. **Prostate** 2001; 47(1): 59–65.

SR023 Ishii, K., S. Usui, Y. Sugimura, H. Yamamoto, K. Yoshikawa, and K. Hiran. Extract from *Serenoa repens* suppresses the invasion activity of human urological cancer cells by inhibiting urokinase-type plasminogen activator. **Biol Pharm Bull** 2001; 24(2): 188–190.

SR024 Vacherot, F., M. Azzouz, S. Gil-Diez-De-Medina, et al. Induction of apoptosis and inhibition of cell proliferation by the lipido-sterolic extract of *Serenoa repens* (LSESr, Permixon) in benign prostatic hyperplasia. **Prostate** 2000; 45(3): 259–266.

SR025 Bayne, C. W., M. Ross, F. Donnelly, and F. K. Habib. The selectivity and specificity of the actions of the lipido-sterolic extract of *Serenoa repens* (Permixon) on the prostate. **J Urol** 2000; 164(3 Pt 1): 876–881.

SR026 Barsanti, J. A., D. R. Finco, M. M. Mahaffey, et al. Effects of an extract of *Serenoa repens* on dogs with hyperplasia of the prostate gland. **Amer J Vet Res** 2000; 61(8): 880–885.

SR027 Ondrizek, R. R., P. J. Chan, W. C. Patton, and A. King. Inhibition of human sperm motility by specific herbs used in alternative medicine. **J Assist Reprod Genet** 1999; 16(2): 87–91.

SR028 Ondrizek, R. R., P. J. Chan, W. C. Patton, and A. King. An alternative medicine study of herbal effects on the penetration of zona-free hamster oocytes and the integrity of sperm deoxyribonucleic acid. **Fertil Steril** 1999; 71(3): 517–522.

SR029   Palin, M. F., M. Faguy, J. G. LeHoux, and G. Pelletier. Inhibitory effects of *Serenoa repens* on the kinetic of pig prostatic microsomal 5alpha-reductase activity. **Endocrine** 1998; 9(1): 65–69.

SR030   Di Silverio, F., S. Monti, A. Sciarra, et al. Effects of long-term treatment with *Serenoa repens* (Permixon) on the concentrations and regional distribution of androgens and epidermal growth factor in benign prostatic hyperplasia. **Prostate** 1998; 37(2): 77–83.

SR031   Gerber, G. S., G. P. Zagaja, G. T. Bales, G. W. Chodak, and B.A. Contreras. Saw palmetto (*Serenoa repens*) in men with lower urinary tract symptoms: effects on urodynamic parameters and voiding symptoms. **Urology** 1998; 51(6): 1003–1007.

SR032   Paubert-Braquet, M., H. Cousse, J. P. Raynaud, J. M. Mencia-Huerta, and P. Braquet. Effect of the lipidosterolic extract of *Serenoa repens* (Permixon) and its major components on basic fibroblast growth factor-induced proliferation of cultures of human prostate biopsies. **Eur Urol** 1998; 33(3):340–347.

SR033   Paubert-Braquet, M., J. M. Mencia Huerta, H. Cousse, and P. Braquet. Effect of the lipidic lipidosterolic extract of *Serenoa repens* (Permixon) on the ionophore A23187-stimulated production of leukotriene B4 (LTB4) from human polymorphonuclear neutrophils. **Prostaglandins Leukot Essent Fatty Acids** 1997; 57(3): 299–304.

SR034   Shimada, H., V. E. Tyler, and J. L. McLaughlin. Biologically active acylglycerides from the berries of saw-palmetto (*Serenoa repens*). **J Nat Prod** 1997; 60(4): 417–418.

SR035   Chevalier, G., P. Benard, H. Cousse, and T. Bengone. Distribution study of radioactivity in rats after oral administration of the lipido/sterolic extract of *Serenoa repens* (Permixon) supplemented with [1-14C]-lauric acid, [1-14C]-oleic acid or [4-14C]-beta-sitosterol. **Eur J Drug Metab Pharmacokinet** 1997; 22(1): 73–83.

SR036   Ravenna, L., F. Di Silverio, M. A. Russo, et al. Effects of the lipidosterolic

extract of *Serenoa repens* (Permixon) on human prostatic cell lines. **Prostate** 1996; 29(4): 219–230.

SR037   Paubert-Braquet, M., F. O. Richardson, N. Servent-Saez, et al. Effect of *Serenoa repens* extract (Permixon) on estradiol/testosterone-induced experimental prostate enlargement in the rat. **Pharmacol Res** 1996; 34(3–4): 171–179.

SR038   Delos, S., J. L. Carsol, E. Ghazarossian, J. P. Raynaud, and P. M. Martin. Testosterone metabolism in primary cultures of human prostate epithelial cells and fibroblasts. **J Steroid Biochem Mol Biol** 1995; 55(3–4): 375–383.

SR039   Iehle, C., S. Delos, O. Guirou, R. Tate, J. P. Raynaud, and P. M. Martin. Human prostatic steroid 5 alpha-reductase isoforms—a comparative study of selective inhibitors. **J Steroid Biochem Mol Biol** 1995; 54(5–6): 273–279.

SR040   Delos, S., C. Iehle, P. M. Martin, and J. P. Raynaud. Inhibition of the activity of 'basic' 5 alpha-reductase (type 1) detected in DU 145 cells and expressed in insect cells. **J Steroid Biochem Mol Biol** 1994; 48(4): 347–352.

SR041   Strauch, G., P. Perles, G. Vergult, et al. Comparison of finasteride (Proscar) and *Serenoa repens* (Permixon) in the inhibition of 5-alpha reductase in healthy male volunteers. **Eur Urol** 1994; 26(3): 247–252.

SR042   Breu, W., M. Hagenlocher, K. Redl, G. Tittel, F. Stadler, and H. Wagner. Antiinflammatory activity of sabal fruit extracts prepared with supercritical carbon dioxide. *In vitro* antagonists of cyclooxygenase and 5-lipoxygenase metabolism. **Arzneimittelforschung** 1992; 42(4): 547–551.

SR043   Di Silverio, F., G. D'Eramo, C. Lubrano, et al. Evidence that *Serenoa repens* extract displays an antiestrogenic activity in prostatic tissue of benign prostatic hypertrophy patients. **Eur Urol** 1992; 21(4): 309–314.

SR044   el-Sheikh, M. M., M. R. Dakkak, and A. Saddique. The effect of Permixon on androgen receptors. **Acta Obstet Gynecol Scand** 1988; 67(5): 397–399.

SR045   Casarosa, C., M. Cosci di Coscio, and M. Fratta. Lack of effects of a lyposterolic extract of *Serenoa repens* on plasma levels of testosterone, follicle-stimulating hormone, and luteinizing hormone. **Clin Ther** 1988; 10(5): 585–588.

SR046 Sultan, C., A. Terraza, C. Devillier, et al. Inhibition of androgen metabolism and binding by a liposterolic extract of "*Serenoa repens* B" in human foreskin fibroblasts. **J Steroid Biochem** 1984; 20(1): 515–519.

SR047 Carilla, E., M. Briley, F. Fauran, C. Sultan, and C. Duvilliers. Binding of Permixon, a new treatment for prostatic benign hyperplasia, to the cytosolic androgen receptor in the rat prostate. **J Steroid Biochem** 1984; 20(1): 521–523.

SR048 Peng, C. C., P. A. Glassman, L. E. Trilli, J. Hayes-Hunter, and C. B. Good. Incidence and severity of potential drug-dietary supplement interactions in primary care patients: an exploratory study of 2 outpatient practices. **Arch Intern Med** 2004; 164(6): 630–636.

SR049 Wadsworth, T. L., J. M. Carroll, R. A. Mallinson, C. T. Roberts Jr, and C. E. Roselli. Saw palmetto extract suppresses insulin-like growth factor-I signaling and induces stress-activated protein kinase/c-Jun N-terminal kinase phosphorylation in human prostate epithelial cells. **Endocrinology** 2004; 145(7): 3205–3214.

SR050 Kaplan, S. A., M. A. Volpe, and A. E. Te. A prospective, 1-year trial using saw palmetto versus finasteride in the treatment of category III prostatitis/chronic pelvic pain syndrome. **J Urol** 2004; 171(1): 284–288.

SR051 Boon, H., K. Westlake, M. Stewart, et al. Use of complementary/alternative medicine by men diagnosed with prostate cancer: prevalence and characteristics. **Urology** 2003; 62(5): 849–853.

SR052 Veltri, R. W., L. S. Marks, M. C. Miller, et al. Saw palmetto alters nuclear measurements reflecting DNA content in men with symptomatic BPH: evidence for a possible molecular mechanism. **Urology** 2002; 60(4): 617–622.

SR053 Goldmann, W. H., A. L. Sharma, S. J. Currier, P. D. Johnston, D. A. Rana, and C.P. Sharma. Saw palmetto berry extract inhibits cell growth and Cox-2

expression in prostatic cancer cells. **Cell Biol Int** 2001; 25(11): 1117–1124.

SR054 Gerber, G. S., D. Kuznetsov, B. C. Johnson, and J.D. Burstein. Randomized, double-blind, placebo-controlled trial of saw palmetto in men with lower urinary tract symptoms. **Urology** 2001; 58(6): 960–964.

SR055 Brown, G. A., M. D. Vukovich, E. R. Martini, et al. Effects of androstenedione-herbal supplementation on serum sex hormone concentrations in 30- to 59-year-old men. **Int J Vitam Nutr Res** 2001; 71(5): 293–301.

SR056 Brown, G. A., M. D. Vukovich, E. R. Martini, et al. Endocrine and lipid responses to chronic androstenediol-herbal supplementation in 30 to 58 year old men. **J Am Coll Nutr** 2001; 20(5): 520–528.

SR057 Cheema, P., O. El-Mefty, and A. R. Jazieh. Intraoperative haemorrhage associated with the use of extract of Saw Palmetto herb: a case report and review of literature. **J Intern Med** 2001; 250(2): 167–169.

SR058 Marks, L. S., D. L. Hess, F. J. Dorey, M. Luz Macairan, P. B. Cruz Santos, and V. E. Tyler. Tissue effects of saw palmetto and finasteride: use of biopsy cores for in situ quantification of prostatic androgens. **Urology** 2001; 57(5): 999–1005.

SR059 Goepel, M., L. Dinh, A. Mitchell, R. F. Schafers, H. Rubben, and M. C. Michel. Do saw palmetto extracts block human alpha1-adrenoceptor subtypes *in vivo*? **Prostate** 2001; 46(3): 226–232.

SR060 Porterfield, H. UsToo PC-SPES surveys: review of studies and update of previous survey results. **Mol Urol** 2000; 4(3): 289–291.

SR061 de la Taille, A., O. R. Hayek, M. Burchardt, T. Burchardt, and A. E. Katz. Role of herbal compounds (PC-SPES) in hormone-refractory prostate cancer: two case reports. **J Altern Complement Med** 2000; 6(5): 449–451.

SR062 Brown, G. A., M. D. Vukovich, T. A. Reifenrath, et al. Effects of anabolic precursors on serum testosterone concentrations and adaptations to resistance training in young men. **Int J**

Sport Nutr Exerc Metab 2000; 10(3): 340–359.

SR063 Goepel, M., U. Hecker, S. Krege, H. Rubben, and M. C. Michel. Saw palmetto extracts potently and non-competitively inhibit human alpha1-adrenoceptors *in vitro*. **Prostate** 1999; 38(3): 208–215.

SR064 Gutierrez, M., A. Hidalgo, and B. Cantabrana. Spasmolytic activity of a lipidic extract from *Sabal serrulata* fruits: further study of the mechanisms underlying this activity. **Planta Med** 1996; 62(6): 507–511.

SR065 Gutierrez, M., M. J. Garcia de Boto, B. Cantabrana, and A. Hidalgo. Mechanisms involved in the spasmolytic effect of extracts from *Sabal serrulata* fruit on smooth muscle. **Gen Pharmacol** 1996; 27(1): 171–176.

SR066 Wagner, H., A. Proksch, I. Riess-Maurer, et al. Immunostimulant action of polysaccharides (heteroglycans) from higher plants. Preliminary communication. **Arzneimittelforschung** 1984; 34(6): 659–661.

SR067 Wagner, H., A. Proksch, I. Riess-Maurer, et al. Immunostimulating action of polysaccharides (heteroglycans) from higher plants. **Arzneimittelforschung** 1985; 35(7): 1069–1075.

SR068 De Bernardi Di Valserra, M., and A. S. Tripodi. Rectal bioavailability and pharmacokinetics in healthy volunteers of *Serenoa repens* new formulation. **Arch Med Interna (Italy)** 1994; 46(2): 77–86.

SR069 Roveda, S., and P. Colombo. Clinical controlled trial on therapeutical bioequivalence and tolerability of *Serenoa repens* oral capsules 160 mg or rectal capsules 640 mg. **Arch Med Interna (Italy)** 1994; 46(2): 61–75.

SR070 Boccafoschi, C., and Annoscia, S. Comparison of *Serenoa repens* extract with placebo by controlled clinical trial in patients with prostatic adenomatosis. **Urologia** 1983; 50: 1257–1268.

SR071 Emili, E., M. Lo Cigno, and U. Petrone. Clinical trial of a new drug for treating hypertrophy of the prostate (Permixon). **Urologia** 1983; 50: 1042–1048.

SR072 Mattei, F. M., M. Capone, and A. Acconcia. *Serenoa repens* extract in the medical treatment of benign prostatic hypertrophy. **Urologia** 1988; 55: 547–552.

SR073 Niederprüm, H. J., H. U. Schweikert, and K. S. Zänker. Testosterone 5μ-reductase inhibition by free fatty acids from *Sabal serrulata* fruits. **Phytomedicine** 1994; 1: 127–133.

SR074 Wagner, H., and H. Flachsbarth. A new antiphlogistic principle from *Sabal serrulata*. I. **Planta Med** 1981; 41: 244–251.

SR075 Bayne, C. W., F. Donnelly, M. Ross, and F. K. Habib. *Serenoa repens* (Permixon): 5-alpha-reductase types I and II inhibitor-new evidence in a coculture model of BPH. **Prostate** 1999; 40(4): 232–241.

SR076 Champault, G., A. M. Bonnard, J. Cauquil, and J. C. Patel. Medical treatment of the prostatic adenoma. A controlled test of PA 109 vs placebo in 110 patients. **J Ann Urol (Paris)** 1984; 6: 407–410.

SR077 Schoepflin, G., H. Timpler, and R. Hansel. Beta sitosterol as an active principle of sabal fruit. **Planta Med** 1966; 14(4): 403–407.

SR078 Hansel, R., G. Schoepflin, and H. Timpler. The occurrence of anthranilic acid in sabal fruit (*Serenoa repens*). **Planta Med** 1966; 14(3): 261–265.

SR079 Hansel, R., H. Timpler, and G. Schoepflin. Thin-layer chromatography of sabal (saw palmetto) fruit. **Planta Med** 1964; 12(2): 169–172.

SR080 Griebel, C., and E. Bames. A palm fruit employed for imparting aroma to brandy. **Z Nahr-Genussm** 1916; 1916: 282–290.

SR081 Feurt, S. D., and L. E. Fox. A note on the effects of feeding saw palmetto berries, *Serenoa repens* (Bartram) small, to rats. **J Amer Pharm Ass Sci Ed** 1954; 43: 636–638.

SR082 Sultan, C., A. Terraza, E. Carilla, M. Briley, and B. Descomps. Antiandrogenic effects of Permixon: *in vitro* studies. **Acta Urol Ital** 1987; 1(4): 23.

SR083 Ragab, A., J. Ragab, A. Delhon, et al. Effects of Permixon on phospholipase A2 activity and on arachidonic acid metabolism in cultured prostatic cells. **Acta Urol Ital** 1987; 1987 (1): 23–24.

SR084 Rhodes, L., R. L. Primka, C. Berman, et al. Comparison of finasteride (Proscar), a 5-alpha reductase inhibitor, and various commercial plant extracts in *in vitro* and *in vivo* 5-alpha reductase inhibition. **Prostate** 1993; 22: 43–51.

SR085 Odenthal, K. P., and H.W. Rauwald. Lipophilic extract from *Sabal serrulata* inhibits contractions in smooth muscular tissue. **Akt Urol** 1996; 27: 152–158.

SR086 De Bernardi Di Valserra, M., A. S. Tripodi, S. Contos, and R. Germogli. *Serenoa repens* capsules; a bioequivalence study. **Acta Toxicol Ter** 1994; 15(1): 21–39.

SR087 Nemecz, G. Saw palmetto berries of this scrubby palm tree of the southeastern U.S. may be an answer to symptoms associated with an enlarged prostate. **US Pharmacist** 1998; 23(1): 97–102.

SR088 Stenger, A., J. P. Tarayre, E. Carilla, et al. Pharmacologic and biochemical study of an hexane extract of *Serenoa repens* B (PA 109). **Gaz Med France** 1982; 89(17): 2041–2048.

SR089 Koch, E., and W. S. Arzneimitel. Pharmacology and modes of action of extracts of palmetto fruit (*Sabal* fructus), stinging nettle roots (*Urticae* radix) and pumpkin seed (*Cucurbitae peponis* semen) in the treatment of benign prostatic hyperplasia. Phytopharm Forsch Klin Anwend, D. Loew, N. Rietbrock, (eds.), Verlag Dietrich Steinkopf, Darmstadt 1995; 1995: 57–79.

SR090 Ziegler, H., and U. Holscher. Efficacy of saw palmetto fruit special extract WS 1473 in patients with alken stage I-II benign prostatic hyperplasia-open multicentre study. **Jatros Urol** 1998; 14: 34–43.

SR091 Derakhshani, P., H. Geerke, K. J. Bohnert, and U. Engelmann. Beeinflussung des internationalen prostate-symptomen-score unter der therapie mit sagepalmenfruchteextrakt bei taglicher einmalgabe. **Urologe** 1997; 37: 384–391.

SR092 Metzker, H., and U. Holscher. Efficacy of a combined *Sabal-Urtica* preparation in the treatment of benign prostatic hyperplasia (BPH). **Urologe** 1996; 36 B: 292–300.

SR093 Schneider, H. J., E. Honold, and T. Masuhr. Treatment of benign prostatic hyperplasia. Results of a surveillance study in the practices of urological specialists using a combined plant-based preparation (*Sabal* extract WS 1473 and *Urtica* extract WS 1031). **Fortschr Med** 1995; 113(3): 37–40.

SR094 Hamid, S., S. Rojter, and H. Vierling. Protracted cholestatic hepatitis after the use of prostate. **Ann Intern Med** 1997; 127(2): 169–170.

SR095 Schneider, H. J., and A. Uysal. Internationaler prostate-symptomen-score (I-PSS) im klinischen alltag. **Urologe** 1994; 34: 443–447.

SR096 Barr, E. I. A composition for the treatment of androgenic alopecia and hirsutism. Patent-PCT Int Appl-98 33,472 198; 21 pp.

SR097 Hirakoshi, J., K. Ishinabe, K. Yatagai, I. Hanada, and H. Iwaki. Urination promoters containing saw-palmetto extracts and lycopene. Patent-Japan Kokai Tokkyo Koho-10 158,182 1998; 4 pp.

SR098 Marandola, P., H. Jallous, E. Bombardelli, and P. Morazzoni. Main phytoderivaties in the management of benign prostatic hyperplasia. **Fitoterapia** 1997; 68(3): 195–204.

SR099 Bombardelli, E., and P. Morazzoni. *Serenoa repens* (Bartram) J.K. Small. **Fitoterapia** 1997; 68(2): 99–133.

SR100 Salinero, R., A. Miguel, A. Sevilla Toral, et al. Extracts of *Sabal serrulata* as adrenergic antagonists and inflammation inhibitors. Patent-Eur Pat Appl-527,101 1993: 8 pp.

SR101 Niederprum, H. J., H. U. Schweikert, and K. S. Zanker. Testosterone 5-alpha-reductase inhibition by free fatty acids from *Sabal serrulata* fruits. **Phytomedicine** 1994; 1(2): 127–133.

SR102 Hagenlocher, M., G. Romalo, and H. U. Schweikert. Specific inhibition of 5-alpha reductase by a new extract of *Sabal serrulata*. **Akt Urol** 1993; 24: 146–149.

SR103 Briley, M., E. Carilla, and F. Furan. Permixon, a new treatment for benign prostatic hyperplasia, acts directly at the cytosolic androgen receptor in rat prostate. **Br J Pharmacol** 1983; 79: 327.

SR104   De Swaef, S. I., J. O. de Beer, and A. J. Vlietinck. Quantitative determination of P-coumaric acid in *Echinacea purpurea* press juice and urgenin. A validated method. **J Liq Chromatogr** 1994; 17(19): 4169–4183.

SR105   Jommi, G., L. Verotta, and M. J. Magistretti. Alcohols isolated from lipophilic *Serenoa repens* extracts and their use for the treatment of prostate pathologies. Patent-Eur Pat Appl-287,000 1988; 9 pp.

SR106   Weisser, H., S. Tunn, B. Behnke, and M. Krieg. Effects of the *Sabal serrulata* extract IDS 89 and its subfractions on 5alpha-reductase activity in human benign prostatic hyperplasia. **Prostate** 1996; 28(5): 300–306.

SR107   Champault, G., J. C. Patel, and A. M. Bonnard. A double-blind trial of an extract of the plant *Serenoa repens* in benign prostatic hyperplasia. **Br J Clin Pharmacol** 1984; 18: 461–462.

SR108   Lowe, F. C., and J. C. Ku. Phytotherapy in treatment of benign prostatic hyperplasia: a critical review. **Urology** 1996; 48(1): 12–20.

SR109   Odenthal, K. P. Phytotherapy of benign prostatic hyperplasia (BPH) with *Cucurbita, Hypoxis, Pygeum, Urtica* and *Sabal serrulata* (*Serenoa repens*). **Phytother Res** 1996; 10: S141–S143.

SR110   Duker, E. M., and L. Kopanski. Inhibition of 5-alpha-reductase activity by extracts from *Sabal serrulata*. **Planta Med** 1989; 55(6): 587.

SR111   Bach, D. and L. Ebeling. Long-term drug treatment of benign prostatic hyperplasia-results of a prospective, 3-year multicenter study using sabal extract IDS 89. **Phytomedicine** 1996; 3(2): 105–111.

SR112   von Kloss, P. Steam vaporizable constituents of pressed juice of *Sabal serrulata* (Roem et. Schult). **Archneimforsch** 1966; 16(1): 95–96.

SR113   Wajda-Dobos, J. P., M. Farines, J. Soulier, and H. Cousse. Comparative study of the lipid fraction of pulp and seeds of *Serenoa repens* (*Palmaceae*). **Ol Corps Gras Lipides** 1996; 3(2): 136–139.

SR114   Caponera, M., G. D'Eramo, G. P. Flammia, et al. Antiestrogenic activity of *Serenoa repens* in patients with BPH. **Acta Urol Ital** 1992; 1992(4): 271–272.

SR115   Ondrizek, R. R., P. J. Chen, W. C. Patton, and A. King. An alternative medicine study of herbal effects on penetration of zonea-free hamster oocytes and the integrity of sperm deoxyribonucleic acid. **Fertil Steril** 1999; 71(3): 517–522.

SR116   Sawaya, M. E. Novel agents for the treatment of alopecia. **Semin Cutaneous Med Surg** 1998; 17(4): 276–283.

SR117   Cristoni, A., P. Morazzoni, and E. Bombardelli. Chemical and pharmacological study on hypercritical CO_2 extracts of *Serenoa repens*. **Fitoterapia** 1997; 68(4): 355–358.

SR118   Bayne, C. W., E. S. Grant, K. Chapman, and F. K. Habib. Characterization of a new co-culture model for BPH which expresses 5 alpha-reductase types I and II: the effects of Permixon on DHT formation. **J Urol** 1999; 157: 755.

SR119   de la Talle, A., O. R. Hayek, R. Buttyan, E. Bagiella, M. Murchardt, and A. E. Katz. Effects of a phytotherapeutic agent, PC-SPES, on prostate cancer; a preliminary investigation on human cell lines and patients. **BJU Int** 1999; 84(7): 845–850.

SR120   Jommi, G., L. Verotta, P. Gariboldi, and B. Gabetta. Constituents of the lipophilic extract of the fruits of *Serenoa repens* (Bart.) Small. **Gazz Cim Ital** 1988; 118(12): 823–826.

SR121   Hiermann, A. About contents of sabal fruits and their anti-inflammatory effect. **Arch Pharm (Weiheim)** 1989; 322(2): 111–114.

SR122   Hatinguais, P. and R. Belle. Stable, deodorized antiprostatic extract of *Sabal serrulatum*. Patent-Fr Demande-2,480,754 1981; 5 pp.

SR123   Hatinguais, P. H., R. Belle, Y. Basso, J. P. Ribet, M. Bauer, and J. L. Pousset. Composition of the hexane extract from *Serenoa repens* fruit. **Trav Soc Pharm (Montpeiller)** 1981; 41: 253–262.

SR124   Anon. Prostatitis inhibitors from *Sabal serrulatum* fruits. Patent-Japan Kokkai Tokkyo Koho-58 67,625 1983; 3 pp.

SR125 Tarayre, J. P., A. Delhon, H. Lauressergues, et al. Anti-edematous action of a hexane extract from *Serenoa repens* Bartr. Drupes. **Ann Pharm Fr** 1983; 41(6): 559–570.

SR126 Novitch, M., and R. S. Schweiker. Orally administered menstrual drug producs for over-the-counter human use, establishment of a monograph. **Fed Regist** 1982; 47: 55,076–55,101.

SR127 Dragendorff, G. Die heilpflanzen der verschiedenen volker und zeiten, Enke, Stuttgart 1898; 885 pp.

SR128 Anon. The herbalist. Hammond Book Company, Hammond, Indiana 1931; 400 pp.

SR129 Breu, W., M. Hagenlocher, K. Redl, G. Tittel, F. Stadler, and H. Wagner. Antiphlogistic activity of an extract from *Sabal serrulata* fruits prepared by supercritical carbon dioxide/*in vitro* inhibition of the cyclooxygenase and 5-lipoxygenase metabolism. **Arzneimforsch** 1992; 42(4): 547–551.

SR130 de Swaef, S. I., and A. J. Vlietinck. Simultaneous quantification of lauric acid and ethyl laureate in *Sabal serrulata* by capillary gas chromatography and derivatisation with trimethyl sulphoniumhydroxide. **J Chromatogr A** 1996; 719(2): 479–482.

15 | Sesamum indicum
L.

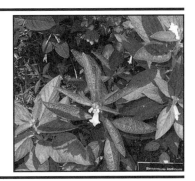

Common Names

Acchellu	India	Sesam	Germany
Ajonjoli	Spain	Sesam	Spain
Ashadital	India	Sesam	Sweden
Bariktil	India	Sesame	France
Bijan	Malaysia	Sesame	United Kingdom
Chaam-kkae	Korea	Sesame	United States
Cycam	Bulgaria	Sesamfre	Iceland
Dee la	Thailand	Sesami	Greece
Ellu	India	Sesamkruid	Netherlands
Gergelim	Brazil	Sesamo	Italy
Gingelly	United Kingdom	Sesamo	Portugal
Goma	Japan	Sesamo	Spain
Harilik seesam	Estonia	Sesamzaad	Netherlands
Hei chih ma	China	Sezam indicky	Slovakia
Karuthellu	India	Sezam	Croatia
Khasa	India	Sezam	Czech Republic
Kkae	Korea	Sezam	Poland
Koba	Japan	Sezam	Russia
Konjed	Iran	Sezam	Ukraine
Kunzhut	Russia	Sezama seklas	Latvia
Kunzuut	Estonia	Sezama	Slovenia
Linga	Philippines	Sezamas	Lithuania
Man nga	Laos	Sezamo	Spain
Mittho-tel	India	Shooshma	Armenia
Moa	China	Shooshmayi good	Armenia
Mua chi	China	Shumshum	Israel
Nga	Laos	Sim-sim	Arabic countries
Ngaa	Thailand	Sim-sim	Netherlands
Nuvvulu	India	Suom	Finland
Rasi	India	Susam	Albania
Sasim	Arabic countries	Susam	Bulgaria
Seesami	Finland	Susam	Turkey
Semsem	United Kingdom	Susan	Romenia
Sesam	Denmark	Sven	Sweden

From: *Medicinal Plants of the World, vol. 3: Chemical Constituents, Traditional and Modern Medicinal Uses*
By: I. A. Ross © Humana Press Inc., Totowa, NJ

Szezam	Hungary	Tisi	India
Szezammag	Hungary	Ufuta	Mozambique
Szezammag	Israel	Ufuta	Tanzania
Tal	India	Vanglo	Germany
Teel	France	Vung	Vietnam
Til	India	Wijen	Indonesia
Til	Pakistan	Yallu	India
Tila	India	Zelzlane	Arabic countries
Till	France	Zi ma zi	China

BOTANICAL DESCRIPTION

Sesame is an erect annual (or occasionally, a perennial) of the PEDALIACEAE family that grows to a height of 0.5–1.5 m, depending on the variety and the growing conditions. Some varieties are highly branched, whereas others are unbranched. Leaves, 7.5–12.5 cm, simple or, when variable, with upper ones narrowly oblong, middle ones ovate and toothed and the lower ones lobate or pedatisect. Flowers are white, pink, or mauve-pink with dark markings, borne in racemes in the leak axils. The fruit is capsular, oblong-quadrangular, slightly compressed, deeply four grooved, 1.5–5 cm long. Seeds are black, brown, or white, 2.5–3 mm long and approx 1.5 mm wide. In general, the unbranched varieties mature earlier. At maturity, leaves and stems tend to change from green to yellow to red. The leaves will begin to fall off the plants. The bell-shaped white to pale-rose flowers begin to develop in the leaf axils 6–8 weeks after planting, and this continues for several weeks. Multiple flowering is favored by opposite leaves. Initiation of flowering is sensitive to photoperiod and varies among varieties. Sesame is normally self-pollinated, although cross-pollination by insects is common. The fruit contains 50–100 or more seeds. The seeds mature 4–6 weeks after fertilization. The growth of sesame is indeterminant; that is, the plant continues to produce leaves, flowers, and capsules as long as the weather permits. The lighter colored seeds are considered higher quality. There is great diversity within the several hundred varieties of sesame. However, the sesame varieties are usually divided into two types: shattering and nonshattering. On ripening, sesame capsules split, releasing the seed (hence the phrase, "open sesame"). Because of this shattering characteristic, sesame has been grown primarily on small plots that are harvested by hand. The discovery of an indehiscent (nonshattering) mutant by Langham in 1943 began the work toward development of a high-yielding, shatter-resistant variety. Although researchers have made significant progress in sesame breeding, harvest losses resulting from shattering continue to limit domestic production.

ORIGIN AND DISTRIBUTION

Sesamum indicum L. is one of the oldest cultivated plants in the world. It was a highly prized oil crop of Babylon and Assyria at least 4000 years ago. Today, India and China are the world's largest producers of sesame, followed by Myanmar, Sudan, Mexico, Nigeria, Venezuela, Turkey, Uganda, and Ethiopia.

TRADITIONAL MEDICINAL USES

Arabic countries. Dried seeds are used externally in the form of a plaster as a contraceptive in Unani medicine. The seed oil is applied on the glans penis before coitus to prevent conception[SI111].

China. Hot water extract of seed is taken orally for impotence[SI028]. Seed oil is taken orally for tuberculosis[SI035].

Cuba. Seed oil is taken orally as a galacto-gogue[SI138].

Europe. Seed oil taken orally is used as an emmenagogue[SI025].

Haiti. Decoction of dried seeds is taken orally for asthma[SI122].

India. The seed oil is taken orally as a purgative[SI139]. A mixture of dried fruits of *Sesamum indicum, Clerodendrum indicum, Moringa pterygosperma,* and *Piper nigrum* is mixed with crude sugar and taken orally for 20 days to produce sterility[SI103]. Leaves are ground with jaggary and taken orally with coconut milk to treat rabies[SI062]. Infusion of the leaf is taken once a day for controlling diabetes[SI069]. Decoction of 25–30 dried leaves is given once a day for 6 months to control diabetes[SI093]. Extract of the seed is taken orally as an abortifacient and an emmenagogue[SI029]. Hot water extract of the seed is taken orally as an emmena-gogue[SI036,SI136] and an abortive[SI136]. Hot water extract of the dried seed is taken orally as an abortifacient[SI123], an emmenagogue[SI123], a tonic, a diuretic, and an aphrodisiac; to promote hair growth; for ulcers, piles, eye diseases, and biliousness; and as a galacto-gogue[SI126]. Dried seeds when taken orally have an abortifacient effect in an over-dose[SI107]. Olive oil extract of *Terminalia arjuna, Aglaia roxburghiana, Jasminum officinalis, Indigofera tinctoria, Tinspora cordifolia, Pterocarpus marsupium, Eclipta alba, Pandanus tectorius, Oroxylum indicum, Valeriana hardwickii, Terminalia chebula, Termianlia bellerica, Emblica officinalis, Punica granatum, Nelumbium speciosum,* and *Sesamum indicum* is used externally to prevent premature graying of hair[SI127]. Paste of *Bridelia scandens* prepared in *Sesamum indicum* oil is applied externally for wounds caused by dog bites[SI115]. Fresh seed oil is used for eye diseases. A decoction of the leaf of *Gymnema silvestre* is heated with sesame seed oil until an emulsion is formed and then used as a drop for the eyes several times a day[SI113].

Iran. Oil of dried seeds is taken orally for its laxative effect[SI045].

Ivory Coast. The juice of new leaves is drunk to expel placenta[SI034].

Jordan. Seed oil is taken orally to induce lactation and as an antitussive[SI075].

Malaysia. Hot water extract of seeds is taken orally as an emmenagogue and in a large dose as an abortifacient[SI038]. Seed oil is taken orally as an emmenagogue and used by males as a tonic for sexual neurasthenia[SI032].

Mexico. Seeds, ground and mixed with masa, are eaten for increasing milk flow in nursing mothers[SI031].

Morocco. Seeds are eaten as a hypnotic and stimulant and taken by females as a stimulant for lactation[SI077].

Mozambique. Juice of the entire plant is taken orally as an aphrodisiac[SI079]. Hot water extract of the seed is taken orally as emmenagogue and abortifacient[SI079].

Nepal. Seed oil smeared around umbilicus and 3–5 mL placed inside the ostium is used as an abortifacient[SI070].

Pakistan. Seeds are taken orally as an emmenagogue[SI026].

Peru. Hot water extract of the dried bark is taken orally for dislocations, chest pains, and contusions[SI125].

Saudi Arabia. Hot water extract of dried plant was used as a contraceptive in the 13th century[SI137].

South Africa. Hot water extract of aerial parts is taken orally by the Bantu as an aphrodisiac[SI036]. Hot water extract of leaves is taken orally by the Transvaal Sotho as a remedy for malaria[SI036].

South Korea. Hot water extract of seed is taken orally to induce menstruation[SI130]. Hot water extract of dried seed is taken orally as an abortifacient and emmenagogue[SI119].

United States. Dried seeds are eaten as an emmenagogue[SI110]. Hot water extract of the seed oil is taken orally to promote menstruation[SI037].

Vietnam. The seed oil is taken orally as an emmenagogue[SI033].

CHEMICAL CONSTITUENTS

(ppm unless otherwise indicated)

Amyrin,α: Sd oil[SI061]

Amyrin, β: Sd oil[SI061]

Anthraquinone, 2-(4-methyl-pent-3-enyl): Hairy Rt Cult 29[SI042]

Anthraquinone, 2-(4-methyl-penta-1-3-dienyl): Hairy Rt Cult 18[SI042]

Arachidonic acid: Sd oil <1%[SI067]

Arginine: Sd cake 3.9%[SI040]

Asarinin, (+): Sd oil[SI112]

Avenasterol, 5-dehydro: Sd oil[SI061]

Avenasterol, 7-dehydro: Sd oil[SI061]

Behenic acid: Sd oil <0.5%[SI067]

Bicyclo(3.3.0)-octane, 3-7-dioxa, 2-(3-4-methylenedioxy-phenyl)-6-(4-hydroxy-3-methoxy-phenyl): Sd[SI059]

Caffeic acid: Lf, Fr[SI132]

Campesterol: Sd oil[SI061]

Campneoside I: Pl 330.9[SI044]

Campneoside II: Pl 49.5[SI044]

Cholesterol: Sd oil[SI061]

Cistanoside F: Pl 217.1[SI044]

Citrostadienol: Sd oil[SI061]

Coumaric acid, ortho: Lf, Fr[SI132]

Coumaric acid, para: Lf, Fr[SI132]

Cycloartanol, 24-methylene: Sd oil[SI061]

Cycloartenol, 24-methylene: Sd oil[SI067]

Cycloartenol: Sd oil[SI061]

Cycloeucalenol: Sd oil[SI061]

Diacetyl: Sd oil[SI067]

Esculentic acid: Call Tiss[SI072], Pl[SI052]

Fatty acids: Sd oil[SI153]

Ferulic acid, *trans*: Sd 5.4–40[SI151,SI120]

Ferulic acid: Lf, Fr[SI132]

Fucosterol, iso: Sd oil[SI067]

Gadoleic acid: Sd oil <0.5%[SI067]

Gentisic acid: Lf[SI132]

Globulin, α: Sd[SI089]

Glyoxal, methyl: Sd oil[SI067]

Glyoxal: Sd oil[SI067]

Gramisterol: Sd oil[SI061]

Kobusin, (+): Sd 1.1[SI151]

Linoleic acid: Sd oil[SI050]

Linolenic acid, α: Sd oil[SI086]

Linolenic acid, γ: Sd oil[SI086]

Linolenic acid: Sd oil <1%[SI067]

Myristic acid: Sd oil[SI067]

Naphthazarin-2-3-epoxide, 2-iso-propenyl: Hairy Rt Cult 550[SI042]

Nepetin: Lf[SI141]

Obtusifoliol: Sd oil[SI061]

Oleic acid: Sd oil[SI050]

Oxalic acid: Sd[SI063]

Palmitic acid: Sd oil[SI050]

Palmitoleic acid: Sd oil <0.5%[SI067]

Pedaliin: Lf 0.3%[SI142]

Pinoresinol 4'-O-β-D-glucopyranosyl (1-2)-β-D-glucopyranoside: Sd 42[SI152]

Pinoresinol 4'-O-β-D-glucopyranosyl (1-6)-β-D-glucopyranoside: Sd 20.6[SI152]

Pinoresinol glycoside: Sd[SI078]

Pinoresinol, (+): Sd 17.9[SI078]

Pinoresinol: Sd 162.5[SI043]

Pinoresinol-4'-O-β-D-glucopyranosyl (1-2)-O-(β-D-glucopyranosyl (1-6))-β-D-glucopyranoside, (+): Sd 52.2[SI156]

Piperitol, (+): Sd 1.5[SI151]

Planteose: Sd[SI104]

Protecatechuic acid: Lf, Fr[SI132]

Protein: Lf[SI102], Sd 29.5%[SI132]

Sesamin analog: Sd 16[SI120], Sd oil 0.17%[SI128], Call Tiss 4807.6[SI051], Rt[SI131], Pod[SI151]

Sesamin, (+): Call Tiss 4903.8[SI059]

Sesamin, epi, (+): Sd 1.5[SI151]

Sesamin, epi: Sd[SI097]

Sesamin: Pl[SI047], Sd oil[SI096], Sd[SI097]

Sesaminol diglucoside: Pl[SI047]

Sesaminol, epi: Sd[SI097]

Sesaminol: Sd[SI053]

Sesaminol-2'-O-β-D-glucopyranoside: Sd 111.2[SI043]

Sesaminol-2'-O-β-D-glucopyranosyl(1-2)-O-[β-D-glucopyranosyl(1-6)]-β-D-glucopyranoside: Sd 237.5[SI043]

Sesaminol-2'-O-β-D-glucopyranosyl(1-2)-O-β-D-glucopyranoside: Sd 1422.5[SI043]

Sesaminone, epi, (+): Pod, Sd 0.78[SI151]

Sesamol: Sd oil[SI108]

Sesamolin: Sd[SI068], Pl[SI047], St[SI131]

Sesamolin analog: Sd 48[SI120]

Sesamolin, (+): Call Tiss 1.01[SI051], Pod, Sd 217.9[SI151]

Sesamolinol: Sd[SI041]

Sesamolinol, (+): 1.9[SI151]

Sesamum compound 10: Pl 59.2[SI044]

Sesamum compound 11: Pl 76.4[SI044]

Sesamum compound 7: Pl 21.1[SI044]

Sesamum compound 8: Pl 23[SI044]

Sesamum compound 9: Pl 26.4[SI044]

Simplexoside aglycone: Sd 16-86.2[SI120,SI043]

Sitosterol, β: Sd oil[SI112]

SOP-1: Sd oil[SI153]

SOP-2: Sd oil[SI153]
SOP-3: Sd oil[SI153]
Squalene: Sd oil[SI144]
Stearic acid: Sd oil[SI086]
Stigmast-7-en-3-β-ol: Sd oil[SI061]
Stigmasterol: Sd oil[SI061]
Sucrose: Sd[SI104]
Tannic acid: Sd[SI063]
Tocopherol, α: Sd oil[SI039]
Tocopherol, β: Sd oil[SI067]
Tocopherol, δ: Sd oil[SI067]
Tocopherol, γ: Sd oil 60-70[SI117]
Urs-12-en-28-oic acid, 3-β-(cis-para-
coumaroyl-oxy)-2-α-23-dihydroxy: Pl[SI052]
Urs-12-en-28-oic acid, 3-β-(trans-para-
coumaroyl-oxy)-2-α-23-dihydroxy: Pl[SI052],
Call Tiss[SI072]
Vanillic acid: Lf[SI132]
Verbascoside: Call Tiss[SI074], Pl 388.09[SI044]
Verbascoside, decaffeoyl: Pl 201.4[SI044]

PHARMACOLOGICAL ACTIVITIES AND CLINICAL TRIALS

Abortifacient effect. Ethanol (50 and 100%) extracts of the dried seed, administered intragastrically to pregnant rats at a dose of 200 mg/kg, was inactive[SI087,SI135]. Acetone extract of the dried seed, on agar plate at a concentration of 0.2 g/plate, was active on *Salmonella typhimurium* TA98 and TA100 vs aflatoxin B1-induced mutagenesis, *Aspergillus ochraceous* extract-induced mutagenesis, and *Aspergillus versicolor* extract-induced mutagenesis[SI101].

Acyl-coenzyme A inhibition. Cholesterol acyl-transferase inhibitor CP-105,191 dissolved in sesame oil was investigated in fed and fasted dogs. Systemic availability of CP-105,191 area-under-the-curve (AUC) was three- to fourfold higher in fed dogs than in fasted dogs when 50-mg doses were administered as aqueous suspension. When CP-105,191 was partially dissolved in 20 mL sesame oil, the availability of CP-105,191 was increased by a factor of 2. Plasma AUCs were similar for fed and fasted dogs after the 12.5-mg dose completely dissolved in sesame oil, indicating that the increased availability of drug when administered with food is related to the presence of lipid[SI019].

Allergenic activity. Seed oil, applied externally on adults at various concentrations, was active[SI143]. Oral administration to female adults at a dose of 10 g/person produced strong activity[SI048]. The seeds, administered by inhalation to male adults, induced allergic reaction. One adult developed occupational hypersensitivity to sesame seeds. This was confirmed by skin prick test[SI082]. Inhalation of seeds by adults induced asthma, rhinitis, and urticaria[SI066]. The seeds, administered orally to male adults at a dose of 2 mg/day, induced allergic reaction. The seed produced generalized urticaria in a male adult[SI080]. The seed, administered orally to female adults at a dose of 10 g/person, induced anaphylaxis[SI048]. In 9070 investigated infants and young children (0–2 years old), the overall prevalence of clinically relevant immunoglobulin (Ig) E-mediated reactions among these patients was estimated at 1.2% (104/9070). Anaphylaxis was the presenting symptom in 6/78 (7.7%) cases[SI005]. Seed oil, applied externally to adults, was inactive. It was applied to skin, hair, nails, eyes, and mucous membranes without irritation[SI067]. Seed oil applied as patch test to adults produced dermatitis[SI096]. Seeds, administered orally to female adults, induced sesame seed anaphylaxis[SI048]. The seed ingested by adults produced a severe allergic reactions in sensitized individuals[SI065].

α-Tocopherol effect. The seed, administered in the ration of male rats at a dose of 20% of low α-tocopherol diet for 8 weeks, produced an increase of α-tocopherol in the blood and tissue. Results were significant at $p < 0.01$[SI046].

Anaphylactic response. Seed oil, administered periodontally to adults, was effective. A 46-year-old male developed recurrent reaction to sesame seed oil. The symptoms were chills, shakiness, cramps, vomiting, fecal incontinence, fainting, flushing, and pruritic welts. Skin test revealed a four-plus multitest response and a marginally positive rast. Significant histamine release was also noted[SI058]. Seeds, administered orally to female adults, induced anaphylaxis[SI048]. The seed, administered orally to female adults, induced anaphylaxis. In a double-blind, placebo-controlled case study of a patient with celiac challenged with sesame seeds, it was indicated that sesame can induce non-IgE-mediated anaphylaxis[SI084]. Ten allergic patients had positive IgE antibodies and skin-prick test to food-containing sesame[SI002]. Four patients with anaphylaxis, angioedema, or urticaria after ingestion of sesame seed or sesame oil-containing products were studied for anti-sesame seed extract IgE by the radioallergosorbent test. Three of four were be positive[SI023].

Antibacterial activity. Ethanol extract of the shade-dried seed, on agar plate at a concentration of 2.5 mg/disc, was inactive on *Escherichia coli*, *Proteus mirabilis*, *Pseudomonas aeruginosa*, *Staphylococcus aureus*, and *Staphylococcus epidermidis*[SI088]. Seed oil, on agar plate at an undiluted dose, was inactive on *Bacillus subtilis*, *Escherichia coli*, *Salmonella typhosa*, *Staphylococcus aureus*, and *Vibrio cholerae*[SI129]. The seeds, on agar plate, were active on *Bacillus subtilis*, *Escherichia coli*, *Pseudomonas cichorii*, and *Salmonella typhimurium*[SI083]. Pretreatment of mice with sesame extract significantly reduced the lethality of bacterial infection, possibly because of its host-mediated action. No apparent acute toxicity was detected in mice by oral administration of 10 g/kg of the extract[SI009].

Anticrustacean activity. Methylene chloride extracts of the dried leaf and root, at a concentration of 500 ppm, were inactive on *Artemia salina*. The assay system was intended to predict for antitumor activity. Methanol extract of the dried root, at a concentration of 500 ppm, was inactive on *Artemia salina*[SI071]. Ethanol extract of the shade-dried seed was inactive on *Artemia salina*[SI088].

Antifungal activity. Seed oil on agar plate was inactive on *Aspergillus niger*[SI129]. Methyl-

ene chloride extract of the dried leaf, on agar plate at a concentration of 100 μg/plate, was inactive on *Cladosporium cucumerinum*. Methanol and methylene chloride extracts of the dried root, at a concentration of 100.0 μg/plate, were active on *Cladosporium cucumerinum*[SI071]. Seed oil, on agar plate at an undiluted dose, was inactive on *Trichophyton mentagrophytes* and *Trichophyton rubrum*[SI129].

Antihemolytic activity. The seed, administered in the ration of male rats at a dose of 5% of diet, was active on red blood cells (RBCs) vs low α-tocopherol diet. Results were significant at $p < 0.01$[SI046].

Antihypercholesterolemic activity. Seed oil, administered by gastric intubation to rabbits at a dose of 1 g/kg, was active[SI149].

Antihypertensive effect. Sesame oil lignan sesamin, in two-kidney, one-clip (2K,1C) renal hypertensive rats fed a sesamin-containing (1% w/w) diet, was investigated. The hypertension was markedly reduced, but the sesame diet ameliorated the vascular hypotrophy. Results indicated that sesamin is useful as prophylactic treatment to combat the development of renal hypertension and cardiac hypertrophy[SI017].

Anti-implantation effect. Ethanol extract of the dried seed, administered intragastrically to female rats at a dose of 200 mg/kg, was inactive vs early pregnancy[SI087].

Anti-inflammatory effect. Sesame oil, present in the injectable gold preparation "Auromyose," was administered at a dose of 18 g/daily for 12 weeks to 11 healthy male volunteers. Tumor necrosis factor (TNF)-α, prostaglandin (PG)-E2, and leukotriene production levels did not indicate any statistically significant changes. This result did not suggest antiinflammatory effect of sesame oil as present in injectable gold preparations used in the treatment of rheumatoid arthritis[SI013].

Anti-irradiation effect. Methanol extract of the dried seed, administered intraperitoneally to mice at a dose of 1 g/kg, was inactive vs soft X-ray irradiation at lethal dose[SI154].

Antimutagenic activity. Ethanol (70%) extract of the dried aerial parts, on agar plate, was inactive on *Escherichia coli* PQ37 vs mitomycin-induced mutagenesis, assessed by the SOS-chromotest method[SI095].

Antioxidant activity. Hexane and methanol extracts of the dried seed, tested on lard at a concentration of 0.06 %, were inactive[SI116]. Seed oil, at undiluted concentration, was active[SI117]. Acetone extract of the seed, at a concentration of 0.2 mg/kg, was active. Linoleic acid was used as a substrate in this test[SI120].

Antitoxic effect. Sesame oil, adiministered to male Wistar rats, ameliorated hepatic and renal damage in a dose-dependent manner and increased survival in lipopolysaccharide-treated rats. It decreased lipid peroxide concentration in serum but not in liver and kidney. Serum nitrite production was unaffected by sesame oil ingestion, and the activity of xanthine oxidase was reduced in the lipopolysaccharide-challenged rats[SI004].

Anti-tumor activity. Water extract of the dried seed, administered intragastrically to mice at a dose of 50 mg/animal daily for 5 days, was active on CA-Ehrlich-ascites, 18% increase in life-span. Intraperitoneal administration was active on Dalton's lyphoma and CA-Ehrlich-ascites, 19 and 39% increase in life-span, respectively[SI094]. Seed oil, administered to rats intraperitoneally with 1,2,5,6-dibenzanthracene or retene, was active on sarcoma[SI150].

Antiviral activity. Ethanol (80%) extract of the dried leaf, in cell culture at a concentration of 0.2 mL/well, was equivocal on poliovirus; inactive on herpes virus, measles, and Semliki Forest virus and produced weak activity on coxsackie virus[SI076]. Pretreatment of mice with sesame extract failed to reduce the cytophatic effect of human immunodeficiency virus 1 (HIV-1) infection in MT-4 cells. No apparent acute toxicity was detected in mice with oral administration of 10 g/kg of the extract[SI009].

Anti-yeast activity. Ethanol extract of the shade-dried seed, on agar plate at a concentration of 2.5 mg/disc, was inactive on *Candida albicans*[SI088]. Undiluted seed oil on agar plate was inactive on *Candida albicans* and *Saccharomyces cerevisiae*[SI129].

Apoptosis induction. The exposure of human lymphoid leukemia Molt 4B cells to sesamolin, a component of sesame seed, produced growth inhibition and the induction of apoptosis[SI010].

Carcinogenic activity. Seed oil, in the ration of rats at a dose of 2% of diet, was active on squamous cell carcinoma of the fore stomach. Seed oil, administered intraperitoneally to mice at a dose of 0.5 mL/animal, was inactive. Pulmonary adenomas in offsprings did not occur with increased incidence. Seed oil, administered subcutaneously to mice at a dose of 0.2 mL/kg dosed daily, was inactive. Increased incidence of mammary adenocarcinoma was observed[SI067].

Cholesterol level and metabolism. Sesame oil, administered to male Wistar rats in the diet at concentrations of 12 or 24% for 4 weeks, produced significantly lower liver cholesterol and liver lipid levels, serum total cholesterol, and low-density lipoprotein (LDL) cholesterol in rats fed the 24% diet. The high degree of unsaturation (85%) of sesame oil and the presence of linoleic acid could be an important factor[SI016]. Sesamin, administered to rats in the diet at a concentration of 0.5% sesame oil for 4 weeks, reduced the concentration of serum and liver cholesterol significantly, irrespective of the presence or absence of cholesterol in the diet. Sesamin inhibited micellar solubility of cholesterol but not bile acids. It did not bound taurocholate nor affected the absorption of fatty acids. Only a marginal proportion (ca 0.15%) of sesamin administered intragastrically was recovered in the lymph. There was significant reduction in the activity of liver microsomal 3-hydroxy-3-methylglutaryl coenzyme A (HMG-CoA) reductase, but the activity of hepatic cholesterol 7 α-hydroxylase and alcohol dehydrogenase remained unaffected[SI021].

Chromotropic effect negative. Methanol (70%) extract of the seed, administered to guinea pigs at a concentration of 100 μg/mL, was active on the atrium. The extract, administered intravenously to rats at dose of 10 mg/kg, produced atropine abolished effect[SI057].

Corticosteroid type activity. Seed oil, administered parenterally to pregnant rats, was active. The survival time of adrenalectomized pregnant rats and their subsequent litters was increased[SI148].

Cytotoxic activity. Ethanol (90%) extract of the dried entire plant, in cell culture at a concentration of 0.25 mg/mL, was active on human lymphocytes; Vero cells, effective dose $(ED)_{50}$ 0.36 mg/mL; Chinese hamster ovary cells, ED_{50} 0.44 mg/mL; and Dalton's lyphoma, ED_{50} 1.2 mg/mL[SI091]. Methylene chloride extract of the dried leaf, in cell culture, produced weak activity on CA-colon-SW 480, inhibitory concentration $(IC)_{50}$ 6.1 μg/mL. A concentration of 500 ppm was inactive on CA-human-colon-CO-115[SI071]. Methylene chloride extract of the dried root, in cell culture at a concentration of 500 ppm, was inactive on CA-human-colon-CO-115 and active on CA-colon-SW 480, IC_{50} 3.6 μg/mL. Methanol extract of the dried root, in cell culture at a concentration of 500 ppm, was inactive on CA-colon-SW 480 and CA-human-colon-CO-115[SI071]. Ethanol (50%) extract of the seed, in cell culture, was inactive on CA-9KB, ED_{50} greater than 20 μg/mL[SI027]. Water extract of the dried seed, in cell culture at a concentration of 500.0 μg/mL, produced weak activity on CA-mammary-microalveolar[SI098]. Water extract of the dried seed, in cell culture at a concentration of 500 μg/mL, was inactive on CA-JTC-26[SI054]. Seed oil, in cell culture at concentrations of 0.01% and 0.1%, was inactive on the rat fibroblasts. A concentration of 1% produced weak activity[SI140]. Seed oil, in cell culture at

a concentration of 100.0 μg/mL, was active on CA-colon-CACO-2, CA-human-colon-CO-115, and human colon cancer cell line HT29[SI100]. Seed oil, in cell culture at a concentration of 300 μg/mL, was inactive on melanoma-NHEM and melanoma-SK-MEL-2[SI055]. Water extract of the dried seed was active on Leuk-P815. Tumor-toxic activity was evaluated by culturing mastocytoma P815 cells with macrophage cells and measured the incorporation of ^{3}H-thimidine radioactivity[SI099]. Ethanol (100%) extract of the shade dried seed, in cell culture at various concentrations, was inactive on CA-A549, CA-mammary-MCF-7, and human colon cancer cell line DLD-1[SI088].

Dermatitis improvement. Seed oil, applied externally twice daily for 2 years to 35 adults with dermatitic lesions, was acitve. The effect was seen only with polymerized oil[SI067].

DNA synthesis inhibition. Ethanol (90%) extract of the dried entire plant, at a concentration of 0.25 mg/mL, was active[SI091].

Early antigen viral induction stimulation. Ether extract of the seed, in cell culture at concentration of 0.1 mg/mL, was inactive on lymphoma-RAJ1[SI105].

Embryotoxic effect. Benzene and petroleum ether extracts of the dried seed, administered by gastric intubation to pregnant rats at a dose of 150 mg/kg, were inactive[SI109]. Ethanol (50%) extract of the seed, administered orally to female rats at a dose of 200 mg/kg, was inactive[SI135].

Estrogenic effect. Seed oil, applied subcutaneously to ovariectomized mice, was inactive[SI134]. The plant, administered orally to immature female rats at a dose of 2 g/kg, was active[SI090].

Fatty acid oxidation. Seeds, administered orally to rats at a dose of 200 g/kg, increased hepatic mitochondrial and the peroxisomal fatty acid oxidation rate[SI003].

Glucosidase inhibition. Ethyl acetate and water soluble fractions of the seed were inactive on the intestine[SI085].

Glutamate–oxaloacetate–transaminase inhibition. Seed oil, administered to mice at a concentration of 0.6% of diet, was active. Biological activity reported has been patented[SI064].

Glutamate–pyruvate–transaminase inhibition. The seed and seed oil, administered to mice at a concentration of 0.6% of diet, were active. Biological activity reported has been patented[SI064].

Generally recognized as safe status. Approved by the US Food and Drug Administration in 1996 (sect. 582.10) as a flavoring agent[SI155].

Hair-stimulant effect. Ethanol (50%) extract of the dried seed, applied externally to mice at a dose of 0.33 g/mL for 10 days, was active[SI092].

Hemotoxic activity. Seed oil, adiministered orally to human adults, produced thrombocytosis in children. the effect was inactivated by ultraviolet radiation[SI146].

Hypercholesterolemic activity. Seed oil, administered by gastric intubation to rabbits at a dose of 0.4 g/kg, was inactive[SI149]. Male Wistar rats fed 12 or 24% sesame oil in the diet for 4 weeks were investigated. The rats on the 24% sesame oil diet had significantly lower lymphatic cholesterol and fatty acids[SI020].

Hyperglycemic activity. Extract of the dried entire plant, administered to rats at a dose 30% of diet, was active[SI121]. Seed oil, adiministered orally to adults at a dose of 60 g/person, produced weak activity[SI147]. Hot water extract (4%) or methanol eluent fraction (0.7%) of the defatted seed, administered orally to genetically diabetic 5 weeks old male KK-Ay-mice, had a reductive effect on the plasma glucose concentration. The effect is suggested to be casused by the delayed glucose absorption[SI001].

Hyperlipidemic activity. Seed oil, adiministered orally to adults at a dose of 60 g/person, was active[SI147]. Seed oil, administered by gastric intubation to rabbits at a dose of 0.4 g/kg, was active[SI149].

Hypocholesterolemic activity. Extract of the dried entire plant, administered to rats at a dose of 30% of diet, was active[SI121]. Lignan fraction of the seed, administered in the ration of 4-week-old rats at a dose of 0.2% of the diet for 3 weeks, was active. Dietary fat sources were safflower and primrose oils[SI097].

Hypoglyceridemic activity. Lignan fraction of the seed, administered to 4-week-old rats at a dose of 0.2% of diet for 3 weeks, was active. Dietary fat sources were safflower and primrose oils[SI097].

Hypophospholipidemic activity. Lignan fraction of the seed administered to 4-week-old rats at a dose of 0.2% of diet for 3 weeks, was active. Dietary fat sources were safflower and primrose oils[SI097].

Hypotensive effect. Methanol (70%) extract of the seed, administered intravenously to rats at dose of 3 mg/kg, was active. The effect was inhibited by pretreatment with atropine[SI057].

Immunoglobulin level. The effect of sesaminol and sesamin on the ethanol-induced immune indices were examined in rats given a low (10%)-casein diet. Sesaminol decreased splenic leukotriene B4 production, whereas sesamin increased the plasma PGE2 concentration. A significant IgG-elevating effect of these lignans was observed. The concentration of plasma IgE was not influenced[SI015].

Inflammation induction. Seed oil, applied externally as a patch test to human adults at a dose of 0.032 mL/person, was inactive[SI147].

Inotropic effect negatve. Methanol (70%) extract of the seed, administered to guinea pigs at dose of 100 μg/mL, was active on the atrium. The effect was abolished by atropine[SI057].

Insecticide activity. Seed oil, applied externally on cattle at a concentration of 0.7%, was active. It was used as a delousing agent[SI067].

Interleukin induction. Water extract of the dried seed produced weak activity.

Interleukin (IL)-1 activity was measured by the IL-1 dependent growth of a T-helper cell line[SI099].

Larvicidal activity. Methylene chloride extract of the dried leaf, at a concentration of 500 ppm, was inactive on *Aedes aegypti*. Methylene chloride extract of the dried root was active on *Aedes aegypti*, lethal concentration (LC)$_{100}$ 12.5 μg/mL. The methanol extract was inactive[SI071].

Lipid metabolism effect. Lignan fraction of the seed, administered to 4-week-old rats at a dose of 0.2% of diet for 3 weeks, was active. Dietary fat source, were evening primrose and safflower oils. Proportion of dihomo-γ-linolenate increased in response to reduction of δ-5-desaturase activity and the proportion of docosapentaenoate decreased in liver phosphatidylcholine. Liver phospholipid level decreased vs control. Lignan fraction of the seed administered to 4-week-old rats at a dose of 0.2% of diet for 3 weeks, was active. The dietary fat source was evening primrose and safflower oils. Liver phospholipid level decreased vs control. With the dietary fat source evening primrose oil, fecal excretion of neutral steroids increased and microbial transformation of cholesterol to coprostanol decreased. The specific activity of liver microsomal δ-5 and δ-6 desaturases were decreased and increased, respectively. Lignan fraction of the seed, administered to 4-week-old rats at a dose of 0.2% of diet for 3 weeks, was inactive. The production of thromboxane A2 (TXA-2) by platelets and PGI-2 by the aorta was not influenced whether dietary fat was evening primrose oil or safflower oil[SI097].

Lipid peroxide formation inhibition. The seed, administered to male rats at a dose of 5% of diet, was active in liver vs low-alpha-tocopherol diet. Results were significant at $p < 0.01$ level[SI046].

Metabolism. Seed oil, administered intraperitoneally to mice at a dose of 160 mg/kg, produced a decrease in the hydroxylation reactions of dimethylaminopyrine and hexobarbital[SI067].

Moluscicidal activity. Methylene chloride extract of the dried leaf, at a concentration of 400 ppm, was inactive on *Biomphalaria glabrata*. Methylene chloride and methanol extracts of the dried root were also inactive[SI071].

Monoamine oxidase activity increase. Seed oil, in cell culture, was active on astrocytes vs chlorgyline-induced monoamine oxidase (MAO) inhibition, IC$_{50}$ 9077 ppm[SI081].

Mutagenic activity. Water extract of the plant, on agar plate at a concentration of 100 mg/plate, was inactive on pig kidney-LLC-PK-1 cells and trophoblastic cells of placenta. The effect was the same with or without metabolic activation[SI106]. Acetone extract of the dried seed, on agar plate at a concentration of 0.2 μg/plate, was inactive on *Salmonella typhimurium* TA100 and TA98. Metabolic activation had no effect on the results[SI101]. Ethanol extract of the shade dried seed, on agar plate at various concentrations, was inactive on *Salmonella typhimurium* T1530[SI088]. Seed oil, on agar plate, was inactive on *Salmonella typhimurium* TA100 and TA98[SI067]. Chloroform/methanol extract (2:1), on agar plate at a concentration of 10 mg/plate, was inactive on *Salmonella typhimurium* TA100 and TA98. The effect was the same with or without metabolic activation[SI106]. Mice fed diets containing various levels of sesame oil for 8 weeks were investigated. Aflatoxin B1-induced chromosomal aberrations in bone narrow cells were statistically higher in mice fed 9 and 12% sesame oil than those fed 3% sesame oil. The data suggested that the metabolism of a mutagen could be influenced by the dietary lipid intake of the test animals[SI022].

Nasal mucosal effect. Pure sesame oil (Nozoil) was tested in 79 subjects with nasal mucosa dryness. Half of them received pure sesame oil for 2 weeks followed by isotonic sodium chloride solution (ISCS) for 2 weeks. The other half received ISCS for 2 weeks, followed by pure sesame oil for 2 weeks. Nasal mucosal dryness improved significantly when pure sesame oil was used compared with ISCS ($p < 0.001$). The improvement in nasal stuffiness was also better with pure sesame oil ($p < 0.001$) as was improvement in nasal crusts ($p < 0.001$). Eight of 10 subjects reported that their nasal symptoms had improved with pure sesame oil compared with 3 of 10 for ISCS ($p < 0.001$). Adverse events were few and temporary[SI006]. Twenty patients with dryness of the nose, and 20 patients who had previously undergone nasal irradiation were investigated. For the 20 days, the patients sprayed sesame oil into each nostril three times a day, the nasal problems decreased significantly. The greatest effect was exerted on dryness and the side effects from using sesame oil were few in number and mild[SI011].

Nematocidal activity. Ethanol (95%) extract of the seed oil, at a concentration of 500 ppm, was active. Petroleum ether extract of the seed oil, at a concentration of 500 ppm, completely controlled rootknot in grape, tomato, and sugar beet without phytotoxicity. The biological activity reported has been patented. The seed oil was also active and the biological activity has been patented[SI114].

Neuromuscular blocking activity. Decoction of the seed oil, administered orally to adults of both sexes at a dose of 4.6 g/person, was active. A mixture of *Piper longum*, *Zingiber officinale*, *Piper cubeba*, *Curcuma zedoaria*, *Juniperus communis*, *Cichorium intybus*, *Mentha arvensis*, *Commiphora mukul*, and *Sesamum indicum* was given. Twenty five patients with laquwa (spastic facial paralysis) were treated with this mixture in divided doses of 4.6 g in 24 hours. Six grams of a decoction of *Lavendula stoechas* was also given in some cases. Seventy six percent of the patients were cured, 16% showed a partial response, and 8% did not improve[SI118].

Pharmacokinetics. Seed oil, administered intramuscularly to dogs at a dose of 1 mL/kg labeled glyceryl trioleate injected with the oil, was distributed primarily to iliac nodes, heart, liver, and lungs[SI067].

Phytotoxic effect. Ethanol (95%) extract of the dried seed oil, at a concentration of 500 ppm, was inactive. The biological activity reported has been patented[SI114].

Prostaglandin induction. Seed oil, administered subcutaneously to rats at a dose of 1 g/day for 14 days, stimulated PGI-2 synthesis in the thoracic aorta[SI124].

Pyruvate kinase inhibition. The seed, administered to male rats at a dose of 5% of diet, was active in plasma vs low-α-tocopherol diet. Results were significant at $p < 0.05$ level[SI046].

Quil-A saponin toxicity. Mice fed Quil-A-supplemented diet (a saponin that emulsifies fats and potentiates the immune responses) showed higher level of docosapentaenoic acid in the liver. These changes were associated with a significant reduction in the plasma PGE1 and PGE2 and thrombohane-B2 levels in response to an intraperitoneal injection of a lethal dose of lipopolysaccharide endotoxin, LD_{50} 20 mg/kg. The data suggest that sesame seed oil and Quil A, when present in the diet, exerted cumulative effects that resulted in a decrease in the levels of dienoic eicosanoids with a reduction in IL-1 β and a concommitant elevation in the levels of IL-10 that were associated with a marked increase survival in mice[SI014].

Radical scavenging effect. Seed oil, in cell culture, was active on astrocytes vs peroxide radical scavenging, IC_{50} 27461 ppm[SI081].

Spasmogenic activity. Methanol (70%) extract of the seed, administered to guinea pigs at a dose of 1 mg/mL, was active on the uterus and ileum. The effect was abolished by atropine. Methanol (70%) extract of the seed, administered to rats at dose of 1 mg/mL, was active on uterus (estrogen)[SI057].

Steroidogenic activity. Seed oil, applied externally to rats, produced 3-oxosteroid level increased on the treated skin[SI067].

Teratogenic activity. Seed oil, administered intragastrically to rats at a dose of 4 mL/animal for 6–10 days of gestation, was inactive[SI067].

Tocopherol level. Consumption of 5 mg of γ-tocopherol per day for a 3-day period from sesame seeds in nine subjects, significantly elevated serum γ-tocopherol levels (19.1% increase, $p = 0.03$) and depressed plasma β-tocopherol (34% decrease, $p = 0.01$). No significant changes in baseline or post-intervention plasma levels of cholesterol, triglycerides, or carotenoids were found[SI007]. In 40 investigated female students (mean age 26 years) after 4 weeks of sesame oil-rich diet, the γ-tocopherol concentrations normalized to serum lipids increased significantly ($p < 0.01$), and the α/γ-tocopherol ratios decreased significantly from baseline concentrations ($p < 0.05$). The α-tocopherol concentrations did not change[SI008]. Rats fed diets low in α-tocopherol and high in γ-tocopherol, differed in content of sesamin (0.25, 0.5, 1, 2, or 4 g/kg) from sesame oil for 4 weeks. Sesamin-feeding increased γ-tocopherol and γ/α-tocopherol ratios in the plasma ($p < 0.05$), liver ($p < 0.001$), and lungs ($p < 0.001$). The increase was not significant for α-tocopherol. Results suggest, that sesamin appears to spare γ-tocopherol in rat plasma and tissues, and the effect persists in the presence of γ-tocopherol. The bioavaliability of γ-tocopherol was enhanced in phenol-containing diet[SI018].

Toxic effect. The seed oil oxidized hemoglobin A to methemoglobin in RBCs[SI067]. Seed oil, administered orally to rats, produced reticulendothelioses[SI145]. A 48-year-old man experienced subcutaneous nodules 9 months after self-injection of sesame seed oil into the pectoral area for muscle augumentation. Excision revealed a cyst filled with oily material, surrounded by granulomatous tissue[SI012]. Miniature swine fed brominated sesame oil at dietary levels of 5, 25, 50, or 500 mg/kg of body weight for 17 weeks showed decreased growth rate and food intake at the high dose of sesame oil. Marked elevations in LDH, SGOT, and SGPT values were seen at the highest dose level, and these enzyme activities were increased at the 50 mg/kg dose level[SI024].

Toxicity assesment. Ethanol (50%) extract, administered intraperitoneally to mice, produced LD_{50} 500 mg/kg[SI027].

Tumor-promotion inhibition. Methanol extract of the dried entire plant, in cell culture at a concentration of 200 μg/mL, was active vs 12-O-hexadecanoylphorbol-13-acetate-induced Epstein–Barr virus activation[SI049].

Tyrosinase inhibition. Methanol (80%) extract of the dried entire plant at a concentration of 100 μg/mL produced weak activity[SI049].

White blood cell-macrophage stimulant. Water extract of the dried seed at a concentration of 2 mg/mL was active on macrophages. Nitrate formation was used as an index of the macrophage stimulating activity to screen effective foods[SI099].

Weight-gain inhibition. Seed oil administered subcutaneously to mice at a dose of 0.05 mL/animal was active. Brain weight also decreased after 210 days of dosing[SI067].

REFERENCES

SI001   Takeuchi, H., L. Y. Mooi, Y. Inagaki, and P. He. Hypoglycemic effect of a hot-water extract from defatted sesame (*Sesamum indicum* L.) seed on the blood glucose level in genetically diabetic KK-Ay mice. **Biosci Biotech Biochem** 2001; 65(10): 2318–2321.

SI002   Pastorello, E. A., E. Varin, L. Farioli, et al. The major allergen of sesame seeds (*Sesamum indicum*) is a 2S albumin. **J Chromatogr B, Biomed Sci Appl** 2001; 756(1–2): 85–93.

SI003 Sirato-Yasumoto, S., M. Katsuta, Y. Okuyama, Y. Takahashi, and T. Ide. Effect of sesame seeds rich in sesamin and sesamolin on fatty acid oxidation in rat liver. **J Agric Food Chem** 2001; 49(5): 2647–2651.

SI004 Hsu, D. Z., and M. Y. Liu. Sesame oil attenuates multiple organ failure and increases survival rate during endotoxemia in rats. **Critic Care Med** 2002; 30(8): 1859–1862.

SI005 Dalal, I., I. Binson, R. Reifen, et al. Food allergy is a matter of geography after all: sesame as a major cause of severe IgE-mediated food allergic reactions among infants and young children in Israel. **Allergy** 2002; 57(4): 362–365.

SI006 Johnsen, J., B. M. Bratt, O. Michel-Barron, C. Glennow, and B. Petruson. Pure sesame oil vs isotonic sodium chloride solution as treatment for dry nasal mucosa. **Arch Otolaryngol Head Neck Surg** 2001; 127(11): 1353–1356.

SI007 Cooney, R. V., L. J. Custer, L. Okinaka, and A. A. Franke. Effect of dietary sesame seeds on plasma tocopherol levels. **Nutr Canc** 2001; 39(1): 66–71.

SI008 Lemcke-Norojarvi, M., A. Kamal-Eldin, L. A. Appelqvist, L. H. Dimberg, M. Ohrvall, and B. Vessby. Corn and sesame oils increase serum gamma-tocopherol concentrations in healthy Swedish women. **J Nutr** 2001; 131(4): 1195–1201.

SI009 Kobayashi, N., S. Unten, H. Kakuta, et al. Diverse biological activities of healthy foods. **In Vivo** 2001; 15(1): 17–23.

SI010 Miyahara, Y., H. Hibasami, H. Katsuzaki, K. Imai, and T. Komiya. Sesamolin from sesame seed inhibits proliferation by inducing apoptosis in human lymphoid leukemia Molt 4B cells. **Int J Mol Med** 2001; 7(4): 369–371.

SI011 Blork-Eriksson, T., M. Gunnarsson, M. Holmstrom, A. Nordqvist, and B. Petruson. Fewer problems with dry nasal mucous membranes following local use of sesame oil. **Rhinology** 2000; 38(4): 200–203.

SI012 Darsow, U., H. Bruckbauer, W. I. Worret, H. Hofmann, and J. Ring. Subcutaneous oleomas induced by self-injection of sesame seed oil for muscle augumentation. **J Amer Acad Derm** 2000; 42(2Pt1): 292–294.

SI013 Wolde, S., F. Engels, A. M. Miltenburg, E. A. Kujipers, G. I. Struijk-Wielinga, and B. A. Dijkmans. Sesame oil in injectable gold: two drugs in one? **Br J Rheumatol** 1997; 36(9): 1012–1015.

SI014 Chavali, S. R., W. W. Zhong, T. Utsunomiya, and R. A. Forse. Decreased production of interleukin-1-beta, prostaglandin-E2 and thromboxane-B2, and elevated levels of interleukin-6 and -10 are associated with increased survival during endotoxic shock in mice consuming diets enriched with sesame seed oil supplemented with Quil-A saponin. **Int Arch Allergy Immunol** 1997; 114(2): 153–160.

SI015 Nonaka, M., K. Yamashita, Y. Iizuka, M. Namiki, and M. Sugano. Effect of dietary sesaminol and sesamin on eicosanoid production and immunoglobulin level in rats given ethanol. **Biosci Biotech Biochem** 1997; 61(5): 836–839.

SI016 Satchithanandam, S., R. Chanderbhan, A. T. Kharroubi, et al. Effect of sesame oil on serum and liver lipid profiles in the rat. **Int J Vitamin Nutr Res** 1996; 66(4): 386–392.

SI017 Kita, S., Y. Matsumura, S. Morimoto, et al. Antihypertensive effect of sesamin. II. Protection against two-kidney, one-clip renal hypertension and cardiovascular hypertrophy. **Biol Pharm Bull** 1995; 18(9): 1283–1285.

SI018 Kamal-Eldin, A., D. Pettersson, and L. A. Appelqvist. Sesamin (compound from sesame oil) increases tocopherol levels in rats fed *ad libitum*. **Lipids** 1995; 30(6): 499–505.

SI019 Inskeep, P. B., K. M. Davis, and A. E. Ree. Pharmacokinetics of the acyl coenzyme A: cholesterol acyl transferase inhibitor CP-105,191 in dogs-the effect of food and sesame oil on systemic exposure following oral dosing. **J Pharm Sci** 1995; 84(2): 131–133.

SI020 Satchithanandam, S., M. Reicks, R. J. Calvert, M. M. Cassidy, and D. Kritchevsky. Coconut oil and sesame oil affect lymphatic absorption of cholesterol and fatty acids in rats. **J Nutr** 1993; 123(11): 1852–1858.

SI021 Hirose, N., T. Inoue, K. Nishihara, et al. Inhibition of cholesterol absorption and synthesis in rats by sesamin. **J Lipid Res** 1991; 32(4): 629–638.

SI022 Krishamurthy, P. B., and G. S. Neelaram. Effect of dietary fat on aflatoxin B1-induced chromosomal aberrations in mice. **Toxicol Lett** 1986; 31(3): 229–234.

SI023 Malish, D., M. M. Glovsky, D. R. Hoffman, L. Ghiekiere, and J. M. Hawking. Anaphylaxis after sesame seed ingestion. **J Allergy Clin Immun** 1981; 67(1): 35–38.

SI024 Farber, T. M., D. L. Ritter, M. A. Weinberger, et al. The toxicity of brominated sesame oil and brominated soybean oil in miniature swine. **Toxicology** 1976; 5(3): 319–336.

SI025 Quisumbing, E. Medicinal plants of the Philippines. Tech Bull 16, Rep Philippines, Dept Agr Nat Resources, Manila 1951; 1.

SI026 Ahmad, Y. S. A note of the plants of medicinal value found in Pakistan. Govt of Pakistan Press, Karachi, 1957.

SI027 Dhar, M. L., M. M. Dhar, B. N. Dhawan, B. N. Mehrotha, and C. Ray. Screening of Indian plants for biological activity. Part 1. **Indian J Exp Biol** 1968; 6: 232–247.

SI028 Anon. The atlas of commonly used Chinese traditional drugs, Revolutionary Committee of the Inst Material Medica, Chinese Acad Sci, Pekin 1970.

SI029 Saha, J. C., E. C. Savini, and S. Kasinathan. Ecbolic properties of Indian medicinal plants. Part I. **Indian J Med Res** 1961; 49: 130–151.

SI030 Kapur, R. D. Action of some indigenous drugs on uterus. Preliminary note. **Indian J Med Res** 1948; 36: 47.

SI031 Steggerda, M. Some ethnological data concerning one hundred Yucatan plants. Anthropological Papers No. 29. Smithson Inst Bur Amer Ethnol 1943; 136; 193.

SI032 Gimlette, J. D. A dictionary of Malayan medicine, Oxford Univ Press., New York, 1939.

SI033 Petelot, A. Les plantes medicinales du Cambodge, du Laos and du Vietnam,

vols. 1–4. Archives des Reserches Agronomiques et Pastorals au Vietnam no. 23. 1954.

SI034 Kerharo, J., and A. Bouquet. Plantes medicinales and toxicues de la Cote-D'Ivoire-Haute-Volta, Vigot Freres, Paris 1950; 297 pp.

SI035 Schramm, G. Plant and animal drugs of the old Chinese material medica in the therapy of pulmonary tuberculosis. **Planta Med** 1956; 4(4): 97–104.

SI036 Watt, J. M., and M. G. Breyer-Brandwik. The medicinal and poisonous plants of Southern and Eastern Africa, 2nd ed., E. S. Livingstone, Ltd., London, 1962.

SI037 Grieve, M., and C. F. Leyel. A modern herbal. The medicinal, culinary, cosmetic and economic properties, cultivation and folk-lore of herbs, grasses, fungi, shrubs and trees with all their modern scientific uses, 1931.

SI038 Burkill, I. H. Dictionary of the economic products of the Malay Peninsula. Ministry of Agriculture and Cooperatives, Kuala Lumpur, Malaysia, vol. II. 1966; 1.

SI039 Mannan, A., and K. Ahmad. Studies on vitamin E in the foods of East Pakistan. **Pak J Biol Agr Sci** 1966; 9: 13.

SI040 Ramachandran, B. V. Arginine content of oilseed cakes. **J Sci Ind Res C** 1957; 16: 70.

SI041 Osawa, T., M. Nagata, M. Namiki, and Y. Fukuda. Sesaminol, a novel antioxidant isolated from sesame seeds. **Agr Biol Chem** 1985; 49(11): 3351–3352.

SI042 Ogasawara, T., K. Chiba, and M. Tada. Production in high yield of naphthoquinone by a hairy root culture of *Sesamum indicum*. **Phytochemistry** 1993; 33(5): 1095–1098.

SI043 Katsuzaki, H., S. Kawakishi, and T. Osawa. Sesaminol glucosides in sesame seeds. **Phytochemistry** 1993; 35(3): 773–776.

SI044 Suzuki, N., T. Miyase, and A. Ufno. Phenylethanoid glycosides of *Sesamum indicum*. **Phytochemistry** 1993; 34(3): 729–732.

SI045 Zargari, A. Medicinal plants, vol. 3, 5th ed., Tehran University Publications, No 1810/3, Tehran, Iran, 1992; 3: 889.

SI046 Yamashita, K., Y. Iizuka, T. Imai, and M. Namiki. Sesame seed and its lignans produce marked enhancement of vitamin E activity in rats fed a low alpha-tocopherol diet. **Lipids** 1995; 30(11): 1019–1028.

SI047 Kuriyama, K., K. Tsuchiya, and T. Murui. Generation of new lignan glucosides during germination of sesame seeds. **Nippon Nogei Kagaku Kaishi** 1995; 69(6): 685–693.

SI048 Stern, A., and B. Wuthrich. Non-IgE-mediated anaphylaxis to sesame. **Allergy** 1998; 53(3): 325–326.

SI049 Shin, N. H., K. S. Lee, S. H. Kang, K. R. Min, S. H. Lee, and Y. S. Kim. Inhibitory effect of herbal extracts of DOPA oxidase activity of tyrosinase. **Nat Prod Sci** 1997; 3(2): 111–121.

SI050 Oezcan, M., and A. Akguel. Some compositional characteristics of sesame seeds and oil. **Turk J Agr For** 1995; 19(1): 59–65.

SI051 Mimura, M., Y. Takahara, A. Ichikawa, and T. Osawa. Lignan compounds and their manufacture with *Sesamum indicum*. Patent-Japan Kokai Tokkyo Koho-63,207,389 1997; 5 pp.

SI052 Okada, N., K. Takebayashi, A. Kawashima, and M. Niwano. A triterpene, its manufacture, and cancer inhibitors containing triterpenes. Patent-Japan Kokai Tokkyo Koho-06,329,590 1994; 9 pp.

SI053 Kuryama, K., and T. Murui. Manufacture of lignan glycosides and lignans from sesame seeds. Patent-Japan Kokai Tokkyo Koho-07,145,066 1995; 10 pp.

SI054 Sato, A. Studies on anti-tumor activity of crude drugs. III. The effect of decreasing resistance of cancer cell in long term in vitro screening test with aqueous extracts of some crude drugs. **Yakugaku Zasshi** 1990; 110(7): 490–497.

SI055 Smith, D. E., and J . W. Salerno. Selective growth inhibition of a human malignant melanoma cell line by sesame oil *in vitro*. **Prostaglandins Essent Fatty Acids** 1992; 46(2):145–150.

SI056 James, C., A. Williams-Akita, Y. A. K. Rao, L. Chiarmonte, and A. T. Schneider. Sesame seed anaphylaxis. **N Y J Med** 1991; 91(10): 457–458.

SI057 Hassan Gilant, A. U., and K. Aftab. Presence of acetylcholine-like substance (S) in *Sesamum indicum*. **Arch Pharm Res** 1992; 15(1): 95–98.

SI058 Chiu, J. T., and I. B. Haydik. Sesame seed oil anaphylaxis. **J Allergy Clin Immunol** 1991; 88(3): 414–415.

SI059 Mimura, M., Y. Takahara, A. Ichikawa, and T. Osawa. Lignan compounds and their manufacture with *Sesamum indicum*. Patent-Japan Kokai Tokkyo Koho-36,207,389 1988; 5 pp.

SI060 Murui, T., and A. Ide. Anticarcinogenic glycosides with aglycones extracted from sesame seeds. Patent-Japan Kokai Tokkyo Koho-62,238,287 1987; 6 pp.

SI061 Kamal-Eldin, A., L. A. Appelquist, G. Yousif, and G. M. Iskander. Seed lipids of *Sesamum indicum* and related wild species in Sudan. The sterols. **J Sci Food Agr** 1992; 59(3): 327–334.

SI062 Reddy, M. B., K. R. Reddy, and M. N. Reddy. A survey of plant crude drugs of Anantapur District, Andhra Pradesh, India. **Int J Crude Drug Res** 1989; 27(3): 145–155.

SI063 Odumodu, C. U. Antinutrients content of some locally available legumes and cereals in Nigeria. **Trop Geograph Med** 1992; 44(3): 260–263.

SI064 Shinmen, Y., K. Akimoto, S. Asami, et al. Dioxabicyclooctane derivatives as liver function improvers. Patent-Eur Pat Apl-409,654 1991; 13 pp.

SI065 Kagi, M. K., and B. Wuthrich. Falafel burger anaphylaxis due to sesame seed allergy. **Ann Allergy** 193; 71(2): 127-129.

SI066 Keskinen, H., P. Ostman, E. Vaherj, et al. A case of occupational asthma, rhinitis and urticaria due to sesame seed. **Clin Exp Allergy** 1991; 21: 523–524.

SI067 Anon. Final report on the safety assessment of sesame oil. **J Amer Coll Toxicol** 1993; 12(3): 261–277.

SI068 Kang, S. S., J. S. Kim, J. H. Jung, and Y. H. Kim. NMR assessments of two furofan lignans from sesame seeds. **Arch Pharm Res** 1955; 18(5): 361–363.

SI069 Anis, M., and M. Iqbal. Medicinal plantlore of Aligard, India. **Int J Pharmacog** 1994; 32(1): 59–64.

SI070 Bhattarai, N. K. Folk herbal remedies for gynaecological complaints in central Nepal. **Int J Pharmacog** 1994; 32(1): 13–26.

SI071 Cepleanu, F., M. O. Hamburger, B. Sordat, et al. Screening of tropical medicinal plants for Molluscicidal, larvicidal, fungicidal and cytotoxic activities, and brine shrimp toxicity. **Int J Pharmacog** 1994; 32(3): 294–307.

SI072 Okada, N., K. Takebayashi, J. Kawashima, et al. Inhibition of Epstein-Barr virus (EBV) activation by triterpenes in *Sesamum indicum* L. callus. **Shokubutsu Soshiki Baiyo** 1994; 11(2): 145–149.

SI073 Johns, T., E. B. Mhoro, and P. Sanaya. Food plants and masticants of the Batemi of Ngorongoro district, Tanzania. **Econ Bot** 1996; 50(1): 115–121.

SI074 Richaado, H., K. Janetsuto, G. Uiriamu, A. Kawashima, M. Niwano, and M. Mimura. A-2 inhibitors containing acteoside. Patent-Japan Kokai Tokkyo Koho-07,223,964 1995; 7 pp.

SI075 Al-Khalil, S. A survey of plants used in Jordanian traditional medicine. **Int J Pharmacog** 1995; 33(4): 317–323.

SI076 Vlietinck, A. J., L. van Hoof, J. Totte, et al. Screening of hundred Rwandese medicinal plants for antimicrobial and antiviral properties. **J Ethnopharmacol** 1995; 46(1): 31–47.

SI077 Bellakhdar, J., R. Claisse, J. Fleurentin, and C. Younos. Repertory of standard herbal drugs in the Moroccan pharmacopoea. **J Ethnopharmacol** 1991; 35(2): 123–143.

SI078 Kawagishi, S., T. Oosawa, and H. Katsuzaki. Pinoresinol glycoside, sesame seed extract containing the glycoside, and its use for preventing oxidation of lipids. Patent-Japan Kokai Tokkyo Koho-06,116,282 1994; 5 pp.

SI079 Amico, A. Medicinal plants of southern Zambesia. **Fitoterapia** 1977; 48: 101–139.

SI080 Eberlein-Konig, B., F. Rueff, and B. Przybilla. Generalized urticaria caused by sesame seeds with negative prick test result and without demonstrable specific IgE antibodies. **J Allergy Clin Immunol** 1995; 94(4): 560–561.

SI081 Mazzio, E. A., N. Harris, and K. F. A. Soliman. Food constituents attenuate monoamine oxidase activity and peroxidase levels in C6 astrocyte cells. **Planta Med** 1998; 64(7): 603–606.

SI082 Alday, E., G. Curiel, M. J. Lopez-Gil, D. Carreno, and I. Moneo. Occupa-

tional hypersensitivity to sesame seeds. **Allergy** 1996; 51(1): 69–70.

SI083 Kumar, S., G. D. Bagchi, and M. P. Darokar. Antibacterial activity observed in the seeds of some coprophilous plants. **Int J Pharmacog** 1997; 35(3): 179–184.

SI084 Pajno, G. B., G. Passalacqua, G. Magazzu, G. Barberio, D. Vita, and G. W. Canonica. Anaphylaxis to sesame. **Allergy** 2000; 55(2): 199–201.

SI085 Toda, M., J. Kawabata, and T. Kasai. Alpha-glucosidase inhibitors from glove (*Syzygium aromaticum*). **Biosc Biotech Biochem** 2000; 64(2): 294–298.

SI086 Engler, M. M., and M. B. Engler. Dietary borage oil alters plasma, hepatic and vascular tissue fatty acid composition in spontaneously hypertensive rats. **Prostaglandins Leukotrienes Essent Fatty Acids** 1998; 59(1): 11–15.

SI087 Runnebaum, B., T. Rabe, L. Kiesel, and A. O. Prakash. Biological evaluation of some medicinal plants extracts for contraceptive efficacy in females. Future aspects in contraception. Part 2. Female contraception, MTP Press, LTD, Boston, 1984, 115–128.

SI088 Alkofahi, A., R. Batshoun, W. Owais, and N. Najib. Biological activity of some Jordanian medicinal plant extracts. **Fitoterapia** 1996; 67(5): 435–442.

SI089 Prakash, V., and P. K. Nandi. Isolation and characterization of alpha-globulin of sesame seed (*Sesamum indicum*). **J Agr Food Chem** 1978; 26(2): 320.

SI090 Tewari, P. V., H. C. Mapa, and C. Chaturvedi. Experimental study on estrogenic activity of certain indigenous drugs. **J Res Indian Med Yoga Homeopathy** 1976; 11: 7–12.

SI091 Unnikrishnan, M. C., and R. Kuttan. Cytoxicity of extracts of spices to cultured cells. **Nutr Cancer** 1988; 11(4): 251–257.

SI092 Kubo, M., H. Matsuda, M. Fukui, and Y. Nakai. Development studies of cuticle drugs from natural resources. I. Effects of crude drugs extracts on hair growth in mice. **Yakugaku Zasshi** 1988; 108(10): 871–978.

SI093 Singh, V. K. and Z. A. Ali. Folk medicines of Aligarh (Uttar Pradesh), India. **Fitoterapia** 1989; 60(6): 483–490.

SI094   Unnikrishnan, M. C., and R. Kuttan. Tumour reducing and nutricarcinogenic activity of selected spices. **Cancer Lett** 1990; 51(1): 85–89.

SI095   Seo, J. S., Y. W. Lee, N. J. Suh, and I. M. Chang. Assay of antimutagenic activities of vegetable plants. **Korean J Pharmacog** 1990; 21(1): 88–91.

SI096   Neering, H., B. E. J. Vitanyl., K. E. Malten, W. G. Van Ketel, and E. Van Dijk. Allergens in sesame oil contact dermatitis. **Acta Derm** 1975; 55: 31–34.

SI097   Sugano, M., T. Inoue, K. Koba, et al. Influence of sesame lignans on various lipid parameters in rats. **Agr Biol Chem** 1990; 54(10): 2669–2673.

SI098   Sato, A. Studies on anti-tumor activity of crude drugs. I. The effects of aqueous extracts of some crude drugs in short-term screening test. **Yakugaku Zasshi** 1989; 109(6): 407–423.

SI099   Vyas, S. P., and N. Sankhla. Role of bio-regulants in growth and productivity of desert plants. II. Effect of morphactins on growth flowering protein and phosphorus content in *Sesamum indicum*. **Trans Indian Soc Desert Technol Univ Cent Desert Stud** 977; 2: 246.

SI100   Salerno, J. W., and D. E. Smith. The use of sesame oil and other vegetable oils in the inhibiting of human colon cancer growth *in vitro*. **Anticancer Res** 1991; 11(1): 209–215.

SI101   Ruan, C. C., Y. Liang, J. L. Liu, W. S. Tu, and Z. H. Liu. Antimutagenic effect of eight natural foods on moldy foods in a high liver cancer incidence area. **Mutat Res** 1992; 279(1): 35–40.

SI102   Vyas, S. P., and N. Sankhla. Role of bio-regulants in growth and productivity of desert plants. II. Effect of morphactins on growth flowering protein and phosphorus content in *Sesamum indicum*. **Trans Indian Soc Desert Technol Univ Cent Desert Stud** 977; 2: 246.

SI103   Lal, S. D., and K. Lata. Plants used by the Bhat community for regulating fertility. **Econ Bot** 1980; 34: 273–275.

SI104   Dey, P. M. Biosynthesis of planteose in *Sesamum indicum*. **FEBS Lett** 1980; 114: 153–156.

SI105   Ito, Y., S. Yanase, J.Fujita, T. Harayama, M. Takashima, and H. Imanaka. A short-term *in vitro* assay for promoter substances using human lymphoblastoid cells latently infected with Epstein Barr virus. **Cancer Lett** 1981; 13: 29–37.

SI106   Rockwell, P., and I. Raw. A mutagenic screening of various herbs, spices and food additives. **Nutr Cancer** 1979; 1: 10–15.

SI107   Oommachan, M., and S. S. Khan. Plants in aid of family planning programme. **Sci Life** 1981; 1: 64–66.

SI108   Yoshida, M., and T. Kashimoto. Determination of sesamolin, sesamin and sesamol in sesame oil by high-performance liquid chromatography. **Shokuhin Eiseigaku Zasshi** 1982; 23: 142–148.

SI109   Prakash, A. O., R. B. Gupta, and R. Mathur. Effect of oral administration of forty-two indigenous plant extracts on early and late pregnancy in albino rats. **Probe** 1978; 17(4): 315–323.

SI110   Krag, K. J. Plants used as contraceptives by the North American Indians, an ethnobotanical study. **Thesis BS Harvard University** 196; 117 pp

SI111   Razzack, H. M. A. The concept of birth control in Unani medical literature. Unpublished manuscript of the author 1980; 64 pp.

SI112   Kato, Y., E. Ueda, T. Kyoko, A. Yukiyo Nagaoka, S.Iwashita, S. Ninomiya, and N. Kato. Asarinin in sesame oil. **Pharmazie** 1980; 35(12): 808–809.

SI113   Dixit, R. S., And H. C. Pandey. Plants used as folk medicine in Jhansi and Lalitpur sections of Bundelkhand, Uttar Pradesh. **Int J Crude Drug Res** 1984; 22(1): 47–51.

SI114   MC Brayer, B. W. Sesame nematocidal composition. Patent-US-4,442,092 1982; 4 pp.

SI115   John, D. One hundred useful raw drugs of the Kani tribes of Trivandrum Forest Division, Kerala, India. **Int J Crude Drug Res** 1984; 22(1): 17–39.

SI116   Lee, C. Y., J. W. Chiou, and W. H. Chang. Studies on the antioxidative activities of spices grown in Taiwan. (2). **Chung-Kuo Nung Yeh Hua Hsueh Hui Chin** 1982; 20(1/2): 61–66.

SI117   Fukuda, Y., T. Oosawa, and M. Namiki. Antioxidants in sesame seed.

Nippon Shokuhin Kogyo Gakkaishi 1981; 28: 461–464.

SI118 Siddiqui, N. A., and M. Z. Hasan. Therapeutic response of Arab medicines in cases of laquwa. **Bull Islamic Med** 1981; 1: 366–374.

SI119 Woo, W. S., E. B. Lee, K. H. Shin, S. S. Kang, and H. J. Chi. A review of research on plants for fertility regulation in Korea. **Korean J Pharmacog** 1981; 12(3): 153–170.

SI120 Fukuda, Y., T. Osawa, M. Namiki and T. Ozaki. Studies on antioxidative substances in sesame seed. **Agr Biol Chem** 1985; 49(2): 301–306.

SI121 Singhal, P. C., and L. D. Joshi. Glycemic and cholesterolemic role of ginger and til. **J Sci Res Pl Med** 1983; 4(3): 32–34.

SI122 Weniger, B., M. Rouzier, R. Daguilh, D. Henrys, J. H. Henrys, and R. Anton. Popular medicine of the central plateau of Haiti. 2. Ethnopharmacological inventory. **J Ethnopharmacol** 1986; 17(1): 13–30.

SI123 Kamboj, V. P. A review of Indian medicinal plants with interceptive activity. **Indian J Med Res** 1988; 1988(4): 336–355.

SI124 El-Tahir, K. E. H., E. A. Hamad, A. M. Ageel, M. A. A. Nasif, and E. A. Gadkarim. Effects of sesame and cod liver oils on prostacyclin synthesis by the rat thoracic aorta. **Arch Int Pharmacodyn Ther** 1988; 292(1): 182–188.

SI125 Ramirez, V. R., L. J. Mostacero, A. E. Garcia, et al. Vegetales empleados en medicina tradicional Norperuana. Banco Agrario del Peru, NACL Univ Trujillo, Trujillo, Peru, June, 1988; 54 pp.

SI126 Singh, V. P., S. K. Sharma, and V. S. Khare. Medicinal plants from Ujjain district Madhya Pradesh. Part II. **Indian Drugs Pharm Ind** 1980; 1980(5): 7–12.

SI127 Kumar, D. S., and Y. S. Prabhakar. On the ethnomedical significance of the arjun tree, *Terminalia arjuna* (Roxb.) Wight and Arnot. **J Ethnopharmacol** 1987; 20(2): 173–190.

SI128 Heiduschka, A. Unsaponifiable matter of sesame oil. Orig Com 8th Intern Congr Appl Chem 1912; 11: 13.

SI129 Ray, P. G., and S. K. Majumdar. Antimicrobial activity of some Indian plants. **Econ Bot** 1976; 30: 317–320.

SI130 Lee, E. B., H. S. Yun, and W. S. Woo. Plants and animals used for fertility regulation in Korea. **Korean J Pharmacog** 1977; 8: 81–87.

SI131 Nagabhushanan, A., M. Srinivasan, and V. Subrahmanyan. Breakdown and synthesis of sesamolin in the sesame seed (*Sesamum indicum*). **J Sci Ind Res-C** 1956; 15: 283.

SI132 Das, V. S., K. N. Rao, and J. V. Rao. Phenolic acids in some members of *Pedaliaceae*. **Curr Sci** 1966 35: 160.

SI133 Lopez, C., V. L. Villegas, M. De La Paz, J. Silva Lara, and P. Cattaneo. *Sesamum indicum* seeds. II. Chemical composition of the extracted oil. **An Asoc Quim Argent** 1974; 62; 301.

SI134 Vague, J., J. C. Garrigues, J. Berthet, and G. Favier. The oestrogenic effect of several plants oil. **Ann Endocrinol** 1959; 18: 745–751.

SI135 Prakash, A. O., and R. Mathur. Screening of Indian plants for antifertility activity. **Indian J Exp Biol** 1976; 14: 623–626.

SI136 Dragendorff, G. Die heilpflanzen der verschieden volker und zeiten, F. Enke, Stuttgard. 1898; 885 pp.

SI137 Jochle, W. Biology and biochemistry of reproduction and contraception. **Angew Chem Int Ed Engl** 1962; 1: 537–549.

SI138 Roig Y., and J. T. Mesa. Plantas medicinales, aromaticas o venenosas de Cuba, Ministerio de Agricultura, Republica de Cuba, Havana. 1945; 872 pp.

SI139 Nayar, S. L. Poisonous seeds of India. Part II. **J Bombay Nat Hist Soc** 1954 52(2/3): 1–18.

SI140 Saito, K. Fibroblast cultures. **Nippon Yakugaku Zasshi** 1936; 23: 1–5.

SI141 Harborne, J. B., and C. A. Willliams. Comparative biochemistry of flavonoids. XIII. 6-hydroxyluteolin and scutellarein as phyletic markers in higher plants. **Phytochemistry** 1971; 10: 367–378.

SI142 Morita, N. The flavonoid of sesame leaves. I. The structure of the glycoside, pedalin. **Chem Pharm Bull** 1960; 8: 59–65.

SI143　Malten, K. E., J. P. Kuiper, and W. B. J. M. Van der Staak. Contact allergic investigations in 100 patients with ulcus cruris. **Dermatologica** 1973; 147(4): 241–254.

SI144　Fitelson, J. The occurrence of squalene in natural fats. **J Ass Offic Agr Chem** 1943; 26: 506–511

SI145　Diquattro, C., and T. Mercadante. Reticuloendothelioses due to estrogens and sesame oil, their morphological identity. II. **Sez Med** 1955; 62: 171–188.

SI146　Schiff, E., and C. Hirscheberger. Thrombocytosis produced by a hitherto unknown substance the "fat-soluble T factor". **Amer J Dis Child** 1937; 53: 32–38.

SI147　Kabelitz, G. Comparative studies on the behavior of the alimentary lipemia, cholesterol, and blood sugar after loading with one synthetic and two natural food fats. **Arch Ges Physiol** 1944; 247: 593–599

SI148　Tobin, C. E. Effect of adrenalectomy on pregnancy and survival of untreated and sesame oil-treated rats. **Endocrinology** 1941; 28: 419–425.

SI149　Yanagisawa, F., K. Ogasawara, and K. Bushimata. Biochemical studies on plant oils. II. Hypocholesterolemic action. **Tokyo Toritsu Eisei Kenkyusho Kenkyu Nempo** 1967; 1967(19): 90–96

SI150　Pollia, J. A. 1,2,5,6-dibenzanthracene on certain organs and a transplantable rat sarcoma in animals of pure breed. **Radiology** 1937; 29: 683–694.

SI151　Marchand, P. A., M. J. Kato, and N. G. Lewis. (+)-Episesaminone, A *Sesamum indicum* furofuran lignan. Isolation and hemisynthesis. **J Nat Prod** 1997; 60 (11): 1189–1192.

SI152　Katsuzaki, H., M. Kawasumi, S. Kawakishi, and T. Osawa. Structure of novel antioxidative lignan glucosides isolated from sesame seed. **Biosci Biotech Biochem** 1992; 56(12): 2087–2088.

SI153　Chen, E. C. F., S. S. K. Tai, C. C. Peng, and J. T. C. Tzen. Identification of three novel unique proteins in seed oil bodies of sesame. **Plant Cell Physiol** 1998; 39(9): 935–941.

SI154　Ohta, S., N. Sakurai, T. Inoue and M. Shinoda. Studies on chemical protectors against radiation. XXV. Radioprotective activities of various crude drugs. **Yakugaku Zasshi** 1987; 107(1): 70–75.

SI155　Anon. GRAS status of foods and food additives. **Fed Regist** 1976; 41: 38,644.

SI156　Katsuzaki, H., S. Kawakishi, and T. Osawa. Structure of novel antioxidant lignan triglucoside isolated from sesame seed. **Heterocycles** 1993; 36(5): 933–936.

16 | Zingiber officinale

Roscoe.

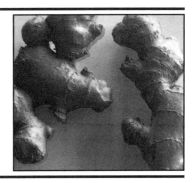

Common Names

Aale	India	Chitta	Africa
Ada	India	Chnay	Cambodia
Adarak	India	Djae	Indonesia
Adhu	India	Djahe	Netherlands
Adi	India	Dumber	Croatia
Adraka	Pakistan	Dumbier lekarstvy	Slovakia
Adruka	India	Dzhindzhifil	Bulgaria
Aduva	Nepal	Engifer	Iceland
Afifindi	Ecuador	Gamug	Tibet
Afu	Africa	Gan jinang	China
Agnimanth	Nepal	Gember	Indonesia
Ajenjibre	Cuba	Gember	Netherlands
Ajenjibre	Mexico	Gengibre	Brazil
Ajijilla	Ecuador	Gengibre	Portugal
Ajilla	Ecuador	Gengibre	Spain
Ajinibre	Mexico	Gengibre	Venezuela
Ajirinrin	Ecuador	Ghimbir	Romania
Akakur	China	Gin	Myanmar
Alha	India	Gingebre	Mauritius
Aliah	Indonesia	Gingebre	Spain
Alla	India	Gingebre	Vietnam
Allam	India	Gingembre	France
Ardak	India	Ginger	Tanzania
Ardakam	India	Ginger	Brazil
Arstniecibas ingvers	Latvia	Ginger	China
Asgumetakui	Africa	Ginger	Greece
Asunglasemtong	India	Ginger	Guyana
Atuja	Malaysia	Ginger	India
Baojiang	China	Ginger	Jamaica
Beuing	Indonesia	Ginger	Japan
Cay gung	Vietnam	Ginger	Nepal
Chapepnomen ba	Ecuador	Ginger	Nicaragua
Chiang	China	Ginger	Philippines
Chichambara	Nicaragua	Ginger	Sri Lanka

From: *Medicinal Plants of the World, vol. 3: Chemical Constituents, Traditional and Modern Medicinal Uses*
By: I. A. Ross © Humana Press Inc., Totowa, NJ

Ginger	Taiwan	Keong	China
Ginger	United States	Kerati	Papua New Guinea
Ginger	Venezuela	Khing	Laos
Gojabghbegh	Armenia	Khing	Thailand
Gung	Vietnam	Khing-daen	Thailand
Gyin sein	Myanmar	Khnehey	Cambodia
Gyin	Myanmar	Khnhei phlung	Cambodia
Gyomber	Hungary	Khuong	Vietnam
Halia bara	Malaysia	Khyen-seing	Myanmar
Halia	Malaysia	Kinkh	Thailand
Haliya merah	Malaysia	Kintoki	Japan
Haliya	Indonesia	Kion	Peru
Harilik ingver	Estonia	Konga	Papua New Guinea
Hli	Papua New Guinea	Kunyit terus	Malaysia
Imberias	Lithuania	Lahja	Indonesia
Imbir	Poland	Lao jiang	China
Imbir	Russia	Lei	Admiralty Islands
Imbyr	Ukraine	Lia	Indonesia
Inber	Israel	Luya	Philippines
Inbwer	Germany	Mtangwizi	Tanzania
Inchi	India	Myoga	Japan
Ingee	India	Nagara	India
Ingefara	Sweden	Ngesnges	Papua New Guinea
Ingefer	Denmark	Nkrabo	Africa
Ingefer	Norway	Nkrama	Africa
Inguru	Japan	Nkrawusa	Africa
Inguru	Sri Lanka	Oshoga	Japan
Ingver	Croatia	Palana	Papua New Guinea
Ingver	Slovenia	Pia di udi	Ecuador
Ingverijuur	Estonia	Pia nuni	Ecuador
Ingwer	Germany	Piperoriza	Greece
Ingwer	Tanzania	Quing jiang	China
Inkivaari	Finland	Rhizoma, zingiberis	Japan
Isiot	Bulgaria	Saeng gang	Korea
Jae	Indonesia	San geung	China
Jahe	Indonesia	Sang keong	China
Jahi	Malaysia	Sga smug	Tibet
Jamaica ginger	United States	Shen jiang	China
Jamveel	Iran	Shengijang	China
Janzabeil	Sudan	Shohkyoh	Japan
Jenegibre	Venezuela	Shokyo	Japan
Jengibre	Cuba	Shokyo	Taiwan
Jengibre	Spain	Shouga	Japan
Jenibre	Guatemala	Shoukyo	Japan
Jenjibre	Ecuador	Shoukyo	Taiwan
Jenjibre	Nicaragua	Shringaveran	India
Jeung	China	Shukku	India
Jiang	China	Shuntya	India
Jinjaa	Japan	Sinh khuong	Vietnam
Kai	China	Sinziminli	Africa
Kallamu	India	Skenjabil	Morocco
Kan chiang	Vietnam	Skenjbir	Morocco
Kanga	Papua New Guinea	Sman-sga	Tibet

Sonth	India	Zanjabil	Arabic countries
Sringaaran	India	Zanjabil	Iran
Sunth	India	Zazvor	Czech Republic
Sunthi	India	Zazvor	Slovakia
Sutho	Nepal	Zencebil	Turkey
Tangauzi	Tanzania	Zencefil	Turkey
Tangawizi	Tanzania	Zenzero	Italy
Tertuyagas	Ecuador	Zenzevero	Italy
Tsinstsimin	China	Zi jiang	China
Tsintsimir	China	Zingiber	Spain
Wai	Papua New Guinea	Zingibil	Oman
Zangbil	Israel	Zinjabil	Yemen
Zangvil	Israel	Zinjibil	Ethiopia
Zanjabeel	India	Zinzam	Mauritius
Zanjabeel	Saudi Arabia		

BOTANICAL DESCRIPTION

Zingiber officinale is a perennial herb belonging to the ZINGIBERACEAE family. The rhizome is horizontal, branched, fleshy, aromatic, white or yellowish to brown. Stem is leafy, thick, to 60 cm high. Leaves are pointed, narrowly or linear-lanceolate, approx 20 cm long and 1.5–2 cm wide, clasping the stem by long sheaths. The inflorescences, rarely produced by cultivated plants, are separate, approx 20 cm high, consisting of threefold flowers subtending with bracts and bracteoles. Bracts are ovate, approx 2.5 cm long, closely pressed against each other, pale green. Calyx is short, three-lobed. Corolla has two yellow-green, pointed segments and shorter, an oblong-ovate, dark-purple lip spotted and striped with yellow. Each flower has only one short-stalked, fertile stamen and solitary stigma. The fruit, which is rarely formed, is a dehiscent capsule containing relatively large seeds.

ORIGIN AND DISTRIBUTION

Native to southern Asia, it is widely distributed through the tropics and subtropics. Requires a rather hot, moist climate and rich, well-drained soil. It is now cultivated in Indonesia, Jamaica, Sri Lanka, and China.

TRADITIONAL MEDICINAL USES

Admiralty Islands. The rhizome is taken orally as a contraceptive[ZO245].

Brazil. Hot water extract of the dried root is used externally for bronchitis and rheumatism[ZO253].

China. Ash of the burned leaves of *Pongamia pinnata*, *Citrullus colocynthis*, *Piper retrofractum*, *Plumbago zeylanica*, *Zingiber officinale*, and *Piper longum*, mixed with molasses and rock salt, is taken orally to treat abdominal diseases, anemia, and phantom tumors[ZO280]. For choleric diarrhea and chronic fever, powdered *Ferula asafoetida*, *Acorus calamus*, *Zingiber officinale*, *Cuminum*, *Terminalia chebula*, *Inula racemosa*, and *Saussurea lappa*, are taken orally[ZO280]. The oils of *Zingiber officinale*, *Saussurea lappa*, *Sansevieria roxburghiana*, *Curcuma longa*, and *Rubia cordifolia*, mixed with salt buttermilk, and rice, are massaged on the patient for cold and cough[ZO280]. For heaviness of the stomach, powdered *Ferula asafoetida*, *Acorus calamus*, *Zingiber officinale*, *Cuminum cyminum*, *Terminalia chebula*, *Inula racemosa*, and *Saussurea lappa*, are taken orally. For skin diseases, decoction of *Tinospora cordifolia*, *Cyperus rotundus*, and *Zingiber officinale*, mixed with equal quantity of decoction of *Aconitum heterophyllum*, is taken orally[ZO280].

China. Decoction of the dried rhizome is taken orally as an antiemetic[ZO133]. Hot water extract of the rhizome, in combination with *Prunus persica* (Sd), *Carthamus tinctorius* (Fl), *Angelica sinensis* (Rt), *Saliva miltiorrhiza* (Rt), *Ligusticum wallichii* (Rt, St), *Gardenia jasminoides* (Fr), *Sanguisorba officinalis* (Rt), *Corydalis ambigua* (Tu), *Glycyrrhiza uralensis* (Rt), *Commiphora myrrha* (resin), *Boswellia carteri* (resin), *Cyperus rotundus* (Rh), *Citrus tangerina* (fruit peel), *Pyrola japonica* (Lf), *Agrimonia pilosa* (Pl), *Lonicera japonica* (Pl), *Panax sanchi* (Rt), *Codonopsis pilosula* (Rt), *Astragalus membranaceus* (Rt), *Atractylodes macrocephala* (Rh), *Curcumina aromatica* (Rh), and *Caesalpinia sappan* (heartwood), and the scales of the *Manis pentadactyla*, is used to treat ectopic pregnancies. Dosing for up to 8 days produced a pain relief, the tumors disappeared in 100% of the cases, and bleeding stopped in 100% of the cases[ZO355]. Decoction of the fresh rhizome is taken orally for excruciating headache. It is taken in combination with *Evodia rutaecarpa*, *Zizyphus jujuba*, and *Panax ginseng*[ZO174]. Hot water extract of the rhizome is taken orally to suppress or retard the menstrual cycle[ZO165]. The dried root, mixed with *Campanumoea pilosula* (Rt), *Astragalus hiroshimanus* (Rh), *Araliacordata* (Rt), and *Paeonia albiflora* (Rt), is administered intravaginally for leucorrhea with backache, fever, and weak pulse in patients with vaginal cancer. For menorrhagia in patients with vaginal cancer, the dried root, mixed with *Typha* species (pollen) and *Agrimonia pilosa* (twig), is administered intravaginally[ZO299].

Cuba. Hot water extract of the rhizome is taken orally as an emmenagogue and for its stimulating and aphrodisiac properties by men[ZO354]. The fresh rhizome is taken orally as an antispasmodic[ZO154].

East Africa. The fresh root, with scrapings of *Ocimum suave*, is taken orally for inflamed tonsils and angina[ZO260].

Ecuador. Decoction of the rhizome is taken orally for migraines, diarrhea, and stomachache[ZO152].

England. Dried rhizome is taken in combination with *Mentha pulegium* (essential oil), *Aloe vera*, *Ipomoea purga*, *Glycyrrhiza glabra*, and *Canella alba* for amenorrhea[ZO302]. Infusion of the fresh rhizome is taken orally in Chinese herbal formulations to reduce nausea and vomiting during pregnancy. The peeled young ginger rhizome is simmered with sweet malt vinegar for several hours[ZO297].

Europe. Hot water extract of the fresh rhizome is taken orally for delayed menstruation and for all forms of motion sickness[ZO300].

Fiji. Dried root, ground with *Vitex negundo* leaves, is applied to the forehead for headache. For colds, seeds of *Elettaria cardamomum*, *Zingiber officinale* rhizome, and *Piper nigrum* seeds, are ground in water, mixed with honey, and taken orally[ZO266]. Fresh rhizome juice, together with the juice of *Allium cepa*, is taken orally to stop vomiting. The fresh juice is taken with honey or sugar for coughs, colds, stomachache, and asthma[ZO266]. Fresh root juice is administered as eardrop for earache[ZO266].

Greece. Wine extract of the rhizome, with pomegranate and oak gall, is used as a vaginal spermicidal suppository[ZO065].

Guatemala. Decoction of the rhizome is taken orally for fever[ZO149].

Honduras. Decoction of the rhizome is taken orally for cold[ZO159].

India. Hot water extract of the dried rhizome is administered orally as a remedy for whooping cough[ZO242] and hemorrhoids in Ayurvedic medicine[ZO255]. The rhizome, in combination with 25 g each of *Prunus amygdalus* and *Pistacia vera*, 10 g of *Piper nigrum*, 100 g of *Hedychium spicatum*, and 200 g of *Elastrus paniculatus*, is taken orally for rheumatism. For dysentery and stomachache, 250 g of dried rhizome is taken with 500 g dried stem bark of *Holarrhena anti-*

dysenterica and 100 g of dried *Piper nigrum*, powdered and mixed with butter oil into pills about the size of a pea. Two to three pills are taken daily[ZO256]. Hot water extract of the rhizome is taken orally for amenorrhea[ZO063]. The decoction is taken orally for diabetes[ZO169], and paste mixed with salt is used externally as an antivenin[ZO148]. The dried root with leaves of *Adhatoda vasica* and *Piper nigrum* and *Piper longum*, are powdered and administered orally to treat bronchitis. The powder is sometimes mixed with honey[ZO119]. The fresh rhizome is taken orally with honey to treat ulcerative gingivitis[ZO119]. Hot water extract of the fresh rhizome is administered subcutaneously to treat filariasis[ZO193]. The fresh rhizome juice is administered to pregnant women just before childbirth to ease delivery. The fresh rhizome is eaten for tuberculosis and throat pain[ZO246] and for stomachache[ZO248]. For anemia, *Tinospora cordifolia*, alone, or in combination with *Strobilanthes auriculatus* roots and the dried rhizome of *Zingiber officinale*, is made into a decoction and taken orally[ZO248]. For digestive complaints, the leaf juice of *Piper betel* and leaf juice of *Zingiber officinale* are taken orally. A decoction of *Andrographis paniculata*, *Ocimum sanctum*, and *Zingiber officinale* is taken orally for malaria. Rhizome, made into a paste, is applied to the forehead for headache. For toothache, black pepper and ginger are used as a tooth powder; combined with charcoal, freshens the mouth. For the common cold, a decoction of coffee prepared with black pepper and ginger is taken orally. To relieve swellings and boils, a paste of *Zingiber officinale* rhizome and *Santalum album* stem is applied to the affected area[ZO248].

Indonesia. Hot water extract of the rhizome is taken orally to aid in childbirth[ZO071]. As an abortifacient, the rhizome, in combination with cinnamon, *Capsicum annuum*, a piece of black cane stalk pound with half of an unripe pineapple and rag (rice, garlic, and *Alpinia galanga*, aromatics, and spices such as cinnamon, ginger, *Capsicum annuum*), is diluted with water and taken twice daily. The rhizome juice is taken orally for colic and used externally in the form of a poultice for swelling of rheumatic areas and on snakebite[ZO241].

Japan. Fresh rhizome is used externally to promote hair growth[ZO239].

Malaysia. The rhizome, mixed with *Piper nigrum* and honey, is taken orally as an abortifacient[ZO064]. Hot water extract of the rhizome is administered orally after childbirth and as an abortifacient[ZO071].

Mauritius. Hot water extract of the dried root is taken orally as an emmenagogue[ZO223].

Mexico. Decoction of the entire plant is taken orally with honey as an emmenagogue and to soothe colic[ZO132]. Hot water extract of the rhizome is taken orally for stomachache[ZO228].

Morocco. Rhizome is taken orally as a calefacient[ZO160].

Nepal. Decoction of the rhizome, mixed with *Artemisia dubia*, is taken orally as an antipyretic. The juice is mixed with butter and massaged on the chest and throat to cure cough. The juice is taken orally for throat infection[ZO168]. Decoction of the rhizome, mixed with the *Justicia adhatoda*, is mixed in warm water and salt and then taken orally twice a day for 2–3 days to treat abdominal pain[ZO155].

Nicaragua. Decoction of the root is taken orally by women during childbirth, as a digestive, and for colds[ZO156]. The rhizome is taken orally for belly pain, fever, and gas[ZO151].

Nigeria. The rhizome is taken orally as a blood purifier, febrifuge, carminative, and stimulant, and for malaria, stomachache, headache, and indigestion[ZO102]. Water extract of the dried rhizome is taken orally to treat malaria[ZO097] and schistosomiasis[ZO224].

Oman. Infusion of the rhizome is taken orally as an expectorant and for bronchitis.

The infusion is administered ophthalmically for cataract[ZO116].

Papua New Guinea. Fresh rhizome juice is taken orally for colds and cough. The fresh rhizome is chewed for malaria, stomach worms, and the temporary relief of toothache[ZO191]. The fresh rhizome is taken orally for pneumonia, tuberculosis, fever, and rheumatism and externally for topical ulcers[ZO254]. Hot water extract of the dried root is taken orally for stomach complaints[ZO254]. The chewed rhizome and leaf are used externally to treat knee pain and swallowed to treat cough[ZO134]. The dried rhizome is chewed, and the juice applied externally for migraine and to treat stingray stings[ZO277]. The juice is taken orally to treat vomiting and stomachache. For head lice, the rhizome is mixed with bark of *Galbulimima belgraveana* and leaves of *Nicotiana tabacum* and the juice is applied externally[ZO294].

Peru. Hot water extract of the dried rhizome is taken orally as a carminative[ZO288] and contraceptive[ZO289].

Philippines. Hot water extract of the dried root is taken orally by pregnant women to minimize the pain of early labor[ZO261].

Rodrigues Islands. Decoction of the rhizome juice, mixed with *Citrus aurantifolia*, is taken orally for pulmonary disorders. The juice, mixed with lemon juice, honey, and hot water extract of *Cymbopogon citratus*, is taken orally for colds[ZO153].

Saudi Arabia. Hot water extract of the dried rhizome is taken orally as a stomachic, a diuretic, a carminative, and an antiemetic[ZO178,ZO184] and used externally as an antiseptic, anesthetic, and astringent[ZO178].

South Korea. Hot water extract of the dried rhizome is taken orally as an abortifacient[ZO264]. Hot water extract of the rhizome, together with *Bupleurum falcatum*, *Scutellaria baicalensis*, *Panax ginseng*, *Glycyrrhiza glabra*, *Zizyphus jujuba*, and *Pinellia tuberosa*, is taken orally for tonsillitis, otitis media, tuberculosis, common cold, liver disorders, chills, fevers, and chest pains[ZO267].

Sudan. Hot water extract of the dried rhizome is taken orally for colds, pneumonia, and rheumatism[ZO227].

Tanzania. Rhizome is pound with the root of *Pteridium aquilinum*, and the juice taken orally as an aphrodisiac. Hot water extract of the rhizome is taken orally as a galactagogue[ZO069,ZO070].

Thailand. Hot water extract of the dried rhizome is taken orally as a carminative[ZO211,ZO212], an antiemetic, an anticolic, a hypnotic, a cardiotonic[ZO212], an emmenagogue, and a stomachic[ZO213]. The fresh rhizome is taken orally as an antiemetic and a gastrointestinal sedative[ZO158]. Hot water extract of the fresh rhizome is taken orally for fever, headache, and diarrhea and as an emmenagogue, a carminative[ZO215], and an aromatic stimulant[ZO216]. The powdered fresh rhizome, together with cloves, are mixed with water and rubbed on the body for the relief of rheumatism[ZO216].

Trinidad. Hot water extract of the rhizome is taken orally for diabetes[ZO101,ZO103].

United States. Hot water extract of the dried rhizome is taken orally as a carminative in flatulent colic and when a warming effect is needed[ZO304]. Wine extract of the dried rhizome, together with *Viburnum opulus*, *Scutellaria lateriflora*, *Symplocarous foetidus*, and *Syzygium aromaticum*, is taken as an antispasmodic[ZO304].

Venezuela. Hot water extract of the rhizome is taken orally to stimulate the menstrual flow[ZO090].

Vietnam. Hot water extract of the rhizome is taken orally as an emmenagogue[ZO066].

Yemen. Hot water extract of the rhizome is taken orally as an aphrodisiac and is used as an aromatic stimulant[ZO234].

CHEMICAL CONSTITUENTS

(ppm unless otherwise indicated)
Acetaldehyde: Rh[ZO305]
Acetic acid: Rh[ZO295]
Acetone: Rh[ZO305]
Aframodial: Sd 0.04%[ZO082]

Angelicoidenol-2-O-β-D-glucopyranoside: Rh 14[ZO084]

Arginine: Tu[ZO247]

Aromadendrene: Rh EO[ZO195]

Aromadendrene, allo: Rh EO 0.14%[ZO290]

Asparagine: Rh 0.05%[ZO308]

Aspartic acid: Aer, Tu[ZO247]

Benzaldehyde: Rh[ZO295]

Benzaldehyde, 3-phenyl: Rh EO[ZO195]

Benzaldehyde, 4-phenyl: Rh EO[ZO195]

Bisabolene: Rh EO[ZO068]

Bisabolene, β: Rh 17.2-30.0[ZO131,ZO079], Rh EO 10.51%[ZO140]

Bisabolene, γ: Rh EO 2.5%[ZO122]

Bisabolol, β: Rh EO 0.59%[ZO290]

Borneol: Rh EO 1.8%[ZO290]

Borneol acetate: Rh EO 0.21%[ZO290]

Borneol methyl ethyl: Rh[ZO144]

Borneol, (+): Rh EO[ZO306]

Borneol, 5-hydroxy-O-β-D-glucopyranoside: Rh 8.5[ZO170]

Borneol, iso: Rh[ZO144]

Butyraldehyde, *N*: Rh[ZO305]

Cadinene, α: Rh EO[ZO195]

Cadinene, δ: Rh EO 0.13%[ZO290]

Cadinol, α: Rh EO[ZO195]

Caffeic acid: Rh[ZO226]

Calamenene: Rh EO[ZO195]

Camphene: Rh EO 12.6%[ZO290]

Camphene hydrate: Rh[ZO144]

Camphor: Rh EO 0.12%[ZO290]

Caprylic acid: Rh EO[ZO306]

Capsaicin: Rh[ZO311]

Car-3-ene: Rh EO[ZO219]

Caryophyllene: EO[ZO068]

Caryophyllene, β: Rh EO 0.09%[ZO290]

Cedorol: Rh EO[ZO195]

Cedrol, α: Rh EO[ZO121]

Chavicol: Rh EO[ZO306]

Chrysanthemin: Rh[ZO129]

Cineol, 1-8: Rh EO 2.6-10%[ZO290,ZO229]

Cineol, 1-8, 2-hydroxy: Rh[ZO295]

Citral: Rh EO 13.0%[ZO067]

Citronellal: Rh EO 0.29%[ZO290]

Citronellol: Rh EO 0.3-13.0%[ZO290,ZO067]

Citronellol acetate: Rh EO[ZO121]

Citronellyl acetate: Rh EO[ZO195]

Copaene, α: Rh EO[ZO293]

Coumaric acid, para: Rh 19[ZO226]

Cubebene, α: Rh EO[ZO121]

Curcumene, α: Rh EO 1.94%[ZO140]

Curcumin: Rh[ZO130]

Curcumin, hexahydro: Rh 21.3[ZO109]

Curcumin, hexahydrodemethyl: Rh[ZO179]

Cyclobutane, *cis*-1-2-*bis*-(*trans*-3-4-dimethoxy styryl): Rh 13.9[ZO081]

Cyclohexene, *cis*-3-(3-4-dimethoxy phenyl)-4-(*trans*-3-4-dimethoxy styryl): Rh 50.6[ZO081]

Cyclohexene, *trans*-3-(2-4-5-trimethoxy phenyl)-4-(*trans*-3-4-dimethoxy styryl): Rh 13.9[ZO081]

Cyclohexene, *trans*-3-(3-4-dimethoxy phenyl)-4-(*trans*-3-4-dimethoxy styryl): Rh 55.8[ZO081]

Cymen-8-ol, para: Rh EO 0.07%[ZO290]

Cymene, para: Rh EO 2.6%[ZO290]

Cysteine: Aer[ZO247]

Dec-*trans*-2-en-1-al: Rh[ZO144]

Deca-3-5-diene, 3-6-epoxy-1-(hydroxy-3-methoxy phenyl): Rh[ZO080]

Decan-1-al: Rh[ZO144]

Decane, 3(R)-5(S)-diacetoxy-1-(3-4-dimethoxy phenyl): Rh[ZO077]

Decane, 3(R)-5(S)-diacetoxy-1-(4-hydroxy-3-methoxy phenyl): Rh 41.8[ZO077]

Decane, 3(R)-acetoxy-5(S)-hydroxy-1-(4-hydroxy-3-methoxy phenyl): Rh 53.1[ZO077]

Decane, 5(S)-acetoxy-3(R)-hydroxy-1-(4-hydroxy-3-methoxy phenyl): Rh 15.8[ZO077]

Diethyl sulfide: Rh[ZO305]

Dodec-*trans*-2-en-1-al: Rh[ZO144]

Elemene, β: Rh EO 0.3%[ZO290]

Elemol: Rh EO 0.38%[ZO290]

Essential oil: Rh 0.08-0.21%[ZO229]

Ethyl acetate: Rh[ZO305]

Ethyl myristate: Rh EO[ZO195]

Eudesmol, β: Rh EO 0.93%[ZO290]

Eudesmol, γ: Rh EO 0.23%[ZO290]

Eugenol: Rh EO[ZO121]

Eugenol, iso: Rh[ZO144]

Eugenol, iso methyl ether: Rh EO 0.08%[ZO290]

Farnesal: Rh EO 0.20%[ZO290]

Farnesene: EO[ZO068]

Farnesene, α: Rh EO 2.5%[ZO290]

Farnesene, α *trans*-*trans*: Rh[ZO201]

Farnesene, β: Rt EO[ZO225]
Farnesene, β *trans*: Rh EO 0.12%[ZO290]
Farnesol: Rh EO[ZO121]
Fluoride: Rh 7.9[ZO291]
Furan, 2-(2-3-epoxy-3-methyl-butyl)-3-methyl: Rh[ZO144]
Furan, 2-(3-methyl-2-butenyl)-3-methyl: Rh[ZO144]
Furanogermenone: Rh[ZO279]
Furfural: Rh EO[ZO290]
Galanolactone: Rh[ZO117]
Geranial: Rh EO 15.9-40.0% [ZO290,ZO229]
Geranic acid, *cis*: Rh[ZO295]
Geranic acid, *trans*: Rh[ZO295]
Geraniol: Rh EO 0.69%[ZO290]
Geraniol acetate: Rh EO 0.20%[ZO290]
Geraniol, β-D-glucopyranoside: Rh 15[ZO170]
Geranium: Rh 87-169[ZO232,ZO236]
Gingediol, 10: Rh[ZO313]
Gingediol, 12: Rh[ZO098]
Gingediol, 12, methyl: Rh[ZO098]
Gingediol, 6: Rh 21-30[ZO109,ZO079]
Gingediol, 6, diacetate: Rh 3.3[ZO109]
Gingediol, 6, diacetate methyl ether: Rh[ZO313]
Gingediol, 6, methyl ether: Rh[ZO313]
Gingediol, 8: Rh[ZO313]
Gingerdiol, 6: Rh[ZO130]
Gingerdione, 10-dihydro: Rh 6.3[ZO109]
Gingerdione, 10: Rh 11[ZO109]
Gingerdione, 10, dehydro: Rh[ZO180]
Gingerdione, 6-10-dehydro: Rt[ZO214]
Gingerdione, 6-10: Rt[ZO214]
Gingerdione, 6: Rh 3.3-10[ZO109,ZO079]
Gingerdione, 6, dehydro: Rh 25.3[ZO109,ZO124]
Gingerdione, 6, dihydro: Rh[ZO180]
Gingerenone A: Rh 118-136[ZO074,ZO075]
Gingerenone B: Rh 4.7[ZO074]
Gingerenone B, iso: Rh 4.7[ZO074]
Gingerenone C: Rh 14.2[ZO074]
Gingerglycolipid A: Rh 13[ZO078,ZO084]
Gingerglycolipid B: Rh 15[ZO078]
Gingerglycolipid C: Rh 14[ZO078,ZO084]
Gingerol: Rh[ZO278]
Gingerol methyl ether: Rh[ZO313]
Gingerol, 10: Rh 2.6-1862[ZO109,ZO233]
Gingerol, 10, methyl: Rh[ZO271]

Gingerol, 12: Rh[ZO309]
Gingerol, 12, methyl: Rh[ZO271]
Gingerol, 14: Rh[ZO271]
Gingerol, 16: Rh[ZO309]
Gingerol, 4: Rh EO[ZO310]
Gingerol, 6: Rh 0.04%-0.71%[ZO147,ZO233]
Gingerol, 6, (+): Rt[ZO109]
Gingerol, 6, (S)(+): Pl[ZO107]
Gingerol, 6, 5-methoxy: Rh[ZO135]
Gingerol, 6, acetyl: Rh 6.6[ZO109]
Gingerol, 6, methyl: Rh[ZO271]
Gingerol, 7: Rh[ZO309]
Gingerol, 8: Rh 110-1069[ZO079, ZO233]
Gingerol, 8, methyl: Rh[ZO271]
Gingerol, 9: Rh[ZO309]
Gingerol, dihydro: Rt EO[ZO225]
Gingerol, methyl: EO[ZO068]
Gingesulfonic acid, 6: Rh 13[ZO084]
Glanolactone: Rh 120[ZO198]
Glycine: Aer, Tu[ZO247]
Guaiol: Rh EO[ZO195]
Hept-4-en-3-one, 7-(3-4-dihydroxy-phenyl)-1-(4-hydroxy-3-methoxy-phenyl): Rh 1.4[ZO076]
Hept-5-en-1-al, 2-6-dimethyl: Rh[ZO144]
Hept-5-en-2-ol, 6-methyl: Rh[ZO295]
Hept-5-en-2-one, 6-methyl: Rh EO[ZO195]
Heptan-2-ol: Rh 0.27%[ZO290]
Heptan-2-ol-β-D-glucopyranoside: Rh 71.6[ZO170]
Heptan-2-one: Rh EO[ZO290]
Heptan-3-one, 5-hydroxy-1-(4-hydroxy-3-5-dimethoxy-phenyl)-7-(4-hydroxy-3-methoxy-phenyl): Rh 0.52[ZO076]
Heptan-3-one, 5-hydroxy-7-(4-hydroxy-3-5-dimethoxy-phenyl)-1-(4-hydroxy-3-methoxy-phenyl): Rh 5.2[ZO076]
Heptan-3-one, 5-hydroxy-7-(4-hydroxy-phenyl)-1-(4-hydroxy-3-methoxy-phenyl): Rh 5.2[ZO076]
Heptane, 1-5-epoxy-3-epi-hydroxy-1-3-4-dihydroxy-5-methoxy-phenyl)-7-(4-hydroxy-3-methoxy-phenyl): Rh[ZO083]
Heptane, 1-5-epoxy-3-hydroxy-1-(3-4-dihydroxy-5-methoxy-phenyl)-7-(4-hydroxy-3-methoxy-phenyl): Rh[ZO083]

Heptane, 1-5-epoxy-3- hydroxy-1- (4-dihydroxy-3-5-dimethoxy-phenyl)-7-(4-hydroxy-3-methoxy-phenyl): Rh[ZO083]

Heptane, 2(R)-5(S)-dihydroxy-1-7-*bis*- (4-hydroxy-3-methoxy-phenyl): Rh 0.00056%[ZO076]

Heptane, 2-2-4-trimethyl: Rh EO[ZO195]

Heptane, 3(S)-5(S)-diacetoxy-1-(4'-hydroxy-3'-5'-dimethoxy-phenyl)-7-(4''-hydroxy-3'-methoxy-phenyl): Rh 20[ZO079]

Heptane, 3(S)-5(S)-diacetoxy-1-7-*bis*-(3-4-dihydroxy-phenyl): Rh 15.7[ZO076]

Heptane, 3(S)-5(S)-dihydroxy-1-(4'-hydroxy-3'-5'-dimethoxy-phenyl)-7-(4'-hydroxy-3'-methoxy-phenyl): Rh 2[ZO079]

Heptane, 3(S)-5(S)-dihydroxy-1-7-*bis*-(4-hydroxy-3- methoxy-phenyl):Rh 0.00053%[ZO076]

Heptane, 3-5-diacetoxy-1-(4-hydroxy-3-5-dimethoxy-henyl)-7-(4-hydroxy-3-methoxy-phenyl): Rh 30.3[ZO075]

Heptane, 3-5-diacetoxy-1-7-*bis*-(4-hydroxy-3-methoxy-phenyl, MeSO: Rh 40.8[ZO075]

Heptane, 3-5-diacetoxy-7-(3-4-dihydroxy-phenyl)-1-(4-hydroxy-3-methoxy-phenyl): Rh 3.5[ZO076]

Heptane, 3-acetoxy-1-5-epoxy-1- (3-4-dihydroxy-5-methoxy-phenyl)-7-(4-hydroxy-3-methoxy-phenyl): Rh[ZO083]

Heptane, 3-epi-acetoxy-1-5-epoxy-1-(3-4-dihydroxy-5-methoxy-phenyl)-7-(4-hydroxy-3-methoxy-phenyl): Rh[ZO083]

Heptane, *N*: Rh[ZO305]

Heptane-3(S)-diol, 1-7-*bis*- (4-hydroxy-3-methoxy-phenyl): Rh 4[ZO079]

Heptenone, methyl: Rh EO[ZO306]

Hexan-1-al: Rh EO 700[ZO290]

Hexan-1-ol: Rh[ZO295]

Hexan-3-ol, *cis*: Rh EO[ZO195]

Himachalene, β: Rh EO[ZO195]

Humulene epoxide 1: Rh[ZO145]

Humulene epoxide 2: Rh[ZO145]

Ionone, β: Rh EO[ZO195]

Juniper camphor: Rh EO[ZO195]

Labda-*trans*-12-ene-15-16-dial, 8-β-17-epoxy: Rh[ZO126]

Labda-*trans*-6(17)-12-diene-15-16-dial: Rh[ZO135]

Lauric acid: Rh EO 900[ZO290]

Leucine: Tu[ZO247]

Leucine, iso: Tu[ZO247]

Limonene: Rh EO 2.1%[ZO290]

Linalool: Rh EO 1–3%[ZO229]

Linalool, oxide: Rh[ZO295]

Linalool, propionate: Rh EO[ZO121]

Linalool, *trans*, oxide: Rh EO[ZO195]

Linalool-β-D-glucopyranoside: Rh 11.6[ZO170]

Melatonin: Rh[ZO295]

Mentha-1-5-dien-7-ol, para: Rh[ZO295]

Mentha-2-8-dien-1-ol, para: Rh[ZO295]

Mentha-1-5-dien-8-ol, para: Rh[ZO295]

Menthan-3-ol, 1-8-epoxy-para-glucopyranoside: Rh 5.8[ZO170]

Menthol acetate: Rh EO[ZO195]

Metha-1-8-dien-7-ol, para: Rh[ZO295]

Methyl acetate: Rh[ZO305]

Methyl nonyl ketone: Rh EO[ZO195]

Muurolene, α: Rh EO[ZO195]

Muurolene, γ: Rh EO 0.91%[ZO290]

Myrcene: Rh[ZO175], Rh EO 1.9%[ZO290]

Myrcene, β: Rh EO[ZO195]

Myrtenal: Rh EO 0.06%[ZO290]

Neral: Rh EO 8.10%-26.0%[ZO290,ZO229]

Nerol: Rh EO[ZO219]

Nerol, oxide: Rh[ZO295]

Nerol-β-D-glucopyranoside: Rh 0.2[ZO170]

Nerolidol: Rh EO[ZO121], Rh[ZO295]

Nerolidol, 9-oxo: Rh EO[ZO195]

Nerolidol, *cis*: Rh EO[ZO140]

Nerolidol, *trans*: Rh EO 0.70%[ZO290]

Nonal-1-al: Rh[ZO144]

Nonal-2-ol: Rh[ZO295], Rh EO 0.2%[ZO290]

Nonane, *N*: Rh[ZO305]

Nonanol, *N*: Rh[ZO305]

Nonanone, *N*: Rh EO[ZO229]

Nonyl aldehyde: Rh EO[ZO306]

Octan-1-ol acetate: Rh[ZO144]

Oct-*trans*-2-en-1-al: Rh[ZO144]

Octa-2-6-diene-1-8-diol, 2-6-dimethyl: Rh[ZO295]

Octa-3-7-diene-1-6-diol, 2-6-dimethyl: Rh[ZO295]

Octa-3-*cis*-6-dien-1-al, 3-7-dimethyl: Rh[ZO144]

Octa-3-*trans*-6-dien-1-al, 3-7-dimethyl: Rh[ZO144]

Octa-*trans*-2-*cis*-6-dien-1-ol, 3-7-dimethyl-8-hydroxy, β-D-glucopyranoside: Rh 5.2[ZO170]

Octa-*trans*-2-*trans*-6-dien-1-ol, 3-7-dimethyl-8-hydroxy, β-D-glucopyranoside: Rh 10.1[ZO170]

Octan-1-al: Rh EO 800[ZO290]

Octan-2-ol: Rh[ZO295]

Octane, N: Rh[ZO305]

Octanol, N: Rh[ZO295]

Octen-2-al, *trans*: Rh EO[ZO195]

Oxalic acid: Rt 0.50%[ZO312]

Paradol: Rh[ZO313]

Paradol, 6: Rh[ZO177]

Patchouli alcohol: Rh EO[ZO195]

Pentan-2-ol: Rh[ZO295]

Perilla aldehyde: Rh EO[ZO140]

Perillen: Rh EO[ZO195]

Perillene: RH EO[ZO114]

Phellandrene, α: Rh EO 0.40%[ZO290]

Phellandrene, β: Rh EO 5.70%[ZO290]

Pin-2-en-5-ol, Rh[ZO144]

Pinene, α: Rh EO 3.90%[ZO290]

Pinene, β: Rh EO 0.53%[ZO290]

Pipecolic acid: Rh 0.032%[ZO308]

Propanol, N: Rh[ZO305]

Propionaldehyde: Rh[ZO305]

Protease: Rh[ZO125]

Pulegole, iso, neo: Rh EO[ZO195]

Rose oxide, *cis*: Rh[ZO144]

Rose oxide, *trans*: Rh[ZO144]

Rosefuran: Rh EO 0.18%[ZO290]

Sabinene: Rh[ZO305]

Santalol, β: Rh EO 16.20%[ZO140]

Selina-3-7(11)-diene: Rh EO 0.13%[ZO290]

Selinen-4-ol, *cis*: Rh[ZO295]

Selinene, α: Rh EO[ZO195]

Selinene, β: Rh EO[ZO195]

Serine: Aer, Tu[ZO247]

Sesquiabinene, *cis*, hydrate: Rh EO[ZO195]

Sesquiphellandrene: Rh EO[ZO195]

Sesquiphellandrene, β: Rh EO[ZO122]

Sesquiphellandrol, β: Rh[ZO175]

Sesquiphellandrol, β, *cis*: Rh EO[ZO088]

Sesquiphellandrol, β, *trans*: Rh EO 0.72%[ZO290]

Sesquisabinene, *cis*, hydrate: Rh[ZO089]

Sequiterpene hydrocarbon: Rh EO[ZO195]

Sesquithujene: Rh[ZO089]

Shikimic acid: Lf[ZO086]

Shogaol: Rh[ZO230]

Shogaol, 10: Rh 73.5[ZO147]

Shogaol, 10, *cis*: Rh[ZO269]

Shogaol, 10, dehydro: Rh 0.031[ZO085]

Shogaol, 10, methyl, anti: Rh[ZO269]

Shogaol, 10, methyl, syn: Rh[ZO269]

Shogaol, 10, *trans*: Rh[ZO269]

Shogaol, 12, *cis*: Rh[ZO269]

Shogaol, 12, *trans*: Rh[ZO269]

Shogaol, 6: Rh 278.5-400[ZO147,ZO198]

Shogaol, 6, *cis*: Rh[ZO269]

Shogaol, 6, methyl: Rh[ZO098]

Shogaol, 6, methyl, anti: Rh[ZO269]

Shogaol, 6, methyl, syn: Rh[ZO269]

Shogaol, 6, *trans*: Rh[ZO269]

Shogaol, 8: Rh 48-130[ZO147]

Shogaol, 8, *cis*: Rh[ZO269]

Shogaol, 8, dehydro: Rh 0.046[ZO085]

Shogaol, 8, methyl, anti: Rh[ZO269]

Shogaol, 8, methyl, syn: Rh[ZO269]

Shogaol, 8, *trans*: Rh[ZO269]

Starch: Rh 12.3%[ZO231]

Sulfide, ethyl iso-propyl: Rh[ZO305]

Sulfide, methyl allyl: Rh[ZO305]

Terpine, 1-8, hydrate: Rh[ZO295]

Terpinen-4-ol: Rh[ZO144]

Terpinene, α: Rh EO 0.07%[ZO290]

Terpinene, γ: Rh EO[ZO195]

Terpineol, 4: Rh[ZO295]

Terpineol, α: Rh EO1.00%[ZO290]

Terpinolene: Rh EO 0.18%[ZO290]

Threonine: Aer, Tu[ZO247]

Thujone, β: Rh EO[ZO195]

Tricyclene: Rh EO 0.23%[ZO290]

Undecan-2-ol: Rh EO 0.05%[ZO290]

Undecan-2-one: Rh EO[ZO121]

Undecanone, N: Rh EO[ZO229]

Uridine: Rh 11[ZO084]

Valeraldehyde, iso: Rh[ZO305]

Valine: Aer, Tu[ZO247]

Xanthorrhizol: Rh EO 0.10%[ZO290]

Ylangene, α: Rh[ZO295]

Zerumbodienone: Rh[ZO145]

Zingerberone: EO[ZO068]

Zingerone: Rh[ZO176], Rt EO[ZO225]

Zingibenene, α: Rh EO 9.2%[ZO290]

Zingiberene: Rh 0.06%[ZO181], Rt EO[ZO087]

Zingiberene, α: Rh EO 44.26%[ZO140]
Zingiberenol: Rh[ZO089]
Zingiberine: Rt[ZO173]
Zingiberol: Rh EO 0.29%[ZO140]
Zingiberone: Rh 0.04%[ZO307]

PHARMACOLOGICAL ACTIVITIES AND CLINICAL TRIALS

Adrenocorticotropic hormone induction. Dried rhizome, in a mixture of 7 g *Bupleurum falcatum*, 5 g *Pinellia ternata*, 3 g *Scutellaria baicalensis*, 4 g *Zingiber officinale*, 3 g *Zizyphus inermis*, 3 g *Panax ginseng*, and 2 g *Glycyrrhiza glabra*, increased plasma adrenocorticotropic hormone (ACTH) level in plasma relative to controls. The increase was not found in adrenalectomized or dexamethasone-treated animals[ZO283].

Acyl-coenzyme A cholesterol acyltransferase inhibition. Decoction of the dried rhizome, administered intragastrically to mice at a dose of 1.2 g/kg, inhibited the incorporation of oleic acid into cholesteryl oleate. The study was conducted with prescription know as shosaikoto, which consists of *Bupleurum falcatum Bupleurum falcatum* (Rt), *Scutellaria baicalensis Scutellaria baicalensis* (Rt), *Pinellia ternata* (Tu), *Zizyphus jujuba* (Fr), *Panax ginseng* (Rt), and *Glycyrrhiza glabra* (Rh)[ZO111].

Alanine aminotransferase inhibition. Decoction of dried rhizome, taken orally by human adults of both sexes at a dose of 7.5 g/day for 6 months, was active on 80 patients with hepatitis B antigen-positive chronic hepatitis. The study was conducted with a prescription that consists of *B.upleurum falcatum Bupleurum falcatum* (Rt), *Scutellaria baicalensis Scutellaria baicalensis* (Rt), *Pinellia ternata* (Tu), *Zizyphus jujuba* (Fr), *Panax ginseng* (Rt), and *Glycyrrhiza glabra* (Rh)[ZO123].

Allergenic effect. A food industry worker developed asthma in inhalation of dust from spices. Skin prick test from ginger was strongly positive. With radioallergosorbent test (RAST), specific immunoglobulin (Ig) E antibodies could be demonstrated in the serum. Leukocytes from a normal donor, after passive sensitization with serum from the patient, released a substantial ($\geq$50%) amount of histamine on challenge with ginger indicating an IgE-mediated allergy toward ginger[ZO058].

Analgesic activity. Ethanol (80%) extract of the rhizome, administered intragastrically to rats at a dose of 100 mg/kg, was inactive vs writhing-induced by acetic acid injection[ZO292]. Hydroalcoholic extract of the dried rhizome, administered intragastrically to mice at a dose of 200 mg/kg, was active vs hot-plate method, tail flick response to radiant heat, and capsaicin-induced algesia and produced weak activity vs acetic acid-induced writhing and formalin-induced algesia[ZO093]. Rhizome juice, administered intragastrically to mice at a dose of 199.8 mg/animal, was active vs tail flick response to radiant heat. The activity produced was equivalent to 10 mg/kg body weight of aspirin[ZO110]. Decoction of the dried rhizome, administered intragastrically to mice at a dose of 1.2 g/kg on days 1–7, was active vs hot-plate method. A dose of 300 mg/kg on days 1–8 was active vs cold stress-induced hyperalgesia, and a dose of 100 mg/kg on days 1–22 was active vs adjuvant-induced hyperalgesia. A mixture of *Cinnamomum cassia* (Bk), *Zingiber officinale* (Rz), *Glycyrrhiza glabra* (Rt), *Zizyphus jujuba* (Fr), *Ephedra sinica* (St), *Asarum* species (Rt), and *Aconitum* species (Rt) was used[ZO199]. Methanol (50%) extract of the rhizome, administered subcutaneously to mice at a dose of 10 g/kg, was active vs inhibition of acetic acid-induced writhing and inactive vs hot-plate method. A dose of 3 g/kg was inactive vs inhibition of acetic acid-induced writhing[ZO237]. Water extract of the dried rhizome, in combination with *Bupleurum falcatum*, *Scutellaria baicalensis*, *Paeonia alba*, *Rheum tanguticum*, *Citrus aurantium*, *Pinellia ter-*

nata, and *Zizyphus inermis,* administered by gastric intubation to mice at a dose of 200 mg/kg, was active vs acetic acid-induced writhing and pressure pain threshold test[ZO323].

Anesthetic activity. Hot water extract of the rhizome, at a concentration of 1%, was active on the sciatic nerve[ZO220].

Angiotensin-II inhibition. Methanol extract of the rhizome, at a concentration of 200 µg/mL, was inactive on rat liver membrane[ZO324].

Anthelmintic activity. Saline extract of the dried rhizome, at a concentration of 2.5%, was 100% effective on *Anisakis* species larvae[ZO143].

Anti-5-hydroxytryptamine effects. Galanolactone, a diterpenoid and one of the active constituents of ginger, was investigated on the guinea pig ileum, rat stomach fundus, and rabbit aortic strips. In the guinea pig ileum, galanolactone inhibited contractile responses to 5-hydroxytryptamine with a pIC_{50} value of 4.93. The concentration-response curve of 5-hydroxytryptamine was shown as a biphasic curve, and galanolactone produced a selective shift to the right of the second phase. In the same preparations, the pIC_{50} value of galanolactone against the response to carbamylcholine was 4.45. The inhibitory effect of galanolactone on the 5-hydroxytryptamine responses in the stomach fundus and aortic strips was less than that in the ileum. In addition, in the thoracic aorta precontracted with 50 mM K^+, the relaxing effect of galanolactone was approx 10% of that of papaverine[ZO039].

Anti-allergenic activity. Hot water extract of the of the dried rhizome, administered by gastric intubation to mice at a dose of 100 mg/kg, was inactive vs type IV reaction with contact dermatitis induced by picryl chloride and type I reaction induced by antidinitrophenylated ascaris-IgE serum in 48 hours homologous PCA in rats. Dosing

was immediately before and 16 hours after challenge. The extract, in a mixture of *Pinellia ternata* (Tu), *Bupleurum falcatum* (Rt), *Pachyma hoelen* (Rt), *Scutellaria baicalensis* (Rt), *Panax ginseng* (Rt), *Glycyrrhiza glabra* (Rt), *Zizyphus vulgaris* (Fr), *Magnolia officinalis* (Bk), and *Perilla frutescens* (Pl) in ratios 9:4:3:2:1.5:1.5:1.5:1.5:1.5:1, was active vs type IV reaction with contact dermatitis induced by picryl chloride and inactive vs type I reaction induced by antidinitrophenylated ascaris-IgE serum in 48 hours homologous passive cutaneous anaphylaxis (PCA) in rats. The results were significant to $p < 0.05$ level. A mixture of *Bupleurum falcatum* (Rt), *Pinellia ternata* (Tu), *Scutellaria baicalensis* (Rt), *Panax ginseng* (Rt), *Glycyrrhiza glabra* (Rt), *Zizyphus vulgaris* (Fr), and *Zizyphus bulgaris* (Rh) (8:8:3:3:3:3:1), was inactive vs type IV reaction with contact dermatitis induced by picryl chloride and active vs type I reaction induced by antidinitrophenylated ascaris-IgE serum in 48 hours homologous PCA in rats[ZO240].

Anti-amoebic activity. Ethanol (80%) extract of the dried rhizome was inactive on *Entamoeba histolytica,* minimum inhibitory concentration (MIC) greater than 1 mg/mL[ZO136]. The extract, administered intragastrically to male hamsters at a dose of 800 mg/kg, was active vs experimentally induced hepatic amebiasis[ZO105]. A dose of 250 mg/kg, administered intragastrically to rats on days 1–5, produced weak activity and a dose of 500 mg/kg was active[ZO136].

Anti-atherosclerotic activity. Ethanol (50%) extract of the dried rhizome, administered intragastrically to male rabbits at a dose of 500 mg/kg, reduced atherogenic index from 4.7 to 1.2 on the aorta[ZO091].

Antibacterial activity. Decoction of the dried entire plant, on agar plate, was inactive on *Proteus vulgaris, Staphylococcus aureus,* and *Staphylococcus epidermidis;* MIC 125 mg/mL. *Bacillus subtilis, Bordetella* *bronchiseptica*, *Sarcina lutea*, and *Pseudomonas aeruginosa*, MIC 250 mg/mL. The decoction produced weak activity on *Bacillus cereus* and *Micrococcus flavus*; MIC 31.25 mg/mL[ZO287]. The essential oil, on agar plate at room temperature, was active on *Lactobacillus acidophilus* and inactive at 37°C. The treatment was inactive on *Bacillus cereus*. No difference was observed in antibacterial activity at room temperature (25–30°C) or at 37°C. Acetone extract of the dried leaf, on agar plate, was active on *Escherichia coli*, *Pseudomonas aeruginosa*, *Salmonella* B, *Salmonella typhi*, *Sarcina lutea*, and *Shigella flexneri* and inactive on *Salmonella newport*, *Serratia marcescens*, *Staphylococcus albus*, and *Staphylococcus aureus*. Ethanol (95%) extract of the dried leaf on agar plate was inactive on *Escherichia coli*, *Pseudomonas aeruginosa*, *Salmonella* B, *Salmonella newport*, *Salmonella typhi*, *Sarcina lutea*, *Serratia marcescens*, *Shigella flexneri*, *Staphylococcus albus*, and *Staphylococcus aureus*. The water extract was active on *Escherichia coli*, *Pseudomonas aeruginosa*, and *Shigella flexneri* and inactive on *Salmonella* B, *Salmonella newport*, *Salmonella typhi*, *Sarcinia lutea*, *Serratia marcescens*, *Staphylococcus albus*, and *Staphylococcus aureus*[ZO296]. The leaf essential oil was active on *Staphylococcus aureus* and inactive on *Escherichia coli* and *Pseudomonas aeruginosa*[ZO222]. Ethanol (80%) extract of the rhizome, on agar plate at a concentration of 50 µg/disc was active on *Bacillus anthracis*, *Bacillus subtilis*, *Escherichia coli* (strains 7075 and BB), *Proteus mirabilis*, *Pseudomonas aeruginosa*, *Salmonella typhi* (strain H), *Staphylococcus aureus*, *Staphylococcus epidermidis*, and *Staphylococcus haemolyticus*[ZO292]. Decoction of the rhizome, on agar plate, was inactive on *Streptococcus mutans*, MIC 250 mg/mL[ZO189]. Water extract of the rhizome, on agar plate at a concentration of 5 mg/mL, was inactive on *Helicobacter pylori*[ZO167]. Powdered-dried rhizome, in broth culture at a concentration of 4.5%, was inactive on

Yersinia enterolitica[ZO325]. Ethanol (90%) extract of the dried rhizome, on agar plate at a concentration of 500 mg/disc, produced weak activity on *Bacillus subtilis*, *Escherichia coli*, *Streptococcus aureus*, and *Streptococcus faecalis*[ZO318]. Hot water extract of the dried rhizome, on agar plate at a concentration of 50 mg/disc, was inactive on *Salmonella typhimurium* TA100 and TA98[ZO326].

Antibody formation enhancement. Decoction of the dried rhizome, in cell culture at a concentration of 100 µg/mL, was active. Peripheral lymphocytes from eight patients with chronic active hepatitis, four with hepatits B e antigen (HbeAg) and four with anti-Hbe, were cultured. Anti-hepatits B cove (HBc) and anti-Hbe antibodies produced by HbcAg stimulation were enhanced by the treatment, which consisted of *Zingiber officinale* (Rh), *Bupleurum falcatum* (Rt), *Scutellaria baicalensis* (Rt), *P. ternata* (Tu), *Zizyphus jujuba* (Fr), *Panax ginseng* (Rt), and *Glycyrrhiza glabra* (Rh)[ZO108]. The decoction was also active on peripheral blood monocytes from healthy adults treated with pokeweed mitogen. The treatment enhanced plaque cell formation in response to sheep red blood cells[ZO123].

Anticathartic effect. Acetone extract of ginger, administered orally to rats at a dose of 75 mg/kg, significantly inhibited 5-hydroxytryptamine-induced diarrhea. To clarify the active constituents responsible, extract was fractionated into four fractions by silica gel chromatography. Fractions two and three, which were effective, were further purified and [6]-shogaol, [6]-dehydrogingerdione, and [8]- and [10]-gingerol had an anticathartic action. [6]-shogaol was more potent than [6]-dehydrogingerdione and [8]- and [10]-gingerol[ZO041].

Anticholesterolemic activity. Ginger, administered orally to rats, significantly elevated the activity of hepatic cholesterol-7

α-hydroxylase, the rate-limiting enzyme of bile acid biosynthesis. The results indicated that ginger could stimulate the conversion of cholesterol to bile acids, an important pathway of elimination of cholesterol from the body[ZO040]. Standardized ginger extracts were evaluated for their effects on the development of atherosclerosis in apolipoprotein E (apo E)-deficient mice, in relation to plasma cholesterol levels and resistance of the low-density lipoprotein (LDL) to oxidation and aggregation. Sixty apo E-deficient mice, 6 weeks of age, were divided into three groups of 20 each and administered via the drinking water the following treatment for 10 weeks: group 1, placebo (control group); 1.1% alcohol; group 2, 25 µg of ginger extract in 1.1% alcohol; and group 3, 250 µg of ginger extract in 1.1% alcohol. Aortic atherosclerotic lesion areas were reduced 44% ($p < 0.01$) in mice that consumed 250 µg of extract/day. It also resulted in reductions ($p < 0.01$) in plasma triglycerides and cholesterol by 27 and 29%, respectively, in very low-density lipoprotein (VLDL) by 36 and 53%, respectively, and in LDL by 58 and 33%, respectively. These results were associated with a 76% reduction in cellular cholesterol biosynthesis rate in peritoneal macrophages derived from the apo E-deficient mice that consumed the high dose. Peritoneal macrophages harvested from apo E-deficient mice after consumption of 25 or 250 µg of the extract daily had a lower ($p < 0.01$) capacity to oxidize LDL (45 and 60%, respectively) and to take up and degrade oxidized LDL (43 and 47%, respectively). Consumption of 250 µg of ginger also reduced ($p < 0.01$) the basal level of LDL-associated lipid peroxides by 62%. In parallel, a 33% inhibition ($p < 0.01$) in LDL aggregation (induced by vortexing) was obtained[ZO015]. Ethanol (50%) extract of the dried rhizome, administered intragastrically to male rabbits at a dose of 500 mg/kg, reduced total cholesterol and LDL cholesterol in cholesterol-fed animals[ZO091].

Anticonvulsant activity. Hot water extract of the rhizome, at a concentration of 0.15%, was active vs inhibition of Metrazol-induced bursting of snail neurons[ZO218]. Decoction of the dried rhizome, taken orally by human adults at a concentration of 4 g/person, was active. The study involved 24 patients with frequent uncontrollable epileptic seizures. The treatment resulted in six cases that were well controlled (no seizure 10 months), 13 that were improved (marked decrease or grand mal was eliminated), and three that showed no effect. No patients had their condition worsen. The treatment also contained *Bulleurum falcatum* (Rt), *Cinnamomum cassia* (Bk), *Paeonia albiflora* (Rt), *Glycyrrhiza glabra* var. glandulifera (Rt), *Panax ginseng* (Rt), *Scutellaria baicalensis* (Rt), *Pinellia ternata* (Tu), and *Zizyphus jujuba* (Fr)[ZO249]. Water extract of the dried rhizome, administered by gastric intubation to mice at a dose of 4 g/kg, was active vs supramaximal electroshock-induced convulsions and audiogenic seizures and inactive vs strychnine- and pentlenetetrazide-induced convulsions. The results significant were at $p < 0.05$ level. The extract was used in combination with *Glycyrrhiza glabra*, *Panax ginseng*, *Scutellaria baicalensis*, *Zizyphus jujuba*, *Pinellia ternata*, *Bulleurum falcatum*, *Cinnamomum cassia*, and *Paeonia albiflora*[ZO250]. Decoction of *Zingiber officinale*, *Glycyrrhiza glabra*, *Panax ginseng*, *Scutellaria baicalensis*, *Zizyphus jujuba*, *Pinellia ternata*, *Bupleurum falcatum*, *Cinnamomum cassia*, and *Paeonia albiflora*, administered intragastrically to mice at a dose of 1 mg/kg[ZO208] and intravenously to rats at a dose of 1 mg/kg[ZO210], was active vs metrazole-induced convulsions. Water extract of *Bupleurum falcatum*, *Scutellaria baicalensis*, *Paeonia alba*, *Rheum tanguticum*, *Citrus aurantium*, *Pinellia ternata*, *Zingiber officinale*, and *Zizyphus inermis*, administered by gastric intubation to mice at a dose of 800 mg/kg, was inactive vs strychnine- and picrotoxin-induced convulsions and active vs caffeine-induced convulsions[ZO323].

Anticrustacean activity. Ethanol (95%) extract of the dried rhizome was active on *Artemia salina*, lethal dose (LD)$_{50}$ 100 µg/mL[ZO327].

Antidiarrheal activity. Decoction of the dried rhizome, taken orally by children, was active. Infantile diarrhea was treated with kexieding capsule composed of 5 plant materials, including roasted ginger, clove, and fruit peel of *Punica granatum*. Of the 234 infants and 71 children treated, 281 (92%) were cured in 1–3 days and 9 (3%) were significantly improved. The total effective rate was 95%[ZO206]. Water extract of the dried rhizome, administered by gastric intubation to mice at a dose of 0.5 mg/g, was active vs castor oil-induced diarrhea[ZO328].

Anti-edema activity. Methanol extract of the rhizome, applied topically to mice at a dose of 2 mg/ear, was active vs 12-O-tetradecanoyl-13-acetate-induced ear inflammation. The inhibition ratio was nine[ZO118].

Anti-emetic effect. Patients scheduled to have gynecological diagnostic laparoscopy as day cases were randomly allocated into placebo, droperidol, ginger, and ginger plus droperidol groups to receive either 2 g of ginger or 1.25 mg droperidol or both. There were no significant differences in the incidences of postoperative nausea, which were 32, 20, 22, and 33%; and vomiting, which were 35, 15, 25, and 25% in the four groups, respectively[ZO025]. In a double-blind, randomized, controlled trial in 108 ASA 1 or 2 patients undergoing gynecological laparoscopic surgery under general anesthesia, the efficacy of ginger for the prevention of postoperative nausea and vomiting was studied. The patients received oral placebo, ginger BP 0.5 g, or ginger BP 1 g, all with oral diazepam premedication, 1 hour before surgery and were assessed at 3 hours postoperatively. The incidence of nausea and vomiting increased slightly but not significantly with increasing dose of ginger. The incidence of moderate or severe nausea was 22, 33, and 36%, whereas the incidence of vomiting was 17, 14, and 31% in groups receiving 0.5 and 1 g ginger, respectively[ZO028]. Water extract of the dried rhizome, administered intragastrically to male rats at a dose of 50 mg/kg, was active. The dose blocked the lithium chloride-induced conditioned place aversion, indicating antiemetic activity comparable with metoclopramide. A mixture of 50% ginger, 20% gingko, and 30% water was used[ZO142]. Powdered-dried rhizome, taken orally by human adults at a dose of 1 g/person, was active in a double-blind, placebo-controlled study on nausea in 120 patients undergoing gynecological laparoscopic same-day surgery[ZO120]. Rhizome, administered orally to female human adults at a dose of 1 g/day, was active in a crossover study in 27 women suffering from hyperemesis gravidarum. The patients received 250 mg of ginger powder or placebo four times daily for 4 days. Sickness was assessed using a symptom score. The results suggested a significantly ($p < 0.05$) greater symptomatic benefit after administration of ginger compared with placebo. In a randomized, double-blind controlled clinical study, 60 women received 1 g of rhizome per day. The patients were allocated randomly to receive ginger, 10 mg metoclopramide, or placebo as a single dose given with preoperative medication. The severity of postoperative nausea was assessed on a four-point scale. The incidence of nausea during the first 24 hours after surgery was 28%, 30%, and 51% in the ginger, metoclopramide, and placebo, respectively. A statistically significant ($p < 0.05$) difference in favor of ginger compared with placebo was reported for the total number of incidents of nausea. In a study of 120 patients, the rhizome, metoclopramide, and placebo were given 1 hour before surgery and the incidence of nausea and vomiting was 21%, 27%, and 41% in the ginger, metoclopramide, and placebo groups, respectively. Significantly fewer patients with nausea were reported in the ginger group compared with the placebo group[ZO072]. The rhizome, taken orally by pregnant human adults at a dose of 1 g/day in a double-blind randomized, crossover study, was more effective than placebo in diminishing or eliminating emesis during pregnancy[ZO329]. Acetone extract of the dried rhizome, administered intragastrically to dogs of both sexes at a dose of 200 mg/kg, was active vs cisplatin-induced emesis and inactive vs apomorphine-induced emesis. The water extract was inactive vs cisplatin-induced emesis[ZO330].

Antifungal activity. 6-Dehydrozingerone isolated by steam distillation from fresh rhizome exhibited antifungal activity against *Rhizoctonia solani*, effective concentration $(EC)_{50}$ 86.49 mg/L[ZO005]. The essential oil, on agar plate, was active on *Aspergillus niger* at 37°C and inactive at room temperature. The undiluted essential oil was active on *Alternaria* species, *Aspergillus candidus*, *Aspergillus flavus*, *Aspergillus fumigatus*, *Aspergillus nidulans*, *Aspergillus niger*, *Cladosporium herbarium*, *Cunninghamella echinulata*, *Helminthosporium sacchari*, *Microsporum gypseum*, *Mucor mucedo*, *Penicillium digitatum*, *Rhizopus nigricans*, *Trichophyton rubrum*, and *Trichothecium roseum* and inactive on *Fusarium oxysporum*[ZO113]. Acetone and ethanol (95%) extracts of the dried leaf, on agar plate at a concentration of 50%, were active on *Neurospora crassa*. The water extract, at a concentration of 50%, was inactive[ZO252].

Antigen expression. Decoction of the rhizome, in cell culture at a concentration of 100 μg/mL, was active on lymphocytes from patients who were human immunodeficiency virus (HIV)-positive asymptomatic and had acquired immunodeficiency syndrome (AIDS). The study was conducted with a prescription that contained *Bupleurum falcatum* (Rt), *Zingiber officinale* (Rh), *Scutellaria baicalensis* (Rt), *Pinellia ternata*(Tu), *Zizyphus jujuba* (Fr), *Panax ginseng* (Rt), and *Glycyrrhiza glabra* (Rh)[ZO204].

Antihepatotoxic activity. Hot water extract of the rhizome, administered by gastric intubation to rats at dosages of 100 and 400 mg/kg, was active vs CCl_4-induced hepatotoxicity. Methionine (100 mg/kg) was added to the 100 mg/kg dose. The treatment also consisted of *Bupleurum falcatum* (Rt), *Scutellaria baicalensis*(Rt), *Pinellia ternata* (Tu), *Zizyphus jujuba* (Fr), *Panax ginseng* (Rt), and *Glycyrrhiza glabra* (Rh)[ZO267]. Ethanol (50%) and water extracts of the dried rhizome, in cell culture at a concentration of 1 mg/mL, were inactive on hepatocytes vs complement-mediated cytotoxicity[ZO190]. Hot water extract of the dried rhizome, administered intragastrically to mice for 1 month, was active vs CCl_4-induced hepatotoxicity. The test agent consisted of 7 g *Bupleurum falcatum*, 5 g *Pinellia ternata*, 3 g *Scutellaria baicalensis*, 2 g *Glycyrrhiza glabra*, 1 g *Zingiber officinale*, 3 g *Panax ginseng*, and 3 g *Zizyphus jujuba* in 100 mL water[ZO185]. Hot water extract of the dried rhizome, administered intraperitoneally to rats at a dose of 200 mg/kg, was active vs D-galactosamine-induced hepatotoxicity. A mixture of 5 g *Bupleurum falcatum*, 4 g *Pinellia ternata*, 3 g *Scutellaria baicalensis*, 4 g *Zingiber officinale*, 3 g *Zizyphus inermis*, 3 g *Paeonia albiflora*, 2 g *Citrus aurantium*, and 1 g *Rheum* species was used. A mixture of 7 g *Bupleurum falcatum*, 5 g *Pinellia ternata*, 3 g *Scutellaria baicalensis*, 4 g *Zingiber officinale*, 3 g *Zizyphus inermis*, 3 g *Panax ginseng*, and 2 g *Glycyrrhiza glabra*, suppressed hyaline degeneration of liver induced by D-galactosamine[ZO282]. Methanol extract of a mixture of *Machilus* and *Alisma* species, *Amomum xanthiodes*, *Bulboschoenus maritimus*, *Artemisia iwayomogis*, *Atractylodes japonica*, *Crataegus cuneata*, *Hordeum vulgare*, *Citrus sinensis*, *Polyporus umbellatus*, *Agastache rugosa*, *Raphanus sativus*, *Poncirus trifoliatus*, *Curcuma zedoaria*, *Citrus aurantium*, *Saussurea lappa*, *Glycyrrhiza glabra*, and *Zingiber officinale*, administered by gastric intubation to rabbits at a dose of 0.5 g/kg, was active vs CCl$_4$-induced hepatox-icity[ZO331].

Antihypercholesterolemic activity. Oleo-resin, administered orally to rats, was active vs cholesterol-primed animals[ZO217]. Ethanol (95%) extract of the dried rhizome, admin-istered intragastrically to male rabbits at a dose of 200 mg/kg, was active vs cholesterol-fed animals[ZO104].

Antihyperglycemic activity. Rhizome ash, administered intragastrically to albino rats at doses of 90 and 250 mg/kg, was inactive vs glucose tolerance tests (GTT)[ZO169].

Antihypothermic effect. Acetone extract of ginger, administered orally to rats at a dose of 100 mg/kg, inhibited 5-hydrox-ytryptamine-induced hypothermia. The ac-tive constituent of the extract was further examined. Four fractions were isolated by column chromatography. Fractions 1 and 2 produced significant activity. When frac-tion 2 was further purified, [6]-shogaol was obtained. A dose of 10 mg/kg, administered orally, also produced inhibition of 5-hydrox-ytryptamine-induced hypothermia[ZO041].

Anti-inflammatory effect. Powdered gin-ger was evaluated in 56 patients (28 with rheumatoid arthritis, 18 with osteoarthritis, and 10 with muscular discomfort). Among the patients with arthritis, more than 75% experienced, to varying degrees, relief in pain and swelling. All the patients with muscular discomfort experienced relief in pain. None of the patients reported adverse effects during the period of ginger consump-tion that ranged from 3 months to 2.5 years[ZO036]. Ethanol (80%) extract of the rhi-zome, administered intragastrically to rats at a dose of 50 mg/kg, was active vs edema-in-duced in the paw by carrageenan inject-ion[ZO292]. Water extract of the rhizome, administered intragastrically to rats at a dose of 2 g/kg was active vs formalin-induced pedal edema[ZO150]. Hot water extract of the dried rhizome, administered by gastric intu-bation to rats at a dose of 1 g/kg, was active

vs carrageenan-induced pedal edema and cotton pellet granuloma. A mixture of 8 g *Bupleurum* species, 3 g *Glycyrrhiza glabra*, 3 g *Zizyphus jujuba*, 1 g *Zingiber officinale*, 3 g *Panax ginseng*, 8 g *Pinellia ternata*, and 3 g *Scutellaria baicalensis* was used[ZO259]. Dried rhizome in combination with *Commiphora mukul*, taken orally by 24 patients with rheumatoid arthritis, produced complete relief in 8 patients and partial relief in 7 patients[ZO243]. Decoction of the dried rhi-zome, administered intragastrically to rats at a dose of 100 mg/kg on days 1–22, was inactive vs adjuvant-induced arthritis. The decoction was used in combination with *Cinnamomum cassia* (Bk), *Glycyrrhiza glabra* (Rt), *Zizyphus jujuba* (Fr), *Ephedra sinica* (St), *Asiasarum* species (Rt), and *Aconitum* species (Rt)[ZO199]. Ethyl acetate extract of the dried rhizome, applied externally to the mouse at a dose of 20 µL/animal, produced weak activity vs tetradecanoyl phorbol acetate-induced acetate phospholipid synthesis and 12-O-tetradecanoylphorbol-13-acetate-induced ear inflammation. The hexane extract was equivocal[ZO095]. Hot wa-ter extract of the dried rhizome, at variable concentrations, was inactive on the rat red blood cell (RBC) vs resistance of heat-induced hemolysis. A mixture of 6 g *Bupleurum falcatum*, 4.7 g *Pinellia ternata*, 2.7 g *Scutellaria baicalensis*, 3.3 g *Zingiber officinale*, and 2.7 g *Zizyphus inermis* was used. The extract, administered by gastric intubation to rats at a concentration of 500 mg/kg for 30 days, reduced swelling 23.2% on day 24 vs adjuvant-induced arthritis. Dosing at 1 hour before and 1 and 2 hours after was inactive vs carrageenan- and dextran-induced pedal edema and inflam-mation induced by paw immersion in hot water. A mixture of 6 g *Bupleurum falcatum*, 4 g *Pinellia ternata*, 3 g *Scutellaria baicalensis*, 4 g *Zingiber officinale*, 3 g *Zizyphus inermis*, 3 g *Paeonia albiflora*, 2 g *Citrus aurantium*, and 1 g *Rheum* species, administered by gastric intubation at a dose of 500 mg/kg for 30 days, reduced swelling 36% on day 24 vs adjuvant-induced arthritis. When administered 1 hour before and 1 and 2 hours after immersion, reduced swelling by 12.5% vs inflammation induced by paw immersion in hot water, reduced swelling 22.1% after 5 hours after dextran injection vs dextran-induced pedal edema, and was active vs carrageenan-induced pedal edema. A mixture of 5 g *Bupleurum falcatum*, 1.5 g *Glycyrrhiza glabra*, 2 g *Zizyphus inermis*, 2 g *Zingiber officinale*, 2 g *Panax ginseng*, 4 g *Pinellia ternata*, 2 g *Cinnamomum cassia*, 2 g *Paeonia albiflora*, and 2 g *Scutellaria baicalensis*, administered by gastric intubation at a dose of 500 mg/kg 1 hour before and 1 and 2 hours after injection of dextran, reduced swelling 25.5% at 5 hours vs dextran-induced pedal edema and 32.5% on day 24 vs adjuvant-induced arthritis. The treatment was inactive vs inflammation induced by paw immersion in hot water and carrageenan-induced pedal edema. A mixture of 7 g *Bupleurum falcatum*, 2 g *Glycyrrhiza glabra*, 3 g *Zizyphus inermis*, 4 g *Zingiber officinale*, 3 g *Panax ginseng*, 5 g *Pinellia ternata*, and 3 g *Scutellaria baicalensis*, administered by gastric intubation to rats at a dose of 500 mg/kg, was inactive vs adjuvant-induced arthritis, dextran- and carrageenan-induced pedal edema, and inflammation induced by paw immersion in hot water[ZO332]. Hot water extract of the dried rhizome, administered intraperitoneally to rats at doses of 100 and 200 mg/kg, were active vs carrageenan-induced pedal edema. The effect was not seen in adrenalectomized rats[ZO333]. Methanol extract of the dried rhizome, applied topically to mice at a dose of 20 µL/animal, was active vs tetradecanoyl phorbol acetate-induced acetate phospholipid synthesis and 12-O-tetradecanoylphorbol-13-acetate-induced ear inflammation[ZO095].

Antimotion sickness effect. Ginger and other medications were compared with scopolamine and d-amphetamine for effectiveness in prevention of motion sickness. The subjects were given the medications 2 hours before they were rotated in a chair until a symptom total short of vomiting was reached. The three doses of ginger administered were all at the placebo level of efficacy. Amitriptyline, ethopropazine, and trihexyphenidyl increased the tolerated head movements, but the increase was not statistically significant. Significant levels of protection were produced by dimenhydrinate, promethazine, scopolamine, and D-amphetamine. Efficacy was greatest, as the dose was increased[ZO003]. Powdered rhizome, taken orally by human adults at a dose of 1 g/person, was active vs seasickness[ZO284]. A dose of 940 mg/kg was active vs motion sickness in 36 susceptible volunteers[ZO141]. The ground rhizome, taken orally by 80 male adults at a dose of 1 g/day, was active. Those who received the powder suffered less seasickness compared with those who received placebo. The difference was statistically significant, $p < 0.05$, 4 hours after receiving the treatment[ZO072].

Antimutagenic activity. Aqueous high-speed supernatant of the plant juice, on agar plate at a concentration of 0.1 mL/plate, was active on *Salmonella typhimurium* TA98 vs tryptophan pyrolysate mutagenicity. S9 mix was added[ZO273]. Infusion of the rhizome, on agar plate at a concentration of 100 µL/disc was inactive on *Salmonella typhimurium* TA100 and TA98 vs ethyl methanesulfonate and 2-amino-anthracene-induced mutagenicity, respectively. Metabolic activation was not required for activity[ZO161].

Anti-nauseant effect. The rhizome, taken orally by pregnant women at a dose of 250 mg/person for 4 days, was active. Thirty women participated in the double-blind randomized crossover study of the efficacy of the powdered rhizome in hyperemesis gravidarum. Each participant swallowed a 250 mg capsule containing ginger or lactose four times daily for the first 4 days of treatment. This was interrupted by a 2-day washout period, and the alternative medication was given in the second 4-day period. Two scoring systems evaluated the severity and relief of the symptoms before and after each period. The scores indicated that 70.4% of the participants indicated preference to the period in which ginger was given[ZO298].

Anti-nematodal activity. Water extract of the rhizome, at a concentration of 10 mg/mL, was inactive on *Toxocara canis*. The methanol extract, at a concentration of 1 mg/mL, was active[ZO209].

Anti-neurotoxic activity. Hot water extract of the dried rhizome at a concentration of 75 µg/mL, was active vs cytochalasin B-induced neurite distortion[ZO281].

Anti-osteoarthritic effect. Ginger extract was compared to placebo and ibuprofen in patients with osteoarthritis of the hip and knee in a controlled, double-blind, double-dummy, crossover study with a washout period of 1 week followed by three treatment periods in a randomized sequence, each of 3 weeks' duration. The ranking of efficacy of the three treatment periods were ibuprofen more than ginger extract greater than placebo for visual analogue scale of pain (Friedman test: 24.65, $p < 0.00001$) and the Lequesne-index (Friedman test: 20.76, $p < 0.00005$). In the crossover study, no significant difference between placebo and ginger extract could be demonstrated (Siegel-Castellan test), whereas explorative tests of differences in the first treatment period showed a better effect of both ibuprofen and ginger extract than placebo ($p < 0.05$). There were no serious adverse events reported during the periods with active medications[ZO020].

Antioxidant effect. Alcohol (50%) extract of the ginger produced significant effect on enzymatic lipid peroxidation. The extract dose-dependently inhibited oxidation of fatty acid and linoleic acid in the presence of soybean lipoxygenase. Ginger, onion and ginger, and garlic and ginger produced cumulative inhibition of lipid peroxidation this exhibiting their synergistic antioxidant activity. The antioxidant activity of the extract were retained even after boiling for 30 minutes at 100°C, indicating that the constituents were resistant to thermal denaturation[ZO016]. The effect of ginger (1%, w/w) on exposure of rats to subchronic malathion (O,O-dimethyl-S-1,2,bisethoxy-carbonyl-ethyl phosphorodithioate) was evaluated. Administration of malathion (20 ppm) for 4 weeks increased the malondialdehyde levels in serum, activities of superoxide dismutase, catalase, and glutathione peroxidase in erythrocytes and glutathione reductase and glutathione S-transferase in serum. It decreased the glutathione level in whole blood. Concomitant dietary feeding of ginger significantly attenuated malathion-induced lipid peroxidation and oxidative stress in the rats. The results indicated the possible involvement of free radicals in organophosphate-induced toxicity and highlighted the protective action of ginger[ZO017]. Ginger (1% w/w) significantly lowered lipid peroxidation by maintaining the activities of the antioxidant enzymes superoxide dismutase, catalase, and glutathione peroxidase in rats. The blood glutathione content was significantly increased in ginger-fed rats. Similar effects were also observed after natural antioxidant ascorbic acid (100 mg/kg, body weight) treatment[ZO010]. The glucosides, 1-(4-O-β-D-glucopyranosyl-3-methoxyphenyl)-3,5-dihydroxydecane and 5-O-β-D-glucopyranosyl-3-hydroxy-1-(4-hydroxy-3-methoxyphenyl)decane, incubated with acetone, were hydrolyzed to 6-gingerdiol. Their antioxidative activities were investigated and compared to that of their aglycon, 6-gingerdiol, by a linoleic acid model system and by their 1,1-diphenyl-2-picrylhydrazyl (DPPH) radical-scavenging ability. 1-(4-O-β-D-glucopyranosyl-3-methoxyphenyl)-3,5-dihydroxydecane did not indicate any activity, 5-O-β-D-glucopyranosyl-3-hydroxy-1-(4-hydroxy-3-methoxyphenyl)decane had as strong activity as the aglycon in both measurements[ZO019]. Amrita Bindu, a salt-spice mixture, with pepper and ginger being the main ingredients, was investigated for its effect in maintaining antioxidant defense systems in blood and liver when exposed to a carcinogenic nitrosamine, N-methyl-N'-nitrosoguanidine (MNNG). The mixture prevented MNNG-induced depletion of the antioxidant enzymes and the scavenger antioxidants glutathione and vitamins A, C, and E. It provides protection against free radical- and reactive oxygen species-induced tissue lipid peroxidation and the resultant tissue degeneration[ZO030]. Polyunsaturated fatty acids are vulnerable to peroxidative attack. Protecting from peroxidation is essential to use their beneficial effects in health and in preventing disease. The antioxidants vitamin E, t-butylhydroxy toluene, and t-butylhydroxy anisole inhibited ascorbate/Fe^{2+}-induced lipid peroxidation in rat liver microsomes. Zingerone from ginger-inhibited lipid peroxidation at high concentrations (>150 μM). The inhibition was not affected by the addition of high Fe^{2+} concentration[ZO037]. Aqueous high-speed supernatant of the rhizome, at a concentration of 0.04 mL and hot water extract and juice at concentration of 0.02 mL, was active[ZO073]. Methanol extract of the rhizome, administered intragastrically to mice at a dose of 0.16 g/kg, was active vs ethanol-induced lipid peroxidation in the mouse liver[ZO182].

Antioxytocic effect. Water extract of the dried rhizome, at a concentration of 0.01 g/mL, produced weak activity on the rat uterus vs oxytocin-induced contractions[ZO328].

Antipyretic activity. Ethanol (80%) extract of the rhizome, administered intragastrically to rats at a dose of 100 mg/kg, was active vs hyperthermia induced by yeast injection[ZO292]. Water extract of a mixture of Bupleurum falcatum, Scutellaria baicalensis, Paeonia alba, Rheum tanguticum, Citrus aurantium, Pinellia ternata, Zingiber officinale, and Zizyphus inermis, administered by gastric intubation to mice and rabbits at a dose of 200 mg/kg, was active vs typhoid vaccine-induced pyrexia[ZO323].

Anti-radiation effect. Methanol extract of the dried rhizome, administered intraperitoneally to mice at a dose of 400 mg/kg, was inactive vs soft X-ray irradiation at lethal dose[ZO334].

Anti-rheumatic effect. Ginger oil, administered orally at a dose of 33 mg/kg to male Sprague–Dawley rats with arthritis induced in the knee and paw by injecting 0.05 mL of fine suspension of dead Mycobacterium tuberculosis bacilli in liquid paraffin (5 mg/mL, produced a significant suppression of both paw and joint swelling[ZO029]. Hot water extract of the dried rhizome, administered intragastrically to female mice at a dose of 20 mg/mL, was active in influenza virus-infected animals[ZO099].

Antischistosomal activity. Hot water extract of the dried rhizome, taken orally by human adults at variable dosage levels, was active. A mixture of Rehmannia glutinosa (Rt), Dioscorea batatas (Tu), Dolichos lablab (Sd), Glycyrrhiza uralensis (Rt), Zingiber officinale (Rh), Evodiarutae carpa (Fr), Atractylodes macrocephala (Rh), and Panax ginseng (Rt) was used[ZO301].

Antispasmodic activity. Ethanol (95%) extract of the dried rhizome, at a concentration of 200 μg/mL, was active on the guinea pig ileum vs histamine- and barium-induced contractions. The water extract was active vs barium-induced contractions and inactive vs histamine-induced contractions[ZO335]. The hot water extract, at a concentration of 1 mg/mL, was active vs barium- and acetylcholine (ACh)-induced contractions. A concentration of 3 mg/mL was active vs histamine-induced contractions and on the vas deferens vs norepinephrine-induced contractions[ZO336]. Water extract of the dried rhizome, in combination with *Pinellia ternata, Citrus aurantium, Pachyma hoelen,* and *Glycyrrhiza glabra,* at a concentration of 0.01 g/mL, was active on the guinea pig ileum and rabbit small intestine vs ACh- and barium-induced contractions[ZO328]. Water extract of a mixture of *Bupleurum falcatum, Scutellaria baicalensis, Paeonia alba, Rheum tanguticum, Citrus aurantium, Pinellia ternata, Zingiber officinale,* and *Zizyphus inermis,* administered to mice at a concentration of 1–5 mg/mL, was active vs histamine-induced contractions. A concentration of 10 mg/mL was active vs barium- and ACh-induced contractions[ZO323].

Anti-tumor activity. Ginger rhizome was investigated for antitumor promoter activity using the short-term assay of inhibition of 12-O-tetradecanoyl phorbol-13-acetate (TPA)-induced Epstein-Barr virus early antigen (EBV-EA) in Raji cells. The inhibition of TPA-induced EBV-EA was detected using the indirect immunofluorescence assay (IFA) and Western blot technique. The indirect IFA detected the expression/inhibition of EBV-EA-D (diffused EA), whereas the Western blot technique detected the expression/inhibition of both EBV-EA-D and EA-R (restricted EA). The rhizome possesses inhibitory activity toward EBV activation, induced by TPA. The cytotoxicity assay was conducted to determine the toxicity of the rhizome extract[ZO023]. Water extract of *Zingiber officinale, Bupleurum falcatum, Pinellia ternata, Scutellaria baicalensis, Zizyphus jujuba, Panax ginseng,* and *Glycyrrhiza glabra,* administered by gastric intubation to mice at a dose of 300 mg/kg, was active on Leuk-L1210. Cytarabine or 5-fluorouracil was also administered. Water extract of the dried rhizome, administered intraperitoneally at doses of 100 and 300 mg/kg, in combination with *Bupleurum falcatum, Pinellia ternata, Scutellaria*

baicalensis, Zizyphus jujuba, Panax ginseng, and *Glycyrrhiza glabra* on days 1 to 10, were inactive[ZO268]. Ethanol (95%) extract of the dried rhizome, administered intraperitoneally to mice at a dose of 100 mg/kg, was inactive on Sarcoma 180 (ASC)[ZO194]. Ethanol (90%) extract of the dried rhizome, administered intraperitoneally to mice at a dose of 500 mg/kg, was inactive on CA-Ehrlich ascites, Sarcoma 180 (ASC), and Leuk-SN36[ZO318].

Anti-ulcer effect. Acetone extract of ginger, administered orally to rats with HCl/ethanol-induced gastric ulcers at a dose of 1 g/kg, significantly inhibited gastric lesions by 97.5%. Zingiberene and 6-gingerol, at a dose of 100 mg/kg, also inhibited gastric lesions by 53.6 and 54.5%, respectively[ZO050]. Decoctions of dried and roasted ginger were investigated on four experimental gastric ulcer models. The decoction was administered orally at a dose of 4.5 g/kg to rats. The roasted ginger had a significant inhibiting tendency on three gastric ulcer models, except the indomethacin-induced model. The dried ginger had no such effects[ZO042]. The rhizome, administered to rats at a dose of 150 mg/kg, produced 57.5% inhibition of gastric ulcers induced by HCl and ethanol. The acetone/ethanol extract, at a dose of 500 mg/kg, produced 91.9% inhibition. Butanol extract, at a dose of 285 mg/kg, produced 12.4% inhibition and water extract at a dose of 640 mg/kg, produced 45.8% inhibition[ZO079]. Acetone and methanol extracts of the dried rhizome, administered intragastrically to rats at a dose of 1 g/kg, were active vs HCl/ethanol-induced ulcers. Chromatographic fraction of the dried rhizome, administered intragastrically to rats at a dose of 40 mg/kg, was active vs HCl/ethanol-induced ulcers[ZO181]. Hot water extract of the dried rhizome, administered by gastric intubation to mice at a dose of 1.766 g/kg, was inactive vs stress induced ulcers[ZO337]. Methanol (50%) extract of the dried rhizome, administered by gastric intubation to mice at a dose of 10 g/kg, was inactive vs stress-induced (restraint) ulcers[ZO237]. Water extract of the dried rhizome, administered intraperitoneally to rats at a dose of 1 mg/g, was active vs Shay ulcers. The results were significant at $p < 0.001$ level[ZO328]. Ethanol (95%) extract of the dried rhizome, administered by gastric intubation to rats at a dose of 500 mg/kg, significantly lowered ulcer index of necrotizing agents (80% ethanol, 0.6% HCl, 0.2 M NaOH, and 25% NaCl), and was active vs aspirin-, indomethacin-, and cold stress-induced ulcers. The extract was inactive vs reserpine- and Shay-induced ulcers[ZO184]. Water extract of the dried rhizome in a preparation containing *Atractylodes macrocephala*, *Amomum* species, *Magnolia officinalis*, *Citrus aurantium* ssp. *nobilis*, *Pachyma hoelen*, *Elettaria cardamomum*, *Panax ginseng*, *Saussurea lappa*, *Glycyrrhiza* species, and *Zizyphus vulgaris*, administered intraduodenally to rats at a dose of 1 g/kg, was active vs aspirin-, histamine-, stress-(water immersion), and pylorus ligation-induced ulcers[ZO338].

Antivertigo effect. Powdered rhizome, administered orally to human adults at a dose of 1 g/person, was active vs seasickness[ZO284]. Rhizome, administered orally to adults of both sexes at a dose of 1 g/person, was inactive. The treatment was administered 2 hours before the subjects were rotated in a chair making head movement until a symptom short of vomiting was reached[ZO183].

Antiviral activity. Aqueous low-speed supernatant of the rhizome, at a concentration of 1% and the rhizome juice, produced strong activity on virus-top necrosis[ZO172]. Decoction of the rhizome together with *c* at a concentration of 250 µg/mL, was active on HIV-1 and Rauscher murine leukemia viruses. Reverse transcriptase activity was inhibited[ZO209]. Water extract of the rhizome, in cell culture at a concentration of 10%, was inactive on herpes virus type 2, A2-

Virus (Manheim 57), poliovirus II, vaccinia virus[ZO257], and LPPI virus[ZO274]. Hot water extract of the dried rhizome, in cell culture at a concentration of 500 µg/mL, was inactive on herpes simplex I virus. A dose of 300 mg/kg, administered intragastrically to female mice, was active on herpes simplex I virus[ZO138]. Hexane extract of the dried rhizome, in cell culture, was active on rhinovirus type 1-B virus[ZO131]. Hot water extract of the dried rhizome, in cell culture at a concentration of 0.5 mg/mL, was inactive on herpes simplex I virus, measles virus, and poliovirus I[ZO339].

Anti-yeast activity. The essential oil, on agar plate, was inactive on *Saccharomyces cervisiae*[ZO127]. Ethanol (95%) extract of the dried rhizome, in broth culture at a concentration of 10%, was inactive on *Candida albicans*, *Candida glabrata*, and *Candida tropicalis*[ZO340]. Ethanol (90%) extract of the dried rhizome, on agar plate at a concentration of 500 mg/disc, was inactive on *Candida albicans*[ZO318].

Arachidonate metabolism inhibition. Decoction of the dried rhizome, at a concentration of 0.3 mg/plate, was active on sheep vesicular gland microsomal fraction[ZO315]. Decoction of the dried rhizome, administered intraperitoneally to rats at a dose of 0.74 g/animal, was inactive. Serum from rats fed the decoction was added to sheep vesicular gland microsomal fraction. Arachidonic acid metabolism in gland enzyme mixture was measured. The system was not affected by rat serum lipids[ZO315]. Hot water extract of the dried rhizome in a mixture containing 7 g *Bupleurum falcatum*, 5 g *Pinellia ternata*, 3 g *Scutellaria baicalensis*, 3 g *Panax ginseng*, 4 g *Zingiber officinale*, 3 g *Zizyphus vulgaris*, and 2 g *Glycyrrhiza glabra* in 700 mL water, administered intragastrically to mice on days 1–3, was active[ZO341]. A mixture of *Zingiber officinale* (Rh), *Bupleurum falcatum* (Rt), *Scutellaria baicalensis* (Rt), *Pinellia ternata* (Tu), *Zizyphus jujuba* (Fr), *Panax ginseng* (Rt), and *Glycyrrhiza* *glabra* (Rh), in cell culture, was active on macrophages[ZO123].

Aspartate transaminase effect. Decoction of the dried rhizome, taken orally by 80 adults of both sexes with hepatitis B antigen-positive chronic hepatitis at a dose of 7.5 g/day for 6 months, was active[ZO123]. The treatment consisted of *Zingiber officinale* (Rh), *Bupleurum falcatum* (Rt), *Scutellaria baicalensis* (Rt), *Pinellia ternata* (Tu), *Zizyphus jujuba* (Fr), *Panax ginseng* (Rt), and *Glycyrrhiza glabra* (Rh)[ZO123].

Bacterial stimulant activity. Powdered rhizome, in broth culture at a concentration of 2 g/L, was active on *Lactobacillus plantarum*[ZO285].

Barbiturate potentiation. Ethanol (95%) and methanol (75%) extracts of the rhizome, administered intraperitoneally to male mice at a dose of 500 mg/kg, were inactive[ZO221]. Methanol extract of the rhizome, administered intraperitoneally to mice at a dose of 500 mg/kg on days 1–3, was inactive[ZO265]. Water extract of the dried rhizome, administered by gastric intubation to mice at a dose of 4 g/kg, was active. A mixture of *Zingiber officinale*, *Glycyrrhiza glabra*, *Panax ginseng*, *Scutellaria baicalensis*, *Zizyphus jujuba*, *Pinellia ternata*, *Bupleurum falcatum*, *Cinnamomum cassia*, and *Paeonia albiflora* was used[ZO250]. Hot water extract of the dried rhizome, administered by gastric intubation to male mice at a dose of 1 g/kg, was inactive. A mixture of *Pinellia ternata* (Tu), *Magnolia obovata* (Bk), *Perilla frutescens* (Aer), *Zibngiber officinale* (Rh), and *Poria cocos* (Fr) (6, 3, 2, 1, and 5 g, respectively) was used. A dose of 2 g/kg was active[ZO342]. Hot water extract of the dried rhizome, administered by gastric intubation to male mice at a dose of 4 g/kg, was inactive[ZO342]. Methanol (50%) extract of the dried rhizome, administered subcutaneously to mice at a dose of 10 g/kg, was active and a dose of 3 g/kg was inactive[ZO237].

Capillary permeability. Methanol (50%) extract of the dried rhizome, administered

subcutaneously to mice at a dose of 10.0 g/kg, had no effect[ZO237].

Carcinogenesis inhibition. Decoction of the dried rhizome, in the ration of rats at a concentration of 20% of the diet, was equivocal vs azoxymethane-induced aberrant crypt foci[ZO343].

Cardiac depressant activity. Hot water extract of the dried rhizome, at a concentration of 3 mg/mL, was active on the guinea pig[ZO336].

Cardiotonic activity. Gingerol, a constituent of ginger, tested in the guinea pig isolated atrial cells at a concentration of 3×10^{-6} M, produced an increase in the degree and the rate of longitudinal contractions. In the guinea pig left atria, gingerol produced little influence on the action potential, although it increased the contractile force of the atria. The whole-cell patch-clamp experiments showed that the slow inward current was little affected by gingerol in the voltage-clamped guinea pig cardiac myocytes. The measurement of extravesicular Ca^{2+} uptake of fragmented sarcoplasmic reticulum prepared from canine cardiac muscle in a concentration-dependent manner[ZO049]. Gingerol, isolated from the rhizome, stimulated the Ca^{2+}-pumping activity of fragmented sarcoplasmic reticulum prepared from the rabbit skeletal and dog cardiac muscles. The extravesicular Ca^{2+} concentrations of the heavy fraction of the fragmented sarcoplasmic reticulum were measured directly with a Ca^{2+} electrode to examine the effect. Gingerol, at a concentration of 3–30 µM, accelerated the Ca^{2+}-pumping rate of skeletal and cardiac sarcoplasmic reticulum in a concentration-dependent manner. Gingerol also activated Ca^{2+}-adenosine triphosphatase (ATPase) activities of skeletal and cardiac sarcoplasmic reticulum (EC_{50}, 4 µM). The activation of the Ca^{2+}-ATPase activity was completely reversed by 100-fold dilution with the fresh saline solution. Kinetic analysis of the activating effects of gingerol suggests that the activation of sarcoplasmic reticulum Ca^{2+}-ATPase is uncompetitive and competitive regarding Mg. Adenosine triphosphate (ATP) at concentrations of 0.2–0.5 mM and above 1 mM, respectively. Kinetic analysis also suggested that the activation by gingerol in mixed-type with respect to free Ca^{2+} and this enzyme is activated probably resulting from the acceleration of enzyme-substrate complex breakdown. Gingerol had no significant effect on sarcolemma Ca^{2+}-ATPase, myosin Ca^{2+}-ATPase, actin-activated myosin ATPase and cyclic adenosine monophosphate (cAMP)-phosphodiesterase activities[ZO051].

Cardiovascular effect. [6]-shogaol, administered intravenously to rats at a dose of 0.5 mg/kg, produced a rapid fall in blood pressure, bradycardia, and apnea. There was a marked pressure pressor response in blood pressure that occurred after the rapid fall. A dose of 3.6 μM produced inotropic and chronotropic actions on isolated atria in rats. The effect disappeared by repeated injections or pretreatment of 100 mg/kg administered subcutaneously[ZO054]. Intravenous doses of 0.1 to 0.5 μg produced a pressor response in a dose dependent manner. The response was markedly reduced by spinal destruction at the sacral cord level. Norepinephrine (10 μg/kg, intravenously) induced pressor response that was not affected by spinal destruction. In rats in which the spinal cord was destroyed at the thoracic cord level, [6]-shogaol-induced pressor response was reduced by hexamethonium (10 mg/kg, intravenously) and phentolamine (10 mg/kg, intravenously). When the spinal cord was destroyed at the sacral level, the pressor response was not affected by these blockades. In the hindquarters of rats that were perfused with rat's blood, [6]-shogaol produced two pressor responses on the perfusion pressure. The first was accompanied by a rise in systemic blood pressure, was re-

duced by hexamethonium but was not entirely eliminated by phentolamine. The pressure response disappeared with spinal destruction at the sacral cord level. The second response that occurred when the systemic blood pressure regained its original pressure was not affected by hexamethonium, phentolamine, or spinal destruction. Pressor response induced by the injection of [6]-shogaol (10 μg) into the perfusion circuit was not affected by phentolamine and spinal destruction[ZO056]. Ethanol (95%) extract of the rhizome, administered by iv infusion to dogs at a dose of 5 mL/animal at a rate of 1 mL/minute, increased the heart rate[ZO314].

Cell proliferation inhibition. The rhizome, in cell culture at a concentration of 3.75%, was active on human fibroblast[ZO096]. Decoction of the dried rhizome, at a concentration of 50 μg/mL, produced weak activity on the mouse mesangial cells[ZO139].

Chemopreventitive effect. The antitumor promotional activity of [6]-gingerol, a major pungent principle of the rhizome, was investigated using a two-stage mouse skin carcinogenesis model. Topical application of the extract onto shaven backs of female mice before each topical dose of 12-O-tetradecanoylphorbol-13-acetate significantly inhibited 7,12-dimethylbenz[a]-anthracene-induced skin papilloma genesis. The extract also suppressed TPA-induced epidermal ornithine decarboxylase activity and inflammation[ZO024].

Cholagogic effect. The effect of ginger on bile secretion was examined to clarify the stomachic action of ginger and to investigate its active constituents. The results indicated that the acetone extracts, which contain the essential oils and pungent principles, produced an increase in the bile secretion. Further analyses for the active constituents of the acetone extracts through column chromatography indicated that [6]-gingerol and [10]-gingerol, which are the pungent principles, are mainly responsible for the cholagogic effect[ZO059].

Choleretic activity. Acetone extract of the dried rhizome, administered intraduodenally to rats at a dose of 500 mg/kg, was active. The water extract was inactive, and the chromatographic fraction, at a dose of 150 mg/kg, was active[ZO344].

Cholesterol absorption inhibition. Oleoresin, administered orally to rats, was active on cholesterol-primed animals[ZO217].

Cholesterol ester formation. Decoction of the dried rhizome, administered intragastrically to mice at a dose of 1.2 g/kg, produced no effect. The study was conducted with a mixture of *Zingiber officinale* (Rh), *Bupleurum falcatum* (Rt), *Scutellaria baicalensis* (Rt), *Pinellia ternata* (Tu), *Zizyphus jujuba* (Fr), *Panax ginseng* (Rt), and *Glycyrrhiza glabra* (Rh)[ZO111].

Choline acetyltransferase induction. Water extract of the rhizome, in cell culture at a concentration of 200 µg/mL and a dose of 500 mg/kg administered intragastrically to male rats, were active on astroglial cells. The extract was used in combination with dried *Pinellia ternata*, *Citrus aurantium*, *Poria cocos*, *Citrus unshiu*, *Glycyrrhiza glabra*, *Polygala tenuifolia*, *Scrophularia ningpoensis*, *Panax ginseng*, *Rhemannia glutinosa*, and *Zizyphus jujuba*[ZO106].

Circulation stimulation. Hot water extract of the dried rhizome, administered intravenously to rabbits at a dose of 4.5 mg/kg, was equivocal[ZO345].

Clastogenic effect. Crude aqueous extract of the rhizome, administered by gavage at doses of 0.5, 1, 2, 5, and 10 g/kg body weight and ginger oil, administered intraperitoneally at doses of 1.25 and 2.50 mL/kg body weight, were evaluated in mice. Attention was drawn to the weakness of the clastogenic activity expressed by ginger extract. In comparison, ginger oil produced a higher frequency of chromosomal aberrations[ZO013].

CNS effects. Water extract of the rhizome, administered to mice by gastric intubation at a dose of 4 g/kg, produced no change in the electroencephalogram (EEG), behavior, or active and resting cycles. A mixture of *Zingiber officinale*, *Glycyrrhiza glabra*, *Panax ginseng*, *Scutellaria baicalensis*, *Zizyphus jujuba*, *Pinellia ternata*, *Bupleurum falcatum*, *Cinnamomum cassia*, and *Paeonia albiflora* was used[ZO250]. Ethanol (95%) extract of the rhizome, administered intraperitoneally to male mice at a dose of 500 mg/kg, did not produce any depressant activity[ZO221]. Ethanol (95%) extract of the rhizome, administered intravenously to rabbits at a dose of 1.5 mL/animal, produced a stimulating activity[ZO314].

Coagulation effect. The decoction, ether extraction and suspension liquid of roasted ginger and charcoal of ginger, had markedly shortened the blood coagulation time in mice. The decoction, ether extraction of fresh ginger and dried ginger, did not have any effect. The decoction of ginger charcoal has stronger effect than roasted ginger in shortening the blood coagulation time in mice. The effect of the decoction of ginger charcoal on blood coagulation time increases when the dosage is increased[ZO035].

Corticosterone induction. Hot water extract of the rhizome, administered by gastric intubation to rats at a dose of 1.1 g/kg, was active. The dose also increased the plasma level of prednisolone. A mixture of 8 g *Bupleurum* species, 3 g *Glycyrrhiza glabra*, 3 g *Zizyphus jujuba*, 1 g *Zingiber officinale*, 3 g *Panax ginseng*, 8 g *Pinellia ternata*, and 3 g *Scutellaria baicalensis* was used. Results were significant at $p < 0.01$ level[ZO259]. Hot water extract of a mixture of 7 g *Bupleurum falcatum*, 2 g *Glycyrrhiza glabra*, 3 g *Zizyphus inermis*, 4 g *Zingiber officinale*, 3 g *Panax ginseng*, 5 g *Pinellia ternata*, and 3 g *Scutellaria baicalensis*, administered intraperitoneally to rats at a dose of 200 mg/kg, produced an increase in serum adrenal corticosterone vs carrageenan-induced pedal edema. The mixture, at a concentration of 0.1 mg/mL, was inactive on the adrenal gland vs basal and ACTH-induced corticosterone release from rat adrenal gland slices[ZO283].

cAMP stimulation. A mixture of 7 g *Bupleurum falcatum*, 2 g *Glycyrrhiza glabra*, 3 g *Zizyphus inermis*, 4 g *Zingiber officinale*, 3 g *Panax ginseng*, 5 g *Pinellia ternata*, and 3 g *Scutellaria baicalensis*, administered intraperitoneally to rats at a dose of 200 mg/kg, increased cAMP levels in pituitary and adrenal gland but not in the hypothalamus. The increases were inhibited by dexamethasone[ZO283].

Cyclo-oxygenase-2 inhibition. Seventeen pungent oleoresins of ginger and synthetic analogs were evaluated for inhibition on cyclooxygenase-2 enzyme activity in the intact cell. The compounds exhibited a concentration and structure dependent inhibition of the enzyme, with IC_{50} values in the range of 1–25 μM. Ginger constituents, 8-paradol and 8-shogaol, as well as two synthetic analogs, 3-hydroxy-1-(4-hydroxy-3-methoxyphenyl)decane and 5-hydroxy-1-(4-hydroxy-3-methoxyphenyl)dodecane, showed strong inhibitory effects on cyclooxygenase enzyme activity. The SAR analysis of these compounds revealed that the features that affect cyclooxygenase inhibition are lipophilicity of the alkyl side chain, substitution pattern of hydroxy and carbonyl groups on the side chain, and substitution pattern of hydroxy and methoxy groups on the aromatic moiety[ZO006].

Cytotoxic activity. Water extract of the rhizome, in cell culture at a concentration of 10% was inactive on HeLa cells[ZO257]. Ethanol (95%), petroleum ether, and methyl chloride extracts of the dried rhizome, at a concentration of 320 μg/mL, were inactive on Raji cells[ZO319].

Degranulation inhibition. Hot water extract of the rhizome, in cell culture at a concentration of 0.1 mg/mL, was active vs compound 48/40-induced degranulation of mast cells. A mixture of *Bupleurum falcatum*, *Pinellia ternata*, *Poria cocos*, *Scutellaria bai-*

calensis, *Zizyphus vulgaris*, *Panax ginseng*, *Magnolia obovata*, *Glycyrrhiza glabra*, and *Perilla frutescens* was used[ZO259].

Desmutagenic activity. Aqueous high-speed supernatant of the fresh fruit juice, on agar plate at a concentration of 0.5 mL/plate, was active on *Salmonella typhimurium* TA98 vs mutagenicity of l-tryptophane pyrolysis products. The assay was done in the presence of S9 mix[ZO275]. Fresh fruit juice, at a concentration of 0.5 mL/plate, was active on *Salmonella typhimurium* TA98[ZO276].

Digestive effect. The fresh rhizome, administered orally to rats at a dose of 50 mg%, significantly enhanced intestinal lipase activity and also the disaccharidases sucrase and maltase[ZO027].

Diuretic activity. Ethanol (50%) extract of the dried aerial parts, administered intraperitoneally to rats at a dose of 45 mg/kg, was active[ZO262]. Methanol (50%) extract of the dried rhizome, administered subcutaneously to mice at a dose of 10 g/kg, was inactive[ZO237].

DNA polymerase inhibition. Decoction of the rhizome, at a concentration of 500 μg/mL, was active on α and β inhibition and inactive on gamma inhibition. This study was conducted with a mixture of *Bupleurum falcatum* (Rt), *Scutellaria baicalensis* (Rt), *Pinellia ternata* (Tu), *Zizyphus jujuba* (Fr), *Panax ginseng* (Rt), and *Glycyrrhiza glabra* (Rh)[ZO203]. Water extract of the mixture, at a concentration of 500 μg/mL, was active on α, β, and γ inhibition when reverse transcriptase activity from HIV was assayed[ZO203].

Enzymatic activity. A reductive metabolism of S-(+)-[6]-gingerol [1-(4'-hydroxy-3'-methoxyphenyl)-5-hydroxydecan-3-one], was investigated in vitro with phenobarbital-induced rat liver 10,000g supernatant containing the NADPH-generating system. The ethyl acetate-extractable products were isolated and two metabolites were identified as disatereomers of [6]-gingerdiol by gas chromatography/mass spectrometry. The ratio of the two isomers formed was about 1:5, suggesting the stereospecific reduction of S-(+)-[6]-gingerol by carbonyl reductase activity present in the postmitochondrial supernatant fraction of rat liver[ZO031]. Ginger oil, administered orally to Swiss albino mice at a dose of 10 µL/day for 14 days, significantly elevated aryl hydrocarbon hydroxylase and glutathione S-transferase activities. There was no significant effect on cytochrome P450 and acid soluble sulfhydryl glutathione S-transferase[ZO033].

Epstein–Barr virus early antigen activation. Ether extract and the decoction, in cell culture at a concentration of 5 µg/mL, inhibited antigen activation[ZO346].

Fibrinolytic activity. The administration of 50 g of fat to 30 healthy adult volunteers decreased fibrinolytic activity from a mean of 64.20 to 52.10 units ($p < 0.001$). Supplementation of 5 g of ginger powder with the fatty meal not only prevented the fall in fibrinolytic activity but actually increased it significantly ($p < 0.001$)[ZO004].

Gastric exfoliation effect. DNA content of gastric aspirates was determined after intragastric infusions of 2, 4, and 6 g of ginger daily. The mean changes of DNA-p/minute in the gastric aspirates after the 2- and 4-g doses were 1.37 ± 2.3 and 6.74 ± 3.06, respectively. Doses of 0.6 g or more produced a significant increase in exfoliation of gastric surface epithelial cells in human subjects[ZO043].

Gastric secretory inhibition. Water extract of the entire plant, administered by gastric intubation to rabbits at a dose of 169 mg/kg, was active. The methanol extract at a concentration of 114 mg/kg was also active[ZO187].

Gastrointestinal effect. Ginger root, in combination with ginseng, *Zanthoxylum* fruit, and malt sugar, administered orally to guinea pigs at a concentration of 10–300 mg/kg, significantly improved carbachol-accelerated small intestinal transit in a dose-dependent manner[ZO001]. Dai-Kenchu-To,

used as the treatment of paralytic ileus, was investigated in vitro. A dose of 30–300 µg/mL produced a significant inhibition on carbachol-induced contraction in a concentration dependent manner of the rat distal colon. The treatment contained 20% *Zanthoxylum* fruit, 30% ginseng root, and 50% ginger rhizome. Although each of them had no effect on carbachol-induced contraction, the combination of three ingredients produced significant inhibition[ZO007]. Acetone extract of the rhizome, administered intragastrically to mice at a dose of 75 mg/kg, increased gastric motility[ZO192]. Acetone extract of ginger, administered orally to mice at a dose of 75 mg/kg, [6]-shogaol at 2.5 mg/kg, or a [6]-, [8]- or [10]-gingerol at 5 mg/kg enhanced the transport of charcoal meal. The effects of these substances were similar to or slightly weaker than metoclopramide and donperidone[ZO044]. Dried rhizome, taken orally by adults at a dose of 1 g/person, did not reduce gastric motility[ZO115]. Dai-Kenchu-To and each ingredient were investigated on upper gastrointestinal motility and mechanism of action. Five dogs were equipped with four-strain gauge-force transducers on the gastric body, antrum, duodenum, and jejunum to measure contractile activity of the circular muscle. Dai-Kenchu-To (1.5 g) or the separate ingredients *Zanthoxylum* fruit, ginseng root, or dried ginger rhizome (1 g each) was administered by bolus into the gastric lumen. *Zanthoxylum* fruit elicited phasic contractions mainly in the duodenum and jejunum, whereas dried ginger rhizome induced phasic contractions in the antrum. Ginseng root had no effect. Phasic contractions induced by intragastric Dai-Kenchu-To were inhibited by atropine and hexamethonium at all sites, although ondansetron inhibited these contractions in the antrum and duodenum[ZO021]. Ginger rhizome extract (2×100 mg) was investigated in fasting and postprandial gastroduodenal motility with stationary manometry in 12 healthy volunteers. The interdigestive antral motility was significantly increased by ginger during phase III of the migrating motor complex. The volunteers also had a significantly increased motor response to a test meal in the corpus; a trend to an increased motor response during ginger treatment was seen in all other regions of interest. The treatment improved gastroduodenal motility in the fasting state and after the standard test meal[ZO022]. Methanol (50%) extract of the dried rhizome, administered subcutaneously to mice at a dose of 10 g/kg, inhibited gastric secretion. The extract had no effect on gastric motility[ZO237].

Glucose metabolism stimulation. Ethanol (95%) extract of the rhizome, administered in the drinking water of mice at a concentration of 5%, was active. The extract, in combination with *Hordeum vulgare*, *Rhizoma zingiberis*, *Ligusticum chuanxiong*, *Lilium brownii*, *Nephelium longa*, and *Polygonum multiflorum*, increased glucose oxidation in epididymal fat pads of obese C57BL/6J mice[ZO137].

Glucosidase inhibition. Ethanol extract of the dried rhizome produced 26% inhibition of α-glucosidase on the rat intestine[ZO100].

Glutamate oxaloacetate transaminase inhibition. Hot water extract of the rhizome, administered by gastric intubation to rats at dosages of 100 and 400 mg/kg, was active vs CCl_4-induced hepatotoxicity. Methionine (100 mg/kg) was added to the 100 mg/kg dose. The results were significant at $p < 0.01$ level. The treatment also consisted of *Bupleurum falcatum* (Rt), *Scutellaria baicalensis*(Rt), *Pinellia ternata* (Tu), *Zizyphus jujuba* (Fr), *Panax ginseng* (Rt), and *Glycyrrhiza glabra* (Rh)[ZO267]. Hot water extract of a mixture of 7 g *Bupleurum falcatum*, 2 g *Glycyrrhiza glabra*, 3 g *Zizyphus inermis*, 4 g *Zingiber officinale*, 3 g *Panax ginseng*, 5 g *Pinellia ternata*, and 3 g *Scutellaria baicalensis*, administered intraperitoneally to rats at a dose of 200 mg/kg, suppressed

increase in serum glutamate pyruvate transaminase (GPT) resulting from D-galactosamine-induced liver injury[ZO282].

GPT inhibition. Hot water extract of the rhizome, administered by gastric intubation to rats at dosages of 100 and 400 mg/kg, was active vs CCl_4-induced hepatotoxicity. Methionine (100 mg/kg) was added to the 100 mg/kg dose. The results were significant at $p < 0.01$ level. The treatment also contained *Bupleurum falcatum* (Rt), *Scutellaria baicalensis* (Rt), *Pinellia ternataPinellia ternata* (Tu), *Zizyphus jujuba* (Fr), *Panax ginseng* (Rt), and *Glycyrrhiza glabra* (Rh)[ZO267]. Hot water extract of the rhizome, administered intragastrically to mice for a period of 1 month, was active vs CCl_4- and galactosamine-induced toxicity. The extract was used in combination with 7 g *Bupleurum falcatum*, 5 g *Pinellia ternata*, 3 g *Scutellaria baicalensis*, 2 g *Glycyrrhiza glabra*, 1 g *Zingiber officinale*, 3 g *Panax ginseng*, and 3 g *Zizyphus jujuba* in 700 mL water[ZO185].

Hair-stimulant effect. Decoction of the rhizome, applied topically to human adults, was active. A mixture of *Polygonum multiflorum*, *Allium sativum*, *Zingiber officinale*, *Panax ginseng*, *Carthamus tinctorius*, *Platycodon grandiflorum*, *Biota orientalis*, *Ligusticum wallichii*, *Salvia miltiorrhiza*, *Angelica sinensis*, and *Tetrapanax papyrifera*. The biological activity has been patented[ZO112].

Hepatic oxygenase activity. Ginger, administered orally to rats, significantly stimulated liver microsomal cytochrome P450-dependent aryl hydroxylase and cytochrome b5[ZO045].

Hepatitis antigen expression. Decoction of mixture of *Zingiber officinale* (Rt), *Bupleurum falcatum* (Rt), *Scutellaria baicalensis* (Rt), *Pinellia ternata* (Tu), *Zizyphus jujuba* (Fr), *Panax ginseng* (Rt), and *Glycyrrhiza glabra* (Rh), taken orally by 80 patients with hepatitis B antigen-positive chronic hepatitis at a dose of 7.5 g/day for 6 months, produced seroconversion to antihepatitis B antibody in eight patients, 15 became seronegative, and 11 had a decrease of hepatitis B antigen levels of more than 50%[ZO123].

Histamine-release inhibition. Hot water extract of the rhizome, in cell culture at a concentration of 0.1 mg/mL, was active vs compound 48/40-induced histamine release. A mixture of *Bupleurum falcatum*, *Pinellia ternata*, *Poria cocos*, *Scutellaria baicalensis*, *Zizyphus vulgaris*, *Panax ginseng*, *Magnolia obovata*, *Glycyrrhiza glabra*, and *Perilla frutescens* was used[ZO205].

Hydrogen peroxide inhibition. The volatile oil, taken as a scavenger, inhibited the production of hydrogen peroxide in chondrocytes induced by fulvic acid from Kashin-Beck disease area[ZO014].

Hypertensive activity. Ethanol (95%) extract of the rhizome, administered intravenously to dogs at a dose of 5 mL/animal and a rate of 1 mL per minute, was active[ZO314].

Hyperthermic effect. Water extract of the rhizome, administered by gastric intubation to mice at a dose of 4 g/kg, was inactive. The extract was used in combination with *Glycyrrhiza glabra*, *Panax ginseng*, *Scutellaria baicalensis*, *Zizyphus jujuba*, *Pinellia ternata*, *Bupleurum fatcatum*, *Cinnamomum cassia*, and *Paeonia albiflora*[ZO250].

Hypoglycemic activity. Ethanol (50%) extract of the aerial parts, administered by gastric intubation to rats at a dose of 45 mg/kg, was active[ZO262]. Ethanol (80%) extract of the rhizome, administered intragastrically to rabbits at a dose of 100 mg/kg, was active[ZO292].

Hypotensive activity. Methanol (50%) extract of the dried rhizome, administered intravenously to rats at doses of 0.25 and 0.5 g/kg (dry weight of plant), was active[ZO237].

Hypothermic activity. Hot water extract of a mixture of *Pinellia ternata* (Tu), *Magnolia obovata* (Bk), *Perilla frutescens* (Aer), *Zingiber officinale* (Rh), and *Poria cocos* (Fr) (6, 3, 2, 1, and 5 g, respectively), adminis-

tered by gastric intubation to male rats at a dose of 4 g/kg, was inactive[ZO342].

Immunomodulatoy activity. Water extract of a mixture of *Glycyrrhiza glabra* (Rt), *Panax ginseng* (Rt), *Bupleurum falcatum* (Rt), *Scutellaria baicalensis* (Rt), *Zingiber officinale* (Rh), *Angelica acutiloba* (Rt), *Atractylodes japonica* (Rh), *Astragalus membranaceus* (Rt), *Citrus unshiu* (Pericarp), and *Cimifuga simplex* (Rh), administered to mice in the diet at a dose of 115.6 mg/kg, elevated the mitogenic activity of concavalin A (Con A), lipopolysaccharide, phorbol myristate acetate, and phytohemagglutinin. Water extract of *Glycyrrhiza glabra* (Rt), *Panax ginseng* (Rt), *Bupleurum falcatum* (Rt), *Scutellaria baicalensis* (Rt), *Zingiber officinale* (Rh), *Pinellia ternata* (Tu), and *Zizyphus vulgaris* (Fr), in the diet of mice at a dose of 178 mg/kg, suppressed the mitogenic activity of phytohemagglutinin and phorbol myristate acetate. Water extract of *Bupleurum falcatum* (Rt), *Scutellaria baicalensis* (Rt), *Zingiber officinale* (Rh), *Paeonia albiflora* (Rt), *Pinellia ternata* (Tu), *Zizyphus vulgaris* (Fr), *Rheum tanguticum* (Rh), and *Citrus aurantium* (Fr), in the diet of mice at a dose of 192.6 mg/kg, suppressed the mitogenic activity of phytohemagglutinin and phorbol myristate acetate[ZO347].

Immunostimulant activity. Hot water extract of the rhizome, administered intraperitoneally to mice at a dose of 2 mg/kg, was active. The extract was used in combination with *Astragalus membranaceus*, *Atractylodes lancea*, *Panax ginseng*, *Angelica acutiloba*, *Glycyrrhiza glabra*, *Bupleurum falcatum*, *Zizyphus vulgaris*, *Citrus unshiu*, and *Cimicifuga simplex*[ZO196]. Ethanol (80%) extract of the dried rhizome, administered intragastrically to male rats at a dose of 800 mg/kg, was active vs sheep erythrocyte-induced hemagglutination and inactive vs sheep erythrocyte-induced B- and T-cell proliferation[ZO105].

Insect growth inhibition. 6-Dehydroshogaol isolated by steam distillation from fresh rhizome exhibited moderate insect growth regulatory and antifeedant activity against *Spilosoma obliqua*[ZO005].

Interferon-induction stimulation. Hot water extract of the rhizome, at a concentration of 6 μg/mL, was active. A dose of 2 g/kg, administered intragastrically to mouse, was active, and 100 mg/kg, administered intraperitoneally to mice, was active vs polymyxin-B induced interferon secretion inhibition. The extract used was in combination with *Bupleurum chinense, Pinellia ternata, Scutellaria baicalensis, Zizyphus jujuba, Panax ginseng,* and *Glycyrrhiza glabra*[ZO197]. Decoction of *Zingiber officinale* (Rh), *Bupleurum falcatum* (Rt), *Scutellaria baicalensis* (Rt), *Pinellia ternata* (Tu), *Zizyphus jujuba* (Fr), *Panax ginseng* (Rt), and *Glycyrrhiza glabra* (Rh), in cell culture at a concentration of 100 μg/mL, was active. Peripheral lymphocytes from eight patients with chronic active hepatitis, four with HbeAg and four with anti-Hbe were cultured. RHbeAg or HbeAg both stimulated interferon (IFN)-γ production, which was enhanced[ZO108].

Interleukin-1-α release inhibition. Hot water extract of the rhizome, administered intragastrically to female mice at a dose of 20 mg/mL, was active vs influenza virus infected animals. Results significant at $p <$ 0.001 level[ZO099].

Intestinal absorption inhibition. Methanol extract of the dried rhizome at a concentration of 1% and water extract at a concentration of 0.01%, administered by perfusion on the rat, were active vs absorption of sulfaguanidine[ZO348].

Larvicidal activity. Water and acetone extracts of the rhizome were inactive on *Aedes aegypti*[ZO303].

Leukocyte migration inhibition. Ethanol (80%) extract of the dried rhizome, administered intragastrically to rats at a dose of 800 mg/kg, was active vs sheep erythrocyte-induced leucocyte migration[ZO105].

Lipid peroxide formation inhibition. Methylene chloride extract of the rhizome, at a concentration of 0.02%, was active[ZO130].

Lipolytic effect. Ethanol (95%) extract of the rhizome, in the drinking water of obese mice at a concentration of 5%, was active. The extract was used in combination with *Hordeum vulgare, Rhizoma zingiberis, Ligusticum chuanxiong, Lilium brownii, Nephelium longa,* and *Polygonum multiflorum*[ZO137].

Lymphocyte blastogenesis stimulant. Water extract of the heartwood, administered intraperitoneally to mice at a dose of 250 mg/kg, induced an accumulation of B lymphocytes in the peritoneal cavity and spleen, and functional maturation of B cells was observed as indicated by antibody responses[ZO349].

Macrophage cytotoxicity enhancement. Hot water extract of the rhizome, administered by gastric intubation to mice at a dose of 600 mg/kg, was inactive on LEUK-L1210. The preparation used also contained *Bupleurum falcatum, Pinellia ternata, Scutellaria baicalensis, Zizyphus jujuba, Panax ginseng,* and *Glycyrrhiza glabra*[ZO268].

Memory retention impairment. Acetone/water extract of the rhizome, administered intragastrically to male rats at a dose of 1 mg/kg, was inactive vs inhibitory avoidance conditioning and water maze performance[ZO094].

Memory retention improvement. Decoction of the rhizome, administered intragastrically to male mice at a dose of 1 g/kg, produced amelioration of memory registration impairment induced by ethanol in step through and step down tests. The decoction was used in combination with *Glycyrrhiza glabra* (Rt), *Saussurea lappa* (Rt), *Zizyphus jujuba* (Fr), *Zizyphus jujuba* (Sd), and *Euphoria longana* (Aril)[ZO202]. The powdered rhizome, administered intragastrically to rats, increased passive avoidance test latency in aged animals. The rhizome was used in combination with *Pinellia ternata, Phyllostachys* *nigra, Citrus aurantium, Poria cocos, Citrus unshiu, Glycyrrhiza glabra, Polygala tenuifolia, Scrophularia ningpoensis, Panax ginseng, Rhemannia glutinosa,* and *Zizyphus jujuba*[ZO350].

Metabolism. Zingerone, 4-(4-hydroxy-3-methoxyphenyl) butan-2-one, a pungent principle of ginger, has been investigated in rats. Oral or intraperitoneal dosage of 100 mg/kg resulted in urinary excretion of most metabolites within 24 hours, mainly as glucuronide and/or sulphate conjugates. Although zingerone itself accounted for roughly 50–55% of the dose, reduction to the corresponding carbinol (11–13%) also occurred. Side chain oxidation took place at all three available sites and oxidation at the three-position, giving rise to C6-C2 metabolites, predominated. Appreciable biliary excretion occurred (40% in 12 hours). Biliary studies and studies in vitro using cecal microorganisms indicated that several O-demethylated metabolites found in the urine are of bacterial origin[ZO062].

Mitogenic activity. Alcohol insoluble fraction and the water extract of rhizome, at a concentration of 200 µg/mL, were inactive on the mouse thymus. The alcohol soluble fraction, at a concentration of 100 µg/mL, was active[ZO166].

Molluscicidal activity. Methanol extract of the dried rhizome, at a concentration of 100 ppm, produced 20% mortality on *Bulinus globosus*[ZO351].

Mutagenic activity. Ginger extract and the constituents gingerol, shogaol, and zingerone were tested in *Salmonella typhimurium* strains TA100, TA98, TA1535, and TA1538 in the presence of S9 mix. Gingerol and shogaol were mutagenic in metabolic activation in strains TA100 and TA1535. Zingerone was nonmutagenic in all of the four strains with or without S9 mix. When the mutagenicity of gingerol and shogaol was tested in the presence of different concentrations of zingerone, it was observed that zingerone suppressed the mutagenic activity in both of the compounds in a dose-dependent manner[ZO052]. Water extract of the rhizome, on agar plate at a concentration of 100 mg/mL, was inactive on *Bacillus subtilis* H-17(Rec+) and produced weak activity on *Salmonella typhimurium* TA100[ZO244]. The hot water extract, at a concentration of 12.5 mg of dried rhizome/disc, was active on *Salmonella typhimurium* TA100. A concentration of 50 mg/disc was inactive on *Salmonella typhimurium* TA98. Histidine was removed from the extract before testing and metabolic activation had no effect on the results[ZO238]. Methanol extract of the rhizome, on agar plate at a concentration of 100 mg/mL, was inactive on *Bacillus subtilis* H-17(Rec+)[ZO244]. Ethanol (70%) extract of the rhizome, on agar plate at a concentration of 4 mg/mL, was inactive on *Escherichia coli* PQ37 when assayed by SOS Chromotest, and inactive on *Salmonella typhimurium* TA1535 when assayed by SOS UMU test[ZO207]. Ethanol (95%) extract of the rhizome, on agar plate at a concentration of 100 µg/plate, was active on *Salmonella typhimurium* TA100 and TA1535, and inactive on TA98 and TA1538[ZO278]. Ethanol (95%) extract of the dried rhizome, on agar plate at a concentration of 10 mg/plate, produced strong activity on *Salmonella typhimurium* TA102[ZO327]. Ethanol (70%), and water and chloroform extracts of the ethanol extract of the dried rhizome, on agar plate at a concentration of 50 mg/mL, were inactive on *Escherichia coli* PQ 37. Metabolic activation had no effect on the results[ZO352]. Hot water extract of the dried rhizome, on agar plate at a concentration of 50 mg/disc, was inactive on *Salmonella typhimurium* TA100 and TA98[ZO326].

Natural-killer cell enhancement. Polysaccharide fraction of the rhizome, administered intragastrically to female mice at a dose of 1 g/kg, produced weak activity vs mononuclear cell incubated with YAC-1 cells[ZO092].

Nausea inhibitory effect. Women with nausea and vomiting during pregnancy were treated within a randomized double-masked design to receive either 1 g of ginger per day or an identical placebo for 4 days. During the 5-month period, 70 women participated. They were graded by the severity of their nausea using visual analog scales and recording the number of vomiting episodes in the previous 24 hours before treatment and again during 4 consecutive days while taking the treatment. The visual analog scores of posttherapy minus baseline nausea decreased significantly in the ginger group (2.1 compared with 0.9, $p = 0.14$). The number of vomiting episodes also decreased significantly in the ginger group (1.4) compared with the placebo group (0.3, $p < 0.001$). Likert scales showed that 28 of 32 in the ginger group had improvement in nausea symptoms compared with 10 of 35 in the placebo group ($p < 0.001$). No adverse effect of ginger on pregnancy outcome was detected[ZO008].

Nematocidal activity. Decoction of the rhizome, at a concentration of 10 mg/mL, was inactive on *Toxocara canis*[ZO200]. Water extract of the rhizome, in cell culture at a concentration of 10 mg/mL was inactive on *Toxacara canis*. The methanol extract at a concentration of 1 mg/mL was active[ZO157].

Nerve growth factor stimulation. Powdered rhizome, administered intragastrically to rats, was active on the brain. A Kampo medicine "Kami-Untan-To," with *Pinellia ternata*, *Phykllostachys nigra*, *Citrus aurantium*, *Poria cocos*, *Citrus unshiu*, *Glycyrrhiza glabra*, *Polygala tenuifolia*, *Scrophularia ningpoensis*, *Panax ginseng*, *Rhemannia glutinosa*, *Zizyphus jujuba*, and *Zingiber officinale* was used[ZO350].

Neuromuscular blocking activity. Decoction of the dried rhizome, taken orally by human adults of both sexes at a dose of 4.6 g/person, was active on 25 patients with spastic facial paralysis. The patients were treated with a mixture of *Piper longum*, *Zingiber officinale*, *Piper cubeba*, *Curcuma zedoaria*, *Juniperus communis*, *Cichorium intybus*, *Mentha arvensis*, *Commiphora mukul*, and *Sesamum indicum* given in divided doses of 4.6 g in 24 hours. Six g of a decoction of *Lavandula stoechas* was also given in some cases. Seventy-six percent of the patients were cured, 16% showed a partial response, and 8% did not show any improvement[ZO263].

Pancreatic effect. Ginger (50 mg%), administered orally to rats, significantly enhanced pancreatic lipase activity and significantly stimulated trypsin and chymotrypsin. The stimulatory influence was not observed when the treatment was restricted to a single dose[ZO018].

Passive cutaneous anaphylaxis inhibition. Acetone extract of the dried rhizome, administered intragastrically to rats at a dose of 200 mg/kg, was active vs IgE-sensitized animals[ZO353].

Pepsin inhibition. Water extract of the rhizome, administered by gastric intubation to rabbits at a dose of 125 mg/kg, was active. Results significant at $p < 0.05$ level. The extract also contained *Pinellia ternata* (Rh), *Atractylis* species (Rh), *Citrus aurantium* (Pl), *Pachyma hoelen* fruit body, *Panax ginseng* (Rt), *Glycyrrhiza glabra* (Rt), *Zingiber officinale* (Rh), and *Zizyphus jujuba* (Fr)[ZO258].

Phagocytosis activity. Ethanol (80%) extract of the rhizome, in cell culture at a concentration of 500 μg/mL, did not decrease the rate of activity on mouse spleen lymphocytes (DBA/2)[ZO292].

Pharmacokinetics. [6]-Gingerol, the pungent constituent of ginger, was studied after bolus intravenous injection at a dose of 3 mg/kg to rats. Quantitative analysis with high reproducibility was achieved over the concentration range of 0.2–40 μg/mL. A two-compartment open model described the plasma concentration-time curve. [6]-Gingerol was rapidly cleared from plasma with a terminal half-life of 7.23 minutes and a total body clearance of 16.8 mL/minutes/kg. Serum protein binding of [6]-gingerol was 92.4%[ZO038].

Phosphodiesterase inhibition. Hot water extract of the rhizome, at a concentration of 1 mg/mL, was inactive[ZO163].

Plaque formation suppressant. Water extract of the rhizome was inactive on *Streptococcus mutans*. The methanol and methanol/water extracts were active; IC_{50} were greater than 1000, 60, and 230 µg/mL, respectively[ZO272].

Platelet aggregation inhibition. Gingerol was evaluated for its ability to inhibit human platelet activation, as compared to aspirin, by measuring the effect on arachidonic acid-induced platelet serotonin release and aggregation in vitro. The IC_{50} for arachidonic acid-induced (at EC_{50} was 0.75 mM) serotonin release by aspirin was 23.4 µM. Gingerol inhibited the arachidonic acid-induced platelet reaction in a similar dose range as aspirin, with IC_{50} values between 45.3 and 82.6 µM. The analogues (G1-G7), were also effective inhibitors of arachidonic acid-induced platelet aggregation. Maximum inhibitory values of 10.5 and 10.4 µM for G3 and G4, respectively, were approximately twofold greater than aspirin (IC_{max} 6 µM). The other analogues maximally inhibited arachidonic acid-induced platelet aggregation at approx 20–25 µM[ZO002]. Aqueous extract of ginger was found to inhibit aggregation induced by ADP, epinephrine, collagen, and arachidonate in a dose-dependent manner in vitro. A correlation was found between the amounts of ginger extract needed to inhibit platelet aggregation and those to inhibit platelet thromboxane synthesis. The extract reduced platelet prostaglandin-endoperoxides. A dose-related inhibition of platelet thromboxane and prostaglandin (PGF_2-α, PGE_2 and PGD_2) synthesis was affected by ginger extract. The extract inhibited biosynthesis of prostacyclin in rat aorta from labeled arachidonate. It mildly inhibited the synthesis of prostacyclin from endogenous pool of AA in the rat aorta[ZO060]. The extract

inhibited platelet aggregation induced by several aggregation agents, including arachidonate, in a dose-dependent manner. It inhibited the platelet cyclooxygenase products, and this effect correlated well with its inhibitory effects on platelet aggregation induced by the agents. The effects were dose-dependent. Although it inhibited the biosynthesis of 6-keto-F1-α in rat aortic rings from labeled arachidonate, it did not reduce prostacyclin production from endogenous arachidonate pool in aortic rings. The extract was further extracted into three organic solvents in order of increasing polarity (*N*-hexane, chloroform, and ethyl acetate). An analysis of the *N*-hexane extract revealed at least three clearly separated TLC bands containing constituents that inhibited platelet thromboxane generation simultaneously increasing lipoxygenase products[ZO061]. Chloroform, *N*-hexane, and ethyl acetate extracts of the rhizome reduced platelet thromboxane formation from exogenous arachidonate and inhibited platelet aggregation induced by arachidonate, epinephrine, ADP, and collagen. The aqueous extract reduced the formation of thromboxane from arachidonate-labeled platelets without showing effects on platelet phospholipase activity. Thromboxane formation in labeled platelets on activation with calcium ionophore A23187 was reduced by ginger components isolated from 2 TLC bands, in a dose-dependent manner. At the higher dose, lipoxygenase products were also reduced. The incorporation of arachidonate into platelet phospholipids increased in platelets treated with aqueous ginger extract[ZO053]. [6]-Shogaol, extracted from semidried ginger inhibited carrageenan-induced swelling of the hind paw in rats and arachidonic acid-induced platelet aggregation in rabbits; it prevented PGI 2 release from the aorta of rats when tested as an inhibitor of platelet aggregation. The results indicated that shogaol might have an inhibitory action on cyclo-oxygenase in both platelets and aorta. Investigation of the effects of shogaol on cyclo-oxygenases in rabbit platelets and microsome fractions of rat aorta indicated that shogaol inhibited cyclo-oxygenase activities of both tissues in a concentration-dependent manner. The effect of shogaol on 5-lipoxygenase from RBL-1 cells indicated that shogaol produced an inhibitory action on 5-lipoxygenase activity[ZO055]. Dried ginger was investigated in eight healthy male volunteers in a randomized double-blind study of the effects of 2 g dried ginger or placebo capsules. Bleeding time, platelet count, thromboelastography, and whole blood platelet aggregometry were performed 3 hours and 24 hours after the treatment. There were no differences between ginger and placebo in any of the variables measured. The effect of ginger on thromboxane synthetase activity is dose dependent, or only occurs with fresh ginger, and that up to 2 g of dried ginger is unlikely to cause platelet dysfunction when used therapeutically[ZO032]. Dried ginger, administered orally in two doses of 2.5 g each to male volunteers who consumed 100 g of butter in 7 days, significantly ($p < 0.001$) inhibited the platelet aggregation induced by ADP and epinephrine. Serum lipids, however, remained unchanged in both ginger treated and control groups[ZO034]. Powdered rhizome, administered orally to human adults at a dose of 5 g/person, was active vs ADP- and epinephrine-induced aggregations[ZO162]. The rhizome, taken orally by human adults at a dose of 2 g/person, was inactive[ZO032]. Water extract of the dried rhizome, at a concentration of 5 mg/mL, was active vs arachidonic acid-, collagen-, and ADP-induced aggregation[ZO322].

PG inhibition. Ethanol (80%) extract of the rhizome, in cell culture at a concentration of 100 µg/mL, was active on leukocytes[ZO292]. Hot water extract of the rhizome, at a concentration of 750 µg/mL, pro- duced weak activity on the rabbit microsomes[ZO251]. Decoction of the dried rhizome, administered intraperitoneally to rats at a dose of 0.74 g/animal, was inactive. Serum from rats fed the decoction was added to sheep vesicular gland microsomal fraction and the proportion of PGH_2 in arachidonic acid metabolites measured. The system was not affected by rat serum lipids[ZO315].

Proteolytic activity. Hot water extract of the rhizome, at a concentration of 1 mg/mL, was inactive[ZO235].

Prothrombin time decrease. Hot water extract of the rhizome, administered intragastrically to mice for 1 month, was active. The extract was used in combination with 7 g *Bupleurum falcatum*, 5 g *Pinellia ternata*, 3 g *Scutellaria baicalensis*, 2 g *Glycyrrhiza glabra*, 1 g *Zingiber officinale*, 3 g *Panax ginseng*, and 3 g *Zizyphus jujuba* in 700 mL water[ZO185].

Renal function improvement. Decoction of the dried rhizome, taken orally by 15 patients with chronic renal failure resulting from chronic glomerulonephritis, polycystic disease, tuberculosis, or diabetes, at variable dosage levels, was active. The patients were dosed three times daily for 3 months with a combination of *Zingiber officinale* and *Panax ginseng*. Improvements were seen in blood urea nitrogen, edema, fatigue, nausea, and constipation without effect on hematocrit or albumin. The effect decreased after 6 months[ZO316].

Respiratory stimulant effects. Ethanol (95%) extract of the rhizome, administered intravenously to dogs at a dose of 3 mL/animal, was active[ZO314].

Reverse transcriptase activity. Water extract of *Zingiber officinale* (Rh), *Bupleurum falcatum*, *Scutellaria baicalensis* (Rt), *Pinellia ternata* (Tu), *Zizyphus jujuba* (Fr), *Panax ginseng* (Rt), and *Glycyrrhiza glabra* (Rh), at a concentration of 200 µg/mL, was active on Moloney murine leukemia virus and HIV[ZO203].

Reverse transcriptase inhibition. Decoction of the rhizome, in cell culture, was active on Rauscher murine leukemia virus. The study was conducted with a prescription consisted of *Bupleurum falcatum* (Rt), *Scutellaria baicalensis* (Rt), *Pinellia ternata* (Tu), *Zizyphus jujuba* (Fr), *Panax ginseng* (Rt), and *Glycyrrhiza glabra* (Rh)[ZO203].

Serotonin antagonist activity. Acetone extract of the rhizome, at a concentration of 25 µg/mL, was active on the guinea pig ileum vs serotonin-induced contractions[ZO186].

Smooth muscle relaxant activity. The essential oil was active on the guinea pig trachea and ileum, ED_{50} 171 and 36 mg/L, respectively[ZO270].

Superoxide dismutase stimulation. Ethanol (95%) extract of the fresh aerial parts, administered intraperitoneally to mice at a dose of 0.5 g/kg, was inactive[ZO164].

Tachyphylactic activity. Zingerone, a natural pungent-tasting compound in ginger, was evaluated by whole cell patch-clamp studies performed on rat trigeminal ganglion. The inward currents activated by zingerone (30 mM) had peak times of approx 2 seconds, and all currents exhibited marked desensitization. Capsaicin (1 µM) activated a variety of inward currents having peak times ranging from 2 to 46 seconds that desensitized to various extents ranging from 0 to 100%. The inward currents activated by piperine (100 µM) had peak times of approx 25 seconds, and all exhibited a small desensitization. Piperine- and zingerone-induced currents were found only in cells that could be activated by capsaicin. Capsazepine (10 µM), an established antagonist of capsaicin-induced currents, inhibited the current evoked by piperine and zingerone, suggesting that all three compounds activate vanilloid receptors. Dose-response relationships for capsaicin, piperine, and zingerone obtained at a holding potential of 60 mV had threshold and apparent dissociation constants of 0.1 and 0.68 µM, 3 and 35 µM, and 1 and 15 mM, respectively. After seven 30-second applications of 1 µM capsaicin or 100 µM piperine (in a buffer with 2 mM Ca^{2+}), each interspersed with 2-minute 50-second washes, the peak currents were inhibited by approx 60 and 40%, respectively. In contrast, 30 mM zingerone failed to evoke a current after six applications. After complete tachyphylaxis produced by 30 mM zingerone, 1 µM capsaicin failed to evoke a current, suggesting that these two compounds cross-desensitize. The physiological responses produced by these compounds can be rationalized, in part, by their different activation and sensitization kinetics, and perhaps by the existence of different subtypes of vanilloid receptors[ZO026].

Taste-modifying effect. Water extract of the dried rhizome, administered intragastrically to male rats at a dose of 50 mg/mL, increased activity of vagal gastric nerve. The extract also blocked the suppression of vagal gastric nerve activity induced by *Pinellia ternata*[ZO317].

Teratogenic effect. A patented extract of garlic, administered by gavage to 22 pregnant rats at concentrations of 100, 333, and 1000 mg/kg from days 6 to 15 of gestation, produced no maternal or developmental toxicity. The rats were sacrificed on day 21 of gestation and examined for standard parameters of reproductive performance. The fetuses were examined for signs of teratogenic and toxic effects. No deaths or treatment related adverse effects were observed[ZO009]. Ginger tea, administered to Sprague–Dawley rats from gestation day 6–15 at a dose of 20 or 50 g/L and then sacrificed at day 20, produced no maternal toxicity. However, embryonic loss in the treatment groups was two times that of controls ($p < 0.05$). No gross morphological malformations were seen in the treated fetuses. Fetuses exposed to the ginger tea were significantly heavier than controls, an effect that was greater in female fetuses and was not correlated with increased placental size. Treated fetuses also had more advanced skeletal development as determined by measurement or sternal and metacarpal ossification centers[ZO011].

Thermogenic activity. Chloroform extract of the dried rhizome, at concentrations of 5 and 50 μg/mL administered by perfusion to the hind limb of rats, stimulated oxygen uptake[ZO128].

Thromboxane A2 inhibition. Rhizome, taken orally by human adults at a dose of 70 g/person for 7 days, was active[ZO188].

Thromboxane effect. The effect of raw ginger, taken orally by women at a dose of 5 g daily for 7 days, was investigated. Thromboxane determination was made in serum obtained after blood clotting. The values obtained were 782 ± 482 pmol/mL serum before ginger consumption and after consumption 498 ± 164 pmol/mL[ZO048].

Thromboxane synthetase inhibition. Ginger has been found to act as a potent inhibitor of thromboxane synthetase, raising levels of prostacyclin, without a concomitant rise in PGE2 or PGF2-α[ZO057].

Toxic effect. Decoctions of dried and roasted ginger were investigated on four experimental gastric ulcer models. The acute toxicity test has shown that the LD_{50} of the roasted ginger decoction administered orally was 170.6 ± 1.1 g/kg and the LD_{50} of the dried ginger decoction was over 250 g/kg[ZO042]. Ethanol (80%) extract of the rhizome, administered intragastrically to mice at a dose of 3 g/kg, was active[ZO292]. Ether extract of the rhizome adulterated with phenol ester-triorthocresyl phosphate produced paralysis in human adults who ingested 1–20 ounces of the extract. The symptoms appeared 4–35 days after the ingestion. Four to 6 years after the onset of the paralysis, only three of the patients had recovered enough to walk without support. Most of the patients had made good improvement in the arms but very little in the legs. Four of the patients were unable to stand or walk[ZO320].

Toxicity assessment. Ethanol (50%) extract of the aerial parts, administered intraperitoneally to mice, produced LD_{50} 178 mg/kg[ZO262].

Toxicity assessment. Ethanol (90%) extract of the dried rhizome, administered intraperitoneally to mice, produced LD_{50} of 1 g/kg[ZO318].

Toxicological evaluation. The effect of a patented standardized ginger extract, EV.EXT 33, was studied in rats. The extract had no significant effect on blood glucose levels at the doses used. It also had no significant effects on coagulation parameters or on warfarin-induced changes in blood coagulation, indicating that it did not interact with warfarin. It did not decrease systolic blood pressure or increase heart rate in the rat[ZO012].

Tryptophan pyrrolase stimulation. Hot water extract of 7 g *Bupleurum falcatum*, 5 g *Pinellai ternata*, 3 g *Scutellaria baicalensis*, 4 g *Zingiber officinale*, 3 g *Panax ginseng*, 3 g *Zizyphus inermis*, and 2 g *Glycyrrhiza glabra*, administered intraperitoneally to rats at a dose of 200 mg/kg, suppressed decrease in hepatic tryptophan pyrrolase resulting from D-galactosamine-induced liver injury[ZO282].

Tumor necrosis factor inhibition. Ethanol (95%) extract of the rhizome, in cell culture at a concentration of 100 μg/mL, was inactive on macrophage cell line RAW 264.7 vs LPS induction of TNF-α[ZO171].

Tumor promotion inhibition. Ethyl acetate and methanol extracts of the dried rhizome, in cell culture at a concentration of 50 μg/mL, produced weak activity on C3H/10T1/2 cells vs tetradecanoyl phorbol acetate-induced acetate phospholipid synthesis. The hexane extract was inactive[ZO095]. Ethanol (95%) and petroleum ether extracts of the dried rhizome, in cell culture at a concentration of 160 and 80 μg/mL, respectively, produced weak activity on Raji cells vs 12-O-tetradecanoylphorbol-13-acetate-induced EBV-EA activation. The methyl chloride extract, at a concentration of 40 µg/mL, was active[ZO319].

Tumor promotion inhibition. Methanol extract of the fresh aerial parts, in cell culture at a concentration of 200 µg, was active on EBV vs 12-O-hexadecanoylphorbol-13-acetate-induced virus activation[ZO286].

Turgal stimulant activity. Hot water extract of 7 g *Bupleurum falcatum*, 5 g *Pinellai ternata*, 3 g *Scutellaria baicalensis*, 4 g *Zingiber officinale*, 3 g *Panax ginseng*, 3 g *Zizyphus inermis*, and 2 g *Glycyrrhiza glabra*, administered intraperitoneally to rats at a dose of 200 mg/kg, decreased the volume of exudate in carrageenan-induced pleurisy[ZO282].

Urease inhibition. Water extract of the rhizome, at a concentration of 0.3 mg/mL, was inactive[ZO167].

Vasoconstrictive effect. Gingerols were evaluated on the isolated mouse and rat blood vessels. Leukotrienes C4 and D4, a thromboxane A2, PGF2-α, PGI2-Na, PGE2, the stable PGI2 derivative TRK-100, and PGD2, induced contraction in longitudinal segments of mouse mesenteric veins in that order of potency. Exogenous arachidonic acid did not cause contraction. The mesenteric veins also contracted in response to norepinephrine and phenylephrine but not to clonidine. The gingerols alone relaxed the muscle transiently and then augmented response to prostaglandin F2-α, prostaglandin E2, prostaglandin I2-Na, and TRK-100, but suppressed the response to prostaglandin D2. [6]-gingerols also potentiated the PGF2-α-induced contraction in longitudinal segments of the rat mesenteric vein and vena cava, but inhibited it in circular segments of rat aorta and longitudinal segments of the mouse mesenteric arteries[ZO046]. Crude and processed ginger extracts and pungent components, S-(+)-[6]-gingerol and [6]-shogaol were investigated

on norepinephrine and PGF2-α-induced contraction using mouse mesenteric veins. Both constituents inhibited the contractile responses to norepinephrine. The crude extract and S-(+)-[6]-gingerol potentiated the PGF2-α-induced contraction, whereas processed ginger extract and [6]-shogaol inhibited the contraction[ZO047].

WBC stimulant. Decoction of *Zingiber officinale* (Rh), *Bupleurum falcatum*, *Scutellaria baicalensis* (Rt), *Pinellia ternata* (Tu), *Zizyphus jujuba* (Fr), *Panax ginseng* (Rt), and *Glycyrrhiza glabra* (Rh), in cell culture at a concentration of 20 µg/mL, produced an average enhanced response of 40%. Response was enhanced 34% when pokeweed mitogen-induced peripheral mononuclear cell proliferation was assayed. The treatment was inactive vs enhancement of phytohemagglutinin-induced peripheral mononuclear cell proliferation, enhancement of Con A-induced peripheral mononuclear cell proliferation, leukocytes obtained from patients with AIDS, Con A-induced proliferation in leukocytes obtained from patients with AIDS, phytohemagglutinin-induced proliferation in leukocytes obtained from patients with AIDS, and 23% increased vs pokeweed mitogen-induced proliferation in leukocytes obtained from patients with AIDS[ZO320].

Weight-gain inhibition. Ethanol (95%) extract of the rhizome, in the drinking water of obese (C57BL/6J) mice, was active. The extract was used in combination with *Hordeum vulgare*, *Zingiberis rhizoma*, *Ligisticum chuanxiong*, *Lilium brownii*, *Nephelium longa*, and *Polygonum multiflorum*[ZO137].

REFERENCES

ZO001 Satoh, K., Y. Kase, T. Hayakawa, P. Murata, A. Ishige, and H. Sasaki. Dai-kenchu-to enhances accelerated small intestinal movement. **Biol Pharm Bull** 2001; 24(10): 1122–1126.

ZO002 Koo, K. L., A. J. Ammit, V. H. Tran, C. C. Duke, and B. D. Roufogalis. Gingerols and related analogues inhibit arachidonic acid-induced human platelet serotonin release and aggregation. **Thromb Res** 2001; 103(5): 387–397.

ZO003 Wood, C. D., J. E. Manno, M. J. Wood, B. R. Manno, and M. E. Mims. Comparison of efficacy of ginger with various antimotion sickness drugs. **Clin Res Pr Drug Regul Aff** 1988; 6(2): 129–136.

ZO004 Verma, S. K., and A. Bordia. Ginger, fat and fibrinolysis. **Indian J Med Sci** 2001; 55(2): 83–86.

ZO005 Argawal, M., S. Walia, S. Dhingra, and B. P. Khambay. Insect growth inhibition, antifeedant and antifungal activity of compounds isolated/derived from *Zingiber officinale* Roscoe (ginger) rhizomes. **Pest Manag Sci** 2001; 57(3): 289–300.

ZO006 Tjendraputra, E., V. H. Tran, D. Liu-Brennan, B. D. Roufogalis, and C. C. Duke. Effect of ginger constituents and synthetic analogues on cyclo-oxygenase-2 enzyme in intact cells. **Bioorg Chem** 2001; 29(3): 156–163.

ZO007 Tulimat, M. A., T. Ishiguchi, S. Kurosawa, T. Nakamura, and T. Takahashi. The inhibitory effect of herbal medicine—Dai Kenchu To (DKT)—on the colonic motility in rats *in vitro*. **Am J Chim Med** 2001; 29(1): 111–118.

ZO008 Vutyavanich, T., T. Kraisarin, and R. Ruangsri. Ginger for nausea and vomiting in pregnancy: randomized, double-masked, placebo-controlled trial. **Obstet Gynecol** 2001; 97(4): 577–582.

ZO009 Weidner, M. S., and K. Sigwart. Investigation of the teratogenic potential of *Zingiber officinale* extract in the rat. **Reprod Toxicol** 2001; 15(1): 75–80.

ZO010 Ahmed, R. S., V. Seth, and B. D. Banerjee. Influence of dietary ginger (*Zingiber officinale* Roscoe) on antioxidant defense system in rat: comparison with ascorbic acid. **Indian J Exp Biol** 2000; 38(6): 604–606.

ZO011 Wilkinson, J. M. Effect of ginger tea on fetal development of Sprague-Dawley rats. **Reprod Toxicol** 2000; 14(6): 507–512.

ZO012 Weidner, M. S., and K. Sigwart. The safety of a ginger extract in the rat. **J Ethnopharmacol** 2000; 73(3): 513–520.

ZO013 Mukhopadhyay, M. J. and A. Mukherjee. Clastogenic effect of ginger rhizome in mice. **Phytother Res** 2000; 14(7): 555–557.

ZO014 Guo, P., J. Xu, S. Xu, and K. Wang. **Zhongguo Zhong Yao Za Zhi** 1997; 22(9): 559–561.

ZO015 Fuhrman, B., M. Rosenblat, T. Hayek, R. Coleman, and M. Aviram. Ginger extract consumption reduces plasma cholesterol, inhibits LDL oxidation and attenuates development of atherosclerosis in atherosclerotic, apolipoprotein E-deficient mice. **J Nutr** 2000; 130(5): 1124–1131.

ZO016 Shobana, S., and K. A. Naidu. Antioxidant activity of selected Indian spices. **Prostaglandins Leukot Essent Fatty Acids** 2000; 62(2): 107–110.

ZO017 Ahmed, R. S., V. Seth, S. T. Pasha, and B. D. Banerjee. Influence of dietary ginger (*Zingiber officinale* Roscoe) on oxidative stress induced by malathion in rats. **Food Chem Toxicol** 2000; 38(5): 443–450.

ZO018 Platel, K., and K. Srinivasan. Influence of dietary spices and their active principles on pancreatic digestive enzymes in albino rats. **Nahrung** 2000; 44(1): 42–46.

ZO019 Sekiwa, Y., K. Kubota, and A. Kobayashi. Isolation of novel glucosides related to gingerdiol from ginger and their antioxidative activities. **J Agri Food Chem** 2000; 48(2): 373–377.

ZO020 Bliddal, H., A. Rosetzsky, P. Schlichting, et al. A randomized, placebo-controlled, cross-over study of ginger extracts and ibuprofen in osteoarthritis. **Osteoarthritis Cartilage** 2000; 8(1): 9–12.

ZO021 Shibata, C., I. Sasaki, H. Naito, T. Ueno, and S. Matsuno. The herbal medicine Dai-Kenchu-Tou stimulates upper gut motility through cholinergic and 5-hydroxytryptamine 3 receptors in conscious dogs. **Surgery** 1999; 126(5): 918–924.

ZO022 Micklefield, G. H., Y. Redeker, V. Meister, O. Jung, I. Greving, and B. May. Effects of ginger on gastroduodenal motility. **Int J Clin Pharmacol** 1999; 37(7): 341–346.

ZO023 Lee, E. and Y. J. Surh. Induction of apoptosis in HL-60 cells by pungent vanilloids, [6]-gingerol and [6]-pardol. **Cancer Lett** 1998; 134-2: 163–168.

ZO024 Park, K. K., K. S. Chum, J. M. Lee, S. S. Lee, and Y. J. Surh. Inhibitory effects of [6]-gingerol, a major pungent principle of ginger, on phorbol ester-induced inflammation, epidermal ornithine decarboxylase activity and skin tumor promotion in ICR mice. **Cancer Lett** 1998; 129(2): 139–144.

ZO025 Visalyaputra, S., N. Petchpaisit, K. Somcharoen, and R. Choavaratana. The efficacy of ginger root in the prevention of postoperative nausea and vomiting after outpatient gynaecological laparoscopy. **Anaesthesia** 1998; 53(5): 506–510.

ZO026 Liu, L., and S. A. Simon. Similarities and differences in the currents activated by capsaicin, piperine and zingerone in rat trigeminal ganglion cells. **J Neurophysiol** 1996; 76(3): 1858–1869.

ZO027 Platel, K., and K. Srinivasan. Influence of dietary spices or their active principles on digestive enzymes of small intestinal mucosa in rats. **Int J Food Sci Nutr** 1996; 47(1): 55–59.

ZO028 Arfeen, Z., H. Owen, J. L. Plummer, A. H. Ilsey, R. A. Sorby-Adams, and C. J. Doecke. A double-blind randomized controlled trial of ginger for the prevention of postoperative nausea and vomiting. **Anaesth Intensive Care** 1995; 23(4): 449–452.

ZO029 Sharma, J. N., K. C. Srivastava, and E. K. Gan. Suppressive effects of eugenol and ginger oil on arthritic rats. **Pharmacology** 1994; 49(5): 314–318.

ZO030 Shanmugasundaram, K. R., S. Ramanujam, and E. R. Shanmugasundaram. Amrita Bindu—a salt-spice herbal health food supplement for the prevention of nitrosamine induced depletion of antioxidants. **J Ethnopharmacol** 1994; 42(2): 83–93.

ZO031 Surh, Y. J., and S. S. Lee. Enzymatic reduction of [6]-gingerol, a major pungent principle of ginger, in the cell-free preparation of rat liver. **Life Sci** 1994; 54(19): PL 321–326.

ZO032 Lumb, A. B. Effect of dried ginger on human platelet function. **Thromb Haemost** 1994; 71(1): 110–111.

ZO033 Banerjee, S., R. Sharma, R. K. Kale, and A. R. Rao. Influence of certain

essential oils on carcinogen-metabolizing enzymes and acid-soluble sulfhydryls on mouse liver. **Nutr Cancer** 1994; 21(3): 263–269.

ZO034 Verma, S. K., J. Singh, R. Khamesra, and A. Bordia. Effect of ginger on platelet aggregation in man. **Indian J Med Res** 1993; 98: 240–242.

ZO035 Wu, H., D. J. Ye, Y. Z. Zhao, and S. L. Wang. Effect of different preparations of ginger on blood coagulation time in mice. **Zhongguo Zhong Yao Za Zhi** 1993; 18(3): 147–149.

ZO036 Srivastava, K. C., and T. Mustafa. Ginger (*Zingiber officinale*) in rheumatism and musculoskeletal disorders. **Med Hypotheses** 1992; 39(4): 342–348.

ZO037 Reddy, A. C., and B. R. Lokesh. Studies on spice principles as antioxidants in the inhibition of lipid peroxidation of rat liver microsomes. **Mol Cell Biochem** 1992; 111(1–2): 117–124.

ZO038 Ding, G. H., K. Naora, M. Hayashibara, Y. Katagiri, Y. Kano, and K. Iwamoto. Pharmacokinetics of [6]-gingerol after intravenous administration in rats. **Chem Pharm Bull (Tokyo)** 1991; 39(6): 1612–1614.

ZO039 Huang, Q. R., M. Iwamoto, S. Aoki, et al. Anti-5-hydroxytryptamine effect of galanolactone, diterpenoid isolated from ginger. **Chem Pharm Bull (Tokyo)** 1991; 39(2): 397–399.

ZO040 Srinivasan, K., and K. Sambaiah. The effect of spices on cholesterol 7 alpha-hydroxylase activity and on serum and hepatic cholesterol levels in the rat. **Int J Vitam Nutr Res** 1991; 61(4): 364–369.

ZO041 Huang, Q., H. Matsuda, K. Sakai, J. Yamahara, and Y. Tamai. The effect of ginger on serotonin induced hypothermia and diarrhea. **Yakugaku Zasshi** 1990; 110(12): 936–942.

ZO042 Wu, H., D. Ye, Y. Bai, and Y. Zhao. Effect of dry ginger and roasted ginger on experimental gastric ulcers in rats. **Zhongguo Zhong Yao Za Zhi** 1990; 15(5): 278-280, 317–318.

ZO043 Desai, H. G., R. H. Kalro, and A. P. Choksi. Effect of ginger and garlic on DNA content of gastric aspirate. **Indian J Med Res** 1990; 92: 139–141.

ZO044 Yamahara, J., Q. R. Huang, Y. H. Li, L. Xu, and H. Fujimura. Gastrointestinal motility enhancing effect of ginger and its active constituents. **Chem Pharm Bull (Tokyo)** 1990; 38(2): 430–431.

ZO045 Sambaiah, K., and K. Srinvasan. Influence of spices and spice principles on hepatic mixed function oxygenase system in rats. **Indian J Biochem Biophys** 1989; 26(4): 254–258.

ZO046 Kimuru, I., M. Kimuru, and L. R. Pancho. Modulation of eicosanoid-induced contraction of mouse and rat blood vessels by gingerols. **Jpn J Pharmacol.** 1989; 50(3): 253–261.

ZO047 Pancho, L. R., I. Kimura, R. Unno, M. Kurono, and M. Kimura. Reverse effects between crude and processed ginger extracts on PGF2 alpha-induced contraction in mouse mesenteric veins. **Jpn J Pharmacol** 1989; 50(2): 243–246.

ZO048 Srivastava, K. C. Effect of onion and ginger consumption on platelet thromboxane production in humans. **Prostaglandins Leukot Essent Fatty Acids** 1989; 35(3): 183–185.

ZO049 Kobayashi, M., Y. Ishida, N. Shoji, and Y. Ohizumi. Cardiotonic action of [8]-gingerol, an activator of the Ca^{++}-pumping adenosine triphosphate of sarcoplasmic reticulum, in guinea pig atrial muscle. **J Pharmacol Exp Ther** 1988; 246(2): 667–673.

ZO050 Yahamara, J., M. Mochizuki, H. Q. Rong, H. Matasuda, and H. Fujimura. The anti-ulcer effect in rats of ginger constituents. **J Ethnopharmacol** 1988; 23(2-3): 299–304.

ZO051 Kobayashi, M., N. Shoji, and Y. Ohizumi. Gingerol, a novel cardiotonic agent, activates the Ca^{2+}-pumping ATPase in skeletal and cardiac sarcoplasmic reticulum. **Biochim Biophys Acta** 1987; 903(1): 96–102.

ZO052 Nagabhushan, M., A. J. Amonkar, and S. V. Bhide. Mutagenicity of gingerol and shogaol and antimutagenicity of zingerone in *Salmonella*/microsome assay. **Cancer Lett** 1987; 36(2): 221–233.

ZO053 Srivastava, K. C. Isolation and effect of some ginger component of platelet aggregation and eicosanoid biosynthesis. **Prostaglandins Leukot Med** 1986; 25(2-3): 187–198.

ZO054 Suekawa, M., H. Sone, I. Sakakibara, Y. Ikeya, M. Aburada, and E. Hosoya.

Pharmacological studies on ginger. V. Pharmacological comparison between (6)-shogaol and capsaicin. **Nippon Yakugaku Zasshi** 1986; 88(5): 339–347.

ZO055 Suekawa, M., K. Yuasa, M. Isono, et al. Pharmacological studies on ginger. IV. Effect of (6)-shogaol on arachidonic cascade. **Nippon Yakurigaku Zasshi** 1986; 88(4): 263–269.

ZO056 Suekawa, M., M. Aburada, and E. Hosoya. Pharmacological studies on ginger. III. Effect of the spinal destruction on (6)-shogaol-induced pressor response in rats. **J Pharmacobiodyn** 1986; 9(10): 853–860.

ZO057 Backon, J. Ginger: Inhibition of thromboxane synthetase and stimulation of prostacyclin: relevance for medicine and psychiatry. **Med Hypotheses** 1986; 20(3): 271–278.

ZO058 Van Toorenenbergen, A. W., and P. H. Dieges. Immunoglobulin E antibodies against coriander and other spices. **J Allergy Clin Immunol** 1985; 76(3): 477–481.

ZO059 Yamahara, J., K. Miki, T. Chisaka, et al. Cholagogic effect of ginger and its active constituents. **J Ethnopharmacol** 1985; 13(2): 217–225.

ZO060 Srivas, K. C. Effects of aqueous extracts of onion, garlic and ginger on platelet aggregation and metabolism of arachidonic acid in the blood vascular system: *in vitro* study. **Prostaglandins Leukot Med** 1984; 13(2): 227–235.

ZO061 Srivastava, K. C. Aqueous extracts of onion, garlic and ginger inhibit platelet aggregation and alter arachidonic acid metabolism. **Biomed Biochim Acta** 1984; 43(8–9): S335–S346.

ZO062 Monge, P., R. Scheline, and E. Solheim. The metabolism of zingerone, a pungent principle of ginger. **Xenobiotica** 1976; 6(7): 411–423.

ZO063 Jain, S. K., and C. R. Tarafder. Medicinal plant-lore of the santals. **Econ Bot** 1970; 24: 241–278.

ZO064 Gimlette, J. D. Malay poisons and charm cures. J. & A. Churchill, London, 3rd edition, 1929.

ZO065 Jochle, W. Biology and pathology of reproduction in Greek mythology. **Contraception** 1971; 4: 1–13.

ZO066 Petelot, A. Les plantes medicinales du Cambodge, du Laos et du Vietnam, vols. 1–4. Archives des Reserches Agronomiquest Pastorales au Vietnam no. 23 1954.

ZO067 Haginiwa, J., M. Harada, and I. Morishita. Pharmacological studies on crude drugs. VII. Properties of essential oil components of aromatics and their pharmacological effect on mouse intestine. **Yakugaku Zasshi** 1963; 83: 624.

ZO068 Schermerhorn, J. W. and M. W. Quimby. Orders *Scitamineae* and *Microspermae*. Lynn Index 1958; 3.

ZO069 Haerdi, F. Native medicinal plants of Ulanga district of Tanganyika (east Africa). Dissertation, Verlag fur Recht und Gessellschaft AG, Basel, Switzerland, 1964.

ZO070 Watt, J. M., and M. G. Breyer-Brandwijk. The medicinal and poisonous plants of southern and eastern Africa. 2nd ed. E & S Livingstone Ltd., London, 1962.

ZO071 Burkill, I. H. Dictionary of the economic products of the Malay peninsula. Ministry of Agriculture and Cooperatives, Kuala Lumpur, Malaysia, vol II, 1966.

ZO072 Ernst, E., and M. H. Pittler. Efficacy of ginger for nausea and vomiting: a systematic review of randomized clinical trials. **Br J Anaesth** 2000; 84(3): 367–371.

ZO073 Lee, Y. B., Y. S. Kim, and C. R. Ashmore. Antioxidant property in ginger rhizome and its application to meat products. **J Food Sci** 1986; 51(1): 20–23.

ZO074 Endo, K., E. Kanno, and Y. Oshima. Structures of antifungal diarylheptenones, gingerenones A, B, C and isogingerenone B, isolated from the rhizomes of *Zingiber officinale*. **Phytochemistry** 1990; 29(3): 797–799.

ZO075 Kikuzaki, H., J. Usuguchi, and N. Nakatani. Constituents of Zingiberaceae. 1. Diarylheptanoids from the rhizomes of ginger (*Zingiber officinale* Roscoe). **Chem Pharm Bull** 1991; 39(1): 120–122.

ZO076 Kikuzaki, H., M. Kobayashi, and N. Natakani. Diarylheptanoids from rhizomes of *Zingiber officinale*. **Phytochemistry** 1991; 30(11): 2647–3651.

ZO077 Kikuzaki, H., S. M. Tsai, and N. Nakatani. Gingerdiol related compounds from the rhizomes of *Zingiber*

officinale. **Phytochemistry** 1992; 31(5): 1783–1786.

ZO078 Yoshikawa, M., S. Hatakeyama, K. Taniguchi, H. Matuda, and J. Yamahara. 6-Gingesulfonic acid, a new anti-ulcer principle, and gingerglycolipds A, B and C, three new monoacyldigalactosylglycerols from *Zingiberis rhizoma* originating in Taiwan. **Chem Pharm Bull** 1992; 40(8): 2239–2241.

ZO079 Yamahara, J., S. Hatakeyama, K. Taniguchi, M. Kawamura, and M. Yoshikawa. Stomachic principles in ginger. II. Pungent and anti-ulcer effects of low polar constituents isolated from ginger, the dried rhizoma of *Zingiber officinale* Roscoe, cultivated in Taiwan. The absolute stereostructure of a new diarylheptanoid. **Yakugaku Zasshi** 1992; 112(9): 645–655.

ZO080 Nakatani, N., and H. Kikuzaki. New phenolic compounds of ginger (*Zingiber officinale* Roscoe). **Chem Exp** 1992; 7(3): 221–224.

ZO081 Jitoe, A., T. Masuda, and N. Nakatani. Phenylbutenoid dimers from the rhizomes of *Zingiber cassumunar*. **Phytochemistry** 1993; 32(2): 357–363.

ZO082 Ayafor, J. F., M. H. K. Tchuendem, B. Nyasse, F. Tillequin, and H. Anke. Aframodial and other bioactive diterpenoids from *Aframomum* species. **Pure Appl Chem** 1994; 66(10/11): 2327–2330.

ZO083 Kikuzaki, H., and N. Nakatani. Cyclic diarylheptanoids from rhizomes of *Zingiber officinale*. **Phytochemistry** 1996; 43(1): 272–277.

ZO084 Yoshikawa, M., S. Yamaguchi, K. Kunimi, H. Matsuda, Y. Okuno, J. Yamahara, and N. Murakami. Stomachic principles in ginger. III. An anti-ulcer principle, 6-gingesulfonic acid, and three monoacyldigalactosylglycerols, gingerglycolipids A, B and C, from *Zingiberis* rhizoma originating in Taiwan. **Chem Pharm Bull** 1994; 42(6): 1226–1230.

ZO085 Wu, T. S., Y. C. Wu, P. L. Wu, C. Y. Chern, Y. L. Leu, and Y. Y. Chan. Structure and synthesis of [N]-dehydroshogaols from *Zingiber officinale*. **Phytochemistry** 1998; 48(5): 889–891.

ZO086 Yoshida, S., K. Tazaki, and T. Minamikawa. Occurrence of shikimic and quinic acids in Angiosperms. **Phytochemistry** 1975; 14: 195–197.

ZO087 Mitra, C. R. Important Indian spices. III. Ginger (*Zingiberaceae*). **Riechst Aromen Koerperpflegem** 1975; 25: 170.

ZO088 Bednarczyk, A. A., W. G. Galetto, and A. Kramer. Cis- and trans-beta-sesquiphellandrol. Two new sesquiterpene alcohols from oil of ginger *Zingiber officinale*. **J Agr Food Chem** 1975; 23(3): 499–501.

ZO089 Terhune, S. J., J. W. Hogg, A. C. Bromstein, and B. M. Lawrence. Four new sesquiterpene analogs of common monoterpenes. **Can J Chem** 1975; 23(3): 3283–3295.

ZO090 Morton, J. F. Current folk remedies of northern Venezuela. **Q J Crude Drug Res** 1975; 13: 97-121.

ZO091 Sharma, I., D. Gusain, and V. P. Dixit. Hypolpidaemic and antiatheroscolerotic effects of *Zingiber officinale* in cholesterol fed rabbits. **Phytother Res** 1996; 10(6): 517–518.

ZO092 Yamaoka, Y., T. Kawakita, M. Kaneko, and K. Nomoto. A polysaccharide fraction of *Zizyphus fructus* in augmenting natural killer activity by oral administration. **Biol Pharm Bull** 1996; 19(7): 936–939.

ZO093 Vaz, Z. R., L. V. Mata, and J. B. Calixto. Analgesic effect of the herbal medicine catuama in thermal and chemical models of nociception in mice. **Phytother Res** 1997; 11(2): 101–106.

ZO094 Hasenohrl, R. U., B. Topic, C. Frisch, R. Hacker, C. M. Mattern, and J. P. Huston. Dissociation between anxiolytic and hypomnestic effects for combined extracts of *Zingiber officinale* and *Ginkgo biloba*, as opposed to diazepam. **Pharmacol Biochem Behav** 1998; 59(2): 527–535.

ZO095 Okuyama, T., M. Matsuda, Y. Masuda, et al. Studies on cancer bio-chemoprevention of natural resources. X. Inhibitory effect of spices on TPA-enhanced ^{3}H-choline incorporation in phospholipid of C3H10T1/2 cells and on TPA-induced ear edema. **Zhonghua Yaoxue Zazhi** 1995; 47(5): 421–430.

ZO096 Surarit, R., S. Autayapamonvat, and T. Triratana. Effect of some plant extracts of human gingival fibroblasts. **Abstr 19th Congr Sci Technol Thailand** 1993; 27(29): 434.

ZO097 Etkin, N. L. Antimalarial plants used by Hausa in northern Nigeria. **Trop Doctor** 1997; 27(1): 12–16.

ZO098 He, X. G., M. W. Bernart, L. Z. Lian, and L. Z. Lin. High performance liquid chromatography –electrospray mass spectrometric analysis of pungent constituents of ginger. **J Chromatogr A** 1998; 796(2): 327–334.

ZO099 Kurokawa, M., C. A. Kumeda, J. Yamamura, T. Kamiyama, and K. Shiraki. Antipyretic activity of cinnamyl derivatives and related compounds in influenza virus-infected mice. **Eur J Pharmacol** 1998; 348(1): 45–51.

ZO100 Nishioka, T., J. Kawaba, and Y. Aoyama. Baicalein, an alpha-glucosidase inhibitor from *Scutelaria baicalensis*. **J Nat Prod** 1998; 61(11): 1413–1415.

ZO101 Mahabir, D., and M. C. Gulliford. Use of medicinal plants for diabetes in Trinidad and Tobago. **Pan Am J Public Health** 1997; 1(3): 174–178.

ZO102 Gill, L. S., and C. Akinwumi. Nigerian folk medicine: practices and beliefs of the Ondo people. **J Ethnopharmacol** 1986; 18(3): 259–266.

ZO103 Mahabir, D., and M. C. Gulliford. Use of medicinal plants for diabetes in Trinidad and Tobago. **Rev Panam Salud Publ/Pan Am J Publ Health** 1997; 1(3): 174–179.

ZO104 Bhandari, U., J. N. Sharma, J. N. Sharma, and R. Zafar. The protective action of ethanolic ginger (*Zingiber officinale*) extract in cholesterol fed rabbits. **J Ethnopharmacol** 1998; 61(2): 167–171.

ZO105 Sohni, Y. R., and R. M. Bhatt. Activity of a crude extract formulation in experimental hepatic amoebiasis and in immunomodulation studies. **J Ethnopharmacol** 1996; 54(2/3): 119–124.

ZO106 Yabe, T., S. Iizuka, Y. Komatsu, and H. Yamada. Enhancement of choline acetyltransferase activity and nerve growth factor secretion of *Polygalae radix*-extract containing active ingredients in kami-untan-to. **Phytomedicine** 1997; 4(3): 199–205.

ZO107 Denniff, P., and D. A. Whiting. Biosynthesis of (6)-gingerol, pungent principle of *Zingiber officinale*. **Chem Commun** 1976; 711.

ZO108 Kakumu, S., K. Yoshioka, T. Wakita, and T. Ishikawa. Effects of TJ09 shosaiko-to (kampo medicine) on interferon gamma and antibody production specific for hepatitis B virus antigen in patients with type B chronic hepatitis. **Int J Immunopharmacol** 1990; 13(2/3): 141–146.

ZO109 Kiuchi, F., S. Iwakami, M. Shibuya, F. Hanaoka, and U. Sankawa. Inhibition of prostaglandin and leukotriene biosynthesis by gingerols and diarylheptanoids. **Chem Pharm Bull** 1992; 40(2): 387–391.

ZO110 Latifah. Analgesic effect of *Zingiber officinale* Roxb. juice on mice. Thesis MS, Dept Pharm-Fac Math & Sci-Univ Padjadjaran-Indonesia 1987.

ZO111 Nagatsu, Y., M. Inoue, and Y. Ogihara. Effects of shosaikoto (kampo medicine) on lipid metabolism in macrophages. **Chem Pharm Bull** 1992; 40(7): 1828–1830.

ZO112 Huang, M. F., W. J. Hang, and Q. Zhong. Hair growth stimulating preparations containing medicinal plant extracts. Patent-faming Zhuanli Shenquing Gongkai Shuomingshu-1,043,624 1990; 6 pp.

ZO113 Sharma, S. K., and V. P. Singh. The antifungal activity of some essential oils. **Indian Drug Pharm Ind** 1979; 14(1): 3–6.

ZO114 Tanabe, M., M. Yasuda, Y. Adachi, and Y. Kano. Capillary GC-MS analysis of volatile components in Japanese gingers. **Shoyakugaku Zasshi** 1991; 45(4): 321–326.

ZO115 Phillips, S., S. Hutchinson, and R. Ruggier. *Zingiber officinale* does not affect gastric emptying rate. A randomised, placebo-controlled, cross-over trial. **Anaesthesia** 1993; 48(5): 393–395.

ZO116 Ghazanfar, S. A., and M. A. Al-Sabahi. Medicinal plants of northern and central Oman (Arabia). **Econ Bot** 1993; 47(1): 89–98.

ZO117 Yoshikawa, M., S. Hatakeyama, N. Cahtani, Y. Nishino, and J. Yamahara. Qualitative and quantitative analysis of bioactive principles in *Zingiberis rhizoma* by means of high performance liquid chromatography and gas liquid chromatography on the evaluation of *Zingiberis rhizoma* and chemical change of constituents. **Yakugaku Zasshi** 1993; 113(4): 307–315.

ZO118 Yasukawa, K., A. Yamaguchi, J. Arita, S. Sakurai, A. Ikeda, and M. Takido. Inhibitory effect of edible plant extracts on 12-0-tetradecanoylphorbol-13-acetate-induced ear oedema in mice. **Phytother Res** 1993; 7(2): 185–189.

ZO119 Reddy, M. B., K. R. Reddy, and M. N. Reddy. A survey of plant crude drugs of Anantapur district, Andhra Pradesh, India. **Int J Crude Drug Res** 1989; 27(3): 145–155.

ZO120 Phillips, S., R. Ruggier, and S. E. Hutchinson. *Zingiber officinale* (ginger)-an antiemetic for day case surgery. **Anaesthesia** 1993; 48(8): 715–717.

ZO121 Kawamura, F., and M. Okada. Antioxidative effect of ginger on the peroxidation of lard in boiled water. I. Effect of the essential oils and sliced ginger. **Nippon Kasei Gakkaishi** 1992; 43(1): 31–35.

ZO122 Kim, J. S., M. S. Koh, Y. H. Kim, M. K. Kim, and J. S. Hong. Volatile flavor components of Korean ginger (*Zingiber officinale* Roscoe). **Han'guk Sikp'um Kwahakhoe Chi** 1991; 23(2): 141–149.

ZO123 Mizoguchi, Y., Y. Komats, and Y. Okhura. Effects of sho-saiko-to on cytokine cascade and arachidonic cascade. **Adv Exp Med Biol** 1992; 319: 309–317.

ZO124 Yoshikawa, M., N. Chatani, S. Hatakeyama, Y. Nishino, J. Yamahara, and N. Murakami. Crude drug processing by far-infrared treatment. II. Chemical fluctuation of the constituents during the drying of *Zingiber* rhizoma. **Yakugaku Zasshi** 1993; 113(10): 712–717.

ZO125 Thompson, E. H., I. D. Wolf, and C. E. Allen. Ginger rhizome: a new source of proteolytic enzyme. **J Food Sci** 1973; 38: 652–655.

ZO126 Tanabe, M., Y. D. Chen, K. I. Saito, and Y. Kano. Cholesterol biosynthesis inhibitory component from *Zingiber officinale* Roscoe. **Chem Pharm Bull** 1993; 41(4): 710–713.

ZO127 Meena, M. R., and V. Sethi. Antimicrobial activity of essential oils from spices. **J Food Sci Technol** 1994; 31(1): 68–70.

ZO128 Eldershaw, T. P. D., E. Q. Colquhoun, K. A. Dora, Z. C. Peng, and M. G. Clark. Pungent principles of ginger (*Zingiber officinale*) are thermogenic in the perfused rat hindlimb. **Int J Obesity** 1992; 16: 755–763.

ZO129 Fu, H. Y., T. C. Huang, C. T. Ho, and H. Daun. Characterization of the major anthyocyanin in acidified green ginger (*Zingiber officinale* Roscoe). **Zhongguo Nongye Huaxue Huizhi** 1993; 31(5): 587–595.

ZO130 Kikuzaki, H., and N. Nakatani. Antioxidant effects of some ginger constituents. **J Food Sci** 1993; 58(6): 1407–1410.

ZO131 Denyer, C. V., P. Jackson, D. M. Loakes, M. R. Ellis, and D. A. B. Young. Isolation of antirhinoviral sesquiterpenes from ginger (*Zingiber officinale*). **J Nat Prod** 1994; 57(5): 658–662.

ZO132 Zamora-Martinez, M. C., and C. N. P. Pola. Medicinal plants used in some rural populations of Oaxaca, Puebla and Veracruz, Mexico. **J Ethnopharmacol** 1992; 35(3): 229–257.

ZO133 Kawai, T., K. Kinoshita, K. Koyama, and K. Takahashi. Anti-emetic principles of *Magnolia obovata* bark and *Zingiber officinale* rhizome. **Planta Med** !994; 60(1): 17.

ZO134 Holdsworth, D., and L. Balun. Medicinal plants of the east and west Sepik provinces, Papua New Guinea. **Int J Pharmacog** 1992; 30(3): 218–222.

ZO135 Kawakishi, S., Y. Morimitsu, and T. Osawa. Chemistry of ginger components and inhibitory factors of the arachidonic acid cascade. **Asc Symp Ser** 1994; 547: 244–250.

ZO136 Sohni, Y. R., P. Kaimal, and R. M. Bhatt. The antiamoebic effect of a crude drug formulation of herbal extracts against *Entamoeba histolytica in vitro* and *in vivo*. **J Ethnopharmacol** 1995; 45(1): 43–52.

ZO137 Wijaya, E., Z. M. Wu, and F. Ng. Effect of "Slimax", a Chinese herbal mix-

ture, on obesity. **Int J Pharmacog** 1995; 33(1): 41–46.

ZO138 Nagasaka, K., M. Kurokawa, M. Imakita, K. Terasawa, and K. Shiraki. Efficacy of kakkon-to, a traditional herb medicine, in herpes simplex virus type 1 infection in mice. **J Med Virol** 1995; 46(1): 28–34.

ZO139 Yokozawa, T., H. Oura, M. Hattori, M. Iwano, and K. Dohi. Effect of wen-pi-tang and its crude drug extracts on proliferation of cultured mouse mesangial cells. **Phytother Res** 1994; 8(3): 170–173.

ZO140 Lin, Z. K., and Y. F. Hua. Chemical constituents of the essential oil from *Zingiber officinale* Roscoe of Sichuan. **You-ji Hua Hsueh** 1987; 1987(6): 444–448.

ZO141 Mowrey, D. B., and D. E. Clayson. Motion sickness, ginger and psychophysics. **Lancet** 1982; 655–657.

ZO142 Frisch, C., R. U. Hasenohri, C. M. Mattern, R. Hacker, and J. P. Huston. Blockade of lithium chloride-induced conditioned place aversion as a test for antiemetic agents: comparison of metoclopramide with combined extracts of *Zingiber officinale* and *Ginkgo biloba*. **Pharmacol Biochem Behav** 1995; 52(2): 321–327.

ZO143 Kasuya, S., C. Goto, and H. Ohtomo. Studies on prophylaxis against anisakiasis-A screening of killing effects of extracts from foods on the larvae. **Kansensh Ogaku Zasshi** 1988; 62(12): 1152–1156.

ZO144 Nishimura, O. Identification of the characteristic odorants in fresh rhizomes of ginger (*Zingiber officinale* Roscoe) using aroma extract dilution analysis and modified multidimensional gas chromatography-mass spectroscopy. **J Agr Food Chem** 1995; 43(11): 2941–2945.

ZO145 Fujimoto, Y., K. Maruno, and S. Made. Antitumor sesquiterpene extraction from ginger roots. Patent-Japan Kokai Tokkyo Koho-01 221,344 1989; 6 pp.

ZO146 Yabe, T., K. Toriizuka, and H. Yamada. Kami-untan-to (Kut) improves cholinergic deficits in aged rats. **Phytomedicine** 1996; 2(3): 253–258.

ZO147 Nishimura, K., Y. Kitada, and T. Fukuda. Phenols for moisture-increasing of skin horny layers and compositions containing the phenols. Patent-Japan Kokai Tokkyo Koho-06 239, 729 1994; 5 pp.

ZO148 Selvanyahgam, Z. E., S. G. Gnanevendhan, K. Balakrishna, and R. B. Rao. Antisnake venom botanicals from ethnomedicine. **J Herbs Spices Med Plants** 1994; 2(4): 45–100.

ZO149 Giron, L. M., V. Freire, A. Alonzo, and A. Caceres. Ethnobotanical survey of the medicinal flora used by the Caribs of Guatemala. **J Ethnopharmacol** 1991; 34(2/3): 173–187.

ZO150 Basavarajaiah, C. R., D. S. Lucas, R. Anadarajashekhar, and R. R. Parmesh. Fundamentals of Ayurvedic pharmaceuticals: anti-inflammatory activity of different preparations of three medicinal plants. **J Res Edu Ind Med** 1990; 9(3): 25–30.

ZO151 Barrett, B. Medicinal plants of Nicaragua's Atlantic coast. **Econ Bot** 1994; 48(1): 8–20.

ZO152 Russo, E. B. Headache treatments by native peoples of the Ecuadorian Amazon: a preliminary cross-disciplinary assessment. **J Ethnopharmacol** 1992; 36(3): 193–206.

ZO153 Gurib-Fakim, A., M. D. Sweraj, J. Gueho, and E. Dulloo. Medicinal plants of Rodrigues. **Int J Pharmacog** 1996; 34(1): 2–14.

ZO154 Ruiz, A. R., R. A. de la Torre, N. Alonso, A. Villaescusa, J. Betancourt, and A. Vizoso. Screening of medicinal plants for induction of somatic segregation activity in *Aspergillus nidulans*. **J Ethnopharmacol** 1996; 52(3): 123–127.

ZO155 Bhattarai, N. K. Medical ethnobotany in the Rapti zone, Nepal. **Fitoterapia** 1993; 64(6): 483–493.

ZO156 Coee, F. G., and G. J. Anderson. Ethnobotany of the Garifuna of eastern Nicaragua. **Econ Bot** 1996; 50(1): 71–107.

ZO157 Kiuchi, F. Studies on the nematocidal constituents of natural medicines. **Nat Med** 1995; 49(4): 364–372.

ZO158 Bignall, J. Postoperative *Zingiber*. **Lancet** 1993; 342 8868: 429.

ZO159 Lentz, D. L. Medicinal and other economic plants of the Paya of Honduras. **Econ Bot** 1993; 47(4): 358–370.

ZO160 Bellakhdar, J., R. Claisse, J. Fleurentin and C. Younos. Repertory of standard herbal drugs in the Moroccan pharmacopoea. **J Ethnopharmacol** 1991; 35(2): 123–143.

ZO161 Badria, F. A. Is man helpless against cancer? An environmental approach: antimutagenic agents from Egyptian food and medicinal preparations. **Cancer Lett** 1994; 84(1): 1–5.

ZO162 Verma, S. K., J. Singh, R. Khanesra, and A. Bordia. Effect of ginger on platelet aggregation in man. **Indian J Med Res** 1993; 98(5): 240–242.

ZO163 Thein, K., W. Myin, M. M. Myint, et al. Preliminary screening of medicinal plants for biological activity based on inhibition of cyclic AMP phospodiesterase. **Int J Pharmaceut** 1995; 33(4): 330–333.

ZO164 Yoshizaki, F., T. Komatsu, K. Inoue, R. Kanari, T. Ando, and S. Hisamichi. Survey of crude drugs effective in eliminating superoxides in blood plasma of mice. **Int J Pharmacog** 1996; 34(4): 277–282.

ZO165 Lucas, R. Secrets of the Chinese herbalists. Parker Publishing Co., New York, 1977.

ZO166 Terawaki, K., M. Nose, and Y. Ogihara. The role of crude polysaccharide fractions on the mitogenic activity by Shosaikoto. **Phytomedicine** 1998; 5(5): 347–352.

ZO167 Bae, E. A., M. J. Han, N. J. Kim, and D. H. Kim. Anti-*Helicobacter pylori* activity of herbal medicines. **Biol Pharm Bull** 1998; 21(9): 990–992.

ZO168 Bhattarai, N. K. Herbal folk medicines of Kabhrepalanchok district, central Nepal. **Int J Crude Drug Res** 1990; 28(3): 225–231.

ZO169 Kar, A., B. K. Choudhary, and N. G. Bandyopadhyay. Preliminary studies on the inorganic constituents of some indigenous hypoglycemic herbs on oral glucose tolerance test. **J Exp Bot** 1999; 64(2): 179–184.

ZO170 Sekiwa, Y., Y. Mizuno, Y. Yamamoto, K. Kubota, A. Kobayashi, and H. Koshino. Isolation of some glucosides as aroma precursors from ginger. **Biosci Biotech Biochem** 1999; 63(2): 384–389.

ZO171 Cho, J. Y., J. Park, P. S. Kim, et al. Inhibitory effect of oriental herbal medicines on tumor necrosis factor-alpha production in lipopolysaccharide-stimulated RAW264.7 cells. **Nat Prod Sci** 1999; 5(1): 12–19.

ZO172   Roy, A. N., B. P. Sinha, and K. C. Gupta. The inhibitory effect of plant juices on the infectivity of top necrosis virus of pea. **Indian J Microbiol** 1979; 19: 198–201.

ZO173   Mc Gaw, D. R., I. C. Yen, and V. Dyal. The effect of drying conditions on the yield and composition of the essential oil of West Indian ginger. Proc Int Drying Symp 4th 1984; 2: 612–615.

ZO174   Kong, Y. C. Wu chu-yu (*Evodia rutaecarpa*) from Pen-ts-ao to action mechanism (the action mechanism of dehydroevodiamine). Scientific basis of traditional Chinese medicine, Y. Lau and J. P. Fowler (eds.) 1982; 45–49.

ZO175   Sakamura, F., K. Ogihara, T. Suga, K. Taniguchi, and R. Tanaka. Volatile constituents of *Zingiber officinale* rhizomes produced by *in vitro* shoot tip culture. **Phytochemistry** 1986; 25(6): 1333–1335.

ZO176   Chen, C. C., M. C. Kuo, C. M. Wu, and C. T. Ho. Pungent compounds of ginger (*Zingiber officinale* Roscoe) extracted by liquid carbon dioxide. **J Agr Food Chem** 1986; 34(3): 477–480.

ZO177   Smith, R. M. Analysis of the pungent principles of ginger and grains of paradise by high-performance liquid chromatography using electrochemical detection. **Chromatographia** 1982; 16: 155–157.

ZO178   Al-Yahya, M. A. Phytochemical studies of the plants used in traditional medicine of Saudi Arabia. **Fitoterapia** 1986; 57(3): 179–182.

ZO179   Harvey, D. J. Gas chromatographic and mass spectrometric studies of ginger constituents. Identification of gingerdiones and new hexahydrocurcumin analogues. **J Chromatogr** 1981; 212(1): 75–84.

ZO180   Kiuchi, F., M. Shibuya, and U. Sankawa. Inhibitors of prostaglandin biosynthesis from ginger. **Chem Pharm Bull** 1982; 30(2): 754–757.

ZO181   Yamahara, J., M. Mochizuki, H. Q. Rong, H. Matsuda, and H. Fujimura. The anti-ulcer effect in rats of ginger constituents. **J Ethnopharmacol** 1988; 23(2/3): 299–304.

ZO182   Han, B. H., Y. N. Han, and M. H. Park. Chemical and biochemical studies on antioxidant components of ginseng. Advances in Chinese medicinal materials research H. M. Chang, H. W. Yeung, W. W. Tso, and A. Koo (eds.), World Scientific Press Philadelphia, PA, 1984; pp. 485–498.

ZO183   Wood, C. D., J. E. Manno, M. J. Wood, B. R. Manno, and M. E. Mims. Comparison of efficacy of ginger with various antimotion sickness drugs. **Clin Res Pract Drug Reg Affairs** 1988; 6(2): 129–136.

ZO184   Al-Yahya, M. A., S. Rafatullah, J. S. Mossa, A. M. Ageel, N. S. Parmar, and M. Tariq. Gastroprotective activity of ginger, *Zingiber officinale* Rosc., in albino rats. **Amer J Chinese Med** 1989; 17(1/2): 51–56.

ZO185   Amagaya, S., M. Hayakawa, Y. Ogihara, et al. Treatment of chronic liver injury in mice by oral administration of Xiao-Chai-Hu-Tang. **J Ethnopharmacol** 1989; 25(2): 181–187.

ZO186   Yamahara, J., H. Q. Rong, M. Iwamoto, G. Kobayashi, H. Matsuda, and H. Fujimura. Active components of ginger exhibiting antiserotonergic action. **Phytother Res** 1989; 3(2): 70–71.

ZO187   Sakai, K., Y. Miyazaki, T. Yamane, Y. Saiton, C. Ikwaw, and T. Nishihata. Effect of extracts of *Zingiberaceae* herbs on gastric secretion in rabbits. **Chem Pharm Bull** 1989; 37(1): 215–217.

ZO188   Srivastava, K. C. Effect of onion and ginger consumption on platelet thromboxane production in humans. **Prostoglandins Leukotrienes Essent Fatty Acids** 1989; 35(3): 183–185.

ZO189   Chen, C. P., C. C. Lin, and T. Namba. Screening of Taiwanese crude drugs for antibacterial activity against *Streptococcus* mutants. **J Ethnopharmacol** 1989; 27(3): 285–295.

ZO190   Kiso, Y., M. Suzuki, M. Yasuda, et al. Antihepatotoxic actions of traditional Chinese medicines. 2. The pharmacological interaction of components of a dai-saiko-to-employing complement-mediated cytotoxicity in primary cultured mouse hepatocytes. **Phytother Res** 1990; 4(1): 36–38.

ZO191   Holdsworth, D., and T. Rali. A survey of medicinal plants of the southern

Highlands, Papua New Guinea. **Int J Crude Drug Res** 1989; 27(1): 1–8.

ZO192 Yamahara, J., Q. R. Huang, Y. H. LA, L. Xu, and H. Fujimura. Gastrointestinal motility enhancing effect of ginger and its active constituents. **Chem Pharm Bull** 1990; 38(2): 430–431.

ZO193 Comley, J. C. W. New macrofilaricidal leads from plants? **Trop Med Parasitol** 1990; 41(1): 1–9.

ZO194 Itokawa, H., F. Hirayama, S. Tsuruoka, K. Mizuno, K. Takeya, and A. Nitta. Screening test for antitumor activity of crude drugs (III). Studies on antitumor activity of Indonesian medicinal plants. **Shoyakugaku Zasshi** 1990; 44(1): 58–62.

ZO195 Miyazawa, M., and H. Kameoka. Volatile flavor components of *Zingiberis rhizoma* (*Zingiber officinale* Roscoe). **Agr Biol Chem** 1988; 52(11): 2961–2963.

ZO196 Toda, S., M. Kimura, and M. Ohnishi. Induction of neutrophil accumulation by Chinese herbal medicines "hochu-etsuki-to" and "jyuzen-daiho-to". **J Ethnopharmacol** 1990; 30(1): 91–95.

ZO197 Kawakita, T., S. Nakai, Y. Kumazawa, O. Miur, E. Yumioka, and K. Nomoto. Induction of interferon after administration of a traditional Chinese medicine. Xiao-Chai-Hu-Tang (Shosaiko-To). **Int J Immunopharmacol** 1990; 12(5): 515–521.

ZO198 Kano, Y., M. Tanabe, and M. Yasuda. On the evaluation of the preparation of Chinese medicinal prescriptions (V). Diterpenes from Japanese ginger "kintoki". **Shoyakugaku Zasshi** 1990; 44(1): 55–57.

ZO199 Kuraishi, Y., T. Nanayama, T. Yamaguchi, T. Hotani, and M. Satoh. Antinociceptive effects of Oriental medicine kei-kyoh-zoh-soh-oh-shin-bu-toh in mice and rats. **J Pharmacobio Dyn** 1990; 13(1): 49–56.

ZO200 Kiuchi, F., M. Hioki, N. Nakamura, N. Miyashita, Y. Tsuda, and K. Kondo. Screening of crude drugs used in Sri Lanka for nematocidal activity on the larva of *Toxocaria canis*. **Shoyakugaku Zasshi** 1989; 43(3): 288–293.

ZO201 Van Beek, T. A., and G. P. Lelyveld. Isolation and identification of five major sesquiterpene hydrocarbons of ginger. **Phytochem Anal** 1991; 2(1): 26–34.

ZO202 Nishizaza, K., H. Saito, and N. Nishiyama. Effects of kamikihi-to, a traditional Chinese medicine, on learning and memory performance in mice. **Phytother Res** 1991; 5(3): 97–102.

ZO203 Ono, K., H. Nakane, M. Fukushima, J. C. Chernmann, and F. Barre-Sinoussi. Differential inhibition of the activities of reverse transcriptase and various cellar DNA polymerases by a traditional Kampo drug, Sho-Saiko-To. **Biomed Pharmacother** 1990; 44: 13–16.

ZO204 Buimovici-Klein, E., V. Mohan, M. Lang, E. Fenamore, Y. Inada, and L. Z. Cooper. Inhibition of HIV replication in lymphocyte cultures of virus-positive subjects in the presence of shosaiko-to, an oriental plant extract. **Antiviral Res** 1990; 14(4/5): 279–286.

ZO205 Toda, S., M. Kimura, M. Ohnishi, and K. Nakashima. Effect of Chinese herbal medicine "saiboku-to" on histamine release from and the degranulation of mouse peritoneal mast cells induced by compound 48/80. **J Ethnopharmacol** 1988; 24(2/3): 303–309.

ZO206 Zheng, Y. Z., and N. Zhang. Treatment of 305 cases of infantile diarrhea with kexieding capsule. **Fujian J Trad Chinese Med** 1988; 19(3): 13–14.

ZO207 Chang, I. M., I. C. Guest, J. Lee-Chang, N. W. Paik, J. W. Jhoun, and R. Y. Ryun. Assay of potential mutagenicity and antimutagenicity of Chinese herbal drugs by using SOS chromotest (*E. coli* PQ37) and SOS UMU test (*S. typhimurium* TA 1535/PSK1002). Proc First Korea-Japan Toxicology Symposium Safety Assessment of Chemicals *in vitro* 1989; 133–145.

ZO208 Sugaya, E., A. Ishige, K. Sekiguchi, et al. Inhibitory effect of a mixture of herbal drugs (TJ-960, SK) on pentylenetetrazol-induced convulsion in EL mice. **Epilepsy Res** 1988; 2(5): 337–339.

ZO209 Kiuchi, F., N. Nakamura, N. Miyashita, S. Nishizawa, Y. Tsuda, and K. Kondo. Nematocidal activity of some anthelmints, traditional medicines, and spices by a new assay method using larvae of *Toxocara canis*. **Shoyakugaku Zasshi** 1989; 43(4): 279–287.

ZO210 Sugaya, E., A. Ishige, K. Sekiguchi, et al. Inhibitory effect of TJ-960 (SK) on pentylenetetrazol-induced EEG power spectrum changes. **Epilepsy Res** 1988; 2(1): 27–31.

ZO211 Panthong, A., and P. Tejasen. Study of the effect and the mechanism of action of ginger (*Zingiber officinale* Roscoe) on motility of the intact intestine in dogs. **Cheng Mai Med Bull** 1975; 14(3): 221–231.

ZO212 Hantrakul, M., and P. Tejason. Study of the acute toxicity and cardiovascular effects of ginger (*Zingiber officinale* Roscoe). **Thai J Pharm Sci** 1976; 1(6): 517–530.

ZO213 Loewsoponkul, P. Effect of Thai emmenagogue drugs on rat uterine. Thesis-Master, 1982; 96 pp.

ZO214 Sankawa, U. Modulators of arachidonate cascade contained in medicinal plants used in traditional medicine. Abstr 3rd Congress of the Federation of Asian and Oceanian Biochemists Bangkok Thailand 1983; pp. 28.

ZO215 Ketusinh, O., S. Wimolwattanapun, and N. Nilvises. Smooth muscle actions of some Thai herbal carminatives. **Thai J Pharmacol** 1984; 6(1): 11–19.

ZO216 Pathong, A., and P. Sivamogstham. Pharmacological study of the action of ginger (*Zingiber officinale* Roscoe) on the gastrointestinal tract. **Chieng Mai Med Bull** 1974; 13(1): 41–53.

ZO217 Gujral, S., H. Bhumra, and M. Swaroop. Effect of ginger (*Zingiber officinale*) oleoresin on serum, and hepatic cholesterol levels in cholesterol fed rats. **Nutr Exp Int** 1978; 17: 183.

ZO218 Sugaya, A., T. Tsuda, E. Sugaya, M. Takato, and K. Takamura. Effects of Chinese medicine saiko-keishi-to on the abnormal bursting activity of snail neurons. **Planta Med** 1978; 34: 294–298.

ZO219 Sakamura, F., and S. Hayashi. Studies on constituents of essential oil from *Zingiber officinale*. Part I. Constituents of essential oil from rhizomes of *Zingiber officinale*. **Nippon Nogei Kagaku Kaishi** 1978; 52: 207–211.

ZO220 Sugaya, A., T. Tsuda, E. Sugaya, M. Usami, and K. Takamura. Local anaesthetic action of the Chinese medicine saiko-keishi-to. **Planta Med** 1979; 37: 274–276.

ZO221 Woo, W. S., K. H. Shin, and I. C. Kim. The effect of irritating spices on drug metabolizing activity: effects on hexobarbital hypnosis in mice. **Korean J Pharmacog** 1977; 8: 115–119.

ZO222 Sinha, A. K., M. S. Mehra, G. K. Sinha, and R. C. Pathak. Antibacterial study of some essential oils. **Indian Parfum** 1979; 20: 25–27.

ZO223 Sussman, L. K. Herbal medicine on Mauritius. **J Ethnopharmacol** 1980; 2(3): 259–278.

ZO224 Sofowora, A. The present status of knowledge of the plants used in traditional medicine in western Africa: a medical approach and a chemical evaluation. **J Ethnopharmacol** 1980; 2(2): 109–118.

ZO225 Chen, Y. H., and H. Z. Guo. A survey of raw and dry ginger produced in Szechuan (China). **Planta Med** 1980; 39: 57–65.

ZO226 Schultz, J. M., and K. Herrmann. Occurrence of hydrohybenzoic acid and hydroxycinnamic acid in spices. IV. Phenolics of spices. **Z Lebensm-Unters Forsch** 1980; 171: 193–199.

ZO227 Hussein Ayoub, S. M., and A. Baerheim-Suendsen. Medicinal and aromatic plants in the Sudan: usage and exploration. **Fitoterapia** 1981; 52: 243–246.

ZO228 Ishikura, N. Flavonol glycosides in the flowers of *Hibiscus mutabilis f. versicolor*. **Agr Biol Chem** 1982; 46: 1705–1706.

ZO229 Smith, R. M., and J. M. Robinson. The essential oil of ginger from Fiji. **Phytochemistry** 1981; 20: 203–206.

ZO230 Anon. Analgesic formulations containing shogaol and gingerol. Patent-Japan Kokai Tokkyo Koho-82 46,914 1982; 5 pp.

ZO231 Reyes, F. G. R., B. L. D'Appolonia, C. F. Ciacco, and M. W. Montgomery. Characterization of starch from ginger roots (*Zingiber officinale*). **Starch (Weinheim)** 1982; 34(2): 40–44.

ZO232 Paik, N. H., M. K. Park, S. H. Choi, D. C. Moon, and T. L. Kang. Studies of germanium in herbal drugs. II. Extracting effect of germanium of different solvents in *Zingiberis rhizoma*. **Seoul Taehakkyo Yakhak Nonmunjip** 1980; 5; 75–79.

ZO233 Shoji, N., A. Iwasa, T. Takemoto, Y. Ishida, and Y. Ohizumi. Cardiotonic principles of ginger (*Zingiber officinale* Roscoe). **J Pharm Sci** 1982; 71: 1174–1175.

ZO234 Fleurentin, J., and J. M. Pelt. Repertory of drugs and medicinal plants of Yemen. **J Ethnopharmacol** 1982; 6(1): 85–108.

ZO235 Yamasaki, K., H. Yokohama, Y. Nunoura, C. Umezawa, and K. Yoneda. Studies on effect of crude drugs on enzyme activities. I. Influence of cinnamon bark upon protein digestive action by pancreatin. **Shoyakugaku Zasshi** 1982; 36: 11–16.

ZO236 Paik, N. H., W. K. Lee, M. K. Park, and J. I. Park. Determination of germanium in botanical drugs by flameless atomic absorption. **Yakhak Hoe Chi** 1979; 23: 141–146.

ZO237 Kasahara, Y., E. Saito, and H. Hikino. Pharmacological actions of *Pinellia* tubers and *Zingiber* rhizomes. **Shoyakugaku Zasshi** 1983; 37(1): 73–83.

ZO238 Yamamoto, H., T. Mizutani, and H. Nomura. Studies on the mutagenicity of crude drug extracts. I. **Yakugaku Zasshi** 1982; 102: 596–601.

ZO239 Tanaka, S., M. Saito, and M. Tabata. Bioassay of crude drugs for hair growth promoting activity in mice by a new simple method. **Planta Med Suppl** 1980; 40: 84–90.

ZO240 Koda, A., T. Nishiyori, H. Nagai, N. Matsuura, and H. Tsuchiya. Anti-allergic actions of crude drugs and blended Chinese traditional medicines. Effects on type I and type IV allergic reactions. **Nippon Yakurigaku Zasshi** 1982; 80: 31–41.

ZO241 Hirschhorn, H. H. Botanical remedies of the former Dutch East Indies (Indonesia). I. *Eumycetes, Pteridophyta, Gymnospermae, Angiospermae* (Monocotyledones only). **J Ethnopharmacol** 1983; 7(2): 123–156.

ZO242 Ikram, M. A review on the medicinal plants. **Hamdard** 1981; 24(1/2): 102–129.

ZO243 Kishore, P., K. V. Devidas, and S. Banarjee. Clinical studies on the role of sunthiguggulu yoga in the treatment of amavata-rheumatoid arthritis. **Rheumatism** 1982; 17(3): 103–110.

ZO244 Morimoto, Y., F. Watanabe, T. Osawa, T. Okitsu, and T. Kada. Mutagenicity screening of crude drugs with *Bacillus subtilis* Rec-assay and *Salmonella*/microsome reversion assay. **Mutat Res** 1982; 97: 81–102.

ZO245 Holdsworth, D., and B. Wamoi. Medicinal plants of the Admiralty Islands, Papua New Guinea. Part I. **Int J Crude Drug Res** 1982; 20(4): 169–181.

ZO246 Rao, R. R., and N. S. Jamir. Ethnobotanical studies in Nagaland. I. Medicinal plants. **Econ Bot** 1982; 36: 176–181.

ZO247 Takahashi, M., K. Osawa, T. Sato, and J. Ueda. Components of amino acids on *Zingiber officinale* Roscoe. **Ann Rep Tohoku Coll Pharm** 1982; 29: 75–76.

ZO248 John, D. One hundred useful raw drugs of the Kani tribes of Trivandrum Forest division, Kerala, India. **Int J Crude Drug Res** 1984; 22(1): 17–39.

ZO249 Narita, Y., H. Satowa, T. Kokubu, and E. Sugaya. Treatment of epileptic patients with the Chinese herbal medicine "saiko-keishi-to" (SK). **IRCS Libr Compend** 1982; 10(2): 88–89.

ZO250 Takato, M., K. Takamura, A. Sugaya, T. Tsuda, and E. Sugaya. Effect of the Chinese medicine "saiko-keishi-to" on audiogenic seizure mice, kindling animals and conventional pharmacological screening procedures. **IRCS Libr Compend** 1982; 10(2): 86–87.

ZO251 Kiuchi, F., M. Shibuya, T. Kinoshita, and U. Sankawa. Inhibition of prostaglandin biosynthesis by the constituents of medicinal plants. **Chem Pharm Bull** 1983; 31(10): 3391–3396.

ZO252 Lopez Abraham. A. N., N. M. Rojas Hernandez, and C. A. Jimenez Misas. Potential antineoplastic activity of Cuban plants. IV. **Rev Cubana Farm** 1981; 15(1): 71–77.

ZO253 Van Den Berg, M. A. Ver-o-peso: the ethnobotany of an amazonian market. Advances in Economic Botany Ethnobotany in the Neotropics G. T. France and J. A. Kallunki (eds.), New York Botanical Garden Bronx, 1984; 1: 140–149.

ZO254 Holdsworth, D. Phytomedicine of the Madang province, Papua New Guinea part I. Karkar Island. **Int J Crude Drug Res** 1984; 22(3): 111–119.

ZO255   Sircar, N. N. Pharmaco-therapeutics of Dasemani drugs. **Ancient Sci Life** 1984; 3(3): 132–135.

ZO256   Jain, S. P., and H. S. Puri. Ethnomedical plants of Jaunsar-Bawar Hills, Uttar Pradesh, India. **J Ethnopharmacol** 1984; 12(2): 213–222.

ZO257   May, G., and G. Willuhn. Antiviral activity of aqueous extracts from medicinal plants in tissue cultures. **Arzneim-Forsch** 1978; 28(1): 1–7.

ZO258   Chang, I. K., and S. I. L. Park. Effects of Yukgunja-tang on secretion of gastric juice and movements of isolated stomach. **Korean J Pharmacog** 1984; 15(3): 128–133.

ZO259   Shimizu, K., S. Amagaya, and Y. Ogihara. Combination effects of shosaikoto (Chinese traditional medicine) and prednisolone on the anti-inflammatory action. **J Pharmacobio Dyn** 1984; 9(1): 105–127.

ZO260   Hedberg, I., O. Hedbrg, P. J. Madati, K. E. Mshigeni, E. N. Mshiu, and G. Samuelsson. Inventory of plants used in traditional medicine in Tanzania. II. Plants of the families *Dilleniaceae-Opiliaceae*. **J Ethnopharmacol** 1983; 9(1): 105–127.

ZO261   Velazco, E. A. Herbal and traditional practices related to maternal and child health care. **Rural Reconstruction Review** 1980; 35–39.

ZO262   Aswal, B. S., D. S. Bhakuni, A. K. Goel, K. Kar, B. N. Mehrotra, and K. C. Mukherjee. Screening of Indian plants for biological activity, part X. **Indian J Exp Biol** 1984; 22(6): 312–332.

ZO263   Siddiqui, N. A., and M. Z. Hasan. Therapeutic response of Arab medicines in cases of Laquwa. **Bull Islamic Med** 1981; 1: 366–374.

ZO264   Woo, W. S., E. B. Lee, K. H. Shin, S. S. Kang, and H. J. Chi. A review of research on plants for fertility regulation in Korea. **Korean J Pharmacog** 1981; 12(3): 153–170.

ZO265   Shin, K. H., and W. S. Woo. A survey of the response of medicinal plants on drug metabolism. **Korean J Pharmacog** 1980; 11: 109–122.

ZO266   Singh, Y. N. Traditional medicine in Fiji: Some herbal folk cures used by Fiji Indians. **J Ethnopharmacol** 1986; 15(1): 57–88.

ZO267   Kim, J. S., G. H. Kim, and I. H. Kim. Studies on the concurrent administrations of sosiho-tang extract and methionine. Effects on the liver lesion induced by carbon tetrachloride in rats. **Korean J Pharmacog** 1986; 17(2): 148–152.

ZO268   Ito, H., and K. Shimura. Effects of a blended Chinese medicine, xiao-chai-hu-tang, on Lewis lung carcinoma growth and inhibition of lung metastasis, with special reference to macrophage activation. **Jap J Pharmacol** 1986; 41: 307–314.

ZO269   Chen, C. C., R. T. Rosen, and C. T. Ho. Chromatographic analyses of isomeric shogaol compounds derived from isolated gingerol compounds of ginger (*Zingiber officinale* Roscoe). **J Chromatogr** 1986; 360: 175–184.

ZO270   Reiter, M., and W. Brandt. Relaxant effects on tracheal and ileal smooth muscles of the guinea pig. **Arzneim-Forsch** 1985; 35(1): 408–414.

ZO271   Chen. C. C., R. T. Rosen, and C. T. Ho. Chromatographic analyses of gingerol compounds in ginger (*Zingiber officinale* Roscoe). **J Chromatogr** 1986; 360: 163–173.

ZO272   Namba, T., M. Tsunezuka, D. M. R. B. Dissanayake, et al. Studies on dental caries prevention by traditional medicines (part VII) screening of ayurvedic medicines for anti-plaque action. **Shoyakugaku Zasshi** 1985; 39(2): 146–153.

ZO273   Kada, T., K. Morita, and T. Inoue. Anti-mutagenic action of vegetable factor(s) on the mutagenic principle of tryptophan pyrolysate. **Mutat Res** 1978; 53: 351–353.

ZO274   Dean, M. A., A. S. Dhaliwal, and W. R. Jones. Effects of *Zingiberaceae* rhizome extract of the infectivity of cyanophage LPP-1. **Trans Ill State Acad Sci Suppl** 1987; 80: Abstr 83.

ZO275   Morita, K., M. Hara, and T. Kada. Studies on natural desmutagens: screening for vegetable and fruits factors active in inactivation of mutagenic pyrolysis products from amino acids. **Agr Biol Chem** 1978; 42(6): 1235–1238.

ZO276   Yamaguchi, T., Y. Yamashita, and T. Abe. Desmutagenic activity of peroxidase on autoxidized linolenic acid. **Agr Biol Chem** 1980; 44(4): 959–961.

ZO277 Holdsworth, D., B. Pilokos, and P. Lambes. Traditional medicinal plants of New Ireland, Papua New Guinea. **Int J Crude Drug Res** 1983; 21(4): 161–168.

ZO278 Nagabhushan, M., A. J. Amonkar, and S. V. Bhide. Mutagenicity of gingerol and shogaol and antimutagenicity of zingerone in *Salmonella*/microsome assay. **Cancer Lett** 1987; 36(2): 221–233.

ZO279 Shiba, M., A. Myata, M. Okada, and K. Watanabe. Antiulcer furanogermenone extraction from ginger. Patent-Japan Kokai Tokkyo Koho-61 227,523 1986; 4 pp.

ZO280 Lama, S., and S. C. Santra. Development of Tibetan plant medicine. **Sci Cult** 1979; 45: 262–265.

ZO281 Sugaya, A., M. Yuzurihara, T. Tsuda, et al. Normalizing effect of Saiko-Keishi-To commercial formula on cytochalasin-B distorted neurites using primary cultured neurons of rat cerebral cortex. **J Ethnopharmacol** 1987; 21(2): 193–199.

ZO282 Kato, M., M. Marumoto, M. Hayashi, T. Maeda, and E. Hayashi. Pharmacological studies on saiko-prescriptions. VI. Effect of Shosaiko-To on liver injury induced by D-galactosamine in rats. **Yakugaku Zasshi** 1984; 104(7): 798–804.

ZO283 Kato, M., M. Marmoto, M. Hayashi, T. Maeda, and E. Hayashi. Pharmacological studies on saiko-prescriptions. V. Mechanisms of actions of shosaiko-to on swelling of rat hind paws induced by carrageenan. **Yakugaku Zasshi** 1984; 104(5): 516–523.

ZO284 Grontved, A., T. Brask, J. Kambskard, and E. Hentzer. Ginger root against seasickness. A controlled trial on the open sea. **Acta Otolaryngol (Stockholm)** 1988; 105(1/2): 45–49.

ZO285 Nes, I. F., R. Skjelkvale, O. Olsvik, and B. P. Berdal. The effect of natural spices and oleoresins on *Lactobacillus plantarum* and *Staphylococcus aureus*. Microb Assoc Interact Food Proc Int IUMS-ICFMH Sym 12th 1984; 1983 (1984): 435–440.

ZO286 Koshimizu, K., H. Ohigashi, H. Tokuda, A. Kondo, and K. Yamaguchi. Screening of edible plants against possible anti-tumor promoting activity. **Cancer Lett** 1988; 39(3): 247–257.

ZO287 Chen, C. P., C. C. Lin, and T. Namba. Development of Natural Crude Drug Resources from Taiwan. VI. In vitro studies of the inhibitory effect on 12 microorganism. **Shoyakugaku Zasshi** 1987: 41(3): 215–225.

ZO288 Ramirez, V. S., L. J. Mostacero, A. E. Garcia, et al. Vegetales Empleados en Medicina Tradicional Norperuana. Banco Agrario del Peru & NACL Univ Trujillo, Peru, June 1988; 54 pp.

ZO289 Gonzalez, F., and M. Silva. A survey of plants with antifertility properties described in the South American folk medicine. Abstr. Princess Congress I Bangkok Thailand 10–13 Dec 1987; 20 pp.

ZO290 Van Beek, T. A., M. A. Posthumus, G. P. Lelyveld, H. V. Phiet, and B. T. Yen. Investigation of the essential oil of Vietnamese ginger. **Phytochemistry** 1987; 26(11): 3005–3010.

ZO291 Sakai, T., K. Kobashi, M. Tsunezuka, M. Hattori, and T. Namba. Studies on dental caries prevention by tradicional Chinese medicines. Part VI. On the fluoride content in crude drugs. **Shoyakugaku Zasshi** 1985; 39(2): 165–169.

ZO292 Mascolo, N., R. Jain, S. C. Jain, and F. Capasso. Ethnopharmacologic Investigation of Ginger (*Zingiber officinale*). **J Ethnopharmacol** 1989; 27(1/2): 129–140.

ZO293 Hou, W., and L. L. Wu. Essential oil of *Zingiber officinale*. **Huaxue Shijie** 1989; 30(9): 240–243.

ZO294 Holdsworth, D., and H. Sakulas. Medicinal plants of the Morobe province part II. The Aseki Valley. **Int J Crude Drug Res** 1986; 24(1): 31–40.

ZO295 Wu, P., M. C. Kuo, and C. T. Ho. Glycosidically bound aroma compounds in ginger (*Zingiberis officinale* Roscoe). **J Agr Food Chem** 1990; 38(7): 1553–1555.

ZO296 Misas, C. A. J., N. M. R. Hernandez, and A. N. L. Abraham. Contribution to the biological evaluation of Cuban plants. II. **Rev Cub Med Trop** 1979; 31: 13–19.

ZO297 Liu, W. H. D. Ginger root, a new antiemetic. **Anaesthesia** 1991; 45(12): 1085.

ZO298 Fischer-Rasmussen, W., S. K. Kjaer, C. Dahl, and U. Asping. Ginger treatment of *Hyperemesis gravidarum*. **Eur J Obstet Gynecol Reprod Biol** 1991; 38(1): 19–24.

ZO299   Pan, P. C. The application of Chinese traditional medicine in the treatment of vaginal cancer. **Chin J Obstet Gynecol** 1960; 8: 156–162.

ZO300   De Bairacli Levy, J. Common herbs for natural health. Schocken Books, New York 1974; 200 pp.

ZO301   Kuo, C. L. Use of "Wi-Kuan-Chien" in treatment of acute schistosomiasis diarrhea and febrility. **Shang Hai Chung I Yao Tsa Chih** 1965; 4: 16.

ZO302   Anon. More Secret Remedies. What they cost and what they contain. British Medical Association, London 1912; 185–209.

ZO303   Jacobson, M. Insecticides from plants. A review of the literature, 1941-1953. Agr Handbook no 154, USDA 1958; 299 pp.

ZO304   Anon. The herbalist. Hammond Book Company, Hammond, IN, 1931; 400 pp.

ZO305   Kami, T., M. Nakayama, and S. Hayashi. Volatile constituents of *Zingiber officinale*. **Phytochemistry** 1972; 11(11): 3377–3381.

ZO306   Brooks, B. T. Zingiberol-a new sesquiterpene alcohol occurring in the essential oil of ginger. **J Amer Chem Soc** 1916; 38: 430–432.

ZO307   Nomura, H. Pungent principles of ginger. I. A new ketone, zingiberone, occuring in ginger. **Sci Rep Tohoku Imp Univ** 1917; 6: 41–52.

ZO308   Murakami, T., F. Inugai, M. Nagasawa, H. Inatomi, and N. Mori. Water-soluble constituents of crude drugs. III. Free amino acids isolated from ginger rhizome. **Yakugaku Zasshi** 1965; 85(9): 845–846.

ZO309   Masada, Y., T. Inoue, K. Hashimoto, M. Fujioka, and K. Shiraki. Studies on the pungent principles of ginger (*Zingiber officinale*) by GC-MS (gas chromatography-mass spectrometry). **Yakugaku Zasshi** 1973; 93(3): 318–321.

ZO310   Hartman, M. Chemical composition of certain products from ginger (*Zingiber officinale*). **Zivocisna Vyroba** 1971; 16(10/11): 805–812.

ZO311   Nelson, E.K. Constitution of capsaicin, the pungent principle of ginger. II. **J Amer Chem Soc** 1920; 42: 597–599.

ZO312   Nakahara, K. Oxalic acid content of vegetable foods. **Eiyo To Shokuryo** 1974; 27(1): 33–36.

ZO313   Masada, Y., T. Inoue, K. Hashimoto, M. Fujioka, and C. Uchino. Studies on the constituents of ginger (*Zingiber officinale* Roscoe) by GC-MS. **Yakugaku Zasshi** 1974; 87(6): 735–738.

ZO314   Emig, H. M. The pharmacological action of ginger. **J Amer Pharm Ass** 1931; 20: 114–116.

ZO315   Umeda, M., S. Amagaya, and Y. Ogihara. Effects of certain herbal medicines on the biotransformation of arachidonic acid: A new pharmacological testing method using serum. **J Ethnopharmacol** 1988; 23(1): 91–98.

ZO316   Nishio, S., S. Hayashi, and H. Yoshihara. The effects of ginseng and ginger combination and rhubarb & licorice combination on patients with chronic renal failure. **Int J Orient Med** 1993; 18(3): 148–155.

ZO317   Niijima, A., M. Kubo, K. Hashimoto, Y. Komatsu, M. Maruno, and M. Okada. Effect of oral administration of *Pinella ternata*, *Zingiberis rhizoma* and their mixture on the efferent activity of the gastric branch of the vagus nerve in the rat. **Neurosci Lett** 1998; 258(1): 5–8.

ZO318   Woo, W. S., E. B. Lee, and B. H. Han. Biological evaluation of Korean medicinal plants. III. **Arch Pharm Res** 1979; 2: 127–131.

ZO319   Vimala, S., A. W. Norhahnom, and M. Yadav. Anti-tumor promoter activity in Malaysian ginger rhizobia used in traditional medicine. **Brit J Cancer** 1999; 80(1/2): 110–116.

ZO320   Inada, Y., K. Watanabe, M. Kamiyama, T. Kanemitsu, W. S. Clark, and M. Lange. In vitro immunomodulatory effects of traditional kampo medicine (Sho-Saiko-To: SST) on peripheral mononuclear cells in patients with AIDS. **Biomed Pharmacother** 1990; 44(1): 17–19.

ZO321   Weber, M. L. A follow-up study of thirty-five cases of paralysis caused by adulterated Jamaica-ginger extract. **Med Bull Vet Admin** 1937; 13: 228–242.

ZO322   Kim, J. H., Y. S. Yoo, M. I. Mang, and H. S. Yun-Choi. Effects of some combined crude drug preparations against platelet aggregations. **Korean J Pharmacog** 1990; 21(2): 126–129.

ZO323   Hung, N. D., I. K. Chang, H. C. Jung, and N. J. Kim. Studies on the efficacy of combined preparation of crude drugs (XII). **Korean J Pharmacog** 1983; 14(1): 9–16.

ZO324   Oh, W. K., D. O. Kang, C. S. Park, et al. Screening of the angiotensin II antagonists from medicinal plants. **Korean J Pharmacog** 1997; 28(1): 26–34.

ZO325   Bara. M. T. F., and M. C. D. Vanetti. Antimicrobial effect of spices on the growth of *Yersina enterocolitica*. **J Herbs Spices Med Plants** 1995; 3(4): 51–58.

ZO326   Lee, H. K., Y. K. Kim, Y. H. Kim, and J. K. Roh. Effect of bacterial growth-inhibiting ingredients on the Ames mutagenicity of medicinal herbs. **Mutat Res** 1987; 192: 99–104.

ZO327   Mahmoud, I., A. Alkofahi, and A. Abdelaziz. Mutagenic and toxic activities of several spices and some Jordanian medicinal plants. **Int J Pharmacog** 1992; 30(2): 81–85.

ZO328   Hong, N. D., I. K. Chang, J. W. Kim, S. K. Ryu, and N. J. Kim. Studies on the efficacy of combined preparation of crude drugs (XXII). **Korean J Pharmacog** 1985; 16(2): 73–80.

ZO329   Fischer-Rasmussem, W., S. K. Kjaer, C. Dahl, and U. Asping. Ginger treatment of hyperemesis gravidarum. **Eur J Obstet Gynecol Reprod Biol** 1990; 38: 19–24.

ZO330   Sharma, S. S., V. Kochupillai, S. K. Gupta, S. D. Seth, and Y. K. Gupta. Antiemetic efficacy of ginger (*Zingiber officinale*) against cisplatin-induced emesis in dogs. **J Ethnopharmacol** 1997; 57(2): 93–96.

ZO331   Hong, N. D., J. W. Kim, B. W. Kim, and J. G. Shon. Studies on the efficacy of the combined preparation of crude drugs. 6. Effect of "Saengkankunbi-Tang" on activities of liver enzyme, protein contents and the excretory action of bile juice in the serum of CCl4-intoxicated rabbits. **Korean J Pharmacog** 1982; 13: 33–38.

ZO332   Kato, M., M. Hayashi, M. Hayashi, and T. Maeda. Pharmacological studies on Saiko-prescriptions. III. Inhibitory effects of Saiko-presctiptions on experimental inflammatory actions in rats. **Yakugaku Zasshi** 1983; 103(4): 466–472.

ZO333   Kato, M., Marumoto, M. Hayashi, T. Maeda, and E. Hayashi. Pharmacological studies on Saiko-prescriptions. VI. Effect of Shosaiko-To on swelling of rat hind paws induced by carrageenin. **Yakugaku Zasshi** 1984; 104(5): 509–514.

ZO334   Ohta, S., N. Sakurai, T. Inoue, and M. Shinoda. Studies on the chemical protectors against radiation. XXV. Radioprotective activities of various crude drugs. **Yakugaku Zasshi** 1987; 107(1): 70–75.

ZO335   Itokawa, H., S. Mihashi, K. Watanabe, H. Natsumoto,, and T. Hamanaka. Studies on the constituents of crude drugs having inhibitory activity against contraction of the ileum caused by histamine or barium chloride (1) screening test for the activity of commercially available crude drugs and the related plant materials. **Shoyakugaku Zasshi** 1983; 37(3): 223–228.

ZO336   Kato, M., J. Nagao, M. Hayashi, and E. Hayashi. Pharmacological studies on saiko-prescriptions. I. Effects of saiko-prescriptions on the isolated smooth muscles. **Yakugaku Zasshi** 1982; 102: 371–380.

ZO337   Yamazaki, M., and H. Shirota. Application of experimental stress ulcer test in mice for the survey of neurotropic naturally occurring drug materials. **Shoyakugaku Zasshi** 1981; 35: 96–102.

ZO338   Hong, N. D., I. K. Chang, N. J. Kim, and I. S. Lee. Studies on the efficacy of combined preparations of crude drug (XXXIX). Effects of Hyangsayangwee-Tang on the stomach and intestinal disorder. **Korean J Pharmacog** 1989; 20(3): 188–195.

ZO339   Kurokawa, M., H. Ochiai, K. Nagasaka, et al. Antiviral traditional medicines against herpes simplex (HSV-1), poliovirus, and measles virus *in vitro* and their therapeutic efficacies for HSV-1 infection in mice. **Antiviral Res** 1993; 22(2/3): 175–188.

ZO340   Nakamoto, K., S. Sadamorei, and T. Hamada. Effects of crude drugs and berberine hydrochloride on the activities of fungi. **J Prost Dent** 1990; 64(6): 691–694.

ZO341   Nagatsu, Y., M. Inoue, and Y. Ogihara. Modification of macrophage functions by shosaikoto (Kampo medicine) leads to enhancement of immune response. **Chem Pharm Bull** 1989; 37(6): 1540–1542.

ZO342   Sugaya, A., T. Tsuda, T. Obuchi, and E. Sugaya. Effect of Chinese herbal medicine "Hange-Koboku-To" on laryngeal reflex of cats and in other pharmacological tests. **Planta Med** 1983; 47(1):59–62.

ZO343   Fukutake, M., S. Yokota, H. Kawamura, A. Iizuka, S. Amagaya, K. Fukuda, and Y. Komatsu. Inhibitory effect of *Coptidis rhizoma* and *Scutellariae radix* on azomethane-induced aberrant crypt foci formatin in rat colon. **Biol Pharm Bull** 1998; 21(8): 814–817.

ZO344   Yamahara, J., K. Miki, T. Chisaka, et al. Cholagogic effect of ginger and its active constituents. **J Ethnopharmacol** 1985; 13(2): 217–225.

ZO345   Ohmoto, T., Y. I. Sung, K. Koife, and T. Nikaido. Effect of alkaloids of simaroubaceous plants on the local blood flow rate. **Shoyakuga Zasshi** 1985; 39(1): 28–34.

ZO346   Furukawa, M., H. Sakashita, M. Kamide, and R. Umeda. Inhibitory effects of Kampo medicine on Epstein-Barr virus antigen induction by tumor promotor. **Auris-Nasus Larynx (Tokyo)** 1990; 17(1): 49–54.

ZO347   Iwama, H., S. Amagaya, and Y. Ogihara. Effects of five Kampohozais on the mitogenic activity of lipopolysaccharide, concanavalin A, Phorbol Myristate acetate and phytohemagglutinin in vivo. **J Ethnopharmacol** 1986; 18(2): 193–204.

ZO348   Sakai, K., N. Oshima, T. Kutsuna, et al. Pharmaceutical studies on crude drugs. I. Effect of *Zingiberaceae* crude drug extracts on sulfaguanidine ab-

sorption from the rat small intestine. **Yakugaku Zasshi** 1986; 106(10): 947–950.

ZO349   Kawakita, T., A. Yamada, Y. Kumazawa, and K. Nomoto. Functional maturation of immature B cells accumulated in the periphery by an intraperitoneal administration of a traditional Chinese medicine, Xiao-Chia-Hu-Tang (Japanese name: Shosaiko-To). **Immunopharmacol Immunotoxicol** 1987; 9(2/3): 299–317.

ZO350   Yabe, T., K. Toriizuka, and H. Yamada. Kami-Untan-To (KUT) improves cholinergic deficits in aged rats. **Phytomedicine** 1996; 2(3): 253–258.

ZO351   Sofowara, E. A., and C. O. Adewunmi. Preliminary screening of some plant extracts for mulluscicidal activity. **Planta Med** 1980: 39: 57–65.

ZO352   Pang, H. A., Y. W. Lee, N. J. Sun, and I. M. Chang. Toxicological study on Korean tea materials: Screening of potential mutagenic activities by using SOS-Chromotest. **Korean J Pharmacog** 1990; 21(1): 83–87.

ZO353   Yamahara, J., H. Matsuda, S. Yamaguchi, H. Shimoda, N. Murakami, and M. Yoshikawa. Pharmacological studty on ginger processing. I. Antiallergenic activity and cardiotonic action of gingerols and shogaols. **Nat Med** 1995; 49(1): 76–83.

ZO354   Roig, Y., and J. T. Mesa. Plantas medicinales, aromaticas O Venenosas De Cuba. Ministero De Agricultura, Republica De Cuba, Havana. Book 1945: 872 pp.

ZO355   Zhu, F. Q., W. J. Zhang, and J. X. Xu. Experience of treating 42 cases of ectopic pregnancy by the method of combining TCM and western medicine. **Zhejiang-Zhongyi Zazhi** 1982; 17: 102.

Glossary

Abdominal. Pertaining to the part of trunk that lies between the thorax and the pelvis.

Abortifacient. An agent that induces the premature expulsion of a fetus.

Abortion. Giving birth to an embryo or fetus prior to the stage of viability.

Abscess. A circumscribed collection of pus; a cavity formed by liquefaction necrosis within the solid tissue.

Aconitine. A poisonous drug from the dried tuberous root of *Aconitum napellus*. It was once given internally as a febrifuge and gastric anesthetic.

Ad libitum. At pleasure.

Adenocarcinoma. Carcinoma derived from glandular tissue or in which the tumor cells form recognizable glandular structures; may be classified according to the predominant pattern of cell arrangement, as papillary, alveolar, etc., or according to a particular products of the cells, as mucinous adenocarcinoma.

Adenoma. A benign epithelial tumor in which the cells form recognizable glandular structures or in which the cells are clearly derived from glandular epithelium.

Adrenalectomize. To excise one or both adrenal glands.

Agglutination. Clumping; the process of union in the healing of a wound; the clumping together in suspension of antigen-bearing cells, microorganisms, or particles in the presence of specific antibodies (agglutinins).

Agrobacterium tumefaciens. A species of bacteria of the family *Rhizobiaceae*. It is a small, Gram-negative, aerobic, flagellated rod that is found in the soil or in the roots or stems of plants. Most species produce hypertrophies (galls) in plant stems.

Ailment. Any disease or affection of the body; usually refers to slight or mild disorder.

Aleurone. The outermost layer of the endosperm.

α-Tocopherol. Vitamin E.

Alkaloid. A large, varied group of complex nitrogen-containing compounds, usually alkaline, that reacts with acids to form soluble salts, many of which have physiological effect on humans, e.g., nicotine and, caffeine, etc.

Allergen. A compound that produces an allergic reaction.

Allergy. A state of hypersensitivity induced by exposure to a particular antigen (allergen) resulting in harmful immunological reactions on subsequent exposures.

Alopecia. Baldness; absence of the hair from skin in areas where it normally is present.

From: *Medicinal Plants of the World, vol. 3: Chemical Constituents, Traditional and Modern Medicinal Uses*
By: I. A. Ross © Humana Press Inc., Totowa, NJ

Amastigote. Any of the bodies representing the morphologic (leishmanial) stage in the life cycle of all trypanosomatic protozoa resembling the typical adult form of members of the genus *Leishmania*.

Amenorrhea. Absence or abnormal stoppage of menstruation.

Analgesic. An agent that relieves pain without causing loss of consciousness.

Anaphrodisiac Antiaphrodisiac; an agent suppressing sexual desire.

Anaphylactic. Related to anaphylaxis; manifesting extremely great sensitivity to foreign protein or other material.

Ancylostomiasis. Infection with hookworms of the genus *Ancyclostoma*.

Androgenetic alopecia. A progressive, diffuse, symmetric loss of scalp hair in the 20s and early 30s with hair loss from the vertex and frontoparietal regions. In females beginning somewhat later, with less severe hair loss in the frontocentral area of the scalp.

Anemia. A reduction below normal in the number of erythrocytes per cu mm, in the quantity of hemoglobin, or in the volume of the packed red cells per 100 mL of blood, which occurs when equilibrium between blood loss and blood production is disturbed.

Anesthetic. An agent that is used to abolish the sensation of pain.

Angina. Spasmodic, choking, or suffocative pain.

Angioedema. A vascular reaction involving the deep dermis, subcutaneous, or submucosal tissues, representing localized edema caused by dilatation and increased permeability of the capillaries, and characterized by development of giant wheals.

Angiotensin. Any of a family of polypeptide vasopressor hormones formed by the catalytic action of rennin on rennin substrate.

Anodyne. A medicine that relieves pain through reducing nerve excitability, milder than analgesic.

Anthelmintic. Vermifuge; an agent that destroys and expels worms from the intestine.

Anti-acne. Preventing the inflammatory disease of the pilosebaceous unit.

Anti-amoebic. Destroying or suppressing the growth of amoebae.

Anti-ancylostomiasis. Preventing the infection with hookworms of the genus *Ancyclostoma*.

Anti-atherogenic. Preventing the formation of atheromatous lesions in the arterial intima.

Anti-atherosclerotic. Preventing the formation of plaques containing cholesterol, lipoid material, and lipophages within the intima and inner media of large- and medium-sized arteries.

Antibacterial. Destroys or stops the growth of bacteria.

Antibody. Sensitize; substance evoked in humans or animals by an antigen, and characterized by reacting specifically with the antigen in some demonstrable way.

Anticarcinogen. An agent to counteract cancer.

Anticathartic. An agent that prevents evacuation of the bowels.

Anticholesterolemic. Promoting a reduction in cholesterol levels in the blood.

Anticlastogenic. Preventing disruption or breakage, as of chromosomes.

Anticonvulsant. An agent that prevents or relieves convulsions or cramps.

Anticrustacean. Antiparasitical; an agent that prevents parasite infections or diseases caused by parasites.

Antidiabetic. An agent that prevents or alleviates diabetes.

Antidiarrheal. An agent to relieve diarrhea.

Antidysrrhythmic. Preventing arrhythmia.

Anti-emetic. Prevents or alleviates nausea and vomiting.

Anti-epileptic. An agent that combats the convulsions or seizures of epilepsy.

Antifebrile. Antipyretic.

Antifungal. An agent that inhibits the growth or multiplication of fungi, or kills them outright.

Antigalactogogue. Prevents or decreases secretion of milk.

Antigen. Any substance that, under appropriate conditions, induces a specific immune response and reacts with the products of that response.

Antiglaucomic. Preventing the eye diseases characterized by an increase in intraocular pressure, which causes pathological changes in the optic disk and typical defects in the field of vision (glaucoma).

Antihalitosis. An agent that prevents offensive breath.

Antihemolytic. Preventing hemolysis.

Antihistaminic. Neutralizing the effect or inhibiting production of histamine.

Antihypercholesterolemic. Effective in decreasing or preventing an excessively high level of cholesterol in the blood.

Antihyperglycemic. An agent that counteracts high levels of glucose in the blood.

Antihyperlipemic. An agent that prevents an elevated concentration of triglycerides in the blood; reduces arterial plaques.

Antihypertensive. An agent that reduces abnormally high blood pressure.

Anti-implantation. Preventing the attachment of the blastocyst to the epithelial lining of the uterus, its penetration through the epithelium, and in humans, its embedding in the compact layer of the endometrium, beginning 6 or 7 days after fertilization.

Anti-inflammatory. An agent that reduces or neutralizes inflammation.

Antimicrobial. An agent that inhibits the growth or multiplication of micro-organisms, or kills them.

Antimitogenic. An agent that prevents mitosis (indirect division of a cell) or cell transformation.

Antimutagenic. A substance that antagonizes the mutagenic effects of other substances.

Antimycobacterial. An agent that is effective against Mycobacteria; a genus of bacteria occurring as Gram-positive, aerobic, mostly slow-growing, slightly curved or straight rods, sometimes branching and filamentous, and distinguished by acid-fast staining. It contains many species, including the highly pathogenic that cause tuberculosis or leprosy.

Anti-nematodal. An agent that is effective against nematode (roundworm); a class of tapered cylindrical helminthes, many species of which are parasites.

Anti-nociceptive. Having an analgesic effect; reducing sensitivity to painful stimuli.

Antioxidant. An agent that prevents or delays deterioration by the action of oxygen.

Antioxytocic. An agent that prevents uterine contractions during childbirth.

Antiparasitical. Destructive to parasites.

Antiphlogistic. An agent that counteracts inflammation and fever.

Antiprogesterone. An agent that reduces the progesterone level.

Antiproteinemic. An agent that reduces an excess of protein in the blood.

Antiprotozoan. Antiprotozoal; destroying protozoa, or checking their growth or reproduction.

Antipyretic. An agent to reduce fever; febrifuge.

Antiradiation. An agent capable of counteracting the effects of radiation; effective against radiation injury.

Antirheumatic. An agent that relieves or cures rheumatism.

Antischistosomal. Effective against a genus of trematode parasites or flukes (schistosomes).

Antisecretory. Inhibiting or diminishing gastric secretion.

Antiseptic. Preventing sepsis, decay, and putrefaction; also an agent that kills germs, microbes.

Antispasmodic. An agent that relieves spasms, usually of smooth muscle, as in arteries, bronchi, intestine, bile duct, ureters, or sphincters, but also of voluntary muscle; spasmolytic.

Antithrombotic. Preventing or interfering with the formation of thrombi (an aggregation of blood factors).

Antithyroid. Counteracting the functioning of the thyroid, especially in its synthesis of thyroid hormone.

Antitumor. Preventing or effective against tumors or cancer formation. Anticarcinogen.

Antitussive. Preventing or relieving cough.

Antiulcerative. Preventing or promoting the healing of ulcers.

Antiulcerogenic. Preventing the production of ulcers.

Antivertigo. Counteracting an illusory sense that either the environment or the body is revolving; it may result from disease of the inner ear or may be due to disturbances of the vestibular centers or pathways in the central nervous system.

Antiviral. An agent that inhibits growth or multiplication of viruses, or kills them.

Anti-yeast. An agent that inhibits the growth or , multiplication of or kills yeasts.

Aphrodisiac. Any drug that arouses the sexual instinct; increasing or exciting the sexual desire.

Apoliprotein. Any of the protein constituents of lipoproteins, grouped by function in four classes A, B, C, and E (the former apolipoprotein [apo] D is now apo A-III).

Apoptosis. Fragmentation of a cell into membrane-bound particles that are eliminated by phagocytosis. Programmed cell death.

Arrhythmia. Any variation from the normal rhythm of the heartbeat; it may be an abnormality of either the rate, regularity, or site of impulse origin or the sequence of activation.

Arterial thrombosis. The formation of an aggregate of blood factors (thrombus), primarily platelets and fibrin, with entrapment of cellular elements in the arteries.

Arthritis. Inflammation of a joint.

Ascaris. Roundworm (maw-worm; eelworm) found in the small intestine, causing colicky pains and diarrhea, especially in children.

Ascites. Excessive accumulation of serious fluid in the peritoneal (abdominal) cavity.

Asthenia. Lack or loss of strength, usually involving muscular system.

Asthma. A condition marked by recurrent attacks of paroxysmal dyspnea, with wheezing resulting from spasmodic contraction of the bronchi. Some cases of asthma are allergic manifestations in sensitized persons.

Astringent. An agent that causes tissue to contract.

Astrocyte. One of the large neuroglia cells of nervous tissue.

Atopic. Allergic; related to atopy (a genetic predisposition toward the development of immediate hypersensitivity reactions against common environmental allergens.

Atractyloside. A highly poisonous steroid from *Atractylis gummifera* with a strychnine-like action, producing convulsion of a hypoglycemic nature. Atractyloside interferes with oxidative reactions, the citric acid cycle, and nerve conduction.

Atrium. The upper chamber of each half of the heart; the portion of nasal cavity; in the lung, a subdivision of the alveolar duct from which alveolar sacs open.

Aural. Within the ear (auris).

Baldness. Alopecia; absence of hair from the scalp.

Benign prostatic hyperplasia. Age-associated enlargement of the prostate, resulting from proliferation of both glandular and stromal elements, beginning generally in the fifth decade of life. It may cause urethral compression and obstruction.

Biliary. Pertaining to the bile, to the bile ducts, or to the gallbladder.

Biliousness. An imprecisely delineated congestive disturbance with anorexia, coated tongue, constipation, headache, dizziness, pasty complexion, and rarely, slight jaundice; assumed to result from hepatic dysfunction.

Blennorrhagia. Discharge from mucus surfaces.

Blistering. The formation of a blister; vesication.

Bradycardia. Brachycardia; bradyrhythmia; oligocardia; slowness of the heartbeat under 60 beats per minute.

Bradypnea. Abnormal slowness of breathing.

Bronchoconstrictor. Constricting or narrowing the lumina of the air passages of the lungs.

Bronchodilator. An agent that causes expansion of the lumina of the air passages of the lung.

Cachexia. A general lack of nutrition and wasting occurring in the course of a chronic disease or emotional disturbance.

Calculi. Abnormal concretion occurring within the animal boy and usually composed of mineral salts.

Calefacient. An agent causing a sense of warmth in the part to which it is applied.

Carcinogen. A substance that predisposes cancer development.

Carcinogenesis. The production of carcinoma.

Carcinoma. A malignant new growth made up of epithelial cells tending to infiltrate the surrounding tissues and give rise to metastases.

Cardiac. Pertaining to the heart.

Cardiovascular. Pertaining to the heart and blood vessels.

Cardiotonic. An agent that has a tonic effect on the heart.

Carminative. An agent that relieves the presence of an excessive amount of gas in the stomach and intestine; preventing the formation or causing the expulsion of flatus.

Carrageenan. Carrageenin; a polysaccharide obtained from Irish moss; a galactosan sulfate resembling agar in molecular structure.

Catalase. An enzyme (EC 1.11.1.6; a hemoprotein), catalyzing the decomposition of hydrogen peroxide to water and oxygen.

Cataleptic. Pertaining to, characterized by, or inducing the condition of maintaining whatever body posture one is placed in (catalepsy).

Cataract. A loss of transparency of the crystalline lens of eye, or of its capsule.

Cecolectomy. Excision of a segment or all of cecum.

Cercaria. The free-swimming trematode larva that emerges from its host snail, in humans it penetrates the skin directly.

Cerebral ischemia. Infarction; an ischemic condition of the brain, producing a persistent focal neurological deficit in the area of distribution of one of the cerebral arteries.

Chalazion. An eyelid mass that results from chronic inflammation of a meibomian gland and shows a granulomatous reaction to liberated fat when subjected to histopathological examination.

Charcoal. Carbon prepared by charring wood or other organic material.

Chemiluminescence. Luminescence produced by the direct transformation of chemical energy into light energy.

Chilblain. A recurrent localized erythema and doughy subcutaneous swelling caused by exposure to cold associated with dampness, and accompanied by pruritus and a burning sensation, usually involving the hands, feet, ears, and face in children; the legs and toes in women; and the hands and fingers in men.

Cholagogue. An agent that stimulates the bile flow to the intestines.

Cholecystectomy. Surgical removal of the gallbladder.

Cholelithiasis. The presence or formation of gallstones.

Cholestatic. Pertaining to or characterized by suppression or stopping of the flow of bile (cholestasis), having intrahepatic or extrahepatic causes.

Cholesterogenesis. Synthesis of cholesterol.

Cholinergic. Relating to nerve fibers that cause effects similar to those induced by acetylcholine.

Chronotropic. Affecting the time or rate, as the rate of contraction of the heart.

Clara cells. Unciliated cells occurring at the boundary where alveolar ducts branch from the bronchioles.

Clastogenic. Giving rise to or inducing disruption or breakages, as of chromosomes.

Clofibrate. An antihyperlipidemic agent used to reduce elevated serum lipids when administered orally.

CNS. Central nervous system.

Colic. Pertaining to the colon; acute abdominal pain; characteristically, intermittent visceral pain with fluctuations corresponding to smooth muscle peristalsis.

Conjunctivitis. Inflammation of the delicate membrane that lines the eyelids and covers the exposed surface of the sclera (conjunctiva), generally consisting of conjunctival hyperemia associated with a discharge.

Constipation. Infrequent or difficult evacuation of feces.

Contraceptive. An agent that diminishes the likelihood of or prevents conception.

Corpus luteum. A yellow glandular mass in the ovary formed by an ovarian follicle that has matured and discharged its ovum. If the ovum has been impregnated, the *corpus luteum* increases in size and persist for several months.

Corticosterone. A natural corticoid ‚with moderate glucocorticoid activity and some mineralocorticoid activity, possessing life-maintaining properties in adrenalectomized animals and several other activities peculiar to the adrenal cortex. Its actions closely resemble those of cortisol, except that it is not anti-inflammatory.

Counter-irritant. An agent that produces inflammation or irritation when applied locally to affect another, usually irritated, surface to stimulate circulation, e.g., liniment.

Cytochrome P450. Trivial name (P for pigment, 450 nm for the absorption maximum of the carbon monoxide derivative) for a cytochrome occurring in most tissues and containing a protoheme IX prosthetic group. It serves as the oxygenating catalyst in a wide variety of reactions catalyzed by monooxygenases. Cytochrome P450 activates molecular oxygen for an attack on the substrate.

Cytophatic. Pertaining to, or characterized by, pathological changes in cells.

Cytotoxic. An agent that is toxic to certain organs, tissues, or cells.

Decoction. A preparation made by boiling a plant part in water; a boiled extract.

Dental enamel. A hard, thin, transcluent layer of calcified substance that envelops and protects the dentin of the crown of the tooth. It is the hardest substance in the body and is almost entirely composed of calcium salts.

Denture stomatitis. Generalized inflammation of the oral mucosa observed sometimes in patient with new dentures or with old, ill-fitting ones, caused by *Candida albicans*, characterized by redness, swelling, and painfulness of the mucosa coming in contact with the denture.

Dermatitis. Inflammation of the skin.

Diabetes mellitus. A chronic syndrome of impaired carbohydrate, protein, and fat metabolism owing to insufficient secretion of insulin or to target tissue insulin resistance.

Diabetes. A general term referring to disorders characterized by excessive urine excretion (polyuria), as in diabetes mellitus and diabetes insipidus.

Diuretic. An agent promoting urination.

DMBA. 7,12-dimethylbenz[a]anthracene; a humorigenic agent.

Dopaminergic. Pertaining to neurons that release dopamine and to the effects exerted thereby; activated or transmitted by dopamine.

Dopamine. A catecholamine formed in the body by the decarboxylation of dopa; an intermediate product in the synthesis of norepinephrine; acts as a neurotransmitter in the central nervous system. It is also produced peripherally and acts on peripheral receptors, e.g., in blood vessels.

Down syndrome. A chromosome disorder characterized by a small, antheroposteriorly flattened skull; short, flat-bridge nose; epicanthal fold; short phalanges; widened spaces between the first and second digits of hands and feet; and moderate to severe mental retardation.

Dromotropic. Affecting the conductivity of a nerve fiber.

Dysentery. Any of various disorders marked by inflammation of the intestines, especially of the colon, and attended by pain in the abdomen, tenesmus, and frequent stools containing blood and mucus.

Dysmenorrhea. Painful menstruation.

Dyspnea. Sense of difficulty in breathing, often associated with lung or heart disease.

Dysuria. Painful or difficult urination.

Eccentric hypertophy. Hypertrophy of a hollow organ, with dilatation of this cavity.

Eczema. A pruritic papulovesicular dermatitis occurring as a reaction to many exogenous and endogenous agents, characterized in a acute stage by erythema, edema associated with a serious exudates between the cells of the epidermis and an inflammatory infiltrate in the dermis, oozing and vesiculation, and crusting and scaling. In the chronic stage by the lichenification or thickening or both, signs of excoriations, and hyperpigmentation or hypopigmentation or both.

Edema. The presence of abnormally large amounts of fluid in the intercellular tissue of the body; usually applied to demonstrable accumulation of excessive fluid in the subcutaneous tissues.

Embryopathy. A morbid condition of the embryo or a disorder resulting from abnormal embryonic development.

Emesis. Vomiting.

Emetic. An agent that induces vomiting.

Emmenagogue. A substance that promotes or assists the flow of menstrual fluid.

Emollient. An agent that smoothes and protects the skin when applied locally.

Emphysema. A pathological accumulation of air in tissues or organs; applied especially to such a condition of the lungs.

Endometrium. The inner mucous membrane of the uterus, the thickness and structure of which vary with the phase of the menstrual cycle.

Endothelium. The layer of epithelial cells that lines the cavities of the heart and of the blood and lymph vessels and the serous cavities of the body, originating from the mesoderm.

Endotoxin. A heat-stable bacterial toxin not freely liberated into the surrounding medium. Endotoxins are released only when the integrity of the cell wall is disturbed, are less potent than most exotoxins, are less specific, and do not form toxoids. When injected in large quantities, endotoxins produce hemorrhagic shock and severe diarrhea. Smaller amounts cause fever, altered resistance to bacterial infections, leukopenia followed by leukocytosis, and numerous other biological effects.

Endovenous. Intravenous.

Enema. A liquid injected or to be injected into the rectum.

Enteropathy. An intestinal disease.

Enterotoxin. A toxin specifically affecting cells of the intestinal mucosa, causing vomiting and diarrhea, e.g., those elaborated by species of *Bacillus*, *Clostridium*, *Escherichia*, *Staphylococcus*, and *Vibrio*.

Epididymal. Pertaining to the epididymis; the elongated cord-like structure along the posterior border of the testis, whose elongated coiled duct provides for the storage, transit, and maturation of spermatozoa, and is continuous with the ductus deferens.

Epstein–Barr virus. A herpes-like virus found in cell cultures of Burkitt lymphoma; also, antibodies reactive with Epstein–Barr

B virus have been reported in cases of infectious mononucleosis.

Erysipelas. A specific, acute, inflammatory disease caused by a hemolytic *Streptococcus*. The eruption, limited to the skin and sharply defined, is usually accompanied by severe constitutional symptoms.

Erythema. Redness of the skin, inflammation.

Estrogens. A substance that induces female hormonal activity.

Expectorant. An agent that induces the removal (coughing up) of mucous secretion from the lungs.

Fatty acids. Hydrolysis products of fats.

Febrifuge. That which reduces fever; antipyretic.

Fibrinolysis. The hydrolysis of an elastic, filamentous protein (fibrin) derived from fibrinogen by the action of thrombin, which releases fibrinopeptides A and B (co-fibrins A and B) from fibrinogen in co-agulation of the blood.

Filariasis. The presence of parasites filariae in the blood and tissues of the body. May be asymptomatic, and living worms cause minimal tissue reaction. Death of the adult worms causes marked inflammation and lymphatic obstruction.

Flatulent colic. Tympanites; distention of the abdomen, resulting from the presence of gas or air in the intestine or in the peritoneal cavity, as in peritonitis and typhoid fever.

Flavonoids. A class of tricyclic molecules, usually occurring in glycosidic form and widely distributed in plants, often as a pigment.

Foam cells. Cells with a peculiar vacuolated appearance owing to the presence of complex lipoids; such cells are seen notably in xanthoma.

Follicular. Pertaining to the lymph nodule.

Follicular cells. Cells located in the epithelium of follicles.

Foot-and-mouth disease. An acute, extremely contagious disease caused by pi-cornavirus, affecting wild and domestic animals, chiefly cattle, pigs, sheep, goats, and other ruminants, and very rarely humans. It is marked by an eruption of vesicles on the lips, buccal cavity, pharynx, legs, and feet; sometimes the skin of the udder or teats is involved.

FSH. Follicle-stimulating hormone.

Furuncle. A painful nodule formed in the skin by circumscribed inflammation of the corium and subcutaneous tissue, enclosing a central slough or "core." It is caused by staphylococci.

Galactogogue. An agent that promotes secretion of milk.

Gallbladder (cholecyst; *vesica biliaris; vesica fellea*). The pear-shaped reservoir for the bile in the postinferior surface of he liver, between the right and quadrate lobe; the cystic duct projects to join the common bile duct.

Gallstone. A concretion, usually of cholesterol, formed in the gallbladder or bile duct.

Gargle. A solution used for rinsing in medicating the mouth and throat.

Gastroenteritis. Inflammation of the stomach and intestinal tract.

Gastroesophageal reflux. Reflux of the stomach and duodenal contents into the esophagus, which may sometimes occur normally, particularly in the distended stomach postprandially, or as a chronic pathological condition.

Gastroesophageal. Pertaining to the stomach and esophagus, as the gastroesophageal junction.

Genotoxic. Damaging to DNA, causing mutations or cancer.

GI. Gastrointestinal.

Glomerular. Pertaining to, or of the nature of tuft or cluster (glomerulus), composed of blood vessels or nerve fibers, especially a renal glomerulus.

Glutathione. A tripeptide, widely distributed in animal and plant tissues. It exists in reduced (GSH) and oxidized (GSSH) forms, and it functions in various redox reactions, in the formation and maintenance of disulfide bonds in proteins and in transport of amino acids across cell membranes. In erythrocytes, these reactions prevent oxidative damage by reduction of methemoglobin, and peroxides.

Glycosides. Sugar esters.

Goitrogenic. Producing an enlargement of the thyroid gland, causing a swelling in the front part of the neck.

Gonorrhea. A contagious catarrhal inflammation of the genital mucous membrane, transmitted chiefly by coitus, and resulting from *Neisseria gonorrhoeae*.

Gout. An inherited metabolic disorder occurring especially in men, characterized by a raised but variable blood uric acid level, recurrent acute arthritis of sudden onset, deposition of crystalline sodium urate in connective tissues and articular cartilage, and progressive chronic arthritis.

Gum. Water swellable carbohydrate derivatives.

HDL cholesterol. High-density lipoprotein cholesterol.

Hematopoiesis. The formation and development of blood cells.

Hemolysis. Disruption of the integrity of the red cell membrane causing release of hemoglobin.

Hemorrhage. Bleeding; a flow of blood, especially if it is very profuse.

Hemorrhoid. A varicose dilatation of a vein of the superior or inferior hemorrhoidal plexus, resulting from a persistent increase in venous pressure.

Hemostat. An agent that checks hemorrhage when properly applied to a bleeding point.

Hemostatic. A compound that retards bleeding.

Hemotoxic. Poisonous to the blood and hematopoietic system (system pertaining to or effecting the formation of blood cells).

Hepatectomy. Removal of a part of the liver.

Hepatic. An agent that promotes the well-being of the liver and increases the secretion of bile.

Hepatitis. Inflammation of the liver, usually from the viral infection, sometimes from toxic agents.

Hepatoblastoma. A malignant intrahepatic tumor occurring in infants and young children and consisting chiefly of embryonic hepatic tissue.

Herpes. Any inflammatory skin disease caused by a herpesvirus and characterized by the formation of clusters of small vesicles. When used alone, the term may refer to herpes simplex or *Herpes zoster*.

HMG-CoA reductase. 3-Hydroxy-3-methylglutaryl coenzyme A-reductase.

Hoarseness. A rough or noisy quality of voice.

Homocysteine. A sulfur-containing amino acid, a homologue of cysteine, produced by the demethylation of methionine, and an intermediate in the biosynthesis from methionine via cystathionine.

Husk. The shell; the outer covering of some fruits as of corn and many other cereals.

Hypercholesterolemic. An agent that pertains to, is characterized by, or tends to produce an excess of cholesterol in the blood.

Hyperemesis gravidorum. Pernicious vomiting of pregnancy.

Hyperemia. An excess of blood in a part; engorgement.

Hyperglycemic. Pertaining to, characterized by, or causing an increase in the level of glucose in the blood.

Hyperkeratosis. Hypertrophy of the corneous layer of the skin, or any disease characterized by it.

Hyperlipemic. Pertaining to, characterized by, or causing an elevated concentration of any or all of the lipids in the plasma.

Hypertension. High arterial pressure. Various criteria for its threshold have been suggested, from 140 mmHg systolic and 90 mmHg diastolic, to 200 mmHg systolic and 110 mmHg diastolic. Hypertension may have no known cause (idiopathic or idiopathic) or may be associated with other primary diseases (secondary).

Hypertensive. Causing or marking a rise in blood pressure.

Hyperthermia. Abnormally high body temperature, especially that induced for therapeutic purposes.

Hypertriglyceridemic. Pertaining to, characterized by, or causing an increase in the level of triglyceride in the blood.

Hyperventilation. Increased pulmonary ventilation beyond that needed to maintain the blood gases within the normal ranges.

Hypnotic. A drug that acts to induce sleep.

Hypocholesterolemic. Pertaining to, characterized by, or producing an abnormally diminished amount of cholesterol in the blood.

Hypofertile. Having diminished reproductive capacity.

Hypogammaglobulinemia. A condition characterized by abnormally low levels of all classes of immunoglobulins.

Hypoglycemic. Causing a deficiency of blood glucose.

Hypotensive. Causing or marking a lowering of blood pressure.

Hypouricemia. Deficiency of uric acid in the blood, along with xanthinuria, resulting from deficiency of xanthineoxidase, the enzyme required for conversion of hypoxanthine to xanthine and of xanthine to uric acid.

Hypoxia. Reduction of oxygen supply to tissue below physiological levels despite adequate perfusion of the tissue by blood.

Hypoventilation. Underventilation; reduced alveolar ventilation in relation to the oxygen consumption.

Hysteria. A diagnostic term, referrable to a wide variety of psychogenic symptoms that may be mental, sensory, motor, or visceral.

Idiopathy. A morbid state of spontaneous origin; one neither sympathetic nor traumatic.

Immunogenicity. The property that endows a substance with the capacity to provoke an immune response, or the degree to which a substance possesses this property.

Immunoglobulin. Immunoprotein; glycoprotein of animal origin with known antibody activity, or protein related by chemical structure, which may or may not have antibody activity. Divided into five classes: IgM, IgG, IgA, IgD, and IgE on the basis of structure and biological activity.

Immunostimulant. Stimulating various functions or activities of the immune system.

Immunosuppressant. An agent capable of suppressing immune responses.

Inebriation. The condition of being drunk.

Infestation. Parasitic attack or subsistence on the skin and its appendages, as by insects, mites, or ticks.

Infusion. A preparation made by soaking a plant part in hot or cold water, e.g., tea.

Inotropic. Affecting the force or energy of muscular contractions. Negatively inotropic—weakening the force of muscular contractions. Positively inotropic—increasing the strength of muscular contractions.

Insecticidal. An agent selectively poisonous to insects.

Interferon. Any of a family of glycoproteins that exert virus-nonspecific but host-specific antiviral activity by inducing the transcription of cellular genes coding for antiviral proteins that selectively inhibit the synthesis of viral RNA and proteins. Interferons have immunoregulatory functions and can inhibit the growth of nonviral intracellular parasites.

Interleukin. A generic term for a group of multifunctional cytokines that are produced by a variety of lymphoid and nonlymphoid cells and whose effects occur at least partly within the lymphopoietic system.

Intragastric. Situated or occurring within the stomach.

Intraperitoneal. Within the peritoneal cavity.

Ischemia. Deficiency of blood in a part, usually results from functional constriction or actual obstruction of a blood vessel.

Isotype. An immunoglobulin heavy- or light-chain class or subclass characterized by antigenic determinants in the constant region.

Jaundice. A syndrome characterized by hyperbilirubinemia (excessive concentrations of bilirubin in the blood) and deposition of bile pigment in the skin, mucous membranes, and sclera with resulting yellow appearance of the patient.

Karyotype. The chromosome characteristics of an individual or of a cell line, usually presented as a systematized array of metaphase chromosomes from a photomicrograph of a single cell nucleus arranged in pairs in descending order of size and according to the position of centromere.

Labor. The function of the female organism by which the product of conception is expelled from the uterus through the vagina to the outside world.

Larvicidal. Destructive to insect larvae.

Laxative. An agent that promotes evacuation of the bowels. A mild purgative.

LDL cholesterol. Low-density lipoprotein cholesterol.

Leprosy. A slowly progressive, chronic infectious disease caused by *Mycobacterium leprae* and characterized by the development of granulomatous or neurotropic lesions in the skin, mucous membranes, nerves, bones, and viscera.

Lesion. Any pathological or traumatic discontinuity of tissue or loss of function of a part.

Leucorrhea. A whitish, viscid discharge from the vagina and uterine cavity.

Leukocyte. White blood cells.

Leukocytosis. A transient increase in the number of leukocytes in the blood, resulting from hemorrhage, fever, infection, inflammation, etc.

Leukotriene. Biologically active compound functions as regulators of allergic and inflammatory reactions. They are identified by the letters A, B, C, D, and E, with subscripts indicating the number of double bonds in the molecule.

LH. Luteinizing hormone.

Libido. Conscious or unconscious sexual desire; creative energy. Any passionate form of life force.

Lipogenetic. Lipogenic; forming, producing or caused by fat.

Lipolytic. Pertaining to, characterized by, or causing the decomposition or splitting up of fat (lipolysis).

Lithiasis. A condition characterized by the formation of calculi and concretions.

Lobar pneumonia. An acute febrile disease produced by *Streptococcus pneumoniae*, and marked by inflammation of one or more lobes of the lung, together with consolidation. It is attended with chill, followed by sudden elevation of temperature, dyspnea, rapid breathing, pain in the side, and cough, with blood-stained expectoration. The symptoms abate after 1 week.

Luteal. Pertaining to or having the properties of the *corpus luteum* or its active principle.

Lymphoblast. A morphologically immature lymphocyte; an activated lymphocyte that has been transformed in response to antigenic stimulation.

Lymphohistiocytic. Involving lymphocytes and histiocytes.

Lymphopoietic. Pertaining to, characterized by, or causing the development of lymphatic tissue (lymphopoiesis).

Malaria. An infectious disease endemic in parts of Africa, Asia, Turkey, the West Indies, Central and South America, and Oceania, caused by protozoa of the genus *Plasmodium*, and usually transmitted by the bites of infected anopheline mosquitoes. It is characterized by prostration associated with paroxysms of high fever, shaking chills, sweating, anemia, and splenomegaly, which may lead to death.

Malignancy. The property or condition of being resistant to treatment (malignant).

Mastocytoma. A nodular cutaneous mast cell infiltrate, which is usually present at birth or soon after as a solitary nodule, although three to four lesions may occur. Lesions typical of urticaria pigmentosa may occur later.

Measles. A highly contagious infectious disease caused by paramyxovirus, common among children and seen in the unimmune of any age. Characteristically, coryza, cervical lymphadentitis, Koplik's spotspalpebral conjunctivitis, photophobia, malagia, malaise, and a harassing cough with steadily mounting fever precede the skin eruption.

Melanoid. Resembling melanin.

Menorrhagia. Hypermenorrhea; excessive uterine bleeding occurring at regular intervals, the period of blood being of usual duration.

Methemoglobinemia. The presence of methemoglobin in the blood, resulting in cyanosis and headache, dizziness, fatigue, ataxia, dyspnea, tachycardia, nausea, vomiting, drowsiness, stupor, coma, and sometimes death.

Miscarriage. Loss of products of conception from the uterus before the fetus is viable; spontaneous abortion.

Mitogenic. An agent that affects cell division.

Molluscacidal. Destructive to snails and other mollusks.

Monocytic. Pertaining to or, characterized by a mononuclear phagocytic leukocytes, formed in bone marrow and transported to tissues, as of the lung and liver, where they develop into macrophages.

Morbidity. A disease condition or state, the incidence or prevalence of a disease or of all diseases in a population.

Mutagenic. Causing change or inducing genetic mutation.

Myocardial infarction. An area of coagulation necrosis in a tissue resulting from local ischemia in the heart.

Nausea. Sickness at the stomach; an inclination to vomit.

Nematocidal. Destroying nematode worms.

Neoplasia. The formation of a new tissue, with uncontrolled and progressive growth.

It would cause cessation of, multiplication of normal cells.

Nephritis. Inflammation of the kidney.

Nephropathy. Disease of the kidneys.

Nephrotoxic. Toxic or destructive to kidney cells.

Neuralgia. Pain extending along the course of one or more nerves. Many varieties of neuralgia are distinguished according to the part affected, as brachial, facial, occipital, or supraorbital, or to the case, as anemic, diabetic, gouty, malarial, or syphilitic.

Neurasthenia. A syndrome of chronic mental and physical weakness and fatigue, which was supposed to be caused by exhaustion of the nervous system.

Neutrophil. A granular leukocyte, having a nucleus with three to five lobes connected by slender threads of chromatin, and cytoplasm containing fine inconspicuous granules. Neutrophils have the properties of chemotaxis: adherence to immune complexes, and phagocytosis.

Nigrostratial. Projecting from the substantia nigra to the corpus striatum; said of a bundle of nerve fibers.

Non-Hodgkin's lymphoma. A heterogenous group of a malignant lymphomas, the only common feature being an absence of the giant Reed-Sternberg cells characteristic of Hodgkin's disease. They arise from the lymphoid components of the immune system, and present a clinical picture broadly similar to that of Hodgkin's disease, except the disease is initially more widespread, with the most common manifestation being painless enlargement of one or more peripheral lymph nodes.

Occlusion. The act of closure or state of being closed; an obstruction or a closing off.

Oleoresins. Natural mixtures of resins and volatile oils.

Ophthalmic. Healing for disorders and diseases of the eye.

Osteoarthritis. Noninflammatory degenerative joint disease occurring chiefly in older persons, characterized by degeneration of the articular cartilage, hypertophy of bone at the margins, and changes in the synovial membrane, accompanied by pain and stiffness.

Osteoclast. A large multinuclear cell associated with the absorption and removal of bone, osteoclasts become highly active in the presence of parathyroid hormone, causing increased bone resorption and release of bone salts (phosphorus, and especially calcium) into the extracellular fluid.

Ovalbumin. An albumin obtainable from the whites of eggs.

Oviposition. The act of laying or depositing eggs.

PAC. Premature atrial complex; a single ectopic atrial beat arising prematurely, manifests electrocardiographically as an abnormally shaped premature P wave, usually with a slightly increased PR interval. It occurs in normal hearts, sometimes associated with the use of stimulants, but may be associated with structural heart disease.

Pancreatic. Pertaining to the pancreas; a large, elongated, racemose gland situated transversely behind the stomach, between the spleen and duodenum, producing insulin, glucagons, somatostatin, polypeptide (the endocrine part), and a pancreatic juice that contains enzymes essential to protein digestion (the exocrine part).

Papilloma. A benign epithelial neoplasm producing finger-like or verrucous projections from the epithelial surface.

Parakeratosis. Persistence of the nuclei of the keratinocytes into the stratum corneum (horny layer) of the skin. Parakeratosis is normal in the epithelium of true mucous membrane of the mouth and vagina.

Parkinson's disease. Neurological disorder characterized by hypokinesia, tremor, and muscular rigidity.

Pectoral. Pertaining to the thorax or chest; relieving disorders of the respiratory tract, as an expectorant.

Pediculicide. An agent that destroys parasitic insects (lice).

Pepsin. A general name for several names of the gastric juice that catalyze the hydrolysis of the protein to form polypeptides.

Per rectum. By the way of rectum.

Periodontosis. Juvenile periodontitis; a rare form that has an onset at puberty, is more common in females, and is manifested by deep periodontal pockets, usually involving the first molars and incisors.

Pessary. An instrument placed in the vagina to support the uterus or rectum or as a contraceptive device; a medicated vaginal suppository.

Phagocytosis. Ingestion and digestion of bacteria and particles by phagocytes.

Pheromone. A substance secreted to the outside of the body by an individual and perceived (as by smell) by a second individual, releasing a specific reaction of behavior in the percipient.

Phospholipidemia. The presence of phospholipids in the blood.

Phytotoxic. Pertaining to phytotoxin, or plant poison; inhibiting the growth of plants.

Phytotoxin. An exotoxin produced by certain species of higher plants; they are resistant to proteolytic digestion, and are effective when taken by mouth.

Platelet aggregation. Clumping together of platelets as part of a sequential mechanism leading to the initiation and formation of a thrombus or hemostatic plug.

Platelet. Disc-like structure, 2–4 mm in diameter, found in the blood of all mammals and chiefly known for its role in blood coagulation.

Pleural empyema. Accumulation of a liquid inflammation product made up of leukocytes (pus) in a cavity of the lungs.

Pleurisy. Inflammation of the pleura, with exudation into its cavity and on its surface.

Pneumonia. Inflammation of the lungs with consolidation.

Pneumonitis. Inflammation of the lungs.

Pneumothrax. An accumulation of air or gas in the pleural space, which may occur spontaneously or as a result of trauma or a pathological process, or be introduced deliberately.

Poliovirus. A virus of the genus *Enterovirus* that is the etiological agent of poliomyelitis, separable on the basis of specificity of neutralizing antibody into three serotypes, designated types 1, 2, and 3.

Pollinosis. Allergic reaction in the body to the airborne pollen of plants, resulting in the seasonal type of hay fever or rose cold.

Polymorphonuclear cells. Cells having a nucleus deeply lobed or so divided that it appears to be multiple.

Poultice. A moist, usually warm or hot mass of plant material applied to the skin, or with cloth between the skin and plant material, to effect a medicinal action.

Prolactin. A hormone secreted by special cells of the anterior pituitary gland that stimulates and sustains lactation in postpartum mammals, the mammary glands having been prepared by other hormones, including estrogens, progesterone, growth hormone, corticosteroids, and insulin.

Promastigote. Any of the bodies representing the morphological stage in the life cycle of certain tryptanosomatid protozoa resembling the typical adult form of members of the genus *Leptomonas*.

Prostaglandin (PG). Components derived from unsaturated 20-carbon fatty acids, primarily arachidonic acid, via the cyclooxygenase pathway. They are extremely potent mediators of a diverse group of physiological processes.

Proteinemia. An excess of proteins in the blood.

Proteolytic. Pertaining to, characterized by, or promoting the splitting of proteins by hydrolysis of the peptide bonds with formation of smaller polypeptides (proteolysis).

Psoriatic. Pertaining to, affected with, or of the nature of a common chronic, squamous dermatosis with polygenic inheritance and a fluctuating course (psoriasis).

Purgative. An agent that causes cleansing or watery evacuation of the bowels, usually with griping (painful cramps).

Pus. A liquid inflammation product composed made up of cells (leukocytes) and a thin protein-rich fluid called liquor puris.

PVC. Pulmonary venous congestion; premature ventricular contraction.

Pyretic. Pertaining to or of the nature of fever.

Rabies. An acute infectious disease of the central nervous system affecting most mammals including humans, caused by rhabdovirus. Typical symptoms include paresthesia and a burning sensation or pain at the site of inoculation, periods of hyperexcitability, agitation, delirium, hallucinations, and bizarre behavior, between which the person is often cooperative and lucid.

Rage. A state of violent anger; a total discharge of the sympathetic portion of the autonomic system.

RBBB. Right bundle branch block.

Reflux. A backward or return flow.

Gastroesophageal reflux. Reflux of the stomach and duodenal contents into the esophagus, which may sometimes occur normally, particularly in the distended stomach postprandially, or as a chronic pathological condition.

Renal. Pertaining to the kidney.

Resins. Water-insoluble mixtures of resins, their acids, and alcohols.

Reticulocyte. A young red blood cell showing a basophilic reticulum under vital staining.

Rhinitis. Inflammation of nasal mucosa.

Salivary. Pertaining to the clear, alkaline, somewhat viscid secretion from the parotid, submaxillary, sublingual, and smaller mucous glands of the mouth.

Saponin. A glycoside compound in plants, which, when shaken with water, has a foaming or "soapy" action.

Sarcolemma. The delicate plasma membrane thatwhich invests every striated muscle fiber.

Sarcoma. Any of the group of tumors usually arising from the connective tissue, although the term now includes some of epithelial origin; most are malignant. Many types have prefixes denoting the type of tissue or structure involved, e.g., fibrosarcoma.

Schistosomiasis. The state of being infected with flukes of the genus *Schistosoma*.

Scorbutic. Concerning or affected with scurvy.

Scrofula. Tuberculosis involving the lymph nodes of the neck, usually occurs in early life, now rarely seen.

Scabies. A contagious dermatitis of humans and various animals, caused by the itch mite, *Sarcoptes scabiei*, and characterized by a popular eruption over tiny, raised sinuous burrows produced by digging into the upper layer of the epidermis by the egg-laying female mite, which is accompanied by intense pruritus and sometimes associated with eczema and secondary bacterial infection.

Seasonal rhinoconjunctivitis (SRC). Inflammation of the mucus membranes of the nose and eyes.

Sedative. An agent that allays excitement.

Semliki Forest virus. A species of viruses of the genus *Alphavirus*, originally isolated from *Aedes* mosquitoes in Western Uganda; it is widespread in Africa, where it appears to be nonpathogenic, although infections of laboratory workers have occurred.

Sp. Abbreviation for species (singular).

Spp. Abbreviation for species (plural).

Spasmogenic. Relating to the production of, or causing spasms.

Spasmolytic. An agent to lessen muscle spasms or cramps; antispasmodic.

Speech. The utterance of vocal sounds conveying ideas.

Spermatogonium. An undifferentiated germ cell of a male, originating in a seminiferous tubule and dividing into two primary spermatocytes.

Spermicidal. Destructive to spermatozoa.

Suppository. A medicated mass adapted for introduction into the rectal, vaginal, or urethral orifice of the body.

Sphincter. A ring-like band of muscle fibers that constricts a passage or closes a natural orifice.

Splenomegaly. Enlargement of a large, gland-like, ductless organ situated in the upper part of the abdominal cavity on the left side and lateral to the cardiac end of the stomach (spleen).

SRBC. Sheep red blood cells.

Steroidogenic. Producing steroids.

Sterols. Molecules related to cholesterol and some hormones.

Stimulant. An agent to increase body metabolism.

Stimulant, CNS. A compound that excites mental function.

Sting. An injury caused by the venom of a plant or animal (biotoxin) introduced into the individual or with which he or she has come in contact, together with the mechanical trauma caused by the organ responsible for its introduction.

Stomachic. A preparation that gives strength and tone to the stomach. Also used to stimulate the appetite.

Stupor. A lowered level of consciousness manifested by the subject's responding only to vigorous stimulation.

Subcutaneous. Beneath the skin.

Submandibular. Below the bone of the lower jaw (mandible).

Sudorific. Diaphoretic; a compound that increases perspiration.

Suspension. A preparation of a finely divided drug intended to be incorporated in some suitable liquid vehicle before it is used, or already incorporated in such a vehicle.

Sympathomimetic. Mimicking the effects of impulses conveyed by adrenergic postganglionic fibers of the sympathetic nervous system.

Synovial fluid. A transparent alkaline viscid fluid, resembling the white of an egg, secreted by the synovial membrane, and contained in joint cavities, bursae, and tendon sheaths.

Tachycardia. A raised heart beat rate.

Tachyphylaxis. Rapid immunization against the effect of toxic doses of an extract of serum by previous injection of small doses; rapidly decreasing response to a drug or physiologically active agent after administration of a few doses.

Tannin. Bitter principle of plant containing plant polyphenols.

Tapeworm. A parasitic intestinal cestode worm having a flattened, band-like form. The eggs of tapeworms are ingested by the intermediate host, they produce the larval stage in tissues. When the flesh of intermediate host is eaten, the larvae develop within the alimentary canal of the definitive host into adult tapeworms.

T-cells. T-lymphocytes; thymus-dependent lymphocytes; the cells primarily responsible for cell-mediated immunity.

Tenifuge. Taeniafuge; an agent that expels tapeworms.

Teratogen. A substance that can cause the deformity of a fetus.

Terpenes. Hydrocarbon volatile oils, often with a strong smell.

Tetanus. An acute, often fatal, infectious disease caused by anaerobic, spore-forming bacillus *Clostridium tetani*. The clinical manifestations are the result of tetanospasmin, a potent neurotoxin elaborated by the germinating spores.

Thermogenic. Producing heat.

Thrombocytosis. Increased numbers of platelets in the peripheral blood.

Thyroid gland. One of the endocrine glands, normally situated in the lower part of the front of the neck and consisting two lobes, one on either side of the trachea and joined in front by a narrow isthmus. It excretes, stores, and liberates the thyroid hormones, which play major endocrine roles in regulating the metabolic rate.

Tincture. An alcoholic or hydroalcoholic solution prepared from biological substances or from chemical substances.

Tocopherol. Any of a series of structurally similar compounds, methyl-substituted tocols.

Tonic. An ambiguous term referring to a substance thought to have overall positive medicinal effect of an unspecified nature.

Tonsil. A small, rounded mass of tissue, especially of lymphoid tissue.

Tourette's syndrome. A syndrome of facial and vocal tics with onset in childhood, progressing to generalized jerking movements in any part of the body, with echolalia and coprolalia.

Toxic. Pertaining to, resulting from, or of the nature of a poison or toxin. Manifesting the symptoms of severe infections.

Trabecula. A general term for a supporting or anchoring strand of a connective tissue, such as a strand extending from a capsule into the substance of the enclosed organ.

Tranquilizer. An agent that reduces psychotic behavior.

Triacylglycerol. Triglyceride; a compound consisting of three molecules of fatty acids esterified to glycerol. It is a neutral fat synthesized from carbohydrates for storage in animal adipose cells. On enzymatic hydrolysis, it releases free fatty acids in the blood.

Tuberculosis. Any of the infectious diseases of man and animals caused by species *Mycobacterium* and characterized by the formation of tubercles and caseous necrosis in the tissues.

Ulcerative gingivitis (acute necrotizing ulcerative gingivitis; ANUG). A progressive painful infection, also occurring in subacute and recurrent forms, marked by crateriform lesions of the interdental papillae that are covered by pseudomembranous slough and circumscribed by linear erythema; fetid breath, increased salivation, and spontaneous gingival hemorrhage are additional features.

Ulcerogenic. Leading to the production of ulcers.

Urease. An enzyme of the hydrolase class that catalyzes the hydrolysis of urea to CO_2 and ammonia. It is nickel protein found in micro-organisms and plant that is frequently used in clinical assays of plasma urea concentrations.

Urticaria. A vascular reactions, usually transient, involving the upper dermis, representing localized edema, caused by dilatation and increased permeability of capillaries, and marked by the development of wheals.

Vaccine. A suspension of attenuated or killed micro-organisms or of antigenic proteins derived from them.

Vaginitis. Inflammation of the vagina marked by pain and by a purulent discharge.

Vasoconstrictor. An agent that causes blood vessels to constrict, or narrow the caliber.

Vasodilator. An agent that causes blood vessels to relax and dilate.

Vermicidal. Having worm-killing properties.

Vermifuge. Anthelmintic; an agent that kills worms.

VLDL cholesterol. Very low-density lipoprotein cholesterol.

Vulnerary. An agent used for healing wounds, fresh cuts, etc., usually used as a poultice.

Waxes. Esters of fatty acids with high-molecular-weight alcohols.

WBC. White blood cells.

Cross Reference

Common Names	Country	Latin bionomial
'O:yz	Laos	*Saccharum officinarum*
A´-li	Colombia	*Nicotiana tabacum*
Aale	India	*Zingiber officinale*
Aankha	India	*Saccharum officinarum*
Acchellu	India	*Sesamum indicum*
Aceituna	Spain	*Olea europaea*
Aco	Wales	*Nicotiana tabacum*
Ada	India	*Zingiber officinale*
Adarak	India	*Zingiber officinale*
Adhu	India	*Zingiber officinale*
Adi	India	*Zingiber officinale*
Adraka	Pakistan	*Zingiber officinale*
Adruka	India	*Zingiber officinale*
Aduva	Nepal	*Zingiber officinale*
Afifindi	Ecuador	*Zingiber officinale*
Afu	Africa	*Zingiber officinale*
Agnimanth	Nepal	*Zingiber officinale*
Aisiksikimi	United States	*Camellia sinensis*
Aisskssiinainikimm	United States	*Oryza sativa*
Ajenjibre	Cuba	*Zingiber officinale*
Ajenjibre	Mexico	*Zingiber officinale*
Ajijilla	Ecuador	*Zingiber officinale*
Ajilla	Ecuador	*Zingiber officinale*
Ajinibre	Mexico	*Zingiber officinale*
Ajirinrin	Ecuador	*Zingiber officinale*
Ajonjoli	Spain	*Sesamum indicum*
Ak	Pakistan	*Saccharum officinarum*
Akakur	China	*Zingiber officinale*
Akeita	France	*Coffea arabica*
Aleysi	Suriname	*Oryza sativa*
Alha	India	*Zingiber officinale*
Aliah	Indonesia	*Zingiber officinale*

From: *Medicinal Plants of the World, vol. 3: Chemical Constituents, Traditional and Modern Medicinal Uses*
By: I. A. Ross © Humana Press Inc., Totowa, NJ

Alla	India	*Zingiber officinale*
Allam	India	*Zingiber officinale*
Almindelig hamp	Denmark	*Cannabis sativa*
Almindelig	Denmark	*Hordeum vulgare*
Aloruz	Arabic countries	*Oryza sativa*
Alyvos	Lithuania	*Olea europaea*
American dwarf palm tree	United States	*Serenoa repens*
Ampeu	Cambodia	*Saccharum officinarum*
Anaargeel	Iran	*Cocos nucifera*
Anjadana	Pakistan	*Ferula assafoetida*
Araabia kohvipuu	Estonia	*Coffea arabica*
Araisa	Samoa	*Oryza sativa*
Ardak	India	*Zingiber officinale*
Ardakam	India	*Zingiber officinale*
Arisi	India	*Oryza sativa*
Arlysen	Cornwall	*Hordeum vulgare*
Aros	Netherlands Antilles	*Oryza sativa*
Aroz	France	*Oryza sativa*
Arpa	Hungary	*Hordeum vulgare*
Arpa	Turkey	*Hordeum vulgare*
Arpa	Turkmenistan	*Hordeum vulgare*
Arre kokosi	Albania	*Cocos nucifera*
Arros	Spain	*Oryza sativa*
Arroz colorado	Argentina	*Oryza sativa*
Arroz macho	Argentina	*Oryza sativa*
Arroz preto	Brazil	*Oryza sativa*
Arroz rojo	Bolivia	*Oryza sativa*
Arroz rojo	Colombia	*Oryza sativa*
Arroz rojo	Costa Rica	*Oryza sativa*
Arroz rojo	Cuba	*Oryza sativa*
Arroz rojo	Ecuador	*Oryza sativa*
Arroz rojo	Honduras	*Oryza sativa*
Arroz rojo	Mexico	*Oryza sativa*
Arroz rojo	Nicaragua	*Oryza sativa*
Arroz rojo	Panama	*Oryza sativa*
Arroz rojo	Paraguay	*Oryza sativa*
Arroz rojo	Peru	*Oryza sativa*
Arroz rojo	Puerto Rico	*Oryza sativa*
Arroz rojo	Venezuela	*Oryza sativa*
Arroz vermelho	Brazil	*Oryza sativa*
Arroz	Portugal	*Oryza sativa*
Arroz	Spain	*Oryza sativa*
Arstniecibas ingvers	Latvia	*Zingiber officinale*
Aruz	Ecuador	*Oryza sativa*
Asa	Japan	*Cannabis sativa*
Asafetida	England	*Ferula assafoetida*
Asafetida	Croatia	*Ferula assafoetida*
Asafetida	Finland	*Ferula assafoetida*
Asafetida	Germany	*Ferula assafoetida*
Asafetida	Guyana	*Ferula assafoetida*
Asafetida	Iceland	*Ferula assafoetida*
Asafetida	Lithuania	*Ferula assafoetida*

Asafetida	Netherlands	*Ferula assafoetida*
Asafetida	Poland	*Ferula assafoetida*
Asafetida	Russia	*Ferula assafoetida*
Asafetida	Spain	*Ferula assafoetida*
Asafetida	Sweden	*Ferula assafoetida*
Asafetida	United States	*Ferula assafoetida*
Asafetide	France	*Ferula assafoetida*
Asafootida	Estonia	*Ferula assafoetida*
Asafotida	Germany	*Ferula assafoetida*
Asant	Germany	*Ferula assafoetida*
Aseituna	Netherlands Antilles	*Olea europaea*
Asgumetakui	Africa	*Zingiber officinale*
Ashadital	India	*Sesamum indicum*
Ashwagolam	India	*Plantago ovata*
Assa Foetida	France	*Ferula assafoetida*
Assafetida	Italy	*Ferula assafoetida*
Asunglasemtong	India	*Zingiber officinale*
Atuja	Malaysia	*Zingiber officinale*
A-wei	China	*Ferula assafoetida*
Aza	Greece	*Ferula assafoetida*
Azeitona	Portugal	*Olea europaea*
Azucar, cane de	Canary Islands	*Saccharum officinarum*
Azucar, cane de	Guatemala	*Saccharum officinarum*
Babka	Poland	*Plantago ovata*
Baco	Wales	*Nicotiana tabacum*
Bagasse	China	*Saccharum officinarum*
Bahia coconut palm	Brazil	*Cocos nucifera*
Bang	Egypt	*Cannabis sativa*
Baojiang	China	*Zingiber officinale*
Barhanj	Arabic countries	*Plantago ovata*
Bariis	Somalia	*Oryza sativa*
Bariktil	India	*Sesamum indicum*
Barley	Guyana	*Hordeum vulgare*
Barley	United Kingdom	*Hordeum vulgare*
Barley	United States	*Hordeum vulgare*
Barlysyn	Wales	*Hordeum vulgare*
Beras	Malaysia	*Oryza sativa*
Beuing	Indonesia	*Zingiber officinale*
Bhaang	India	*Cannabis sativa*
Bhaango	Nepal	*Cannabis sativa*
Bidr qtn	Arabic countries	*Plantago ovata*
Bijan	Malaysia	*Sesamum indicum*
Birhni	India	*Oryza sativa*
Black bush	United States	*Larrea tridentata*
Blond psyllium	Arabic countries	*Plantago ovata*
Boko	Philippines	*Cocos nucifera*
Boktel	Malaysia	*Daucus carota*
Bokti	Indonesia	*Daucus carota*
Bortol	Sudan	*Daucus carota*
Bugas	Philippines	*Oryza sativa*
Buko	Philippines	*Cocos nucifera*
Bunna	Ethiopia	*Coffea arabica*

Buzar qatona	Arabic countries	*Plantago ovata*
Byg	Denmark	*Hordeum vulgare*
Bygg	Faeroe Islands	*Hordeum vulgare*
Bygg	Iceland	*Hordeum vulgare*
Bygg	Norway	*Hordeum vulgare*
Cabbage palm	United States	*Serenoa repens*
Ca-fae	Thailand	*Coffea arabica*
Café	Africa	*Coffea arabica*
Café	Argentina	*Coffea arabica*
Café	Bolivia	*Coffea arabica*
Café	Brazil	*Coffea arabica*
Café	Catalonia	*Coffea arabica*
Café	Chile	*Coffea arabica*
Café	Ecuador	*Coffea arabica*
Café	France	*Coffea arabica*
Café	Peru	*Coffea arabica*
Café	Portugal	*Coffea arabica*
Café	Spain	*Coffea arabica*
Café	Vietnam	*Coffea arabica*
Cafea	Romania	*Coffea arabica*
Caffe	Finland	*Coffea arabica*
Caffe	Italy	*Coffea arabica*
Caife	Ireland	*Coffea arabica*
Cairead	Ireland	*Daucus carota*
Caj	Albania	*Camellia sinensis*
Caj	Croatia	*Camellia sinensis*
Caj	Czech Republic	*Camellia sinensis*
Caj	Hawaii	*Camellia sinensis*
Caj	Serbia	*Camellia sinensis*
Cana comun	Spain	*Saccharum officinarum*
Cana de assucar	Portugal	*Saccharum officinarum*
Cana de azucar	Canary Islands	*Saccharum officinarum*
Cana de azucar	Guatemala	*Saccharum officinarum*
Cana de azucar	Mexico	*Saccharum officinarum*
Cana de azucar	Spain	*Saccharum officinarum*
Cana dulce	Canary Islands	*Saccharum officinarum*
Cana dulce	Spain	*Saccharum officinarum*
Canaduz	Spain	*Saccharum officinarum*
Canamiel	Spain	*Saccharum officinarum*
Canamo indico	Spain	*Cannabis sativa*
Canapa indica	Italy	*Cannabis sativa*
Cane, sugar	India	*Saccharum officinarum*
Canhamo	Portugal	*Cannabis sativa*
Canna da zucchero	Italy	*Saccharum officinarum*
Canna mele	Italy	*Saccharum officinarum*
Canne de sucre	France	*Saccharum officinarum*
Cares	Nepal	*Cannabis sativa*
Caretysen	Cornwall	*Daucus carota*
Carot	Cambodia	*Daucus carota*
Carot	Vietnam	*Daucus carota*
Carota	Italy	*Daucus carota*
Carota salvatica	Italy	*Daucus carota*

Carota	Italy	*Daucus carota*
Carote	Italy	*Daucus carota*
Carotola	Germany	*Daucus carota*
Carotte sauvage	Mauritius	*Daucus carota*
Carotte	France	*Daucus carota*
Carradje	The Isle of Man (Manx)	*Daucus carota*
Carrot sauvage	Belgium	*Daucus carota*
Carrot sauvage	Canada	*Daucus carota*
Carrot sauvage	France	*Daucus carota*
Carrot sauvage	Tunisia	*Daucus carota*
Carrot	Guyana	*Daucus carota*
Carrot	United Kingdom	*Daucus carota*
Carrot	United States	*Daucus carota*
Cay gung	Vietnam	*Zingiber officinale*
Cay mia	Vietnam	*Saccharum officinarum*
Cay	Turkey	*Camellia sinensis*
Ceai	Romania	*Camellia sinensis*
Cebada	Spain	*Hordeum vulgare*
Cenoura brava	Portugal	*Daucus carota*
Cenoura selvagem	Brazil	*Daucus carota*
Cenoura	Portugal	*Daucus carota*
Cevada	Portugal	*Hordeum vulgare*
Cha	Brazil	*Camellia sinensis*
Cha	China	*Camellia sinensis*
Cha	Hawaii	*Camellia sinensis*
Cha	Pacific Islands	*Camellia sinensis*
Cha	Portugal	*Camellia sinensis*
Cha'ncat	Mexico	*Saccharum officinarum*
Chaam-kkae	Korea	*Sesamum indicum*
Chai	Bulgaria	*Camellia sinensis*
Chai	Georgia	*Coffea arabica*
Chai	Mozambique	*Camellia sinensis*
Chai	Russia	*Camellia sinensis*
Chai	Tanzania	*Camellia sinensis*
Chai	Ukraine	*Camellia sinensis*
Chai	Zaire	*Camellia sinensis*
Chaj	Macedonia	*Camellia sinensis*
Chanvre cultive	France	*Cannabis sativa*
Chanvre de l'Inde	France	*Cannabis sativa*
Chanvre	France	*Cannabis sativa*
Chanvrier sauvage	France	*Cannabis sativa*
Chaparral	England	*Larrea tridentata*
Chaparral	United States	*Larrea tridentata*
Chapepnomen ba	Ecuador	*Zingiber officinale*
Charas	India	*Cannabis sativa*
Chayna roslina	Ukraine	*Camellia sinensis*
Ch-chientzu	China	*Plantago ovata*
Chiang	China	*Zingiber officinale*
Chichambara	Nicaragua	*Zingiber officinale*
Chinesischer tea	Germany	*Camellia sinensis*
Chitta	Africa	*Zingiber officinale*
Chnay	Cambodia	*Zingiber officinale*

Chou palmiste	France	*Serenoa repens*
Churras	India	*Cannabis sativa*
Cno coco	England	*Cocos nucifera*
Cno coco	Ireland	*Cocos nucifera*
Cocco	Italy	*Cocos nucifera*
Coco da Bahia	Brazil	*Cocos nucifera*
Coco da India	Portugal	*Cocos nucifera*
Coco fruto	Spain	*Cocos nucifera*
Coco	Portugal	*Cocos nucifera*
Coco	Spain	*Cocos nucifera*
Coconut	Guyana	*Cocos nucifera*
Cocotera	Spain	*Cocos nucifera*
Cocotier	France	*Cocos nucifera*
Cocotier	Romania	*Cocos nucifera*
Coffee	Guyana	*Coffea arabica*
Coffee	United Kingdom	*Coffea arabica*
Coffee	United States	*Coffea arabica*
Com cay lua	Vietnam	*Oryza sativa*
Common plantain	Arabic countries	*Plantago ovata*
Coqueiro da Bahia	Brazil	*Cocos nucifera*
Coqueiro	Portugal	*Cocos nucifera*
Corifa del Malabar	Italy	*Serenoa repens*
Creosote bush	Guyana	*Larrea tridentata*
Creosote bush	England	*Larrea tridentata*
Creosote bush	United States	*Larrea tridentata*
Creosotum	United States	*Larrea tridentata*
Cro bainney	The Isle of Man	*Cocos nucifera*
Cukornad	Hungary	*Saccharum officinarum*
Cukrova trtina	Czech Republic	*Saccharum officinarum*
Culoare masline	Romania	*Olea europaea*
Cunuc yacu	Ecuador	*Camellia sinensis*
Curral	Scotland	*Daucus carota*
Curran	Scotland	*Daucus carota*
Cycam	Bulgaria	*Sesamum indicum*
Da ma cao	China	*Cannabis sativa*
Da ma ren	China	*Cannabis sativa*
Da ma	China	*Cannabis sativa*
Daab	India	*Cocos nucifera*
Dafu	Kenya	*Cocos nucifera*
Dafu	Mozambique	*Cocos nucifera*
Dafu	Tanzania	*Cocos nucifera*
Dafu	Zaire	*Cocos nucifera*
Dagga	South Africa	*Cannabis sativa*
Dansk pot	Denmark	*Cannabis sativa*
Dauco marino	Italy	*Daucus carota*
Daucus carotte	France	*Daucus carota*
Dee la	Thailand	*Sesamum indicum*
Dege e ullirit	Albania	*Olea europaea*
Dé-oo-wé	Colombia	*Nicotiana tabacum*
Devil's dung	United States	*Ferula assafoetida*
Djae	Indonesia	*Zingiber officinale*
Djahe	Netherlands	*Zingiber officinale*

Djoflatao	Iceland	*Ferula assafoetida*
Dohány	Hungary	*Nicotiana tabacum*
Driveldrikis	Latvia	*Ferula assafoetida*
Dua	Vietnam	*Cocos nucifera*
Duhan	Albania	*Nicotiana tabacum*
Duhan	Croatia	*Nicotiana tabacum*
Duivelsdrek	Netherlands	*Ferula assafoetida*
Dulce, cana	Canary Islands	*Saccharum officinarum*
Dumber	Croatia	*Zingiber officinale*
Dumbier lekarstvy	Slovakia	*Zingiber officinale*
Duvan	Serbia	*Nicotiana tabacum*
Duvn	Serbia	*Nicotiana tabacum*
Dwarf Evergreen Oak	United States	*Larrea tridentata*
Dybaco	Wales	*Nicotiana tabacum*
Dyvelsdrak	Denmark	*Ferula assafoetida*
Dyvelsdrekk	Norway	*Ferula assafoetida*
Dyvelstrack	Sweden	*Ferula assafoetida*
Dzhindzhifil	Bulgaria	*Zingiber officinale*
E´-li	Colombia	*Nicotiana tabacum*
Eaj	Czech Republic	*Camellia sinensis*
Eajovnik	Czech Republic	*Camellia sinensis*
Echemik	Bulgaria	*Hordeum vulgare*
Echter hanf	Germany	*Cannabis sativa*
Echter tabak	Germany	*Nicotiana tabacum*
Elb	Albania	*Hordeum vulgare*
Elia	Greece	*Olea europaea*
Ellu	India	*Sesamum indicum*
Engifer	Iceland	*Zingiber officinale*
Eorna	Scotland	*Hordeum vulgare*
Erus	Malaysia	*Oryza sativa*
Esrar	Turkey	*Cannabis sativa*
Euroopa olipuu	Estonia	*Olea europaea*
Eylbert	Israel	*Olea europaea*
Faco	Wales	*Nicotiana tabacum*
Ferule persique	France	*Ferula assafoetida*
Fyglys	Wales	*Nicotiana tabacum*
Ga feh	China	*Coffea arabica*
Gaajara	India	*Daucus carota*
Gaanjaa	Nepal	*Cannabis sativa*
Gafae	Thailand	*Coffea arabica*
Gahzar	India	*Daucus carota*
Gaiweruam	Germany	*Daucus carota*
Gajar	India	*Daucus carota*
Gajiimaa	Nepal	*Cannabis sativa*
Gajjarakkilangu	India	*Daucus carota*
Gajor	India	*Daucus carota*
Gamug	Tibet	*Zingiber officinale*
Gan jinang	China	*Zingiber officinale*
Gan zhe	China	*Saccharum officinarum*
Ganiesi	Nicaragua	*Saccharum officinarum*
Ganja	Guyana	*Cannabis sativa*
Ganja	India	*Cannabis sativa*

Ganna	Nepal	*Saccharum officinarum*
Ganna	Pakistan	*Saccharum officinarum*
Gannaa	India	*Saccharum officinarum*
Gannaa	Pakistan	*Saccharum officinarum*
Garase	South Africa	*Hordeum vulgare*
Gawz el Hindi	Arabic countries	*Cocos nucifera*
Gazar baladi	India	*Daucus carota*
Gazar	India	*Daucus carota*
Gazur	India	*Daucus carota*
Gelbe Rube	Germany	*Daucus carota*
Gele peen	Netherlands	*Daucus carota*
Gele Wortel	Netherlands	*Daucus carota*
Gember	Indonesia	*Zingiber officinale*
Gember	Netherlands	*Zingiber officinale*
Gendari	Pakistan	*Saccharum officinarum*
Gengibre	Brazil	*Zingiber officinale*
Gengibre	Portugal	*Zingiber officinale*
Gengibre	Spain	*Zingiber officinale*
Gengibre	Venezuela	*Zingiber officinale*
Gergelim	Brazil	*Sesamum indicum*
Gerst	Netherlands	*Hordeum vulgare*
Gerste	Germany	*Hordeum vulgare*
Gewone gerst	Netherlands	*Hordeum vulgare*
Ghah'veh	Iran	*Coffea arabica*
Ghimbir	Romania	*Zingiber officinale*
Gin	Myanmar	*Zingiber officinale*
Gingebre	Mauritius	*Zingiber officinale*
Gingebre	Spain	*Zingiber officinale*
Gingebre	Vietnam	*Zingiber officinale*
Gingelly	United Kingdom	*Sesamum indicum*
Gingembre	France	*Zingiber officinale*
Ginger	Brazil	*Zingiber officinale*
Ginger	China	*Zingiber officinale*
Ginger	Greece	*Zingiber officinale*
Ginger	Guyana	*Zingiber officinale*
Ginger	India	*Zingiber officinale*
Ginger	Jamaica	*Zingiber officinale*
Ginger	Japan	*Zingiber officinale*
Ginger	Nepal	*Zingiber officinale*
Ginger	Nicaragua	*Zingiber officinale*
Ginger	Philippines	*Zingiber officinale*
Ginger	Sri Lanka	*Zingiber officinale*
Ginger	Taiwan	*Zingiber officinale*
Ginger	Tanzania	*Zingiber officinale*
Ginger	United States	*Zingiber officinale*
Ginger	Venezuela	*Zingiber officinale*
Gobernadora	England	*Larrea tridentata*
Gobernadora	Spain	*Larrea tridentata*
Gobernadora	United States	*Larrea tridentata*
Godenvoedsel	Netherlands	*Ferula assafoetida*
Gojabghbegh	Armenia	*Zingiber officinale*
Goma	Japan	*Sesamum indicum*

Grand tabac	France	*Nicotiana tabacum*
Grease bush	United States	*Larrea tridentata*
Greasewood	United States	*Larrea tridentata*
Grifa	Spain	*Cannabis sativa*
Grote waaier palm	Netherlands	*Serenoa repens*
Guamis	Spain	*Larrea tridentata*
Gujjur	India	*Daucus carota*
Gujjur-jo-beej	India	*Daucus carota*
Gularot	Faeroe Islands	*Daucus carota*
Gulerod	Denmark	*Daucus carota*
Gullerodder	Denmark	*Daucus carota*
Gulrot	Norway	*Daucus carota*
Gung	Vietnam	*Zingiber officinale*
Guo zhe	China	*Saccharum officinarum*
Gyin sein	Myanmar	*Zingiber officinale*
Gyin	Myanmar	*Zingiber officinale*
Gyomber	Hungary	*Zingiber officinale*
Hab zargah	Arabic countries	*Plantago ovata*
Hachis	Spain	*Cannabis sativa*
Haidd	Wales	*Hordeum vulgare*
Hajupihka	Finland	*Ferula assafoetida*
Halia bara	Malaysia	*Zingiber officinale*
Halia	Malaysia	*Zingiber officinale*
Haliya merah	Malaysia	*Zingiber officinale*
Haliya	Indonesia	*Zingiber officinale*
Hamp	Denmark	*Cannabis sativa*
Hamp	Norway	*Cannabis sativa*
Hampa	Sweden	*Cannabis sativa*
Hampjurt	Iceland	*Cannabis sativa*
Hamppu	Finland	*Cannabis sativa*
Hanf	Germany	*Cannabis sativa*
Harilik ingver	Estonia	*Zingiber officinale*
Harilik kanep	Slovenia	*Cannabis sativa*
Harilik seesam	Estonia	*Sesamum indicum*
Harilik suhkruroog	Estonia	*Saccharum officinarum*
Haschischpflanze	Germany	*Cannabis sativa*
Hash	United Kingdom	*Cannabis sativa*
Hashas	Turkey	*Cannabis sativa*
Hashish	Morocco	*Cannabis sativa*
Have-gulerod	Denmark	*Daucus carota*
Havijk	Iran	*Daucus carota*
Havuc	Turkey	*Daucus carota*
Havupunkit	Finland	*Saccharum officinarum*
Hediondilla	Spain	*Larrea tridentata*
Hei chih ma	China	*Sesamum indicum*
Hemp	United Kingdom	*Cannabis sativa*
Hengu	India	*Ferula assafoetida*
Hennep	Netherlands	*Cannabis sativa*
Hentgagan engouz	Armenia	*Cocos nucifera*
Herbata	Poland	*Camellia sinensis*
Hind kinnabi	Turkey	*Cannabis sativa*
Hindistancevizi	Turkey	*Cocos nucifera*

Hing	Bangladesh	*Ferula assafoetida*
Hing	India	*Ferula assafoetida*
Hingu	India	*Ferula assafoetida*
Hli	Papua-New Guinea	*Zingiber officinale*
Hogesoppu	India	*Nicotiana tabacum*
Hong cai tou	China	*Daucus carota*
Hong da gen	China	*Daucus carota*
Hong gan zhe	China	*Saccharum officinarum*
Hong lu fai	China	*Daucus carota*
Hong luo bo	China	*Daucus carota*
Hu lu fai	China	*Daucus carota*
Hu luo bo	China	*Daucus carota*
Huang luo bo	China	*Daucus carota*
Hu-lo-po-tze	China	*Daucus carota*
Huo ma cao	China	*Cannabis sativa*
Huo ma	China	*Cannabis sativa*
I kokosit	Albania	*Cocos nucifera*
Icayi	Rwanda	*Camellia sinensis*
Iikh	India	*Saccharum officinarum*
Ikherothi	Africa	*Daucus carota*
Ikhhu	Pakistan	*Saccharum officinarum*
Ikhofi	Africa	*Coffea arabica*
Ikofu	South Africa	*Coffea arabica*
Ilayisi	Africa	*Oryza sativa*
Ilikherothi	Africa	*Daucus carota*
Ilitye	Africa	*Camellia sinensis*
Imberias	Lithuania	*Zingiber officinale*
Imbir	Poland	*Zingiber officinale*
Imbir	Russia	*Zingiber officinale*
Imbyr	Ukraine	*Zingiber officinale*
Inber	Israel	*Zingiber officinale*
Inbwer	Germany	*Zingiber officinale*
Inchi	India	*Zingiber officinale*
Indian hemp	United Kingdom	*Cannabis sativa*
Indische hennep	Netherlands	*Cannabis sativa*
Indischer hanf	Germany	*Cannabis sativa*
Indisk hamp	Sweden	*Cannabis sativa*
Ingee	India	*Zingiber officinale*
Ingefara	Sweden	*Zingiber officinale*
Ingefer	Denmark	*Zingiber officinale*
Ingefer	Norway	*Zingiber officinale*
Ingu	India	*Ferula assafoetida*
Inguru	Japan	*Zingiber officinale*
Inguru	Sri Lanka	*Zingiber officinale*
Inguva	India	*Ferula assafoetida*
Ingver	Croatia	*Zingiber officinale*
Ingver	Slovenia	*Zingiber officinale*
Ingverijuur	Estonia	*Zingiber officinale*
Ingwer	Germany	*Zingiber officinale*
Ingwer	Tanzania	*Zingiber officinale*
Inkivaari	Finland	*Zingiber officinale*
Isiot	Bulgaria	*Zingiber officinale*

Isphghol	India	*Plantago ovata*
Itiye	Africa	*Camellia sinensis*
Jae	Indonesia	*Zingiber officinale*
Jahe	Indonesia	*Zingiber officinale*
Jahi	Malaysia	*Zingiber officinale*
Jaitun	India	*Olea europaea*
Jamaica ginger	United States	*Zingiber officinale*
Jamveel	Iran	*Zingiber officinale*
Janzabeil	Sudan	*Zingiber officinale*
Jarilla	Spain	*Larrea tridentata*
Jazar barri	Iraq	*Daucus carota*
Jecam	Croatia	*Hordeum vulgare*
Jecam	Serbia	*Hordeum vulgare*
Jeczmien	Poland	*Hordeum vulgare*
Jeemen	Czech Republic	*Hordeum vulgare*
Jenegibre	Venezuela	*Zingiber officinale*
Jengibre	Cuba	*Zingiber officinale*
Jengibre	Spain	*Zingiber officinale*
Jenibre	Guatemala	*Zingiber officinale*
Jenjibre	Ecuador	*Zingiber officinale*
Jenjibre	Nicaragua	*Zingiber officinale*
Jeung	China	*Zingiber officinale*
Jiang	China	*Zingiber officinale*
Jinjaa	Japan	*Zingiber officinale*
Jitabdoogh	Armenia	*Olea europaea*
Jiteni	Armenia	*Olea europaea*
Ju zhong lu	China	*Serenoa repens*
Julipe	India	*Olea europaea*
Ka'fe	Israel	*Coffea arabica*
Kaafi	India	*Coffea arabica*
Kaapi	Central America	*Coffea arabica*
Kaapi	Mexico	*Coffea arabica*
Kaapiopalmu	Finland	*Serenoa repens*
Kaareti	New Zealand	*Daucus carota*
Kaawa	Uganda	*Coffea arabica*
Kafa	Serbia	*Coffea arabica*
Kafa	Turkey	*Cocos nucifera*
Kafe	Albania	*Coffea arabica*
Kafe	Bulgaria	*Coffea arabica*
Kafe	Czech Republic	*Coffea arabica*
Kafe	Gambia	*Coffea arabica*
Kafe	Greece	*Coffea arabica*
Kafe	Latin America	*Coffea arabica*
Kafe	Senegal	*Coffea arabica*
Ka-fei	China	*Coffea arabica*
Kaffe	Denmark	*Coffea arabica*
Kaffe	Norway	*Coffea arabica*
Kaffe	Sweden	*Coffea arabica*
Kaffee	Germany	*Coffea arabica*
Kaffeeplante	Norway	*Coffea arabica*
Kaffeestrauch	Germany	*Coffea arabica*
Kaffi	Iceland	*Coffea arabica*

Kafija	Latvia	*Coffea arabica*
Kahawa	Africa	*Coffea arabica*
Kahioa	Arabic countries	*Coffea arabica*
Kahva	Bosnia	*Coffea arabica*
Kahve	Turkey	*Coffea arabica*
Kahvi	Finland	*Coffea arabica*
Kai	China	*Zingiber officinale*
Kallamu	India	*Zingiber officinale*
Kama I anguza	Afghanistan	*Ferula assafoetida*
Kama I anguza	Pakistan	*Ferula assafoetida*
Kan chiang	Vietnam	*Zingiber officinale*
Kaneh	Israel	*Saccharum officinarum*
Kanga	Papua-New Guinea	*Zingiber officinale*
Kannabis	Finland	*Cannabis sativa*
Kannabisu	Japan	*Cannabis sativa*
Kansha	Japan	*Saccharum officinarum*
Kanvoc	Greece	*Nicotiana tabacum*
Kape	Philippines	*Coffea arabica*
Kapva	Greece	*Nicotiana tabacum*
Karga	India	*Oryza sativa*
Karida	Greece	*Cocos nucifera*
Karlikova palma	Ukraine	*Serenoa repens*
Karlikovaya palma	Russia	*Serenoa repens*
Karot	Australia	*Daucus carota*
Karot	Cambodia	*Daucus carota*
Karot	Netherlands Antilles	*Daucus carota*
Karot	Philippines	*Daucus carota*
Karote	Albania	*Daucus carota*
Karote	Hawaii	*Daucus carota*
Karoti	Samoa	*Daucus carota*
Karoto	Greece	*Daucus carota*
Karotte	Germany	*Daucus carota*
Karotten	Germany	*Daucus carota*
Karotter	Denmark	*Daucus carota*
Karuthellu	India	*Sesamum indicum*
Karuvathu kelengu	India	*Daucus carota*
Karyda	Greece	*Cocos nucifera*
Kava	Croatia	*Coffea arabica*
Kava	Czech Republic	*Coffea arabica*
Kava	Lithuania	*Coffea arabica*
Kava	Slovakia	*Coffea arabica*
Kava	Slovenia	*Coffea arabica*
Kava	Ukraine	*Coffea arabica*
Kave	Hungary	*Coffea arabica*
Kave	Israel	*Coffea arabica*
Kawa	Poland	*Coffea arabica*
Kayam	India	*Ferula assafoetida*
Kdyuir	Turkmenistan	*Daucus carota*
Ke ke ye zi	Taiwan	*Cocos nucifera*
Kelapa	Indonesia	*Cocos nucifera*
Kelapa	Malaysia	*Cocos nucifera*
Keong	China	*Zingiber officinale*

Kerati	Papua-New Guinea	*Zingiber officinale*
Kerp	Albania	*Cannabis sativa*
Khaerot	Thailand	*Daucus carota*
Khand	Pakistan	*Saccharum officinarum*
Khasa	India	*Sesamum indicum*
Kherm´-ba	Ecuador	*Nicotiana tabacum*
Khing	Laos	*Zingiber officinale*
Khing	Thailand	*Zingiber officinale*
Khing-daen	Thailand	*Zingiber officinale*
Khnehey	Cambodia	*Zingiber officinale*
Khnhei phlung	Cambodia	*Zingiber officinale*
Khokhonate	South Africa	*Cocos nucifera*
Khuong	Vietnam	*Zingiber officinale*
Khyen-seing	Myanmar	*Zingiber officinale*
Kinkh	Thailand	*Zingiber officinale*
Kinnab	Turkey	*Cannabis sativa*
Kintoki	Japan	*Zingiber officinale*
Kion	Peru	*Zingiber officinale*
Kis legyezopalma	Hungary	*Serenoa repens*
Kkae	Korea	*Sesamum indicum*
Klao	Thailand	*Oryza sativa*
Klapper	Netherlands	*Cocos nucifera*
Klapperboom	Netherlands	*Cocos nucifera*
Ko	Hawaii	*Saccharum officinarum*
Koarn	Netherlands	*Hordeum vulgare*
Koba	Japan	*Sesamum indicum*
Kobari	India	*Cocos nucifera*
Kobbai	India	*Cocos nucifera*
Kobbai	Sri Lanka	*Cocos nucifera*
Kobbera	India	*Cocos nucifera*
Kobbera	Sri Lanka	*Cocos nucifera*
Kofe	Russia	*Coffea arabica*
Koffee	India	*Coffea arabica*
Koffi	United Kingdom	*Coffea arabica*
Koffie	Netherlands	*Coffea arabica*
Koffie	South Africa	*Coffea arabica*
Koffieboom	Netherlands	*Coffea arabica*
Kofi	Botswana	*Coffea arabica*
Kofi	South Africa	*Coffea arabica*
Kofii	India	*Coffea arabica*
Kofje	Netherlands	*Coffea arabica*
Kohv	Estonia	*Coffea arabica*
Kok mak phao	Laos	*Cocos nucifera*
Kokas	Ethiopia	*Cocos nucifera*
Kokkofoinika	Greece	*Cocos nucifera*
Koko yashi	Japan	*Cocos nucifera*
Koko	Spain	*Cocos nucifera*
Kokonet	Ethiopia	*Cocos nucifera*
Kokos orekonosnyi	Russia	*Cocos nucifera*
Kokos	Bulgaria	*Cocos nucifera*
Kokos	Croatia	*Cocos nucifera*
Kokos	Czech Republic	*Cocos nucifera*

Kokos	Germany	*Cocos nucifera*
Kokos	Netherlands	*Cocos nucifera*
Kokos	Russia	*Cocos nucifera*
Kokos	Sweden	*Cocos nucifera*
Kokos	Ukraine	*Cocos nucifera*
Kokosa	Slovenia	*Cocos nucifera*
Kokoshneta	Iceland	*Cocos nucifera*
Kokosnoed	Denmark	*Cocos nucifera*
Kokosnoot	Netherlands	*Cocos nucifera*
Kokosnot	Sweden	*Cocos nucifera*
Kokosnus	Israel	*Cocos nucifera*
Kokosnuss	Germany	*Cocos nucifera*
Kokosnut	Netherlands	*Cocos nucifera*
Kokosnut	Spain	*Cocos nucifera*
Kokosov orah	Croatia	*Cocos nucifera*
Kokosov orah	Serbia	*Cocos nucifera*
Kokosov orech	Bulgaria	*Cocos nucifera*
Kokosov	Bulgaria	*Cocos nucifera*
Kokosova palma	Slovenia	*Cocos nucifera*
Kokosovaia pal'ma	Russia	*Cocos nucifera*
Kokosovy orech	Czech Republic	*Cocos nucifera*
Kokosovy orech	Slovakia	*Cocos nucifera*
Kokosovyj orech	Ukraine	*Cocos nucifera*
Kokosovyj orjekh	Russia	*Cocos nucifera*
Kokospalm	Netherlands	*Cocos nucifera*
Kokospalm	Sweden	*Cocos nucifera*
Kokospalme	Denmark	*Cocos nucifera*
Kokospalme	Germany	*Cocos nucifera*
Kokronoto	Suriname	*Cocos nucifera*
Kokus	Israel	*Cocos nucifera*
Kokusnod	Faeroe Islands	*Cocos nucifera*
Kokuszdio	Hungary	*Cocos nucifera*
Konga	Papua-New Guinea	*Zingiber officinale*
Konjed	Iran	*Sesamum indicum*
Konopie siewne	Poland	*Cannabis sativa*
Konopie	Poland	*Cannabis sativa*
Konoplja	Slovenia	*Cannabis sativa*
Koohii	Japan	*Coffea arabica*
Kookospahkina	Finland	*Cocos nucifera*
Kookospalm	Estonia	*Cocos nucifera*
Kookospalmu	Finland	*Cocos nucifera*
Kope	Hawaii	*Coffea arabica*
Kopi	Indonesia	*Coffea arabica*
Kopi	Malaysia	*Coffea arabica*
Ko-pi	Sri Lanka	*Coffea arabica*
Ko-pyi	Korea	*Coffea arabica*
Korn	Sweden	*Hordeum vulgare*
Kreosotestrauch	Germany	*Larrea tridentata*
Kronto	Suriname	*Cocos nucifera*
Kultur hanf	Germany	*Cannabis sativa*
Kunyit terus	Malaysia	*Zingiber officinale*
Kunzhut	Russia	*Sesamum indicum*

Kunzuut	Estonia	*Sesamum indicum*
Kushiar	Pakistan	*Saccharum officinarum*
Lag	Guyana	*Cocos nucifera*
Lahja	Indonesia	*Zingiber officinale*
Lao jiang	China	*Zingiber officinale*
Lee-cah fee	United States	*Coffea arabica*
Lei	Admiralty Islands	*Zingiber officinale*
Lia	Indonesia	*Zingiber officinale*
Linga	Philippines	*Sesamum indicum*
Lisn al kalb	Arabic countries	*Plantago ovata*
Lobak merah	Malaysia	*Daucus carota*
Loso	Congo	*Oryza sativa*
Luama	Vietnam	*Oryza sativa*
Lukux-ri	Colombia	*Nicotiana tabacum*
Luya	Philippines	*Zingiber officinale*
Ma ha hing	Laos	*Ferula assafoetida*
Ma phra on	Thailand	*Cocos nucifera*
Maak muu	Thailand	*Cocos nucifera*
Mach'ca	Ecuador	*Hordeum vulgare*
Maco	Wales	*Nicotiana tabacum*
Maconha	Portugal	*Cannabis sativa*
Mahora	Romania	*Nicotiana tabacum*
Mak un on	Myanmar	*Cocos nucifera*
Man nga	Laos	*Sesamum indicum*
Maphrao	Thailand	*Cocos nucifera*
Mar	India	*Cocos nucifera*
Marchew	Poland	*Daucus carota*
Marihana	Netherlands	*Cannabis sativa*
Marihouava	Greece	*Cannabis sativa*
Marihuana	Bulgaria	*Cannabis sativa*
Marihuana	Croatia	*Cannabis sativa*
Marihuana	Czech Republic	*Cannabis sativa*
Marihuana	Denmark	*Cannabis sativa*
Marihuana	France	*Cannabis sativa*
Marihuana	Germany	*Cannabis sativa*
Marihuana	Hungary	*Cannabis sativa*
Marihuana	Mexico	*Cannabis sativa*
Marihuana	Poland	*Cannabis sativa*
Marihuana	Russia	*Cannabis sativa*
Marihuana	Serbia	*Cannabis sativa*
Marihuana	Spain	*Cannabis sativa*
Marihuana	Ukraine	*Cannabis sativa*
Marihuana	United States	*Cannabis sativa*
Marijuana	France	*Cannabis sativa*
Marijuana	Italy	*Cannabis sativa*
Marijuana	Mexico	*Cannabis sativa*
Marijuana	Portugal	*Cannabis sativa*
Marijuana	Sweden	*Cannabis sativa*
Mashinin	Japan	*Cannabis sativa*
Maslin	Romania	*Olea europaea*
Maslina	Bulgaria	*Olea europaea*
Maslina	Croatia	*Olea europaea*

Maslina	Serbia	*Olea europaea*
Maslina	Ukraine	*Olea europaea*
Masline	Israel	*Olea europaea*
Masliniu	Romania	*Olea europaea*
Maslinov	Croatia	*Olea europaea*
Maslinov	Serbia	*Olea europaea*
Mchele	Mozambique	*Oryza sativa*
Mchele	Tanzania	*Oryza sativa*
Mchele	Zaire	*Oryza sativa*
Meacan dearg	Ireland	*Daucus carota*
Mehrzeilige Gerste	Germany	*Hordeum vulgare*
Merde du diable	France	*Ferula assafoetida*
Mia	Vietnam	*Saccharum officinarum*
Mitmerealine oder	Estonia	*Hordeum vulgare*
Mittho-tel	India	*Sesamum indicum*
Mnazi	Mozambique	*Cocos nucifera*
Mnazi	Southeastern Africa	*Cocos nucifera*
Mnazi	Tanzania	*Cocos nucifera*
Mnazi	Zaire	*Cocos nucifera*
Moa	China	*Sesamum indicum*
Moba	Tanzania	*Saccharum officinarum*
Mohlware	South Africa	*Olea europaea*
Mohre	Germany	*Daucus carota*
Mohrrube	Germany	*Daucus carota*
Monitahoohra	Finland	*Hordeum vulgare*
Morkov	Bulgaria	*Daucus carota*
Morkov	Macedonia	*Daucus carota*
Morkov	Romania	*Daucus carota*
Morkov	Russia	*Daucus carota*
Morkva	Ukraine	*Daucus carota*
Moronen	Wales	*Daucus carota*
Morot	Sweden	*Daucus carota*
Mpunga	Africa	*Oryza sativa*
Mrkva	Yugoslavia	*Daucus carota*
Mtangwizi	Tanzania	*Zingiber officinale*
Mua chi	China	*Sesamum indicum*
Mu-lu´	Colombia	*Nicotiana tabacum*
Mupunga	Botswana	*Oryza sativa*
Mupunga	Zambia	*Oryza sativa*
Mupunga	Zimbabwe	*Oryza sativa*
Mvuje	Mozambique	*Ferula assafoetida*
Mvuje	Tanzania	*Ferula assafoetida*
Mvuje	Zaire	*Ferula assafoetida*
Myglys	Wales	*Nicotiana tabacum*
Myoga	Japan	*Zingiber officinale*
Naarakel	India	*Cocos nucifera*
Naariyal kaa per	India	*Cocos nucifera*
Naariyal kaa per	Pakistan	*Cocos nucifera*
Naariyal	India	*Cocos nucifera*
Naariyal	Pakistan	*Cocos nucifera*
Nadiya	India	*Cocos nucifera*
Nagara	India	*Zingiber officinale*

Naishekar	Iran	*Saccharum officinarum*
Nalikeran	Malaysia	*Cocos nucifera*
Nanivaara	India	*Cocos nucifera*
Naral	India	*Cocos nucifera*
Nargil	Arabic countries	*Cocos nucifera*
Nargil	Iran	*Cocos nucifera*
Narial	India	*Cocos nucifera*
Narikela	India	*Cocos nucifera*
Narikol	India	*Cocos nucifera*
Narival	Nepal	*Cocos nucifera*
Nariyal	India	*Cocos nucifera*
Narkel	India	*Cocos nucifera*
Nasi	Indonesia	*Oryza sativa*
Natsume yashi	Japan	*Cocos nucifera*
Navadna konoplja	Slovenia	*Cannabis sativa*
Navadni tobak	Slovenia	*Nicotiana tabacum*
Nazi	Mozambique	*Cocos nucifera*
Nazi	Tanzania	*Cocos nucifera*
Nazi	Zaire	*Cocos nucifera*
Nga	Laos	*Sesamum indicum*
Ngaa	Thailand	*Sesamum indicum*
Ngesnges	Papua-New Guinea	*Zingiber officinale*
Ngjyre ulliri	Albania	*Olea europaea*
Nhybaco	Wales	*Nicotiana tabacum*
Nicotiane	France	*Nicotiana tabacum*
Niistsikapa's	United States	*Daucus carota*
Niska palma	Bulgaria	*Serenoa repens*
Niyog	Philippines	*Cocos nucifera*
Niyok	Hawaii	*Cocos nucifera*
Niyok	Pacific Islands	*Cocos nucifera*
Nkrabo	Africa	*Zingiber officinale*
Nkrama	Africa	*Zingiber officinale*
Nkrawusa	Africa	*Zingiber officinale*
No	China	*Oryza sativa*
Noble cane	United States	*Saccharum officinarum*
Noce di cocco	Italy	*Cocos nucifera*
Noix de coco	France	*Cocos nucifera*
Nora-ninjij	Japan	*Daucus carota*
Noz de coco	Portugal	*Cocos nucifera*
Nuca de cocos	Romania	*Cocos nucifera*
Nuez de coco	Spain	*Cocos nucifera*
Nuvvulu	India	*Sesamum indicum*
Nyior	Malaysia	*Cocos nucifera*
Oarn	The Isle of Man (Manx)	*Hordeum vulgare*
Oastre	Spain	*Olea europaea*
Obeko	Japan	*Plantago ovata*
Ohra	Finland	*Hordeum vulgare*
Oi daeng	Thailand	*Saccharum officinarum*
Oi	Thailand	*Saccharum officinarum*
Olajbogyo	Hungary	*Olea europaea*
Olajfa	Hungary	*Olea europaea*
Olbaum	Germany	*Olea europaea*

Oleifi	Netherlands Antilles	*Olea europaea*
Olewydden	England	*Olea europaea*
Oliba	Spain	*Olea europaea*
Olifa	Iceland	*Olea europaea*
Oliif	Spain	*Olea europaea*
Oliivi	Finland	*Olea europaea*
Olijf	Netherlands	*Olea europaea*
Oliondo	Spain	*Olea europaea*
Olipuus	Estonia	*Olea europaea*
Oliv	Sweden	*Olea europaea*
Oliva europska	Slovakia	*Olea europaea*
Oliva	Czech Republic	*Olea europaea*
Oliva	Ethiopia	*Olea europaea*
Oliva	Hungary	*Olea europaea*
Oliva	Italy	*Olea europaea*
Oliva	Portugal	*Olea europaea*
Oliva	Romania	*Olea europaea*
Oliva	Russia	*Olea europaea*
Oliva	Spain	*Olea europaea*
Oliva	Ukraine	*Olea europaea*
Olivas	Latvia	*Olea europaea*
Olive	England	*Olea europaea*
Olive	France	*Olea europaea*
Olive	Germany	*Olea europaea*
Olive	Guyana	*Olea europaea*
Olive	The Isle of Man (Manx)	*Olea europaea*
Olive	United States	*Olea europaea*
Oliveira	Portugal	*Olea europaea*
Oliven	Denmark	*Olea europaea*
Oliven	Norway	*Olea europaea*
Olivenbaum	Germany	*Olea europaea*
Olivera	Spain	*Olea europaea*
Olivgront	Sweden	*Olea europaea*
Olivo	Spain	*Olea europaea*
Olivove drevo	Czech Republic	*Olea europaea*
Olivovnik europsky	Slovakia	*Olea europaea*
Olivovnik	Czech Republic	*Olea europaea*
Olivy	Czech Republic	*Olea europaea*
Oliwka	Poland	*Olea europaea*
Oljka	Slovenia	*Olea europaea*
Oljypuu	Finland	*Olea europaea*
Olyf	Cornwall	*Olea europaea*
Olyva	Ukraine	*Olea europaea*
Ordoggyoker	Hungary	*Ferula assafoetida*
Orez	Romania	*Oryza sativa*
Orge	France	*Hordeum vulgare*
Oriz	Albania	*Oryza sativa*
Oriz	Bulgaria	*Oryza sativa*
Oriz	Macedonia	*Oryza sativa*
Orizen	Bulgaria	*Oryza sativa*
Orizov	Bulgaria	*Oryza sativa*
Orz	Romania	*Hordeum vulgare*

Orzo	Italy	*Hordeum vulgare*
Oshoga	Japan	*Zingiber officinale*
Oti	United States	*Camellia sinensis*
Oulivie	France	*Olea europaea*
Padi ketek	Indonesia	*Oryza sativa*
Pagári-mulé	Colombia	*Nicotiana tabacum*
Pahari gajar	India	*Daucus carota*
Palana	Papua-New Guinea	*Zingiber officinale*
Palma de coco	Spain	*Cocos nucifera*
Palma del cocco	Italy	*Cocos nucifera*
Palma enana Americana	Spain	*Serenoa repens*
Palma kokosowa	Poland	*Cocos nucifera*
Palma nana	Italy	*Serenoa repens*
Palma sabal	Spain	*Serenoa repens*
Palmeen	The Isle of Man (Manx)	*Serenoa repens*
Palmera de coco	Spain	*Cocos nucifera*
Palmet	Netherlands	*Serenoa repens*
Palmetta Della Florida	Italy	*Serenoa repens*
Palmetto de la sierra	Spain	*Serenoa repens*
Palmetto fan palm	United States	*Serenoa repens*
Palmetto, dark	United States	*Serenoa repens*
Palmier nain	France	*Serenoa repens*
Palmier pitic	Romania	*Serenoa repens*
Palmito	Portugal	*Serenoa repens*
Palmito	Spain	*Serenoa repens*
Paloondo	Spain	*Larrea tridentata*
Paparean	Indonesia	*Oryza sativa*
Pastanaga	Spain	*Daucus carota*
Pastenade	France	*Daucus carota*
Pastenaga	France	*Daucus carota*
Pastinaca selvatica	Italy	*Daucus carota*
Peen	Netherlands	*Daucus carota*
Perungayam	India	*Ferula assafoetida*
Perunkaya	India	*Ferula assafoetida*
Perunkayan	Sri Lanka	*Ferula assafoetida*
Petun	Brazil	*Nicotiana tabacum*
Phakchi-daeng	Thailand	*Daucus carota*
Pia di udi	Ecuador	*Zingiber officinale*
Pia nuni	Ecuador	*Zingiber officinale*
Piperoriza	Greece	*Zingiber officinale*
Pirinac	Croatia	*Oryza sativa*
Pirinac	Serbia	*Oryza sativa*
Pirinac	Turkey	*Oryza sativa*
Pirinac	Yugoslavia	*Oryza sativa*
Pirinc	Turkey	*Oryza sativa*
Pirunpaska	Finland	*Ferula assafoetida*
Pirunpihka	Finland	*Ferula assafoetida*
Pitta gajur	India	*Daucus carota*
Pogaku	India	*Nicotiana tabacum*
Pokala	India	*Nicotiana tabacum*
Polgaha	Sri Lanka	*Cocos nucifera*
Porkanchaa	Thailand	*Cannabis sativa*

Porkkana	Finland	*Daucus carota*
Pot	Denmark	*Cannabis sativa*
Psillo indiano	Germany	*Plantago ovata*
Pugaiyilai	India	*Nicotiana tabacum*
Pugas	Hawaii	*Oryza sativa*
Pugas	Pacific Islands	*Oryza sativa*
Qahve	Azerbaijan	*Coffea arabica*
Qahve	Yemen	*Coffea arabica*
Qahwah	Arabic countries	*Coffea arabica*
Qasab al sukkar	Arabic countries	*Saccharum officinarum*
Qasab es sukkar	Arabic countries	*Saccharum officinarum*
Qinnib	Arabic countries	*Cannabis sativa*
Qolli	Boliwia	*Olea europaea*
Qolli	Peru	*Olea europaea*
Qoqus	Israel	*Cocos nucifera*
Queen Anne's lace	Canada	*Daucus carota*
Quing jiang	China	*Zingiber officinale*
Qurayta	Arabic countries	*Plantago ovata*
Raamathan	India	*Ferula assafoetida*
Rabell	Spain	*Olea europaea*
Raihi	New Zealand	*Oryza sativa*
Rasi	India	*Sesamum indicum*
Rebla	Arabic countries	*Plantago ovata*
Rechina fena	Iran	*Ferula assafoetida*
Reesa	India	*Oryza sativa*
Reis	England	*Oryza sativa*
Reis	Germany	*Oryza sativa*
Reise	The Isle of Man (Manx)	*Oryza sativa*
Reisi	South Africa	*Oryza sativa*
Rhizoma, zingiberis	Japan	*Zingiber officinale*
Rice	Guyana	*Oryza sativa*
Rice	India	*Oryza sativa*
Rice	United Kingdom	*Oryza sativa*
Rice	United States	*Oryza sativa*
Riesen hanf	Germany	*Cannabis sativa*
Riisi	Finland	*Oryza sativa*
Rijst	Netherlands	*Oryza sativa*
Ris	Denmark	*Oryza sativa*
Ris	Faroe Islands	*Oryza sativa*
Ris	France	*Oryza sativa*
Ris	Norway	*Oryza sativa*
Ris	Russia	*Oryza sativa*
Ris	Sweden	*Oryza sativa*
Ris	Switzerland	*Oryza sativa*
Ris	Ukraine	*Oryza sativa*
Risch melna	Switzerland	*Daucus carota*
Risgryn	Sweden	*Oryza sativa*
Riso	Italy	*Oryza sativa*
Riz	France	*Oryza sativa*
Riz	Rwanda	*Oryza sativa*
Rizs	Hungary	*Oryza sativa*
Ruokaporkana	Finland	*Daucus carota*

Ruzi	Greece	*Oryza sativa*
Rys	Netherlands	*Oryza sativa*
Rys	South Africa	*Oryza sativa*
Ryz	Poland	*Oryza sativa*
Ryze	Czech Republic	*Oryza sativa*
Saat-Gerste	Germany	*Hordeum vulgare*
Sabal du Mexique	France	*Serenoa repens*
Sabal du Texas	France	*Serenoa repens*
Sabal	United States	*Serenoa repens*
Saccar	Nepal	*Saccharum officinarum*
Saeng gang	Korea	*Zingiber officinale*
Sagapeen	Netherlands	*Ferula assafoetida*
Sagepalme	Germany	*Serenoa repens*
Sagepalmefruchte	Germany	*Serenoa repens*
Sagpalmetto	Sweden	*Serenoa repens*
Sahacar	Nepal	*Saccharum officinarum*
Sahachar	Nepal	*Saccharum officinarum*
Saidun	India	*Olea europaea*
Saidun	Sri Lanka	*Olea europaea*
Sakhara	India	*Saccharum officinarum*
Sakharnyi trostnik kul'turnyi	Russia	*Saccharum officinarum*
Sakharnyi trostnik lekarstvennyi	Russia	*Saccharum officinarum*
Salebyeo	Korea	*Oryza sativa*
San geung	China	*Zingiber officinale*
Sang keong	China	*Zingiber officinale*
Sargarepa	Croatia	*Daucus carota*
Sargarepa	Hungary	*Daucus carota*
Sargarepa	Serbia	*Daucus carota*
Sasim	Arabic countries	*Sesamum indicum*
Satou kibi	Japan	*Saccharum officinarum*
Saw palmetto	Guyana	*Serenoa repens*
Saw palmetto	United Kingdom	*Serenoa repens*
Saw palmetto	United States	*Serenoa repens*
Sechszeilige Gerste	Germany	*Hordeum vulgare*
Seesami	Finland	*Sesamum indicum*
Segwere	South Africa	*Daucus carota*
Semsem	United Kingdom	*Sesamum indicum*
Serenoa palmu	Finland	*Serenoa repens*
Seruma erva	Portugal	*Cannabis sativa*
Sesam	Denmark	*Sesamum indicum*
Sesam	Germany	*Sesamum indicum*
Sesam	Spain	*Sesamum indicum*
Sesam	Sweden	*Sesamum indicum*
Sesame	France	*Sesamum indicum*
Sesame	United Kingdom	*Sesamum indicum*
Sesame	United States	*Sesamum indicum*
Sesamfre	Iceland	*Sesamum indicum*
Sesami	Greece	*Sesamum indicum*
Sesamkruid	Netherlands	*Sesamum indicum*
Sesamo	Italy	*Sesamum indicum*
Sesamo	Portugal	*Sesamum indicum*
Sesamo	Spain	*Sesamum indicum*

Sesamzaad	Netherlands	*Sesamum indicum*
Setan bokosu	Turkey	*Ferula assafoetida*
Seytan tersi	Turkey	*Ferula assafoetida*
Sezam indicky	Slovakia	*Sesamum indicum*
Sezam	Croatia	*Sesamum indicum*
Sezam	Czech Republic	*Sesamum indicum*
Sezam	Poland	*Sesamum indicum*
Sezam	Russia	*Sesamum indicum*
Sezam	Ukraine	*Sesamum indicum*
Sezama seklas	Latvia	*Sesamum indicum*
Sezama	Slovenia	*Sesamum indicum*
Sezamas	Lithuania	*Sesamum indicum*
Sezamo	Spain	*Sesamum indicum*
Sga smug	Tibet	*Zingiber officinale*
Shecerna trska	Croatia	*Saccharum officinarum*
Shecerna trska	Serbia	*Saccharum officinarum*
Sheingho	Myanmar	*Ferula assafoetida*
Shen jiang	China	*Zingiber officinale*
Shengijang	China	*Zingiber officinale*
Shing-kun	Tibet	*Ferula assafoetida*
Shohkyoh	Japan	*Zingiber officinale*
Shokyo	Japan	*Zingiber officinale*
Shokyo	Taiwan	*Zingiber officinale*
Shooshma	Armenia	*Sesamum indicum*
Shooshmayi good	Armenia	*Sesamum indicum*
Shouga	Japan	*Zingiber officinale*
Shoukyo	Japan	*Zingiber officinale*
Shoukyo	Taiwan	*Zingiber officinale*
Shringaveran	India	*Zingiber officinale*
Shukku	India	*Zingiber officinale*
Shumshum	Israel	*Sesamum indicum*
Shuntya	India	*Zingiber officinale*
Sibada	Hawaii	*Hordeum vulgare*
Sibada	Pacific Islands	*Hordeum vulgare*
Sim-sim	Arabic countries	*Sesamum indicum*
Sim-sim	Netherlands	*Sesamum indicum*
Sinh khuong	Vietnam	*Zingiber officinale*
Sinziminli	Africa	*Zingiber officinale*
Skenjabil	Morocco	*Zingiber officinale*
Skenjbir	Morocco	*Zingiber officinale*
Sladkornitrs	Slovenia	*Saccharum officinarum*
Sman-sga	Tibet	*Zingiber officinale*
Sockerror	Sweden	*Saccharum officinarum*
Sokeriruoko	Finland	*Saccharum officinarum*
Solfjaderspalm	Sweden	*Serenoa repens*
Sonth	India	*Zingiber officinale*
Sourdj	Armenia	*Coffea arabica*
Spangur	India	*Plantago ovata*
Speisemohre	Germany	*Daucus carota*
Speisemohren	Germany	*Daucus carota*
Spisegulerod	Denmark	*Daucus carota*
Spogel	Iran	*Plantago ovata*

Sragne	Cambodia	*Oryza sativa*
Sringaaran	India	*Zingiber officinale*
Stinkasant	Germany	*Ferula assafoetida*
Stinking gum	United States	*Ferula assafoetida*
Sugar cane	Barbados	*Saccharum officinarum*
Sugar cane	Guyana	*Saccharum officinarum*
Sugar cane	India	*Saccharum officinarum*
Sugar cane	Indonesia	*Saccharum officinarum*
Sugar cane	Iran	*Saccharum officinarum*
Sugar cane	Jamaica	*Saccharum officinarum*
Sugar cane	Tanzania	*Saccharum officinarum*
Sugar cane	Trinidad	*Saccharum officinarum*
Sugarcane	Hawaii	*Saccharum officinarum*
Sugarcane, blue ribbon	United States	*Saccharum officinarum*
Suikerriet	Netherlands	*Saccharum officinarum*
Sukkerroer	Denmark	*Saccharum officinarum*
Sukkerror	Norway	*Saccharum officinarum*
Sunth	India	*Zingiber officinale*
Sunthi	India	*Zingiber officinale*
Suom	Finland	*Sesamum indicum*
Susam	Albania	*Sesamum indicum*
Susam	Bulgaria	*Sesamum indicum*
Susam	Turkey	*Sesamum indicum*
Susan	Romania	*Sesamum indicum*
Sutho	Nepal	*Zingiber officinale*
Sven	Sweden	*Sesamum indicum*
Szezam	Hungary	*Sesamum indicum*
Szezammag	Hungary	*Sesamum indicum*
Szezammag	Israel	*Sesamum indicum*
T'ha'ari	Tahiti	*Cocos nucifera*
Taa	Germany	*Camellia sinensis*
Tabac	France	*Nicotiana tabacum*
Tabac	Spain	*Nicotiana tabacum*
Tabacco Virginia	Italy	*Nicotiana tabacum*
Tabacni izdelki	Slovenia	*Nicotiana tabacum*
Tabaco	Brazil	*Nicotiana tabacum*
Tabaco	Mexico	*Nicotiana tabacum*
Tabaco	Portugal	*Nicotiana tabacum*
Tabaco	Spain	*Nicotiana tabacum*
Tabaco	Venezuela	*Nicotiana tabacum*
Tabák	Czech Republic	*Nicotiana tabacum*
Tabak	Germany	*Nicotiana tabacum*
Tabak	Netherlands	*Nicotiana tabacum*
Tabak	South Africa	*Nicotiana tabacum*
Tabak	Russia	*Nicotiana tabacum*
Tabaka	Suriname	*Nicotiana tabacum*
Tabako	France	*Nicotiana tabacum*
Tabako	Netherlands Antilles	*Nicotiana tabacum*
Tabako	Philippines	*Nicotiana tabacum*
Tabako	Spain	*Nicotiana tabacum*
Tabaku	Netherlands Antilles	*Nicotiana tabacum*
Tabat	France	*Nicotiana tabacum*

Tae	Ireland	*Camellia sinensis*
Taima	Japan	*Cannabis sativa*
Tal	India	*Sesamum indicum*
Tamaku	India	*Nicotiana tabacum*
Tambaku	India	*Nicotiana tabacum*
Tamrakatu	India	*Nicotiana tabacum*
Tangauzi	Tanzania	*Zingiber officinale*
Tangawizi	Tanzania	*Zingiber officinale*
Tao	China	*Oryza sativa*
Te	Scotland	*Camellia sinensis*
Te	Denmark	*Camellia sinensis*
Te	Faeroe Islands	*Camellia sinensis*
Te	France	*Camellia sinensis*
Te	Italy	*Camellia sinensis*
Te	Norway	*Camellia sinensis*
Te	Spain	*Camellia sinensis*
Te	Suriname	*Camellia sinensis*
Te	Switzerland	*Camellia sinensis*
Te	Wales	*Camellia sinensis*
Tea plant	England	*Camellia sinensis*
Tea	Australia	*Camellia sinensis*
Tea	England	*Camellia sinensis*
Tea	Guyana	*Camellia sinensis*
Tea	Hungary	*Camellia sinensis*
Tea	United States	*Camellia sinensis*
Teboe	Indonesia	*Saccharum officinarum*
Tebu telur	Malaysia	*Saccharum officinarum*
Tebu	Indonesia	*Saccharum officinarum*
Tebu	Malaysia	*Saccharum officinarum*
Tebusk	Denmark	*Camellia sinensis*
Tebuske	Sweden	*Camellia sinensis*
Tee	Finland	*Camellia sinensis*
Tee	Germany	*Camellia sinensis*
Tee	Netherlands	*Camellia sinensis*
Tee	South Africa	*Camellia sinensis*
Teel	France	*Sesamum indicum*
Teepensas	Finland	*Camellia sinensis*
Tembakau	Indonesia	*Nicotiana tabacum*
Tembakau	Malaysia	*Nicotiana tabacum*
Temmdki	Turkmenistan	*Nicotiana tabacum*
Tenkaya	India	*Cocos nucifera*
Tenkaya	Sri Lanka	*Cocos nucifera*
Tennai marama	India	*Cocos nucifera*
Tennai marama	Sri Lanka	*Cocos nucifera*
Tertuyagas	Ecuador	*Zingiber officinale*
Teufelsdreck	Germany	*Ferula assafoetida*
Tey	The Isle of Man (Manx)	*Camellia sinensis*
Teye	South Africa	*Camellia sinensis*
The	France	*Camellia sinensis*
The	Indonesia	*Camellia sinensis*
The	Malaysia	*Camellia sinensis*
Thee	Netherlands	*Camellia sinensis*

Theesoort	Netherlands	*Camellia sinensis*
Theestrauch	Germany	*Camellia sinensis*
Theestruik	Netherlands	*Camellia sinensis*
Theler	France	*Camellia sinensis*
Thenga	India	*Cocos nucifera*
Thenga	Malaysia	*Cocos nucifera*
Thenga	Sri Lanka	*Cocos nucifera*
Thenginkai	India	*Cocos nucifera*
Thengu	India	*Cocos nucifera*
Thengu	Sri Lanka	*Cocos nucifera*
Thenkaii	India	*Cocos nucifera*
Thenkaii	Sri Lanka	*Cocos nucifera*
Thybaco	Wales	*Nicotiana tabacum*
Ti	Congo	*Camellia sinensis*
Ti	Samoa	*Camellia sinensis*
Ti	Scotland	*Camellia sinensis*
Tii	Greenland	*Camellia sinensis*
Tii	New Zealand	*Camellia sinensis*
Tii	Northwest Territories, Canada	*Camellia sinensis*
Til	Arabic countries	*Cannabis sativa*
Til	India	*Sesamum indicum*
Til	Pakistan	*Sesamum indicum*
Tila	India	*Sesamum indicum*
Till	France	*Sesamum indicum*
Tisi	India	*Sesamum indicum*
Tiwu	Sudan	*Saccharum officinarum*
To pi'avare	Rarotonga	*Saccharum officinarum*
Tobac	Ireland	*Nicotiana tabacum*
Tobacco	Australia	*Nicotiana tabacum*
Tobacco	Guyana	*Nicotiana tabacum*
Tobacco	Iceland	*Nicotiana tabacum*
Tobacco	Italy	*Nicotiana tabacum*
Tobacco	Kenya	*Nicotiana tabacum*
Tobacco	New Zealand	*Nicotiana tabacum*
Tobacco	United Kingdom	*Nicotiana tabacum*
Tobacco	United States	*Nicotiana tabacum*
Tobacco	West Indies	*Nicotiana tabacum*
Tobak	Denmark	*Nicotiana tabacum*
Tobak	Sweden	*Nicotiana tabacum*
Tobaken	Sweden	*Nicotiana tabacum*
Tobakk	Norway	*Nicotiana tabacum*
Tobakken	Denmark	*Nicotiana tabacum*
Tombaca	Scotland	*Nicotiana tabacum*
Tombagey	The Isle of Man (Manx)	*Nicotiana tabacum*
Ton oi	Thailand	*Saccharum officinarum*
Too moo	China	*Hordeum vulgare*
Toombak	Sudan	*Nicotiana tabacum*
Tra	Vietnam	*Camellia sinensis*
Tsa	Philippines	*Camellia sinensis*
Tsinstsimin	China	*Zingiber officinale*
Tsintsimir	China	*Zingiber officinale*
Tubbak	Faeroe Islands	*Nicotiana tabacum*

Tubo	Philippines	*Saccharum officinarum*
Tue	Papua-New Guinea	*Saccharum officinarum*
Tumbako	Mozambique	*Nicotiana tabacum*
Tumbako	Tanzania	*Nicotiana tabacum*
Tumbako	Zaire	*Nicotiana tabacum*
Tupakka	Finland	*Nicotiana tabacum*
Tutun	Romania	*Nicotiana tabacum*
Tütün	Turkey	*Nicotiana tabacum*
Twak	South Africa	*Nicotiana tabacum*
Tybaco	Wales	*Nicotiana tabacum*
Tyton szlachetny	Poland	*Nicotiana tabacum*
Tyutyun	Bulgaria	*Nicotiana tabacum*
Tyutyun	Ukraine	*Nicotiana tabacum*
Ufuta	Mozambique	*Sesamum indicum*
Ufuta	Tanzania	*Sesamum indicum*
Ugwayi	Botswana	*Nicotiana tabacum*
Ugwayi	South Africa	*Nicotiana tabacum*
Ugwayi	South Africa	*Nicotiana tabacum*
Ukha	India	*Saccharum officinarum*
Ukhu	Nepal	*Saccharum officinarum*
Uliva	Switzerland	*Olea europaea*
Ullastre	Spain	*Olea europaea*
Ulli	Albania	*Olea europaea*
Ullir	Albania	*Olea europaea*
Umupunga	Africa	*Oryza sativa*
Ungbin	Myanmar	*Cocos nucifera*
Usa	India	*Saccharum officinarum*
Usurp	China	*Hordeum vulgare*
Uuka	India	*Saccharum officinarum*
Vaaristubukas	Estonia	*Nicotiana tabacum*
Vanglo	Germany	*Sesamum indicum*
Vary	Madagascar	*Oryza sativa*
Velna suds	Latvia	*Ferula assafoetida*
Vild gulerod	Benin	*Daucus carota*
Vild gulerod	Denmark	*Daucus carota*
Viljelty porkkana	Finland	*Daucus carota*
Vill gulrot	Norway	*Daucus carota*
Virginiantupakka	Finland	*Nicotiana tabacum*
Virginiatobak	Sweden	*Nicotiana tabacum*
Virginiatobakk	Norway	*Nicotiana tabacum*
Virginischer tabak	Germany	*Nicotiana tabacum*
Virginsk tobak	Denmark	*Nicotiana tabacum*
Vrai chanvre	France	*Cannabis sativa*
Vung	Vietnam	*Sesamum indicum*
Wai	Papua-New Guinea	*Zingiber officinale*
Warak sabun masasah	Arabic countries	*Plantago ovata*
Weed	Guyana	*Cannabis sativa*
Wijen	Indonesia	*Sesamum indicum*
Wild carrot	Canada	*Daucus carota*
Wild carrot	England	*Daucus carota*
Wild carrot	New Zealand	*Daucus carota*
Wild gulerod	Denmark	*Daucus carota*

Wild rice	Australia	*Oryza sativa*
Wilde mohre	Germany	*Daucus carota*
Wilde peen	Belgium	*Daucus carota*
Wilde peen	Netherlands	*Daucus carota*
Wilde wortel	Belgium	*Daucus carota*
Wildmorot	Sweden	*Daucus carota*
Wortel	Indonesia	*Daucus carota*
Wortel	Netherlands	*Daucus carota*
Wortel	South Africa	*Daucus carota*
Xian ma	China	*Cannabis sativa*
Yachmen	Russia	*Hordeum vulgare*
Yachmin	Ukraine	*Hordeum vulgare*
Yaku-q'oniwan	Ecuador	*Camellia sinensis*
Yallu	India	*Sesamum indicum*
Yang hua luo bo	China	*Daucus carota*
Ye hu luo bo	China	*Daucus carota*
Ye ma	China	*Cannabis sativa*
Ye shu	China	*Cocos nucifera*
Ye zi	China	*Cocos nucifera*
Ye´-ma	Brazil	*Nicotiana tabacum*
Zaitun	Indonesia	*Olea europaea*
Zanahoria Silvestre	Dominican Republic	*Daucus carota*
Zanahoria silvestre	Chile	*Daucus carota*
Zanahoria silvestre	Peru	*Daucus carota*
Zanahoria silvestre	Spain	*Daucus carota*
Zanahoria silvestre	Venezuela	*Daucus carota*
Zanahoria	Puerto Rico	*Daucus carota*
Zanahoria	Spain	*Daucus carota*
Zangbil	Israel	*Zingiber officinale*
Zangvil	Israel	*Zingiber officinale*
Zanjabeel	India	*Zingiber officinale*
Zanjabeel	Saudi Arabia	*Zingiber officinale*
Zanjabil	Arabic countries	*Zingiber officinale*
Zanjabil	Iran	*Zingiber officinale*
Zapaliczka cuchnaca	Poland	*Ferula assafoetida*
Zaya	Turkmenistan	*Camellia sinensis*
Zayit	Israel	*Olea europaea*
Zaytun	Arabic countries	*Olea europaea*
Zaz	Iran	*Ferula assafoetida*
Zazvor	Czech Republic	*Zingiber officinale*
Zazvor	Slovakia	*Zingiber officinale*
Zebbug	Malta	*Olea europaea*
Zeituni	Mozambique	*Olea europaea*
Zeituni	Tanzania	*Olea europaea*
Zeituni	Zaire	*Olea europaea*
Zelzlane	Arabic countries	*Sesamum indicum*
Zencebil	Turkey	*Zingiber officinale*
Zencefil	Turkey	*Zingiber officinale*
Zenzero	Italy	*Zingiber officinale*
Zenzevero	Italy	*Zingiber officinale*
Zetis	Georgia	*Olea europaea*
Zetiskhili	Georgia	*Olea europaea*

Zeyatin	Turkmenistan	*Olea europaea*
Zeytin	Turkey	*Olea europaea*
Zeytoon	Armenia	*Olea europaea*
Zi jiang	China	*Zingiber officinale*
Zi ma zi	China	*Sesamum indicum*
Zingiber	Spain	*Zingiber officinale*
Zingibil	Oman	*Zingiber officinale*
Zinjabil	Yemen	*Zingiber officinale*
Zinjibil	Ethiopia	*Zingiber officinale*
Zinzam	Mauritius	*Zingiber officinale*
Zuckerrohr	Germany	*Saccharum officinarum*

Index

About the Author

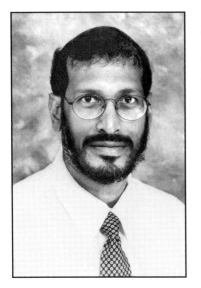

A native of Guyana, Ivan A. Ross is a biologist at the United States Food and Drug Administration. At the age of seventeen he was awarded a scholarship by the United States Agency for International Development to study agriculture at Tuskegee University. After completing his studies he returned to Guyana and was appointed to the Guyana Ministry of Agriculture. During this tour of duty, most of his time was spent in the isolated communities of the Aboriginal populations, incorporating modern agriculture and health care methods with the traditional system. Dr. Ross' interest in traditional medicine originated at this time. He later entered the University of Maryland, College Park, where he studied animal science and biochemistry. In 1987 he joined the United States Department of Health and Human Services, Food and Drug Administration, as a biologist in the Division of Toxicological Research. He is an active investigator and has published several research articles, primarily dealing with food safety. Other areas of his wide-ranging experience include Lecturer of Agricultural and Rural Development at Gambia College, Gambia, West Africa, and seminars throughout Gambia on food safety, health awareness, and agricultural techniques. When not in the laboratory, Dr. Ross is either farming or writing.

.